Red Book® ATLAS

of Pediatric Infectious Diseases

3rd Edition

Editor: Carol J. Baker, MD, FAAP

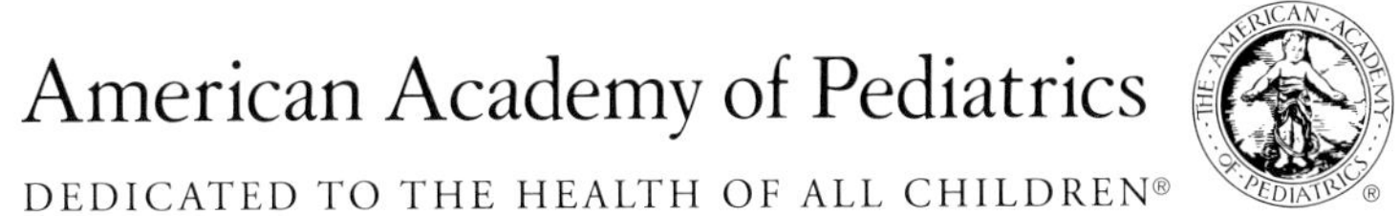

American Academy of Pediatrics Publishing Staff

Mark Grimes, *Director, Department of Publishing*

Peter Lynch, *Manager, Digital Strategy and Product Development*

Barrett Winston, *Digital Solutions Editor*

Theresa Wiener, *Manager, Publishing and Production Services*

Jason Crase, *Manager, Editorial Services*

Peg Mulcahy, *Manager, Art Direction and Production*

Mary Lou White, *Director, Department of Marketing and Sales*

Linda Smessaert, *Marketing Manager, Professional Publications*

Published by the American Academy of Pediatrics
141 Northwest Point Blvd
Elk Grove Village, IL 60007-1019
Telephone: 847/434-4000
Facsimile: 847/434-8000
www.aap.org

First edition published 2010; second, 2013.

Printed in the United States of America

9-375/1016 1 2 3 4 5 6 7 8 9 10

MA0805
ISBN: 978-1-61002-060-2
eBook: 978-1-61002-061-9
Library of Congress Control Number: 2016942360

Contents

Preface

The American Academy of Pediatrics (AAP) *Red Book® Atlas of Pediatric Infectious Diseases*, 3rd Edition, is a summary of key disease information from the AAP *Red Book®: 2015 Report of the Committee on Infectious Diseases*. It is intended to be a study guide for students, residents, and practitioners.

The visual representations of common and atypical clinical manifestations of infectious diseases provide diagnostic information not found in the print version of the *Red Book*. The juxtaposition of these visuals with a summary of the clinical features, epidemiology, diagnostic methods, and treatment information hopefully will serve as a training tool and a quick reference. The *Red Book Atlas* is not intended to provide detailed treatment and management information but rather a big-picture approach that can be refined by consulting reference texts or infectious disease specialists. Complete disease and treatment information from the AAP can be found at http://redbook.solutions.aap.org, the electronic version of the *Red Book*.

This *Red Book Atlas* could not have been completed without the superb assistance of Peter Lynch, Barrett Winston, Jason Crase, Theresa Wiener, and Peg Mulcahy at the AAP and of those physicians who photographed disease manifestations in their patients and shared these with the AAP. Some diseases are rarely seen today because of improved preventive strategies, especially immunization programs. While photographs can't replace hands-on experience, they have helped me to consider the likelihood of a correct diagnosis, and I hope this will be so for the reader. I also want to thank those individuals at the Centers for Disease Control and Prevention who have generously provided many photographs of the etiologic agents, vectors, and life cycles of parasites and protozoa relevant to these largely domestic infections.

The study of pediatric infectious diseases has been a challenging and ever-changing professional life that has brought me great joy. To gather information with my ears, eyes, and hands (the history and physical examination), to place this into the context of relevant epidemiology and incubation period, and then to select a few appropriate diagnostic studies is still exciting for me. Putting these many pieces together and arriving at the correct diagnosis is akin to solving a crime. On many occasions, just seeing *the* clue (a characteristic rash, an asymmetry, a swelling) will solve the medical puzzle, lead to recovery with the proper management, and bring the satisfaction almost nothing can replace. It is my hope that the readers of the third edition of the *Red Book Atlas* might find a similar enthusiasm for the field.

Carol J. Baker, MD, FAAP
Editor

1

Actinomycosis

Clinical Manifestations

Actinomycosis results from pathogen introduction following a breakdown in mucocutaneous protective barriers. Spread within the host is by direct invasion of adjacent tissues, typically forming sinus tracts that cross tissue planes.

There are 3 common anatomic sites of infection. **Cervicofacial** is most common, often occurring after tooth extraction, oral surgery, or other oral/facial trauma, or even from carious teeth. Localized pain and induration may progress to cervical abscess and "woody hard" nodular lesions ("lumpy jaw"), which can develop draining sinus tracts, usually at the angle of the jaw or in the submandibular region. Infection may contribute to chronic tonsillar airway obstruction. **Thoracic** disease most commonly is secondary to aspiration of oropharyngeal secretions but may be an extension of cervicofacial infection. It occurs rarely after esophageal disruption secondary to surgery or nonpenetrating trauma. Thoracic presentation includes pneumonia, which can be complicated by abscesses, empyema, and, rarely, pleurodermal sinuses. Focal or multifocal mediastinal and pulmonary masses may be mistaken for tumors. **Abdominal** actinomycosis is usually attributable to penetrating trauma or intestinal perforation. The appendix and cecum are the most common sites; symptoms are similar to appendicitis. Slowly developing masses may simulate abdominal or retroperitoneal neoplasms. Intra-abdominal abscesses and peritoneal-dermal draining sinuses occur eventually. Chronic localized disease often forms draining sinus tracts with purulent discharge. **Other sites** of infection include the liver, pelvis (which, in some cases, has been linked to use of intrauterine devices), heart, testicles, and brain (which is usually associated with a primary pulmonary focus). Noninvasive primary cutaneous actinomycosis has occurred.

Etiology

The most common species causing human disease is *Actinomyces israelii*.

A israelii and at least 5 other *Actinomyces* species cause human disease. All are slow-growing, microaerophilic or facultative anaerobic, gram-positive, filamentous branching bacilli. They can be part of normal oral, gastrointestinal tract, or vaginal flora. *Actinomyces* species frequently are copathogens in tissues harboring multiple other anaerobic or aerobic species. Isolation of *Aggregatibacter (Actinobacillus) actinomycetemcomitans*, frequently detected with *Actinomyces* species, may predict the presence of actinomycosis.

Epidemiology

Actinomyces species occur worldwide, being components of endogenous oral and gastrointestinal tract flora. *Actinomyces* species are opportunistic pathogens (reported in patients with HIV and chronic granulomatous disease), with disease usually following penetrating (including human bite wounds) and nonpenetrating trauma. Infection is uncommon in infants and children, with 80% of cases occurring in adults. The male to female ratio in children is 1.5 to 1. Overt, microbiologically confirmed, monomicrobial disease caused by *Actinomyces* species has become rare in the era of antimicrobial agents.

Incubation Period

Several days to several years.

Diagnostic Tests

Only specimens from normally sterile sites should be submitted for culture. Microscopic demonstration of beaded, branched, gram-positive bacilli in purulent material or tissue specimens suggests the diagnosis. Acid-fast staining can distinguish *Actinomyces* species, which are acid-fast negative, from *Nocardia* species, which are variably acid-fast positive. Yellow "sulfur granules" visualized microscopically or macroscopically in drainage or loculations of purulent material also suggest the diagnosis. A Gram stain of "sulfur granules" discloses a dense aggregate of bacterial filaments mixed with inflammatory debris. Immunofluorescent stains for *Actinomyces* species are available, as well as polymerase chain reaction assay and 16s rRNA sequencing for tissue specimens.

Treatment

Initial therapy should include intravenous penicillin G or ampicillin for 4 to 6 weeks followed by high doses of oral penicillin (up to 2 g/d for adults), usually for a total of 6 to 12 months. Exclusively oral therapy has been reported as effective as intravenous therapy for cases of cervicofacial disease. Amoxicillin, erythromycin, clindamycin, doxycycline, and tetracycline are alternative antimicrobial choices. All *Actinomyces* appear resistant to ciprofloxacin and metronidazole. Surgical drainage or debridement is often a necessary adjunct to medical management and may allow for a shorter duration of antimicrobial treatment.

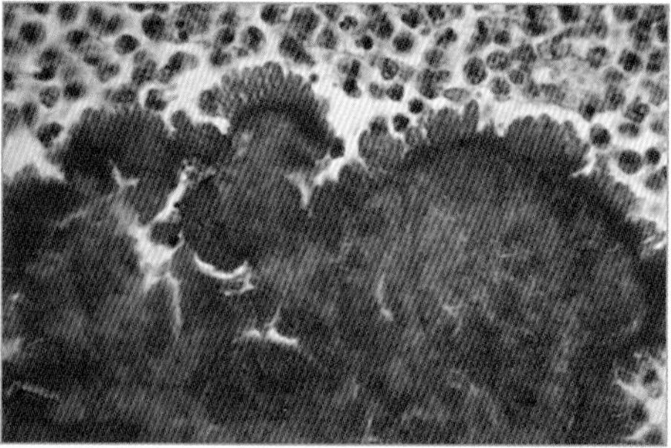

Image 1.1
A sulfur granule from an actinomycotic abscess (hematoxylin-eosin stain). While pathognomonic of actinomycosis, granules are not always present. A Gram stain of sulfur granules shows a dense reticulum of filaments.

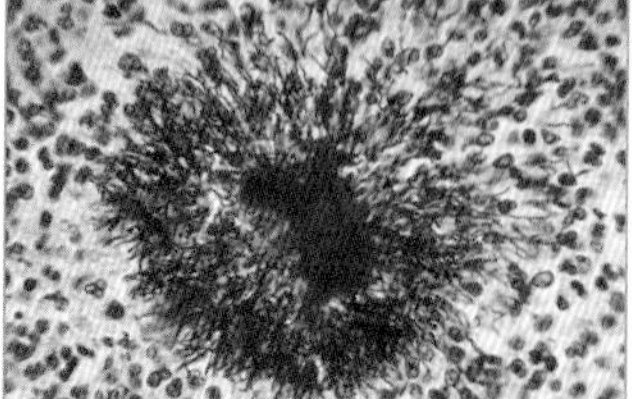

Image 1.2
Tissue showing filamentous branching rods of *Actinomyces israelii* (Brown and Brenn stain). *Actinomyces* species have fastidious growth requirements. Staining of a crushed sulfur granule reveals branching bacilli.

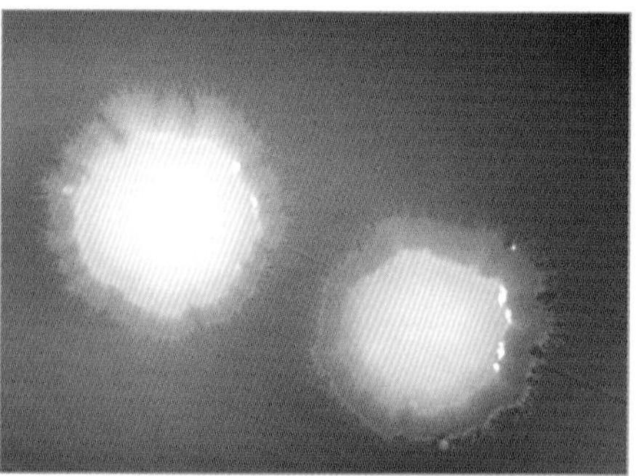

Image 1.3
A brain heart infusion agar plate culture of *Actinomyces* species, magnification x573, at 10 days of incubation. Courtesy of Centers for Disease Control and Prevention.

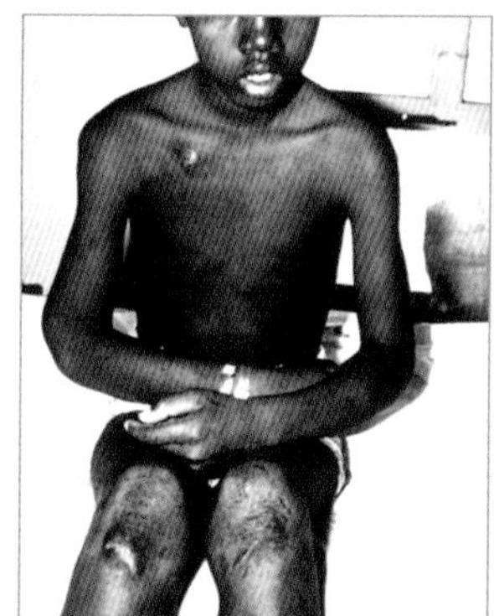

Image 1.4
A 10-year-old boy with chronic pulmonary, abdominal, and lower extremity abscesses with chronic draining sinus tracts from which *Actinomyces israelii* was isolated. Prolonged antimicrobial treatment and surgical drainage were required for resolution of this infectious process.

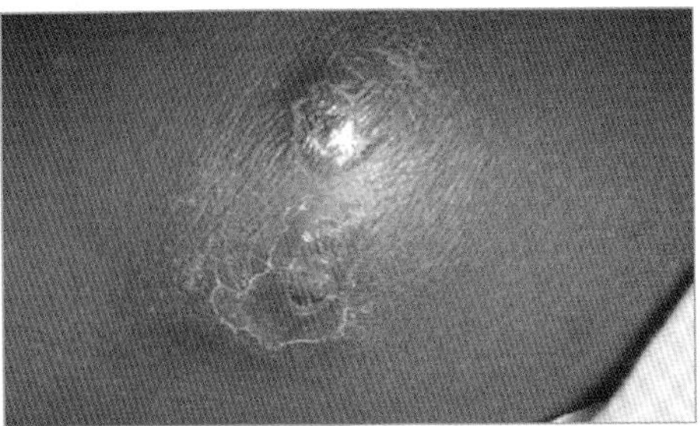

Image 1.5
Actinomycotic abscesses of the thigh of the boy in Image 1.4. Actinomyces infections are often polymicrobial. *Aggregatibacter* (*Actinobacillus*) *actinomycetemcomitans,* one of the HACEK group of organisms, may accompany *Actinomyces israelii* and may cause endocarditis.

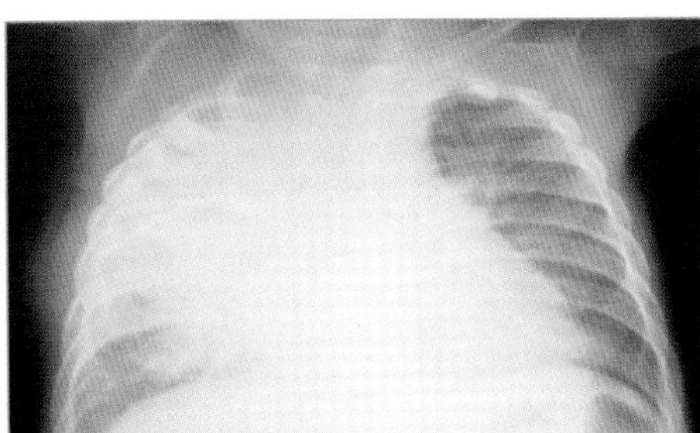

Image 1.6
An 8-month-old boy with pulmonary actinomycosis, an uncommon infection in infancy that may follow aspiration. As in this infant, most cases of actinomycosis are caused by *Actinomyces israelii.*

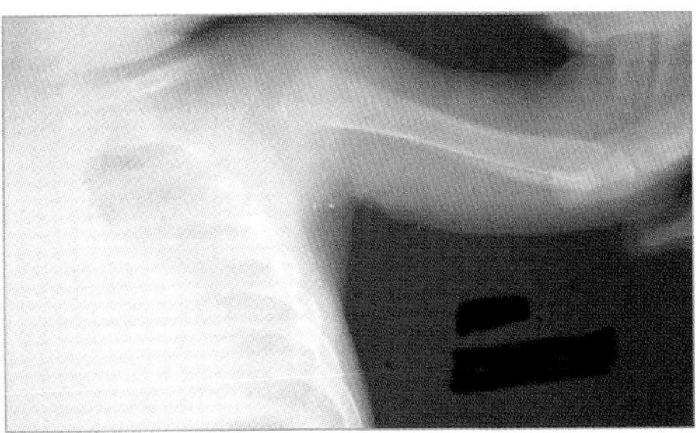

Image 1.7
Periosteal reaction along the left humeral shaft (diaphysis) in the 8-month-old boy in Image 1.6, with pulmonary actinomycosis. The presence of clubbing with this chronic suppurative pulmonary infection and absence of heart disease suggests pulmonary fibrosis contributed to this infant's pulmonary hypertrophic osteoarthropathy. Courtesy of Edgar O. Ledbetter, MD, FAAP.

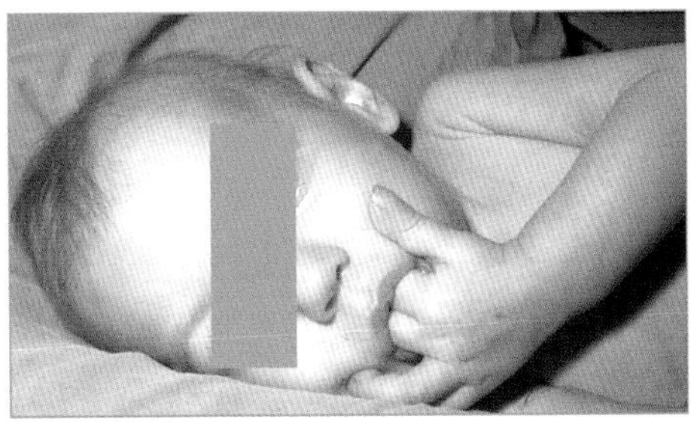

Image 1.8
Clubbing of the thumb and fingers of the 8-month-old boy in images 1.6 and 1.7 with chronic pulmonary actinomycosis. Blood cultures were repeatedly negative without clinical signs of endocarditis. Courtesy of Edgar O. Ledbetter, MD, FAAP.

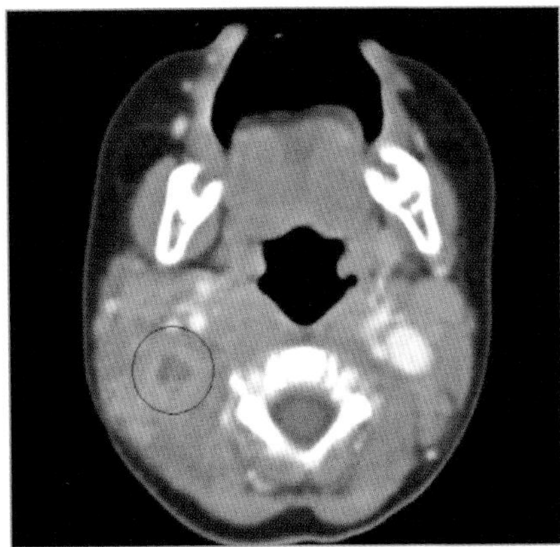

Image 1.9
Actinomyces cervical abscess in a 6-month-old girl. Courtesy of Benjamin Estrada, MD.

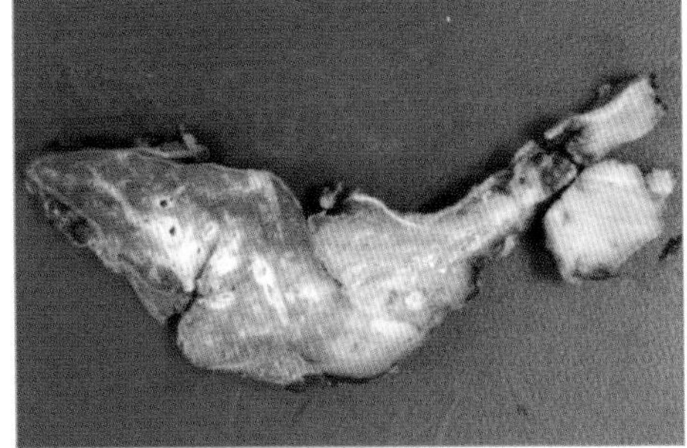

Image 1.10
The resected right lower lobe, diaphragm, and portion of the liver in a 3-year-old previously healthy girl with an unknown source for her pulmonary actinomycosis. Courtesy of Carol J. Baker, MD, FAAP.

2

Adenovirus Infections

Clinical Manifestations

Adenovirus infections of the upper respiratory tract are common and, although often subclinical, can result in symptoms of the common cold, pharyngitis, tonsillitis, otitis media, and pharyngoconjunctival fever. Life-threatening disseminated infection, severe pneumonitis, hepatitis, meningitis, and encephalitis occur occasionally, especially among young infants and people who are immunocompromised. Adenoviruses occasionally cause a pertussis-like syndrome, croup, bronchiolitis, exudative tonsillitis, pneumonia, and hemorrhagic cystitis. Ocular adenovirus infections may present as follicular conjunctivitis or epidemic keratoconjunctivitis. Ophthalmologic illness frequently presents with unilateral inflammation that becomes bilateral; symptoms include photophobia and, sometimes, vision loss. Enteric adenoviruses are an important cause of childhood gastroenteritis.

Etiology

Adenoviruses are double-stranded, nonenveloped DNA viruses; at least 51 distinct serotypes and multiple genetic variants divided into 7 species (A–G) infect humans. Some adenovirus types are associated primarily with respiratory tract disease (types 1–5, 7, 14, and 21), and others are associated primarily with gastroenteritis (types 40 and 41). During 2007, adenovirus type 14 emerged in the United States, where it caused severe and sometimes fatal respiratory tract illness in mostly adults, civilian and military, and has now spread to Europe and Asia.

Epidemiology

Infection in infants and children can occur at any age. Adenoviruses causing respiratory tract infections are usually transmitted by respiratory tract secretions through person-to-person contact, airborne droplets, and fomites. Adenoviruses are hardy viruses, can survive on environmental surfaces for long periods, and are not inactivated by many disinfectants. Conjunctiva can provide a portal of entry. Community outbreaks of adenovirus-associated pharyngoconjunctival fever have been attributed to water exposure from contaminated swimming pools and fomites, such as shared towels. Health care–associated transmission of adenoviral respiratory tract, conjunctival, and gastrointestinal tract infections can occur in hospitals, residential institutions, and nursing homes from exposures to infected health care personnel, patients, or contaminated equipment. Adenovirus infections in transplant recipients can occur from donor tissues. Epidemic keratoconjunctivitis commonly occurs by direct contact, has been associated with equipment used during eye examinations, and is caused principally by serotypes 8, 19, and 37. Enteric strains of adenoviruses are transmitted by the fecal-oral route. Adenoviruses do not demonstrate the marked seasonality of other respiratory tract viruses and circulate throughout the year. Enteric disease occurs year-round and primarily affects children younger than 4 years. Adenovirus infections are most communicable during the first few days of an acute illness, but persistent and intermittent shedding for longer periods, even months, is common. Asymptomatic infections are common. Reinfection can occur.

Incubation Period

Respiratory tract infection, 2 to 14 days; gastroenteritis, 3 to 10 days.

Diagnostic Tests

Methods for diagnosis of adenovirus infection include isolation in cell culture, antigen detection, and molecular detection. Adenoviruses associated with respiratory tract disease can be isolated from pharyngeal and eye secretions and from feces by inoculation of specimens into susceptible cell cultures. A pharyngeal or ocular isolate is more suggestive of recent infection than is a fecal isolate, which may indicate recent infection or prolonged carriage. Rapid detection of adenovirus antigens is possible in a variety of body fluids by commercial immunoassay, including direct fluorescent assay. These rapid assays can be useful for the diagnosis of respiratory tract infections, ocular disease, and diarrheal disease. Enteric adenovirus types 40 and 41 usually cannot be isolated in standard cell cultures. Adenoviruses can also be identified by electron microscopic examination of respiratory and stool specimens, but this modality lacks sensitivity. Polymerase chain reaction assays for adenovirus DNA are replacing other detection methods because of improved sensitivity and increasing commercial availability; however, the persistent and intermittent shedding that commonly follows an acute adenoviral infection can complicate the clinical interpretation of a positive molecular diagnostic test result. Adenovirus typing is available from some reference and research laboratories.

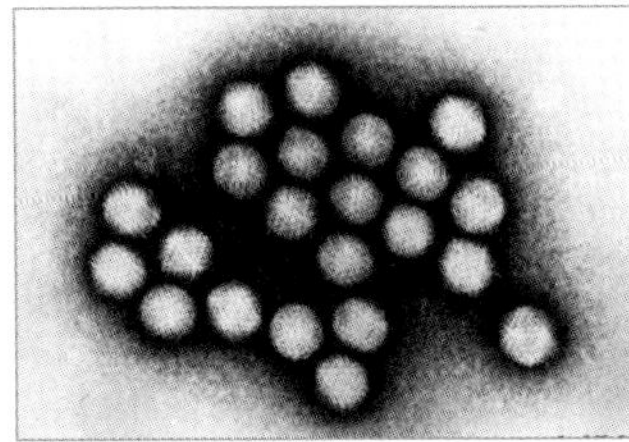

Image 2.1
Transmission electron micrograph of adenovirus. Adenoviruses have a characteristic icosahedral structure. Courtesy of Centers for Disease Control and Prevention/Dr William Gary Jr.

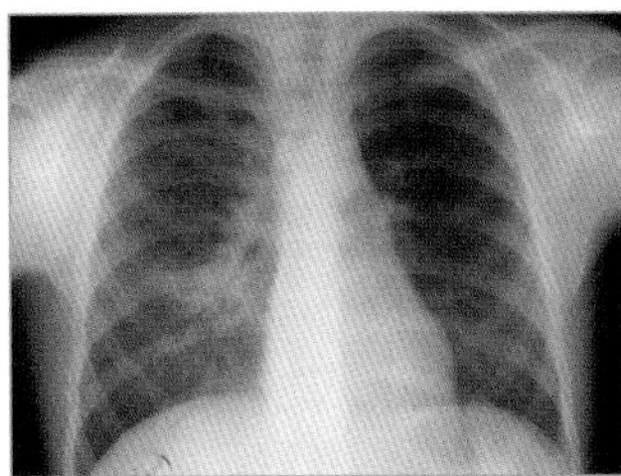

Image 2.3
Adenoviral pneumonia in an 8-year-old girl with diffuse pulmonary infiltrate bilaterally. Most adenoviral infections in the normal host are self-limited and require no specific treatment. Lobar consolidation is unusual.

Treatment

Treatment of adenovirus infection is supportive. Randomized clinical trials evaluating specific antiviral therapy have not been performed. However, case reports of the successful use of cidofovir in immunocompromised patients with severe adenoviral disease have been published, albeit without a uniform dose or dosing strategy. An oral lipid conjugate of cidofovir, brincidofovir (CMX001), is being evaluated for use in patients who are immunocompromised.

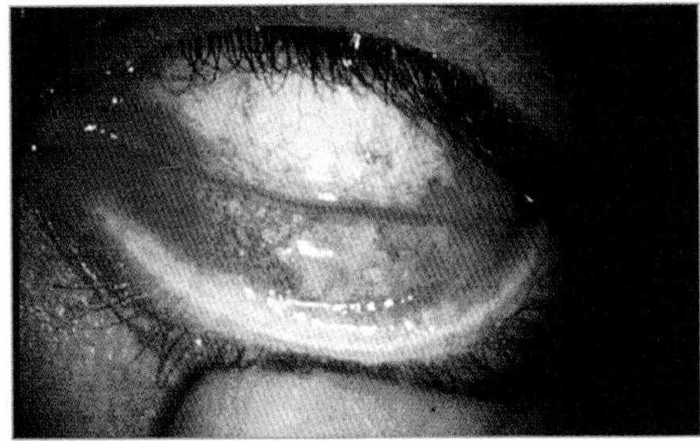

Image 2.2
Acute follicular adenovirus conjunctivitis. Adenoviruses are resistant to alcohol, detergents, and chlorhexidine and may contaminate ophthalmologic solutions and equipment. Instruments can be disinfected by steam autoclaving or immersion in 1% sodium hypochlorite for 10 minutes.

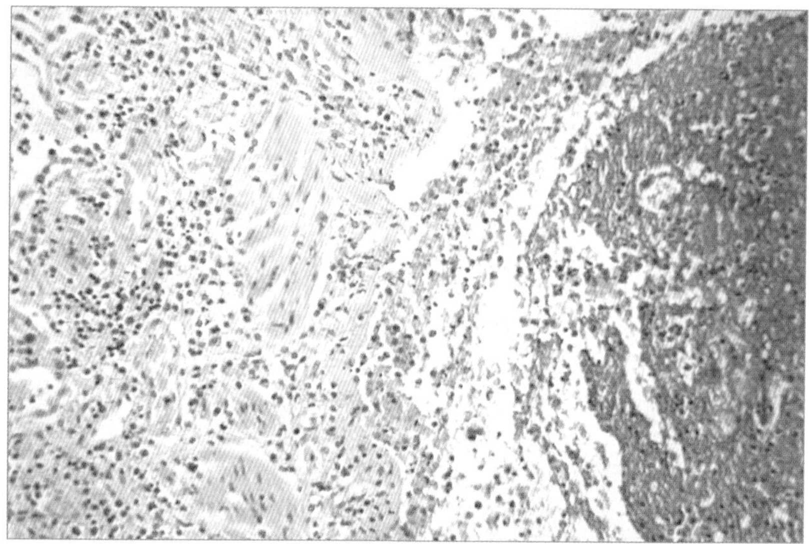

Image 2.4
Histopathology of the lung with bronchiolar occlusion in an immunocompromised child who died with adenoviral pneumonia. Note interstitial mononuclear cell infiltration and hyaline membranes. Adenoviruses types 3 and 7 can cause necrotizing bronchitis and bronchiolitis. Courtesy of Edgar O. Ledbetter, MD, FAAP.

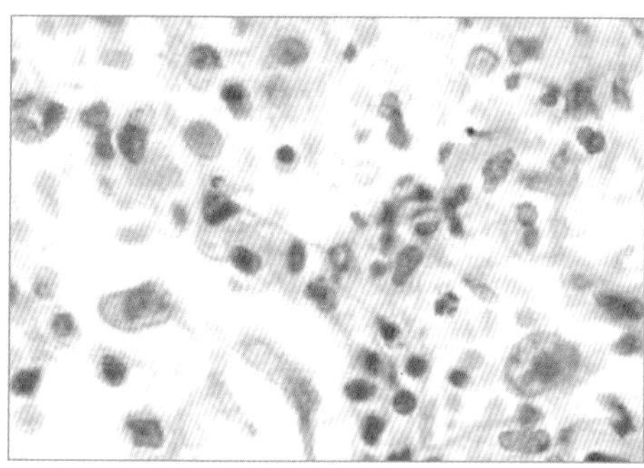

Image 2.5
Pulmonary histopathology of the immunocompromised child in Image 2.4 showing multiple adenovirus intranuclear inclusion cells. Courtesy of Edgar O. Ledbetter, MD, FAAP.

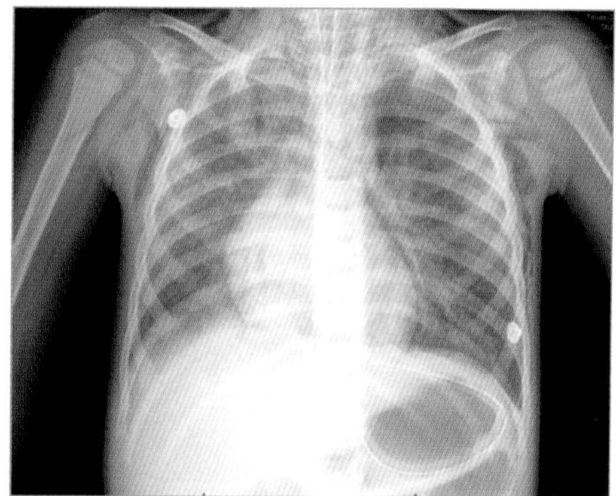

Image 2.6
This previously healthy 3-year-old boy presented with respiratory failure requiring intensive care for adenovirus type 7 pneumonia. He eventually recovered with some mild impairment in pulmonary function studies. Note the pneumomediastinum. Courtesy of Carol J. Baker, MD, FAAP.

3

Amebiasis

Clinical Manifestations

Most individuals with *Entamoeba histolytica* have asymptomatic, noninvasive intestinal tract infection. When symptomatic, clinical syndromes associated with *E histolytica* infection include cramps, watery or bloody diarrhea, and weight loss. Occasionally, the parasite may spread to other organs, most commonly the liver (liver abscess), and cause fever and right upper quadrant pain. Disease is more severe in people who are very young, elderly, or malnourished and pregnant women. People with symptomatic intestinal amebiasis generally have a gradual onset of symptoms over 1 to 3 weeks. The mildest form of intestinal tract disease is nondysenteric colitis. However, amebic dysentery is the most common clinical manifestation of amebiasis and usually includes diarrhea with gross or microscopic blood in the stool, lower abdominal pain, and tenesmus. Weight loss is common, but fever occurs only in a minority of patients (8%–38%). Symptoms can be chronic, with periods of diarrhea and intestinal spasms alternating with periods of constipation, and can mimic inflammatory bowel disease. Progressive involvement of the colon can produce toxic megacolon, fulminant colitis, ulceration of the colon and perianal area, and, rarely, perforation. Colonic progression can occur at multiples sites and carries a high fatality rate. Progression can occur in patients inappropriately treated with corticosteroids or antimotility drugs. An ameboma may occur as an annular lesion of the colon and may present as a palpable mass on physical examination. Amebomas can occur in any area of the colon but are more common in the cecum and may be mistaken for colonic carcinoma. Amebomas usually resolve with antiamebic therapy and do not require surgery.

In a small proportion of patients, extraintestinal disease may occur. The liver is the most common extraintestinal site, and infection can spread from there to the pleural space, lungs, and pericardium. Liver abscess can be acute, with fever, abdominal pain, tachypnea, liver tenderness, and hepatomegaly, or chronic, with weight loss, vague abdominal symptoms, and irritability. Rupture of abscesses into the abdomen or chest may be fatal. Evidence of recent intestinal tract infection usually is absent in extraintestinal disease. Infection can also spread from the colon to the genitourinary tract and skin. The organism rarely spreads hematogenously to the brain and other areas of the body.

Etiology

The genus *Entamoeba* includes 6 species that live in the human intestine. Three of these species are identical morphologically: *E histolytica, Entamoeba dispar,* and *Entamoeba moshkovskii. E dispar* and *E moshkovskii,* generally believed to be nonpathogenic, have recently been associated with intestinal and extraintestinal pathology. *Entamoeba* species are excreted as cysts or trophozoites in stool of infected people.

Epidemiology

E histolytica can be found worldwide but is more prevalent in people of lower socioeconomic status who live in resource-limited countries, where the prevalence of amebic infection can be as high as 50% in some communities. Groups at increased risk of infection in resource-rich countries include immigrants from or long-term visitors to areas with endemic infection, institutionalized people, and men who have sex with men. *E histolytica* is transmitted via amebic cysts by the fecal-oral route. Ingested cysts, which are unaffected by gastric acid, produce trophozoites that infect the colon. Cysts that develop subsequently are the source of transmission, especially from asymptomatic cyst excreters. Infected patients excrete cysts intermittently, sometimes for years if untreated. Transmission has been associated with contaminated food or water. Fecal-oral transmission can also occur in the setting of anal sexual practices or direct rectal inoculation through colonic irrigation devices.

Incubation Period

Variable; commonly 2 to 4 weeks, ranging from a few days to months or years.

Diagnostic Tests

Definitive diagnosis of intestinal tract infection depends on identifying trophozoites or cysts in stool specimens. Examination of serial specimens may be necessary. Specimens of stool can be examined microscopically by wet mount within 30 minutes of collection or may be fixed in formalin or polyvinyl alcohol (available in kits) for concentration, permanent staining, and subsequent microscopic examination. Antigen test kits are available for routine laboratory testing of *E histolytica* directly from stool specimens. Biopsy specimens and endoscopy scrapings (not swabs) can be examined using similar methods. Polymerase chain reaction assay and isoenzyme analysis can differentiate *E histolytica* from *E dispar, E moshkovskii,* and other *Entamoeba* species; some monoclonal antibody-based antigen detection assays can also differentiate *E histolytica* from *E dispar.*

Indirect hemagglutination has been replaced by commercially available enzyme immunoassay kits for routine serodiagnosis of amebiasis. Enzyme immunoassay detects antibody specific for *E histolytica* in approximately 95% or more of patients with extraintestinal amebiasis, 70% of patients with active intestinal tract infection, and 10% of asymptomatic people who are passing cysts of *E histolytica.* Positive serologic test results can persist even after adequate therapy. Diagnosis of an *E histolytica* liver abscess and other extraintestinal infections is aided by serologic testing because stool tests and abscess aspirates frequently are not revealing.

Ultrasonography, computed tomography, and magnetic resonance imaging can identify liver abscesses and other extraintestinal sites of infection. Aspirates from a liver abscess usually show neither trophozoites nor leukocytes.

Treatment

Treatment involves elimination of the tissue-invading trophozoites as well as organisms in the intestinal lumen. *E dispar* and *E moshkovskii* infections often are considered to be nonpathogenic and do not always require treatment. Corticosteroids and antimotility drugs administered to people with amebiasis can worsen symptoms and the disease process. The following regimens are recommended:

- **Asymptomatic cyst excreters (intraluminal infections):** Treat with a luminal amebicide, such as iodoquinol or paromomycin. Metronidazole is not effective.
- **Patients with mild to moderate or severe intestinal tract symptoms or extraintestinal disease (including liver abscess):** Treat with metronidazole or tinidazole, followed by a therapeutic course of a luminal amebicide (iodoquinol or, in absence of intestinal obstruction, paromomycin). Nitazoxanide may also be effective for mild to moderate intestinal amebiasis, although it is not US Food and Drug Administration approved for this indication. An alternate treatment for liver abscess is chloroquine phosphate administered concomitantly with metronidazole or tinidazole, followed by a therapeutic course of a luminal amebicide.

Percutaneous or surgical aspiration of large liver abscesses occasionally is required when response of the abscess to medical therapy is unsatisfactory or there is risk of abscess rupture. In most patients, drainage is not required and does not speed recovery.

Follow-up stool examination is recommended after completion of therapy. Household members and other suspected contacts should have stool examinations performed and be treated if results are positive for *E histolytica.*

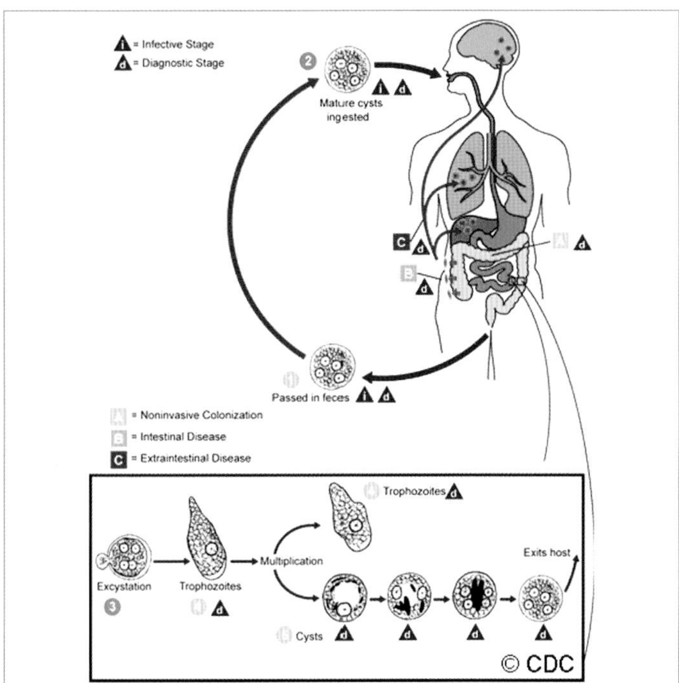

Image 3.1

Cysts are passed in feces (1). Infection by *Entamoeba histolytica* occurs by ingestion of mature cysts (2) in fecally contaminated food, water, or hands. Excystation (3) occurs in the small intestine and trophozoites (4) are released, which migrate to the large intestine. The trophozoites multiply by binary fission and produce cysts (5), which are passed in feces (1). Because of the protection conferred by their walls, the cysts can survive days to weeks in the external environment and are responsible for transmission. (Trophozoites can also be passed in diarrheal stools but are rapidly destroyed once outside the body and, if ingested, would not survive exposure to the gastric environment.) In many cases, trophozoites remain confined to the intestinal lumen (A, noninvasive infection) of individuals who are asymptomatic carriers, passing cysts in their stool. In some patients, trophozoites invade the intestinal mucosa (B, intestinal disease) or, through the bloodstream, extraintestinal sites, such as the liver, brain, and lungs (C, extraintestinal disease), with resultant pathologic manifestations. It has been established that invasive and noninvasive forms represent 2 separate species, *E histolytica* and *Entamoeba dispar,* respectively; however, not all persons infected with *E histolytica* will have invasive disease. These 2 species are morphologically indistinguishable. Transmission can also occur through fecal exposure during sexual contact (in which case not only cysts, but also trophozoites, could prove infective). Courtesy of Centers for Disease Control and Prevention.

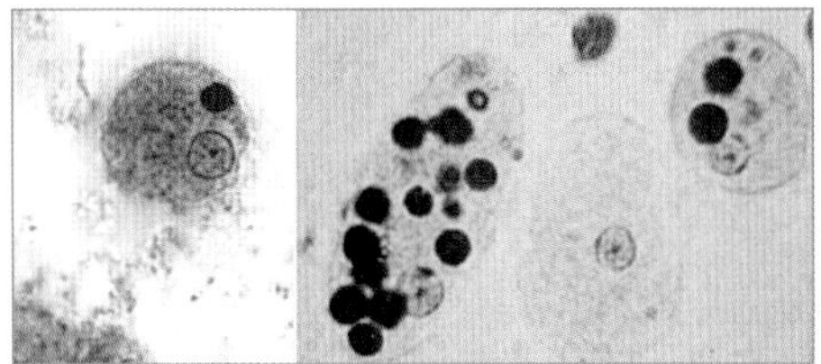

Image 3.2

Trophozoites of *Entamoeba histolytica* with ingested erythrocytes (trichrome stain). The ingested erythrocytes appear as dark inclusions. Erythrophagocytosis is the only characteristic that can be used to differentiate morphologically *E histolytica* from the nonpathogenic *Entamoeba dispar.* In these specimens, the parasite nuclei have the typical small, centrally located karyosome and thin, uniform peripheral chromatin. Courtesy of Centers for Disease Control and Prevention.

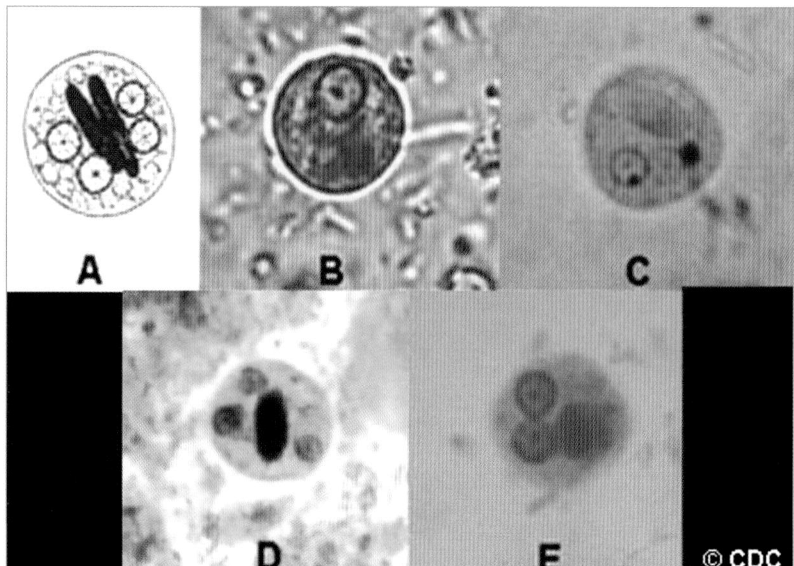

Image 3.3
Cysts of *Entamoeba histolytica* and *Entamoeba dispar.* Line drawing (A), wet mounts (B; iodine, C), and permanent preparations stained with trichrome (D, E). The cysts are usually spherical and often have a halo (B, C). Mature cysts have 4 nuclei. The cyst in B appears uninucleate, while in C, D, and E, 2 to 3 nuclei are visible in the focal plane (the fourth nucleus is coming into focus in D). The nuclei have characteristically centrally located karyosomes and fine, uniformly distributed peripheral chromatin. The cysts in C, D, and E contain chromatoid bodies, with the one in D being particularly well demonstrated, with typically blunted ends. *E histolytica* cysts usually measure 12 to 15 µm. Courtesy of Centers for Disease Control and Prevention.

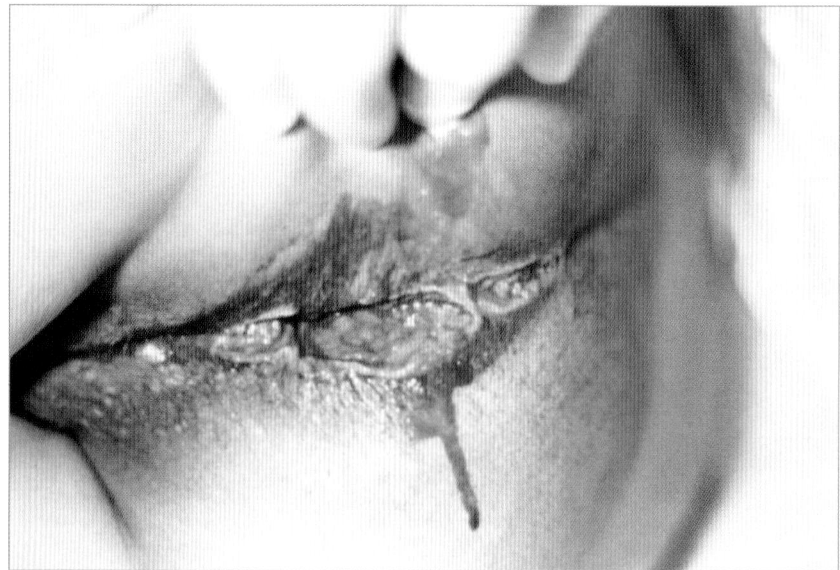

Image 3.4
This patient with amebiasis presented with tissue destruction and granulation of the anoperineal region caused by an *Entamoeba histolytica* infection. Courtesy of Centers for Disease Control and Prevention/Kerrison Juniper, MD; George Healy, PhD, DPDx.

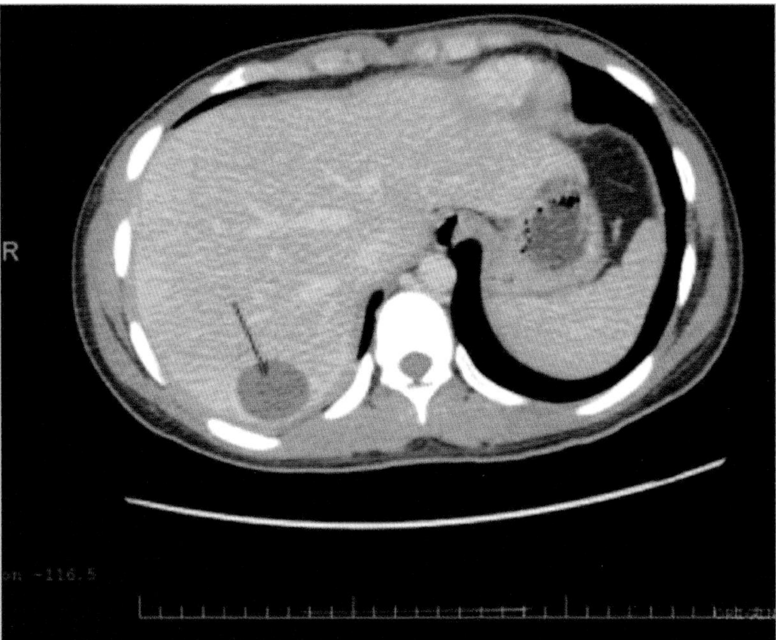

Image 3.5
Computed tomography scan of the abdomen showing a peripherally enhancing low-density lesion in the posterior aspect of the right hepatic lobe. Amebic liver abscess amebiasis, caused by the intestinal protozoal parasite *Entamoeba histolytica,* remains a global health problem, infecting about 50 million people and resulting in 40,000 to 100,000 deaths per year. Prevalence may be as high as 50% in tropical and subtropical countries where overcrowding and poor sanitation are common. In the United States, *E histolytica* infection is seen most commonly in immigrants from developing countries, long-term travelers to endemic areas (most frequently Mexico or Southeast Asia), institutionalized individuals, and men who have sex with men. In 1993, the previously known species *E histolytica* was reclassified into 2 genetically and biochemically distinct but morphologically identical species: the pathogenic *E histolytica* and the nonpathogenic commensal *Entamoeba dispar.* Courtesy of *Pediatrics in Review.*

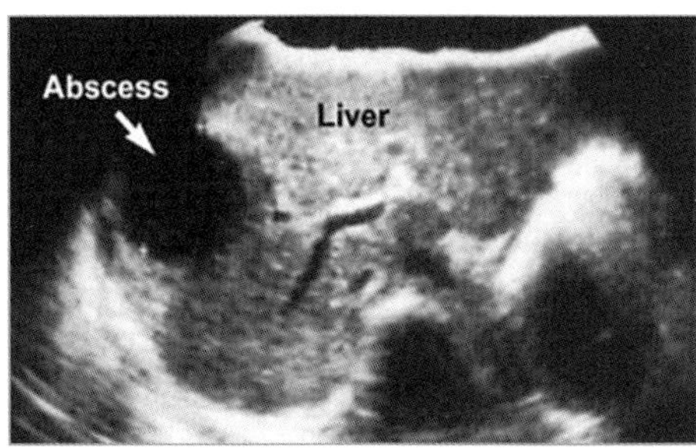

Image 3.6
Abdominal ultrasound showing a liver abscess caused by *Entamoeba histolytica*.

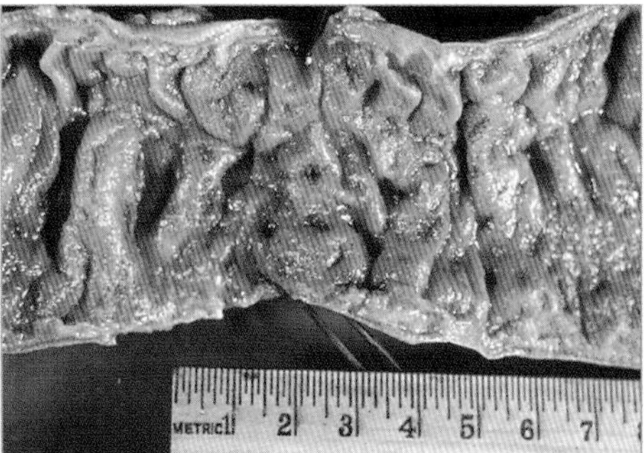

Image 3.7
Gross pathology of intestinal ulcers due to amebiasis. Courtesy of Centers for Disease Control and Prevention/Dr Mae Melvin; Dr E. West.

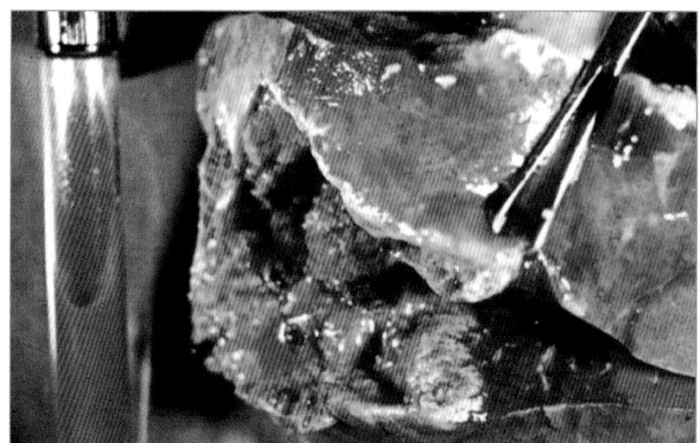

Image 3.8
Gross pathology of amebic (*Entamoeba histolytica*) abscess of liver; tube of "chocolate-like" pus from abscess. Amebic liver abscesses are usually singular and large and in the right lobe of the liver. Bacterial hepatic abscesses are more likely to be multiple. Courtesy of Centers for Disease Control and Prevention/Dr Mae Melvin; Dr E. West.

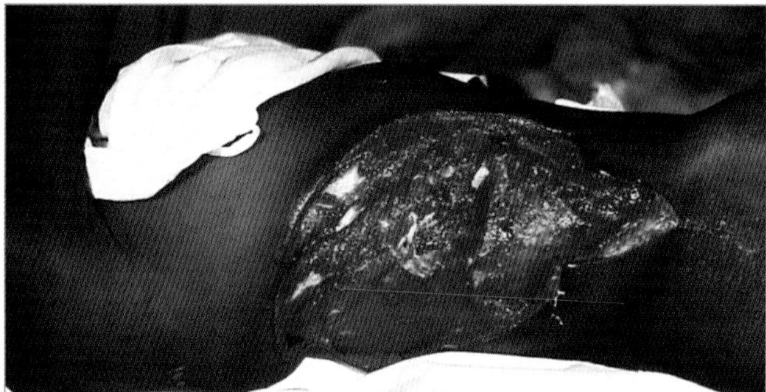

Image 3.9
This patient presented with a case of invasive extraintestinal amebiasis affecting the cutaneous region of the right flank. Courtesy of Centers for Disease Control and Prevention Prevention/Kerrison Juniper, MD, and George Healy, PhD, DPDx.

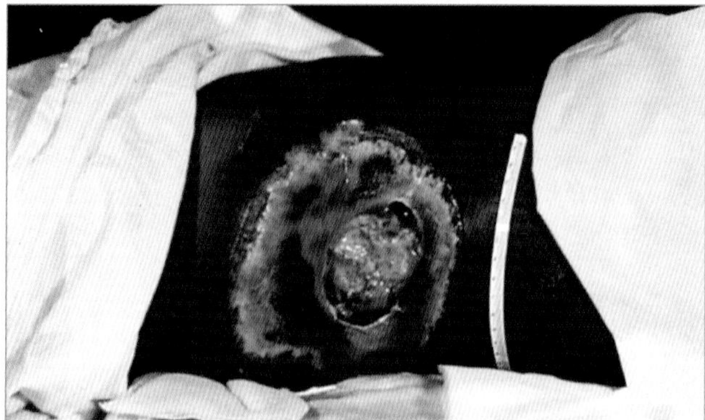

Image 3.10
This patient, also shown in Image 3.9, presented with a case of invasive extraintestinal amebiasis affecting the cutaneous region of the right flank causing severe tissue necrosis. Here we see the site of tissue destruction, predebridement. Courtesy of Centers for Disease Control and Prevention/Kerrison Juniper, MD, and George Healy, PhD, DPDx.

4

Amebic Meningoencephalitis and Keratitis

(*Naegleria fowleri, Acanthamoeba* species, and *Balamuthia mandrillaris*)

Clinical Manifestations

Naegleria fowleri causes a rapidly progressive, almost always fatal, primary amebic meningoencephalitis (PAM). Early symptoms include fever, headache, vomiting, and, sometimes, disturbances of smell and taste. This illness progresses rapidly to signs of meningoencephalitis, including nuchal rigidity, lethargy, confusion, personality changes, and altered level of consciousness. Seizures are common, and death generally occurs within a week of onset of symptoms. No distinct clinical features differentiate this disease from fulminant bacterial meningitis or meningoencephalitis.

Granulomatous amebic encephalitis (GAE) caused by *Acanthamoeba* species and *Balamuthia mandrillaris* has a more insidious onset and develops as a subacute or chronic disease. In general, GAE progresses more slowly than PAM, leading to death several weeks to months after onset of symptoms. Signs and symptoms include personality changes, seizures, headaches, ataxia, cranial nerve palsies, hemiparesis, and other focal neurologic deficits. Fever is often low grade and intermittent. Chronic granulomatous skin lesions (pustules, nodules, ulcers) may be present without central nervous system (CNS) involvement, particularly in patients with AIDS, and lesions may be present for months before brain involvement in immunocompetent hosts.

The most common symptoms of amebic keratitis, a vision-threatening infection usually caused by *Acanthamoeba* species, are pain (often out of proportion to clinical signs), photophobia, tearing, and foreign body sensation. Characteristic clinical findings include radial keratoneuritis and stromal ring infiltrate. *Acanthamoeba* keratitis generally follows an indolent course and initially can resemble herpes simplex or bacterial keratitis; delay in diagnosis is associated with worse outcomes.

Etiology

N fowleri, Acanthamoeba species, and *B mandrillaris* are free-living amebae that exist as motile, infectious trophozoites and environmentally hardy cysts.

Epidemiology

N fowleri is found in warm fresh water and moist soil. Most infections with *N fowleri* have been associated with swimming in natural bodies of warm fresh water, such as ponds, lakes, and hot springs, but other sources have included tap water from geothermal sources and contaminated and poorly chlorinated swimming pools. Disease has been reported worldwide but is uncommon. In the United States, infection occurs primarily in the summer and usually affects children and young adults. Disease has followed inappropriate use of tap water for sinus rinses. The trophozoites of the parasite invade the brain directly from the nose along the olfactory nerves via the cribriform plate. In infections with *N fowleri,* trophozoites, but not cysts, can be visualized in sections of brain or in cerebrospinal fluid (CSF).

Acanthamoeba species are distributed worldwide and are found in soil; dust; cooling towers of electric and nuclear power plants; heating, ventilating, and air-conditioning units; fresh and brackish water; whirlpool baths; and physiotherapy pools. The environmental niche of *B mandrillaris* is not delineated clearly, although it has been isolated from soil. Central nervous system infection attributable to *Acanthamoeba* occurs primarily in people who are debilitated or immunocompromised. However, some patients infected with *B mandrillaris* have had no demonstrable underlying disease or defect. Central nervous system infection by both amebae probably occurs most commonly by inhalation or direct contact with contaminated soil or water. The primary foci of these infections are, most likely, skin or respiratory tract, followed by hematogenous spread to the brain. Fatal encephalitis caused by *Balamuthia* and transmitted by the organ donor has been reported in recipients of organ transplants. *Acanthamoeba* keratitis occurs primarily in people who wear contact lenses, although it also has been associated with corneal trauma. Poor contact lens hygiene or disinfection practices as well as swimming with contact lenses are risk factors.

Incubation Period

N fowleri, 3 to 7 days; *Acanthamoeba* and *Balamuthia* GAE, unknown but thought to be several weeks or months; *Acanthamoeba* keratitis, unknown but thought to be several days to weeks.

Diagnostic Tests

In *N fowleri* infection, computed tomography scans of the head without contrast are unremarkable or show only cerebral edema but, with contrast, might show meningeal enhancement of the basilar cisterns and sulci. However, these changes are not specific for amebic infection. Cerebrospinal fluid pressure usually is elevated (300 to >600 mm water), and CSF indices can show a polymorphonuclear pleocytosis, an increased protein concentration, and a normal to very low glucose concentration. *N fowleri* infection can be documented by microscopic demonstration of the motile trophozoites on a wet mount of centrifuged CSF. Smears of CSF should be stained with Giemsa, trichrome, or Wright stain to identify the trophozoites, if present. Trophozoites can be visualized in sections of the brain. Immunofluorescence and polymerase chain reaction assays performed on CSF and biopsy material to identify the organism are available through the Centers for Disease Control and Prevention (CDC).

In infection with *Acanthamoeba* species and *B mandrillaris*, trophozoites and cysts can be visualized in sections of brain, lungs, and skin; in cases of *Acanthamoeba* keratitis, they can also be visualized in corneal scrapings and by confocal microscopy in vivo in the cornea. In GAE infections, CSF indices typically reveal a lymphocytic pleocytosis and an increased protein concentration, with normal or low glucose concentration. Computed tomography and magnetic resonance imaging of the head reveal single or multiple space-occupying, ring-enhancing lesions that can mimic brain abscesses, tumors, cerebrovascular accidents, or other diseases. *Acanthamoeba* species, but not *Balamuthia* species, can be cultured by the same method used for *N fowleri. B mandrillaris* can be grown using mammalian cell culture. Like *N fowleri*, immunofluorescence and polymerase chain reaction assays can be performed on clinical specimens to identify *Acanthamoeba* species and *Balamuthia* species; these tests are available through the CDC.

Treatment

If meningoencephalitis caused by *N fowleri* is suspected because of the presence of amebic organisms in CSF, therapy should be initiated promptly while awaiting results of confirmatory diagnostic tests. Although an effective treatment regimen for PAM has not been identified, amphotericin B is the drug of choice. However, treatment is usually unsuccessful, with only a few cases of complete recovery having been documented. Two survivors recovered after treatment with amphotericin B in combination with an azole drug (miconazole or fluconazole) plus rifampin. The most up-to-date guidance for treatment of PAM can be found on the CDC Web site (**www.cdc.gov/naegleria**).

Effective treatment for infections caused by *Acanthamoeba* species and *B mandrillaris* has not been established. Several patients with *Acanthamoeba* GAE and *Acanthamoeba* cutaneous infections without CNS involvement have been treated successfully with a multidrug regimen consisting of various combinations of pentamidine, sulfadiazine, flucytosine, either fluconazole or itraconazole, trimethoprim-sulfamethoxazole, and topical application of chlorhexidine gluconate and ketoconazole for skin lesions.

Patients with *Acanthamoeba* keratitis should be evaluated by an ophthalmologist. Early diagnosis and therapy are important for a good outcome.

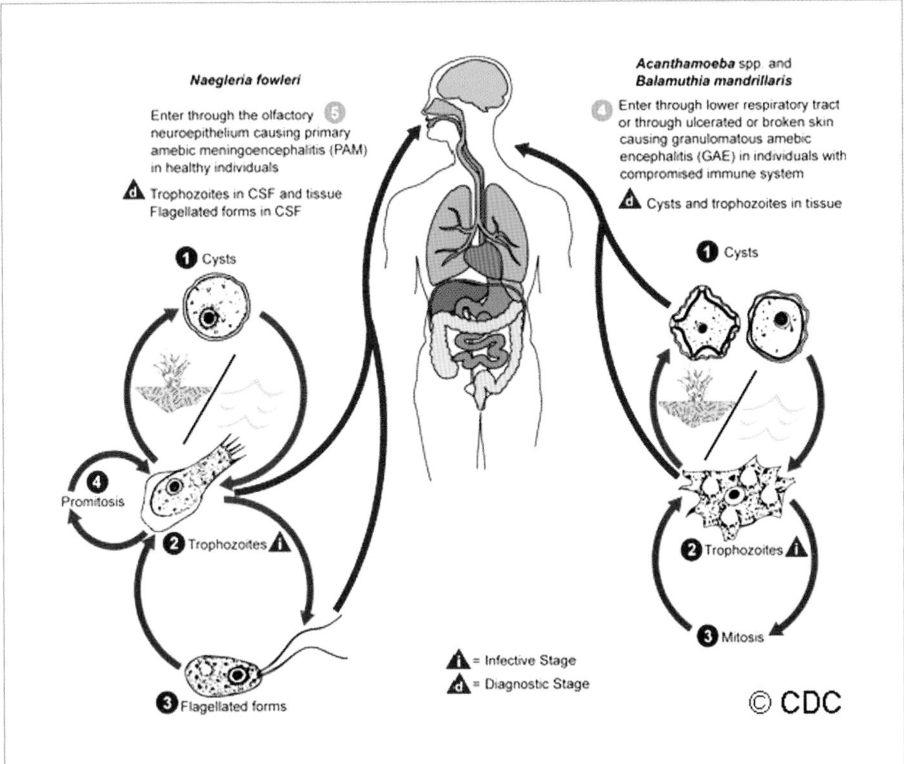

Image 4.1
Free-living amebae belonging to the genera *Acanthamoeba, Balamuthia,* and *Naegleria* are important causes of disease in humans and animals. *Fowleri* produces an acute, and usually lethal, central nervous system disease called primary amebic meningoencephalitis. *Naegleria fowleri* has 3 stages, cysts (1), trophozoites (2), and flagellated forms (3), in its life cycle. The trophozoites replicate by promitosis (nuclear membrane remains intact) (4). *N fowleri* is found in fresh water, soil, thermal discharges of power plants, heated swimming pools, hydrotherapy and medicinal pools, aquariums, and sewage. Trophozoites can turn into temporary flagellated forms, which usually revert back to the trophozoite stage. Trophozoites infect humans or animals by entering the olfactory neuroepithelium (5) and reaching the brain. *N fowleri* trophozoites are found in cerebrospinal fluid and tissue, while flagellated forms are found in cerebrospinal fluid. *Acanthamoeba* species and *Balamuthia mandrillaris* are opportunistic free-living amebae capable of causing granulomatous amebic encephalitis in individuals with compromised immune systems. *Acanthamoeba* species have been found in soil; fresh water, brackish water, and seawater; sewage; swimming pools; contact lens equipment; medicinal pools; dental treatment units; dialysis machines; heating, ventilating, and air-conditioning systems; mammalian cell cultures; vegetables; human nostrils and throats; and human and animal brain, skin, and lung tissues. *B mandrillaris* has not been isolated from the environment but has been isolated from autopsy specimens of infected humans and animals. Unlike *N fowleri, Acanthamoeba* and *Balamuthia* have only 2 stages, cysts (1) and trophozoites (2), in their life cycle. No flagellated stage exists as part of the life cycle. The trophozoites replicate by mitosis (nuclear membrane does not remain intact) (3). The trophozoites are the infective forms and are believed to gain entry into the body through the lower respiratory tract or ulcerated or broken skin and invade the central nervous system by hematogenous dissemination (4). *Acanthamoeba* species and *B mandrillaris* cysts and trophozoites are found in tissue. Courtesy of Centers for Disease Control and Prevention.

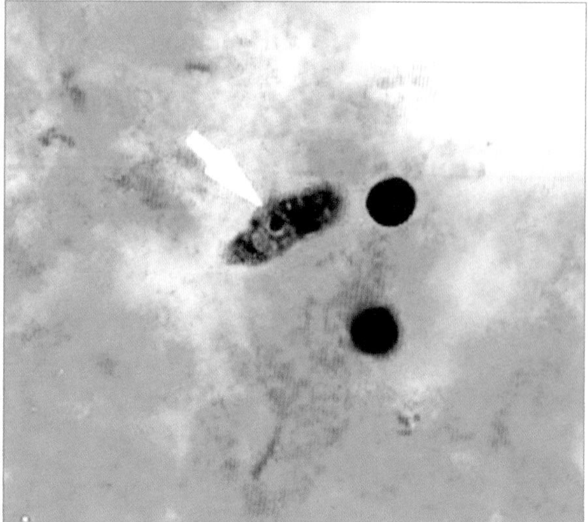

Image 4.2
Naegleria fowleri trophozoite in spinal fluid (trichrome stain). Note the typically large karyosome and monopodial locomotion. Courtesy of Centers for Disease Control and Prevention.

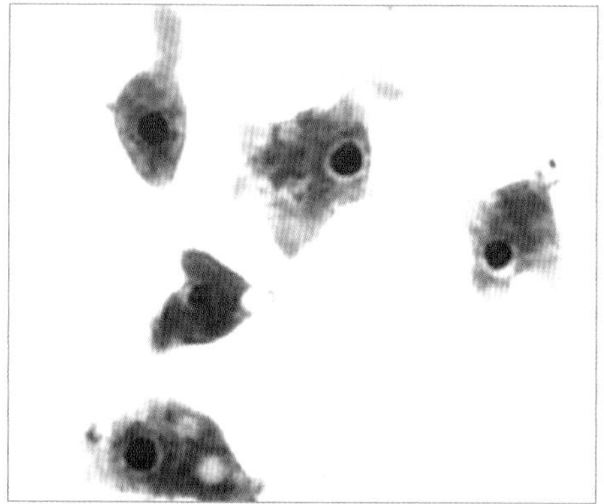

Image 4.3
Naegleria fowleri trophozoites cultured from cerebrospinal fluid. These cells have characteristically large nuclei, with a large, dark-staining karyosome. The amebae are very active and extend and retract pseudopods (trichrome stain). This sample was taken from a patient who died of primary amebic meningoencephalitis in Virginia. Courtesy of Centers for Disease Control and Prevention.

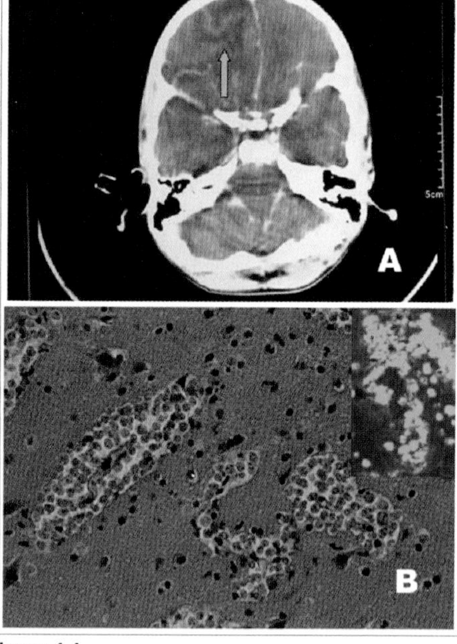

Image 4.4
A, Computed tomographic scan; note the right frontobasal collection (arrow) with a midline shift right to left. B, Brain histology; 3 large clusters of amebic vegetative forms are seen (hematoxylin-eosin stain, magnification x250). Inset: positive indirect immunofluorescent analysis on tissue section with anti–*Naegleria fowleri* serum. Courtesy of *Emerging Infectious Diseases.*

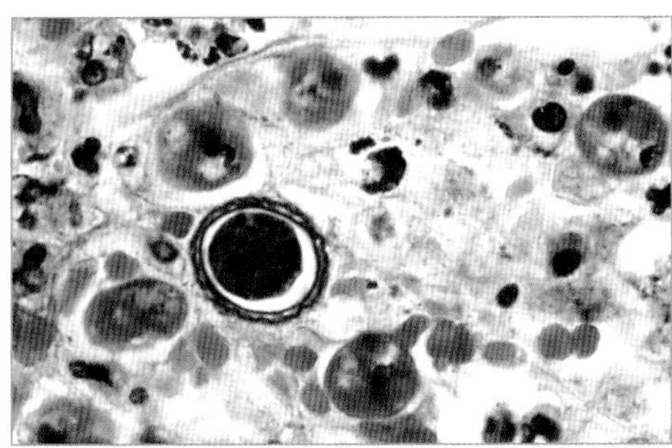

Image 4.5

This photomicrograph depicts a magnified view of brain tissue within which is a centrally located *Acanthamoeba* species cyst. *Acanthamoeba* species are opportunistic free-living amebae, capable of causing granulomatous amebic encephalitis in individuals with compromised immune systems. *Acanthamoeba* species have only 2 stages, cysts and trophozoites, in their life cycle. No flagellated stage exists as part of the life cycle. The trophozoites replicate by mitosis (nuclear membrane does not remain intact). The trophozoites are the infective forms and are believed to gain entry into the body through the lower respiratory tract or ulcerated or broken skin and invade the central nervous system by hematogenous dissemination. *Acanthamoeba* species can also cause severe keratitis in otherwise healthy individuals, particularly contact lens users. These amebae have been found in soil; fresh water, brackish water, and seawater; sewage; swimming pools; contact lens equipment; medicinal pools; dental treatment units; dialysis machines; heating, ventilating, and air-conditioning systems; mammalian cell cultures; vegetables; human nostrils and throats; and human and animal brain, skin, and lung tissues. Courtesy of Centers for Disease Control and Prevention/George Healy, PhD, DPDx.

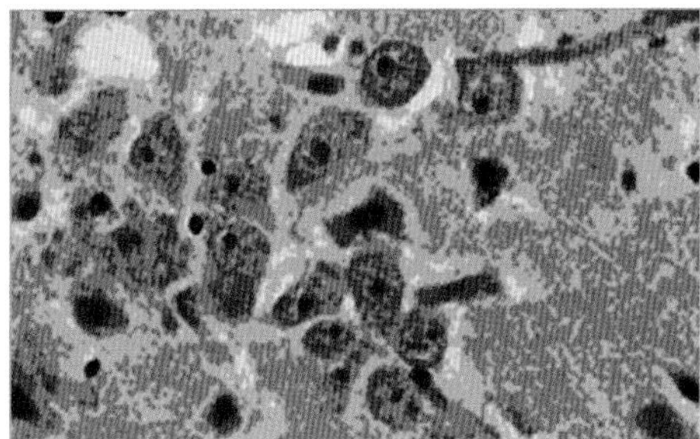

Image 4.6

Balamuthia mandrillaris trophozoites in brain tissue. Courtesy of Centers for Disease Control and Prevention.

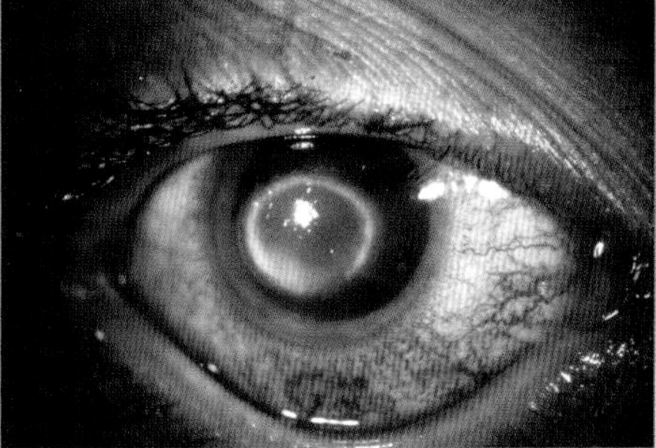

Image 4.7

Acanthamoeba keratitis. Courtesy of Susan Lehman, MD, FAAP.

5

Anthrax

Clinical Manifestations

Anthrax can occur in 4 forms, depending on the route of infection: cutaneous, inhalational, gastrointestinal, and injection.

Cutaneous anthrax begins as a pruritic papule or vesicle and progresses over 2 to 6 days to an ulcerated lesion with subsequent formation of a central black eschar. The lesion itself is characteristically painless, with surrounding edema, hyperemia, and painful regional lymphadenopathy. Patients may have associated fever, lymphangitis, and extensive edema.

Inhalational anthrax is a frequently lethal form of the disease and constitutes a medical emergency. The initial presentation is nonspecific with fever, sweats, nonproductive cough, chest pain, headache, myalgia, malaise, nausea, and vomiting, but illness progresses to the fulminant phase 2 to 5 days later. In some cases, the illness is biphasic with a period of improvement between prodromal symptoms and overwhelming illness. Fulminant manifestations include hypotension, dyspnea, hypoxia, cyanosis, and shock occurring as a result of hemorrhagic mediastinal lymphadenitis, hemorrhagic pneumonia, hemorrhagic pleural effusions, and toxemia. A widened mediastinum is the classic finding on imaging of the chest. Chest radiography may also show pleural effusions or infiltrates, both of which may be hemorrhagic in nature.

Gastrointestinal tract disease can present as one of 2 distinct clinical syndromes—intestinal or oropharyngeal. Patients with the intestinal form have nausea, anorexia, vomiting, and fever progressing to severe abdominal pain, massive ascites, hematemesis, and bloody diarrhea, related to development of edema and ulceration of the bowel, primarily the ileum and cecum. Patients with oropharyngeal anthrax may also have dysphagia with posterior oropharyngeal necrotic ulcers, which can be associated with marked, often unilateral neck swelling, regional adenopathy, fever, and sepsis.

Injection anthrax has not been reported to date in children. Its primary occurrence has been reported among injecting heroin users; however, smoking and snorting of heroin also have been identified as exposure routes. Systemic illness can result from hematogenous and lymphatic dissemination and can occur with any form of anthrax. Most patients with inhalational, gastrointestinal, and injection anthrax have systemic illness. Anthrax meningitis can occur in any patient with systemic illness regardless of origin; it can also occur in patients lacking any other apparent clinical presentation. The case-fatality rate for patients with appropriately treated cutaneous anthrax is usually less than 1%. Even with antimicrobial treatment and supportive care, the mortality rate for inhalational or gastrointestinal tract disease is between 40% and 45% and approaches 100% for meningitis.

Etiology

Bacillus anthracis is an aerobic, gram-positive, encapsulated, spore-forming, nonhemolytic, nonmotile rod. *B anthracis* has 3 major virulence factors: an antiphagocytic capsule and 2 exotoxins, called lethal and edema toxins. The toxins are responsible for the substantial morbidity and clinical manifestations of hemorrhage, edema, and necrosis.

Epidemiology

Anthrax is a zoonotic disease most commonly affecting domestic and wild herbivores that occurs in many rural regions of the world. *B anthracis* spores can remain viable in the soil for decades, representing a potential source of infection for livestock or wildlife through ingestion of spore-contaminated vegetation or water. In susceptible hosts, the spores germinate to become viable bacteria. Natural infection of humans occurs through contact with infected animals or contaminated animal products, including carcasses, hides, hair, wool, meat, and bone meal. Outbreaks of gastrointestinal tract anthrax have occurred after ingestion of undercooked or raw meat from infected animals. Historically, the vast majority (more than 95%) of cases of anthrax in the United States were cutaneous infections among animal handlers or mill workers. The incidence of naturally occurring human anthrax decreased in the United States from an estimated 130 cases annually in the early 1900s to 0 to 2 cases per year from 1979 through 2013. Recent cases of inhalational, cutaneous, and gastrointestinal tract anthrax have occurred in drum makers working with contaminated animal hides and in people participating in events where spore-contaminated drums were played. Severe soft tissue infections among heroin users, including cases with disseminated systemic infection, have been reported, although, to date, such cases have only been reported in Northern Europe.

B anthracis is one of the most likely agents to be used as a biological weapon, because its spores are highly stable, spores can infect via the respiratory route, and the resulting inhalational anthrax has a high mortality rate. In 1979, an accidental release of *B anthracis* spores from a military microbiology facility in the former Soviet Union resulted in at least 68 deaths. In 2001, 22 cases of anthrax (11 inhalational, 11 cutaneous) were identified in the United States after intentional contamination of the mail; 5 (45%) of the inhalational anthrax cases were fatal. In addition to aerosolization, there is a theoretical health risk associated with *B anthracis* spores being introduced into food products or water supplies.

Incubation Period

For cutaneous or gastrointestinal tract disease, typically 1 week or less; range 2 to 43 days in inhalational.

Diagnostic Tests

Depending on clinical presentation, Gram stain, culture, and polymerase chain reaction testing for anthrax should be performed on specimens of blood, pleural fluid, cerebrospinal fluid (CSF), and tissue biopsy specimens and on swabs of vesicular fluid or eschar material from cutaneous or oropharyngeal lesions, rectal swabs, or stool. Whenever possible, specimens should be obtained before initiating antimicrobial therapy. Gram-positive bacilli seen on unspun peripheral blood smears or in vesicular fluid or CSF can be an important initial finding, and polychrome methylene blue-stained smears showing bacilli stained blue with the capsule visualized in red are considered a presumptive identification of *B anthracis*. Traditional microbiologic methods can presumptively identify *B anthracis* from cultures. Definitive identification of suspect *B anthracis* isolates can be performed through the Laboratory Response Network in each state. Additional diagnostic tests for anthrax can be accessed through state health departments, including bacterial DNA detection in blood, CSF, or exudates by polymerase chain reaction assay, tissue immunohistochemistry, an enzyme immunoassay that measures immunoglobulin G antibodies against *B anthracis* protective antigen in paired sera, or a matrix-assisted laser desorption/ionization mass spectrometry assay measuring lethal factor activity in serum samples. The commercially available QuickELISA Anthrax-PA Kit can be used as a screening test.

Treatment

A high index of suspicion and rapid administration of appropriate antimicrobial therapy to people suspected of being infected, along with access to critical care support, are essential for effective treatment of anthrax. No controlled trials in humans have been performed to validate current treatment recommendations for anthrax, and there is limited clinical experience. Case reports suggest that naturally occurring localized or uncomplicated cutaneous disease can be treated effectively with oral ciprofloxacin or an equivalent fluoroquinolone; doxycycline and clindamycin are alternatives, as are penicillins if the isolate is known to be penicillin-susceptible. For bioterrorism-associated cutaneous disease in adults or children, ciprofloxacin or doxycycline are recommended for initial treatment until antimicrobial susceptibility data are available. Because of the risk of concomitant inhalational exposure and subsequent spore dormancy in the lungs, the antimicrobial regimen in cases of bioterrorism-associated cutaneous anthrax or that were exposed to other sources of aerosolized spores should be continued for a total of 60 days.

Ciprofloxacin is recommended as the primary antimicrobial component of an initial multidrug regimen for treatment of all forms of systemic anthrax until results of antimicrobial susceptibility testing are known. Meningitis should be suspected in all cases of inhalational anthrax and other systemic anthrax infections; thus, treatment includes at least 2 other agents with known central nervous system penetration. Meropenem is recommended as the second bactericidal antimicrobial. Linezolid is recommended as the preferred protein synthesis inhibitor if meningeal involvement is suspected.

Treatment should continue for at least 14 days or longer, depending on patient condition. Intravenous therapy can be changed to oral therapy when progression of symptoms cease and it is clinically appropriate. For anthrax with evidence of systemic illness, including fever, shock, and dissemination to other organs, anthrax immune globulin or Raxibacumab (GlaxoSmithKline, Research Triangle Park, NC), a humanized monoclonal antibody, should be considered in consultation with the Centers for Disease Control and Prevention.

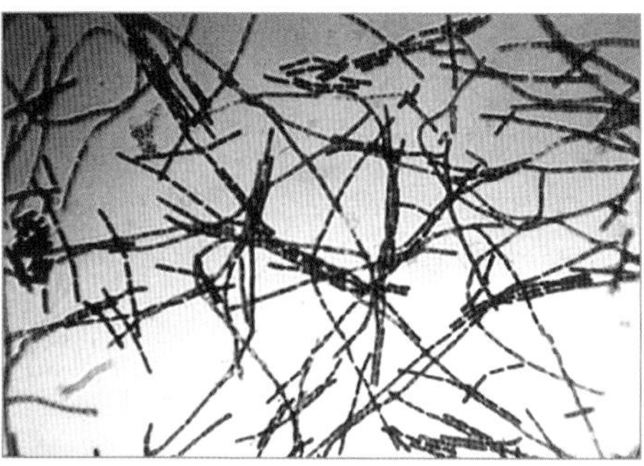

Image 5.1
A photomicrograph of *Bacillus anthracis* bacteria using Gram stain technique. Courtesy of Centers for Disease Control and Prevention.

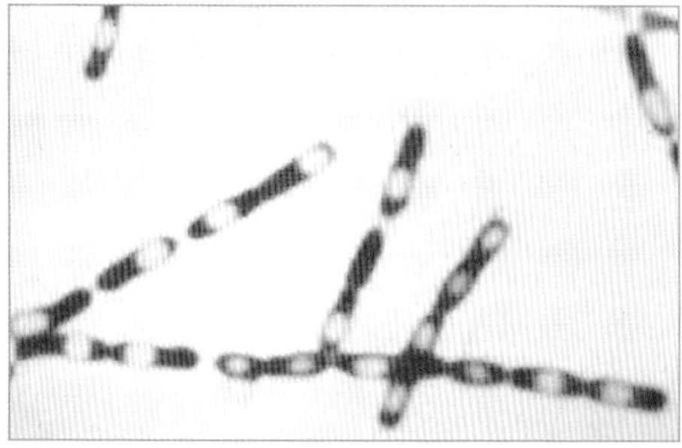

Image 5.2
Sporulation of *Bacillus anthracis,* a gram-positive, nonmotile, encapsulated bacillus.

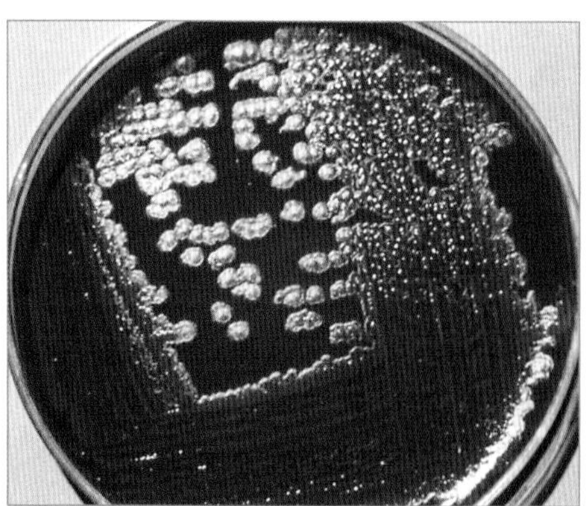

Image 5.3
A 24-hour blood agar plate culture of *Bacillus anthracis.* Courtesy of Robert Jerris, MD.

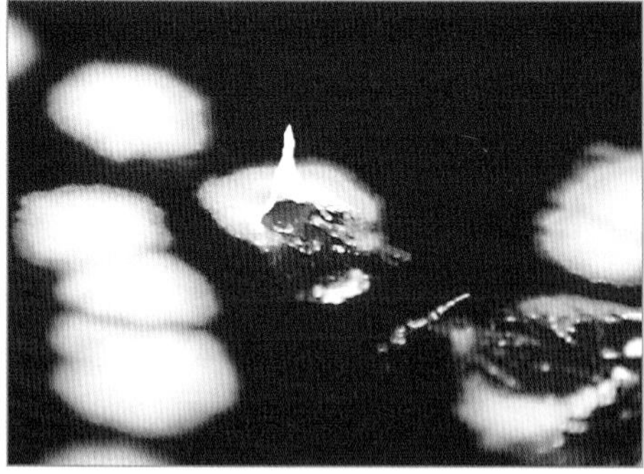

Image 5.4
Bacillus anthracis tenacity positive on sheep blood agar. *B anthracis* colony characteristics: consistency sticky (tenacious). When teased with loop, colony will stand up like beaten egg white. Courtesy of Centers for Disease Control and Prevention/Larry Stauffer, Oregon State Public Health Laboratory.

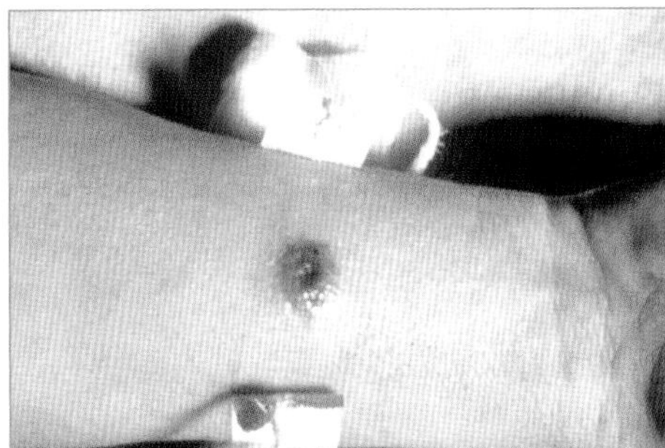

Image 5.5
Anthrax lesion on volar surface of right forearm. Note the rolled-up margin of the lesion with a central area of necrosis (eschar). Courtesy of Centers for Disease Control and Prevention.

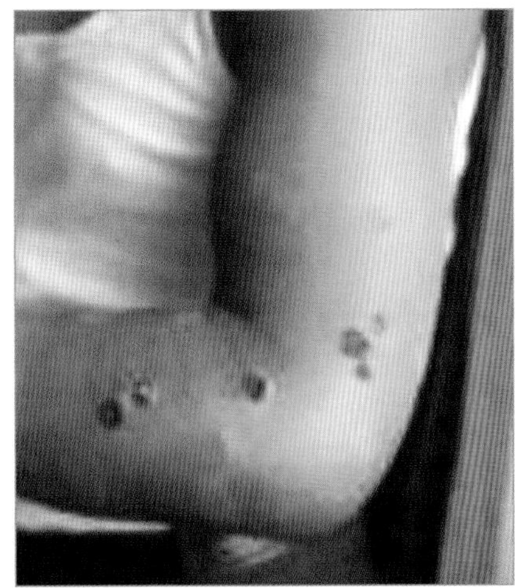

Image 5.6
Cutaneous anthrax. Notice edema and typical lesions. Courtesy of Centers for Disease Control and Prevention.

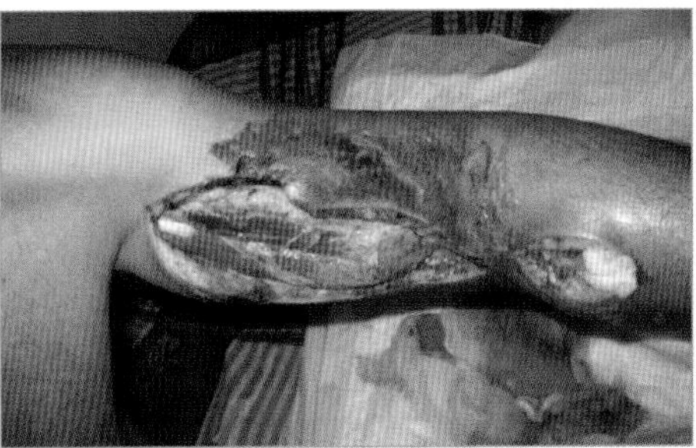

Image 5.7
Generalized cutaneous anthrax infection acquired from an ill cow. The infection began as a papule and was thought to be simple furuncle. Following an attempt at drainage, the infection aggressively spread. Antibiotic therapy was started and the patient survived. Courtesy of Mariam Svanidze, MD.

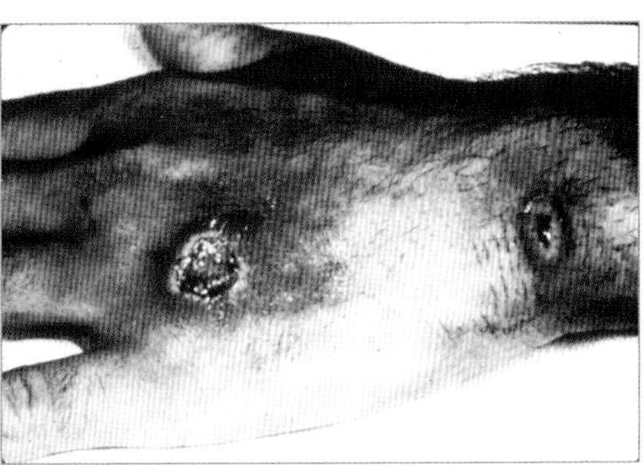

Image 5.8
Anthrax ulcers on hand and wrist of an adult. The cutaneous eschar of anthrax had been misdiagnosed as a brown recluse spider bite. Edema is common and suppuration is absent. Courtesy of Gary Overturf, MD.

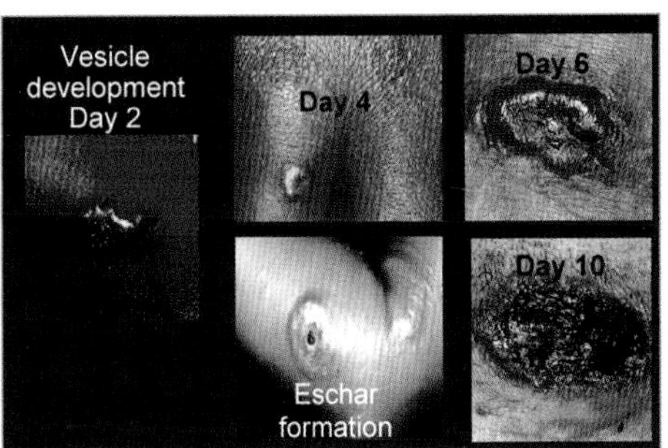

Image 5.9
Cutaneous anthrax. Vesicle development occurs from day 2 through day 10 of progression. Courtesy of Centers for Disease Control and Prevention.

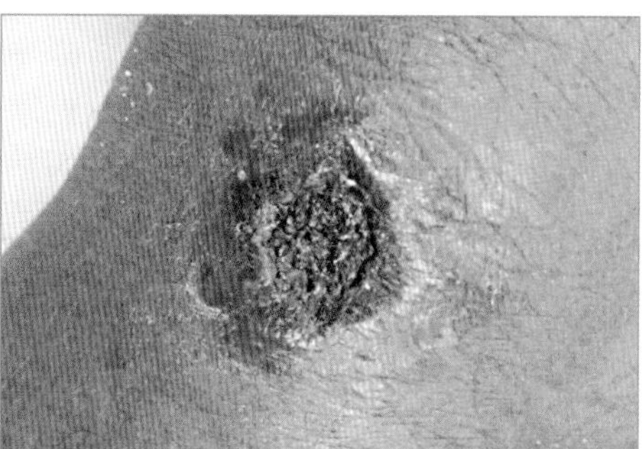

Image 5.10
Cutaneous anthrax lesion on the skin of the forearm caused by the bacterium *Bacillus anthracis*. Here, the disease has manifested itself as a cutaneous ulceration, which has begun to turn black (hence, the origin of the name *anthrax,* after the Greek name for coal). Courtesy of Centers for Disease Control and Prevention.

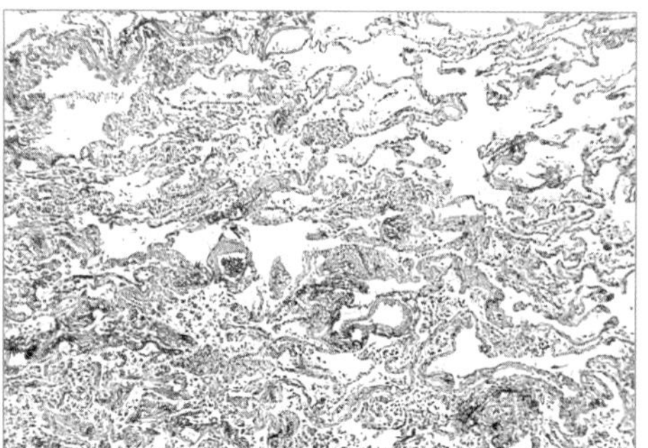

Image 5.12
Photomicrograph of lung tissue demonstrating hemorrhagic pneumonia in a case of fatal human inhalational anthrax (magnification x50). Courtesy of Centers for Disease Control and Prevention/Dr LaForce.

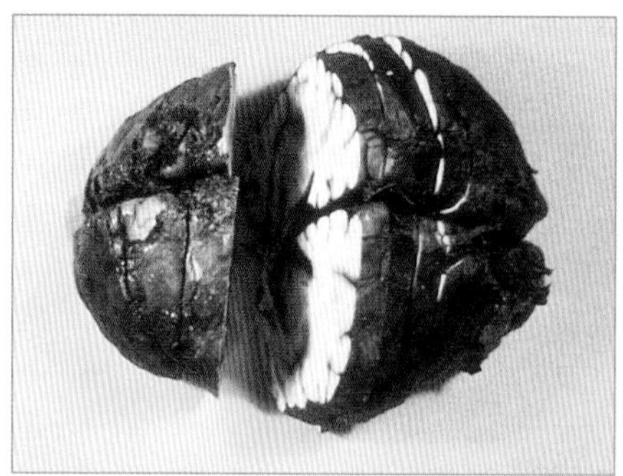

Image 5.14
Gross pathology of fixed, cut brain showing hemorrhagic meningitis secondary to inhalational anthrax. Courtesy of Centers for Disease Control and Prevention.

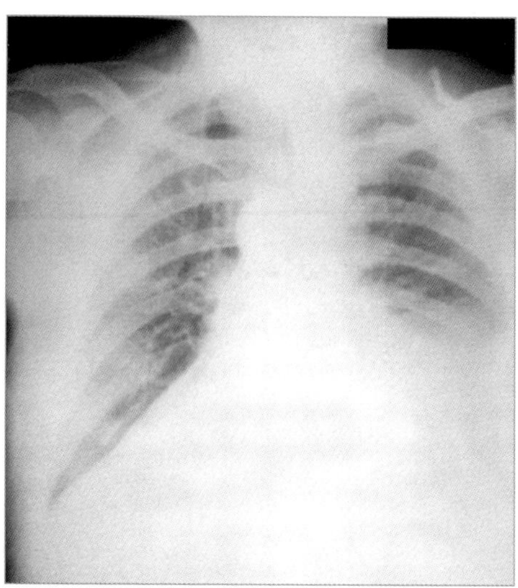

Image 5.11
Posteroanterior chest radiograph taken on the fourth day of illness, which shows a large pleural effusion and marked widening of the mediastinal shadow. Courtesy of Centers for Disease Control and Prevention.

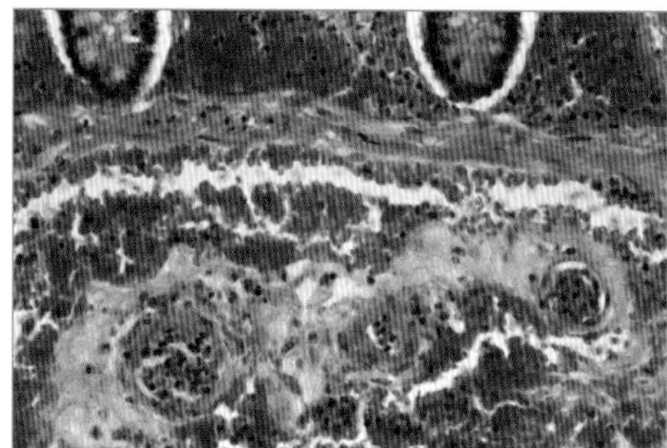

Image 5.13
This micrograph reveals submucosal hemorrhage in the small intestine in a case of fatal human anthrax (hematoxylin-eosin stain, magnification x240). The first symptoms of gastrointestinal tract anthrax are nausea, loss of appetite, bloody diarrhea, and fever, followed by severe stomach pain. One-fourth to more than half of gastro-intestinal tract anthrax cases lead to death. Note the associated arteriolar degeneration. Courtesy of Centers for Disease Control and Prevention/Dr Marshal Fox.

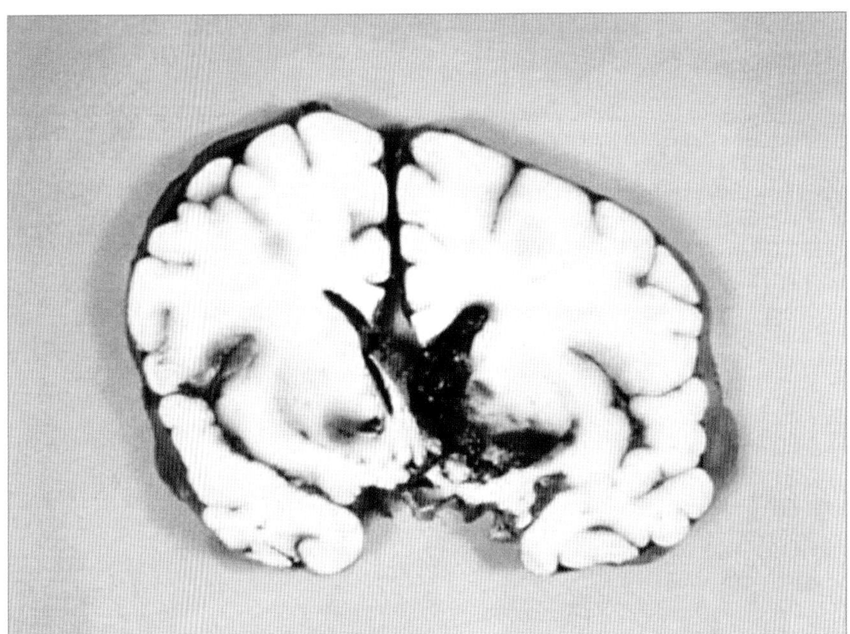

Image 5.15
This is a brain section through the ventricles revealing an interventricular hemorrhage. The 3 virulence factors of *Bacillus anthracis* are edema toxin, lethal toxin, and an antiphagocytic capsular antigen. The toxins are responsible for the primary clinical manifestations of hemorrhage, edema, and necrosis. Courtesy of Centers for Disease Control and Prevention.

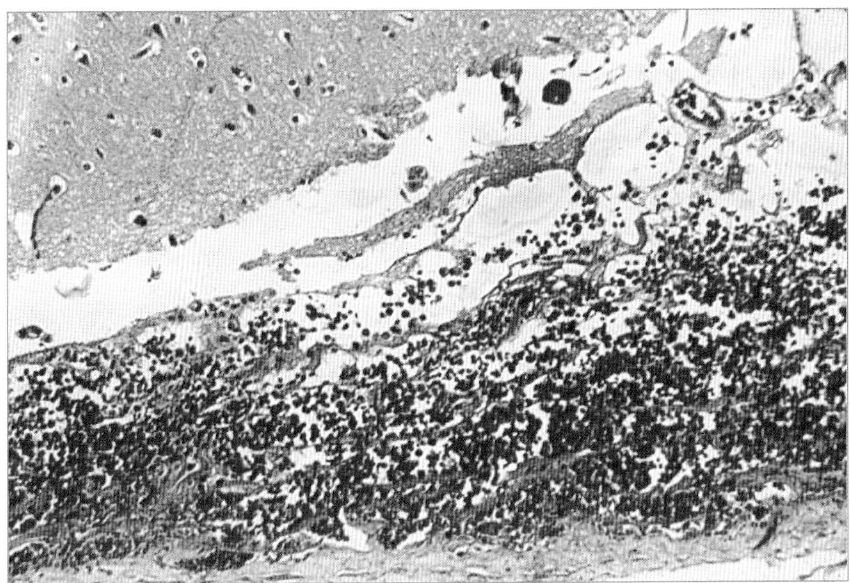

Image 5.16
Photomicrograph of meninges demonstrating hemorrhagic meningitis due to fatal inhalational anthrax (magnification x125). Courtesy of Centers for Disease Control and Prevention/Dr Laforce.

6

Arboviruses

(Including California serogroup, chikungunya, Colorado tick fever, eastern equine encephalitis, Japanese encephalitis, Powassan, St. Louis encephalitis, tick-borne encephalitis, Venezuelan equine encephalitis, western equine encephalitis, and yellow fever viruses)

Clinical Manifestations

More than 100 *ar*thropod-*bo*rne *viruses* (arboviruses) are known to cause human disease. Although most infections are subclinical, symptomatic illness usually manifests as 1 of 3 primary clinical syndromes: generalized systemic febrile illness, neuroinvasive disease, or hemorrhagic fever (Table 6.1).

- **Systemic febrile illness.** Most arboviruses are capable of causing a systemic febrile illness that often includes headache, arthralgia, myalgia, and rash. Some viruses can also cause more characteristic clinical manifestations, such as severe joint pain (eg, chikungunya virus) or jaundice (eg, yellow fever virus). With some arboviruses, fatigue, malaise, and weakness can linger for weeks following initial infection.

Most people infected with chikungunya virus become symptomatic. The incubation period is typically 3 to 7 days (range, 1–12 days). The disease is most often characterized by acute onset of fever (typically >39°C [102°F]) and polyarthralgia. Joint symptoms usually are bilateral and symmetric and can be severe and debilitating. Other symptoms may include headache, myalgia, arthritis, conjunctivitis, nausea/vomiting, or maculopapular rash. Clinical laboratory findings can include lymphopenia, thrombocytopenia, elevated creatinine, and elevated hepatic transaminases. Acute symptoms typically resolve within 7 to 10 days. Rare complications include uveitis, retinitis, myocarditis, hepatitis, nephritis, bullous skin lesions, hemorrhage, meningoencephalitis, myelitis, Guillain-Barré syndrome, and cranial nerve palsies. People at risk for severe disease include neonates exposed intrapartum, older adults (eg, >65 years), and people with underlying medical conditions (eg, hypertension, diabetes, cardiovascular disease). Some patients might have relapse of rheumatologic symptoms (polyarthralgia, polyarthritis, tenosynovitis) in the months following acute

Table 6.1
Clinical Manifestations for Select Domestic and International Arboviral Diseases

Virus	Systemic Febrile Illness	Neuroinvasive Disease[a]	Hemorrhagic Fever
Domestic			
Chikungunya	Yes[b]	Rare	No
Colorado tick fever	Yes	Rare	No
Dengue	Yes	Rare	Yes
Eastern equine encephalitis	Yes	Yes	No
La Crosse	Yes	Yes	No
Powassan	Yes	Yes	No
St. Louis encephalitis	Yes	Yes	No
Western equine encephalitis	Yes	Yes	No
West Nile	Yes	Yes	No
International			
Japanese encephalitis	Yes	Yes	No
Tick-borne encephalitis	Yes	Yes	No
Venezuelan equine encephalitis	Yes	Yes	No
Yellow fever	Yes	No	Yes

[a] Aseptic meningitis, encephalitis, or acute flaccid paralysis.
[b] Most often characterized by sudden onset of high fever and severe joint pain.

illness. Studies report variable proportions of patients with persistent joint pains for months to years. Mortality is rare.

- **Neuroinvasive disease.** Many arboviruses cause neuroinvasive diseases, including aseptic meningitis, encephalitis, or acute flaccid paralysis. Illness usually presents with a prodrome similar to the systemic febrile illness followed by neurologic symptoms. The specific symptoms vary by virus and clinical syndrome but can include vomiting, stiff neck, mental status changes, seizures, or focal neurologic deficits. The severity and long-term outcome of the illness vary by etiologic agent and the underlying characteristics of the host, such as age, immune status, and preexisting medical condition.
- **Hemorrhagic fever.** Hemorrhagic fevers can be caused by dengue or yellow fever viruses. After several days of nonspecific febrile illness, the patient may develop overt signs of hemorrhage (eg, petechiae, ecchymoses, bleeding from the nose and gums, hematemesis, melena) and septic shock (eg, decreased peripheral circulation, azotemia, tachycardia, hypotension). Hemorrhagic fever caused by dengue and yellow fever viruses can be confused with hemorrhagic fevers transmitted by rodents (eg, Argentine hemorrhagic fever, Bolivian hemorrhagic fever, Lassa fever) or those caused by Ebola or Marburg viruses. For information on other potential infections causing hemorrhagic manifestations, see Hemorrhagic Fevers Caused by Arenaviruses, Hemorrhagic Fevers Caused by Bunyaviruses, and Hemorrhagic Fevers Caused by Filoviruses: Ebola and Marburg.

Etiology

Arboviruses are RNA viruses that are transmitted to humans primarily through bites of infected arthropods (mosquitoes, ticks, sand flies, and biting midges). The viral families responsible for most arboviral infections in humans are Flaviviridae (genus *Flavivirus*), Togaviridae (genus *Alphavirus*), and Bunyaviridae (genus *Orthobunyavirus* and *Phlebovirus*). Reoviridae (genus *Coltivirus*) also are responsible for a smaller number of human arboviral infections (eg, Colorado tick fever) (Table 6.2).

Epidemiology

Most arboviruses maintain cycles of transmission between birds or small mammals and arthropod vectors. Humans and domestic animals usually are infected incidentally as "dead-end" hosts. Important exceptions are dengue, yellow fever, and chikungunya viruses, which can be spread from person to arthropod to person (anthroponotic transmission). For other arboviruses, humans usually do not develop a sustained or high enough level of viremia to infect biting arthropod vectors. Direct person-to-person spread of arboviruses can occur through blood transfusion, organ transplantation, intrauterine transmission, and, possibly, human milk. Transmission through percutaneous, mucosal, or aerosol exposure to some arboviruses has occurred rarely in laboratory and occupational settings.

In the United States, arboviral infections primarily occur from late spring through early autumn, when mosquitoes and ticks are most active. The number of domestic or imported arboviral disease cases reported in the United States varies greatly by specific etiology and year (see Table 6.2). Overall, the risk of severe clinical disease for most arboviral infections in the United States is higher among adults than among children. One notable exception is La Crosse virus infection, for which children are at highest risk of severe neurologic disease and long-term sequelae. Eastern equine encephalitis virus causes a low incidence of disease but high case-fatality rate (40%) across all age groups.

Outbreaks of chikungunya have occurred in countries in Africa, Asia, Europe, and the Indian and Pacific oceans. In late 2013, chikungunya virus was found for the first time in the Americas on islands in the Caribbean, with attack rates of up to 80% on some islands. It has spread rapidly throughout the Caribbean, and local transmission has occurred recently in Florida and South America. As of 2014, more than 1 million cases of suspected chikungunya have been reported in the Americas.

Table 6.2
Genus, Geographic Location, Vectors, and Average Number of Annual Cases Reported in the United States for Selected Domestic and International Arboviral Diseases

Virus	Genus	Predominant Geographic Locations: United States	Predominant Geographic Locations: Non–United States	Vectors	Number of US Cases/ Year (Range)[a]
Domestic					
Chikungunya	*Alphavirus*	Imported, and local transmission in Florida[b]	Asia, Africa, Indian Ocean, Western Pacific, Caribbean, South America, North America[c]	Mosquitoes	2006–2013: 28 (5–65) 2014: >1,500[c]
Colorado tick fever	*Coltivirus*	Rocky Mountain states	Western Canada	Ticks	7 (4–14)
Dengue	*Flavivirus*	Puerto Rico, Florida, Texas, and Hawaii	Worldwide in tropical areas	Mosquitoes	273 (2–720)[d]
Eastern equine encephalitis	*Alphavirus*	Eastern and gulf states	Canada, Central and South America	Mosquitoes	9 (4–22)
La Crosse	*Orthobunyavirus*	Midwest and Appalachia	Canada	Mosquitoes	82 (50–130)
Powassan	*Flavivirus*	Northeast and Midwest	Canada, Russia	Ticks	5 (0–16)
St. Louis encephalitis	*Flavivirus*	Widespread	Canada, Caribbean, Mexico, Central and South America	Mosquitoes	14 (1–49)
Western equine encephalitis	*Alphavirus*	Central and West	Central and South America	Mosquitoes	<1
West Nile	*Flavivirus*	Widespread	Canada, Europe, Africa, Asia	Mosquitoes	3,278 (712–9,862)
International					
Japanese encephalitis	*Flavivirus*	Imported only	Asia	Mosquitoes	<1
Tick-borne encephalitis	*Flavivirus*	Imported only	Europe, northern Asia	Ticks	<1
Venezuelan equine encephalitis	*Alphavirus*	Imported only	Mexico, Central and South America	Mosquitoes	<1
Yellow fever	*Flavivirus*	Imported only	South America, Africa	Mosquitoes	<1

[a] Average annual number of domestic or imported cases from 2003 through 2012.
[b] As of December 2, 2014, 11 cases of local transmission documented in Florida.
[c] From 2006 through 2013, studies identified an average of 28 people per year in the United States with positive test results for recent chikungunya virus infection (range, 5–65 per year). All were travelers visiting or returning to the United States from affected areas, mostly Asia. As of December 2, a total of 1,911 chikungunya virus disease cases have been reported during 2014 to ArboNET from US states. Eleven locally transmitted cases have been reported from Florida. All other cases occurred in travelers returning from affected areas in the Americas (n=1,880), the Pacific Islands (n=9), or Asia (n=11). Updated information on chikungunya in the Americas can be found at **www.cdc.gov/chikungunya/geo/united-states.html** and **www.paho.org/hq/index.php?Itemid=40931.**
[d] Domestic and imported cases reported to ArboNET excluding indigenous transmission in Puerto Rico; dengue became nationally notifiable in 2010.

Chikungunya virus primarily is transmitted to humans through the bites of infected mosquitoes, predominantly *Aedes aegypti* and *Aedes albopictus*. Humans are the primary host of chikungunya virus during epidemic periods. Blood-borne transmission is possible; cases have been documented among laboratory personnel handling infected blood and a health care worker drawing blood from an infected patient. Rare in utero transmission has been documented, mostly during the second trimester. Intrapartum transmission has also been documented when the mother was viremic around the time of delivery. Studies have not found chikungunya virus in human milk.

Incubation Period

Typical range, 2 to 15 days. Longer incubation periods can occur in immunocompromised people and for tick-borne viruses, such as tick-borne encephalitis viruses.

Diagnostic Tests

Arboviral infections are confirmed most frequently by measurement of virus-specific antibody in serum or cerebrospinal fluid, usually using an enzyme immunoassay. Acute-phase serum specimens should be tested for virus-specific immunoglobulin (Ig) M antibody. With clinical and epidemiologic correlation, a positive IgM test result has good diagnostic predictive value, but cross-reaction with related arboviruses from the same viral family can occur. For most arboviral infections, IgM is detectable 3 to 8 days after onset of illness and persists for 30 to 90 days, but longer persistence has been documented. Therefore, a positive IgM test result occasionally reflects a past infection. Serum collected within 10 days of illness onset may not have detectable IgM, and the test should be repeated on a convalescent sample. IgG antibody is generally detectable in serum shortly after IgM and persists for years. A plaque-reduction neutralization test can be performed to measure virus-specific neutralizing antibodies and to discriminate between cross-reacting antibodies in primary arboviral infections. A 4-fold or greater increase in virus-specific neutralizing antibodies between acute- and convalescent-phase serum specimens collected 2 to 3 weeks apart may be used to confirm recent infection. In patients who have been immunized against or infected with another arbovirus from the same virus family in the past, cross-reactive antibodies in the IgM and neutralizing antibody assays may make it difficult to identify which arbovirus is causing the patient's illness. For some arboviral infections (eg, Colorado tick fever), the immune response may be delayed, with IgM antibodies not appearing until 2 to 3 weeks after onset of illness and neutralizing antibodies taking up to a month to develop. Immunization history, date of symptom onset, and information on other arboviruses known to circulate in the geographic area that may cross-react in serologic assays should be considered when interpreting results.

Viral culture and nucleic acid amplification tests (NAATs) for RNA can be performed on acute-phase serum, cerebrospinal fluid, or tissue specimens. Arboviruses that are more likely to be detected using culture or NAATs early in the illness include chikungunya, Colorado tick fever, dengue, and yellow fever viruses. For other arboviruses, results of these tests often are negative even early in the clinical course because of the relatively short duration of viremia. Immunohistochemical staining can detect specific viral antigen in fixed tissue.

Antibody testing for common domestic arboviral diseases is performed in most state public health laboratories and many commercial laboratories. Confirmatory plaque-reduction neutralization tests, viral culture, NAATs, immunohistochemical staining, and testing for less common domestic and international arboviruses are performed at the Centers for Disease Control and Prevention.

Treatment

The primary treatment for all arboviral disease is supportive. Although various therapies have been evaluated for several arboviral diseases, none have shown specific benefit.

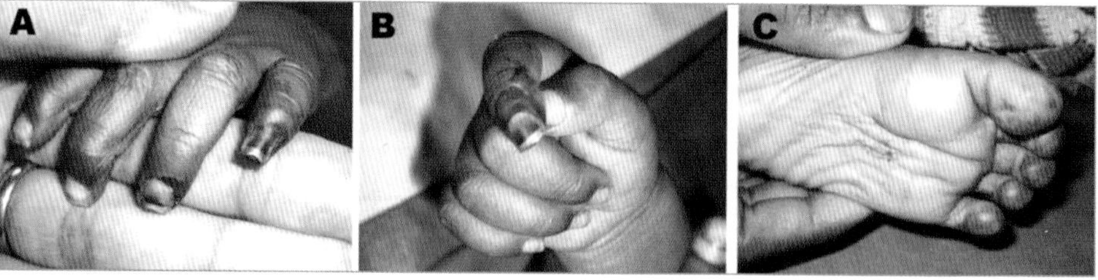

Image 6.1
Digital gangrene in an 8-month-old girl during week 3 of hospitalization. She was admitted to the hospital with fever, multiple seizures, and a widespread rash; chikungunya virus was detected in her plasma. A, Little finger of the left hand; B, index finger of the right hand; C, 4 toes on the right foot. Courtesy of Centers for Disease Control and Prevention/*Emerging Infectious Diseases.*

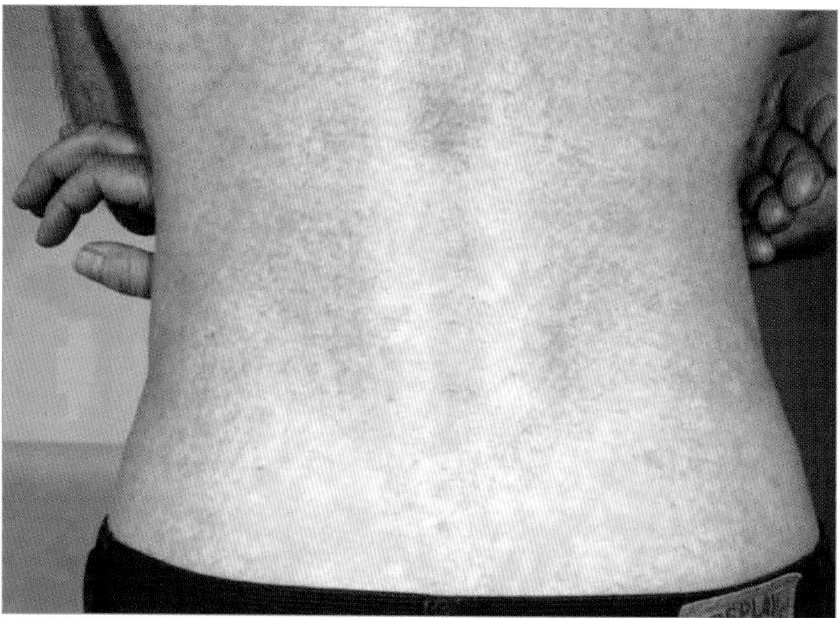

Image 6.2
Cutaneous eruption of chikungunya infection, a generalized exanthema comprising noncoalescent lesions, occurs during the first week of the disease, as seen in this patient with erythematous maculopapular lesions with islands of normal skin. Courtesy of Centers for Disease Control and Prevention/*Emerging Infectious Diseases* and Patrick Hochedez.

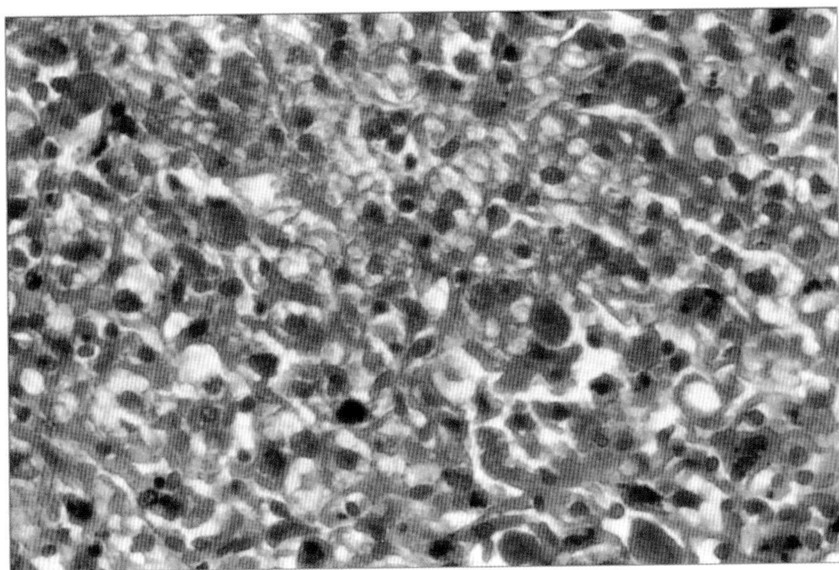

Image 6.3
This image of an autopsy specimen shows characteristic changes in liver tissue from yellow fever infection. Yellow fever is transmitted by the bites of infected mosquitoes. The word "yellow" in the name refers to the jaundice that affects some patients. The virus is endemic in tropical areas of Africa and Latin America. There is no cure for yellow fever. Fortunately, most infected patients improve and their symptoms disappear after 3 to 4 days. However, 15% of patients enter a second, more toxic, phase of the disease. About half of the patients who enter the second phase die within 10 to 14 days; the rest recover. Courtesy of Centers for Disease Control and Prevention.

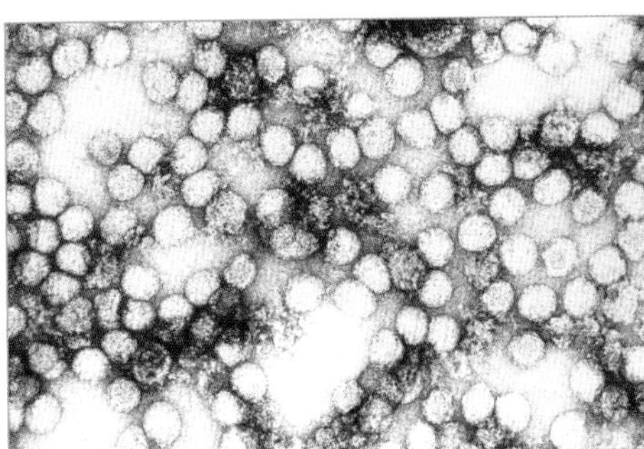

Image 6.4
An electron micrograph of yellow fever virus virions. Virions are spheroidal, uniform in shape, and 40 to 60 nm in diameter. The name "yellow fever" is due to the ensuing jaundice that affects some patients. The vector is the *Aedes aegypti* or *Haemagogus* species mosquito.

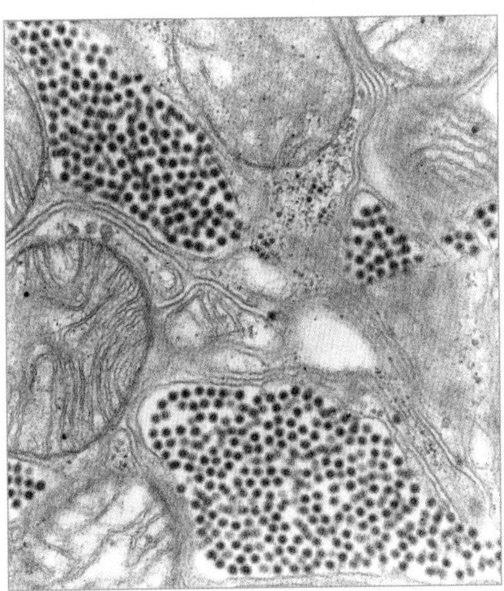

Image 6.5
This colorized transmission electron micrograph depicts a salivary gland that had been extracted from a mosquito, which was infected by the eastern equine encephalitis virus, which has been colorized red (magnification x83,900). Courtesy of Centers for Disease Control and Prevention/Fred Murphy, MD, and Sylvia Whitfield.

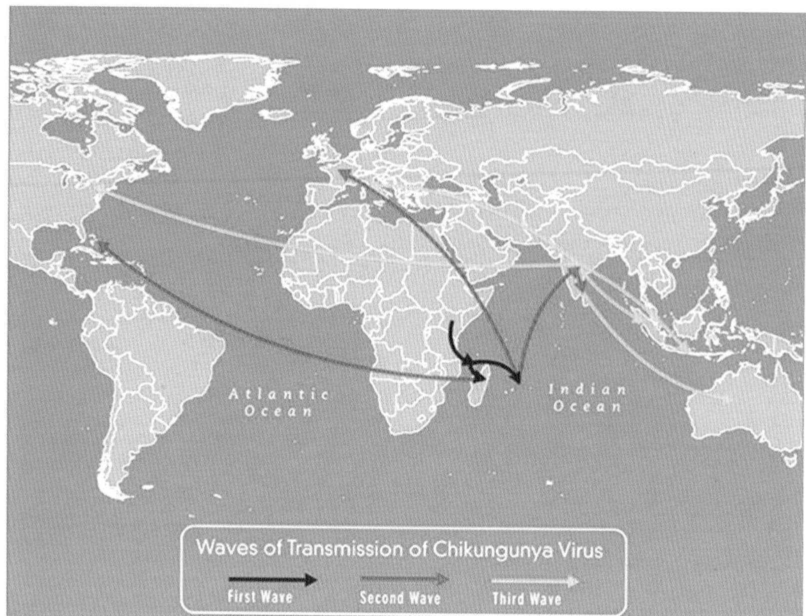

Image 6.6

Global spread of chikungunya virus during 2005 through 2009. Courtesy of *Morbidity and Mortality Weekly Report.*

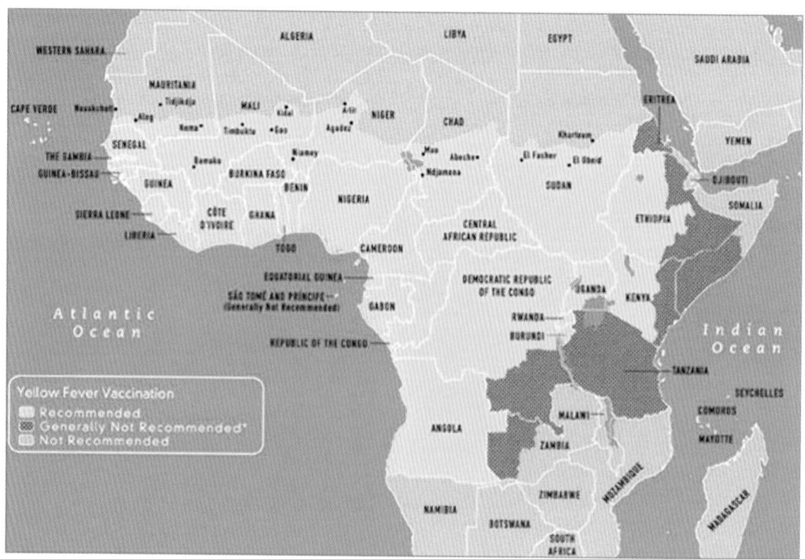

Image 6.7

Yellow fever vaccine recommendations in Africa, 2010. Courtesy of Centers for Disease Control and Prevention.

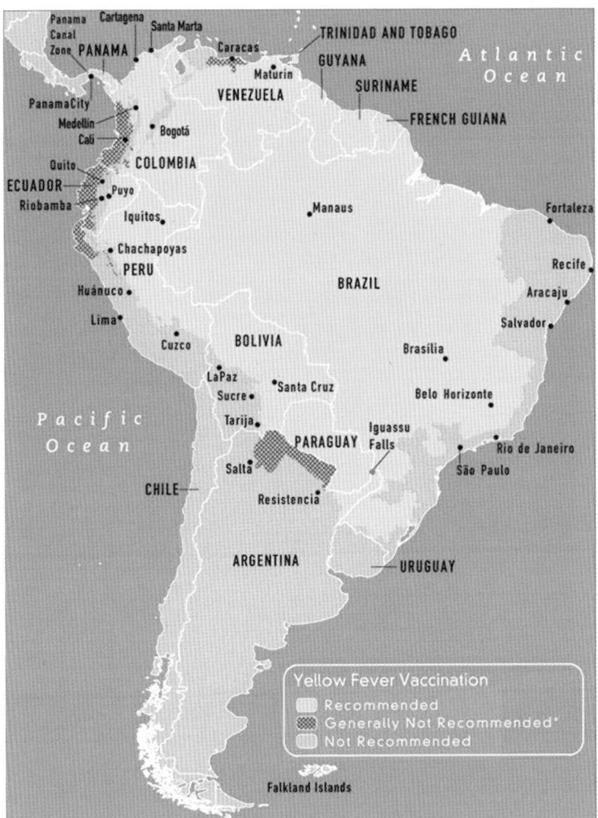

Image 6.8
Yellow fever vaccine recommendations in the Americas, 2010. Courtesy of Centers for Disease Control and Prevention.

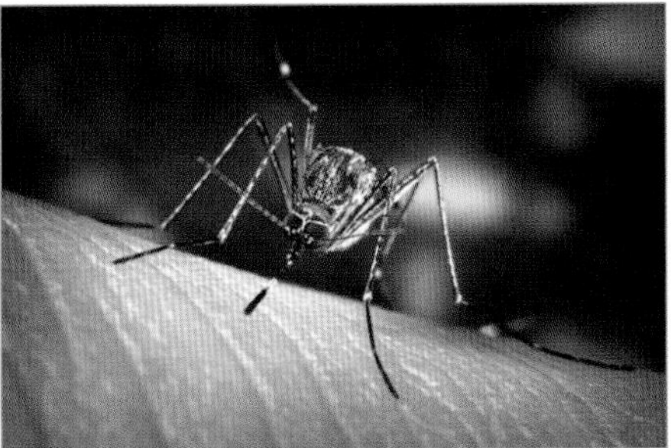

Image 6.9
A close-up anterior view of a *Culex tarsalis* mosquito as it was about to begin feeding. The epidemiologic importance of *C tarsalis* lies in its ability to spread western equine encephalomyelitis, St. Louis encephalitis, and California encephalitis and is currently the main vector of West Nile virus in the western United States. Courtesy of Centers for Disease Control and Prevention/James Gathany.

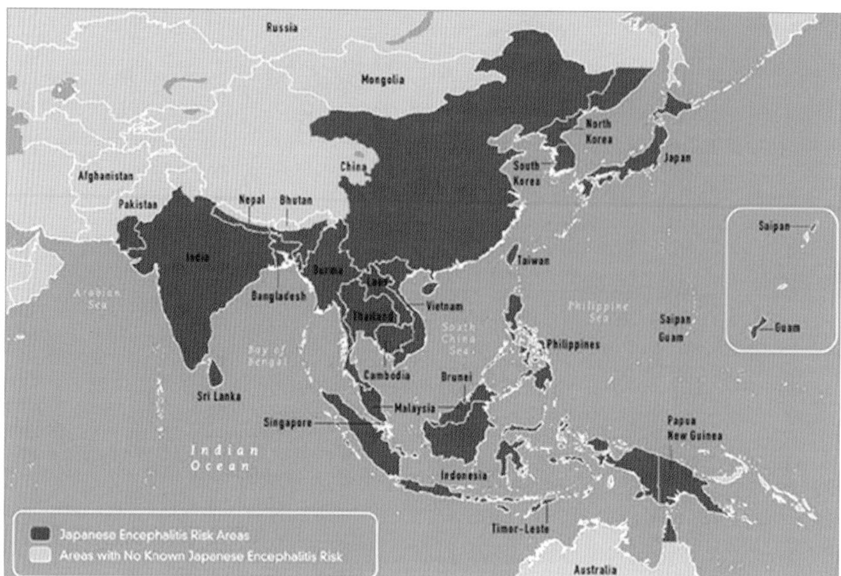

Image 6.10
Geographic distribution of Japanese encephalitis. Courtesy of Centers for Disease Control and Prevention.

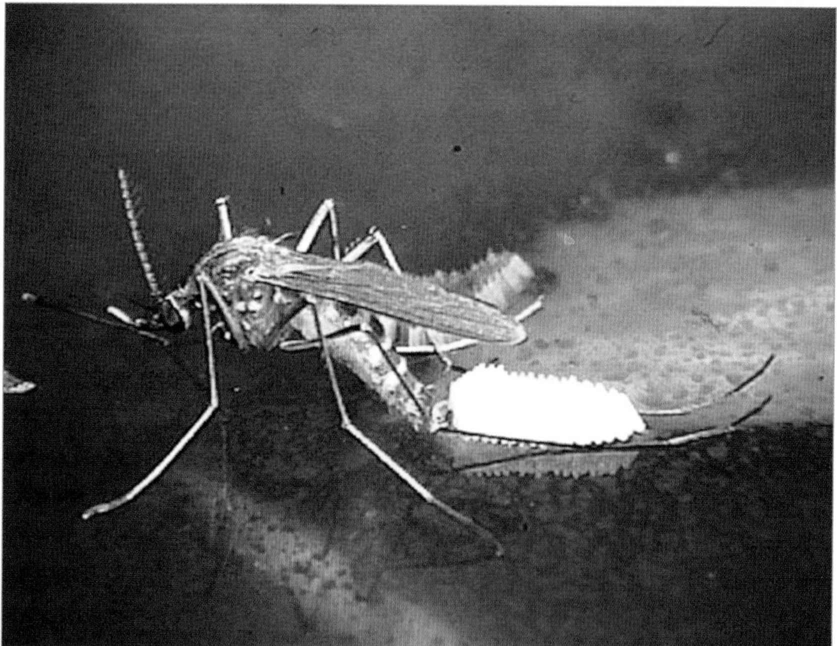

Image 6.11
The virus is transmitted by the bites of infected mosquitoes. This is an image of a *Culex* mosquito laying eggs. Japanese encephalitis is the most common vaccine-preventable cause of encephalitis in Asia. Most infections are mild (eg, fever, headache) or without apparent symptoms. However, about 1 in 200 infections results in severe disease characterized by rapid onset of high fever, headache, neck stiffness, disorientation, coma, seizures, spastic paralysis, and death. Vaccines are available to prevent Japanese encephalitis. Courtesy of Centers for Disease Control and Prevention.

7

Arcanobacterium haemolyticum Infections

Clinical Manifestations

Acute pharyngitis attributable to *Arcanobacterium haemolyticum* is often indistinguishable from that caused by group A streptococci. Fever, pharyngeal exudate, lymphadenopathy, rash, and pruritus are common, but palatal petechiae and strawberry tongue are absent. In almost half of all reported cases, a maculopapular or scarlatiniform exanthem is present, beginning on the extensor surfaces of the distal extremities, spreading centripetally to the chest and back, and sparing the face, palms, and soles. Rash is associated primarily with cases presenting with pharyngitis and typically develops 1 to 4 days after onset of sore throat, although cases have been reported with rash preceding pharyngitis. Respiratory tract infections that mimic diphtheria, including membranous pharyngitis, sinusitis, and pneumonia, and skin and soft tissue infections, including chronic ulceration, cellulitis, paronychia, and wound infection, have been attributed to *A haemolyticum*. Invasive infections, including septicemia, peritonsillar abscess, Lemierre syndrome, brain abscess, orbital cellulitis, meningitis, endocarditis, pyogenic arthritis, osteomyelitis, urinary tract infection, pneumonia, spontaneous bacterial peritonitis, and pyothorax, have been reported. No nonsuppurative sequelae have been reported.

Etiology

A haemolyticum is a catalase-negative, weakly acid-fast, facultative, hemolytic, anaerobic, gram-positive, slender, sometimes club-shaped bacillus formerly classified as *Corynebacterium haemolyticum*.

Epidemiology

Humans are the primary reservoir of *A haemolyticum*, and spread is person to person, presumably via droplet respiratory tract secretions. Severe disease occurs almost exclusively among people who are immunocompromised. Pharyngitis occurs primarily in adolescents and young adults and is very unusual in young children. Although long-term pharyngeal carriage with *A haemolyticum* has been described after an episode of acute pharyngitis, isolation of the bacterium from the nasopharynx of asymptomatic people is rare.

Incubation Period

Unknown.

Diagnostic Tests

A haemolyticum grows on blood-enriched agar, but colonies are small, have narrow bands of hemolysis, and may not be visible for 48 to 72 hours. Detection is enhanced by culture on rabbit or human blood agar rather than sheep blood agar because of larger colony size and wider zones of hemolysis. Presence of 5% carbon dioxide also enhances growth. Pits characteristically form under the colonies on blood agar plates. Two biotypes of *A haemolyticum* have been identified: a rough biotype predominates in respiratory tract infections, and a smooth biotype is most commonly associated with skin and soft-tissue infections.

Treatment

Erythromycin is the drug of choice for treating tonsillopharyngitis attributable to *A haemolyticum*. *A haemolyticum* generally is susceptible to azithromycin, clindamycin, cefuroxime, vancomycin, and tetracycline. Failures in treatment of pharyngitis with penicillin have been reported. Resistance to trimethoprim-sulfamethoxazole is common. In rare cases of disseminated infection, susceptibility tests should be performed. In disseminated infection, parenteral penicillin plus an aminoglycoside may be used initially as empiric treatment.

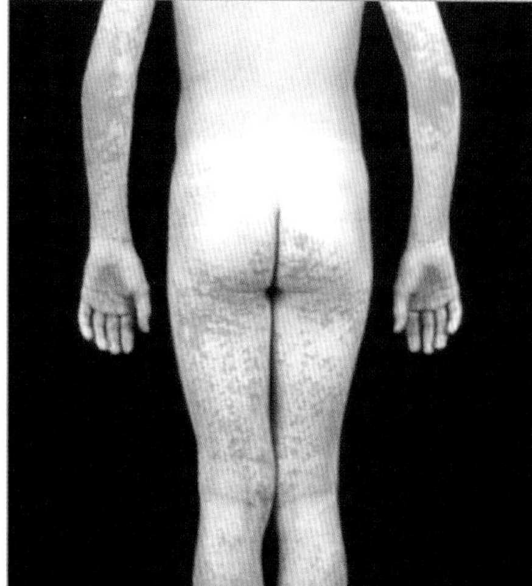

Image 7.1
Arcanobacterium haemolyticum was isolated on pharyngeal culture from this 12-year-old boy with an erythematous rash that was followed by mild desquamation. Copyright Williams/Karofsky.

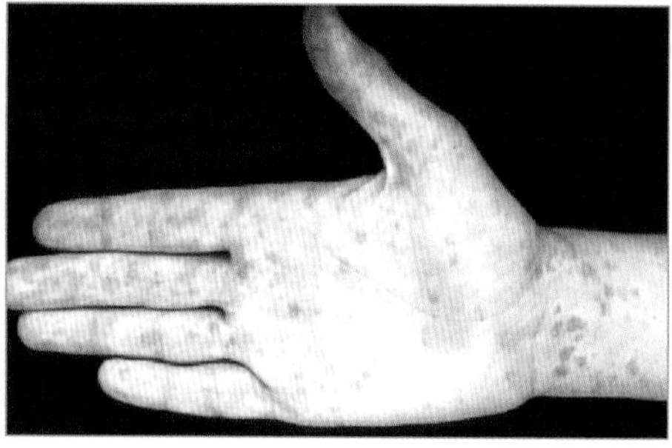

Image 7.3
Note that the palms are affected in this patient, though they are often spared. Copyright Williams/Karofsky.

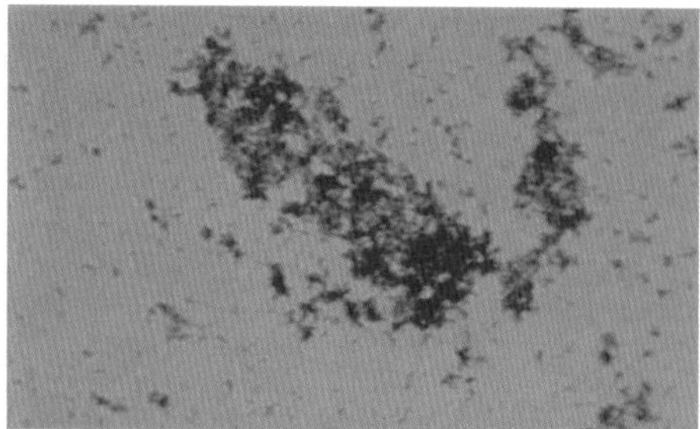

Image 7.5
Arcanobacterium haemolyticum (Gram stain). *A haemolyticum* appears strongly gram-positive in young cultures but becomes more gram-variable after 24 hours of incubation. Copyright Noni MacDonald, MD, FAAP.

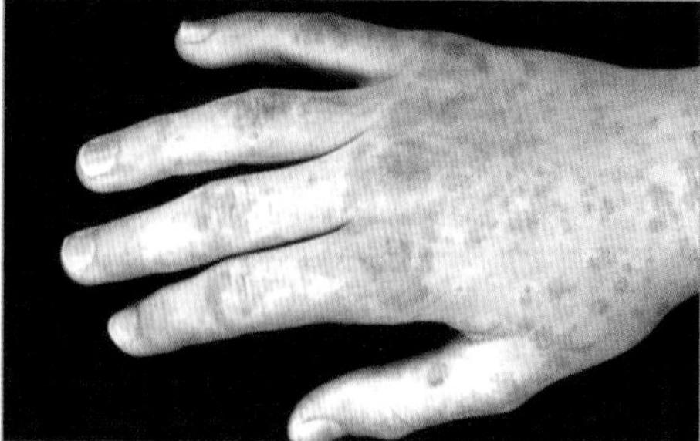

Image 7.2
Arcanobacterium haemolyticum–associated rash on dorsal surface of hand in the 12-year-old boy in images 7.1, 7.3, and 7.4. Copyright Williams/Karofsky.

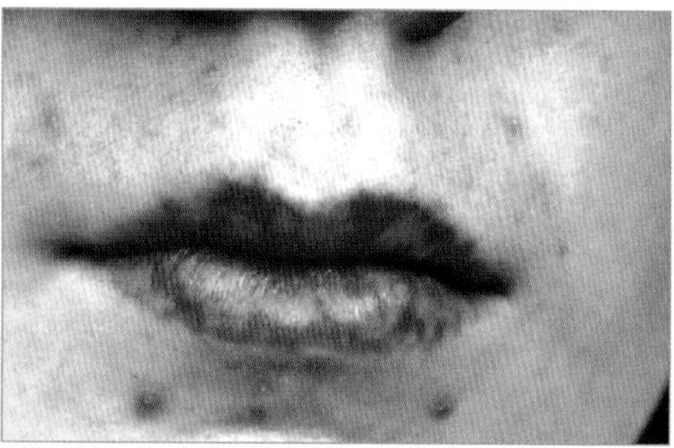

Image 7.4
Although not present in this patient with facial skin lesions associated with *Arcanobacterium haemolyticum* pharyngitis, a pharyngeal membrane similar to that of diphtheria may occur with *A haemolyticum* pharyngeal infection. Copyright Williams/Karofsky.

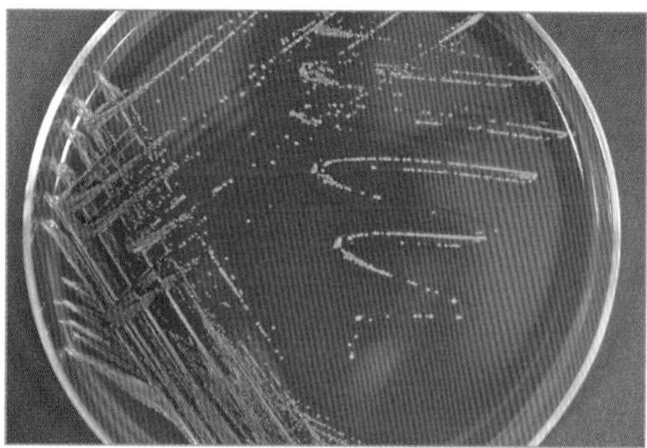

Image 7.6
Arcanobacterium haemolyticum on blood agar. Colonies are small and produce b-hemolysis on blood agar. Courtesy of Julia Rosebush, DO; Robert Jerris, PhD; and Theresa Stanley, M(ASCP).

8

Ascaris lumbricoides Infections

Clinical Manifestations

Most infections with *Ascaris lumbricoides* are asymptomatic, although moderate to heavy infections can lead to malnutrition and nonspecific gastrointestinal tract symptoms. During the larval migratory phase, an acute transient pneumonitis (Löffler syndrome) associated with fever and marked eosinophilia may occur. Acute intestinal obstruction has been associated with heavy infections. Children are prone to this complication because of the small diameter of the intestinal lumen and their propensity to acquire large worm burdens. Worm migration can cause peritonitis secondary to intestinal wall perforation and common bile duct obstruction, resulting in biliary colic, cholangitis, or pancreatitis. Adult worms can be stimulated to migrate by stressful conditions (eg, fever, illness, anesthesia) and by some anthelmintic drugs. *A lumbricoides* has been found in the appendiceal lumen in patients with acute appendicitis.

Etiology

A lumbricoides is the most prevalent of all human intestinal nematodes (roundworms), with more than 1 billion people infected worldwide.

Epidemiology

Adult worms live in the lumen of the small intestine. Female worms produce approximately 200,000 eggs per day, which are excreted in stool and must incubate in soil for 2 to 3 weeks for an embryo to become infectious. Following ingestion of embryonated eggs, usually from contaminated soil, larvae hatch in the small intestine, penetrate the mucosa, and are transported passively by portal blood to the liver and lungs. After migrating into the airways, larvae ascend through the tracheobronchial tree to the pharynx, are swallowed, and mature into adults in the small intestine. Infection with *A lumbricoides* is most common in resource-limited countries, including rural and urban communities characterized by poor sanitation. Adult worms can live for 12 to 18 months, resulting in daily fecal excretion of large numbers of ova. Female worms are longer than male worms and can measure 40 cm in length and 6 mm in diameter. Direct person-to-person transmission does not occur.

Incubation Period

Approximately 8 weeks (from ingestion to egg-laying adults).

Diagnostic Tests

Ova are routinely detected by examination of a fresh stool specimen using light microscopy. Infected people may also pass adult worms from the rectum, from the nose after migration through the nares, and from the mouth, usually in vomitus. Adult worms may be detected by computed tomographic scan of the abdomen or by ultrasonographic examination of the biliary tree.

Treatment

Albendazole (taken with food in a single dose), mebendazole for 3 days, or ivermectin (taken on an empty stomach in a single dose) is recommended for treatment of ascariasis. Nitazoxanide taken twice a day for 3 days is also effective against *A lumbricoides*. Reexamination of stool specimens can be performed 2 weeks after therapy to determine whether the worms have been eliminated.

Conservative management of small bowel obstruction, including nasogastric suction and intravenous fluids, may result in resolution of major symptoms before administration of anthelmintic therapy. Use of mineral oil or diatrizoate meglumine and diatrizoate sodium solution (Gastrografin), orally or by nasogastric tube, may cause relaxation of the bolus of worms. Surgical intervention occasionally is necessary to relieve intestinal or biliary tract obstruction or for volvulus or peritonitis secondary to perforation. Endoscopic retrograde cholangiopancreatography has been used successfully for extraction of worms from the biliary tree.

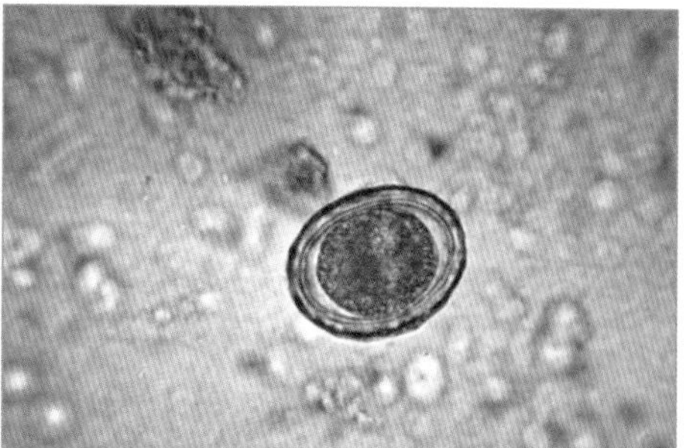

Image 8.1
This micrograph reveals a fertilized egg of the roundworm *Ascaris lumbricoides* (magnification x400). Fertilized eggs are rounded and have a thick shell, while unfertilized eggs are elongated and larger, thinner shelled, and covered by a more visible mammillated layer, which is sometimes covered by protuberances. Courtesy of Centers for Disease Control and Prevention/ Mae Melvin, MD.

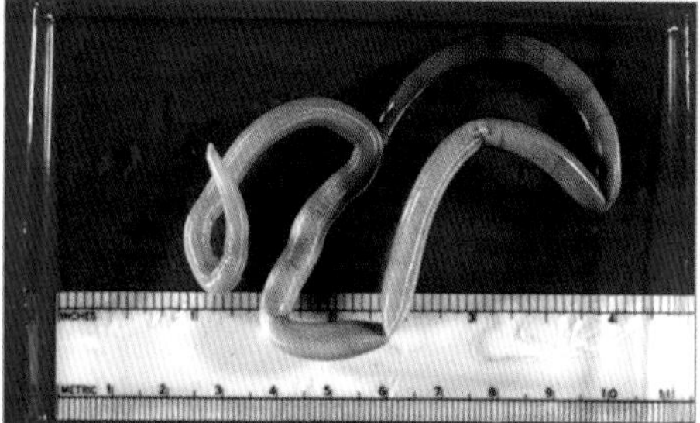

Image 8.3
Adult ascaris.

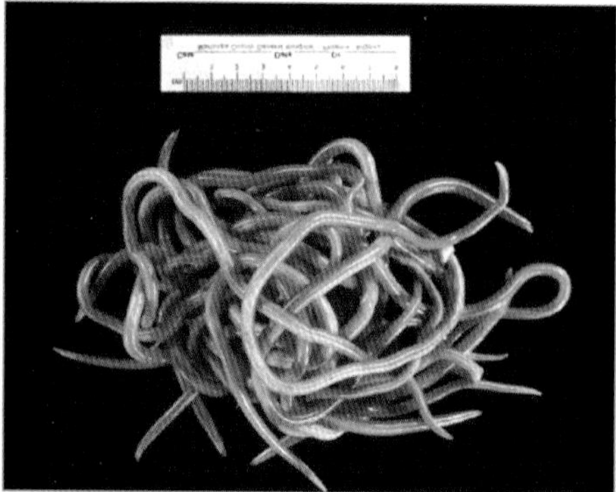

Image 8.5
A mass of large roundworms (*Ascaris lumbricoides*) from a human infestation.

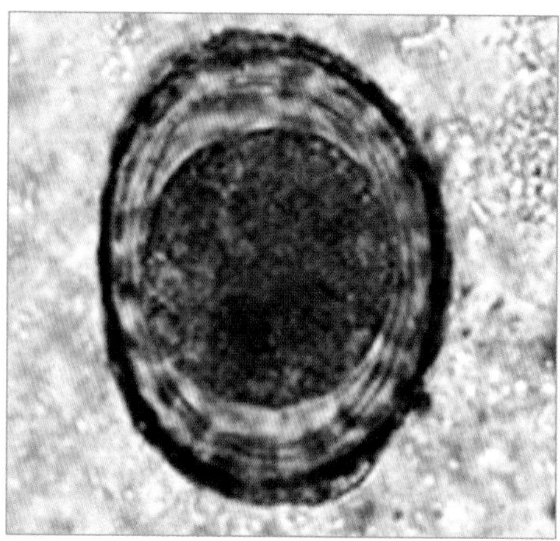

Image 8.2
A fertilized ascaris egg, still at the unicellular stage, which is the usual stage when the eggs are passed in the stool (complete development of the larva requires 18 days under favorable conditions). Courtesy of Centers for Disease Control and Prevention.

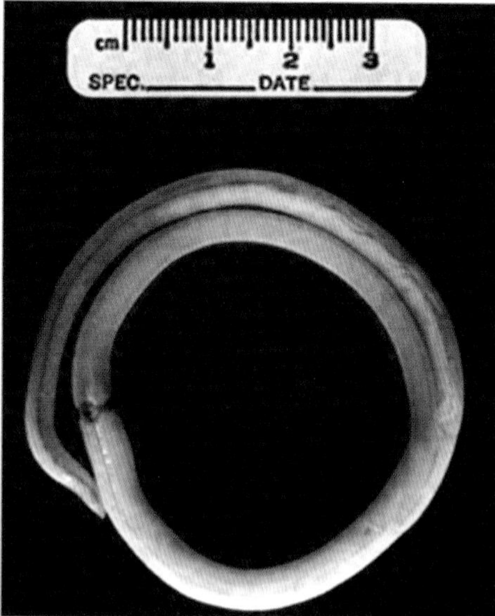

Image 8.4
An adult ascaris. Diagnostic characteristics: tapered ends; length, 15 to 35 cm (females tend to be larger). This worm is a female, as evidenced by the size and genital girdle (the dark circular groove at left side of image). Courtesy of Centers for Disease Control and Prevention.

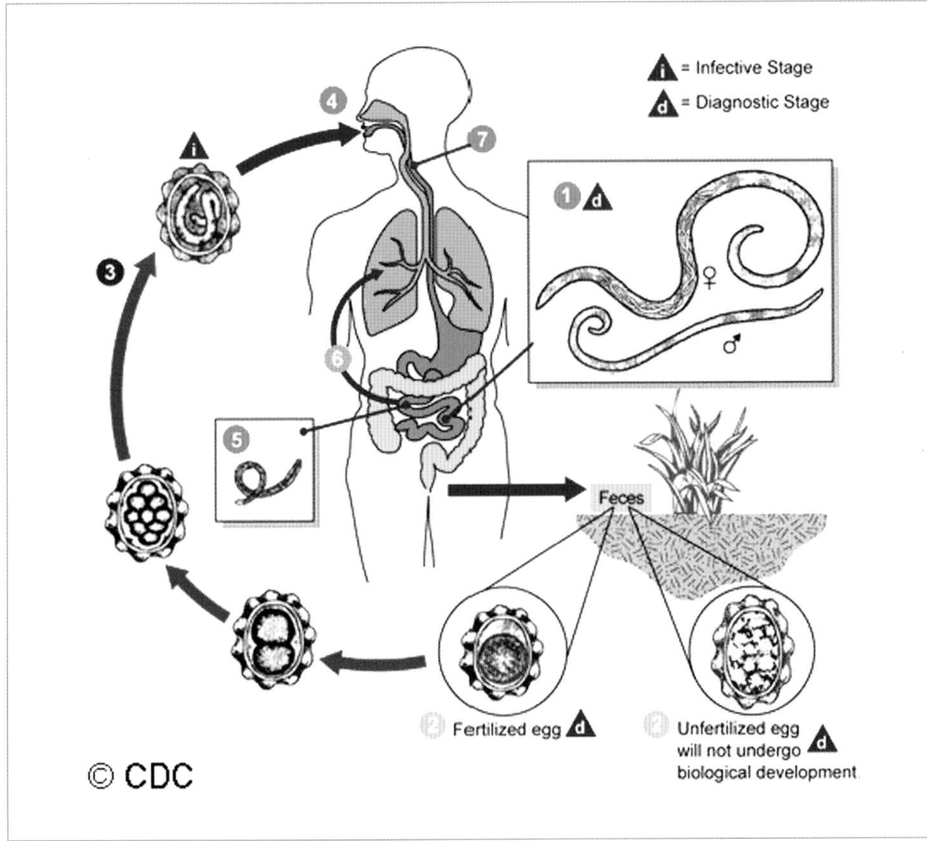

Image 8.6

Adult worms (1) live in the lumen of the small intestine. A female may produce approximately 200,000 eggs per day, which are passed with the feces (2). Unfertilized eggs may be ingested but are not infective. Fertile eggs embryonate and become infective after 18 days to several weeks (3), depending on the environmental conditions (optimum: moist, warm, shaded soil). After infective eggs are swallowed (4), the larvae hatch (5), invade the intestinal mucosa, and are carried via the portal, and then systemic circulation to the lungs (6). The larvae mature further in the lungs (10–14 days), penetrate the alveolar walls, ascend the bronchial tree to the throat, and are swallowed (7). On reaching the small intestine, they develop into adult worms. Between 2 and 3 months are required from ingestion of the infective eggs to oviposition by the adult female. Adult worms can live 1 to 2 years. Courtesy of Centers for Disease Control and Prevention/Courtesy of DPDx.

9

Aspergillosis

Clinical Manifestations

Aspergillosis manifests as 3 principal clinical entities: invasive aspergillosis, pulmonary aspergilloma, and allergic disease. Colonization of the respiratory tract is common. The clinical manifestations and severity depend on the immune status of the host.

- **Invasive aspergillosis** occurs almost exclusively in immunocompromised patients with prolonged neutropenia (eg, cytotoxic chemotherapy), graft-versus-host disease, impaired phagocyte function (eg, chronic granulomatous disease), or receipt of T lymphocyte immunosuppressive therapy. Children at highest risk include those with new-onset acute myelogenous leukemia, with relapse of hematologic malignancy, and recipients of allogeneic hematopoietic stem cell and solid organ transplantation. Invasive infection usually involves pulmonary, sinus, cerebral, or cutaneous sites. Rarely, endocarditis, osteomyelitis, meningitis, infection of the eye or orbit, and esophagitis occur. The hallmark of invasive aspergillosis is angioinvasion with resulting thrombosis, dissemination to other organs, and, occasionally, erosion of the blood vessel wall with catastrophic hemorrhage. Aspergillosis in patients with chronic granulomatous disease rarely displays angioinvasion.
- **Pulmonary aspergillomas and otomycosis** are 2 syndromes of nonallergic colonization by *Aspergillus* species in immunocompetent children. Aspergillomas ("fungal balls") grow in preexisting pulmonary cavities or bronchogenic cysts without invading pulmonary tissue; almost all patients have underlying lung disease, such as cystic fibrosis or tuberculosis. Patients with otomycosis have chronic otitis media with colonization of the external auditory canal by a fungal mat that produces a dark discharge.
- **Allergic bronchopulmonary aspergillosis** is a hypersensitivity lung disease that manifests as episodic wheezing, expectoration of brown mucus plugs, low-grade fever, eosinophilia, and transient pulmonary infiltrates. This form of aspergillosis occurs most commonly in immunocompetent children with asthma or cystic fibrosis and can be a trigger for asthmatic flares.
- **Allergic sinusitis** is a far less common allergic response to colonization by *Aspergillus* species than allergic bronchopulmonary aspergillosis. Allergic sinusitis occurs in children with nasal polyps or previous episodes of sinusitis or who have undergone sinus surgery. Allergic sinusitis is characterized by symptoms of chronic sinusitis with dark plugs of nasal discharge.

Etiology

Aspergillus species are ubiquitous molds that grow on decaying vegetation and in soil. *Aspergillus fumigatus* is the most common cause of invasive aspergillosis, with *Aspergillus flavus* being the next most common. Several other species, including *Aspergillus terreus, Aspergillus nidulans,* and *Aspergillus niger,* also cause invasive human infections.

Epidemiology

The principal route of transmission is inhalation of conidia (spores) originating from multiple environmental sources (eg, plants, vegetables, dust from construction or demolition), soil, and water supplies (eg, showerheads). Incidence of disease in hematopoietic stem cell transplant recipients is highest during periods of neutropenia or treatment for graft-versus-host disease. In solid organ transplant recipients, the risk is highest 1 to 6 months after transplantation or during periods of increased immunosuppression. Health care–associated outbreaks of invasive pulmonary aspergillosis in susceptible hosts have occurred in which the probable source of the fungus was a nearby construction site or faulty ventilation system. Cutaneous aspergillosis occurs less frequently and usually involves sites of skin injury, such as intravenous catheter sites, sites of traumatic inoculation, and sites associated with occlusive dressings, burns, or surgery. Transmission by direct inoculation of skin abrasions or wounds is less likely. Person-to-person spread does not occur.

Incubation Period

Unknown.

Diagnostic Tests

Dichotomously branched and septate hyphae, identified by microscopic examination of 10% potassium hydroxide wet preparations or of Grocott-Gomori methenamine–silver nitrate stain of tissue or bronchoalveolar lavage specimens, are suggestive of the diagnosis. Isolation of *Aspergillus* species or molecular testing with specific reagents is required for definitive diagnosis. The organism is usually not recoverable from blood (except *A terreus*) but is isolated readily from lung, sinus, and skin biopsy specimens when cultured on fungal media. *Aspergillus* species can be a laboratory contaminant, but when evaluating results from ill, immunocompromised patients, recovery of this organism frequently indicates infection. Biopsy of a lesion is usually required to confirm the diagnosis, and care should be taken to distinguish aspergillosis from mucormycosis, which appears similar by diagnostic imaging studies. An enzyme immunosorbent assay serologic test for detection of galactomannan, a molecule found in the cell wall of *Aspergillus* species, from the serum or bronchoalveolar lavage fluid is available commercially and has been found to be useful in children and adults. Monitoring of serum antigen concentrations twice weekly in periods of highest risk (eg, neutropenia, active graft-versus-host disease) may be useful for early detection of invasive aspergillosis in at-risk patients. False-positive test results have been reported and can be related to consumption of food products containing galactomannan (eg, rice, pasta) or cross-reactivity with antimicrobial agents derived from fungi (eg, penicillins, especially piperacillin-tazobactam). A negative galactomannan test result does not exclude diagnosis. A negative galactomannan test result consistently occurs in patients with chronic granulomatous disease. Children frequently do not manifest cavitation or the air crescent or halo signs on chest radiography, and lack of these characteristic signs does not exclude the diagnosis of invasive aspergillosis.

In allergic aspergillosis, diagnosis is suggested by a typical clinical syndrome with elevated total concentrations of immunoglobulin (Ig) E (≥1,000 ng/mL) and *Aspergillus*-specific serum IgE, eosinophilia, and a positive result from a skin test for *Aspergillus* antigens. In people with cystic fibrosis, diagnosis is more difficult because wheezing, eosinophilia, and a positive skin test result not associated with allergic bronchopulmonary aspergillosis are often present.

Treatment

Voriconazole is the drug of choice for invasive aspergillosis, except in neonates, for whom amphotericin B deoxycholate in high doses is recommended. Voriconazole has been shown to be superior to amphotericin B in a large, randomized trial in adults. Therapy is continued for at least 12 weeks, but treatment duration should be individualized. Monitoring of serum galactomannan concentrations in those with significant elevation at onset may be useful to assess response to therapy concomitant with clinical and radiologic evaluation. Voriconazole is metabolized in a linear fashion in children, so the recommended adult dosing is too low for children. Children 12 years and older who weigh 50 kg or more should receive the adult dose. Close monitoring of voriconazole serum trough concentrations when oral voriconazole is used is critical for efficacy and safety and because there is high interpatient variability in metabolism.

Lipid formulations of amphotericin B can be considered as alternative primary therapy in some patients, but *A terreus* is resistant to all amphotericin B products. In refractory disease, treatment could include posaconazole, caspofungin, or micafungin. Caspofungin has been studied in pediatric patients older than 3 months as salvage therapy for invasive aspergillosis. Limited data from a predominantly adult population are available but suggest that micafungin and caspofungin have similar efficacy in treatment of refractory aspergillosis. The pharmacokinetics and safety of posaconazole have not been evaluated in younger children.

The efficacy and safety of combination antifungal therapy for invasive aspergillosis is uncertain, but the most promising combination is a broad-spectrum azole combined with an echinocandin. Immune reconstitution can occur during treatment in some patients. Decreasing immunosuppression, if possible (specifically decreasing corticosteroid dose), is critical to disease control.

Surgical excision of a localized invasive lesion (eg, cutaneous eschars, a single pulmonary lesion, sinus debris, accessible cerebral lesions) is usually warranted. In pulmonary disease, surgery is indicated only when a mass is impinging on a great vessel. Allergic bronchopulmonary aspergillosis is treated with corticosteroids, and adjunctive antifungal therapy is recommended. Allergic sinus aspergillosis is also treated with corticosteroids, and surgery has been reported to be beneficial in many cases. Antifungal therapy has not been found to be useful.

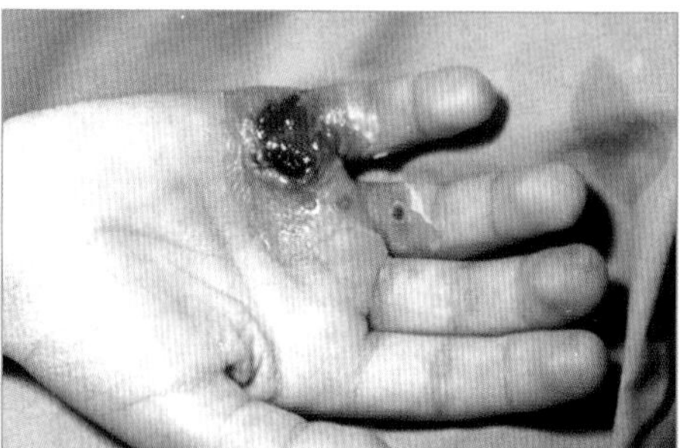

Image 9.1
Aspergilloma of the hand in a 7-year-old boy with chronic granulomatous disease.

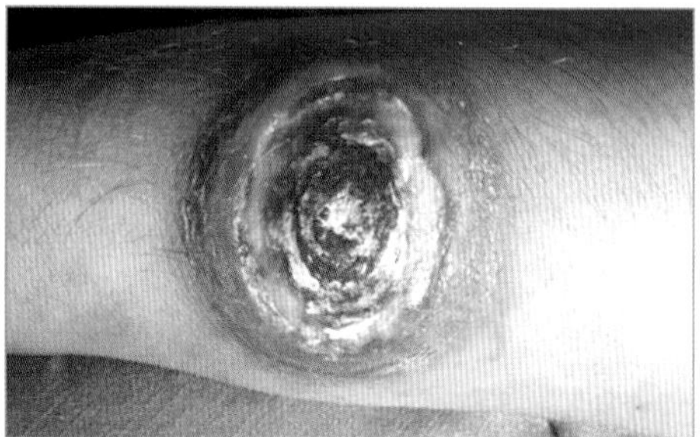

Image 9.2
Aspergilloma at intravenous line site in a 9-year-old boy with acute lymphoblastic leukemia.

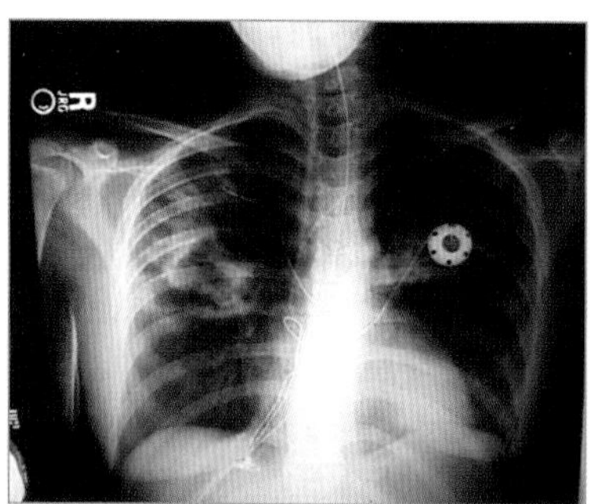

Image 9.3
Aspergillus pneumonia, bilateral, in a 16-year-old boy with acute myelogenous leukemia. Note pulmonary cavitation in the right lung field and perihilar and retrocardiac densities in the left lung field. Copyright Michael Rajnik, MD, FAAP.

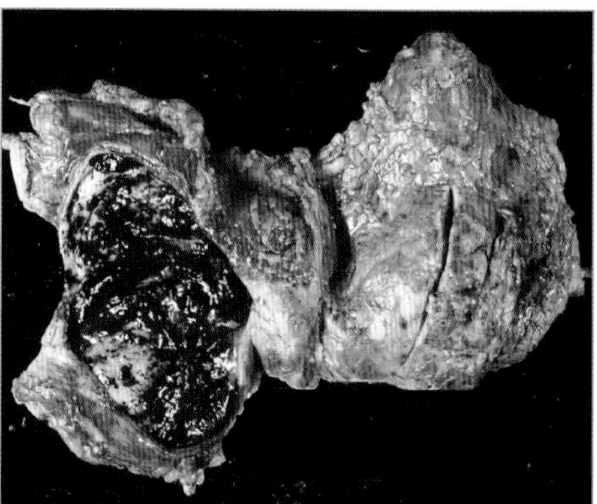

Image 9.4
Pulmonary aspergillosis in a patient with acute lymphatic leukemia. Courtesy of Dimitris P. Agamanolis, MD.

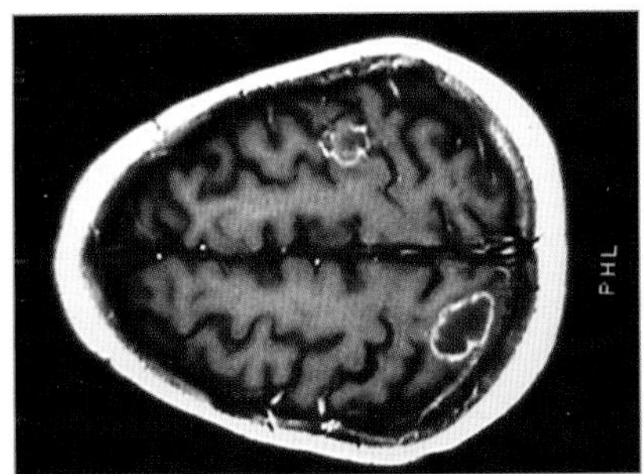

Image 9.5
Aspergillomas in a 10-year-old with Hodgkin-type lymphoma. Courtesy of Benjamin Estrada, MD.

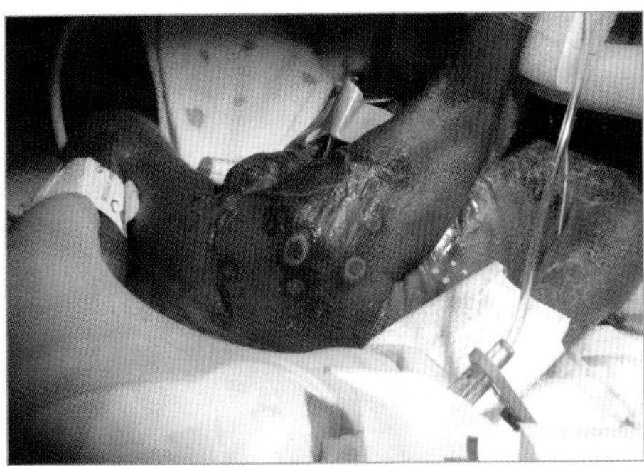

Image 9.6
Cutaneous aspergillosis in a 23-weeks' gestation preterm neonate. Courtesy of David Kaufman, MD.

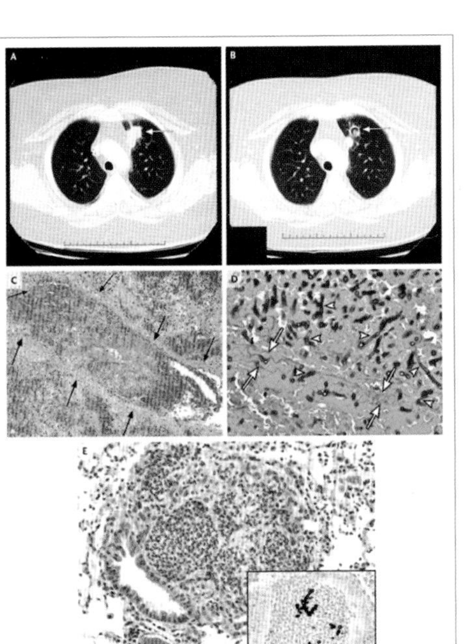

Image 9.7
A, Computed tomographic chest scan of a patient with neutropenia who has invasive aspergillosis in the left upper lung (arrow). A positive serum galactomannan test result established the diagnosis of probable invasive aspergillosis, which averted the need for an invasive diagnostic procedure. B, Cavitation of the lesion after a successful response to therapy and neutrophil recovery (arrow). C, Vascular invasive aspergillosis, which is classically associated with neutropenia but can occur in patients with other conditions, such as in this case of fatal aspergillosis in a recipient of an allogeneic hematopoietic stem-cell transplant who did not have neutropenia but did have severe graft-versus-host disease. A low-power micrograph shows vascular thrombosis (with an arterial vessel outlined by arrows) that is surrounded by extensive coagulative necrosis and hemorrhage (hematoxylin-eosin). D, A high-power micrograph shows hyphae (arrowheads) transverse to the blood vessel wall (outlined by arrows) and intravascular invasion (Grocott-Gomori methenamine–silver nitrate stain, with hyphal walls staining dark). The septated hyphae, some branched at acute angles, are morphologically consistent with *Aspergillus* species. However, other molds can have a similar appearance, so culture or molecular-based analysis at a reference laboratory is required for a definitive diagnosis. E, Experimental aspergillosis in a knockout mouse model of chronic granulomatous disease, an inherited disorder of NADPH oxidase. Densely inflammatory pyogranulomatous pneumonia without vascular invasion or tissue infarction is visible (hematoxylin-eosin), with invasive hyphae in the lung as seen with silver staining (inset). These histologic features are similar to those observed in patients with chronic granulomatous disease and aspergillosis and suggest that NADPH oxidase-independent pathways are able to defend against hyphal invasion of blood vessel walls. From *The New England Journal of Medicine,* Allergic Bronchopulmonary Aspergillosis, 359, e7. Copyright © 2008. Massachusetts Medical Society. Reprinted with permission from Massachusetts Medical Society.

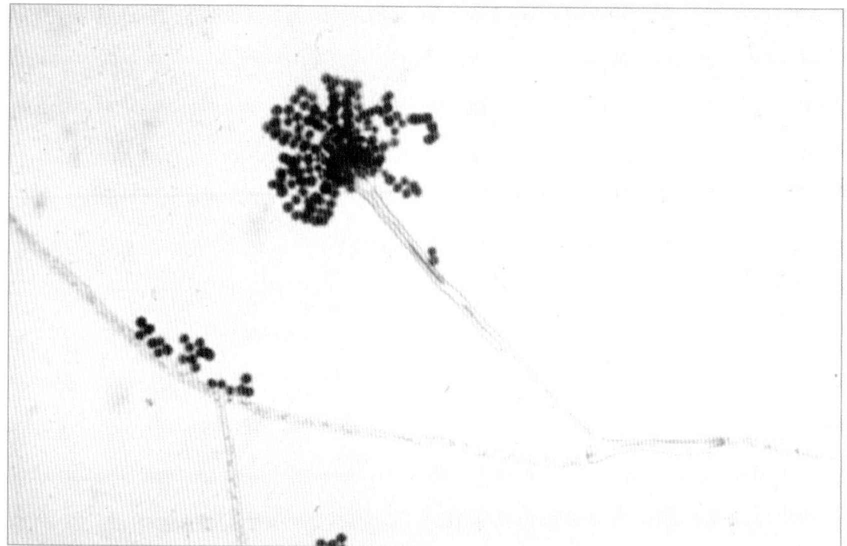

Image 9.8
Conidia and phialospore of *Aspergillus fumigatus*. Courtesy of Centers for Disease Control and Prevention.

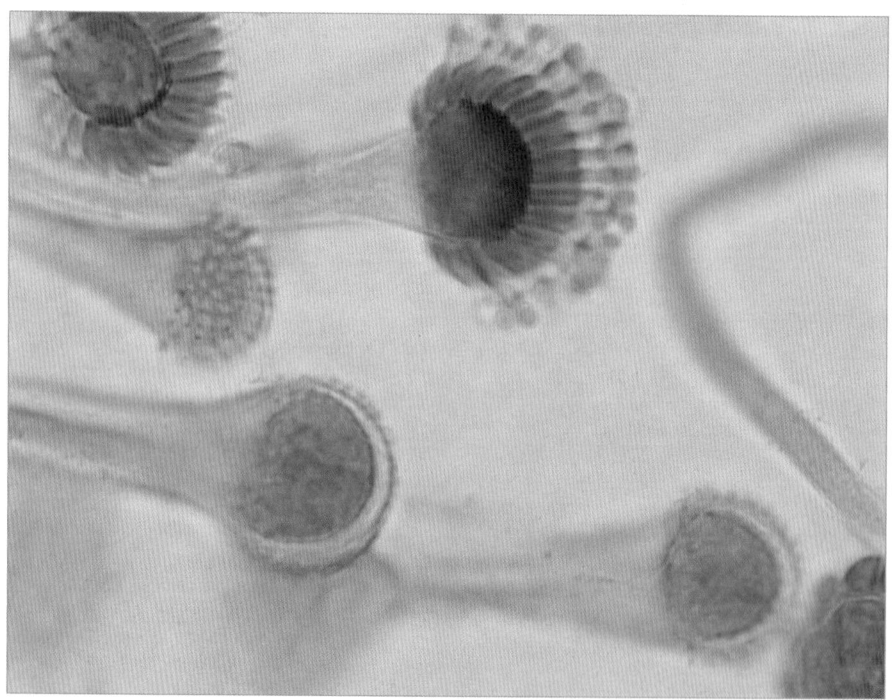

Image 9.9
Aspergillus fumigatus. Courtesy of H. Cody Meissner, MD, FAAP.

10

Astrovirus Infections

Clinical Manifestations

Illness is characterized by diarrhea accompanied by low-grade fever, malaise, and nausea and, less commonly, vomiting and mild dehydration. Illness in an immunocompetent host is self-limited, lasting a median of 5 to 6 days. Asymptomatic infections are common.

Etiology

Astroviruses are nonenveloped, single-stranded RNA viruses with a characteristic starlike appearance when visualized by electron microscopy. Eight human antigenic types originally were described, and several novel species have been identified in recent years.

Epidemiology

Human astroviruses have a worldwide distribution. Multiple antigenic types cocirculate in the same region. Astroviruses have been detected in as many as 5% to 17% of sporadic cases of nonbacterial gastroenteritis among young children in the community but appear to cause a lower proportion of cases of more severe childhood gastroenteritis requiring hospitalization (~3%–9%). Astrovirus infections occur predominantly in children younger than 4 years and have a seasonal peak during the late winter and spring in the United States. Transmission is via the fecal-oral route through contaminated food or water, person-to-person contact, or contaminated surfaces. Outbreaks tend to occur in closed populations of the young and elderly, particularly hospitalized children and children in child care centers. Excretion lasts a median of 5 days after onset of symptoms, but asymptomatic excretion after illness can last for several weeks in healthy children.

Incubation Period

3 to 4 days.

Diagnostic Tests

Commercial tests for diagnosis are not available in the United States, although enzyme immunoassays are available in many other countries. The following tests are available in some research and reference laboratories: electron microscopy for detection of viral particles in stool, enzyme immunoassay for detection of viral antigen in stool or antibody in serum, latex agglutination in stool, and reverse transcriptase-polymerase chain reaction assay for detection of viral RNA in stool. Of these tests, reverse transcriptase-polymerase chain reaction assay is the most sensitive.

Treatment

No specific antiviral therapy is available. Oral or parenteral fluids and electrolytes are given to prevent and correct dehydration.

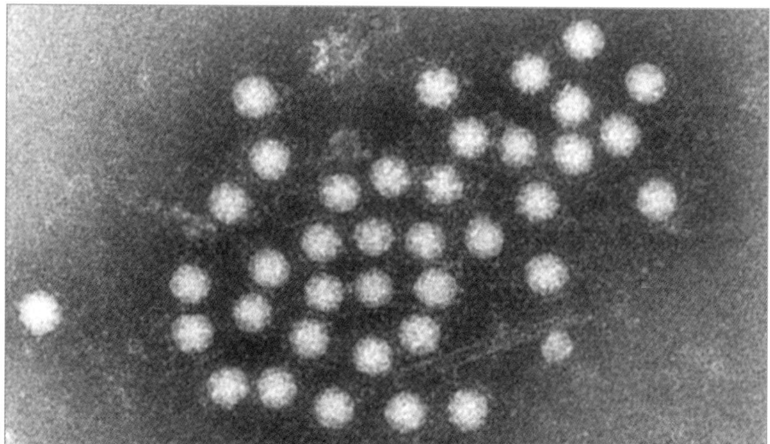

Image 10.1
Electron micrograph of astrovirus obtained from stool of a child with gastroenteritis. Note the characteristic starlike appearance. Courtesy of Centers for Disease Control and Prevention.

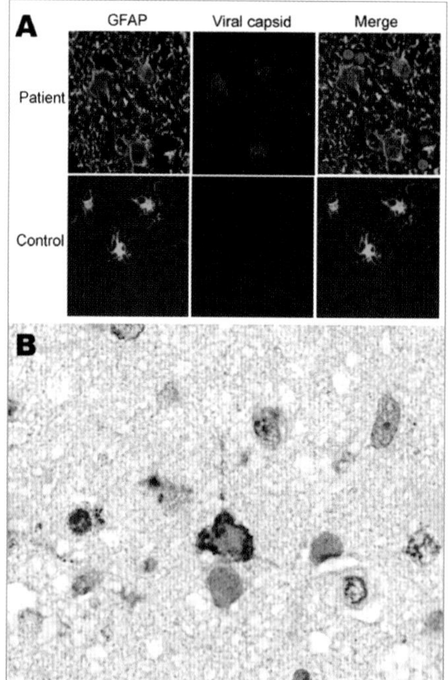

Image 10.2
Astrovirus encephalitis in a boy with X-linked agammaglobulinemia. Panel A: special staining identifies astrovirus in the brain of the patient; Panel B: histopathological changes in brain tissue. Encephalitis is a major cause of death worldwide. Although more than 100 pathogens have been identified as causative agents, the pathogen is not determined for up to 75% of cases. This diagnostic failure impedes effective treatment and underscores the need for better tools and new approaches for detecting novel pathogens or determining new manifestations of known pathogens. Although astroviruses are commonly associated with gastroenteritis, they have not been associated with central nervous system disease. Using unbiased pyrosequencing, astrovirus was determined to be the causative agent for encephalitis in a 15-year-old boy with agammaglobulinemia. Quan PL, Wagner TA, Briese T, et al. Astrovirus encephalitis in boy with X-linked agammaglobulinemia. *Emerg Infect Dis.* 2010;16(6):918–925.

11

Babesiosis

Clinical Manifestations

Babesia infection is often asymptomatic or associated with mild, nonspecific symptoms. The infection also can be severe and life threatening, particularly in people who are asplenic, immunocompromised, or elderly. Babesiosis, like malaria, is characterized by the presence of fever and hemolytic anemia; however, some infected people who are immunocompromised or at the extremes of age (eg, preterm newborns) are afebrile. There can be a prodromal illness, with gradual onset of symptoms, such as malaise, anorexia, and fatigue, followed by development of fever and other influenzalike symptoms (eg, chills, sweats, myalgia, arthralgia, headache, anorexia, nausea). Less common features include sore throat, nonproductive cough, abdominal pain, vomiting, weight loss, conjunctival injection, photophobia, emotional lability, and hyperesthesia. Congenital infection with manifestation as severe sepsis syndrome has been reported.

Clinical signs generally are minimal, often consisting only of fever and tachycardia, although hypotension, respiratory distress, mild hepatosplenomegaly, jaundice, and dark urine may be noted. Thrombocytopenia is common; disseminated intravascular coagulation can be a complication of severe babesiosis. If untreated, illness can last for several weeks or months; even asymptomatic people can have persistent low-level parasitemia, sometimes for longer than 1 year.

Etiology

Babesia species are intraerythrocytic protozoa. The etiologic agents of babesiosis in the United States include *Babesia microti*, which is the cause of most reported cases, and several other genetically and antigenically distinct organisms, such as *Babesia duncani* (formerly the WA1-type parasite).

Epidemiology

Babesiosis predominantly is a tick-borne zoonosis. *Babesia* parasites can also be transmitted by blood transfusion and through perinatal routes. In the United States, the primary reservoir host for *B microti* is the white-footed mouse (*Peromyscus leucopus*), and the primary vector is the tick *Ixodes scapularis*, which also can transmit *Borrelia burgdorferi*, the causative agent of Lyme disease, and *Anaplasma phagocytophilum*, the causative agent of human granulocytic anaplasmosis. Humans become infected through tick bites, which typically are not noticed. The white-tailed deer (*Odocoileus virginianus*) is an important host for blood meals for the tick but is not a reservoir host of *B microti*. An increase in the deer population in some geographic areas, including some suburban areas, during the past few decades is thought to be a major factor in the spread of *I scapularis* and the increase in numbers of reported cases of babesiosis. The reported vector-borne cases of *B microti* infection have been acquired in the Northeast (particularly, but not exclusively, in Connecticut, Massachusetts, New Jersey, New York, and Rhode Island) and in the upper Midwest (Wisconsin and Minnesota). Occasional human cases of babesiosis caused by other species have been described in various regions of the United States; tick vectors and reservoir hosts for these agents typically have not yet been identified. Whereas most US vector-borne cases of babesiosis occur during late spring, summer, or autumn, transfusion-associated cases can occur year-round.

Incubation Period

1 to 5 weeks after a tick bite; 1 week after a contaminated blood transfusion but occasionally is longer (eg, latent infection might become symptomatic after splenectomy).

Diagnostic Tests

Acute, symptomatic cases of babesiosis are typically diagnosed by microscopic identification of the organism on Giemsa- or Wright-stained blood smears. If the diagnosis of babesiosis is being considered, manual (nonautomated) review of blood smears for parasites should be requested explicitly. If seen, the tetrad (Maltese cross) form is pathognomonic. *B microti* and other *Babesia* species can be difficult to distinguish from *Plasmodium falciparum;* examination of blood smears by a reference laboratory should be considered for confirmation of the diagnosis. Adjunctive molecular and serologic testing is performed at the Centers for Disease Control and Prevention. If indicated, the possibility of concurrent *B burgdorferi* or *Anaplasma* infection should be considered.

Treatment

Clindamycin plus oral quinine for 7 to 10 days, or atovaquone plus azithromycin for 7 to 10 days, have comparable efficacy for mild to moderate illness. Therapy with atovaquone plus azithromycin is associated with fewer adverse effects. However, clindamycin and quinine is preferred for severely ill patients. Exchange blood transfusions should be considered for patients who are critically ill (eg, hemodynamically unstable), especially, but not exclusively, for patients with parasitemia levels of 10% or more.

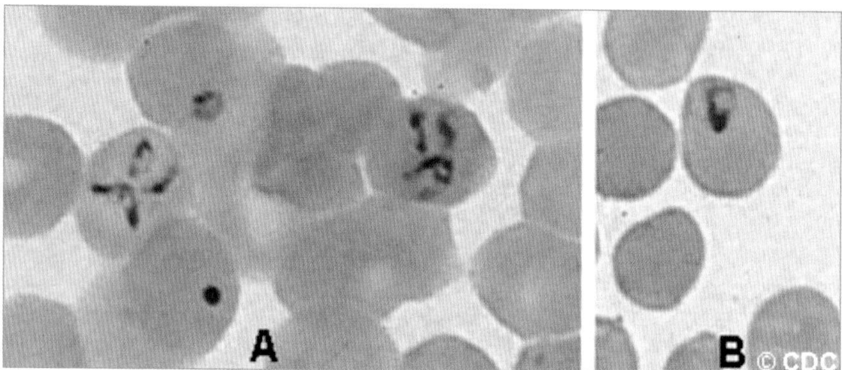

Image 11.1
Infection with *Babesia* in a 6-year-old girl after a splenectomy performed because of hereditary spherocytosis (Giemsa-stained thin smears). A, The tetrad (left side of the image), a dividing form, is pathognomonic for *Babesia*. Note also the variation in size and shape of the ring stage parasites (compare A and B) and absence of pigment. Courtesy of Centers for Disease Control and Prevention.

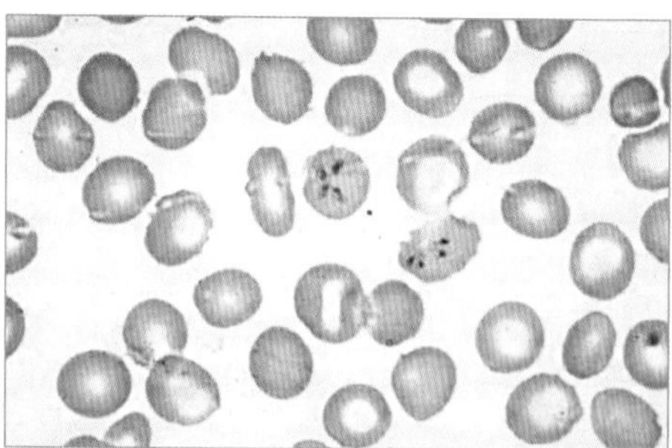

Image 11.2
Babesia microti in a peripheral blood smear. Note the typical intraerythrocytic location of the organisms. Babesiosis is often asymptomatic or associated with mild symptoms. The infection can be life-threatening in people who are asplenic or immunocompromised.

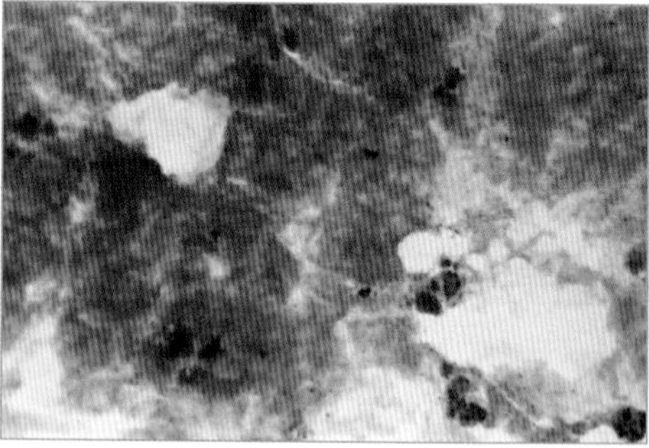

Image 11.3
A Giemsa stain of a blood film from an infected human used to identify the parasite *Babesia microti*. Babesiosis is caused by hemo-protozoan parasites of the genus *Babesia*. While more than 100 species have been reported, *B microti* and *Babesia divergens* have been identified in most human cases. Courtesy of Centers for Disease Control and Prevention/Dr George Healy.

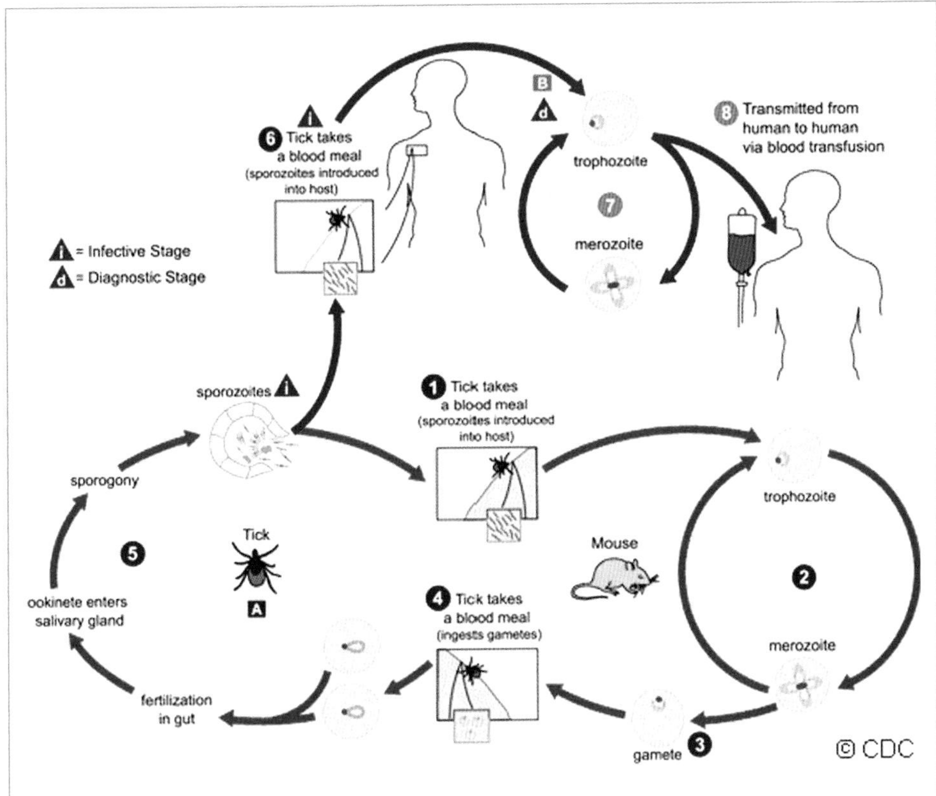

Image 11.4

The *Babesia microti* life cycle involves 2 hosts, which include a rodent, primarily the white-footed mouse (*Peromyscus leucopus*). During a blood meal, a *Babesia*-infected tick introduces sporozoites into the mouse host (1). Sporozoites enter erythrocytes and undergo asexual reproduction (budding) (2). In the blood, some parasites differentiate into male and female gametes, although these cannot be distinguished at the light microscope level (3). The definitive host is a tick, in this case the deer tick (*Ixodes scapularis*). Once ingested by an appropriate tick (4), gametes unite and undergo a sporogonic cycle, resulting in sporozoites (5). Transovarial transmission (also known as vertical, or hereditary, transmission) has been documented for "large" *Babesia* species but not for the "small" *Babesia* species, such as *B microti* (A). Humans enter the cycle when bitten by infected ticks. During a blood meal, a *Babesia*-infected tick introduces sporozoites into the human host (6). Sporozoites enter erythrocytes (B) and undergo asexual replication (budding) (7). Multiplication of the blood stage parasites is responsible for clinical manifestations of the disease. Humans are, for all practical purposes, dead-end hosts, and there is probably little, if any, subsequent transmission that occurs from ticks feeding on infected persons. However, human-to-human transmission is well recognized to occur through blood transfusions (8). Note: Deer are the hosts on which the adult ticks feed and are indirectly part of the *Babesia* cycle, as they influence the tick population. When deer populations increase, tick population also increases, thus heightening the potential for transmission. Courtesy of Centers for Disease Control and Prevention.

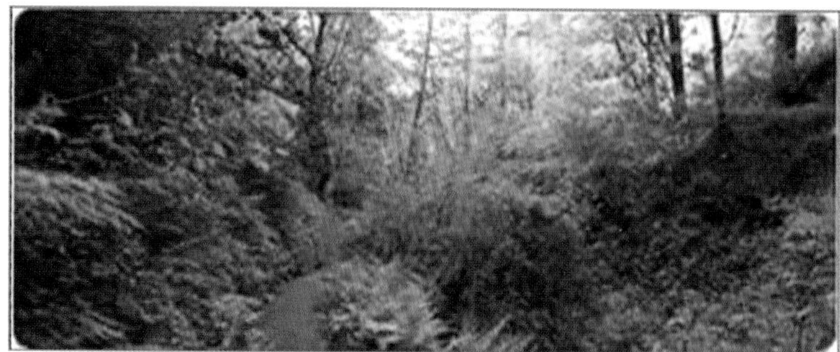

Image 11.5

Babesiosis is caused by parasites that infect red blood cells and are spread by certain ticks. In the United States, tick-borne transmission is most common in parts of the Northeast and upper Midwest, and it usually peaks during the warm months. Although many people who are infected with *Babesia* do not have symptoms, effective treatment is available if symptoms develop. Babesiosis is preventable if simple steps are taken to reduce exposure to ticks. Courtesy of Centers for Disease Control and Prevention.

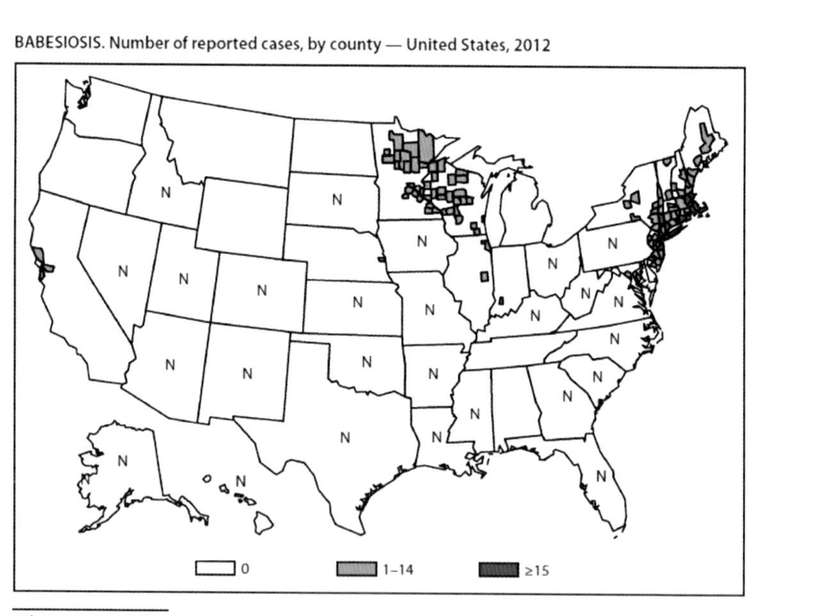

Image 11.6

Number of reported cases, by county—United States, 2012. Courtesy of *Morbidity and Mortality Weekly Report.*

12

Bacillus cereus Infections

Clinical Manifestations

Bacillus cereus is primarily associated with 2 toxin-mediated foodborne illnesses, emetic and diarrheal, but it can also cause invasive extraintestinal infection. The emetic syndrome develops after a short incubation period, similar to staphylococcal foodborne illness. It is characterized by nausea, vomiting, and abdominal cramps, and diarrhea can follow in 30% of patients. The diarrheal syndrome has a longer incubation period, is more severe, and resembles *Clostridium perfringens* foodborne illness. It is characterized by moderate to severe abdominal cramps and watery diarrhea, vomiting in approximately 25% of patients, and, occasionally, low-grade fever. Both illnesses are usually short-lived, but the emetic toxin has been associated with fulminant liver failure.

Invasive extraintestinal infection can be severe and can include a wide range of diseases, including wound and soft tissue infections; bacteremia, including central line–associated bloodstream infection; endocarditis; osteomyelitis; purulent meningitis and ventricular shunt infection; pneumonia; and ocular infections. Along with staphylococci, *B cereus* is a significant cause of bacterial endophthalmitis. Ocular involvement includes panophthalmitis, endophthalmitis, and keratitis.

Etiology

B cereus is an aerobic and facultatively anaerobic, spore-forming, gram-positive bacillus.

Epidemiology

B cereus is ubiquitous in the environment and is commonly present in small numbers in raw, dried, and processed foods. The organism is a common cause of foodborne illness in the United States but may be under-recognized because physicians and clinical laboratories do not routinely test for *B cereus*.

Spores of *B cereus* are heat resistant and can survive pasteurization, brief cooking, or boiling. Vegetative forms can grow and produce enterotoxins over a wide range of temperatures in foods and in the gastrointestinal tract; the latter results in diarrheal syndrome. The emetic syndrome occurs after eating contaminated food containing preformed emetic toxin. The best known association of the emetic syndrome is with ingestion of fried rice made from boiled rice stored at room temperature overnight, but illness has been associated with a wide variety of foods. Foodborne illness caused by *B cereus* is not transmissible from person to person

Risk factors for invasive disease attributable to *B cereus* include history of injection drug use, presence of indwelling intravascular catheters or implanted devices, neutropenia or immunosuppression, and preterm birth. *B cereus* endophthalmitis has occurred after penetrating ocular trauma and injection drug use.

Incubation Period

Emetic syndrome, 0.5 to 6 hours; diarrheal syndrome, 6 to 24 hours.

Diagnostic Tests

For foodborne outbreaks, isolation of *B cereus* from the stool or vomitus of 2 or more ill people and not from control patients, or isolation of 10^5 colony-forming units/g or greater from epidemiologically implicated food, suggests that *B cereus* is the cause of the outbreak. Because the organism can be recovered from stool specimens from some well people, the presence of *B cereus* in feces or vomitus of ill people is not definitive evidence of infection. Food samples must be tested for both enterotoxins because either alone can cause illness.

In patients with risk factors for invasive disease, isolation of *B cereus* from wounds, blood, or other usually sterile body fluids is significant. The common perception of *Bacillus* species as "contaminants" may delay recognition and treatment of serious *B cereus* infections.

Treatment

B cereus foodborne illness usually requires only supportive treatment. Antimicrobial therapy is indicated for patients with invasive disease. Prompt removal of any potentially infected foreign bodies, such as central lines or implants, is essential. For intraocular infections, an ophthalmologist should be consulted about use of intravitreal vancomycin therapy in addition to systemic therapy.

B cereus usually is resistant to β-lactam antibiotics and clindamycin but is susceptible to vancomycin, which is the drug of choice.

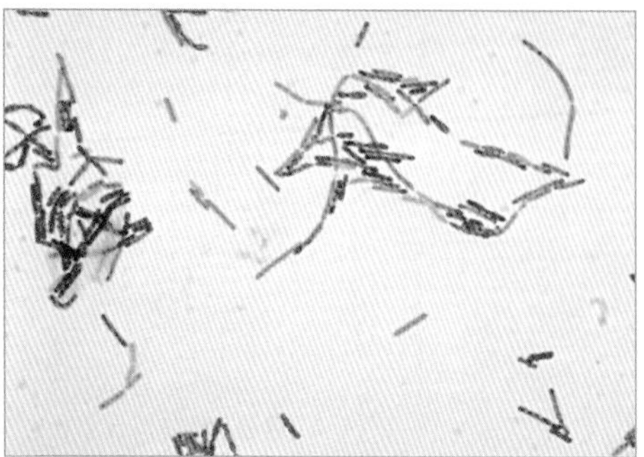

Image 12.1
Bacillus cereus subsp *mycoides* (Gram stain). *B cereus* is a known cause of toxin-induced food poisoning. These organisms may appear gram-variable, as shown here. Courtesy of Centers for Disease Control and Prevention/Dr William A. Clark.

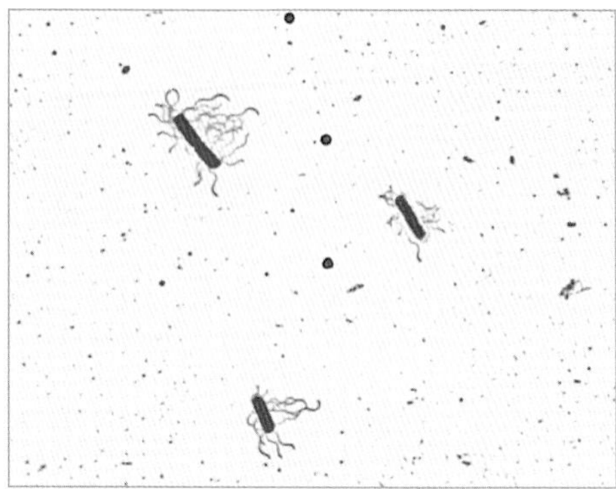

Image 12.2
Leifson flagella stain. *Bacillus cereus* food poisoning is often associated with contaminated rice containing heat-resistant *B cereus* spores. Courtesy of Centers for Disease Control and Prevention/Dr William A. Clark.

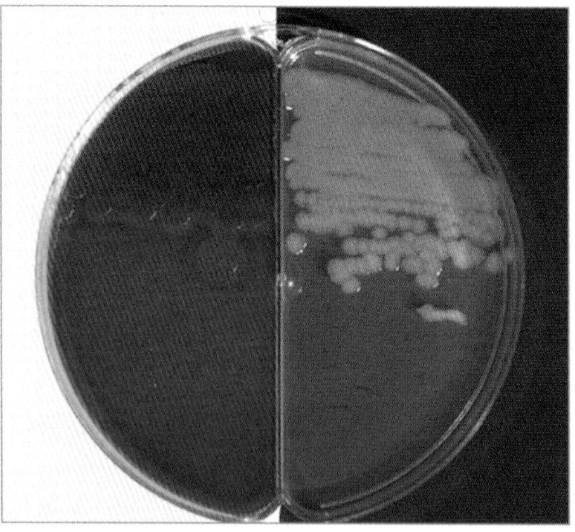

Image 12.3
Blood agar and bicarbonate agar plate cultures of *Bacillus cereus* (negative encapsulation test). Rough colonies of *B cereus* on blood and bicarbonate agars. Courtesy of Centers for Disease Control and Prevention/Dr James Feeley.

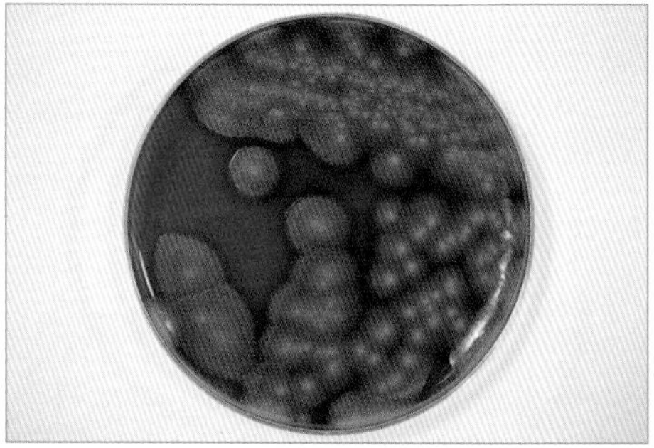

Image 12.4
Bacillus cereus on sheep blood agar. Large, circular, β-hemolytic colonies are noted. The greenish color and ground-glass appearance are typical characteristics of this organism on culture media. Courtesy of Julia Rosebush, DO; Robert Jerris, PhD; and Theresa Stanley, M(ASCP).

13

Bacterial Vaginosis

Clinical Manifestations

Bacterial vaginosis (BV) is a polymicrobial clinical syndrome characterized by changes in vaginal flora, with replacement of normally abundant *Lactobacillus* species by high concentrations of anaerobic bacteria. Bacterial vaginosis is diagnosed primarily in sexually active postpubertal females, but women who have never been sexually active also can be affected. Bacterial vaginosis is asymptomatic in 50% to 75% of females. Symptoms include a thin white or gray, homogenous, adherent vaginal discharge with a fishy odor vaginal discharge. Symptoms of vulvovaginal irritation, pruritus, dysuria, or abdominal pain are not associated with BV. In pregnant women, BV has been associated with adverse outcomes, including chorioamnionitis, premature rupture of membranes, preterm delivery, and postpartum endometritis.

Vaginitis and vulvitis in prepubertal girls rarely, if ever, are manifestations of BV. Vaginitis in prepubertal girls is frequently nonspecific, but possible causes include foreign bodies and infections attributable to group A streptococci, *Escherichia coli,* human herpesvirus, *Neisseria gonorrhoeae, Chlamydia trachomatis, Trichomonas vaginalis,* or enteric bacteria, including *Shigella* species.

Etiology

The microbiologic cause of BV has not been delineated fully. In females with BV, *Lactobacillus* species largely are replaced by commensal anaerobes. Typical microbiologic findings in vaginal specimens show increased concentrations of *Gardnerella vaginalis, Mycoplasma hominis, Prevotella* species, *Mobiluncus* species, and *Ureaplasma* species.

Epidemiology

Bacterial vaginosis is the most common cause of vaginal discharge in sexually active adolescent and adult women. Bacterial vaginosis can be the sole cause of symptoms or accompany other conditions associated with vaginal discharge, such as trichomoniasis or mucopurulent cervicitis secondary to other sexually transmitted infections. Bacterial vaginosis occurs more frequently in females with a new sexual partner or a higher number of sexual partners and in those who engage in douching. Although evidence of sexual transmission of BV is inconclusive, the correct and consistent use of condoms reduces the risk of acquisition. Bacterial vaginosis increases the risk of infectious complications following gynecologic surgery as well as pregnancy complications and the acquisition of HIV, human herpesvirus 2, *N gonorrhoeae,* and *C trachomatis.*

Incubation Period

Unknown.

Diagnostic Tests

Bacterial vaginosis is most commonly diagnosed clinically using the Amsel criteria, requiring that 3 or more of the following symptoms or signs are present:

- Homogenous, thin gray or white vaginal discharge that smoothly coats the vaginal walls
- Vaginal fluid pH greater than 4.5
- A fishy (amine) odor of vaginal discharge before or after addition of 10% potassium hydroxide (ie, the "whiff test")
- Presence of clue cells (squamous vaginal epithelial cells covered with bacteria, which cause a stippled or granular appearance and ragged "moth-eaten" borders) representing at least 20% of the total vaginal epithelial cells seen on microscopic evaluation of vaginal fluid

An alternative method for diagnosing BV is the Nugent score, which is used widely as the gold standard for making the diagnosis in the research setting. Douching, recent intercourse, menstruation, and coexisting infection can alter findings on Gram stain. The BD Affirm VPIII test (BD Diagnostic Systems, Sparks, MD) is a DNA probe test that detects *G vaginalis* and can be used when symptoms and signs are suggestive of BV but microscopy is unavailable. Clinical Laboratory Improvement Amendments–waived rapid tests for BV that measure the activity of sialidase, an enzyme generated by several BV-associated bacteria, such as Diagnosit BVBlue (Gryphus Diagnostics, Knoxville, TN) and OSOM BVBlue Test (Sekisui Diagnostics, Lexington, MA), have strong clinical performance compared with the Nugent criteria. The FemExam *G vaginalis* PIP Activity TestCard (Litmus Concepts Inc, Santa Clara, CA) detects proline iminopeptidase activity of anaerobes and can be performed as a point-of-care test in less than 2 minutes.

Sexually active females with BV should be evaluated for coinfection with syphilis, gonorrhea, chlamydia, trichomoniasis, and HIV. Completion of the hepatitis B and human papillomavirus immunization series should be confirmed.

Treatment

Symptomatic patients should be treated. The goals of treatment are to relieve the symptoms and signs of infection and to potentially decrease the risk of infectious complications. Treatment considerations should include patient preference for oral versus intravaginal treatment, possible adverse effects, and presence of coinfections. Nonpregnant patients may be treated orally with metronidazole or topically with metronidazole gel or clindamycin cream. Alternative regimens include oral tinidazole, oral clindamycin, or clindamycin intravaginally.

Approximately 30% of appropriately treated females have a recurrence within 3 months. Retreatment with the same regimen or an alternative regimen are both reasonable options.

Pregnant or breastfeeding women with symptoms of BV should be treated with oral metronidazole or clindamycin. Oral therapies are preferred in pregnancy to treat possible upper genital tract infection.

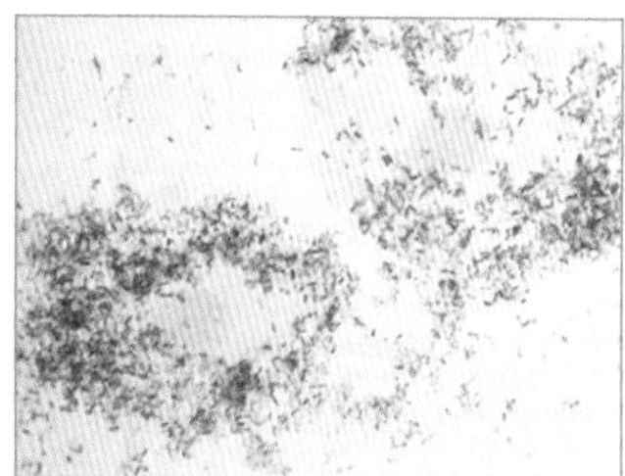

Image 13.1
Clue cells are squamous epithelial cells covered with bacteria found in bacterial vaginosis. Copyright Noni MacDonald, MD.

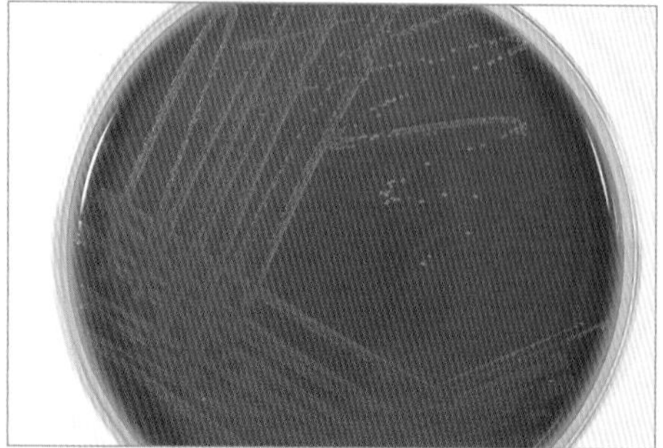

Image 13.3
Gardnerella vaginalis on chocolate agar. Colonies are small, circular, gray, and convex. Courtesy of Julia Rosebush, DO; Robert Jerris, PhD; and Theresa Stanley, M(ASCP).

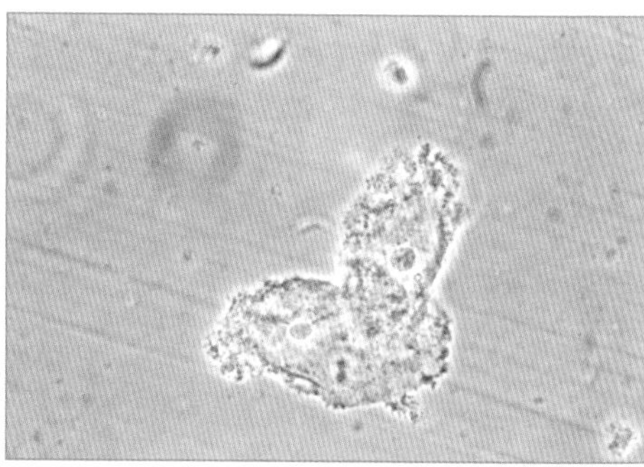

Image 13.2
This photomicrograph reveals bacteria adhering to vaginal epithelial cells known as clue cells. Clue cells are epithelial cells that have had bacteria adhere to their surface, obscuring their borders, and imparting a stippled appearance. The presence of such clue cells is a sign the patient has bacterial vaginosis. Courtesy of Centers for Disease Control and Prevention/ M. Rein.

14

Bacteroides and *Prevotella* Infections

Clinical Manifestations

Bacteroides and *Prevotella* organisms from the oral cavity can cause chronic sinusitis, chronic otitis media, dental infection, peritonsillar abscess, cervical adenitis, retropharyngeal space infection, aspiration pneumonia, lung abscess, pleural empyema, or necrotizing pneumonia. Species from the gastrointestinal tract are recovered in patients with peritonitis, intra-abdominal abscess, pelvic inflammatory disease, postoperative wound infection, or vulvovaginal and perianal infections. Invasion of the bloodstream from the oral cavity or intestinal tract can lead to brain abscess, meningitis, endocarditis, arthritis, or osteomyelitis. Skin and soft tissue infections include synergistic bacterial gangrene and necrotizing fasciitis; omphalitis in newborns; cellulitis at the site of fetal monitors, human bite wounds, or burns; infections adjacent to the mouth or rectum; and infected decubitus ulcers. Neonatal infections, including conjunctivitis, pneumonia, bacteremia, or meningitis, are rare. In most settings where *Bacteroides* and *Prevotella* are implicated, the infections are polymicrobial.

Etiology

Most *Bacteroides* and *Prevotella* organisms associated with human disease are pleomorphic, nonspore-forming, facultatively anaerobic, gram-negative bacilli.

Epidemiology

Bacteroides and *Prevotella* species are part of the normal flora of the mouth, gastrointestinal tract, and female genital tract. Members of the *Bacteroides fragilis* group predominate in the gastrointestinal tract flora; members of the *Prevotella melaninogenica* (formerly *Bacteroides melaninogenicus*) and *Prevotella oralis* (formerly *Bacteroides oralis*) groups are more common in the oral cavity. These species cause infection as opportunists, usually after an alteration in skin or mucosal membranes in conjunction with other endogenous species. Endogenous infection results from aspiration, bowel perforation, or damage to mucosal surfaces from trauma, surgery, or chemotherapy. Mucosal injury or granulocytopenia predispose to infection. Enterotoxigenic *B fragilis* may be a cause of diarrhea. Except in infections resulting from human bites, no evidence of person-to-person transmission exists.

Incubation Period

Usually 1 to 5 days (depending on inoculum and body site).

Diagnostic Tests

Anaerobic culture media are necessary for recovery of *Bacteroides* or *Prevotella* species. Because infections usually are polymicrobial, aerobic cultures should also be obtained. A putrid odor suggests anaerobic infection. Use of an anaerobic transport tube or a sealed syringe is recommended for collection of clinical specimens.

Treatment

Abscesses should be drained when feasible; abscesses involving the brain, liver, and lungs may resolve with effective antimicrobial therapy. Necrotizing soft tissue lesions should be debrided surgically and can require repeated surgeries.

The choice of antimicrobial agent(s) is based on anticipated or known in vitro susceptibility testing. *Bacteroides* infections of the mouth and respiratory tract generally are susceptible to penicillin G, ampicillin, and extended-spectrum penicillins, such as ticarcillin or piperacillin. Clindamycin is active against virtually all mouth and respiratory tract *Bacteroides* and *Prevotella* isolates and is recommended by some experts as the drug of choice for anaerobic infections of the oral cavity and lungs but is not recommended for central nervous system infections. Some species of *Bacteroides* and almost 50% of *Prevotella* species produce β-lactamase. A β-lactam penicillin active against *Bacteroides* species combined with a β-lactamase inhibitor (ampicillin-sulbactam, amoxicillin-clavulanate, ticarcillin-clavulanate, or piperacillin-tazobactam) can be useful to treat these infections. *Bacteroides* species of the gastrointestinal tract usually are resistant to penicillin G but are predictably susceptible to metronidazole, β-lactam plus β-lactamase inhibitors, chloramphenicol, and, sometimes, clindamycin. More than 80% of isolates are susceptible to cefoxitin and meropenem. Cefuroxime, cefotaxime, and ceftriaxone are not reliably effective.

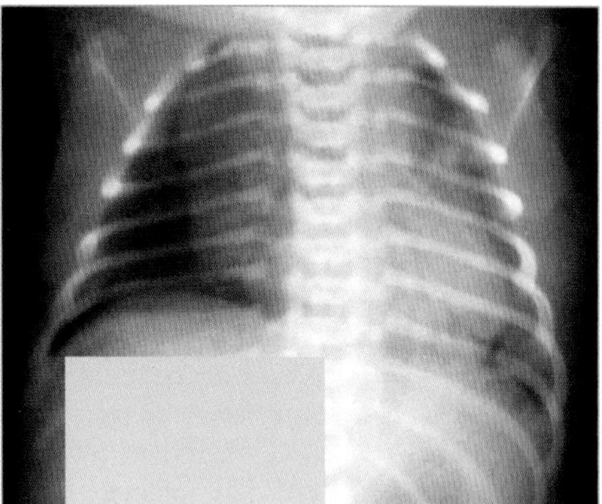

Image 14.1
Bacteroides fragilis pneumonia in a newborn (*B fragilis* isolated from the placenta and blood culture from the newborn). Anaerobic cultures were obtained because of a fecal odor in the amniotic fluid.

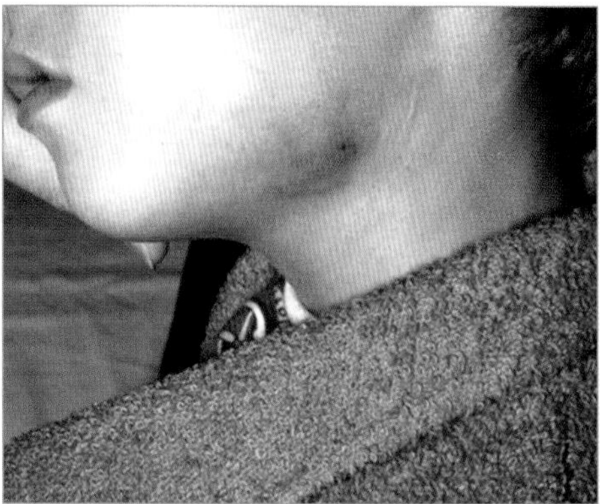

Image 14.2
Prevotella melaninogenica (previously *Bacteroides melaninogenicus*) and group A α-hemolytic streptococcus cultured from a submandibular subcutaneous abscess aspirate from a 12-year-old boy. There was no apparent dental, pharyngeal, or middle ear infection.

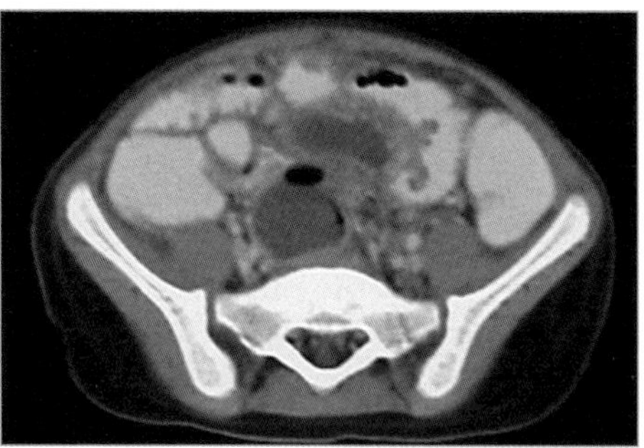

Image 14.3
Bacteroides fragilis abdominal abscess in a 9-year-old boy. Courtesy of Benjamin Estrada, MD.

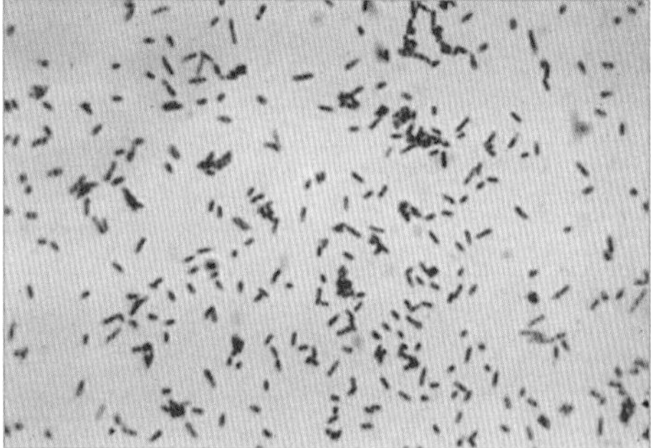

Image 14.4
This photomicrograph shows *Bacteroides fragilis* after being cultured in a thioglycollate medium for 48 hours. *B fragilis* is a gram-negative rod that constitutes 1% to 2% of the normal colonic bacterial microflora in humans. It is associated with extraintestinal infections such as abscesses and soft tissue infections, as well as diarrheal diseases. Courtesy of Centers for Disease Control and Prevention/Dr V. R. Dowell Jr.

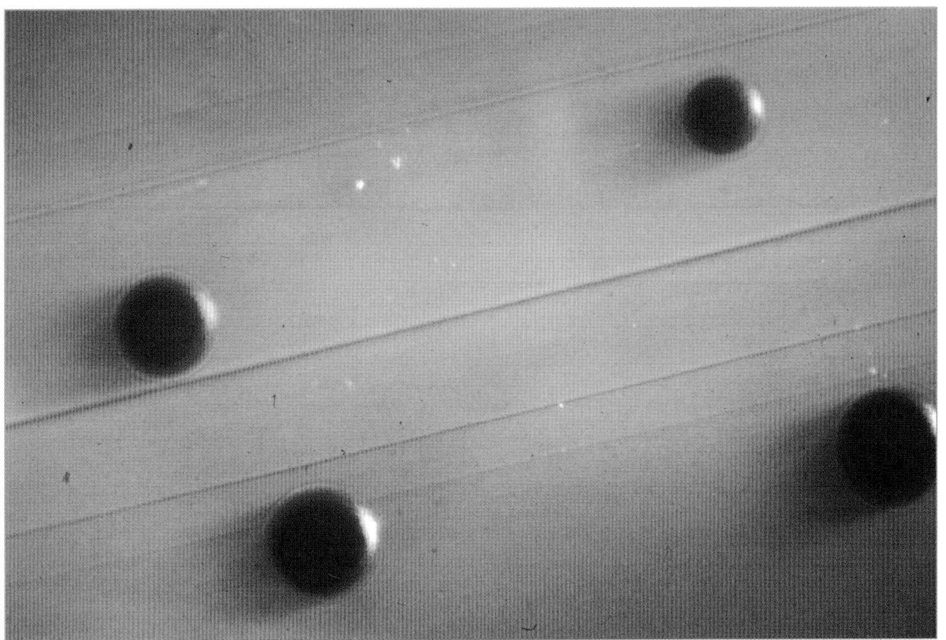

Image 14.5
Prevotella melaninogenica pigmented colonies. Courtesy of Centers for Disease Control and Prevention.

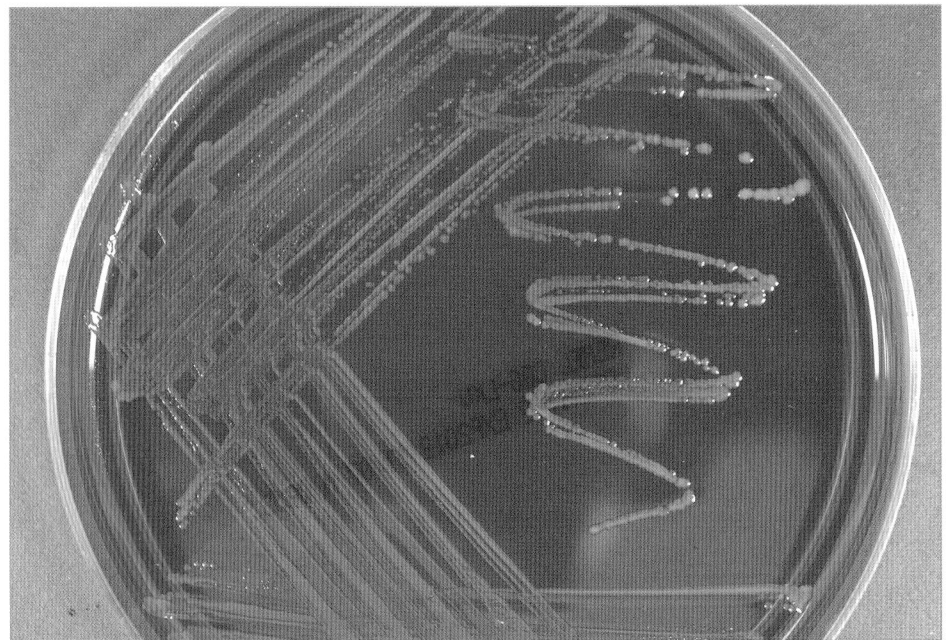

Image 14.6
Bacteroides fragilis on kanamycin-vancomycin–laked blood agar. The organism is not inhibited by kanamycin and vancomycin and, thus, demonstrates good growth on this agar. Courtesy of Julia Rosebush, DO; Robert Jerris, PhD; and Theresa Stanley, M(ASCP).

15

Balantidium coli Infections

(Balantidiasis)

Clinical Manifestations

Most human infections are asymptomatic. Acute symptomatic infection is characterized by rapid onset of nausea, vomiting, abdominal discomfort or pain, and bloody or watery mucoid diarrhea. In some patients, the course is chronic with intermittent episodes of diarrhea, anorexia, and weight loss. Rarely, organisms spread to mesenteric nodes, pleura, lung, liver, or genitourinary sites. Inflammation of the gastrointestinal tract and local lymphatic vessels can result in bowel dilation, ulceration, perforation, and secondary bacterial invasion. Colitis produced by *Balantidium coli* often is indistinguishable from colitis produced by *Entamoeba histolytica*. Fulminant disease can occur in patients who are malnourished or otherwise debilitated or immunocompromised.

Etiology

B coli, a ciliated protozoan, is the largest pathogenic protozoan known to infect humans.

Epidemiology

Pigs are the primary host reservoir of *B coli*, but other sources of infection have been reported. Infections have been reported in most areas of the world but are rare in industrialized countries. Cysts excreted in feces can be transmitted directly from hand to mouth or indirectly through fecally contaminated water or food. Excysted trophozoites infect the colon. A person is infectious as long as cysts are excreted in stool. Cysts may remain viable in the environment for months.

Incubation Period

Unknown but may be several days.

Diagnostic Tests

Diagnosis of infection is established by scraping lesions via sigmoidoscopy, histologic examination of intestinal biopsy specimens, or ova and parasite examination of stool. Diagnosis is usually established by demonstrating trophozoites (or, less frequently, cysts) in stool or tissue specimens. Stool examination is less sensitive, and repeated stool examination is necessary to diagnose infection because shedding of organisms can be intermittent. Microscopic examination of fresh diarrheal stools must be performed promptly because trophozoites degenerate rapidly.

Treatment

The drug of choice is a tetracycline. Alternative drugs are metronidazole and iodoquinol. Successful use of nitazoxanide has also been reported.

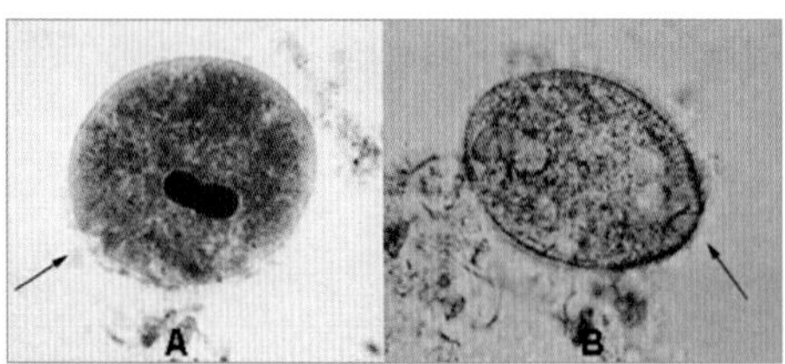

Image 15.1
Balantidium coli trophozoites are characterized by their large size (40–>70 μm); the presence of cilia on the cell surface, which are particularly visible (B); a cytostome (arrows); a bean-shaped macronucleus that is often visible (A); and a smaller, less conspicuous micronucleus. Courtesy of Centers for Disease Control and Prevention.

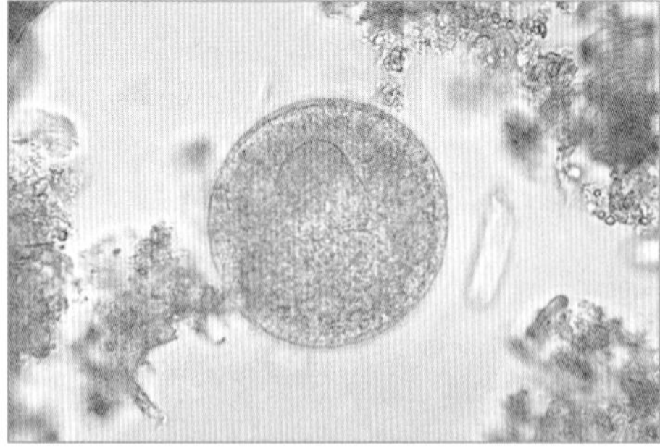

Image 15.2
Balantidium coli cyst in stool preparation. Courtesy of Centers for Disease Control and Prevention/Dr L.L.A. Moore Jr.

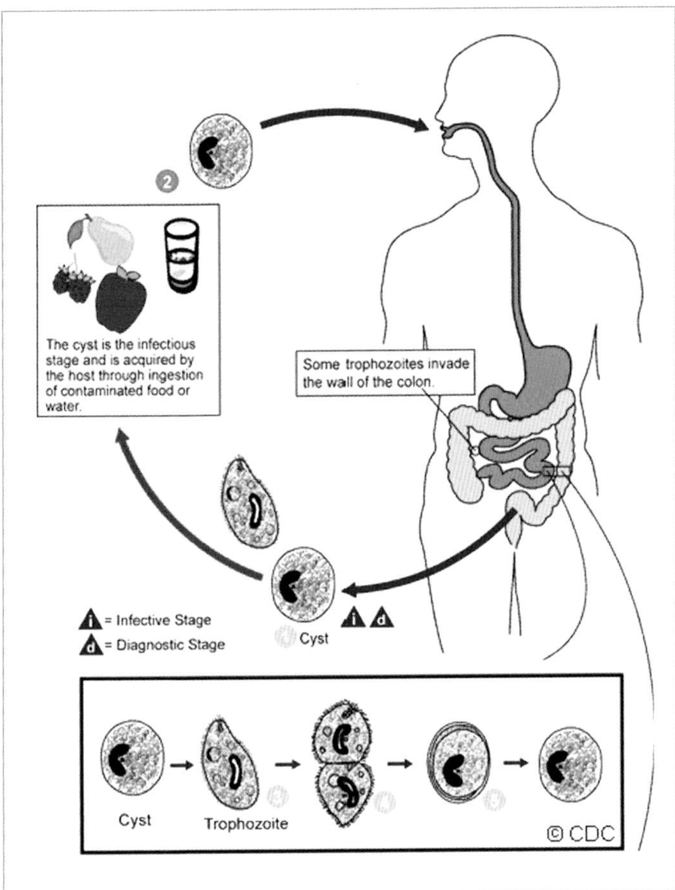

Image 15.3
Cysts are the parasite stage responsible for transmission of balantidiasis (1). The host most often acquires the cyst through ingestion of contaminated food or water (2). Following ingestion, excystation occurs in the small intestine, and the trophozoites colonize the large intestine (3). The trophozoites reside in the lumen of the large intestine of humans and animals, where they replicate by binary fission, during which conjugation may occur (4). Trophozoites undergo encystation to produce infective cysts (5). Some trophozoites invade the wall of the colon and multiply. Some return to the lumen and disintegrate. Mature cysts are passed with feces (1). Courtesy of Centers for Disease Control and Prevention/Alexander J. da Silva, PhD/Melanie Moser.

16

Baylisascaris Infections

Clinical Manifestations

Baylisascaris procyonis, a raccoon roundworm, is a rare cause of acute eosinophilic meningoencephalitis. In a young child, acute central nervous system (CNS) disease (eg, altered mental status, seizures) accompanied by peripheral or cerebrospinal fluid (CSF) eosinophilia occurs 2 to 4 weeks after infection. Severe neurologic sequelae or death are usual outcomes. *B procyonis* is also a rare cause of extraneural disease in older children and adults. Ocular larva migrans can result in diffuse unilateral subacute neuroretinitis; direct visualization of worms in the retina is sometimes possible. Visceral larval migrans can present with nonspecific signs, such as macular rash, pneumonitis, and hepatomegaly. Similar to visceral larva migrans caused by *Toxocara,* subclinical or asymptomatic infection is thought to be the most common outcome of infection.

Etiology

B procyonis is a 10- to 25-cm long roundworm (nematode) with a direct life cycle usually limited to its definitive host, the raccoon. Domestic dogs and some exotic pets, such as kinkajous and ringtails, can serve as definitive hosts and a potential source of human disease.

Epidemiology

B procyonis is distributed focally throughout the United States; in areas where disease is endemic, an estimated 22% to 80% of raccoons can harbor the parasite in their intestine. Reports of infections in dogs raise concern that infected dogs may be able to spread the disease. Embryonated eggs containing infective larvae are ingested from the soil by raccoons, rodents, and birds. When infective eggs or an infected host is eaten by a raccoon, the larvae grow to maturity in the small intestine, where adult female worms shed millions of eggs per day. Eggs become infective after 2 to 4 weeks in the environment and may persist long-term in the soil. Fewer than 25 cases of *Baylisascaris* disease have been document in the United States, although cases may be undiagnosed or underreported.

Risk factors for *Baylisascaris* infection include contact with raccoon latrines (bases of trees, unsealed attics, or flat surfaces such as logs, tree stumps, rocks, decks, and rooftops) and uncovered sandboxes, geophagia/pica, age younger than 4 years, and, in older children, developmental delay. Nearly all reported cases have been in males.

Incubation Period

Unknown.

Diagnostic Tests

Baylisascaris infection is confirmed by identification of larvae in biopsy specimens. Serologic testing (serum, CSF) is available at the Centers for Disease Control and Prevention. A presumptive diagnosis can be made on the basis of clinical (meningoencephalitis, diffuse unilateral subacute neuroretinitis, pseudotumor), epidemiologic (raccoon exposure), and laboratory (blood and CSF eosinophilia) findings. Neuroimaging results can be normal initially, but as larvae grow and migrate through CNS tissue, focal abnormalities are found in periventricular white matter and elsewhere. In ocular disease, ophthalmologic examination can reveal characteristic chorioretinal lesions or, rarely, larvae. Because eggs are not shed in human feces, stool examination is not helpful.

Treatment

On the basis of CNS and CSF penetration and in vitro activity, albendazole, in conjunction with high-dose corticosteroids, has been advocated most widely but may not affect clinical outcome in severe CNS infections. If suspected, treatment should be started while the diagnostic evaluation is being completed. Some experts advocate use of additional anthelmintic agents. Limited data are available on safety and efficacy of these therapies in children. Preventive therapy with albendazole should be considered for children with a history of ingestion of soil potentially contaminated with raccoon feces. Worms localized to the retina may be killed by direct photocoagulation.

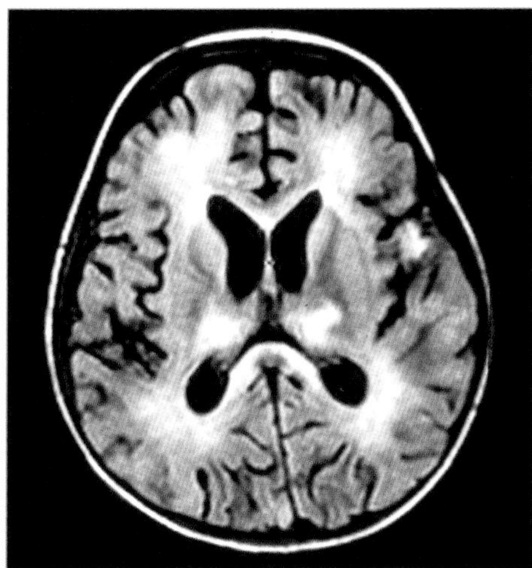

Image 16.1
Neuroimaging of human *Baylisascaris procyonis* neural larval migrans. Axial T2-weighted magnetic resonance image (at the level of the lateral ventricles) demonstrates abnormal patchy hyperintense signal of periventricular white matter and basal ganglia. Courtesy of Gavin.

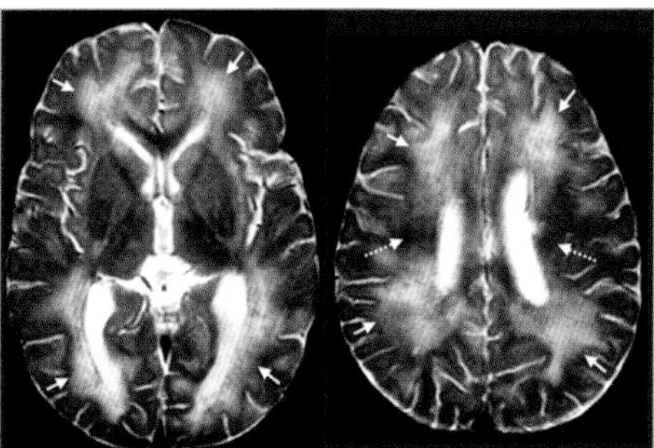

Image 16.2
Biopsy-proven *Baylisascaris procyonis* encephalitis in a 13-month-old boy. Axial T2-weighted magnetic resonance images obtained 12 days after symptom onset show abnormal high signal throughout most of the central white matter (arrows) compared with the dark signal expected at this age (broken arrows). Sorvillo F, Ash LR, Berlin OGW, Yatabe J, Degiorgio C, Morse SA. *Baylisascaris procyonis:* an emerging helminthic zoonosis. *Emerg Infect Dis.* 2002;8(4):355–359.

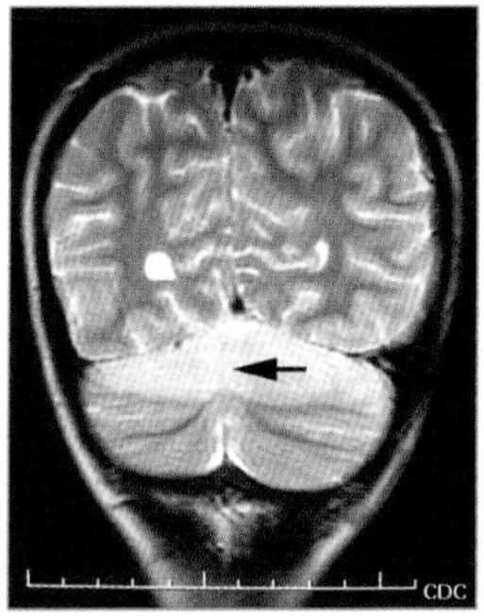

Image 16.3
Coronal T2-weighted magnetic resonance imaging of the brain in a 4-year-old with *Baylisascaris procyonis* eosinophilic meningitis. Arrow shows diffuse edema of the superior cerebellar hemispheres (scale bar increments in centimeters). Courtesy of Centers for Disease Control and Prevention/*Emerging Infectious Diseases* and Poulomi J. Pai.

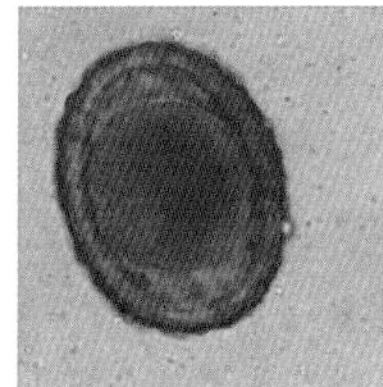

Image 16.4
Unembryonated egg of *Baylisascaris procyonis*. *B procyonis* eggs are 80 to 85 µm by 65 to 70 µm in size, thick-shelled, and usually slightly oval in shape. They have a similar morphology to fertile eggs of *Ascaris lumbricoides*, although eggs of *A lumbricoides* are smaller (55–75 µm x 35–50 µm). The definitive host for *B procyonis* is the raccoon, although dogs may also serve as definitive hosts. As humans do not serve as definitive hosts for *B procyonis,* eggs are not considered a diagnostic finding and are not excreted in human feces. Courtesy of Cheryl Davis, MD, Western Kentucky University.

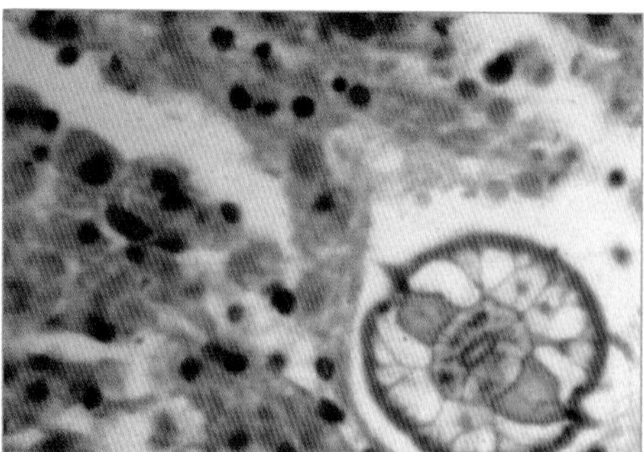

Image 16.5
Baylisascaris procyonis larva in cross-section (at midbody level) (diameter, 60 µm) recovered from the cerebrum of a rabbit with neural larval migrans. Characteristic features include a centrally located (slightly compressed) intestine, flanked on either side by large triangular-shaped excretory columns. Prominent lateral cuticular alae are visible on opposite sides of the body (hematoxylin-eosin stain). Courtesy of Gavin.

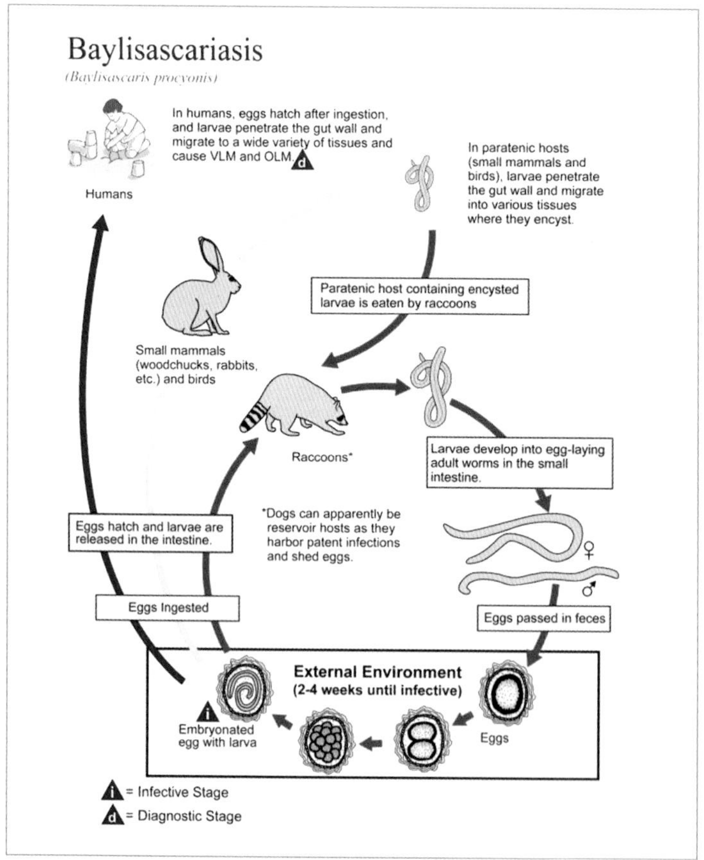

Image 16.6
This illustration depicts the life cycle of *Baylisascaris procyonis*, the causal agent of *Baylisascaris* disease. Courtesy of Centers for Disease Control and Prevention/Alexander J. da Silva, PhD/Melanie Moser.

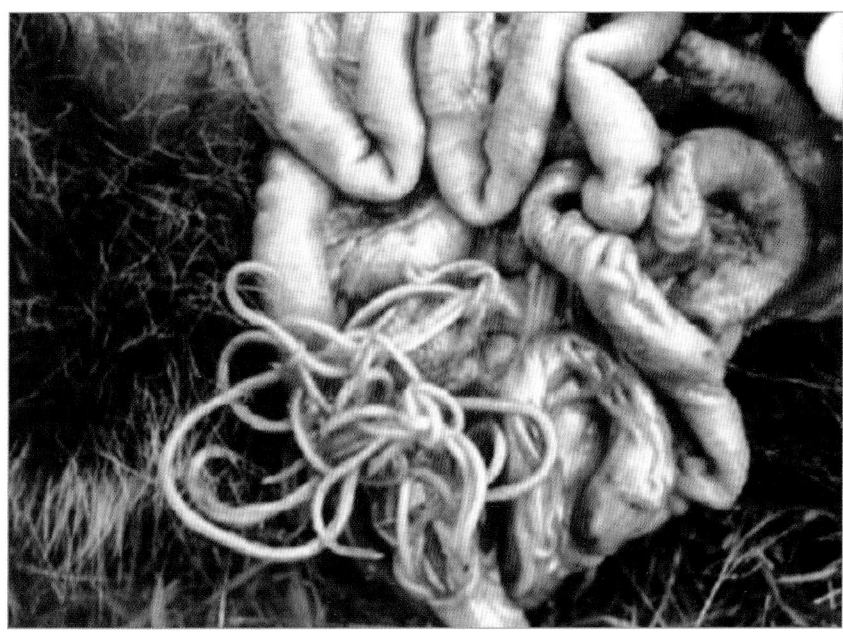

Image 16.7
Baylisascaris is raccoon roundworm, which may cause ocular and neural larval migrans and encephalitis in humans. Photo used with permission of Michigan DNR Wildlife Disease Lab.

17

Infections With *Blastocystis hominis* and Other Subtypes

Clinical Manifestations

The importance of *Blastocystis* species as a cause of gastrointestinal tract disease is controversial. The asymptomatic carrier state is well documented. Clinical symptoms reported include bloating, flatulence, mild to moderate diarrhea without fecal leukocytes or blood, abdominal pain, nausea, and poor growth. When *Blastocystis hominis* is identified in stool from symptomatic patients, other causes of this symptom complex, particularly *Giardia intestinalis* and *Cryptosporidium parvum*, should be investigated before assuming *B hominis* is the cause of the signs and symptoms.

Etiology

B hominis has previously been classified as a protozoan, but molecular studies have characterized it as a stramenopile (a eukaryote). Multiple forms have been described: vacuolar, which is observed most commonly in clinical specimens; granular, which is seen rarely in fresh stools; ameboid; and cystic.

Epidemiology

Blastocystis species are recovered from 1% to 20% of stool specimens examined for ova and parasites. Because transmission is believed to be fecal-oral, presence of the organism may be a marker for presence of other pathogens spread by fecal contamination. Transmission from animals occurs.

Incubation Period

Unknown.

Diagnostic Tests

Stool specimens should be preserved in polyvinyl alcohol and stained with trichrome or iron-hematoxylin before microscopic examination. The parasite may be present in varying numbers, and infections may be reported as light to heavy. The presence of 5 or more organisms per high-power (magnification x400) field can indicate heavy infection with many organisms, which, to some experts, suggests causation when other enteropathogens are absent. Other experts consider the presence of 10 or more organisms per 10 oil immersion fields (magnification x1,000) to represent many organisms.

Treatment

Indications for treatment are not established. Some experts recommend that treatment should be reserved for patients who have persistent symptoms and in whom no other pathogen or process is found to explain the gastrointestinal tract symptoms. Nitazoxanide and metronidazole have demonstrated benefit in symptomatic patients.

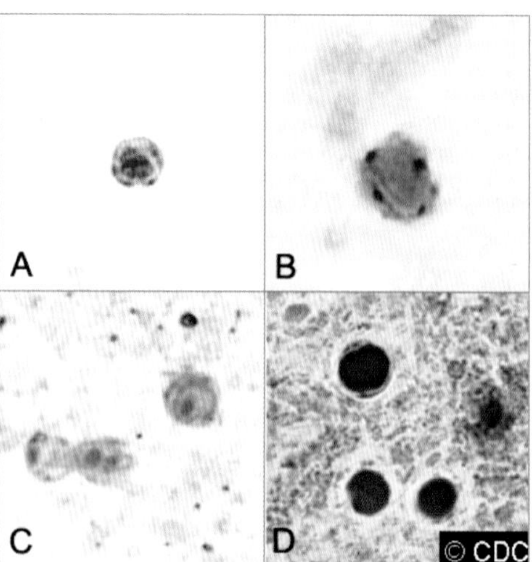

Image 17.1
A–D, *Blastocystis hominis* cystlike forms (trichrome stain). The sizes vary from 4 to 10 µm. The vacuoles stain variably from red to blue. The nuclei in the peripheral cytoplasmic rim are clearly visible, staining purple (B) (4 nuclei). Specimens in figures A through C contributed by Ray Kaplan, MD, SmithKline Beecham Diagnostic Laboratories, Atlanta, GA. D, Courtesy of Centers for Disease Control and Prevention.

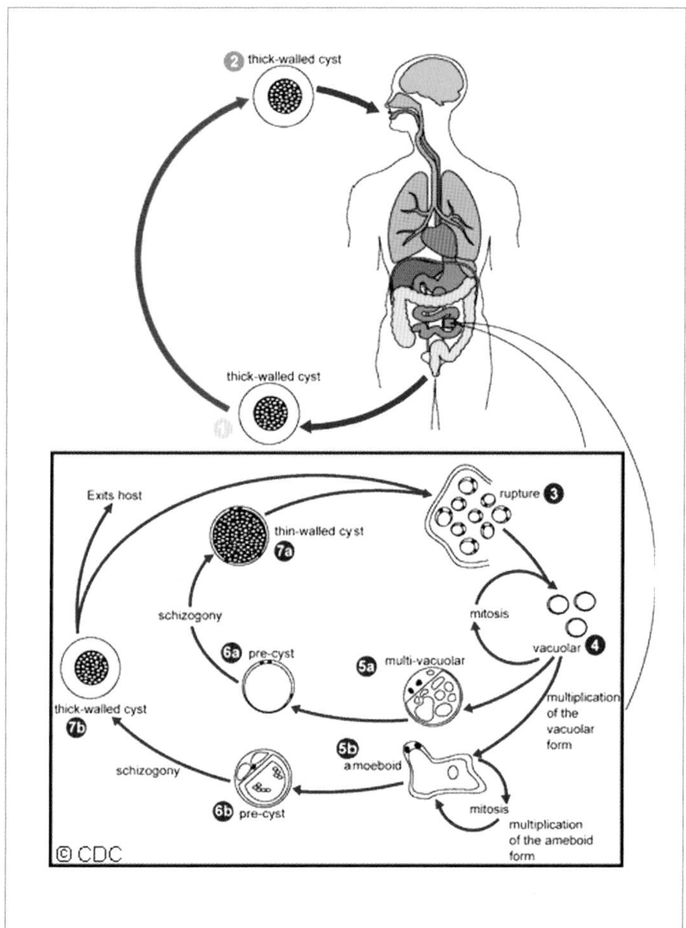

Image 17.2

Knowledge of the life cycle and transmission are still under investigation; therefore, this is a proposed life cycle for *Blastocystis hominis.* The classic form found in human stools is the cyst, which varies tremendously in size from 6 to 40 µm (1). The thick-walled cyst present in the stools (1) is believed to be responsible for external transmission, possibly by the fecal-oral route through ingestion of contaminated water or food (2). The cysts infect epithelial cells of the digestive tract and multiply asexually (3, 4). Vacuolar forms of the parasite give origin to multivacuolar (5a) and ameboid (5b) forms. The multivacuolar form develops into a precyst (6a) that gives origin to a thin-walled cyst (7a) thought to be responsible for autoinfection. The ameboid form gives origin to a precyst (6b), which develops into thick-walled cyst by schizogony (7b). *B hominis* stages were reproduced from Singh M, Suresh K, Ho LC, Ng GC, Yap EH. Elucidation of the life cycle of the intestinal protozoan *Blastocystis hominis. Parasitol Res.* 1995;81(5):449. Life cycle image and information courtesy of DPDx.

18

Blastomycosis

Clinical Manifestations

Infections can be acute, chronic, or fulminant but are asymptomatic in up to 50% of infected people. The most common clinical manifestation of blastomycosis in children is prolonged pulmonary disease, with fever, chest pain, and nonspecific symptoms such as fatigue and myalgia. Rarely, patients may develop acute respiratory distress syndrome. Typical radiographic patterns include patchy pneumonitis, a masslike infiltrate, or nodules. Blastomycosis can be misdiagnosed as bacterial pneumonia, tuberculosis, sarcoidosis, or malignant neoplasm. Disseminated blastomycosis, which can occur in up to 25% of cases, most commonly involves the skin, osteoarticular structures, and genitourinary tract. Cutaneous manifestations can be verrucous, nodular, ulcerative, or pustular. Abscesses are usually subcutaneous but can involve any organ. Central nervous system infection is uncommon, and intrauterine or congenital infection is rare.

Etiology

Blastomycosis is caused by *Blastomyces dermatitidis,* a thermally dimorphic fungus existing in yeast form at 37°C (98°F) in infected tissues and in a mycelial form at room temperature and in soil. Conidia, produced from hyphae of the mycelial form, are infectious.

Epidemiology

Infection is acquired through inhalation of conidia from soil and can occur in immunocompetent and immunocompromised hosts. Increased mortality rates for patients with pulmonary blastomycosis have been associated with advanced age, chronic obstructive pulmonary disease, cancer, and African American ethnicity. Person-to-person transmission does not occur. Blastomycosis is endemic in areas of the central United States, with most cases occurring in the Ohio and Mississippi river valleys, the southeastern states, and states that border the Great Lakes. Sporadic cases also have been reported in Hawaii, Israel, India, Africa, and Central and South America.

Incubation Period

2 weeks to 3 months.

Diagnostic Tests

Definitive diagnosis of blastomycosis is based on identification of characteristic thick-walled, broad-based, single budding yeast cells by culture or in histopathologic specimens. The organism can be seen in sputum, tracheal aspirates, cerebrospinal fluid, urine, or histopathologic specimens from lesions processed with 10% potassium hydroxide or a silver stain. Children with pneumonia who are unable to produce sputum may require bronchoalveolar lavage or open biopsy to establish the diagnosis. Bronchoalveolar lavage is high yield, even in patients with bone or skin manifestations. Organisms can be isolated by culture. Chemiluminescent DNA probes are available for identification of *B dermatitidis.* Because serologic tests (immunodiffusion and complement fixation) lack adequate sensitivity, effort should be made to obtain appropriate specimens for culture. An assay that detects *Blastomyces* antigen in urine is available commercially, but significant cross-reactivity occurs in patients with other endemic mycoses.

Treatment

Amphotericin B is recommended for initial therapy of severe disease. Oral itraconazole is recommended for step-down therapy and mild to moderate infection. Liposomal amphotericin B is recommended for central nervous system infection and may be followed by a prolonged course of azole therapy with fluconazole, voriconazole, or itraconazole. Itraconazole is indicated for treatment of nonlife-threatening infection outside of the central nervous system.

Therapy for severe or central nervous system infections usually is continued for at least 12 months. For mild to moderate pulmonary and extrapulmonary disease, treatment is continued for 6 to 12 months.

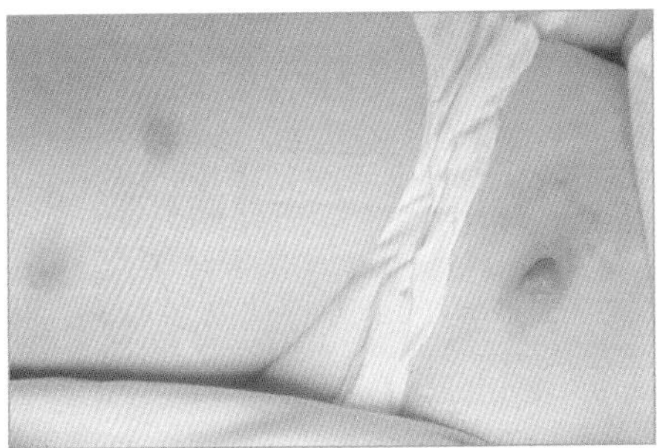

Image 18.1
Nodular skin lesions of blastomycosis, one of which is a bullous lesion on top of a nodule. Aspiration of the bulla revealed yeast forms of *Blastomyces dermatitidis*. Courtesy of Centers for Disease Control and Prevention/Libero Ajello, MD.

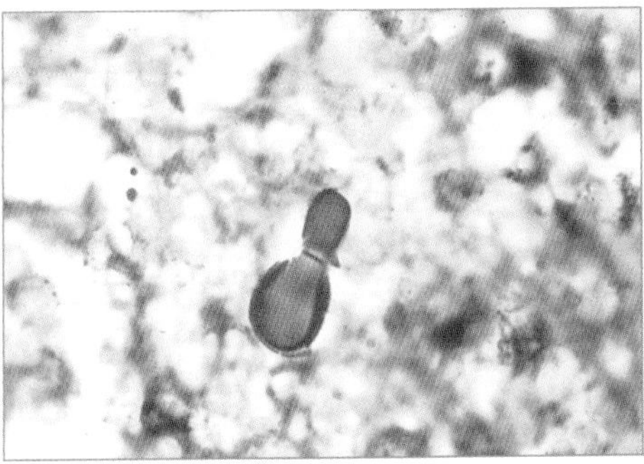

Image 18.3
Histopathology of blastomycosis. Yeast cell of *Blastomyces dermatitidis* undergoing broad-base budding (methenamine silver stain). Courtesy of Centers for Disease Control and Prevention/ Libero Ajello, MD.

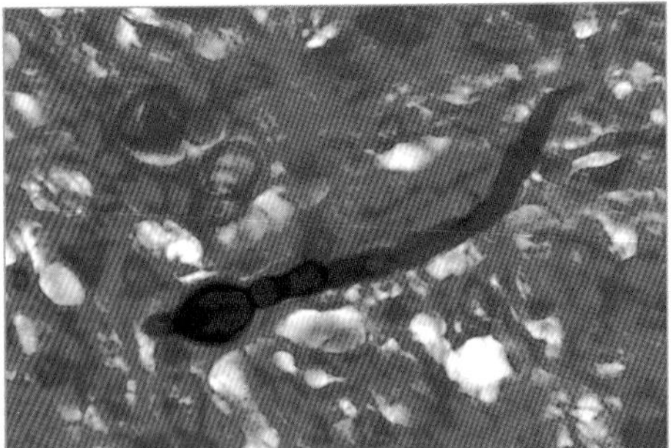

Image 18.5
This micrograph shows histopathologic changes that reveal the presence of the fungal agent *Blastomyces dermatitidis*. Courtesy of Centers for Disease Control and Prevention/Libero Ajello, MD.

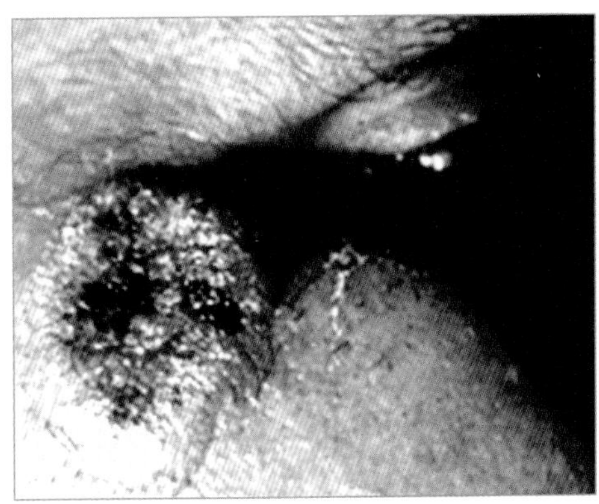

Image 18.2
Cutaneous blastomycosis (face). Cutaneous lesions are nodular, verrucous, or ulcerative, as in this man. Most cutaneous lesions are due to hematogenous spread from a pulmonary infection. Courtesy of Edgar O. Ledbetter, MD, FAAP.

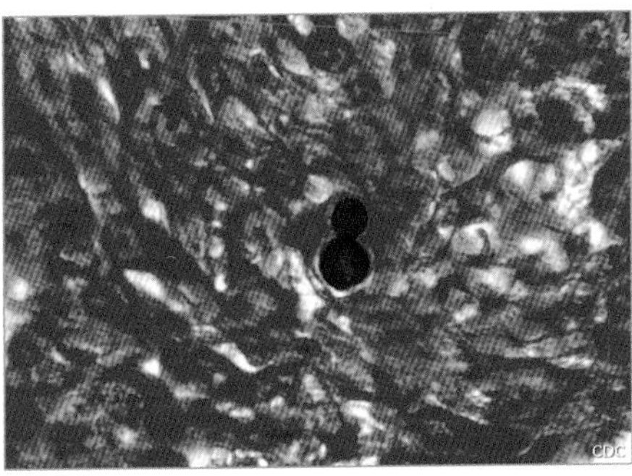

Image 18.4
This photomicrograph depicts the fungal agent *Blastomyces dermatitidis* (hematoxylin-eosin stain). Courtesy of Centers for Disease Control and Prevention/Libero Ajello, MD.

19

Bocavirus

Clinical Manifestations

Human bocavirus (HBoV) was first identified in 2005 from a cohort of children with acute respiratory tract symptoms including fever, rhinorrhea, cough, and wheezing. Human bocavirus has been identified in 5% to 33% of children with acute respiratory tract infections. High rates of HBoV subclinical infection also occur. The role of HBoV as a human pathogen is confounded by simultaneous detection of other viral pathogens in children with HBoV, with coinfection rates as high as 80%. Human bocavirus has been detected in stool samples from children with acute gastroenteritis, but its role in symptoms is uncertain. Nearly all children develop serologic evidence of infection by 5 years of age.

Etiology

Human bocavirus is a nonenveloped, single-stranded DNA virus in the family Parvoviridae, genus *Bocavirus*. Human bocavirus replicates in the respiratory and gastrointestinal tracts.

Epidemiology

Detection of HBoV has been described only in humans. Transmission is presumed to be from respiratory tract secretions, although fecal-oral transmission may be possible. The frequent codetection of other viral pathogens of the respiratory tract in association with HBoV has led to speculations that it may be a true copathogen, it may be shed for long periods after primary infection (up to 75 days), or it may reactivate during subsequent viral infections. Human bocavirus circulates worldwide and throughout the year. In temperate climates, seasonal clustering in the spring has been reported.

Diagnostic Tests

Commercial molecular diagnostic assays for HBoV are available. Human bocavirus polymerase chain reaction and detection of HBoV-specific antibody also are available in research laboratories.

Treatment

No specific therapy is available.

20

Borrelia Infections

(Relapsing Fever)

Clinical Manifestations

Two types of relapsing fever occur in humans: tick-borne and louse-borne. Both are characterized by sudden onset of high fever, shaking chills, sweats, headache, muscle and joint pain, altered sensorium, nausea, and diarrhea. A fleeting macular rash of the trunk and petechiae of the skin and mucous membranes sometimes occur. Findings and complications can differ between types of relapsing fever and include hepatosplenomegaly, jaundice, thrombocytopenia, iridocyclitis, cough with pleuritic pain, pneumonitis, meningitis, and myocarditis. Mortality rates are 10% to 70% in untreated louse-borne relapsing fever (possibly related to comorbidities in refugee-type settings where this disease is typically found) and 4% to 10% in untreated tick-borne relapsing fever. Death occurs predominantly in people with underlying illnesses and extremes of age. Early treatment reduces mortality to less than 5%. Untreated, an initial febrile period of 2 to 7 days terminates spontaneously by crisis. The initial febrile episode is followed by an afebrile period of several days to weeks, and then by one relapse or more (0–13 for tick-borne; 1–5 for louse-born). Relapses typically become shorter and progressively milder, as afebrile periods lengthen. Relapse is associated with expression of new borrelial antigens, and resolution of symptoms is associated with production of antibody specific to those new antigenic determinants. Infection during pregnancy is often severe and can result in spontaneous abortion, preterm birth, stillbirth, or neonatal infection.

Etiology

Relapsing fever is caused by certain spirochetes of the genus *Borrelia*. Worldwide, at least 14 *Borrelia* species cause tick-borne (endemic) relapsing fever, including *Borrelia hermsii*, *Borrelia turicatae*, and *Borrelia parkeri* in North America. *Borrelia recurrentis* is the only species that causes louse-borne (epidemic) relapsing fever, and this organism has no animal reservoir.

Epidemiology

Endemic tick-borne relapsing fever is distributed worldwide, is transmitted by soft-bodied ticks (*Ornithodoros* species), and occurs sporadically and in small clusters, often within families or cohabiting groups. In the United States, tick-borne relapsing fever can be acquired only in western states but has been diagnosed in other states in travelers returning from these areas. Ticks become infected by feeding on rodents or other small mammals and transmit infection via their saliva and other fluids when they take subsequent blood meals. Ticks can serve as reservoirs of infection. Soft-bodied ticks inflict painless bites and feed briefly (15–90 minutes), usually at night, so people are often unaware of bites.

Most tick-borne relapsing fever in the United States is caused by *B hermsii*. Infection typically results from tick exposures in rodent-infested cabins in western mountainous areas, including state and national parks. However, infection has also occurred in primary residences and luxurious rental properties. *B turicatae* infections occur less frequently; most cases have been reported from Texas and are often associated with tick exposures in rodent-infested caves. A single human infection with *B parkeri* has been reported; the tick infected with this *Borrelia* species is associated with arid areas or grasslands in the western United States.

Louse-borne epidemic relapsing fever has been reported in Ethiopia, Eritrea, Somalia, and the Sudan, especially in refugee and displaced populations. Epidemic transmission occurs when body lice (*Pediculus humanus*) become infected by feeding on humans with spirochetemia; infection is transmitted when infected lice are crushed and their body fluids contaminate a bite wound or skin abraded by scratching.

Infected body lice and ticks may remain alive and infectious for several years without feeding. Relapsing fever is not transmitted person to person, but perinatal transmission from an infected mother to her newborn can occur and result in preterm birth, stillbirth, and neonatal death.

Incubation Period

2 to 18 days (mean, 7 days).

Diagnostic Tests

Spirochetes can be observed by darkfield microscopy and in Wright-, Giemsa-, or acridine orange–stained preparations of thin or dehemoglobinized thick smears of peripheral blood or in stained buffy-coat preparations. Organisms can often be visualized in blood obtained while the person is febrile, particularly during initial febrile episodes; organisms are less likely to be recovered from subsequent relapses. Spirochetes can be cultured from blood, although these methods are not widely available. Serum antibodies to *Borrelia* species can be detected by enzyme immunoassay and Western immunoblot analysis at some reference and commercial specialty laboratories; a 4-fold increase in titer is considered confirmatory. These antibody tests are not standardized and are affected by antigenic variations among and within *Borrelia* species and strains. Serologic cross-reactions occur with other spirochetes, including *Borrelia burgdorferi, Treponema pallidum,* and *Leptospira* species.

Treatment

Treatment of tick-borne relapsing fever with a 5- to 10-day course of a tetracycline, usually doxycycline, produces prompt clearance of spirochetes and remission of symptoms. For children younger than 8 years and pregnant women, penicillin or erythromycin are the preferred drugs. Penicillin G procaine or intravenous penicillin G is recommended as initial therapy for people who are unable to take oral therapy, although low-dose penicillin G has been associated with a higher frequency of relapse. A Jarisch-Herxheimer reaction (an acute febrile reaction accompanied by headache, myalgia, respiratory distress in some cases, and an aggravated clinical picture lasting less than 24 hours) is commonly observed during the first few hours after initiating antimicrobial therapy. However, the Jarisch-Herxheimer reaction in children is typically mild and can usually be managed with antipyretic agents alone.

Single-dose treatment using a tetracycline, penicillin, erythromycin, or chloramphenicol is effective for curing louse-borne relapsing fever.

Image 20.1
Borrelia in peripheral blood smear. The spirochetes can be seen with darkfield microscopy and in Wright-, Giemsa-, or acridine orange–stained smears.

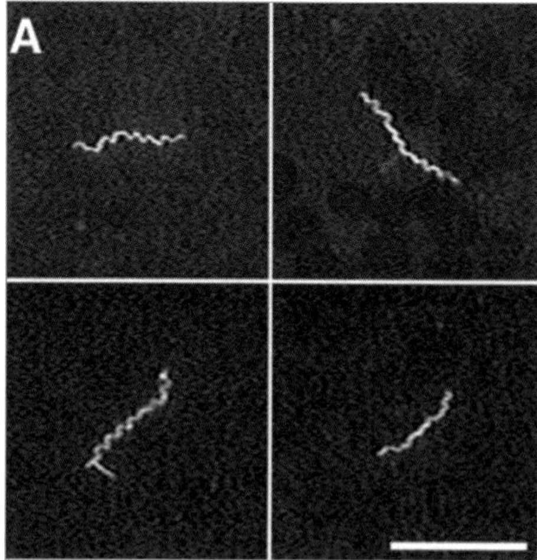

Image 20.2
Borrelia hermsii in the blood of a patient (case 3) stained with rabbit hyperimmune serum and antirabbit fluorescein isothiocyanate (scale bar, 20 mm). Courtesy of *Emerging Infectious Diseases.*

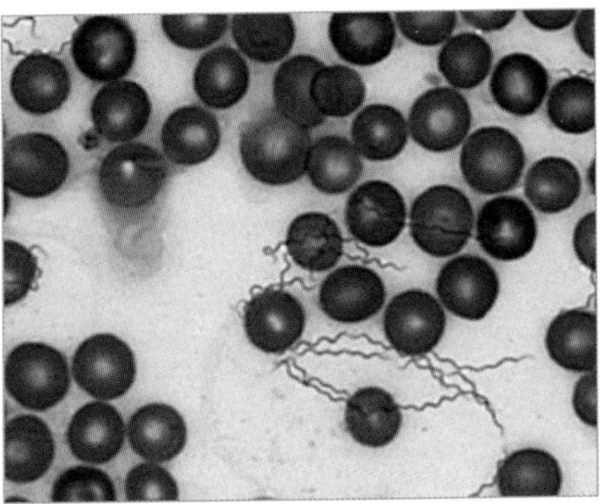

Image 20.3
Borrelia hermsii in a thin smear of mouse blood stained with Wright-Giemsa and visualized with oil immersion bright-field microscopy (magnification x600) for the confirmation of infection with relapsing fever spirochetes in humans and other animals (scale bar, 20 mm). Courtesy of *Emerging Infectious Diseases.*

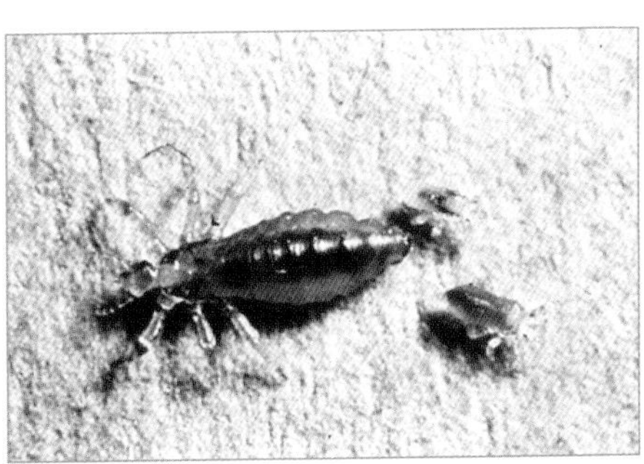

Image 20.4
This image depicts an adult female body louse, *Pediculus humanus,* and 2 larval young. *P humanus* has been shown to serve as a vector for diseases such as typhus, due to *Rickettsia prowazekii,* trench fever caused by *Bartonella* (formerly *Rochalimaea*) *quintana*, and relapsing fever due to *Borrelia recurrentis*. Courtesy of World Health Organization.

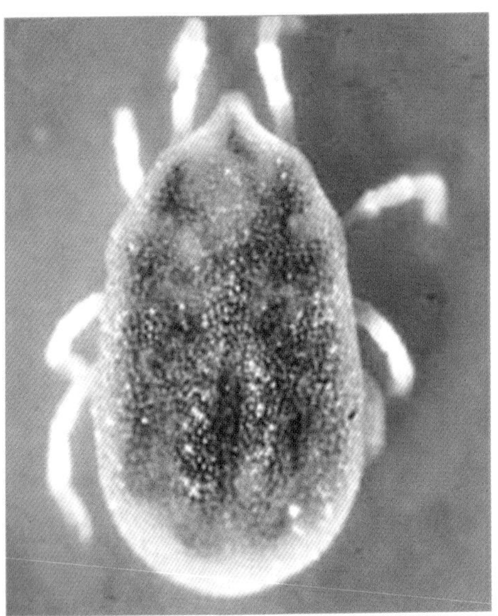

Image 20.5
An *Ornithodoros hermsii* nymph. The length of the soft-bodied tick is 3.0 µm, excluding the legs. It is responsible for transmitting endemic relapsing fever. Schwan TG, Policastro PF, Miller Z, Thompson RL, Damrow T, Keirans JE. Tick-borne relapsing fever caused by *Borrelia hermsii,* Montana. *Emerg Infect Dis*. 2003;9(9):1151–1154.

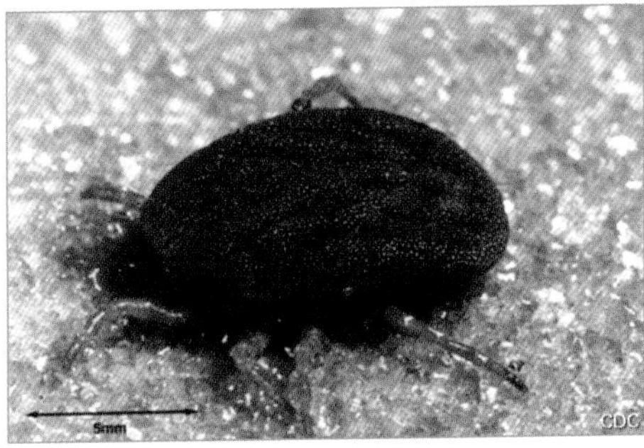

Image 20.6
Ornithodoros moubata ticks frequent traditional homes in sub-Saharan Africa and mainly feed nocturnally. Courtesy of Centers for Disease Control and Prevention/*Emerging Infectious Diseases* and Sally J. Cutler.

21

Brucellosis

Clinical Manifestations

Onset of brucellosis in children can be acute or insidious. Manifestations are nonspecific and include fever, night sweats, weakness, malaise, anorexia, weight loss, arthralgia, myalgia, abdominal pain, and headache. Physical findings can include lymphadenopathy, hepatosplenomegaly, and arthritis. Abdominal pain and peripheral arthritis are reported more frequently in children than in adults. Neurologic deficits, ocular involvement, epididymo-orchitis, and liver or spleen abscesses are reported. Anemia, leukopenia, thrombocytopenia, or, less frequently, pancytopenia are hematologic findings that might suggest the diagnosis. Serious complications include meningitis, endocarditis, osteomyelitis, and, less frequently, pneumonitis and aortic involvement. A detailed history, including travel, exposure to animals, and food habits, including ingestion of raw milk, should be obtained if brucellosis is considered. Chronic disease is less common among children than among adults, although the rate of relapse has been found to be similar. Brucellosis in pregnancy is associated with risk of spontaneous abortion, preterm delivery, miscarriage, and intrauterine infection with fetal death.

Etiology

Brucella bacteria are aerobic small, nonmotile, gram-negative coccobacilli. The species that are known to infect humans are *Brucella abortus, Brucella melitensis, Brucella suis,* and, rarely, *Brucella canis.* Three recently identified species, *Brucella ceti, Brucella pinnipedialis,* and *Brucella inopinata,* are potential human pathogens.

Epidemiology

Brucellosis is a zoonotic disease of wild and domestic animals. It is transmissible to humans by direct or indirect exposure to aborted fetuses or tissues or fluids of infected animals. Transmission occurs by inoculation through mucous membranes or cuts and abrasions in the skin, inhalation of contaminated aerosols, or ingestion of undercooked meat or unpasteurized dairy products. People in occupations such as farming, ranching, and veterinary medicine, as well as abattoir workers, meat inspectors, and laboratory personnel, are at increased risk. Clinicians should alert the laboratory if they anticipate *Brucella* might grow from microbiologic specimens so that appropriate laboratory precautions can be taken. In the United States, approximately 100 to 200 cases of brucellosis are reported annually, and 3% to 10% of cases occur in people younger than 19 years. Most pediatric cases reported in the United States result from ingestion of unpasteurized dairy products. Although human-to-human transmission is rare, in utero transmission has been reported, and infected mothers can transmit *Brucella* to their newborns through breastfeeding.

Incubation Period

Variable (<1 week to several months); most people become ill within 3 to 4 weeks of exposure.

Diagnostic Tests

A definitive diagnosis is established by recovery of *Brucella* species from blood, bone marrow, or other tissue specimens. A variety of media will support growth of *Brucella* species, but the physician should contact laboratory personnel and ask them to incubate cultures for a minimum of 4 weeks. Bactec systems (BD Diagnostic Systems, Sparks, MD) are reliable and can detect *Brucella* species within 5 to 7 days. In patients with a clinically compatible illness, serologic testing using the serum agglutination test can confirm the diagnosis with a 4-fold or greater increase in antibody titers between acute and convalescent serum specimens collected at least 2 weeks apart. The serum agglutination test, the gold standard for serologic diagnosis, will detect antibodies against *B abortus, B suis,* and *B melitensis* but not *B canis,* which requires use of *B canis*–specific antigen. Although a single titer is not diagnostic, most patients with active infection in an area without endemic infection will have a titer of 1:160 or greater within 2 to 4 weeks of clinical disease onset. Lower titers can be found early in the course of infection. Immunoglobulin (Ig) M antibodies are produced within the first week, followed by a gradual increase in IgG synthesis. Low IgM titers may

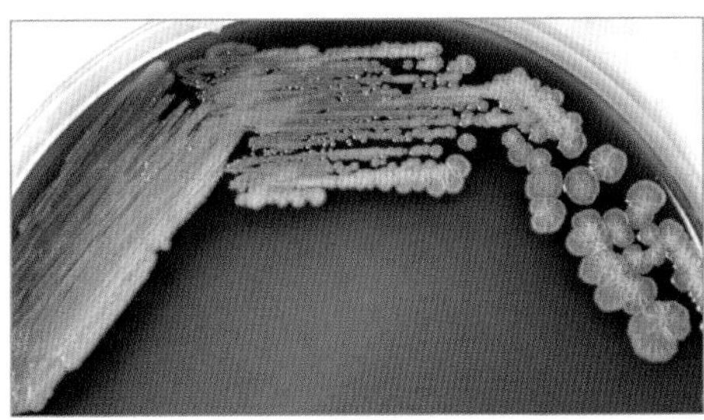

Image 22.2
This photograph depicts the colonial morphology displayed by gram-negative *Burkholderia pseudomallei* bacteria, which was grown on a medium of chocolate agar, for a 72-hour period, at a temperature of 37°C (98.6°F). Courtesy of Centers for Disease Control and Prevention/ Dr Todd Parker, Audra Marsh.

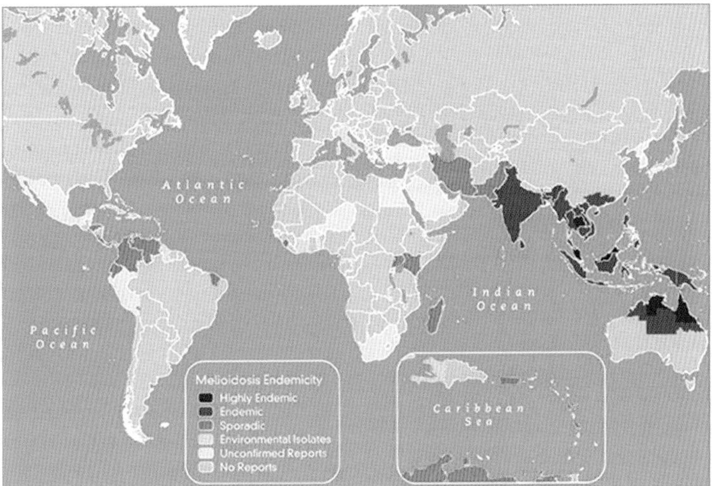

Image 22.3
Endemicity of melioidosis infection. Centers for Disease Control and Prevention National Center for Emerging and Zoonotic Infectious Diseases (NCEZID) Division of Global Migration and Quarantine (DGMQ).

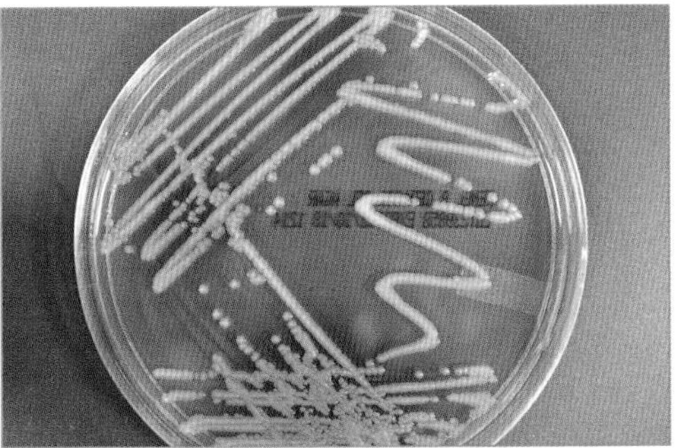

Image 22.4
Burkholderia cepacia on *Burkholderia* selective agar. With vancomycin, gentamicin, and polymyxin B, this agar is used for the isolation of *B cepacia* complex from respiratory secretions of patients with cystic fibrosis. Growth of the organism turns the medium from orange to yellow, and colonies are surrounded by a pink-yellow zone in the medium. Growth may require up to 72 hours of incubation. Courtesy of Julia Rosebush, DO; Robert Jerris, PhD; and Theresa Stanley, M(ASCP).

23

Campylobacter Infections

Clinical Manifestations

Predominant symptoms of *Campylobacter* infections include diarrhea, abdominal pain, malaise, and fever. Stools can contain visible or occult blood. In neonates and young infants, bloody diarrhea without fever can be the only manifestation of infection. Pronounced fevers in children can result in febrile seizures that can occur before gastrointestinal tract symptoms. Abdominal pain can mimic that produced by appendicitis or intussusception. Mild infection lasts 1 or 2 days and resembles viral gastroenteritis. Most patients recover in less than 1 week, but 10% to 20% have a relapse or a prolonged or severe illness. Severe or persistent infection can mimic acute inflammatory bowel disease. Bacteremia is uncommon but can occur in neonates and children. Immunocompromised hosts can have prolonged, relapsing, or extraintestinal infections, especially with *Campylobacter fetus* and other *Campylobacter* species. Immunoreactive complications, such as acute idiopathic polyneuritis (Guillain-Barré syndrome) (occurring in an estimated 1 per 1,000 persons), Miller Fisher variant of Guillain-Barré syndrome (ophthalmoplegia, areflexia, ataxia), reactive arthritis, Reiter syndrome (arthritis, urethritis, and bilateral conjunctivitis), myocarditis, pericarditis, and erythema nodosum, can occur during convalescence.

Etiology

Campylobacter species are motile, comma-shaped, gram-negative bacilli. There are 25 species within the genus *Campylobacter*, but *Campylobacter jejuni* and *Campylobacter coli* are the species isolated most commonly from patients with diarrhea. *C fetus* predominantly causes systemic illness in neonates and debilitated hosts. Other *Campylobacter* species, including *Campylobacter upsaliensis*, *Campylobacter lari*, and *Campylobacter hyointestinalis*, can cause similar diarrheal or systemic illnesses in children.

Epidemiology

Data from the Foodborne Diseases Active Surveillance Network (**www.cdc.gov/foodnet**) indicate that, although incidence decreased in the early 2000s, the 2012 incidence represented a 14% increase over 2006–2008 baseline. Disease incidence has remained stable since 2010–2012, with 13.8 cases per 100,000 population in 2013. The highest rates of infection occur in children younger than 5 years. Most *Campylobacter* infections are acquired domestically, but it is also the most common cause of diarrhea in returning international travelers. In susceptible people, as few as 500 *Campylobacter* organisms can cause infection.

The gastrointestinal tracts of domestic and wild birds and animals are reservoirs of the bacteria. *C jejuni* and *C coli* have been isolated from feces of 30% to 100% of healthy chickens, turkeys, and water fowl. Poultry carcasses commonly are contaminated. Many farm animals and meat sources can harbor the organism and are potential sources of infection. Transmission of *C jejuni* and *C coli* occurs by ingestion of contaminated food or water or by direct contact with fecal material from infected animals or people. Improperly cooked poultry, untreated water, and unpasteurized milk have been the main vehicles of transmission. *Campylobacter* infections usually are sporadic; outbreaks are rare but have occurred among schoolchildren who drank unpasteurized milk, including children who participated in field trips to dairy farms. Person-to-person spread occurs occasionally, particularly among very young children. Uncommonly, outbreaks of diarrhea in child care centers have been reported. Person-to-person transmission has also occurred in neonates of infected mothers and has resulted in health care–associated outbreaks in nurseries. In neonates, *C jejuni* and *C coli* usually cause gastroenteritis, whereas *C fetus* often causes septicemia or meningitis. Enteritis occurs in people of all ages. Excretion of *Campylobacter* organisms typically lasts 2 to 3 weeks without treatment but can be as long as 7 weeks.

Incubation Period

2 to 5 days but can be longer.

Diagnostic Tests

C jejuni and *C coli* can be cultured from feces, and *Campylobacter* species, including *C fetus*, can be cultured from blood. Isolation of *C jejuni* and *C coli* from stool specimens requires selective media, microaerobic conditions, and an incubation temperature of 42°C (107.6°F). Although other *Campylobacter* species are occasionally isolated using routine culture methods, additional methods that use nonselective isolation techniques and increased hydrogen microaerobic conditions are usually required for isolation of species other than *C jejuni* and *C coli*. The presence of motile curved, spiral, or S-shaped rods resembling *Vibrio cholerae* by stool phase contrast or darkfield microscopy can provide rapid, presumptive evidence for *Campylobacter* species infection directly from fresh stool samples. This is less sensitive than culture. *C jejuni* and *C coli* can be detected directly (but not differentiated) by commercially available enzyme immunoassays. False-positive results from these nonculture-based techniques have been reported. Two multiplex nucleic acid amplification tests that detect *Campylobacter* species and other gastrointestinal pathogens, including *Salmonella*, *Shigella*, *Campylobacter*, and Shiga toxin-producing *Escherichia coli*, recently became available commercially, but data on their performance characteristics are limited.

Treatment

Rehydration is the mainstay of treatment for all children with diarrhea. Azithromycin and erythromycin shorten the duration of illness and excretion of susceptible organisms and prevent relapse when given early in gastrointestinal tract infection. Treatment with azithromycin or erythromycin usually eradicates the organism from stool within 2 or 3 days. A fluoroquinolone, such as ciprofloxacin, may be effective, but resistance to ciprofloxacin is common (31% of *C coli* isolates and 22% of *C jejuni* isolates in the United States in 2010 [**www.cdc.gov/NARMS**]) If antimicrobial therapy is given for treatment of gastroenteritis, the recommended duration is 3 to 5 days. Antimicrobial agents for bacteremia should be selected on the basis of antimicrobial susceptibility tests. *C fetus* generally is susceptible to aminoglycosides, extended-spectrum cephalosporins, meropenem, imipenem, and ampicillin. Antimotility agents should not be used because they have been shown to prolong symptoms and may be associated with an increased risk of death.

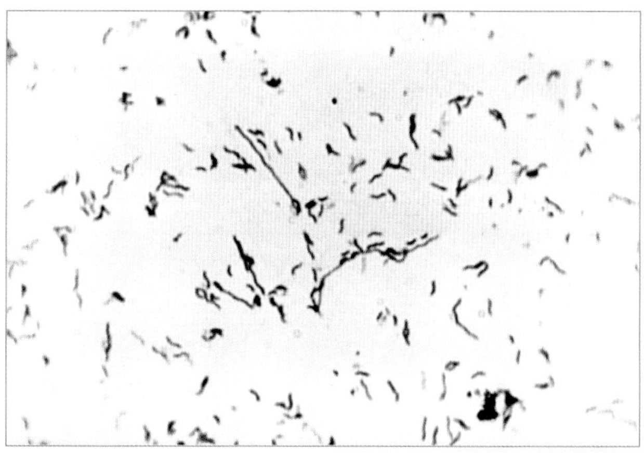

Image 23.1
This photomicrograph depicts findings observed in a 48-hour culture of *Campylobacter jejuni* bacteria revealing characteristic thin-, comma-, or gull winged–shaped forms displayed by this bacterium. *C jejuni* is a slender, curved, motile rod that is microaerophilic (ie, it has a reduced requirement for oxygen). It is a relatively fragile organism, being sensitive to environmental stresses such as drying, heating, disinfectants, and acidic conditions. Courtesy of Centers for Disease Control and Prevention/Robert Weaver, PhD.

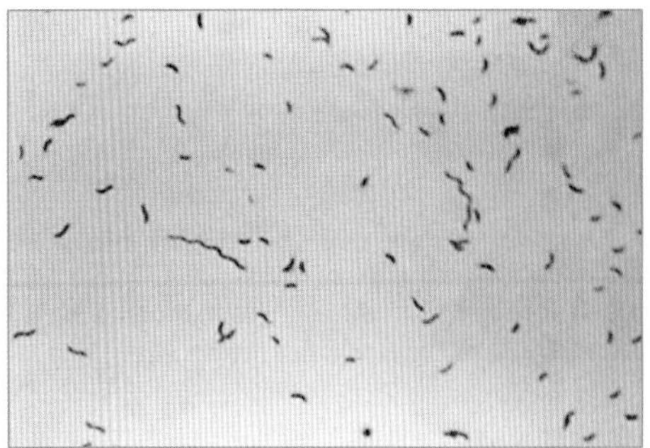

Image 23.2
This image of a Gram-stained specimen shows the spiral rods of *Campylobacter fetus* subsp *fetus* taken from an 18-hour brain-heart infusion with a 7% addition of rabbit blood agar plate culture. Courtesy of Centers for Disease Control and Prevention.

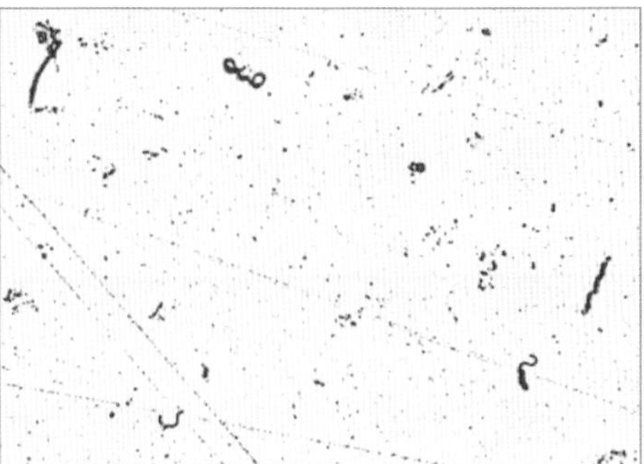

Image 23.3
Campylobacter fetus. Leifson flagella stain (digitally colorized) showing comma-shaped, gram-negative bacilli. Courtesy of Centers for Disease Control and Prevention.

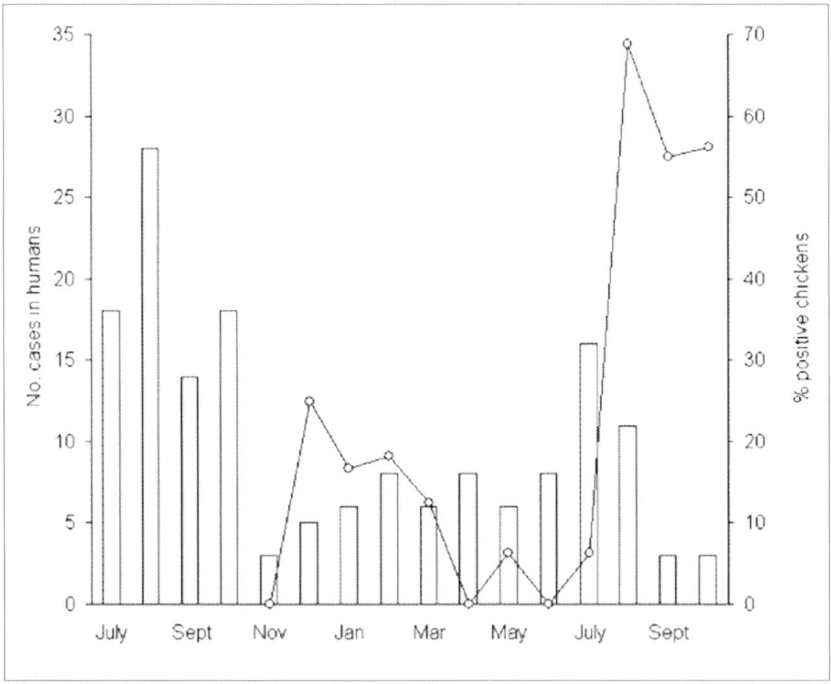

Image 23.4
Monthly distribution of the number of sporadic cases of *Campylobacter* infections in humans from July 2000 to October 2001 (columns) and of the prevalence of *Campylobacter* in whole retail chickens from November 2000 to October 2001 (line graph), Quebec. Courtesy of Michaud S, Ménard S, Arbeit RD. Campylobacteriosis, Eastern Townships, Québec. *Emerg Infect Dis.* 2004;10(10):1844–1847.

24

Candidiasis

Clinical Manifestations

Mucocutaneous infection results in oropharyngeal (thrush) or vaginal or cervical candidiasis; intertriginous lesions of the gluteal folds, buttocks, neck, groin, and axilla; paronychia; and onychia. Dysfunction of T lymphocytes, other immunologic disorders, and endocrinologic diseases are associated with chronic mucocutaneous candidiasis. Chronic or recurrent oral candidiasis can be the presenting sign of HIV infection or primary immunodeficiency. Esophageal and laryngeal candidiasis can occur in patients who are immunocompromised. Disseminated or invasive candidiasis occurs in very low birth weight neonates and, in immunocompromised or debilitated hosts, can involve virtually any organ or anatomic site and be rapidly fatal. Candidemia can occur with or without systemic disease in patients with indwelling central vascular catheters, especially patients receiving prolonged intravenous infusions with parenteral alimentation or lipids. Peritonitis can occur in patients undergoing peritoneal dialysis, especially in patients receiving prolonged broad-spectrum antimicrobial therapy. Candiduria can occur in patients with indwelling urinary catheters, focal renal infection, or disseminated disease.

Etiology

Candida species are yeasts that reproduce by budding. *Candida albicans* and several other species form long chains of elongated yeast forms called pseudohyphae. *C albicans* causes most infections, but in some regions and patient populations, non-*albicans Candida* species now account for more than half of invasive infections. Other species, including *Candida tropicalis, Candida parapsilosis, Candida glabrata* (also called *Torulopsis glabrata*), *Candida krusei, Candida guilliermondii, Candida lusitaniae,* and *Candida dubliniensis,* can also cause serious infections, especially in immunocompromised and debilitated hosts. *C parapsilosis* is second only to *C albicans* as a cause of systemic candidiasis in very low birth weight neonates.

Epidemiology

Like other *Candida* species, *C albicans* is present on skin and in the mouth, intestinal tract, and vagina of immunocompetent people. Vulvovaginal candidiasis is associated with pregnancy, and newborns can acquire the organism in utero, during passage through the vagina, or postnatally. Mild mucocutaneous infection is common in healthy neonates. Person-to-person transmission occurs rarely. Invasive disease typically occurs in people with impaired immunity, with infection usually arising endogenously from colonized sites. Factors such as extreme prematurity, neutropenia, or treatment with corticosteroids or cytotoxic chemotherapy increase the risk of invasive infection. People with diabetes mellitus generally have localized mucocutaneous lesions. In clinical studies, 5% to 20% of newborns weighing less than 1,000 g at birth develop invasive candidiasis. Patients with neutrophil defects, such as chronic granulomatous disease or myeloperoxidase deficiency, are also at increased risk. Patients undergoing intravenous alimentation or receiving broad-spectrum antimicrobial agents, especially extended-spectrum cephalosporins, carbapenems, and vancomycin, or requiring long-term indwelling central venous or peritoneal dialysis catheters have increased susceptibility to infection. Postsurgical patients can be at risk, particularly after cardiothoracic or abdominal procedures.

Incubation Period

Unknown.

Diagnostic Tests

The presumptive diagnosis of mucocutaneous candidiasis or thrush can usually be made clinically, but other organisms or trauma can also cause clinically similar lesions. Yeast cells and pseudohyphae can be found in *C albicans*–infected tissue and are identifiable by microscopic examination of scrapings prepared with Gram, calcofluor white, or fluorescent antibody stains or in a 10% to 20% potassium hydroxide suspension. Endoscopy is useful for diagnosis of esophagitis. Ophthalmologic examination can reveal typical retinal lesions attributable to hematogenous dissemination. Lesions in the brain, kidney, liver, or spleen can be detected by ultrasonography, computed tomography, or magnetic resonance imaging; however, these lesions typically are not detected by imaging until late in the course of disease or after neutropenia has resolved.

A definitive diagnosis of invasive candidiasis requires isolation of the organism from a normally sterile body site (eg, blood, cerebrospinal fluid, bone marrow) or demonstration of organisms in a tissue biopsy specimen. Negative results of culture for *Candida* species do not exclude invasive infection in immunocompromised hosts; in some settings, blood culture is only 50% sensitive. Recovery of the organism is expedited using automated blood culture systems or a lysis-centrifugation method. Special fungal culture media are not needed to grow *Candida* species. A presumptive species identification of *C albicans* can be made by demonstrating germ tube formation, and molecular fluorescence in situ hybridization testing can rapidly distinguish *C albicans* from non-*albicans Candida* species. Patient serum can be tested using the assay for (1,3)-b-D-glucan from fungal cell walls, but this does not distinguish *Candida* species from other fungi.

Treatment

- **Mucous membrane and skin infections.** Oral candidiasis in immunocompetent hosts is treated with oral nystatin suspension or clotrimazole troches applied to lesions. Troches should not be used in infants. Fluconazole may be more effective than oral nystatin or clotrimazole troches and may be considered if other treatments fail. Fluconazole or itraconazole can be beneficial for immunocompromised patients with oropharyngeal candidiasis. Voriconazole or posaconazole are alternative drugs. Although cure rates with fluconazole are greater than with nystatin, relapse rates are comparable.

  Esophagitis caused by *Candida* species is treated with oral fluconazole or itraconazole solution. For patients who cannot tolerate oral therapy, intravenous fluconazole, an echinocandin, or amphotericin B is recommended. The recommended duration of therapy is 14 to 21 days, but duration of treatment depends on severity of illness and patient factors, such as age and degree of immunocompromise.

  Skin infections are treated with topical nystatin, miconazole, clotrimazole, naftifine, ketoconazole, econazole, or ciclopirox. Nystatin is usually effective and the least expensive of these drugs.

  Vulvovaginal candidiasis is treated effectively with many topical formulations, including clotrimazole, miconazole, butoconazole, terconazole, and tioconazole. Such topically applied azole drugs are more effective than nystatin. Oral azole agents (fluconazole, itraconazole, and ketoconazole) are also effective and should be considered for recurrent or refractory cases.

  For chronic mucocutaneous candidiasis, fluconazole, itraconazole, and voriconazole are effective drugs. Low-dose amphotericin B administered intravenously is effective in severe cases. Relapses are common with any of these agents once therapy is terminated, and treatment should be viewed as a lifelong process, hopefully using only intermittent pulses of antifungal agents. Invasive infections in patients with this condition are rare.

  Keratomycosis is treated with corneal baths of voriconazole (1%) in conjunction with systemic therapy. Patients with cystitis caused by *Candida*, especially patients with neutropenia, with renal allographs, and undergoing urologic manipulation, should be treated with fluconazole for 7 days because of the concentrating effect of fluconazole in the urinary tract. An alternative is a short course (7 days) of low-dose amphotericin B intravenously. A urinary catheter in a patient with candidiasis should be removed or replaced promptly.

- **Invasive infections.** Most *Candida* species are susceptible to amphotericin B, although *C lusitaniae* and some strains of *C glabrata* and *C krusei* exhibit decreased susceptibility or resistance. Among patients with persistent candidemia despite appropriate therapy, investigation for a deep focus of infection should be conducted. Lipid-associated or liposomal preparations of amphotericin B can be used as an alternative to amphotericin B deoxycholate in patients who experience significant toxicity during therapy.

Fluconazole is not an appropriate choice for therapy before the infecting *Candida* species has been identified because *C krusei* is resistant to fluconazole and more than 50% of *C glabrata* isolates can also be resistant. Although voriconazole is effective against *C krusei*, it is often ineffective against *C glabrata*. The echinocandins (caspofungin, micafungin, and anidulafungin) all are active in vitro against most *Candida* species and are appropriate first-line drugs for *Candida* infections in patients who are severely ill or neutropenic. The echinocandins should be used with caution against *C parapsilosis* infection because some decreased in vitro susceptibility has been reported. If an echinocandin is initiated empirically and *C parapsilosis* is isolated in a recovering patient, the echinocandin can be continued.

- **Neonates**. Neonates are more likely than older children and adults to have meningitis as a manifestation of candidiasis. Although meningitis can be seen in association with candidemia, approximately half of neonates with candida meningitis do not have a positive blood culture result. Central nervous system disease in the neonate typically manifests as meningoencephalitis and should be assumed to be present in the neonate with candidemia and signs of meningoencephalitis because of the high incidence of this complication. A lumbar puncture is recommended for all neonates with candidemia.

  Amphotericin B deoxycholate is the drug of choice for treating neonates with systemic candidiasis, including meningitis. For susceptible *Candida* species, step-down treatment with fluconazole (12 mg/kg/d administered once daily) may be considered after the patient with *Candida* meningitis has responded to initial treatment. Therapy for central nervous system infection is at least 3 weeks and should continue until all signs and cerebrospinal fluid and radiologic abnormalities have resolved. Echinocandins are not recommended for treatment of central nervous system candidal infections in neonates. The duration of therapy for uncomplicated candidemia is 2 weeks. Lipid formulations of amphotericin B should be used with caution in neonates, particularly in patients with urinary tract involvement. Recent evidence suggests that treatment of neonates with lipid formulations of amphotericin may be associated with worse outcomes when compared with amphotericin B deoxycholate or fluconazole.

- **Older children and adolescents.** In nonneutropenic and clinically stable children and adults, fluconazole or an echinocandin (eg, caspofungin, micafungin, anidulafungin) is the recommended treatment; amphotericin B deoxycholate or lipid formulations are alternative. In nonneutropenic patients with candidemia and no metastatic complications, treatment should continue for 14 days after documented clearance of *Candida* from the bloodstream and resolution of clinical manifestations associated with candidemia.

  In critically ill neutropenic patients, an echinocandin or a lipid formulation of amphotericin B is recommended because of the fungicidal nature of these agents when compared with fluconazole, which is fungistatic. In less seriously ill neutropenic patients, fluconazole is the alternative treatment for patients who have not had recent azole exposure. Avoidance or reduction of systemic immunosuppression is also advised when feasible.

- **Management of indwelling catheters.** In neonates and nonneutropenic children, prompt removal of any infected vascular or peritoneal catheters is strongly recommended. For neutropenic children, catheter removal should be considered. The recommendation in this population is weaker because the source of candidemia in the neutropenic child is more likely to be gastrointestinal, and it is difficult to determine the relative contribution of the catheter. In the situation in which prompt removal of an infected catheter and rapid clearance is established, treatment could be limited for a shorter course.

- **Additional assessments.** Ophthalmologic evaluation is recommended for all patients with candidemia, although the yield is noted to be low. Evaluation should occur once candidemia is controlled, and, in patients with neutropenia, evaluation should be deferred until recovery of the neutrophil count.
- **Chemoprophylaxis.** Invasive candidiasis in neonates is associated with prolonged hospitalization and neurodevelopmental impairment or death in almost 75% of affected neonates with extremely low birth weight (<1,000 g). Four prospective randomized controlled trials and 10 retrospective cohort studies of fungal prophylaxis in neonates with birth weight less than 1,000 g or less than 1,500 g have demonstrated significant reduction of *Candida* colonization, rates of invasive candidiasis, and *Candida*-related mortality in nurseries with a moderate or high incidence of invasive candidiasis. Besides birth weight, other risk factors for invasive candidiasis in neonates include inadequate infection-prevention practices and prolonged use of antimicrobial agents. Adherence to optimal infection-control practices, including "bundles" for intravascular catheter insertion and maintenance and antimicrobial stewardship, can diminish infection rates and should be optimized before implementation of chemoprophylaxis as standard practice in a neonatal intensive care unit. Fluconazole prophylaxis is recommended for extremely low birth weight neonates cared for in neonatal intensive care units with moderate (5%–10%) or high (≥10%) rates of invasive candidiasis. The recommended regimen for extremely low birth weight neonates is to initiate fluconazole treatment intravenously during the first 48 to 72 hours after birth and administer it twice a week for 4 to 6 weeks or until intravenous access is no longer required for care.

Fluconazole prophylaxis can also decrease the risk of mucosal (eg, oropharyngeal, esophageal) candidiasis in patients with advanced HIV disease. However, an increased incidence of infections attributable to *C krusei* (which is intrinsically resistant to fluconazole) has been reported in non–HIV-infected patients receiving prophylactic fluconazole. Prophylaxis should be considered for children undergoing allogenic hematopoietic stem cell transplantation and other highly myelosuppressive chemotherapy during the period of neutropenia. Prophylaxis is not routinely recommended for other immunocompromised children, including children with HIV infection.

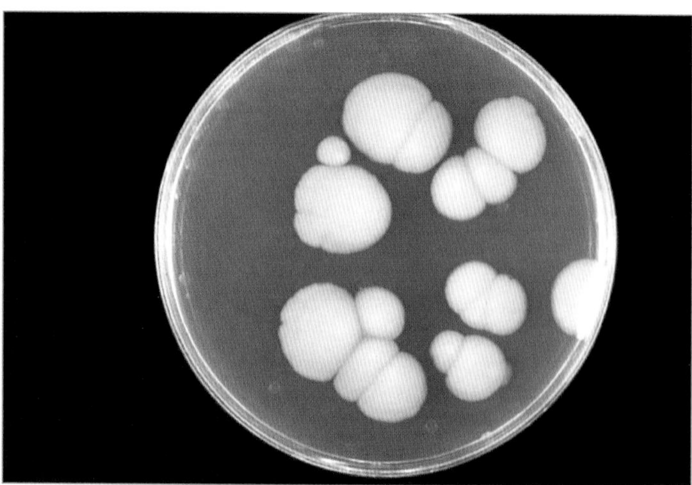

Image 24.1
This is an image of a Sabhi agar plate culture of the fungus *Candida albicans* grown at 20°C (68°F). Courtesy of Centers for Disease Control and Prevention.

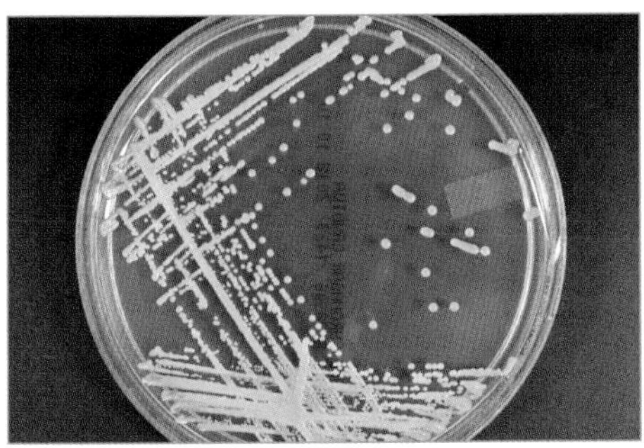

Image 24.2
Candida albicans on chrome agar. Colonies appear light to medium green in color and are smooth and raised. Courtesy of Julia Rosebush, DO; Robert Jerris, PhD; and Theresa Stanley, M(ASCP).

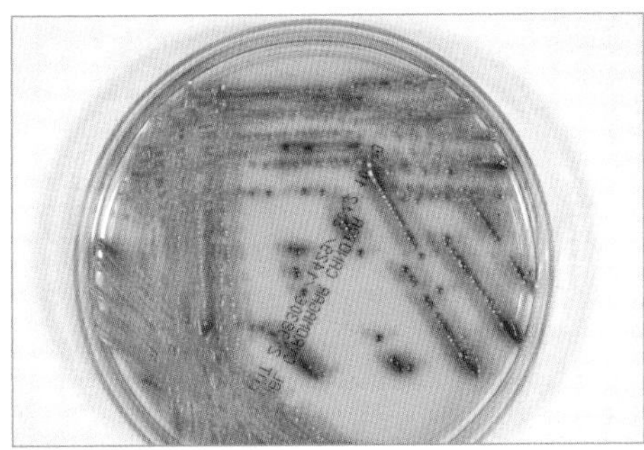

Image 24.3
Candida tropicalis on chrome agar. Colonies appear dark to metallic blue in color with or without a halo and are raised and smooth. Courtesy of Julia Rosebush, DO; Robert Jerris, PhD; and Theresa Stanley, M(ASCP).

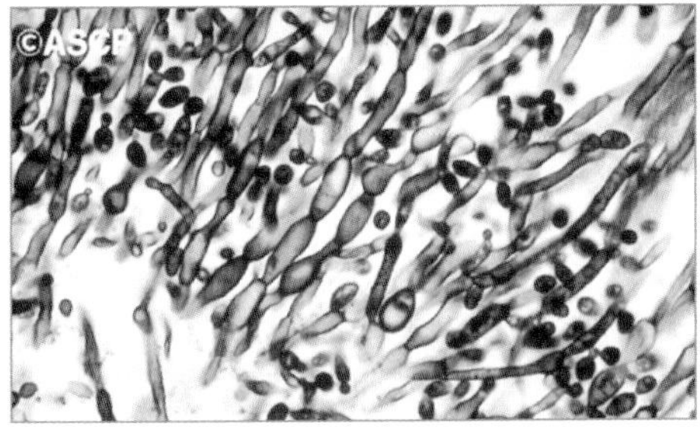

Image 24.4
Histopathologic features of *Candida albicans* infection. Pseudohyphae and true hyphae (methenamine silver stain) found in a tissue biopsy. Copyright American Society for Clinical Pathology.

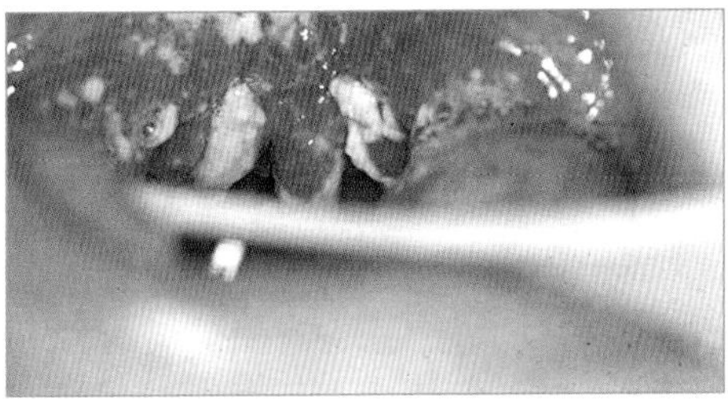

Image 24.5
Candida albicans (thrush) infection of the tonsils and uvula of an otherwise healthy 6-month-old. The white exudate may resemble curds of milk. Copyright Edgar O. Ledbetter, MD, FAAP.

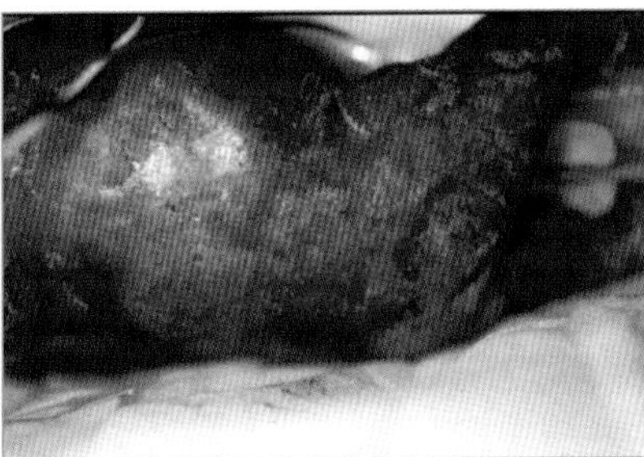

Image 24.6
Photograph of a very low birth weight neonate who developed invasive fungal dermatitis of the back caused by *Candida albicans*. This is an uncommon presentation that is often accompanied by disseminated infection. The diagnosis is established by skin biopsy that reveals invasion of the yeast into the dermis and culture that grows the yeast on routine culture media within 2 to 4 days. Courtesy of Carol J. Baker, MD, FAAP.

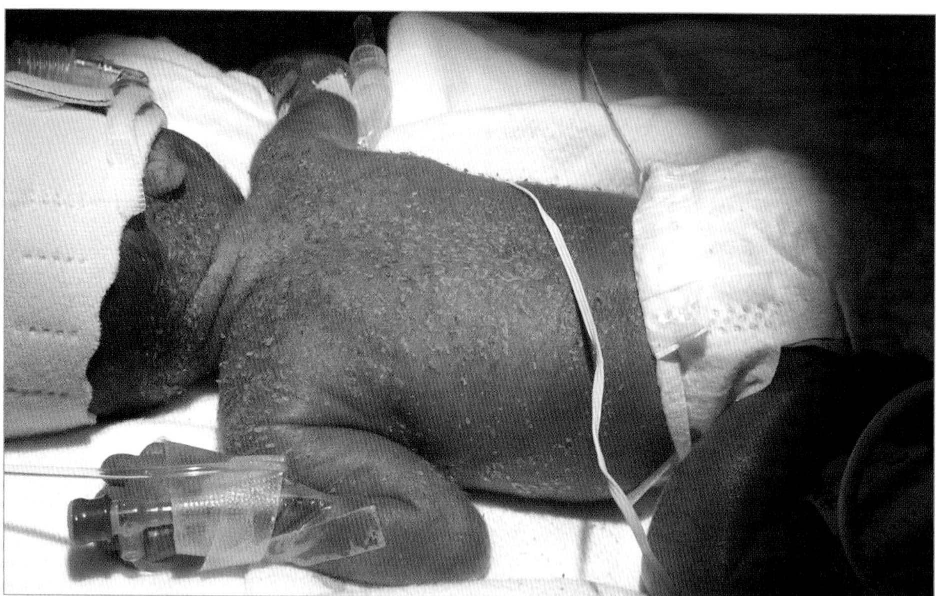

Image 24.7
Flaky skin in an extremely low birth weight neonate (<1,000 g) with congenital cutaneous candidiasis of varying presentations (all skin cultures positive for *Candida albicans*). Courtesy of David Kaufman, MD.

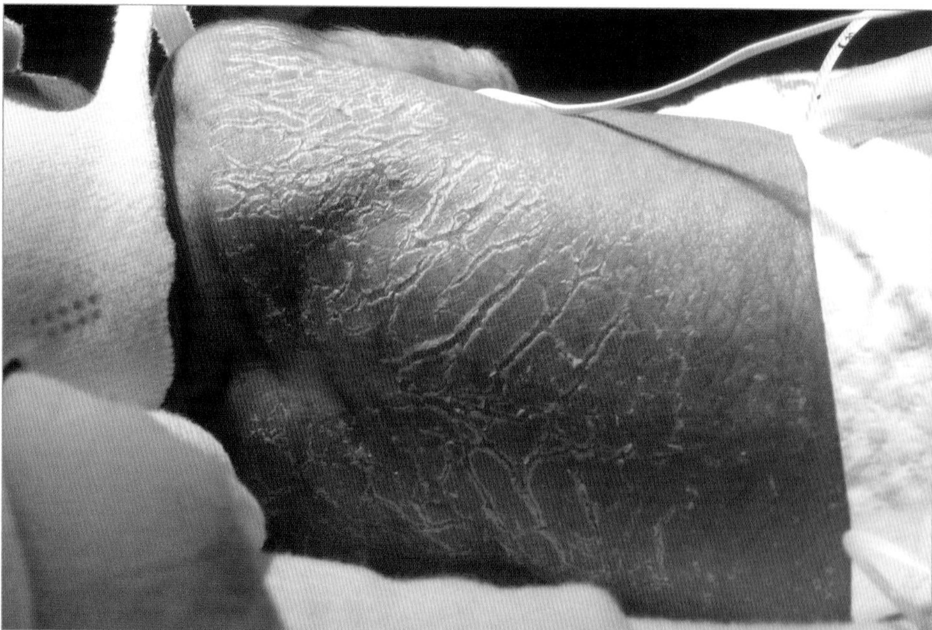

Image 24.8
Extremely low birth weight neonate (<1,000 g) with congenital cutaneous candidiasis of varying presentations (all skin cultures positive for *Candida albicans*). Courtesy of David Kaufman, MD.

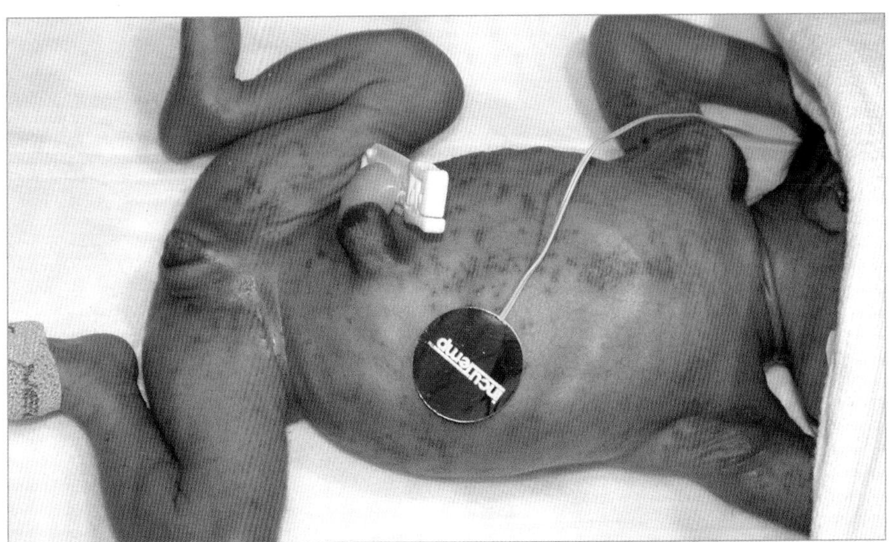

Image 24.9
Extremely low birth weight neonate (<1,000 g) with congenital cutaneous candidiasis (all skin cultures positive for *Candida albicans*). Courtesy of David Kaufman, MD.

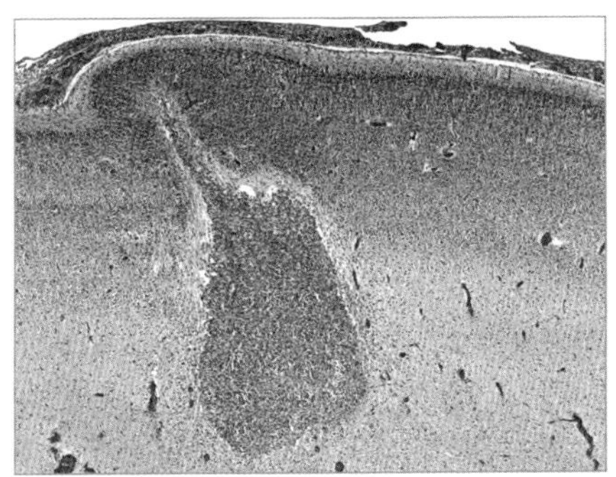

Image 24.10
Disseminated neonatal candidiasis. *Candida* microabscess in the brain. Courtesy of Dimitris P. Agamanolis, MD.

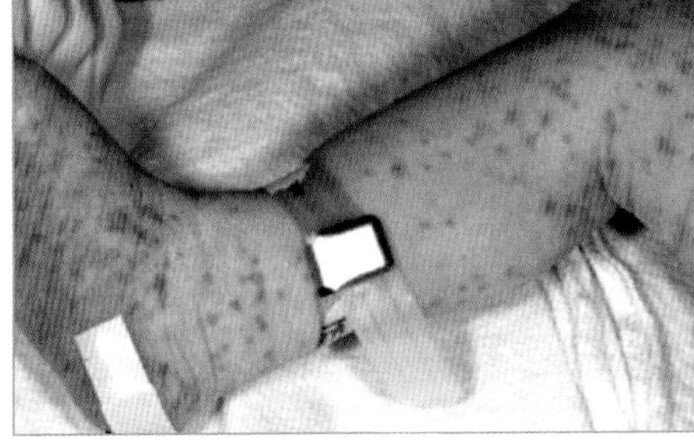

Image 24.11
Congenital candidiasis is characterized by widespread erythematous papules or pustules. Courtesy of Anthony Mancini, MD, FAAP.

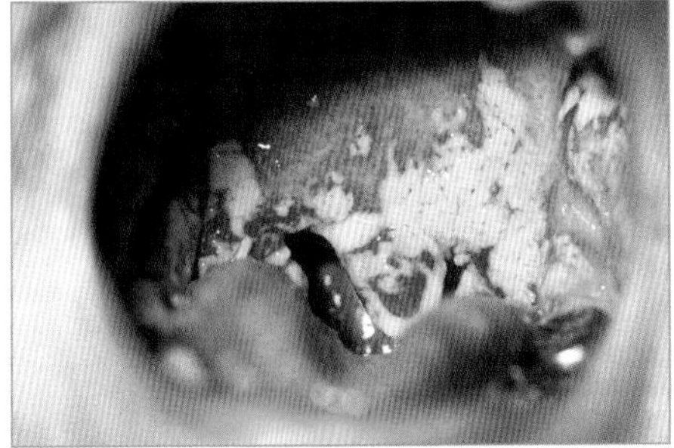

Image 24.12
Oral thrush covering the soft palate and uvula. Courtesy of Centers for Disease Control and Prevention.

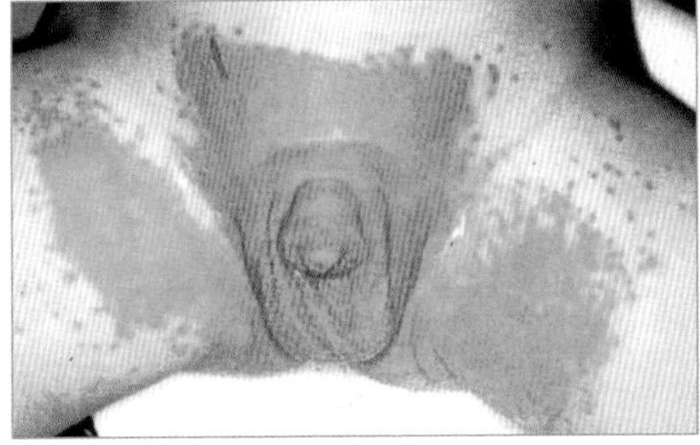

Image 24.13
Candida rash with typical satellite lesions in an infant boy.

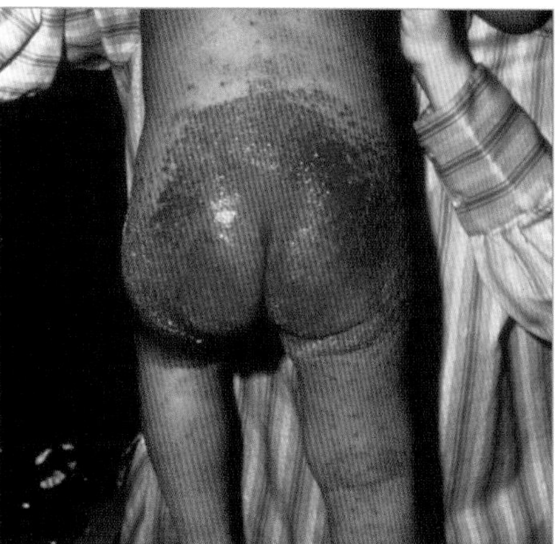

Image 24.14
Severe *Candida* diaper dermatitis with satellite lesions. Courtesy of George Nankervis, MD.

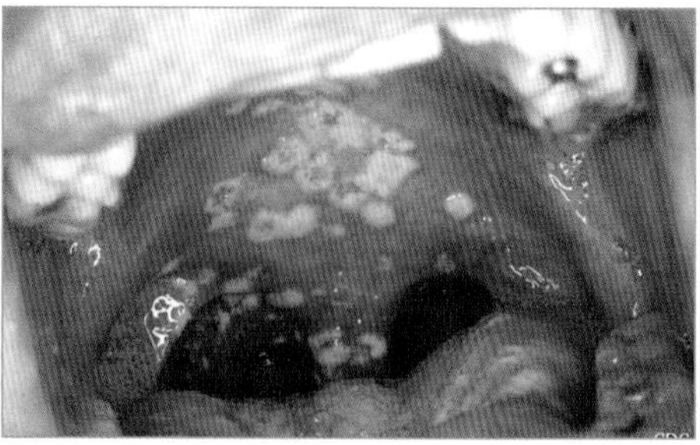

Image 24.15
This patient with HIV/AIDS presented with a secondary oral pseudomembranous candidiasis infection. Courtesy of Centers for Disease Control and Prevention/Sol Silverman Jr, DDS.

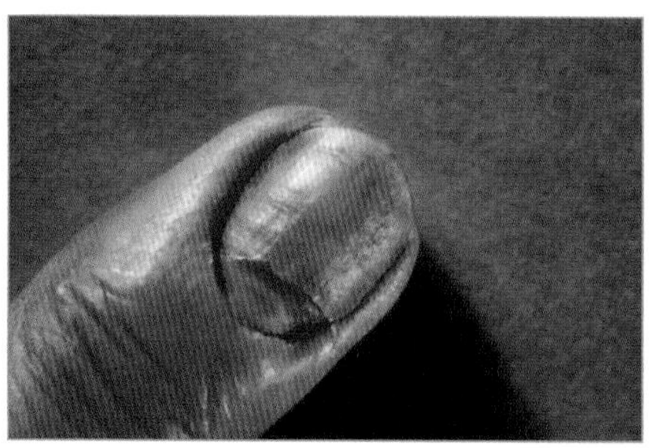

Image 24.16
Candidiasis of the fingernail bed. Courtesy of Centers for Disease Control and Prevention/ Sherry Brinkman.

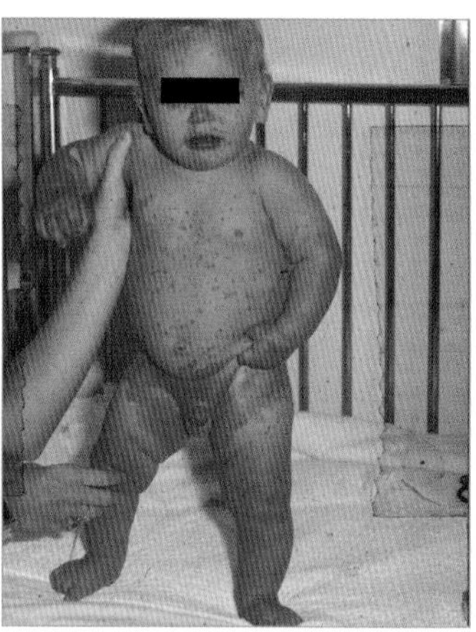

Image 24.17
A 7-month-old white boy with mucocutaneous candidiasis, generalized. Courtesy of Larry Frenkel, MD.

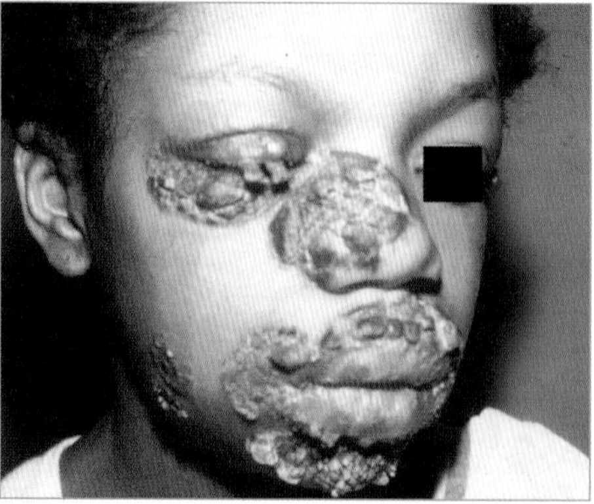

Image 24.18
An immunocompromised 5-year-old boy with multiple *Candida* granulomatous lesions, a rare response to an invasive cutaneous infection. These crusted, verrucous plaques and hornlike projections require systemic candicidal agents for eradication or palliation. Courtesy of George Nankervis, MD.

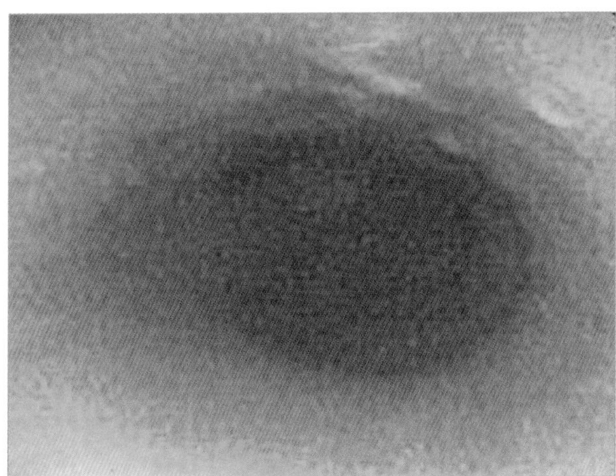

Image 24.19
Candida albicans esophagitis in a 4-year-old girl. Courtesy of Benjamin Estrada, MD.

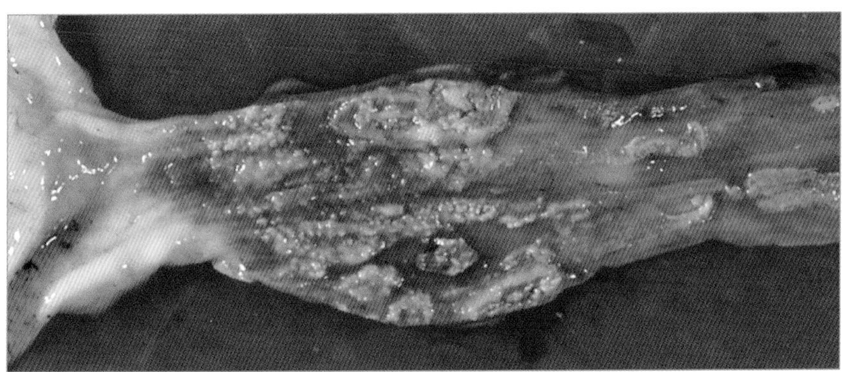

Image 24.20
Candida esophagitis with abscesses and ulceration of the mucosa. Courtesy of Dimitris P. Agamanolis, MD.

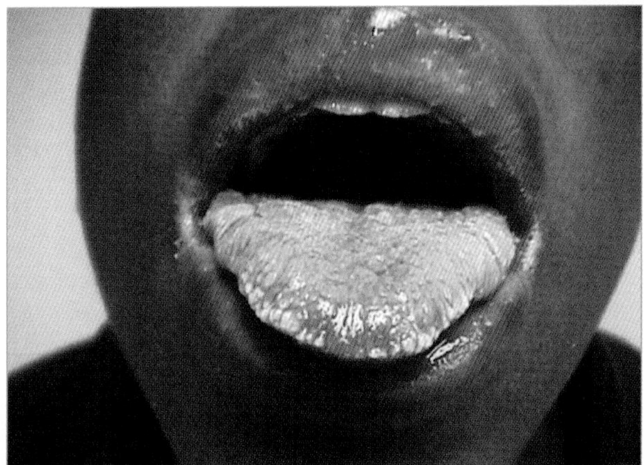

Image 24.21
Candida albicans in a 9-year-old boy with chronic mucocutaneous candidiasis. Courtesy of Benjamin Estrada, MD.

25

Cat-scratch Disease

(*Bartonella henselae*)

Clinical Manifestations

Infections with *Bartonella henselae* can be asymptomatic, but the predominant clinical manifestation of cat-scratch disease (CSD) in an immunocompetent person is regional lymphadenopathy or lymphadenitis. Most people with CSD are afebrile or have low-grade fever with mild systemic symptoms, such as malaise, anorexia, fatigue, and headache. Fever and mild systemic symptoms occur in approximately 30% of patients. A skin papule or pustule is often found at the presumed site of inoculation and usually precedes development of lymphadenopathy by approximately 1 to 2 weeks (range, 7–60 days). Lymphadenopathy involves nodes that drain the site of inoculation, typically axillary, but cervical, submental, epitrochlear, or inguinal nodes can be involved. The skin overlying affected lymph nodes is often tender, warm, erythematous, and indurated. Most *Bartonella*-infected lymph nodes will resolve spontaneously within 4 to 6 weeks, but approximately 10% to 25% of affected nodes suppurate spontaneously. Inoculation of the periocular tissue can result in Parinaud oculoglandular syndrome, which consists of follicular conjunctivitis and ipsilateral preauricular lymphadenopathy. Cat-scratch disease can also present with fevers for 1 to 3 weeks (ie, fever of unknown origin) and be associated with nonspecific symptoms, such as malaise, abdominal pain, headache, and myalgias. Less common manifestations of *B henselae* infection likely reflect blood-borne disseminated disease and include encephalopathy, osteolytic lesions, granulomata in the liver and spleen, glomerulonephritis, pneumonia, thrombocytopenic purpura, and erythema nodosum. Ocular manifestations occur in 5% to 10% of patients. The most frequent presentation of ocular *Bartonella* infection is neuroretinitis, characterized by unilateral painless vision impairment, granulomatous optic disc swelling, and macular edema, with lipid exudates (macular star); simultaneous bilateral involvement has been reported but is less common. Other rare manifestations include retinochoroiditis, anterior uveitis, vitritis, pars planitis, retinal vasculitis, retinitis, branch retinal arteriolar or venular occlusions, and macular hole.

Etiology

B henselae, the causative organism of CSD, is a fastidious, slow-growing, gram-negative bacillus that is also the causative agent of bacillary angiomatosis (vascular proliferative lesions of skin and subcutaneous tissue) and bacillary peliosis (reticuloendothelial lesions in visceral organs, primarily the liver). The latter 2 manifestations of infection are reported among patients who are immunocompromised. *B henselae* is related closely to *Bartonella quintana,* the agent of louse-borne trench fever and the causative agent of bacillary angiomatosis.

Epidemiology

Cat-scratch disease is a common infection, although its true incidence is unknown. *B henselae* is a common causes of regional lymphadenopathy or lymphadenitis in children. Cats are the natural reservoir for *B henselae,* with a seroprevalence of 13% to 90% in domestic and stray cats in the United States. Other animals, including dogs, can be infected and occasionally are associated with human infection. Cat-to-cat transmission occurs via the cat flea (*Ctenocephalides felis*), with feline infection resulting in bacteremia that is usually asymptomatic and lasts weeks to months. Fleas acquire the organism when feeding on a bacteremic cat and then shed infectious organisms in their feces. The bacteria are transmitted to humans by inoculation through a scratch or bite from a bacteremic cat or by hands contaminated by flea feces touching an open wound or the eye. Kittens (more often than cats) and animals from shelters or adopted as strays are more likely to be bacteremic. Most reported cases occur in people younger than 20 years, with most patients having a history of recent contact with apparently healthy cats, typically kittens. No evidence of person-to-person transmission exists.

Incubation Period

From scratch to primary cutaneous lesion, 7 to 12 days; from the appearance of the primary lesion to the appearance of lymphadenopathy, 5 to 50 days (median, 12 days).

Diagnostic Tests

B henselae is a fastidious organism; recovery by routine culture is rarely successful. Specialized laboratories experienced in isolating *Bartonella* organisms are recommended for processing of cultures. The indirect immunofluorescent antibody assay for detection of serum antibodies to antigens of *Bartonella* species is useful for diagnosis of CSD. The indirect immunofluorescent antibody test is available at many commercial laboratories, but because of cross-reactivity with other infections and a high seroprevalence in the general population, clinical correlation is essential. Enzyme immunoassays for detection of antibodies to *B henselae* have been developed. Polymerase chain reaction assays are available in some commercial and research laboratories and at the Centers for Disease Control and Prevention for testing of tissue or body fluids. If tissue (eg, lymph node) specimens are available, bacilli occasionally may be visualized using a silver stain (eg, Warthin-Starry, Steiner); however, this test is not specific for *B henselae.* Early histologic changes in lymph node specimens consist of lymphocytic infiltration with epithelioid granuloma formation. Later changes consist of polymorphonuclear leukocyte infiltration with granulomas that become necrotic and resemble granulomas from patients with tularemia, brucellosis, and mycobacterial infections.

Treatment

Management of localized, uncomplicated CSD is primarily aimed at relief of symptoms because the disease is usually self-limited, resolving spontaneously in 2 to 4 months. Painful suppurative nodes can be treated with needle aspiration for relief of symptoms; incision and drainage should be avoided because this may facilitate fistula formation.

Azithromycin has been shown to have a modest benefit in treating localized CSD, with a significantly greater decrease in lymph node volume after 1 month of therapy compared with placebo. Many experts recommend antimicrobial therapy in acutely or severely ill immunocompetent patients with systemic symptoms, particularly people with retinitis, hepatic or splenic involvement, or painful adenitis. Antimicrobial therapy is recommended for all immunocompromised people. Reports suggest that several oral antimicrobial agents (azithromycin, clarithromycin, ciprofloxacin, doxycycline, trimethoprim-sulfamethoxazole, and rifampin) and parenteral gentamicin are effective. The optimal duration of therapy is not known but may be several weeks for systemic disease.

Antimicrobial therapy for patients with bacillary angiomatosis and bacillary peliosis has been shown to be beneficial and is recommended. Azithromycin or doxycycline is effective for treatment of these condition; therapy should be administered for several months to prevent relapse in people who are immunocompromised.

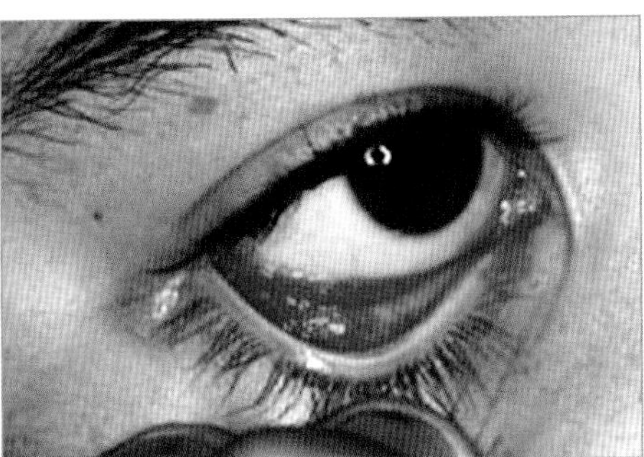

Image 25.1
Clinical manifestations of cat-scratch disease include Parinaud oculoglandular syndrome, which results when inoculation of the eye conjunctiva results in conjunctivitis.

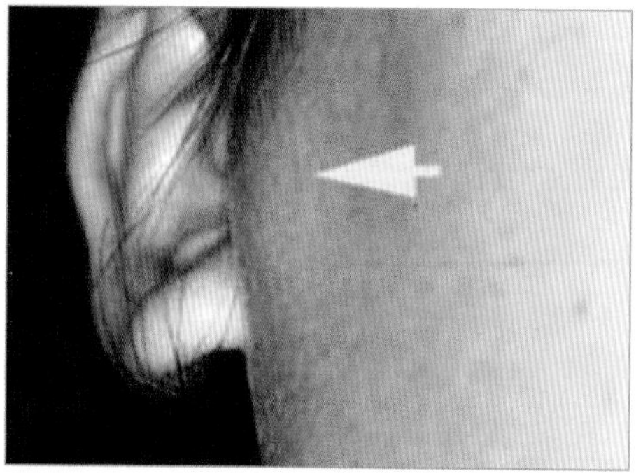

Image 25.2
Boy with signs of Parinaud oculoglandular syndrome, with painless, nonpurulent conjunctivitis and ipsilateral preauricular lymphadenopathy. These findings, combined with the cervical lymphadenopathy and his exposure to a kitten, make cat-scratch disease, or *Bartonella henselae* infection, the most likely possibility. Although most patients who have cat-scratch disease report some contact with kittens or cats, many do not recall being scratched. Cats younger than 1 year are most likely to transmit the organism to humans; human-to-human transmission does not occur.

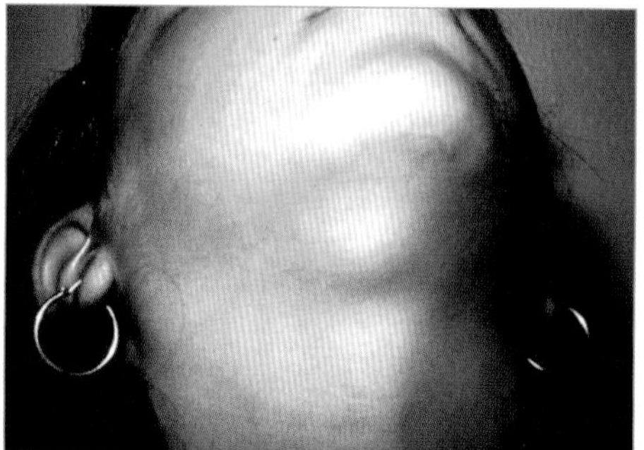

Image 25.3
Submental lymphadenitis due to cat-scratch disease.

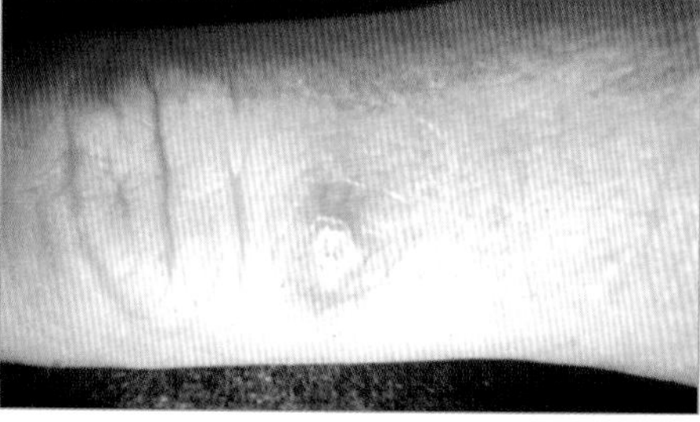

Image 25.4
Cat-scratch granuloma of the finger of a 6-year-old white boy. This is a typical inoculation site lesion, which was noted about 10 days before the development of regional lymphadenopathy.

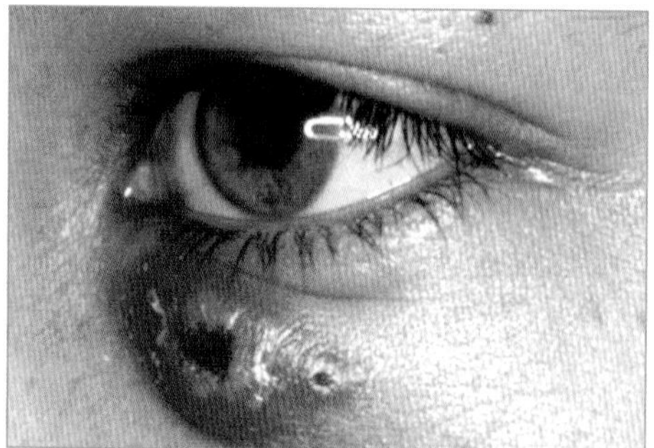

Image 25.5
Papules at inoculation sites on the face of a patient with cat-scratch disease.

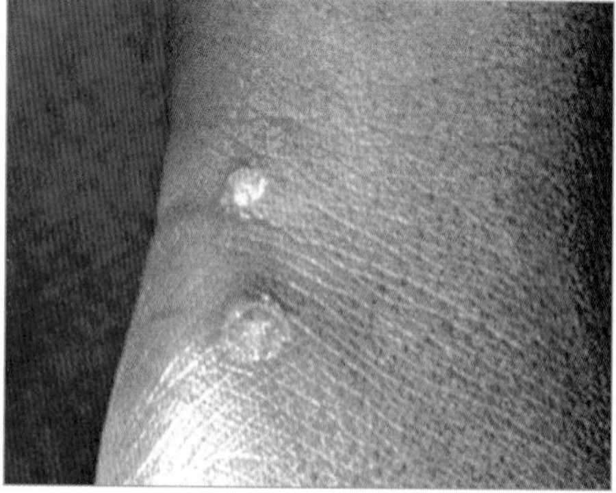

Image 25.6
A papule at each of 2 inoculation sites on the arm of a patient with cat-scratch disease.

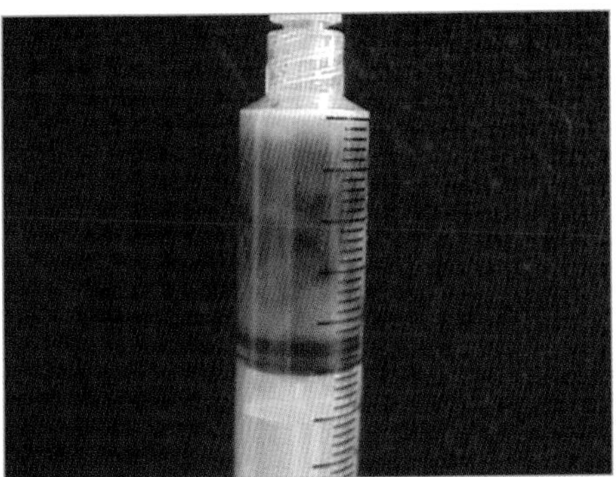

Image 25.7
Sanguinopurulent exudate aspirated from the axillary node of a patient with cat-scratch disease. Copyright Michael Rajnik, MD, FAAP.

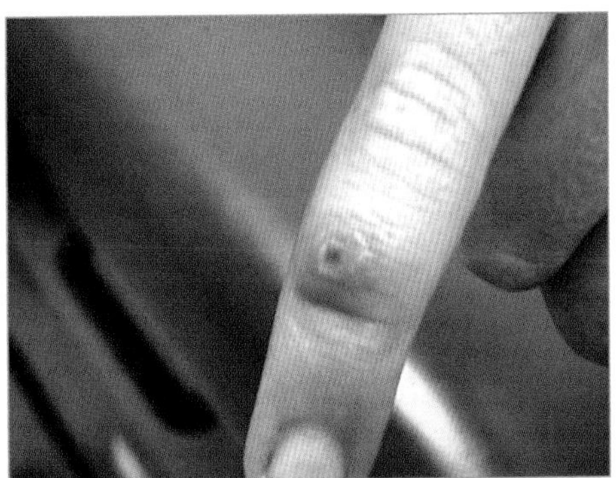

Image 25.8
Cat-scratch disease granuloma of the finger in a 12-year-old white boy with epitrochlear node involvement (see Image 25.10). Copyright Michael Rajnik, MD, FAAP.

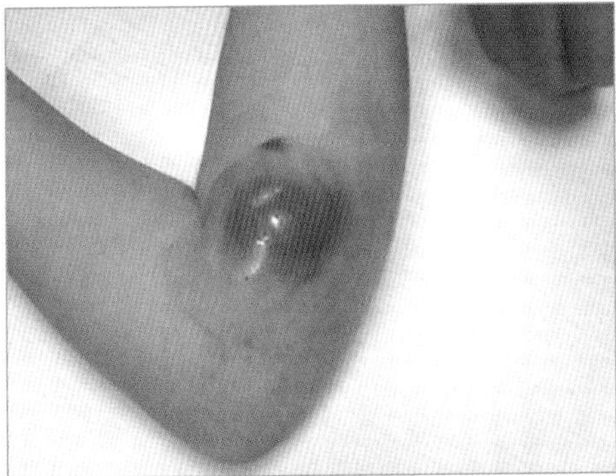

Image 25.9
Epitrochlear suppurative adenitis of cat-scratch disease in the boy in Image 25.9 with a cat-scratch granuloma of the finger. Copyright Michael Rajnik, MD, FAAP.

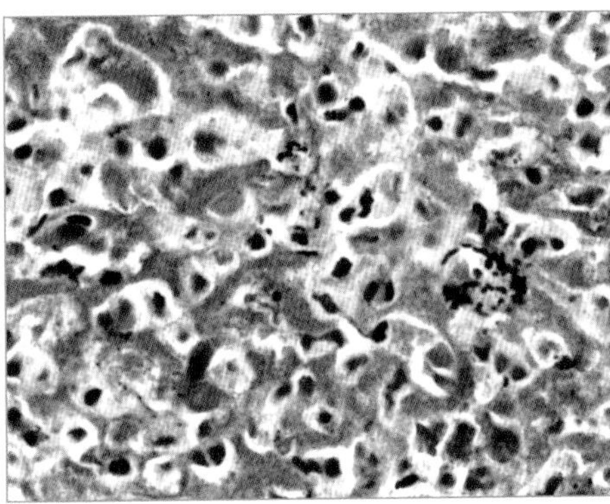

Image 25.10
Stellate microabscess in the lymph node of a patient with cat-scratch disease (Warthin-Starry silver stain; original magnification x158). Courtesy of Christopher Paddock, MD.

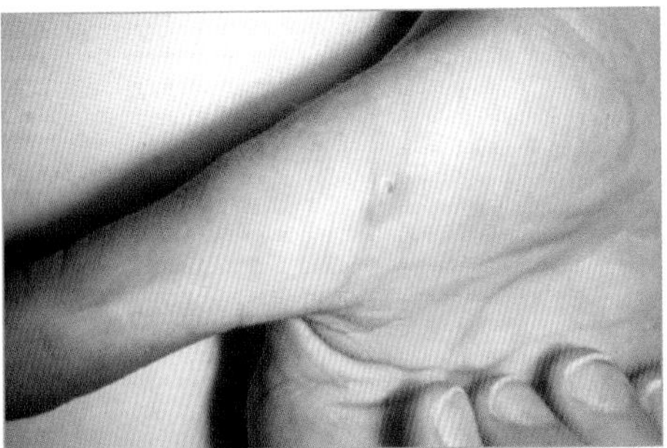

Image 25.11
A granulomatous lesion of cat-scratch disease at the base of the right thumb in a 4-year-old white boy. Courtesy of Centers for Disease Control and Prevention/Dr Thomas F. Sellers; Emory University.

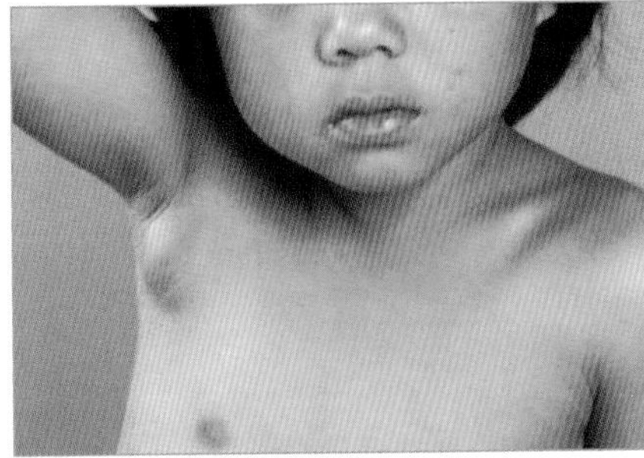

Image 25.12
A 4-year-old Asian boy with right axillary lymphadenopathy due to cat-scratch disease. Courtesy of Ed Fajardo, MD.

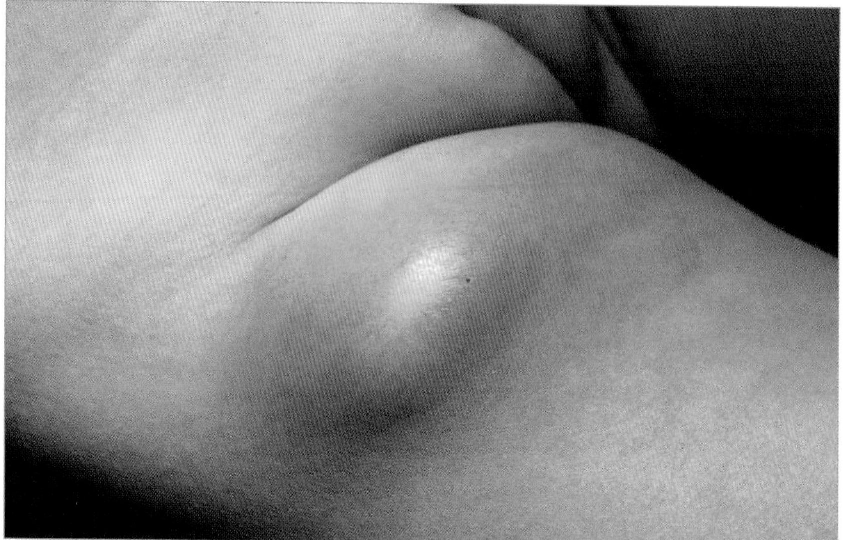

Image 25.13
Inguinal lymphadenitis due to cat-scratch disease in a 3-year-old white girl. Courtesy of Ed Fajardo, MD.

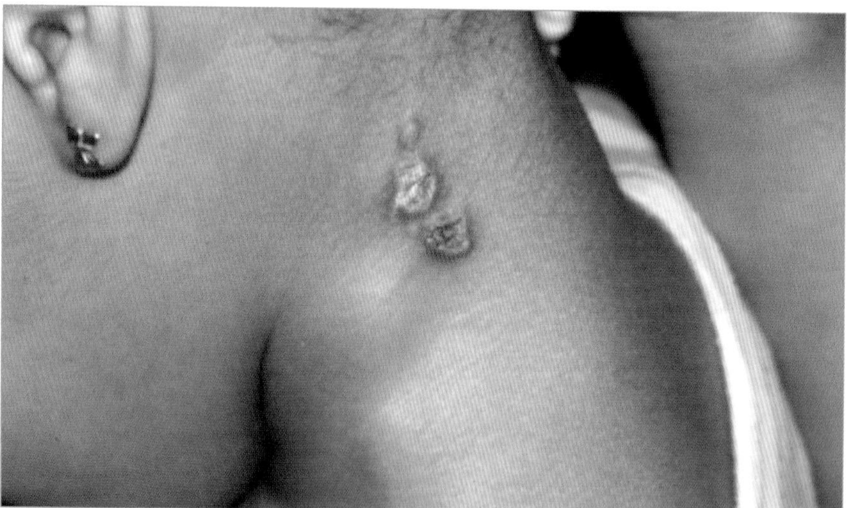

Image 25.14
This 3-year-old was previously scratched on the left side of her neck by a kitten. She developed raised red bumps around the scratch on day 5. This area ulcerated slightly and was slow to heal. No fever was noted, although she was less active for the next several days and complained that her arms and legs were sore. She developed swollen posterior cervical lymph nodes about a week later. Physical examination indicated two 8-mm ulcerations with raised borders and a papule near an enlarged minimally tender posterior cervical node. Serology result was positive for *Bartonella henselae*. She improved with time following a course of azithromycin. Courtesy of Will Sorey, MD.

26

Chancroid

Clinical Manifestations

Chancroid is an acute ulcerative disease of the genitalia. An ulcer begins as an erythematous papule that becomes pustular and erodes over several days, forming a sharply demarcated, somewhat superficial lesion with a serpiginous border. The base of the ulcer is friable and can be covered with a gray or yellow, purulent exudate. Single or multiple ulcers can be present. Unlike a syphilitic chancre, which is painless and indurated, the chancroid ulcer is often painful and nonindurated and can be associated with a painful, unilateral inguinal suppurative adenitis (bubo). Without treatment, ulcer(s) can spontaneously resolve, cause extensive erosion of the genitalia, or lead to scarring and phimosis, a painful inability to retract the foreskin.

In most males, chancroid manifests as a genital ulcer with or without inguinal tenderness; edema of the prepuce is common. In females, most lesions are at the vaginal introitus and symptoms include dysuria, dyspareunia, vaginal discharge, pain on defecation, or anal bleeding. Constitutional symptoms are unusual.

Etiology

Chancroid is caused by *Haemophilus ducreyi*, which is a gram-negative coccobacillus.

Epidemiology

Chancroid is a sexually transmitted infection associated with poverty, prostitution, and illicit drug use. Chancroid is endemic in Africa and the tropics but is rare in the United States; when it does occur, it is usually associated with sporadic outbreaks. Coinfection with syphilis or human herpesvirus occurs in as many as 17% of patients. Chancroid is a well-established cofactor for transmission of HIV. *H ducreyi* also causes a chronic limb ulceration syndrome that is spread by nonsexual contact in older children and adults in the Western Pacific islands. Because sexual contact is the major route of transmission, a diagnosis of chancroid in young children is strong evidence of sexual abuse.

Incubation Period

1 to 10 days.

Diagnostic Tests

Chancroid is usually diagnosed by clinical findings (1 or more painful genital ulcers with tender suppurative inguinal adenopathy) and by excluding other genital ulcerative diseases, such as syphilis, herpes simplex infection, or lymphogranuloma venereum. Confirmation is made by isolation of *H ducreyi* from a genital ulcer or lymph node aspirate, but in less than 80% of patients is this possible. Because special culture media and conditions are required for isolation, laboratory personnel should be informed of the suspicion of chancroid. Buboes are almost always sterile. Polymerase chain reaction assays can provide a specific diagnosis but are not available in most clinical laboratories.

Treatment

H ducreyi has been uniformly susceptible to third-generation cephalosporins, macrolides, and quinolones. Recommended regimens include azithromycin or ceftriaxone. Alternatives include erythromycin or ciprofloxacin. Patients with HIV infection may need prolonged therapy. Syndromic management usually includes treatment for syphilis. Clinical improvement occurs 3 to 7 days after initiation of therapy, and healing is complete in approximately 2 weeks. Adenitis is often slow to resolve and can require needle aspiration or surgical incision. Patients should be reexamined 3 to 7 days after initiating therapy to verify healing. Slow clinical improvement and relapses can occur after therapy, especially in people with HIV infection. Close clinical follow-up is recommended; retreatment with the original regimen is usually effective in patients who experience a relapse.

Patients should be evaluated for other sexually transmitted infections, including syphilis, human herpesvirus, chlamydia, gonorrhea, and HIV, at the time of diagnosis.

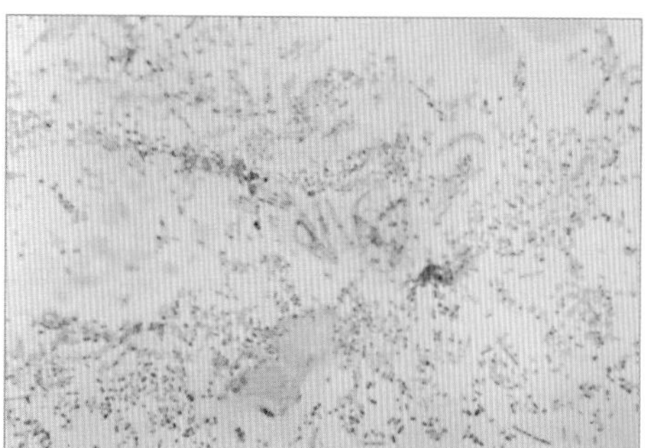

Image 26.1
Haemophilus ducreyi is a gram-negative coccobacillus, as shown in this preparation. Courtesy of Centers for Disease Control and Prevention.

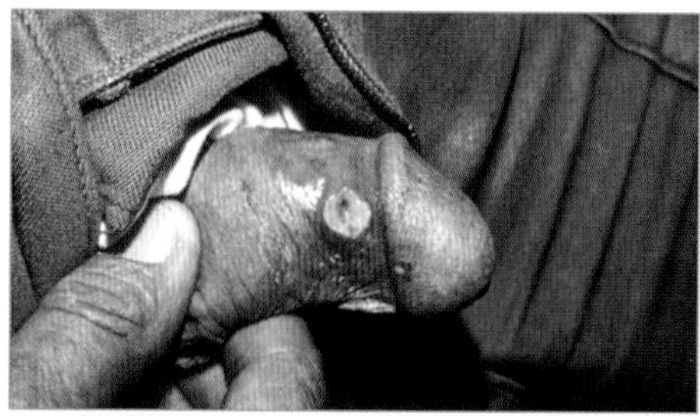

Image 26.2
Ulcerative chancroid lesions with inflammation of the shaft and glans penis caused by *Haemophilus ducreyi*. Chancroid lesions are irregular in shape, painful, and soft (nonindurated) to touch. Courtesy of Hugh Moffet, MD.

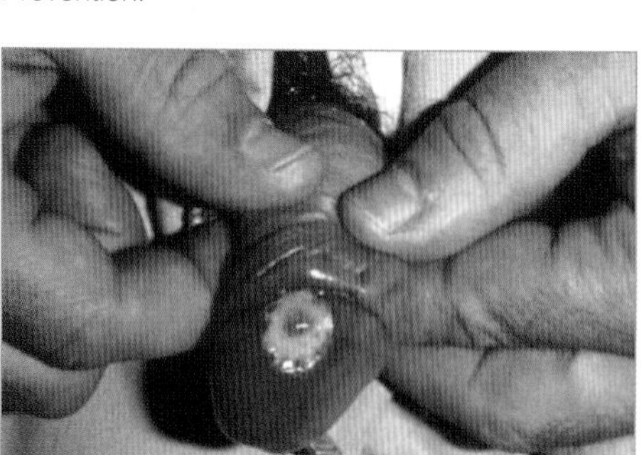

Image 26.3
Chancroid ulcer on the glans penis. Coinfection with syphilis or human herpesvirus occurs in as many as 10% of patients. Courtesy of Hugh Moffet, MD.

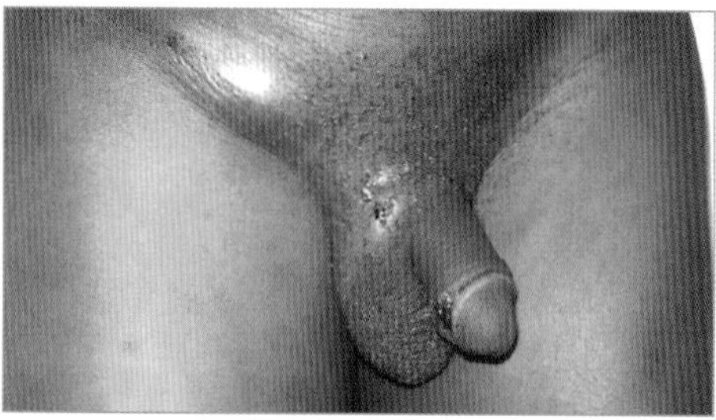

Image 26.4
This adolescent black male presented with a chancroid lesion of the groin and penis affecting the ipsilateral inguinal lymph nodes. First signs of infection typically appear 3 to 5 days after exposure, although symptoms can take up to 2 weeks to appear. Courtesy of Centers for Disease Control and Prevention/J. Pledger.

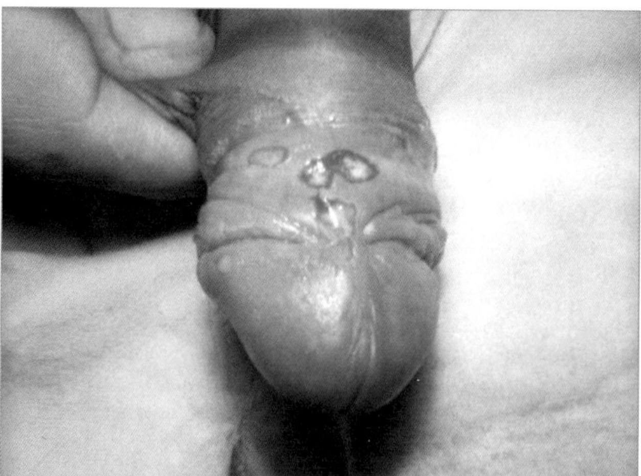

Image 26.5
The penile ulcers on the penis of this adolescent white male proved to be due to chancroid, caused by *Haemophilus ducreyi*, and not syphilis as initially suspected. Chancroid can cause genital ulcers or inguinal buboes in the groin area. Courtesy of Centers for Disease Control and Prevention.

27

Chlamydial Infections

Chlamydophila (formerly *Chlamydia*) *pneumoniae*

Clinical Manifestations

Patients can be asymptomatic or mildly to moderately ill with a variety of respiratory tract diseases, including pneumonia, acute bronchitis, prolonged cough, and, less commonly, pharyngitis, laryngitis, otitis media, and sinusitis. In some patients, a sore throat precedes the onset of cough by a week or more. The clinical course can be biphasic, culminating in atypical pneumonia. *Chlamydophila* pneumoniae can present as severe community-acquired pneumonia in immunocompromised hosts and has been associated with acute exacerbations in patients with cystic fibrosis and acute chest syndrome in children with sickle cell disease.

Physical examination may reveal nonexudative pharyngitis, pulmonary rales, and bronchospasm. Chest radiography may reveal a variety of findings ranging from bilateral infiltrates to a single patchy subsegmental infiltrate. Illness can be prolonged, and cough can persist for 2 to 6 weeks or longer.

Etiology

C pneumoniae is an obligate intracellular bacterium that is distinct antigenically, genetically, and morphologically from *Chlamydia* species, so it is grouped in the genus *Chlamydophila*.

Epidemiology

C pneumoniae infection is presumed to be transmitted from person to person via infected respiratory tract secretions. It is unknown whether there is an animal reservoir. The disease occurs worldwide, but in tropical and low-income countries, disease occurs earlier in life than in industrialized countries in temperate climates. The timing of initial infection peaks between 5 and 15 years of age. In the United States, approximately 50% of adults have *C pneumoniae*–serologic evidence of prior infection by age 20 years. Recurrent infection is common, especially in adults. Clusters of infection have been reported in groups of children and young adults. There is no evidence of seasonality.

Incubation Period

21 days.

Diagnostic Tests

Serologic testing has been the primary means of diagnosing *C pneumoniae* infection but is problematic. The microimmunofluorescent antibody test is the most sensitive and specific serologic test for acute infection. A 4-fold increase in immunoglobulin (Ig) G titer between acute and convalescent sera is preferred to diagnose acute infection, but an IgM titer of 1:16 or greater is also useful. Use of a single IgG titer in diagnosis of acute infection is not recommended because, during primary infection, IgG antibody may not appear until 6 to 8 weeks after onset of illness and increases within 1 to 2 weeks with reinfection. In primary infection, IgM antibody appears approximately 2 to 3 weeks after onset of illness but can be falsely positive because of cross-reactivity with other *Chlamydia* species or falsely negative in cases of reinfection. Early antimicrobial therapy also may suppress antibody response.

C pneumoniae can be isolated from swab specimens obtained from the nasopharynx or oropharynx or from sputum, bronchoalveolar lavage, or tissue biopsy specimens. Specimens should be placed into appropriate transport media and stored at 4°C (39.2°F) until inoculation into cell culture; specimens that cannot be processed within 24 hours should be frozen and stored at −70°C (−94°F). Culturing *C pneumoniae* is difficult and often fails to detect the organism. Nasopharyngeal shedding can occur for months after acute disease, even with treatment. Because of the difficulty of accurately detecting *C pneumoniae* via culture, serologic testing, or immunohistochemistry testing, several types of polymerase chain reaction (PCR) assays have been developed. Sensitivity and specificity of these different PCR techniques remain largely unknown. A multiplex PCR assay has been cleared by the US Food and Drug Administration for diagnosis of *C pneumoniae* using nasopharyngeal samples. The test appears to have high sensitivity and specificity.

Treatment

Most respiratory tract infections thought to be caused by by *C pneumoniae* are treated empirically. For suspected *C pneumoniae* infections, treatment with macrolides (eg, azithromycin, erythromycin, clarithromycin) is recommended. Tetracycline or doxycycline can be used in children older than 7 years. Newer fluoroquinolones (levofloxacin and moxifloxacin) are alternative drugs for patients who are unable to tolerate macrolide antibiotics but should not be used as first-line treatment. Therapy is continued to 10 to 14 days, except for azithromycin, when 5 days is typically adequate.

28

Chlamydophila (formerly *Chlamydia*) *psittaci*

(Psittacosis, Ornithosis, Parrot Fever)

Clinical Manifestations

Psittacosis (ornithosis) is an acute respiratory tract infection with systemic symptoms and signs including fever, nonproductive cough, headache, and malaise. Less common symptoms are pharyngitis, diarrhea, and altered mental status. Extensive interstitial pneumonia can occur, with radiographic changes characteristically more severe than would be expected from chest examination findings. Endocarditis, myocarditis, pericarditis, thrombophlebitis, nephritis, hepatitis, and encephalitis are rare complications. Recent studies have suggested an association with ocular adnexal marginal zone lymphomas involving orbital soft tissue, lacrimal glands, and conjunctiva.

Etiology

Chlamydophila psittaci is an obligate intracellular bacterium that is distinct antigenically, genetically, and morphologically from *Chlamydia* species and, following reclassification, is grouped in the genus *Chlamydophila*.

Epidemiology

Birds are the major reservoir of *C psittaci*. The term **psittacosis** commonly is used, although the term ornithosis more accurately describes the potential for nearly all domestic and wild birds to spread this infection, not just psittacine birds (eg, parakeets, parrots, macaws). In the United States, psittacine birds, pigeons, and turkeys are important sources of human disease. Importation and illegal trafficking of exotic birds is associated with an increased incidence of human disease because shipping, crowding, and other stress factors may increase shedding of the organism among birds with latent infection. Infected birds, whether healthy appearing or obviously ill, can transmit the organism. Infection is usually acquired by inhaling aerosolized excrement or respiratory secretions from the eyes or beaks of infected birds. Handling of plumage and mouth-to-beak contact are the modes of exposure described most frequently, although transmission has been reported through exposure to aviaries, bird exhibits, and lawn mowing. Excretion of *C psittaci* from birds can be intermittent or continuous for weeks or months. Pet owners and workers at poultry slaughter plants, poultry farms, and pet shops are at increased risk of infection. Laboratory personnel working with *C psittaci* are also at risk. Psittacosis is worldwide in distribution and tends to occur sporadically in any season. Although rare, severe illness and abortion have been reported in pregnant women.

Incubation Period

5 to 14 days (may be longer).

Diagnostic Tests

A confirmed diagnosis of psittacosis requires a clinically compatible illness with fever, chills, headache, cough, and myalgias, plus laboratory confirmation by one of the following: isolation of *C psittaci* from respiratory tract specimens or blood, or 4-fold or greater increase in immunoglobulin (Ig) G by complement fixation (CF) or a titer of 1:32 with microimmunofluorescence (MIF) against *C psittaci* between paired acute- and convalescent-phase serum specimens obtained at least 2 to 4 weeks apart. A probable case of psittacosis requires a clinically compatible illness and either supportive serologic test results (eg, *C psittaci* IgM ≥1:16) or detection of *C psittaci* DNA in a respiratory tract specimen by polymerase chain reaction assay. For serologic testing, MIF is more sensitive and specific than CF, but CF and MIF can cross-react with other chlamydial species and should be interpreted cautiously. Additionally, nucleic acid amplification tests have been developed that can distinguish *C psittaci* from other chlamydial species and are under investigation for detection of *C psittaci* from human clinical samples. Treatment with antimicrobial agents may suppress the antibody response. Culturing the organism is recommended; however, it is difficult and should be attempted only by experienced personnel in laboratories where strict containment measures to prevent spread of the organism are used during collection and handling of all specimens because of occupational and laboratory safety concerns.

Treatment

Tetracycline or doxycycline is the drug of choice. Erythromycin and azithromycin are alternative agents and are recommended for children younger than 8 years and pregnant women. Therapy should be for a minimum of 10 days and for 10 to 14 days after fever abates. In patients with severe infection, intravenous doxycycline can be considered.

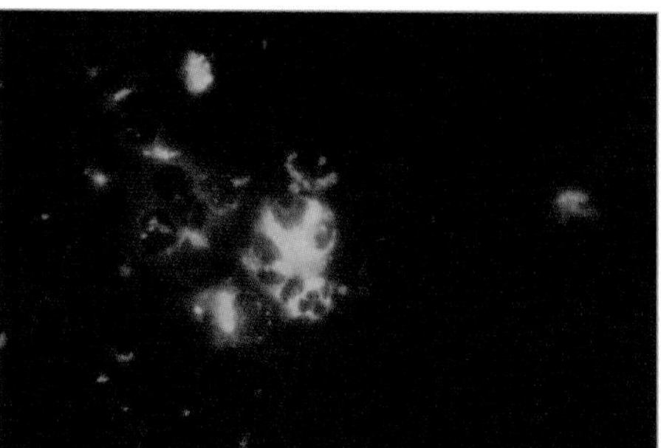

Image 28.1
This direct fluorescent antibody stained mouse brain impression smear reveals the presence of the bacterium *Chlamydophila psittaci.* Psittacosis is acquired by inhaling dried secretions from birds infected with *C psittaci.* Although all birds are susceptible, pet birds and poultry are most frequently involved in transmission to humans. Courtesy of Courtesy of Centers for Disease Control and Prevention/Vester Lewis, MD.

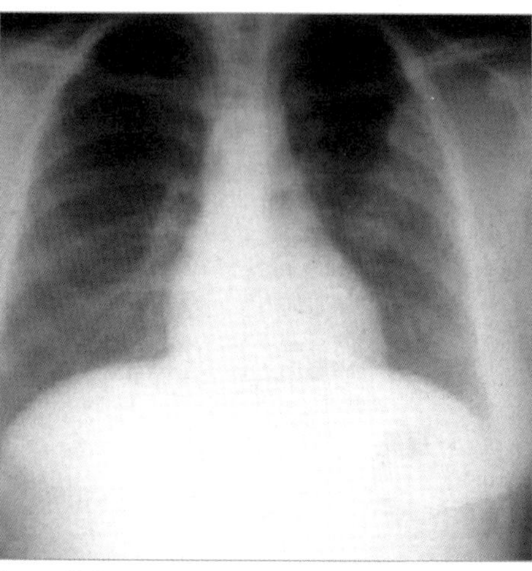

Image 28.2
Chlamydophila psittaci pneumonia in a 16-year-old girl with a cough of 3 weeks' duration. The family had several parrots in the home that were purchased from a roadside stand near the Texas-Mexico border. Interstitial pneumonia, most prominent in the lower lobe of the left lung, is shown. Complement fixation titer for *C psittaci* is 1:128. Copyright David Waagner.

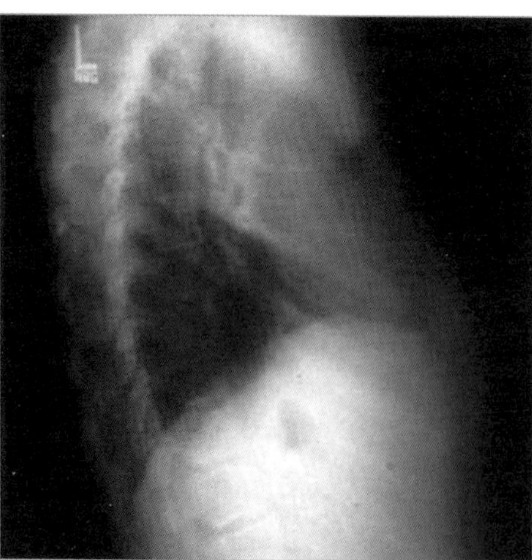

Image 28.3
Lateral chest radiograph of the patient in Image 28.2. Most domestic and wild birds can transmit *Chlamydophila psittaci.* Copyright David Waagner.

29

Chlamydia trachomatis

Clinical Manifestations

Chlamydia trachomatis is associated with a range of clinical manifestations, including neonatal conjunctivitis, nasopharyngitis, and pneumonia in young infants; genital tract infection; lymphogranuloma venereum (LGV); and trachoma.

- **Neonatal chlamydial conjunctivitis** is characterized by ocular congestion, edema, and discharge developing a few days to several weeks after birth and lasting for 1 to 2 weeks and sometimes longer. In contrast to trachoma, scars and pannus formation are rare.
- **Pneumonia** in young infants is usually an afebrile illness of insidious onset occurring between 2 and 19 weeks after birth. A repetitive staccato cough, tachypnea, and rales in an afebrile 1-month-old are characteristic but not always present. Wheezing is uncommon. Hyperinflation usually accompanies infiltrates seen on chest radiographs. Nasal stuffiness and otitis media may occur. Untreated disease can linger or recur. Severe chlamydial pneumonia has occurred in infants and some immunocompromised adults.
- **Genitourinary tract** manifestations, such as vaginitis in prepubertal girls; urethritis, cervicitis, endometritis, salpingitis, proctitis, and perihepatitis (Fitz-Hugh–Curtis syndrome) in postpubertal females; urethritis, epididymitis, and proctitis in males; and Reiter syndrome (arthritis, urethritis, and bilateral conjunctivitis), can occur. Infection can persist for months to years. Reinfection is common. In postpubertal females, chlamydial infection can progress to pelvic inflammatory disease and can result in ectopic pregnancy, infertility, or chronic pelvic pain.
- **Lymphogranuloma venereum** is classically an invasive lymphatic infection with an initial ulcerative lesion on the genitalia accompanied by tender, suppurative inguinal or femoral lymphadenopathy that is typically unilateral. The ulcerative lesion often has resolved by the time the patient seeks care. Proctocolitis may occur in women or men who engage in anal intercourse. Symptoms can resemble those of inflammatory bowel disease, including mucoid or hemorrhagic rectal discharge, constipation, tenesmus, or anorectal pain. Stricture or fistula formation can follow severe or inadequately treated infection.
- **Trachoma** is a chronic follicular keratoconjunctivitis with neovascularization of the cornea that results from repeated and chronic infection. Blindness secondary to extensive local scarring and inflammation occurs in 1% to 15% of people with trachoma.

Etiology

C trachomatis is an obligate intracellular bacterium with at least 18 serologic variants (serovars) divided between the following biologic variants (biovars): oculogenital (serovars A–K) and LGV (serovars L1, L2, and L3). Trachoma usually is caused by serovars A through C, and genital and perinatal infections are caused by B and D through K.

Epidemiology

C trachomatis is the most common reportable sexually transmitted infection in the United States, with high rates among sexually active adolescents and young adult women. A significant proportion of patients are asymptomatic, providing an ongoing reservoir for infection. Prevalence of the organism is consistently highest among adolescent and young adult women. Among all 14- to 25-year-olds participating in the 2008 National Health and Nutrition Examination Survey, prevalence was 3.3% among females and 1.7% among males. Racial disparities are significant. The estimated prevalence among non-Hispanic black people (6.7%) was higher than the estimated prevalence among non-Hispanic white people (0.3%) and Mexican American people (2.4%). Among males who have sex with males screened for rectal chlamydial infection, positivity ranges from 3% to 10%. Oculogenital serovars of *C trachomatis* can be transmitted from the genital tract of infected mothers to their newborns during birth. Acquisition occurs in approximately 50% of neonates born vaginally to infected mothers and in some neonates born by cesarean delivery with membranes intact. The risk of conjunctivitis is 25% to 50% and the risk of pneumonia is 5% to 30% in infants who contract *C trachomatis*. The nasopharynx is the anatomic site most commonly infected.

Genital tract infection in adolescents and adults is transmitted sexually. The possibility of sexual abuse should always be considered in prepubertal children beyond infancy who have vaginal, urethral, or rectal chlamydial infection. Sexual abuse is not limited to prepubertal children, and chlamydial infections can result from sexual abuse or assault in postpubertal adolescents as well.

Asymptomatic infection of the nasopharynx, conjunctivae, vagina, and rectum can be acquired at birth. Nasopharyngeal cultures have been observed to remain positive for as long as 28 months and vaginal and rectal cultures for more than 1 year in infants and children with infection acquired at birth. Infection is not known to be communicable among infants and children. The degree of contagiousness of pulmonary disease is unknown but seems to be low.

Lymphogranuloma venereum biovars are worldwide in distribution but are particularly prevalent in tropical and subtropical areas. Although disease rarely occurs in the United States, outbreaks of LGV have been reported among men who have sex with men. Infection is often asymptomatic in females. Perinatal transmission is rare. Lymphogranuloma venereum is infectious during active disease. Little is known about the prevalence or duration of asymptomatic carriage.

Although rarely observed in the United States since the 1950s, trachoma is the leading infectious cause of blindness worldwide, causing up to 3% of the world's blindness. It generally is confined to poor populations in resource-limited nations of Africa, the Middle East, Asia, Latin America, the Pacific Islands, and remote aboriginal communities in Australia. Trachoma is transmitted by transfer of ocular discharge. Predictors of scarring and blindness for trachoma include increasing age and constant, severe trachoma.

Incubation Period

Variable, depending on infection type; usually at least 1 week.

Diagnostic Tests

C trachomatis urogenital infection in females can be diagnosed by testing first catch urine or swab specimens from the endocervix or vagina. Diagnosis of *C trachomatis* urethral infection in males can be made by testing a urethral swab or first catch urine specimen. Nucleic acid amplification tests (NAATs) are the most sensitive tests for these specimens and are the recommended tests for *C trachomatis* detection.

For detecting *C trachomatis* infections of the genital tract among **postpubescent individuals,** older nonculture tests and non-NAATs, such as DNA probe, direct fluorescent antibody tests, or enzyme immunoassay tests, have inferior sensitivity and specificity characteristics and are no longer recommended for *C trachomatis* testing. In the **evaluation of prepubescent children for possible sexual assault,** the Centers for Disease Control and Prevention recommends culture for *C trachomatis* of a specimen collected from the rectum in boys and girls and from the vagina in girls. A meatal specimen should be obtained from boys for chlamydia testing if urethral discharge is present.

Serum anti–*C trachomatis* antibody concentrations are difficult to determine, and only a few clinical laboratories perform this test. In **children with pneumonia,** an acute microimmunofluorescent serum titer of *C trachomatis*–specific immunoglobulin M of 1:32 or greater is diagnostic. Diagnosis of **LGV** can be supported but not confirmed by a positive result (ie, titer >1:64) on a complement-fixation test for chlamydia or a high titer (typically >1:256, but this can vary by laboratory) on a microimmunofluorescent serologic test for *C trachomatis*. However, most available serologic tests in the United States are based on enzyme immunoassay tests and might not provide a quantitative titer-based result.

Diagnosis of genitourinary tract chlamydial disease in a child should prompt examination for **other sexually transmitted infections,** including syphilis, gonorrhea, and HIV, and investigation of sexual abuse or assault. In the case of a neonate or an infant, because cultures can be positive for at least 12 months after infection acquired at birth, evaluation of the mother is also advisable.

Diagnosis of **ocular trachoma** is usually made clinically in countries with endemic infection.

Treatment

- Newborns and infants with **chlamydial conjunctivitis** or **pneumonia** are treated with oral erythromycin base or ethylsuccinate for 14 days or with azithromycin for 3 days. Because the efficacy of erythromycin therapy is approximately 80% for both of these conditions, a second course may be required, and follow-up of infants is recommended. A diagnosis of *C trachomatis* infection in an infant should prompt treatment of the mother and her sexual partner(s). The need for treatment of infants can be avoided by screening pregnant women to detect and treat *C trachomatis* infection before delivery.

  An association between orally administered erythromycin and infantile hypertrophic pyloric stenosis (IHPS) has been reported in newborns and infants younger than 6 weeks. The risk of IHPS after treatment with other macrolides (eg, azithromycin, clarithromycin) is unknown, although IHPS has been reported after use of azithromycin. Because confirmation of erythromycin as a contributor to cases of IHPS will require additional investigation and alternative therapies are not as well studied, erythromycin remains the drug of choice. Physicians who prescribe erythromycin to newborns should inform parents about the signs and potential risks of developing IHPS.

  Neonates born to mothers known to have untreated chlamydial infection are at high risk of infection; however, prophylactic antimicrobial treatment is not recommended. Neonates should be monitored clinically to ensure appropriate treatment if infection develops. If adequate follow-up cannot be ensured, preemptive therapy should be considered.

- For uncomplicated ***C trachomatis* anogenital tract infection in adolescents or adults,** oral doxycycline for 7 days or single-dose azithromycin is recommended. Alternatives include oral erythromycin base, erythromycin ethylsuccinate, ofloxacin, levofloxacin, or doxycycline delayed-release daily for 7 days. **For children who weigh less than 45 kg,** the recommended regimen is oral erythromycin base or ethylsuccinate for 14 days. **For children who weigh 45 kg or more but who are younger than 8 years,** the recommended regimen is azithromycin, in a single oral dose. **For children 8 years and older,** the recommended regimen is azithromycin as a single oral dose or doxycycline for 7 days. **For pregnant women,** the recommended treatment is azithromycin as a single oral dose. Amoxicillin or erythromycin base for 7 days are alternative regimens. Doxycycline, ofloxacin, and levofloxacin are contraindicated during pregnancy.

- **Follow-up testing.** Test of cure is not recommended for nonpregnant adult or adolescent patients treated for uncomplicated chlamydial infection unless compliance is in question, symptoms persist, or reinfection is suspected. Test of cure (preferably by NAAT) is recommended 3 to 4 weeks after treatment of pregnant women. Because some of these regimens for pregnant women may not be highly efficacious, a second course of therapy may be required. Reinfection is common after initial infection and treatment, and all infected adolescents and adults should be tested for *C trachomatis* 3 months following initial treatment. If retesting at 3 months is not possible, retest whenever patients next present for health care in the 12 months after initial treatment.

- For **LGV**, doxycycline for 21 days is the preferred treatment for children 8 years and older, and erythromycin for 21 days is an alternative regimen; azithromycin for 3 weeks is probably effective but has not been as well studied.

- Treatment of **trachoma** is azithromycin as a single oral dose as recommended by the World Health Organization and includes all household contacts of patients.

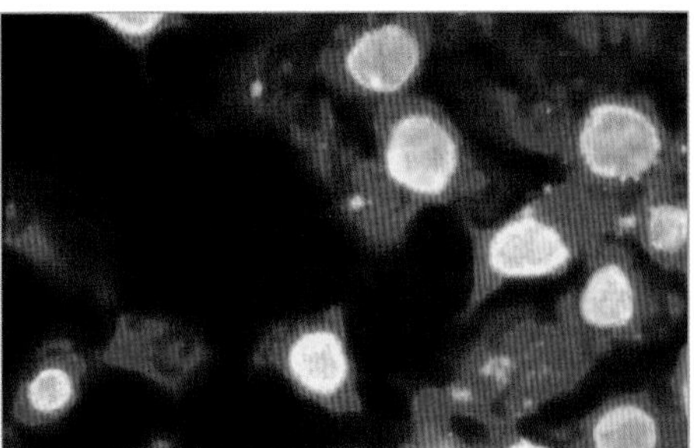

Image 29.1
Infected HeLa cells (fluorescent antibody stain). *Chlamydia trachomatis* is the most common reportable sexually transmitted infection in the United States, with high rates of infection among sexually active adolescents and young adults. Copyright Noni MacDonald, MD.

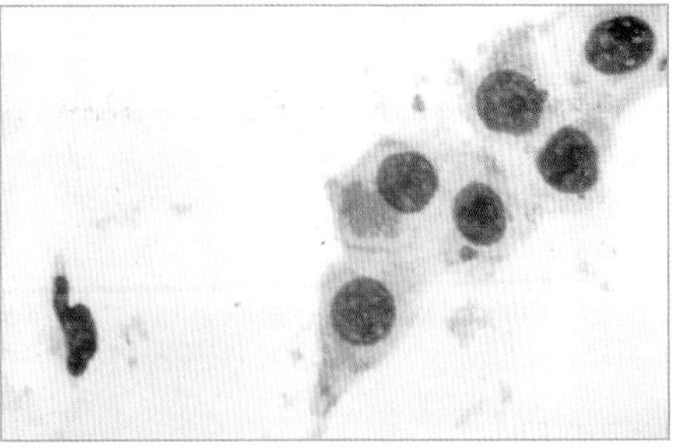

Image 29.2
Photomicrograph of *Chlamydia trachomatis* taken from a urethral scrape (iodine-stained inclusions in McCoy cell line; magnification x200). Untreated, chlamydia can cause severe, costly reproductive and other health problems, including short- and long-term consequences (eg, pelvic inflammatory disease, infertility, potentially fatal tubal pregnancy).

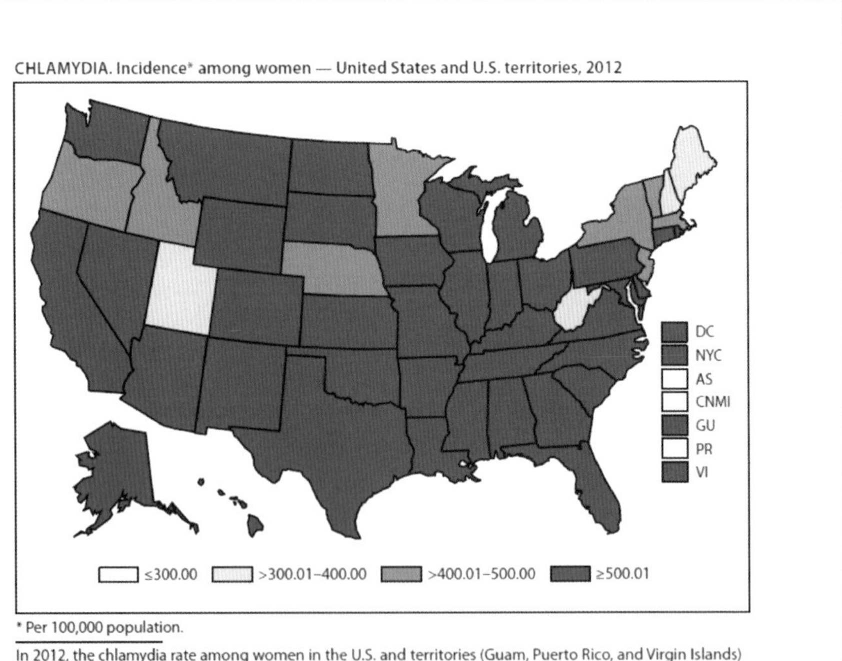

Image 29.3
Chlamydia. Incidence among women—United States and US territories, 2012. Courtesy of *Morbidity and Mortality Weekly Report*.

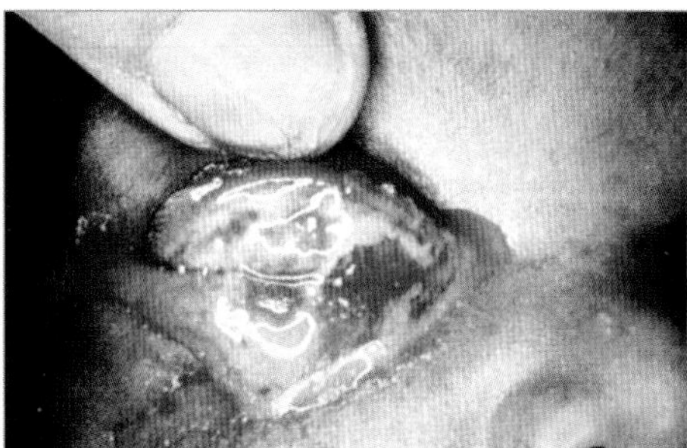

Image 29.4
Conjunctivitis due to *Chlamydia trachomatis*, the most common cause of ophthalmia neonatorum. This is the same infant as in Image 29.6.

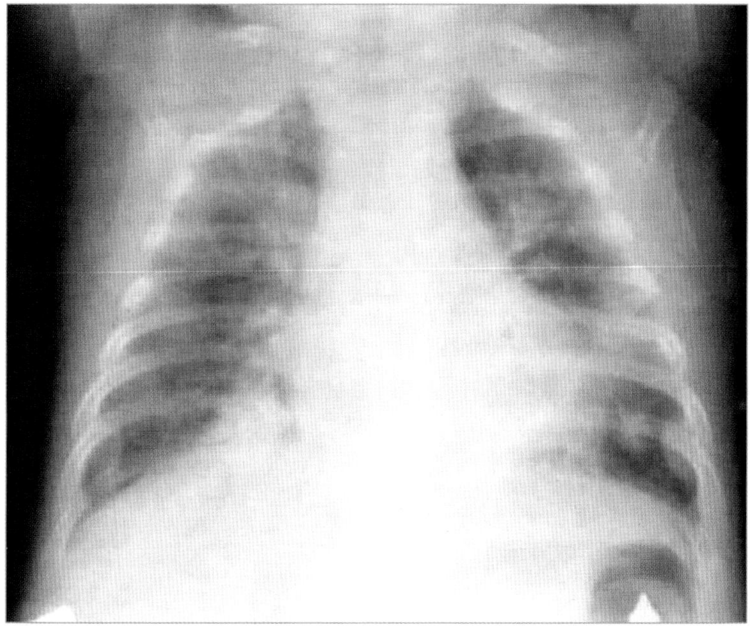

Image 29.5
Chlamydia trachomatis pneumonia, severe and bilateral, in a 5-week-old. Courtesy of Edgar O. Ledbetter, MD, FAAP.

30

Clostridial Infections

Botulism and Infant Botulism

(*Clostridium botulinum*)

Clinical Manifestations

Botulism is a neuroparalytic disorder characterized by an acute, afebrile, symmetric, descending, flaccid paralysis. Paralysis is caused by blockade of neurotransmitter release at the voluntary motor and autonomic neuromuscular junctions. Four naturally occurring forms of human botulism exist: **infant, foodborne, wound,** and adult intestinal colonization. Iatrogenic botulism results from injection of excess therapeutic botulinal toxin. Onset of symptoms occurs abruptly within hours or evolves gradually over several days and includes diplopia, dysphagia, dysphonia, and dysarthria. Cranial nerve palsies are followed by symmetric, descending, flaccid paralysis of somatic musculature in patients who remain fully alert. Infant botulism, which occurs predominantly in infants younger than 6 months (range, 1 day to 12 months), is preceded by or begins with constipation and manifests as decreased movement, loss of facial expression, poor feeding, weak cry, diminished gag reflex, ocular palsies, loss of head control, and progressive descending generalized weakness and hypotonia. Sudden infant death could result from rapidly progressing infant botulism.

Etiology

Botulism occurs after absorption of botulinal toxin into the circulation from a mucosal or wound surface. Seven antigenic toxin types (A–G) of *Clostridium botulinum* have been identified. The most common serotypes of *C botulinum* associated with naturally occurring illness are types A, B, E, and, rarely, F. Non-*botulinum* species of *Clostridium* rarely produce these neurotoxins and cause disease. A few cases of infant botulism have been caused by *Clostridium butyricum* (type E) and *Clostridium baratii* (type F). *C botulinum* spores are ubiquitous in soils and dust worldwide and have been isolated from the home vacuum cleaner dust of patients with infant botulism.

Epidemiology

- **Infant botulism** (annual average, 96 laboratory-confirmed cases from 2006–2011; median age, 16 weeks) results after ingested spores of *C botulinum* or related neurotoxigenic clostridial species germinate, multiply, and produce botulinal toxin in the large intestine through transient colonization of the intestinal microflora. Cases can occur in breastfed infants at the time of first introduction of nonhuman milk substances; the source of spores is usually not identified. Honey has been identified as an avoidable source of spores. No case of infant botulism has been proven to be attributable to consumption of corn syrup. Rarely, intestinal botulism can occur in older children and adults, usually after intestinal surgery and exposure to antimicrobial agents.
- **Foodborne botulism** (annual average, 17 cases from 2006–2010; median age, 53 years) results when food that carries spores of *C botulinum* is preserved or stored improperly under anaerobic conditions that permit germination, multiplication, and toxin production. Illness follows ingestion of the food containing preformed botulinal toxin. Home-processed foods are, by far, the most common cause of foodborne botulism in the United States, followed by rare outbreaks associated with commercially processed and restaurant-associated foods.
- **Wound botulism** (annual average, 26 laboratory-confirmed cases in 2006–2010; median age, 46 years) results when *C botulinum* contaminates traumatized tissue, germinates, multiplies, and produces toxin. Gross trauma or crush injury can be a predisposing event. During the last decade, self-injection of contaminated black tar heroin has been associated with most cases.

Immunity to botulinal toxin does not develop in botulism. Botulism is not transmitted from person to person.

Incubation Period

Infant botulism, 3 to 30 days from ingestion; foodborne botulism, 12 to 48 hours (range, 6 hours–8 days); wound botulism, 4 to 14 days from injury.

Diagnostic Tests

A toxin neutralization bioassay in mice is used to detect botulinal toxin in serum, stool, enema fluid, gastric aspirate, or suspect foods. Enriched selective media is required to isolate *C botulinum* from stool and foods. The diagnosis of infant botulism is made by demonstrating botulinal toxin or botulinal toxin–producing organisms in feces or enema fluid or toxin in serum. Although toxin can be demonstrated in serum in some infants (13% in one large study), stool is the best specimen for diagnosis; enema effluent can also be useful. If constipation makes obtaining a stool specimen difficult, an enema of sterile, nonbacteriostatic water should be given promptly. Wound botulism is confirmed by demonstrating organisms in the wound or tissue or toxin in the serum. To increase the likelihood of diagnosis in foodborne botulism, all suspect foods should be collected, and serum and stool or enema specimens should be obtained from all people with suspected illness. In foodborne cases, serum specimen test results may be positive for toxin as long as 12 days after admission. Because results of laboratory bioassay testing may require several days, treatment with antitoxin should be initiated urgently for all forms of botulism on the basis of clinical suspicion. The most prominent electromyographic finding is an incremental increase of evoked muscle potentials at high-frequency nerve stimulation (20–50 Hz), but this is infrequently needed for diagnosis.

Treatment

- **Meticulous supportive care,** particularly respiratory and nutritional support, constitutes a fundamental aspect of therapy in all forms of botulism. Recovery from botulism may take weeks to months.
- **Antitoxin for infant botulism.** Human-derived antitoxin should be given immediately. Human botulism immune globulin for intravenous use (BabyBIG) is licensed by the US Food and Drug Administration for treatment of infant botulism caused by *C botulinum* type A or B. BabyBIG is produced and distributed by the California Department of Public Health (**www.infantbotulism.org**). BabyBIG significantly decreases days of mechanical ventilation, days of intensive care unit stay, and total length of hospital stay by almost 1 month and leads to cost saving. BabyBIG is first-line therapy for naturally occurring infant botulism. Equine-derived heptavalent botulism antitoxin was licensed by the Food and Drug Administration in 2013 for treatment of adult and pediatric botulism and is available through the Centers for Disease Control and Prevention. Botulism antitoxin has been used to treat patients with type F infant botulism where the antitoxin is not contained in BabyBIG.
- **Antitoxin for noninfant forms of botulism.** Immediate administration of antitoxin is the key to successful therapy because antitoxin treatment ends the toxemia and stops further uptake of toxin. However, because botulinal neurotoxin becomes internalized in the nerve ending, administration of antitoxin does not reverse paralysis. On suspicion of foodborne botulism, the state health department should be contacted immediately to discuss and report. Botulism antitoxin contains antitoxin against all 7 (A–G) botulinal toxin types and is provided by the Centers for Disease Control and Prevention with a treatment protocol.
- **Antimicrobial agents.** Antimicrobial therapy is not prescribed in infant botulism. Aminoglycoside agents can potentiate the paralytic effects of the toxin and should be avoided. Penicillin or metronidazole can be given to patients with wound botulism after antitoxin has been administered. The role of antimicrobial therapy in the adult intestinal colonization form of botulism, if any, has not been established.

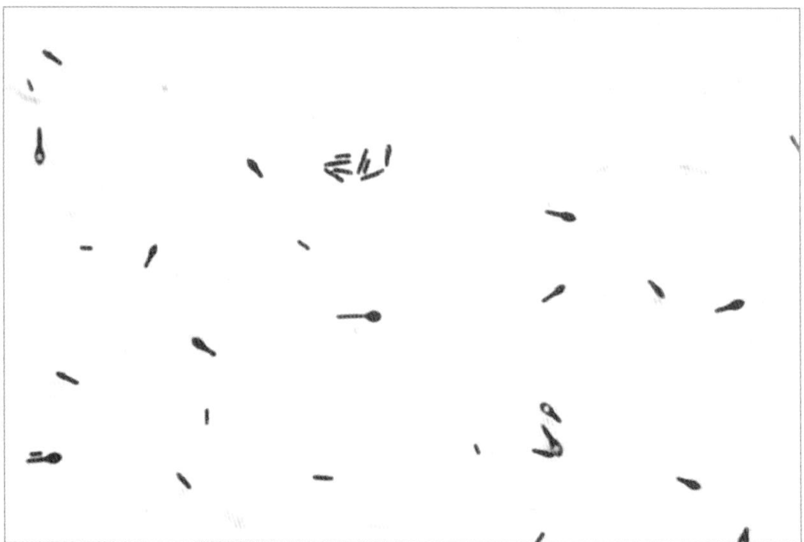

Image 30.1
A photomicrograph of spore forms of *Clostridium botulinum* type A (Gram stain). These *C botulinum* bacteria were cultured in thioglycolate broth for 48 hours at 35°C (95°F). The bacterium *C botulinum* produces a nerve toxin that causes the rare but serious paralytic illness botulism. Courtesy of Centers for Disease Control and Prevention/Dr George Lombard.

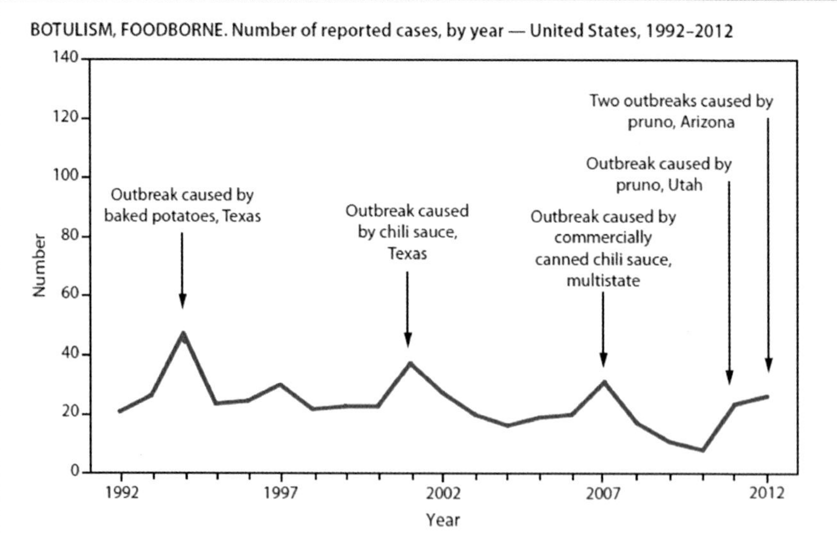

The number of foodborne botulism cases has remained fairly steady, with peaks corresponding to larger outbreaks. In 2012, four outbreaks occurred, two associated with consumption of pruno, an illicit alcoholic brew, in an Arizona prison (4 cases and 8 cases), one associated with home-canned spaghetti and meat sauce (2 cases), and one associated with home-canned beets (3 cases).

Image 30.2
Botulism, foodborne. Number of reported cases, by year—United States, 1992–2012. Courtesy of *Morbidity and Mortality Weekly Report.*

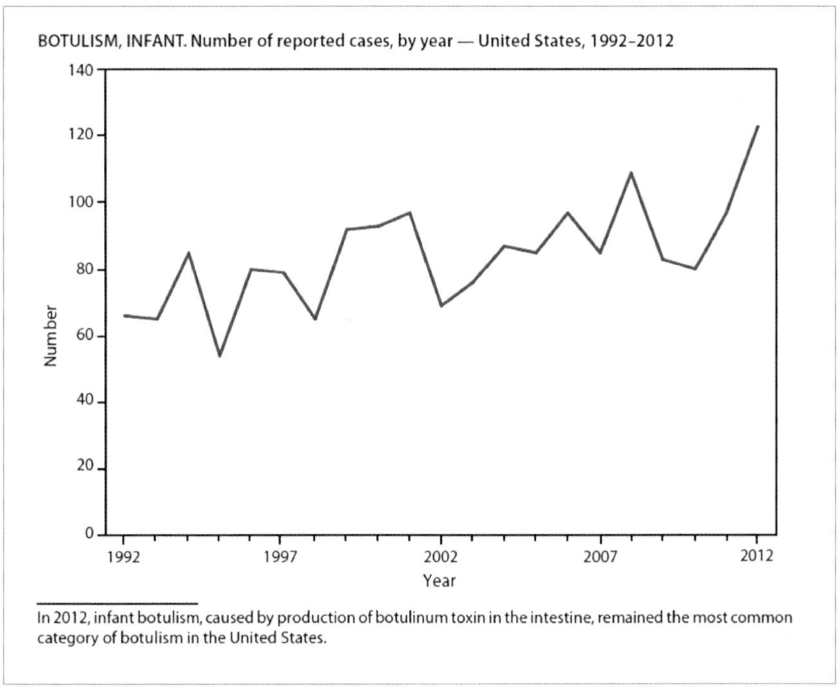

Image 30.3
Botulism, infant. Number of reported cases, by year—United States, 1992–2012. Courtesy of *Morbidity and Mortality Weekly Report.*

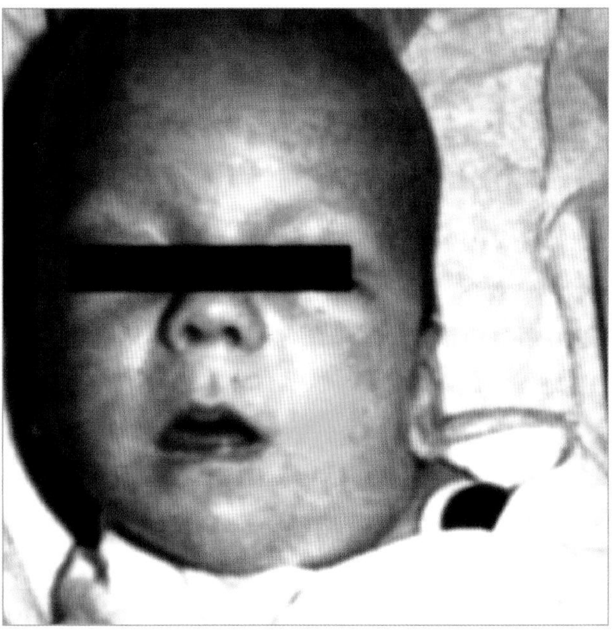

Image 30.4
An infant with mild botulism depicting the loss of facial expression. This infant also had a weak cry, poor feeding, diminished gag reflex, and hypotonia. Infant botulism most often occurs in infants younger than 6 months. Copyright Charles Prober.

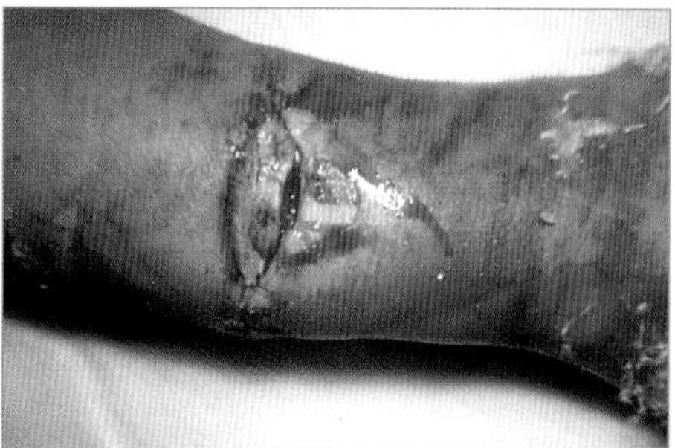

Image 30.5
Wound botulism in the compound fracture of the right arm of a 14-year-old boy. The patient fractured his right ulna and radius and subsequently developed wound botulism. Courtesy of Centers for Disease Control and Prevention.

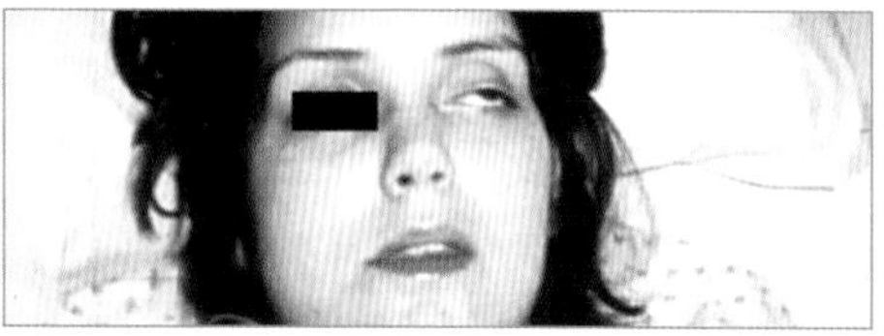

Image 30.7
Botulism with ocular muscle paralysis in a preadolescent girl. She also had respiratory muscle weakness but did not require ventilatory support. Courtesy of Hugh Moffet, MD.

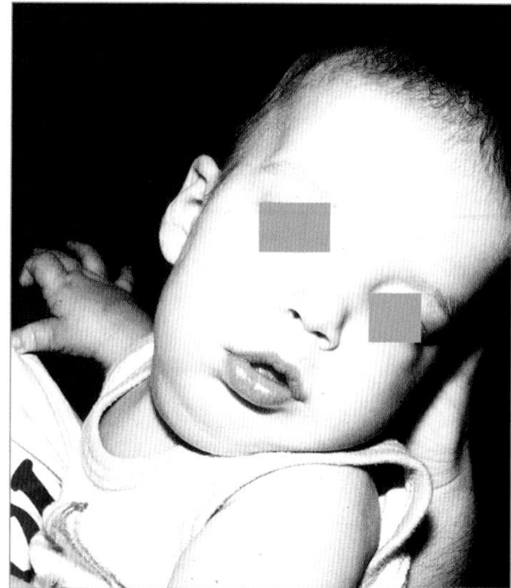

Image 30.6
Infantile botulism in a 4-month-old boy with a 6-day history of progressive weakness, constipation, decreased appetite, and weight loss. The infant had been afebrile, was breastfed, and had not received honey. He was intubated within 24 hours of admission and remained on a ventilator for 26 days. Stool specimens were positive for *Clostridium botulinum* type A. Copyright Larry I. Corman.

31

Clostridial Myonecrosis

(Gas Gangrene)

Clinical Manifestations

Onset is heralded by acute pain at the site of the wound, followed by edema, increasing exquisite tenderness, exudate, and progression of pain. Systemic findings initially include tachycardia disproportionate to the degree of fever, pallor, diaphoresis, hypotension, renal failure, and then, later, alterations in mental status. Crepitus is suggestive but not pathognomonic of *Clostridium* infection and is not always present. Diagnosis is based on clinical manifestations including the characteristic appearance of necrotic muscle at surgery. Untreated gas gangrene can lead to disseminated myonecrosis, suppurative visceral infection, septicemia, and death within hours.

Etiology

Clostridial myonecrosis is caused by *Clostridium* species, most often *Clostridium perfringens*. These organisms are large, gram-positive, spore-forming, anaerobic bacilli with blunt ends. Other *Clostridium* species (eg, *Clostridium sordellii, Clostridium septicum, Clostridium novyi*) have also been associated with myonecrosis. Disease manifestations are caused by potent clostridial exotoxins (eg, *C sordellii* with medical abortion; *C septicum* with malignancy). Mixed infection with other gram-positive and gram-negative bacteria is common.

Epidemiology

Clostridial myonecrosis usually results from contamination of open wounds involving muscle. The sources of *Clostridium* species are soil, contaminated foreign bodies, and human and animal feces. Dirty surgical or traumatic wounds, particularly those with retained foreign bodies or significant amounts of devitalized tissue, predispose to disease. Nontraumatic gas gangrene occurs rarely in people who are immunocompromised, most often in those with underlying malignancy, neutrophil dysfunction, or diseases associated with bowel ischemia.

Incubation Period

From injury, 1 to 4 days.

Diagnostic Tests

Anaerobic cultures of wound exudate, involved soft tissue and muscle, and blood should be performed. Because *Clostridium* species are ubiquitous, their recovery from a wound is not diagnostic unless typical clinical manifestations are present. A Gram-stained smear of wound discharge demonstrating characteristic gram-positive bacilli and few, if any, polymorphonuclear leukocytes suggests clostridial infection. Tissue specimens (not swab specimens) for anaerobic culture must be obtained to confirm the diagnosis. Because some pathogenic *Clostridium* species are exquisitely oxygen sensitive, care should be taken to optimize anaerobic growth conditions. A radiograph of the affected site can demonstrate gas in the tissue, but this is a nonspecific finding. Occasionally, blood culture results are positive and are considered diagnostic.

Treatment

Prompt and complete surgical excision of necrotic tissue and removal of foreign material are essential. Repeated surgical debridement may be required. Management of shock, fluid and electrolyte imbalance, hemolytic anemia, and other complications is crucial. High-dose penicillin G should be administered intravenously. Clindamycin, metronidazole, meropenem, ertapenem, and chloramphenicol can be considered as alternative drugs for patients with a serious penicillin allergy or for treatment of polymicrobial infections. The combination of penicillin G and clindamycin may be superior to penicillin alone because of the theoretical benefit of clindamycin inhibiting toxin synthesis. Hyperbaric oxygen may be beneficial, but efficacy data from adequately controlled clinical studies are not available.

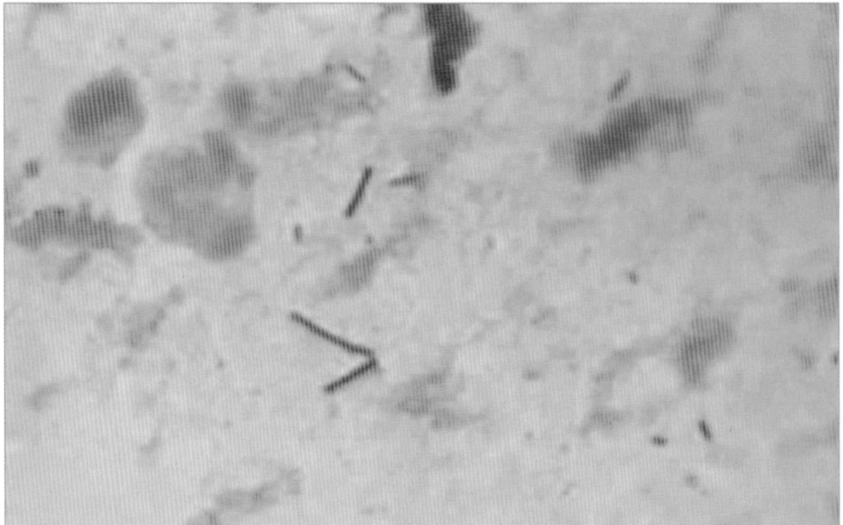

Image 31.1
Gram stain of a tissue aspirate from a patient with clostridial omphalitis showing the characteristic morphology of *Clostridia* bacilli, erroneously stained gram-negative, and sparse polymorphonuclear leukocytes.

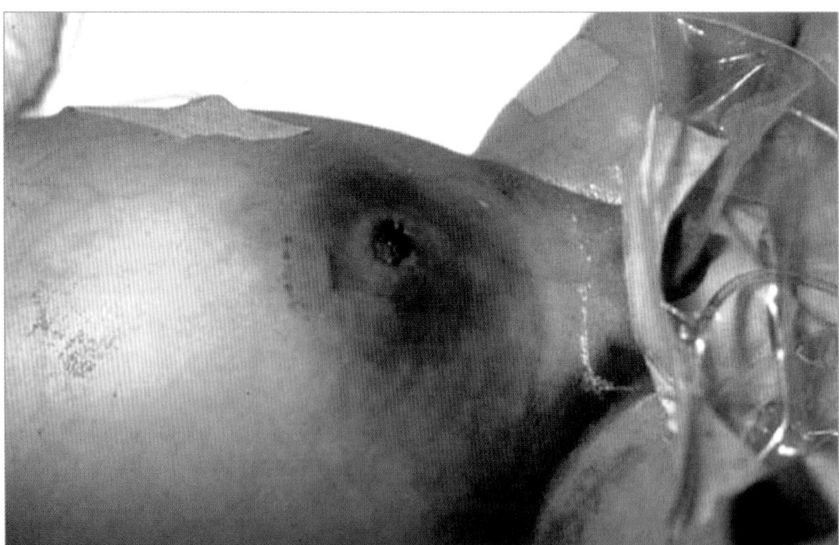

Image 31.2
Clostridial omphalitis in an infant with myonecrosis of the abdominal wall (periumbilical). Early and complete surgical excision of necrotic tissue and careful management of shock, fluid balance, and other complications are crucial for survival.

32

Clostridium difficile

Clinical Manifestations

Clostridium difficile is associated with several syndromes as well as with asymptomatic carriage. Mild to moderate illness is characterized by watery diarrhea, low-grade fever, and mild abdominal pain. Pseudomembranous enterocolitis is characterized by diarrhea with mucus in feces, abdominal cramps and pain, fever, and systemic toxicity. Occasionally, children have marked abdominal tenderness and distention with minimal diarrhea (toxic megacolon). The colonic mucosa often contains 2- to 5-mm, raised, yellowish plaques. Disease often begins while the child is hospitalized receiving antimicrobial therapy but can occur up to 10 weeks after therapy cessation. Community-associated *C difficile* disease is less common but is increasing in frequency. The illness usually, but not always, is associated with antimicrobial therapy or prior hospitalization. Complications, which occur more commonly in older adults, can include toxic megacolon, intestinal perforation, systemic inflammatory response syndrome, and death. Severe or fatal disease is more likely to occur in neutropenic children with leukemia, infants with Hirschsprung disease (congenital megacolon), and patients with inflammatory bowel disease. Colonization with *C difficile,* including toxin-producing strains, occurs in children younger than 5 years and is most common in infants. It is unclear how frequently *C difficile* causes disease in infants younger than 1 year.

Etiology

Clostridium difficile is a spore-forming, obligate anaerobic, gram-positive bacillus. Disease is related to A and B toxins produced by these organisms.

Epidemiology

C difficile can be isolated from soil and is commonly found in the hospital environment. *C difficile* is acquired from the environment or from stool of other colonized or infected people by the fecal-oral route. Intestinal colonization rates in healthy infants can be as high as 50% but usually are less than 5% in children older than 5 years and adults. Hospitals, nursing homes, and child care facilities are major reservoirs for *C difficile*. Risk factors for acquisition of the bacteria include prolonged hospitalization and exposure to an infected person in the hospital or the community. Risk factors for *C difficile* disease include antimicrobial therapy, repeated enemas, gastric acid suppression therapy, prolonged nasogastric tube placement, gastrostomy and jejunostomy tubes, underlying bowel disease, gastrointestinal tract surgery, renal insufficiency, and humoral immunocompromise. *C difficile* colitis has been associated with exposure to almost every antimicrobial agent. Hospitalization of children for *C difficile* colitis is increasing. The NAP1 strain, a more virulent strain of *C difficile* with variations in toxin genes, is associated with severe disease, has emerged as a cause of outbreaks among adults, and has been reported in children.

Incubation Period

Unknown; colitis usually develops 5 to 10 days after initiation of antimicrobial therapy.

Diagnostic Tests

The diagnosis of *C difficile* disease is based on the presence of diarrhea and detection of *C difficile* toxins in a diarrheal specimen. Isolation of the organism or toxin detection from the stool of a patient who is not having liquid stools (unless toxic megacolon is suspected) should not be performed. Endoscopic findings of pseudomembranes and hyperemic, friable rectal mucosa suggest pseudomembranous enterocolitis. The most common testing method for *C difficile* toxins is the commercially available enzyme immunoassay (EIA), which detects toxins A and B. Although EIAs are rapid and performed easily, their sensitivity is relatively low. The cell culture cytotoxicity assay, which also tests for toxin in stool, is more sensitive but requires more labor and has a slow turnaround time, limiting its usefulness in the clinical setting. Two-step testing algorithms that use sensitive but nonspecific (detects toxigenic and nontoxigenic strains) glutamate dehydrogenase EIA combined with confirmatory toxin testing of positive results can also be used. Molecular assays using nucleic acid amplification tests (NAATs) have been developed; NAATs combine good sensitivity and specificity, provide results to clinicians in times comparable with EIAs, and are not required to be part of a 2- or 3-step algorithm. Many children's hospitals are converting to NAAT technology to diagnose *C difficile* infection, but more data are needed in children before this technology can be used routinely as a stand-alone test. The predictive value of a positive NAAT result in a child younger than 5 years is unknown because carriage of toxigenic strains often occurs in these children. Because colonization with *C difficile* in infants is common, testing for other causes of diarrhea is always recommended in these patients. *C difficile* toxin degrades at room temperate and can be undetectable within 2 hours after collection of a stool specimen. Tests of cure should not be performed.

Treatment

Precipitating antimicrobial therapy should be discontinued as soon as possible. Antimicrobial therapy for *C difficile* infection is always indicated for symptomatic patients. *C difficile* is susceptible to metronidazole and vancomycin. Metronidazole, orally, is the drug of choice for initial treatment of children and adolescents with mild to moderate diarrhea and for first relapse. Oral vancomycin or vancomycin administered by enema plus intravenous metronidazole is indicated as initial therapy for patients with severe disease (ie, hospitalized in an intensive care unit, pseudomembranous enterocolitis by endoscopy, or significant underlying intestinal tract disease) and for patients who do not respond to oral metronidazole. Vancomycin for intravenous use can be prepared for oral use. Intravenously administered vancomycin is not effective for *C difficile* infection. Therapy with metronidazole or vancomycin or the combination should be administered for at least 10 days.

Up to 25% of patients experience a relapse after discontinuing therapy, but infection usually responds to a second course of the same treatment. Metronidazole should not be used for treatment of a second recurrence or for chronic therapy because neurotoxicity is possible. Tapered or pulse regimens of vancomycin are recommended under this circumstance. Fidaxomicin and nitazoxanide have been approved for treatment of *C difficile*–associated diarrhea in adults, but no pediatric data are available for fidaxomicin. Nitazoxanide is also an effective therapy in adults. Drugs that decrease intestinal motility should not be administered. Follow-up testing for toxin is not recommended. Fecal transplant (intestinal microbiota transplantation) appears to be effective in adults; there are limited data in pediatrics.

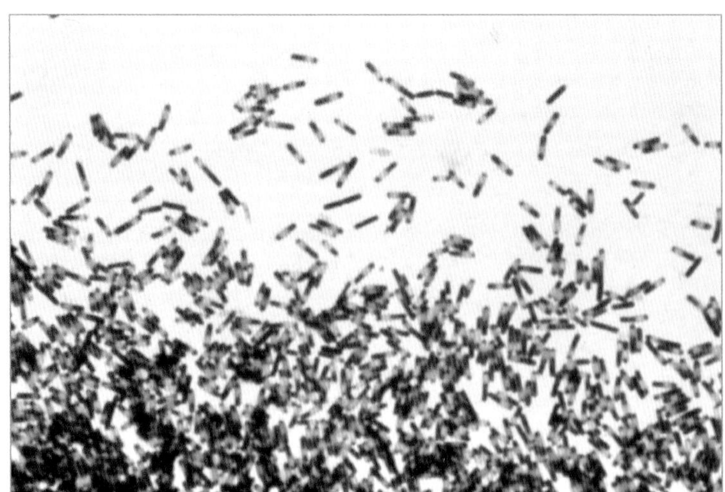

Image 32.1
Clostridium difficile is a gram-positive, spore-forming bacteria that can be part of the normal intestinal flora in as many as 50% of children younger than 2 years. It is a cause of pseudomembranous enterocolitis and antibiotic-associated diarrhea in older children and adults. Courtesy of *AAP News*.

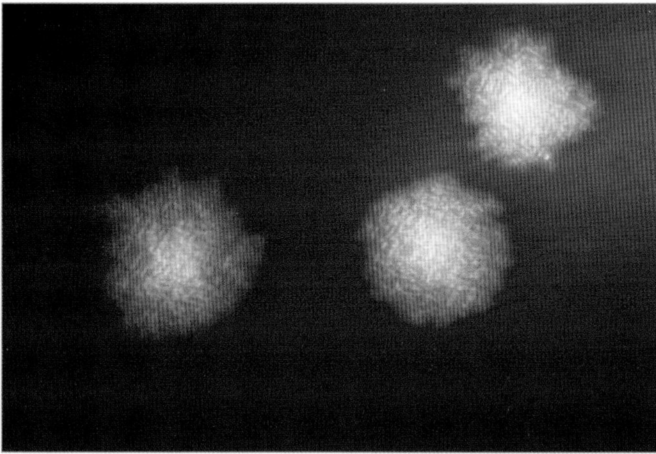

Image 32.2
This photograph depicts *Clostridium difficile* colonies after 48 hours' growth on a blood agar plate (magnification x4.8). Courtesy of Centers for Disease Control and Prevention/Dr Holdeman.

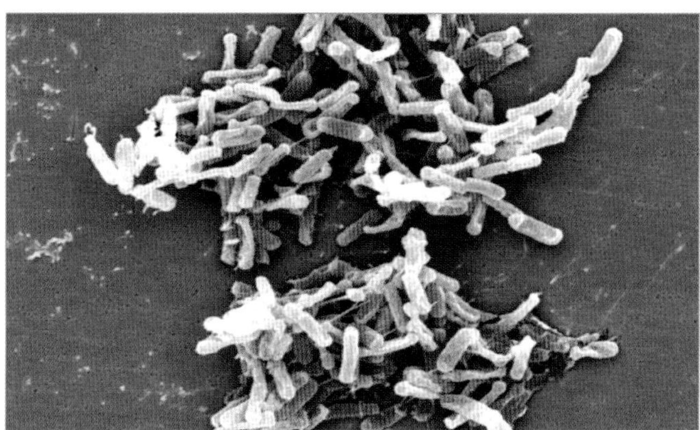

Image 32.3
This micrograph depicts gram-positive *Clostridium difficile* from a stool sample culture obtained using a 0.1-μm filter. People can become infected if they touch items or surfaces that are contaminated with *C difficile* spores and then touch their mouths or mucous membranes. Health care workers can spread the bacteria to other patients or contaminate surfaces through hand contact. Courtesy of Lois Higg/ Courtesy of Centers for Disease Control and Prevention.

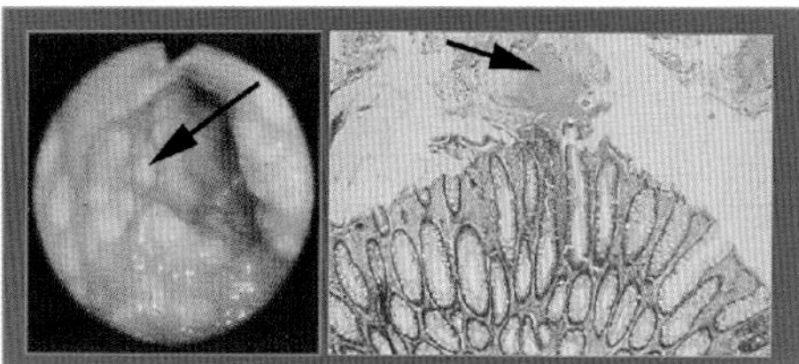

Image 32.4
The right-hand panel shows the typical pseudomembranes of *Clostridium difficile* colitis; the left-hand panel shows the histology, with the pseudomembrane structure at the top middle (arrows). Courtesy of Carol J. Baker, MD, FAAP.

33

Clostridium perfringens Food Poisoning

Clinical Manifestations

Clostridium perfringens foodborne illness is characterized by a sudden onset of watery diarrhea and moderate to severe, cramping, midepigastric pain. Vomiting and fever are uncommon. Symptoms usually resolve within 24 hours. The short incubation period, short duration, and absence of fever in most patients differentiate *C perfringens* foodborne disease from shigellosis and salmonellosis, and the infrequency of vomiting and longer incubation period contrast with the clinical features of foodborne disease associated with heavy metals, *Staphylococcus aureus* enterotoxins, *Bacillus cereus* emetic toxin, and fish and shellfish toxins. Diarrheal illness caused by *B cereus* diarrheal enterotoxins can be indistinguishable from that caused by *C perfringens*. Enteritis necroticans (also known as pigbel) results from hemorrhagic necrosis of the midgut and is a cause of severe illness and death attributable to *C perfringens* food poisoning caused by *Clostridium* β toxin. Rare cases have been reported in the Highlands of Papua, in New Guinea, and in Thailand; malnutrition is an important risk factor.

Etiology

Typical food poisoning is caused by a heat-labile *C perfringens* enterotoxin. *C perfringens* type A, which produces α toxin and enterotoxin, commonly causes foodborne illness. Enteritis necroticans is caused by *C perfringens* type C, which produces α and β toxins and enterotoxin.

Epidemiology

C perfringens is a gram-positive, spore-forming bacillus that is ubiquitous in the environment and the intestinal tracts of humans and animals and is commonly present in raw meat and poultry. Spores of *C perfringens* that survive cooking can germinate and multiply rapidly during slow cooling, when stored at temperatures from 20°C to 60°C (68°F–140°F), and during inadequate reheating. At an optimum temperature, *C perfringens* has one of the fastest rates of growth of any bacterium. Illness results from consumption of food containing high numbers of vegetative organisms (>10^5 colony-forming units [CFU]/g) followed by enterotoxin production in the intestine.

Beef, poultry, gravies, and dried or precooked foods are common sources. Ingestion of the organism is most commonly associated with foods prepared by restaurants or caterers or in institutional settings (eg, schools, camps) where food is prepared in large quantities, cooled slowly, and stored inappropriately for prolonged periods. Illness is not transmissible from person to person.

Incubation Period

6 to 24 hours; usually 8 to 12 hours.

Diagnostic Tests

Because the fecal flora of healthy people commonly includes *C perfringens,* counts of *C perfringens* of 10^6 CFU/g of feces or greater obtained within 48 hours of onset of illness are required to support the diagnosis in ill people. The diagnosis also can be supported by detection of enterotoxin in stool. *C perfringens* can be confirmed as the cause of an outbreak if 10^6 CFU/g are isolated from stool or enterotoxin is demonstrated in the stool of 2 or more ill people or when the concentration of organisms is at least 10^5/g in the epidemiologically implicated food. Although *C perfringens* is an anaerobe, special transport conditions are unnecessary. Stool specimens, rather than rectal swab specimens, should be obtained, transported in ice packs, and tested within 24 hours.

Treatment

Oral rehydration or, occasionally, intravenous fluid and electrolyte replacement may be indicated to prevent or treat dehydration. Antimicrobial agents are not indicated.

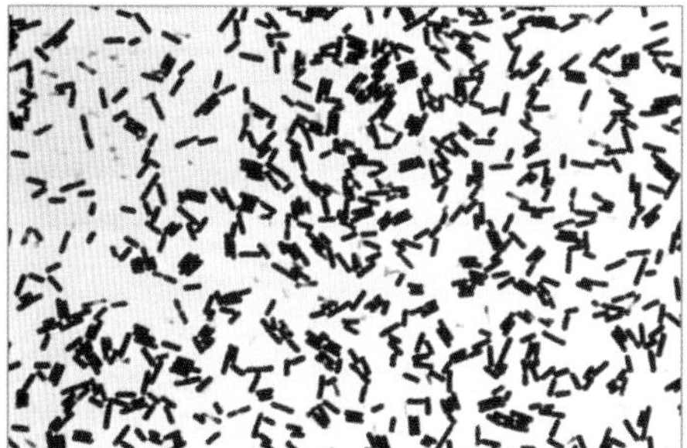

Image 33.1
This photomicrograph reveals numbers of *Clostridium perfringens* bacteria grown in Schaedler broth and subsequently stained using Gram stain (magnification x1,000). *C perfringens* is a spore-forming, heat-resistant bacterium that can cause foodborne disease. The spores persist in the environment and often contaminate raw food materials. These bacteria are found in mammalian feces and soil. Courtesy of Centers for Disease Control and Prevention/Don Stalons.

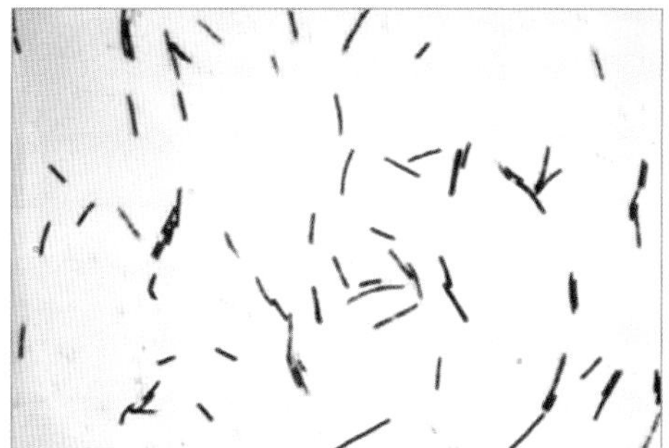

Image 33.2
This photomicrograph reveals *Clostridium perfringens* grown in Schaedler broth using Gram stain. Courtesy of Centers for Disease Control and Prevention/Don Stalons.

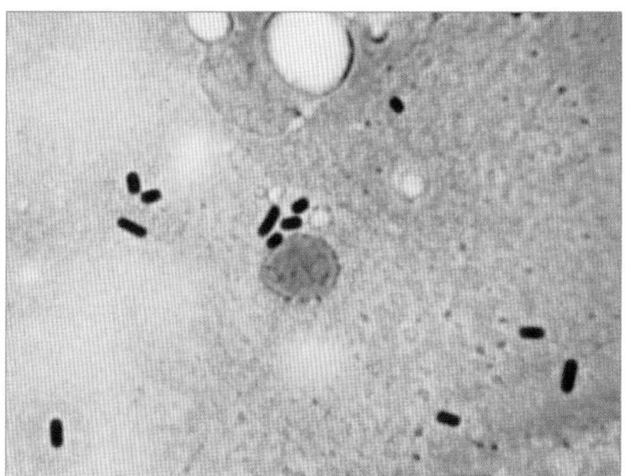

Image 33.3
Clostridium perfringens, an anaerobic, gram-positive, spore-forming bacillus, causes a broad spectrum of pathology, including food poisoning. In Papua New Guinea, *C perfringens* is a cause of severe illness and death called necrotizing enteritis necroticans (locally known as pigbel). Courtesy of Hugh Moffet, MD.

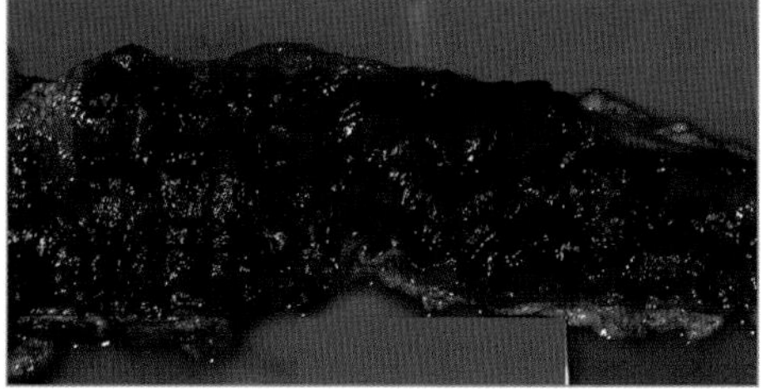

Image 33.4
This slide shows hemorrhagic necrosis of the intestine in a patient with *Clostridium perfringens* sepsis. Courtesy of Dimitris P. Agamanolis, MD.

34

Coccidioidomycosis

Clinical Manifestations

Primary pulmonary infection is acquired by inhaling fungal conidia and is asymptomatic or self-limited in 60% of infected children. Constitutional symptoms, including fatigue and weight loss, are common and can persist for weeks or months. Symptomatic disease can resemble influenza or community-acquired pneumonia, with malaise, fever, cough, myalgia, arthralgia, headache, and chest pain. Pleural effusion, empyema, and mediastinal involvement are more common in children than adults. Acute infection can only be associated with cutaneous abnormalities, such as erythema multiforme, an erythematous maculopapular rash, or erythema nodosum. Chronic pulmonary lesions are rare, but approximately 5% of infected people develop asymptomatic pulmonary radiographic residua (eg, cysts, nodules, cavitary lesions, coin lesions). Nonpulmonary primary infection is rare and usually follows trauma associated with contamination of wounds by arthroconidia. Cutaneous lesions and soft tissue infections often are accompanied by regional lymphadenitis.

Disseminated (extrapulmonary) infection occurs in less than 0.5% of infected people; common sites of dissemination include skin, bones and joints, and the central nervous system (CNS). Meningitis is invariably fatal if untreated. Congenital infection is rare.

Etiology

Coccidioides species are dimorphic fungi. Molecular studies have divided the genus *Coccidioides* into 2 species: *Coccidioides immitis,* confined mainly to California, and *Coccidioides posadasii,* encompassing the remaining areas of distribution of the fungus within certain deserts of the southwestern United States, northern Mexico, and regions of Central and South America.

Epidemiology

Coccidioides species are found mostly in soil in areas of the southwestern United States with endemic infection, including California, Arizona, New Mexico, west and south Texas, southern Nevada, and Utah; northern Mexico; and throughout certain parts of Central and South America. In areas with endemic coccidioidomycosis, clusters of cases can follow dust-generating events, such as storms, seismic events, archaeologic digging, or recreational activities. Most cases occur without a known preceding event. The incidence of reported coccidioidomycosis cases has increased substantially over the past decade and a half, rising from 5.3 per 100,000 population in the area of endemicity (Arizona, California, Nevada, New Mexico, and Utah) in 1998 to 42.6 per 100,000 in 2011. Infection is thought to provide lifelong immunity. Person-to-person transmission of coccidioidomycosis does not occur except in rare instances of cutaneous infection with actively draining lesions, donor-derived transmission via an infected organ, and congenital infection following in utero exposure. Preexisting impairment of T lymphocyte–mediated immunity is a factor for severe primary coccidioidomycosis, disseminated disease, or relapse of past infection. Other people at risk of severe or disseminated disease include people of African or Filipino ancestry, women in the third trimester of pregnancy, and infants.

Incubation Period

Typically 1 to 4 weeks; disseminated infection can develop years after primary infection.

Diagnostic Tests

Diagnosis of coccidioidomycosis is best established using serologic, histopathologic, and culture methods. Serologic tests are useful in the diagnosis and management of infection. The immunoglobulin (Ig) M response can be detected by enzyme immunoassay (EIA) or immunodiffusion methods. In approximately 50% and 90% of primary infections, IgM is detected in the first and third weeks, respectively. IgG response can be detected by immunodiffusion, EIA, or complement fixation (CF) tests. Immunodiffusion and CF tests are highly specific. Complement fixation antibodies in serum are usually of low titer and are transient if the disease is asymptomatic or mild. Persistent high titers (≥1:16) occur with severe disease and almost always in disseminated infection. Cerebrospinal fluid antibodies are also detectable by immunodiffusion or CF testing. Increasing serum and cerebrospinal fluid titers indicate progressive disease, and decreasing titers usually suggest improvement. Complement fixation titers may not be reliable in patients who are immunocompromised. Because clinical laboratories use different diagnostic test kits, positive results should be confirmed in a reference laboratory.

Spherules are as large as 80 μm in diameter and can be visualized with magnification x100 to x400 in infected body fluid specimens (eg, pleural fluid, bronchoalveolar lavage) and biopsy specimens of skin lesions or organs. The presence of a mature spherule with endospores is pathognomonic of infection. Isolation of *Coccidioides* species in culture establishes the diagnosis. Culture of organisms is possible on a variety of artificial media but is potentially hazardous to laboratory personnel because spherules can convert to arthroconidia-bearing mycelia on culture plates. An EIA test for urine, serum, plasma, or bronchoalveolar lavage fluid is available from a US laboratory for detection of *Coccidioides* antigen. Antigen can be detected in more severe forms of disease (sensitivity 71%), but cross-reactions occur in patients with histoplasmosis, blastomycosis, or paracoccidioidomycosis.

Treatment

Antifungal therapy for uncomplicated primary infection in people without risk factors for severe disease is controversial. Although most cases will resolve without therapy, some experts believe treatment may reduce illness duration or risk for severe complications. Most experts recommend treatment of coccidioidomycosis for people at risk of severe disease or people with severe primary infection. Severe primary infection is manifested by CF titers of 1:16 or greater, infiltrates involving more than half of one lung or portions of both lungs, weight loss of greater than 10%, marked chest pain, severe malaise, inability to work or attend school, intense night sweats, or symptoms that persist for more than 2 months. Fluconazole or itraconazole is recommended for 3 to 6 months. Repeated patient encounters every 1 to 3 months for up to 2 years, to document radiographic resolution or to identify pulmonary or extrapulmonary complications, are recommended. For diffuse pneumonia, defined as bilateral reticulonodular or military infiltrates, amphotericin B or high-dose fluconazole is recommended. Amphotericin B is more frequently used in the presence of severe hypoxemia or rapid clinical deterioration. The length of therapy for diffuse pneumonia should be 1 year.

Oral itraconazole or fluconazole is the recommended initial therapy for disseminated infection not involving the CNS. Amphotericin B is recommended as alternative therapy if lesions are progressing or are in critical locations, such as the vertebral column. In patients experiencing failure of conventional amphotericin B deoxycholate therapy or experiencing drug-related toxicities, a lipid formulation of amphotericin B can be substituted.

Consultation with a specialist for treatment of patients with CNS disease caused by *Coccidioides* species is recommended. Oral fluconazole is recommended for treatment of patients with CNS infection. Patients who respond to azole therapy should continue this treatment indefinitely. For CNS infections that are unresponsive to oral azoles or are associated with severe basilar inflammation, intrathecal amphotericin B deoxycholate can be used to augment the azole therapy. A subcutaneous reservoir can facilitate administration into the cisternal space or lateral ventricle. The role of newer azole antifungal agents, such as voriconazole and posaconazole, in treatment of coccidiomycosis has not been established.

The duration of antifungal therapy is variable and depends on the site(s) of involvement, clinical response, and mycologic and immunologic test results. In general, therapy is continued until clinical and laboratory evidence indicates active infection has resolved. Treatment for disseminated coccidioidomycosis is at least 6 months but, for some patients, may be extended to 1 year or longer. The role of subsequent suppressive azole therapy is uncertain, except for patients with CNS infection, osteomyelitis, or underlying HIV infection or solid organ transplant recipients, for whom suppressive therapy is lifelong. Women should be advised to avoid pregnancy while receiving fluconazole, which may be teratogenic.

Surgical debridement or excision of lesions in bone, pericardium, and lung has been advocated for localized, symptomatic, persistent, resistant, or progressive lesions. In some localized infections with sinuses, fistulae, or abscesses, amphotericin B has been instilled locally or used for irrigation of wounds.

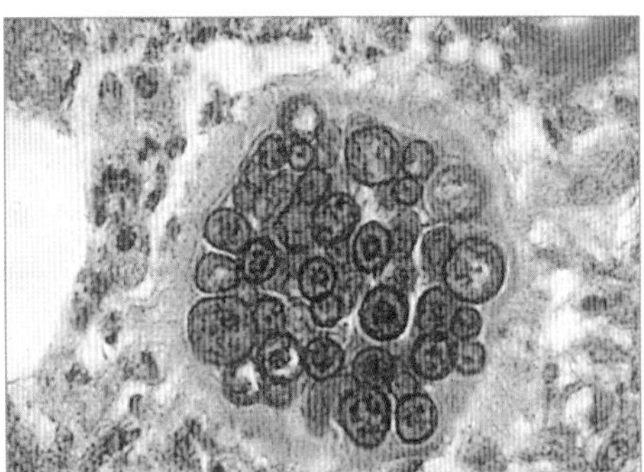

Image 34.1
Spherule with endospores of *Coccidioides immitis* (periodic acid–Schiff reaction). Courtesy of Centers for Disease Control and Prevention.

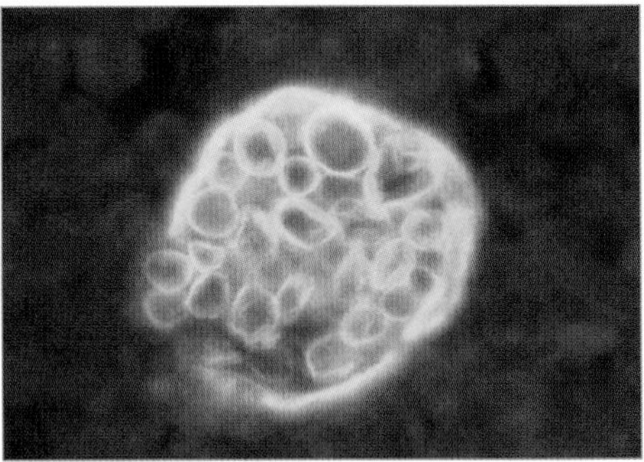

Image 34.2
Spherule of *Coccidioides immitis* with endospores (calcofluor stain). Courtesy of Centers for Disease Control and Prevention.

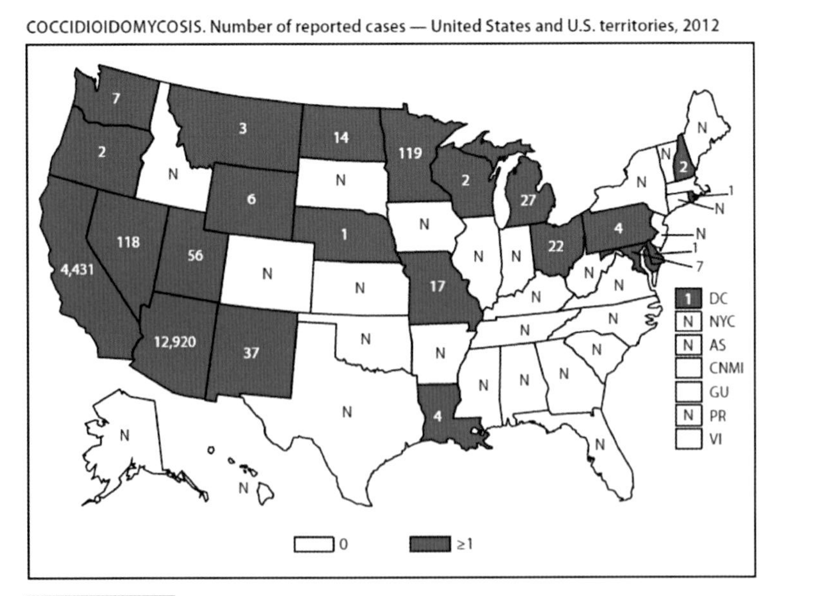

In 2012, 72.6% of reported coccidioidomycosis cases were from Arizona, 24.9% from California, 1.2% from other endemic states (Nevada, New Mexico, and Utah) combined, and 1.3% from nonendemic states.

Image 34.3
Coccidioidomycosis. Number of reported cases—United States and US territories, 2012. Courtesy of *Morbidity and Mortality Weekly Report.*

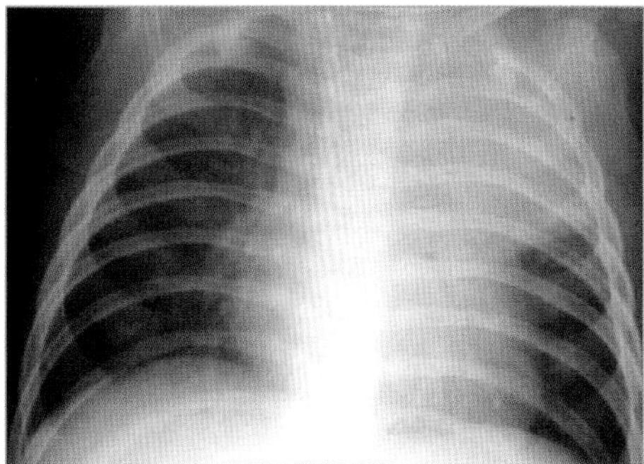

Image 34.4
Pneumonia due to *Coccidioides immitis* in the upper lobe of the left lung of a 5½-month-old. The organism was isolated from gastric aspirate, and complement fixation test result was elevated.

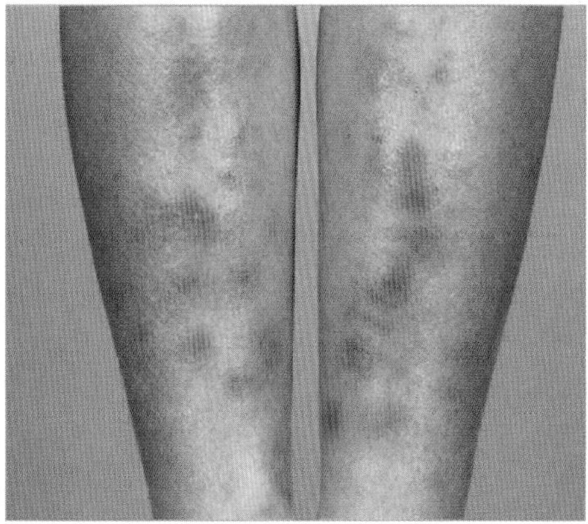

Image 34.6
Erythema nodosum in a preadolescent girl with primary pulmonary coccidioidomycosis.

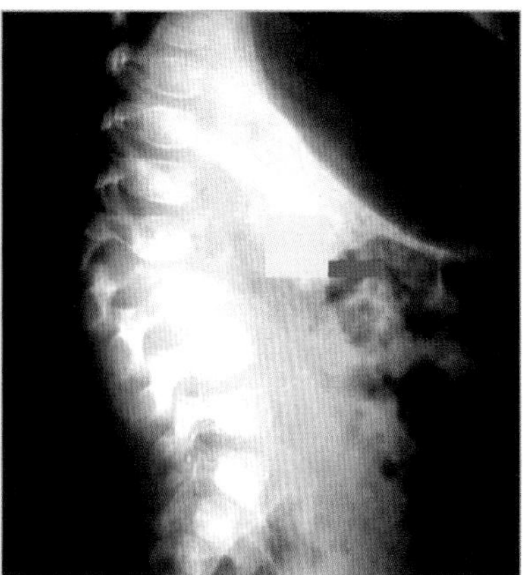

Image 34.8
Spondylitis due to *Coccidioides immitis* in 2-year-old white boy with disseminated disease.

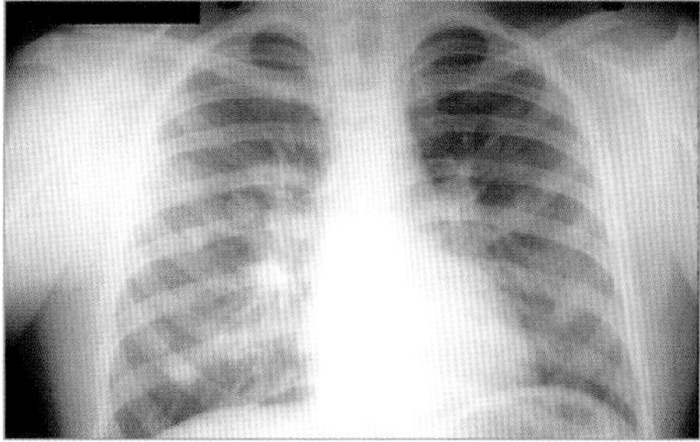

Image 34.5
Primary pulmonary coccidioidomycosis in an 11-year-old boy who recovered spontaneously. The acute disease is usually self-limited in otherwise healthy children. The patient also had erythema nodosum lesions over the tibial area.

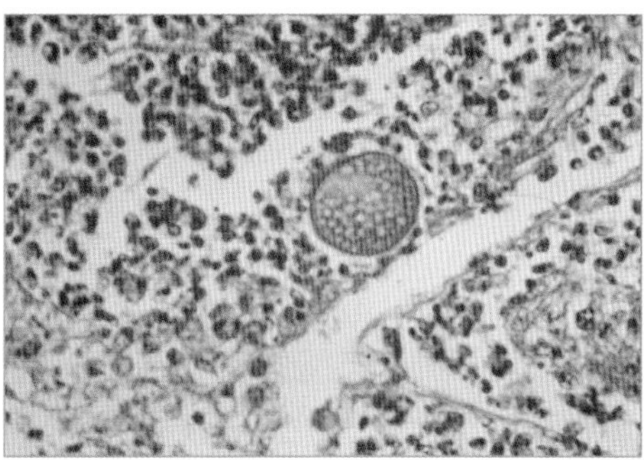

Image 34.7
Histopathology of coccidioidomycosis of lung. Mature spherule with endospores of *Coccidioides immitis* and intense infiltrate of neutrophils (hematoxylin-eosin stain). Courtesy of Centers for Disease Control and Prevention/Dr Lucille K. Georg.

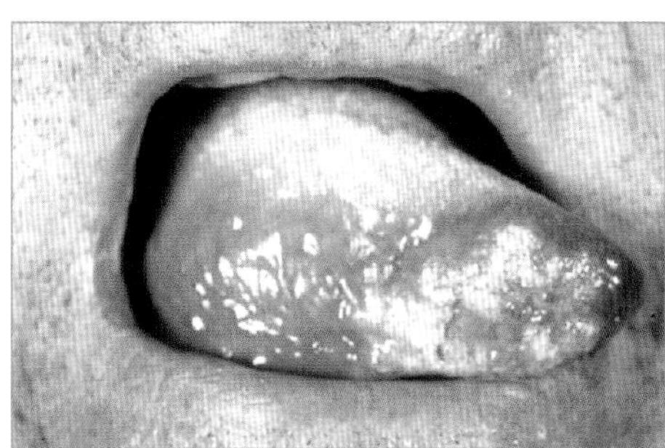

Image 34.9
Coccidioidomycosis of the tongue in an adult male. Courtesy of Edgar O. Ledbetter, MD, FAAP.

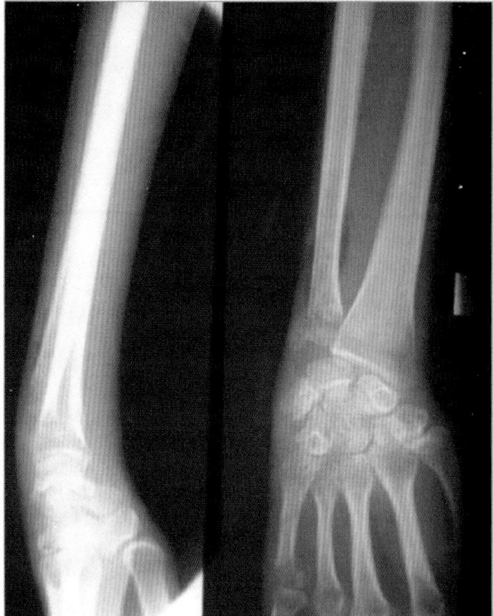

Image 34.10
Disseminated coccidioidomycosis with osteomyelitis of the distal radius and ulna in a preadolescent white boy.

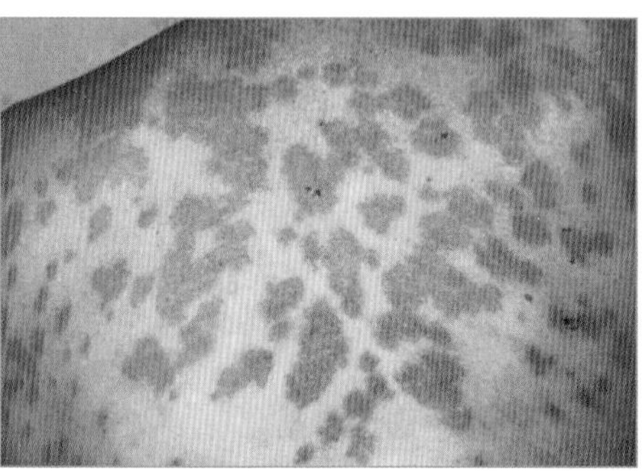

Image 34.12
Erythema nodosum lesions on skin of the back due to hypersensitivity to antigens of *Coccidioides immitis*. Courtesy of Centers for Disease Control and Prevention/Lucille K. Georg, MD.

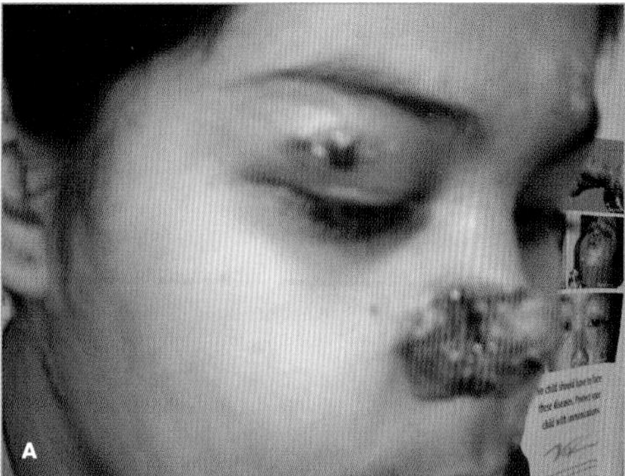

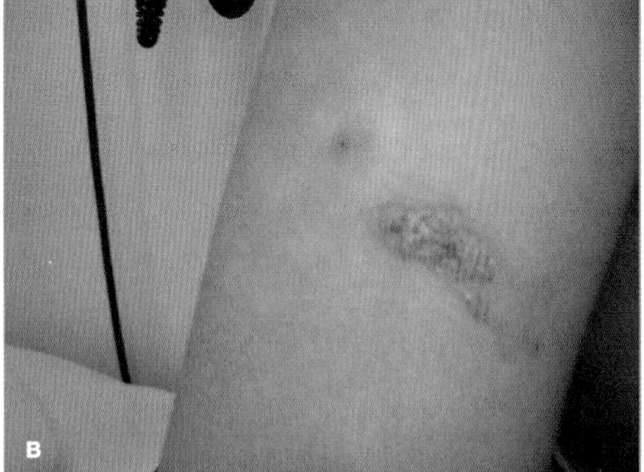

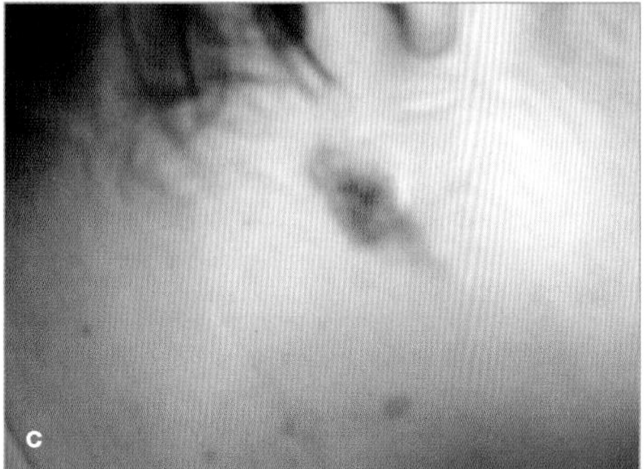

Image 34.11
A 15-year-old Hispanic girl who originally presented with forehead lesions without other symptoms. At the third visit, she had disseminated coccidioidomycosis disease and had developed extensive cutaneous lesions all over her body with severe nasal involvement. Courtesy of Sabiha Hussain, MD.

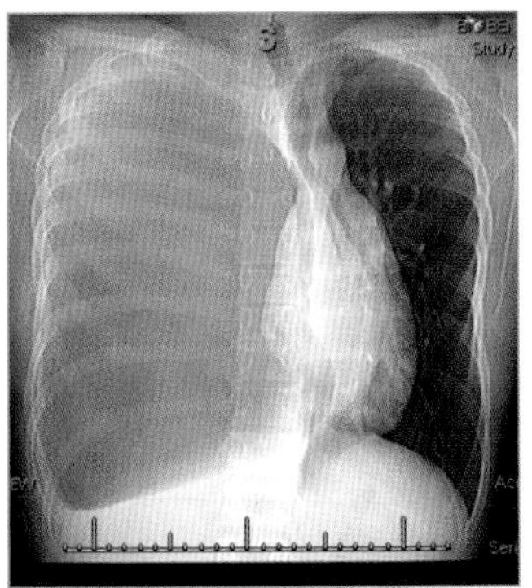

Image 34.13
Chest radiograph of a previously healthy 14-year-old boy who had a several month history of intermittent fever, weight loss, and chest pain and recent onset of exercise intolerance. His pyopneumothorax was caused by *Coccidioides immitis.* He lived in West Texas near the Mexican border. Courtesy of Jeffrey R. Starke, MD.

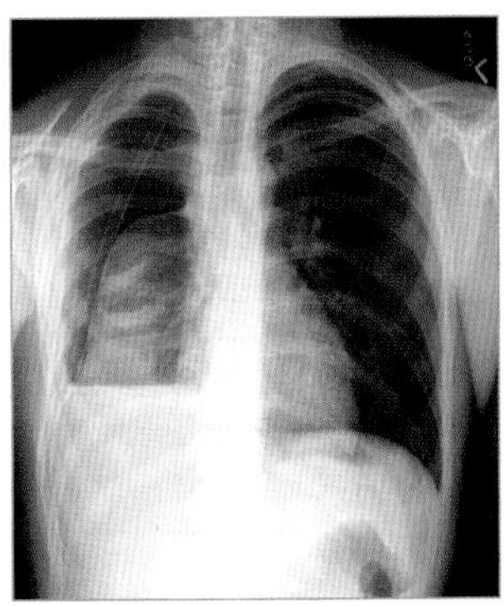

Image 34.14
A chest tube was inserted emergently in the patient in Image 34.15, and his right lung was expanded. Courtesy of Jeffrey R. Starke, MD.

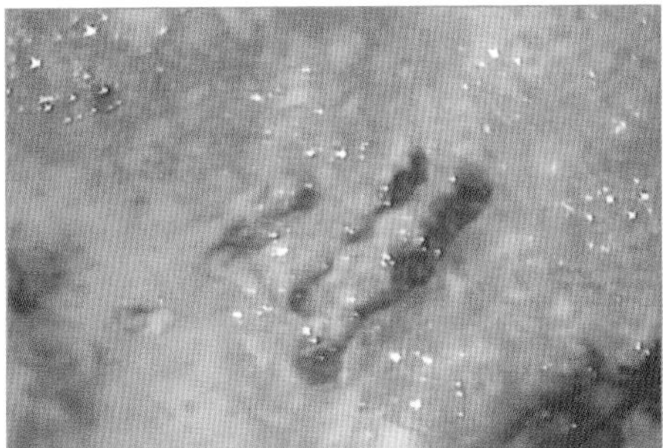

Image 34.15
After 7 days of hospitalization. The patient in images 34.13 and 34.14 had a video-assisted thoracostomy followed by an open thoracotomy for decortication procedure. This photograph demonstrated the copious fluid and thick fibrinous exudate of a chronic empyema found at surgery. Courtesy of Jeffrey R. Starke, MD.

35

Coronaviruses, Including SARS and MERS

Clinical Manifestations

Human coronaviruses (HCoVs) 229E, OC43, NL63, and HKU1 are associated most frequently with the common cold, an upper respiratory tract infection characterized by rhinorrhea, nasal congestion, sore throat, sneezing, and cough that can be associated with fever. Symptoms are self-limiting and typically peak on day 3 or 4 of illness. Human coronavirus infections can also be associated with acute otitis media or asthma exacerbations. Less frequently, they are associated with lower respiratory tract infections, including bronchiolitis, croup, and pneumonia, primarily in infants and immunocompromised children and adults.

SARS-CoV, the HCoV responsible for the 2002–2003 global outbreak of severe acute respiratory syndrome (SARS), was associated with more severe symptoms, although a spectrum of disease, including asymptomatic infections and mild disease, occurred. SARS-CoV disproportionately affected adults, who typically presented with fever, myalgia, headache, malaise, and chills followed by a nonproductive cough and dyspnea generally 5 to 7 days later. Approximately 25% of infected adults developed watery diarrhea. Twenty percent developed worsening respiratory distress requiring intubation and ventilation. The overall associated mortality rate was approximately 10%, with most deaths occurring in the third week of illness. The case-fatality rate in people older than 60 years approached 50%. Typical laboratory abnormalities included lymphopenia and increased lactate dehydrogenase and creatine kinase concentrations. Most had progressive unilateral or bilateral ill-defined airspace infiltrates on chest imaging. Pneumothoraces and other signs of barotrauma were common in critically ill patients receiving mechanical ventilation.

SARS-CoV infections in children are less severe than in adults; notably, no infant or child deaths from SARS-CoV infection were documented in the 2002–2003 global outbreak. Infants and children younger than 12 years who develop SARS typically present with fever, cough, and rhinorrhea. Associated lymphopenia is less severe, and radiographic changes are milder and generally resolve more quickly than in adolescents and adults. Adolescents who develop SARS have clinical courses more closely resembling those of adult disease, presenting with fever, myalgia, headache, and chills. They are also more likely to develop dyspnea, hypoxemia, and worsening chest radiographic findings.

MERS-CoV, the HCoV associated with Middle East respiratory syndrome (MERS), can also cause severe disease. MERS-CoV is associated with a severe respiratory illness similar to SARS-CoV, although a spectrum of disease, including asymptomatic infections and mild disease, can occur. Patients commonly present with fever, myalgia, chills, shortness of breath, and cough. Approximately 25% of patients also experience vomiting, diarrhea, or abdominal pain. Rapid deterioration of oxygenation with progressive unilateral or bilateral airspace infiltrates on chest imaging may follow, requiring mechanical ventilation. The case-fatality rate is high, estimated at nearly 50%. To date, most infections have been reported in male adults with comorbidities, such as diabetes, chronic renal disease, hypertension, and chronic cardiac disease.

Etiology

Coronaviruses are enveloped, nonsegmented, single-stranded, positive-sense RNA viruses named after their corona- or crownlike surface projections observed on electron microscopy that correspond to large surface spike proteins. Coronaviruses are classified in the Nidovirales order. Coronaviruses are host specific and can infect humans as well as a variety of different animals, causing diverse clinical syndromes. Four distinct genera have been described: *Alphacoronavirus*, *Betacoronavirus*, *Gammacoronavirus*, and *Deltacoronavirus*. Human coronaviruses 229E and NL63 belong to the genus *Alphacoronavirus;* HCoVs OC43 and HKU1 belong to lineage A of the genus *Betacoronavirus;* SARS-CoV belongs to lineage B of the genus *Betacoronavirus;* and MERS-CoV belongs to lineage C of the genus *Betacoronavirus.*

Epidemiology

Coronaviruses were first recognized as animal pathogens in the 1930s. Thirty years later, HCoVs 229E and OC43 were identified as human pathogens, along with other coronavirus strains that were not investigated further and for which little is known about their prevalence and associated disease syndromes. In 2003, SARS-CoV was identified as a novel virus responsible for the 2002–2003 global outbreak of SARS, which lasted for 9 months, caused 8,096 reported cases, and resulted in 774 deaths. No SARS-CoV infections have been reported worldwide since early 2004. Most experts believe SARS-CoV evolved from a natural reservoir of SARS-CoV–like viruses in bats through civet cats. Whether or not a large-scale reemergence of SARS will occur is unknown. Finding a novel HCoV sparked a renewed interest in HCoV research, and 2 years later, NL63 and HKU1 were identified as newly recognized HCoVs. Investigations have revealed that NL63 was present in archived human respiratory tract specimens as early as 1981 and HKU1 as early as 1995.

In 2012, MERS-CoV was identified as a novel virus associated with the death of a 60-year-old man from Saudi Arabia with acute pneumonia and renal failure. As of June 11, 2014, 699 laboratory-confirmed cases and 209 deaths had been reported. MERS-CoV is thought to have evolved from a natural reservoir of MERS-CoV–like viruses in bats. An animal source for MERS-CoV has not yet been determined, but recent studies demonstrated MERS-CoV genetic sequences in dromedary camels.

Human coronaviruses 229E, OC43, NL63, and HKU1 can be found worldwide. They cause most disease in the winter and spring months in temperate climates. Seroprevalence data for these HCoVs suggest exposure is common in early childhood, with approximately 90% of adults being seropositive for 229E, OC43, and NL63 and 60% being seropositive for HKU1. In contrast, SARS-CoV infection has not been detected in humans since early 2004. MERS-CoV has been reported in people who reside in or have traveled to the Middle East or who have had contact with a person with the infection from the Middle East, including travel-related cases in the United States. Human-to-human transmission, including clusters of cases, has been observed, but there is no evidence of sustained human-to-human transmission in the community.

The modes of transmission for 229E, OC43, NL63, and HKU1 have not been well studied. However, on the basis of studies of other respiratory tract viruses, it is likely transmission occurs primarily via a combination of droplet and direct and indirect contact spread. For SARS-CoV, studies suggest droplet and direct contact spread are likely the most common modes of transmission, although evidence of indirect contact and aerosol spread also exist. The modes of transmission for MERS-CoV are still being studied.

Human coronaviruses 229E and OC43 are most likely to be transmitted during the first few days of illness, when symptoms and respiratory viral loads are at their highest. Further study is needed to confirm that this holds true for the NL63 and HKU1 viruses. SARS-CoV is most likely to be transmitted during the second week of illness, when symptoms and respiratory viral loads peak. The peak communicable period or kinetics for MERS-CoV are not yet known.

Incubation Period

Human coronaviruses, 2 to 5 days; SARS-CoV, 2 to 10 days; MERS-CoV, 2 to 14 days.

Diagnostic Tests

The 2002–2003 SARS global outbreak garnered renewed interest in better understanding the etiology of respiratory tract infections, and some clinical laboratories have since started offering comprehensive respiratory molecular diagnostic testing for HCoVs using reverse transcriptase-polymerase chain reaction assays. Specimens obtained from the upper and lower respiratory tract are the most appropriate samples for HCoV detection. The yield from lower respiratory tract specimens is higher for SARS-CoV and MERS-CoV. Stool and serum samples are also frequently positive using reverse transcriptase-polymerase chain reaction assays in patients with SARS-CoV and have been positive in some patients with MERS-CoV. For 229E and OC43, specimens are most likely to be positive during the first few days of illness. The optimal timing of specimen collection for MERS-CoV is still being studied.

Serologic testing is a useful tool for diagnosis for SARS and MERS, although these tests are not available widely. Although acute and convalescent sera are optimal, a single serum specimen collected 2 or more weeks from symptom onset may help with the diagnosis of SARS or MERS because these infections are so rare. The CDC should be contacted for additional information on serologic testing.

Treatment

Infections attributable to HCoVs are generally treated with supportive care. SARS-CoV and MERS-CoV infections are more serious. Steroids, type 1 interferons, convalescent plasma, ribavirin, and lopinavir/ritonavir were all used clinically to treat patients with SARS, albeit without evidence of efficacy. In vitro data indicate that cyclosporin A and interferon alfa inhibits MERS-CoV replication. No treatment efficacy of antiviral agent for MERS-CoV has been demonstrated.

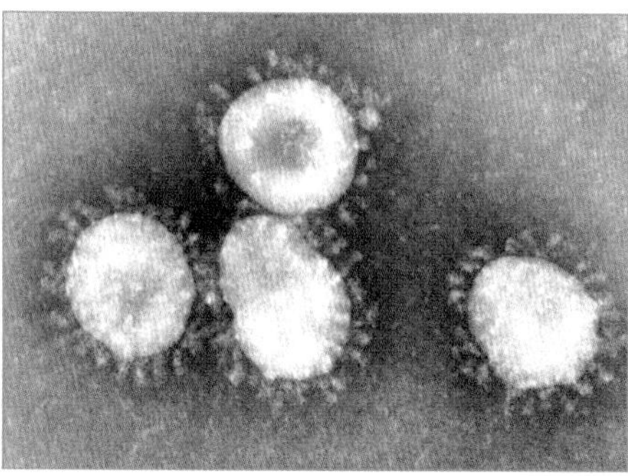

Image 35.1
Coronaviruses are a group of viruses that have a halo or crownlike (corona) appearance when viewed in an electron microscope. SARS-CoV was the etiologic agent of the 2003 severe acute respiratory syndrome (SARS) outbreak. Additional specimens are being tested to learn more about this coronavirus and its etiologic link with SARS. Courtesy of Centers for Disease Control and Prevention/Dr Fred Murphy.

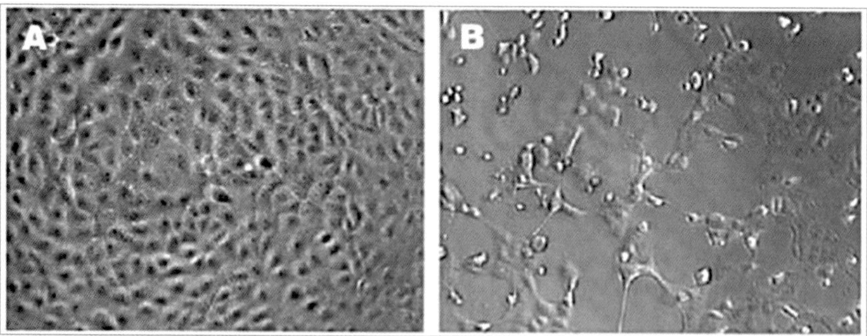

Image 35.2
Microscopic appearance of control (A) and infected (B) Vero E6 cells, demonstrating cytopathic effects. The cytopathic effect of SARS-CoV on Vero E6 was evident within 24 hours after infection. Courtesy of Centers for Disease Control and Prevention/*Emerging Infectious Diseases*.

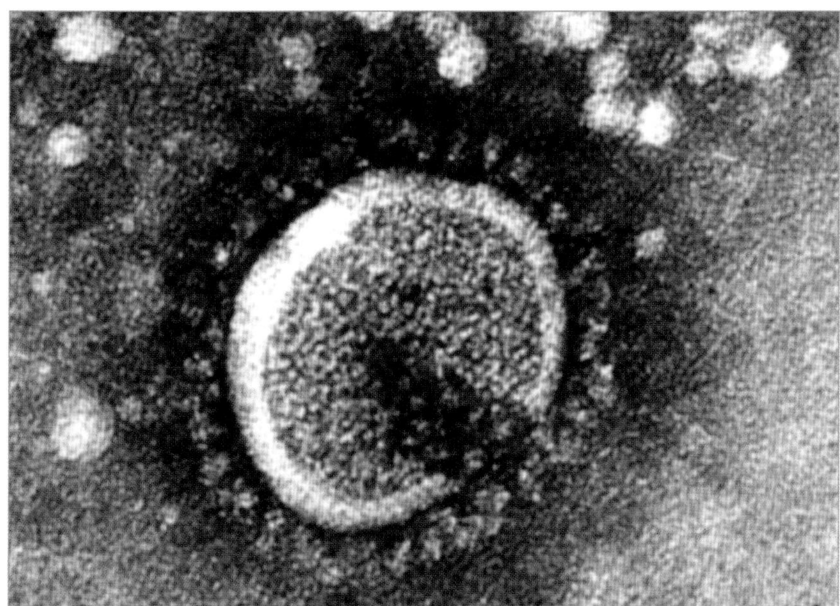

Image 35.3
Electron micrograph of a coronavirus. Pleomorphic virions average 100 nm in diameter and are covered with club-shaped knobs.

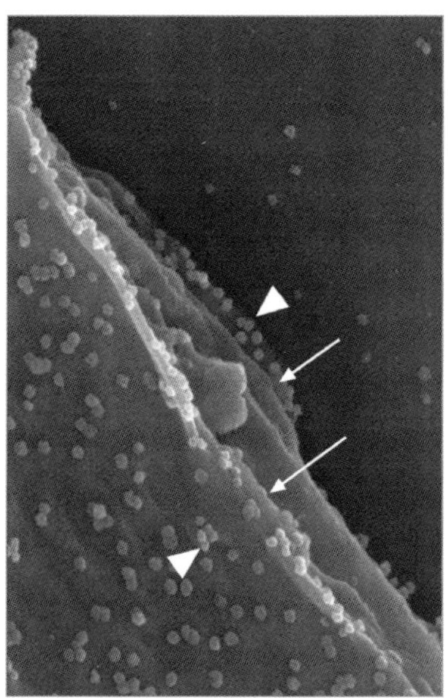

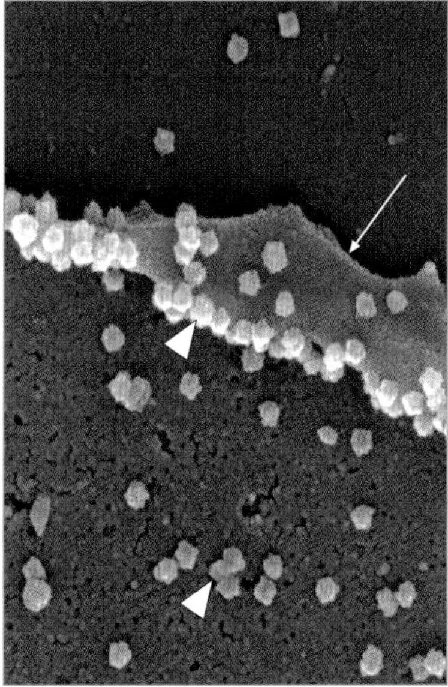

Image 35.4
This scanning electron micrograph (SEM) revealed the thickened, layered edge of severe acute respiratory syndrome–infected Vero E6 culture cells. The thickened edges of the infected cells were ruffled and appeared to comprise layers of folded plasma membranes. Note the layered cell edge (arrows) seen by SEM. Virus particles (arrowheads) are extruded from the layered surfaces. Courtesy of Centers for Disease Control and Prevention/Dr Mary Ng Mah Lee, National University of Singapore.

36

Cryptococcus neoformans and *Cryptococcus gattii* Infections

(Cryptococcosis)

Clinical Manifestations

Primary infection is acquired by inhalation of aerosolized *Cryptococcus* fungal elements found in contaminated soil and is often asymptomatic or mild. Pulmonary disease is characterized by cough, chest pain, and constitutional symptoms. Chest radiographs can reveal solitary or multiple masses; patchy, segmental, or lobar consolidation (often multifocal); or nodular or reticulonodular interstitial changes. Pulmonary cryptococcosis can present as acute respiratory distress syndrome and mimic pneumocystis pneumonia. Hematogenous dissemination to the central nervous system, bones, skin, and other sites can occur, is uncommon, and almost always occurs in children with defects in T lymphocyte–mediated immunity (eg, children with leukemia or lymphoma, congenital immunodeficiency, HIV infection, or AIDS; children taking corticosteroids; children who have undergone solid organ transplantation). Usually, several sites are infected, but manifestations of involvement at one site predominate. Cryptococcal meningitis, the most common and serious form of cryptococcal disease, often follows an indolent course. Clinical findings are characteristic of meningitis, meningoencephalitis, or space-occupying lesions but sometimes can manifest only as subtle, nonspecific findings such as fever, headache, or behavioral changes. Cryptococcal fungemia without apparent organ involvement occurs in patients with HIV infection but is rare in children.

Etiology

Although there are more than 30 species of *Cryptococcus*, only 2 species, *Cryptococcus neoformans* (var *neoformans* and var *grubii*) and *Cryptococcus gattii* are regarded as human pathogens.

Epidemiology

C neoformans var *neoformans* and *C neoformans* var *grubii* are isolated primarily from soil contaminated with pigeon or other bird droppings and cause most human infections, especially infections in immunocompromised hosts. *C neoformans* infects 5% to 10% of adults with AIDS, but infection is rare in HIV-infected children. *C gattii* (formerly *C neoformans* var *gattii*) is associated with trees and surrounding soil and has emerged as a pathogen producing a respiratory syndrome with or without neurologic findings in people from British Columbia, Canada, the Pacific Northwest region of the United States, and, occasionally, other regions of the United States. A high frequency of disease has also been reported in Aboriginal people in Australia and in the central province of Papua New Guinea. *C gattii* causes disease in immunocompetent and immunocompromised people, including children. Person-to-person transmission does not occur.

Incubation Period

C neoformans, unknown; *C gattii,* 8 weeks to 13 months.

Diagnostic Tests

Definitive diagnosis requires isolation of the organism from body fluid or tissue specimens. Blood should be cultured by lysis-centrifugation. Differentiation between *C neoformans* and *C gattii* can be made by the use of the selective medium l-canavanine glycine bromothymol blue agar. Sabouraud dextrose agar is useful for isolation of *Cryptococcus* organisms from sputum, bronchopulmonary lavage, tissue, or cerebrospinal fluid (CSF) specimens. In refractory or relapse cases, susceptibility testing can be helpful, although antifungal resistance is uncommon. A large quantity of CSF is needed to recover the organism because CSF may contain only a few organisms. Cerebrospinal fluid cell count and protein and glucose concentrations can be normal. Encapsulated yeast cells can be visualized using India ink or other stains of CSF and bronchoalveolar lavage specimens, but this method has limited sensitivity. Focal pulmonary or skin lesions can be biopsied for fungal staining and culture.

The latex agglutination test, lateral flow assay, and enzyme immunoassay for detection of cryptococcal capsular polysaccharide antigen in CSF are excellent rapid diagnostic tests for those with suspected meningitis. Antigen is detected in CSF or serum specimens from more than 98% of patients with cryptococcal meningitis; however, antigen test results can be falsely negative when antigen concentrations are low or very high (prozone effect), if infection is caused by unencapsulated strains, or if the patient is less severely immunocompromised.

Treatment

Amphotericin B deoxycholate in combination with oral flucytosine is indicated as initial therapy for patients with meningeal and other serious cryptococcal infections. Serum flucytosine concentrations should be maintained between 30 and 80 mcg/mL. Patients with meningitis should receive combination therapy for at least 2 weeks followed by consolidation therapy with fluconazole for a minimum of 8 weeks or until CSF culture is sterile. Alternatively, the amphotericin B deoxycholate and flucytosine combination can be continued for 6 to 10 weeks. Lipid formulations of amphotericin B can be used as a substitute for amphotericin B deoxycholate in children with renal impairment. If flucytosine cannot be administered, amphotericin B alone is an acceptable alternative and is administered for 4 to 6 weeks. A lumbar puncture should be performed after 2 weeks of therapy to document microbiologic clearance. The 20% to 40% of patients in whom culture result is positive after 2 weeks of therapy will require a more prolonged treatment course. When infection is refractory to systemic therapy, intraventricular amphotericin B can be administered. Monitoring of serum cryptococcal antigen is not useful to monitor response to therapy in patients with cryptococcal meningitis. Patients with less severe disease can be treated with fluconazole or itraconazole, but data on use of these drugs for children with *C neoformans* infection are limited. Another potential treatment option for HIV-infected patients with less severe disease or patients in whom amphotericin B treatment is not possible is combination therapy with fluconazole and flucytosine. The combination of fluconazole and flucytosine has superior efficacy compared with fluconazole alone. Echinocandins are not active against cryptococcal infections and should not be used.

Increased intracranial pressure occurs frequently despite microbiologic response and is often associated with clinical deterioration. Significant elevation of intracranial pressure is a major source of morbidity and should be managed with frequent repeated lumbar punctures or placement of a lumbar drain.

Children with HIV infection who have completed initial therapy for cryptococcosis should receive long-term suppressive therapy with fluconazole. Oral itraconazole daily or amphotericin B deoxycholate, 1 to 3 times weekly, are alternatives. Discontinuing chronic suppressive therapy for cryptococcosis (after 1 year or longer of secondary prophylaxis) can be considered in asymptomatic children 6 years or older who are receiving antiretroviral therapy, have sustained (≥6 months) increases in $CD4^+$ T lymphocyte counts to 100 cells/mm^3 or greater, and have an undetectable viral load for at least 3 months. Most experts would not discontinue secondary prophylaxis for patients younger than 6 years.

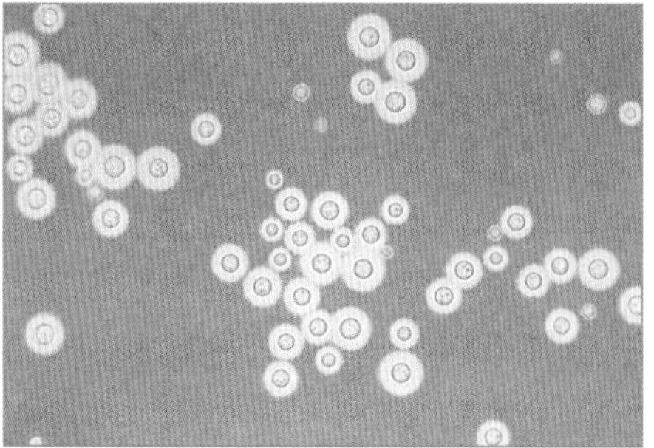

Image 36.1
This photomicrograph depicts *Cryptococcus neoformans* using a light India ink staining preparation. Courtesy of Centers for Disease Control and Prevention/Dr Leanor Haley.

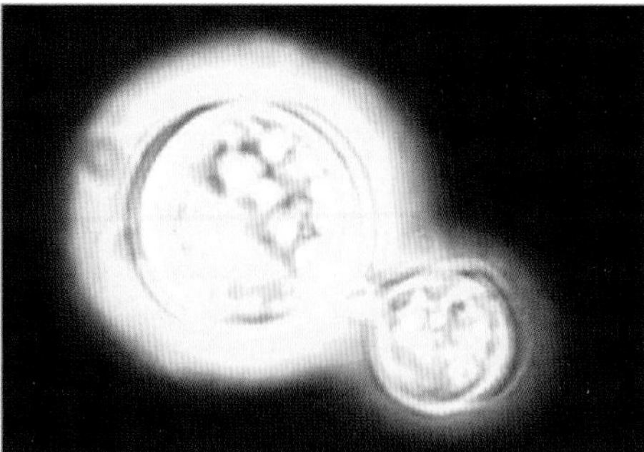

Image 36.2
Cryptococcus neoformans, thin-walled encapsulated yeast in cerebrospinal fluid (India ink preparation, original magnification of cerebrospinal fluid x450).

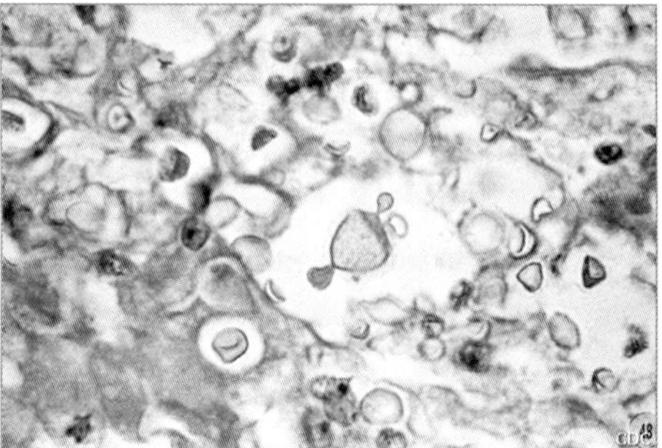

Image 36.3
This photomicrograph depicted numbers of *Cryptococcus neoformans* fungi, the etiologic agents responsible for the disease cryptococcosis. This slide was created from a lung specimen and stained using the hematoxylin-eosin staining technique. Courtesy of Centers for Disease Control and Prevention/Lucille K. Georg, MD.

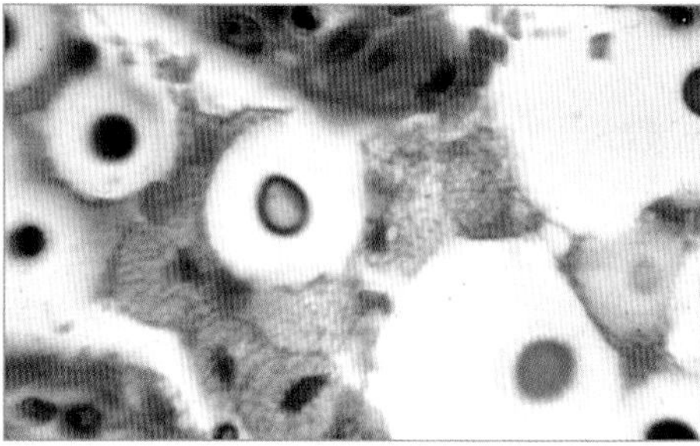

Image 36.4
Cryptococcosis of the liver (original magnification x810) in an immunodeficient patient with disseminated disease. The mucinous capsules are prominent. Courtesy of Edgar O. Ledbetter, MD, FAAP.

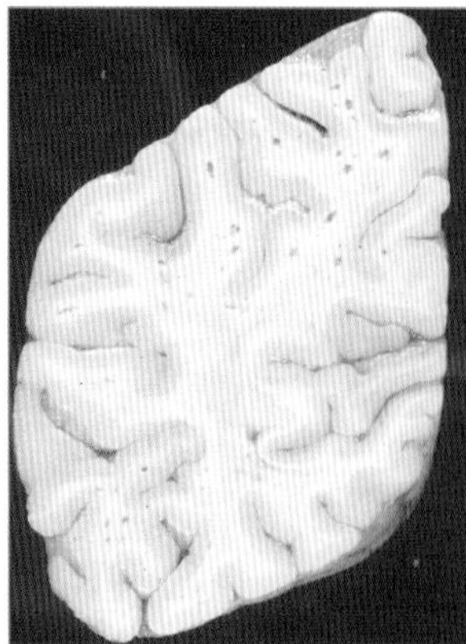

Image 36.5
Cryptococcus meningitis. Cystic lesions resulting from accumulation of organisms in perivascular spaces. Courtesy of Dimitris P. Agamanolis, MD.

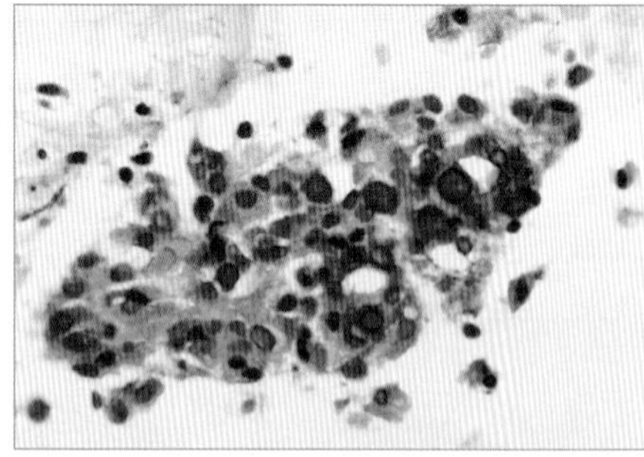

Image 36.6
This micrograph depicts the histopathologic changes associated with cryptococcosis of the lung using mucicarmine stain. Cryptococcosis, caused by the fungal pathogen *Cryptococcus neoformans,* is transmitted through inhalation of airborne yeast cells or biospores. At risk are those who are immunocompromised, especially those with HIV infection. Courtesy of Centers for Disease Control and Prevention/Dr Leanor Haley.

37

Cryptosporidiosis

Clinical Manifestations

Frequent, nonbloody, watery diarrhea is the most common manifestation of cryptosporidiosis, although infection can be asymptomatic. Other symptoms include abdominal cramps, fatigue, fever, vomiting, anorexia, and weight loss. In infected immunocompetent adults and children, diarrheal illness is self-limited, usually lasting 2 to 3 weeks. Infected immunocompromised hosts, such as children with a solid organ transplant or advanced HIV disease, can experience profuse diarrhea lasting weeks to months; this can lead to malnutrition and wasting. Delay in diagnosis and treatment can be associated with death. Elevated tacrolimus concentrations have been reported in solid organ transplant patients, thought to be related to altered drug metabolism in the small intestine and resulting in acute kidney injury. Extraintestinal cryptosporidiosis (ie, disease in the lungs, biliary tract, or, rarely, pancreas) has been reported in people who are immunocompromised.

Etiology

Cryptosporidium species are oocyst-forming coccidian protozoa. Oocysts are excreted in feces of an infected host and transmitted via the fecal-oral route. *Cryptosporidium hominis,* which predominantly infects people, and *Cryptosporidium parvum,* which infects people, preweaned calves, and other mammals, are the primary *Cryptosporidium* species that infect humans.

Epidemiology

Extensive waterborne disease outbreaks have been associated with contamination of drinking water and recreational water (eg, swimming pools, lakes, interactive fountains). The incidence of cryptosporidiosis has been increasing in the United States since 2005; the total (confirmed and probable) number of annually reported cases in 2012 was 7,956. In children, the incidence of cryptosporidiosis is greatest during summer and early fall, corresponding to the outdoor swimming season. Because oocysts are extremely chlorine tolerant, multistep treatment processes are often used to remove (eg, filter) and inactivate (eg, ultraviolet treatment) oocysts to protect public drinking water supplies. Typical filtration systems used for swimming pools are only partially effective in removing oocysts from contaminated water. As a result, *Cryptosporidium* species have become the leading cause of recreational water-associated outbreaks, being associated with 69% of 35 treated recreational water-associated outbreaks with identified infectious causes.

In addition to waterborne transmission, humans can acquire infections from livestock; from animals found in petting zoos, particularly preweaned calves; or from pets. Person-to-person transmission occurs as well and can cause outbreaks in child care centers, in which up to 70% of attendees reportedly have been infected. *Cryptosporidium* species can also cause traveler's diarrhea.

Incubation Period

Usually 3 to 14 days, with oocyst shedding ceasing in immunocompetent people 2 weeks after symptom resolution. In immunocompromised people, oocyst shedding can continue for months.

Diagnostic Tests

Routine laboratory examination of stool for ova and parasites might not include testing for *Cryptosporidium* species, so testing for the organism should be requested specifically. The direct immunofluorescent antibody method for detection of oocysts in stool is the current test of choice for diagnosis of cryptosporidiosis. The detection of oocysts on microscopic examination of stool specimens is also diagnostic. The formalin ethyl acetate stool concentration method is recommended before staining the stool specimen with a modified Kinyoun acid-fast stain. Oocysts generally are small (4–6 µm in diameter). Enzyme immunoassays and immune chromatographic tests (point-of-care rapid tests) for detecting antigen in stool are available commercially, but confirmation of results may be indicated. Because shedding can be intermittent, at least 3 stool specimens collected on separate days should be examined before considering test results to be negative. Organisms can also be identified in intestinal biopsy tissue or sampling of intestinal fluid.

Treatment

Generally, immunocompetent people need no specific therapy. A 3-day course of nitazoxanide oral suspension has been approved by the US Food and Drug Administration for treatment of all people 1 year and older with diarrhea associated with cryptosporidiosis. The nitazoxanide dose for healthy children not infected with HIV is based on age. The appropriate treatment of cryptosporidiosis in children who are solid organ transplant recipients is not known, but longer courses of nitazoxanide (generally >14 days) have been recommended. In HIV-infected patients, improvement in $CD4^+$ T lymphocyte count associated with antiretroviral therapy can lead to symptom resolution and cessation of oocyst shedding. For this reason, administration of combination antiretroviral therapy is the primary treatment for cryptosporidiosis in patients with HIV infection. Given the seriousness of this infection in immunocompromised individuals, use of nitazoxanide can be considered in immunocompromised HIV-infected children in conjunction with combination antiretroviral therapy for immune restoration. The recommended nitazoxanide dosing is the same as for immunocompetent people. Paromomycin, or a combination of paromomycin and azithromycin, might be effective, but few data regarding efficacy are available.

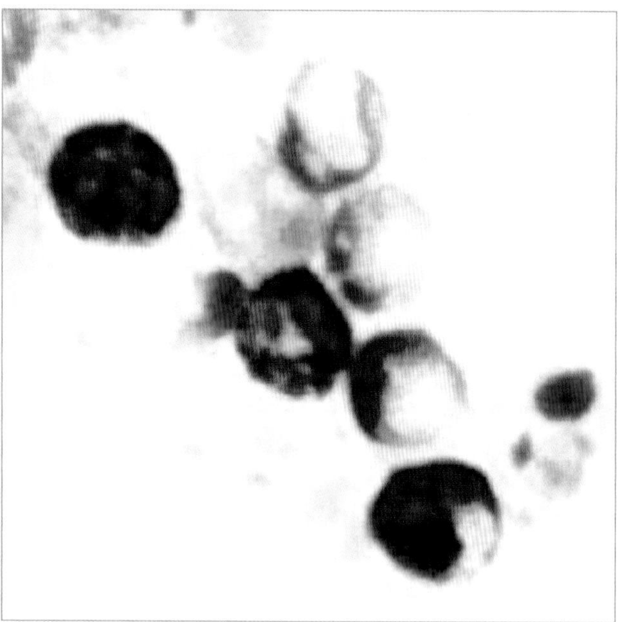

Image 37.1
Oocysts of *Cryptosporidium parvum* (modified Kinyoun acid-fast stain). Monoclonal antibody-based stain for oocytes in stool and an enzyme immunoassay for detecting antigen in stool are available commercially. This image shows that the staining can be variable. In particular, infections that are resolving can be accompanied by increasing numbers of nonacid-fast oocysts or "ghosts." Courtesy of Centers for Disease Control and Prevention.

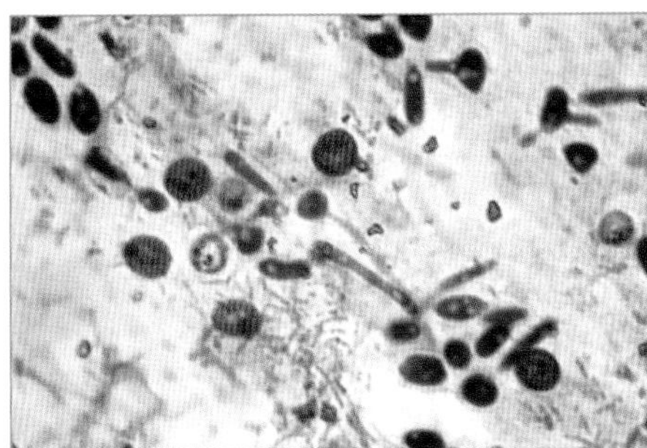

Image 37.2
This micrograph of a direct fecal smear is stained to detect *Cryptosporidium* species, an intracellular protozoan parasite. Using a modified cold Kinyoun acid-fast staining technique and under an oil immersion lens, *Cryptosporidium* species oocysts, which are acid-fast, stain red, and yeast cells, which are not acid-fast, stain green. Ma P, Soave R. Three-step stool examination for cryptosporidiosis in 10 homosexual men with protracted watery diarrhea. *J Infect Dis.* 1983;147(5):824–828. Reprinted with permission from Oxford University Press.

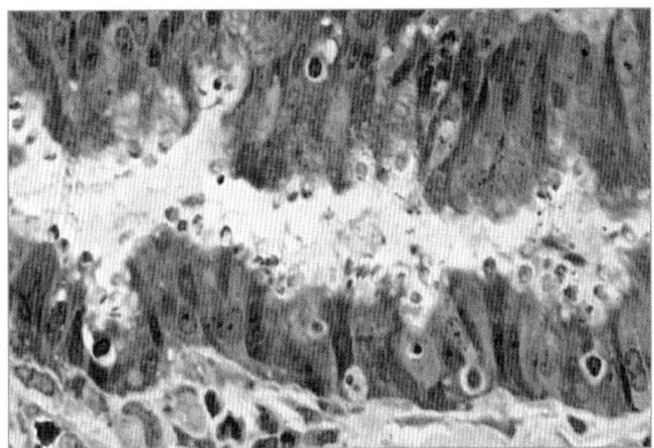

Image 37.3
Histopathology of cryptosporidiosis, intestine. Plastic-embedded, toluidine blue-stained section shows numerous *Cryptosporidium* organisms at luminal surfaces of epithelial cells. Courtesy of Centers for Disease Control and Prevention/Dr Edwin P. Ewing Jr.

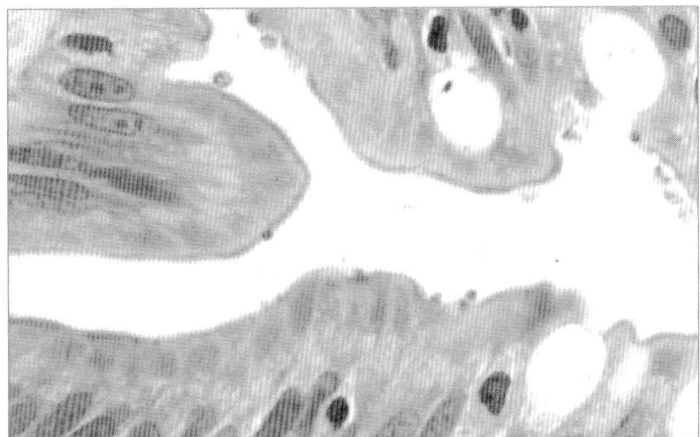

Image 37.4
Cryptosporidium, a spore-forming coccidian protozoan, can be seen on the brush border of intestinal mucosa. *Cryptosporidium* does not invade below the epithelial layer of the mucosa, so fecal leukocytes are absent.

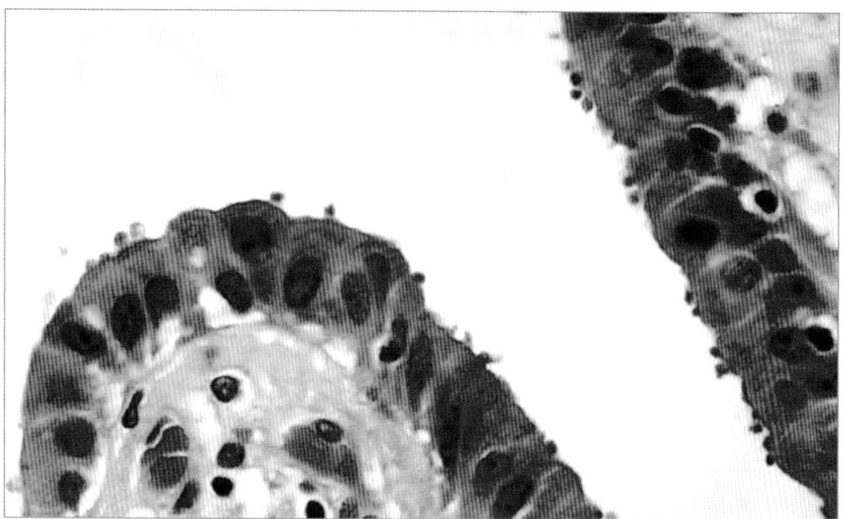

Image 37.5
Cryptosporidiosis of gallbladder in a patient with AIDS. Histopathologic features of gallbladder epithelium include numerous *Cryptosporidium* organisms along luminal surfaces of epithelial cells. Courtesy of Centers for Disease Control and Prevention/Dr Edwin P. Ewing Jr.

CRYPTOSPORIDIOSIS. Incidence* — United States and U.S. territories, 2012

N DC
NYC
N AS
CNMI
GU
N PR
N VI

≤1.50 | >1.51–3.00 | >3.01–4.50 | >4.51–6.00 | ≥6.01

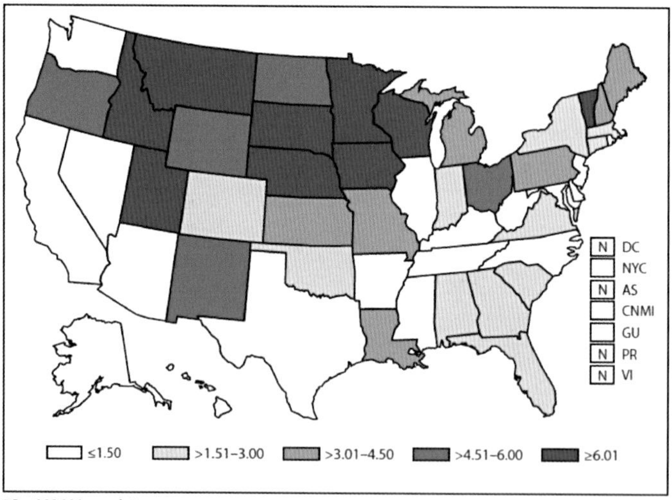

* Per 100,000 population.

Cryptosporidiosis is widespread geographically in the United States. Although incidence appears to be consistently higher in certain states, differences in reported incidence among states might reflect differences in risk factors; the number of cases associated with outbreaks; or in the capacity to detect, investigate, and report cases. Incidence categories have been modified to reflect the recent increase in incidence.

Image 37.6
Incidence—United States and US Territories, 2012. Courtesy of *Morbidity and Mortality Weekly Report.*

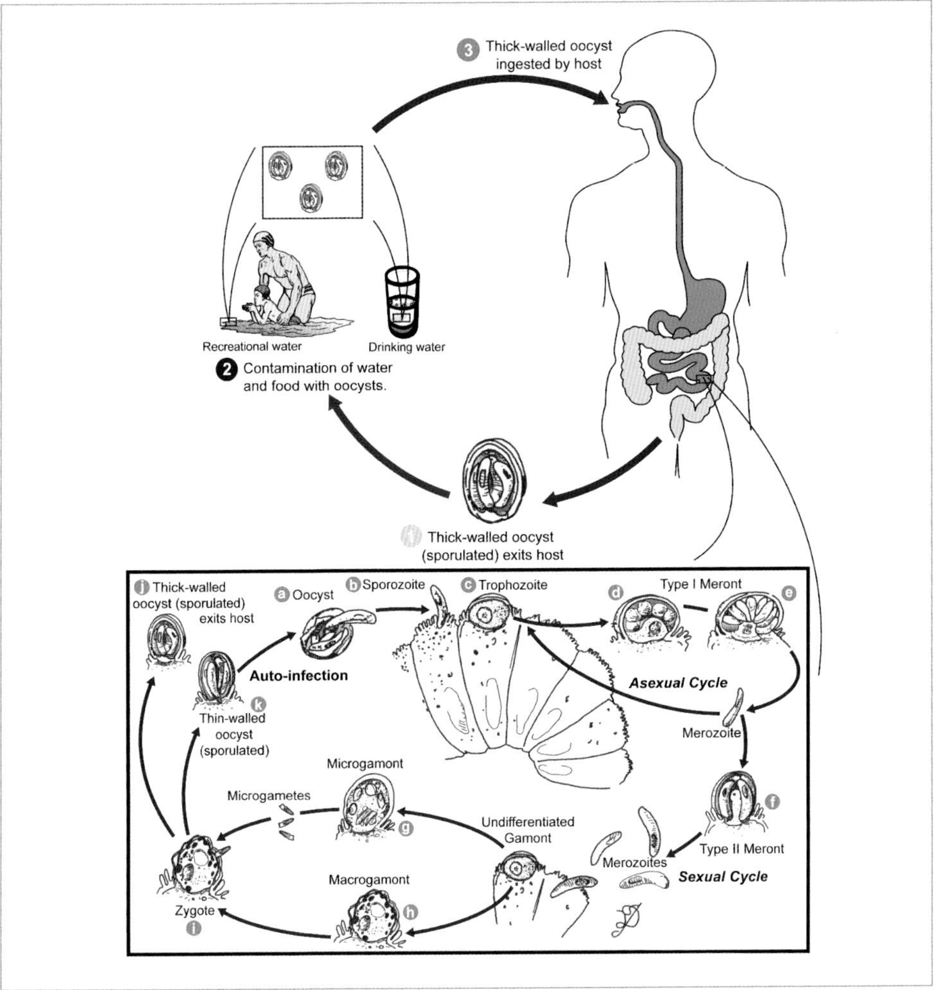

Image 37.7

Life cycle of *Cryptosporidium.* Sporulated oocysts, containing 4 sporozoites, are excreted by the infected host through feces and possibly other routes, such as respiratory secretions (1). Transmission of *Cryptosporidium parvum* occurs mainly through contact with contaminated water (eg, drinking or recreational water). Occasionally, food sources, such as chicken salad, may serve as vehicles for transmission. Many outbreaks in the United States have occurred in water parks, community swimming pools, and child care centers. Zoonotic transmission of *C parvum* occurs through exposure to infected animals or exposure to water contaminated by feces of infected animals (2). Following ingestion (and possibly inhalation) by a suitable host (3), excystation (a) occurs. The sporozoites are released and parasitize epithelial cells (b, c) of the gastrointestinal tract or other tissues. In these cells, the parasites undergo asexual multiplication (schizogony or merogony) (d, e, f) and then sexual multiplication (gametogony), producing microgamonts (male) (g) and macrogamonts (female) (h). On fertilization of the macrogamonts by the microgametes (i), oocysts (j, k) develop that sporulate in the infected host. Two different types of oocysts are produced: the thick-walled, which is commonly excreted from the host (j), and the thin-walled (k), which is primarily involved in autoinfection. Oocysts are infective on excretion, thus permitting direct and immediate fecal-oral transmission. Note that oocysts of *Cyclospora cayetanensis*, another important coccidian parasite, are unsporulated at the time of excretion and do not become infective until sporulation is completed. Refer to the life cycle of *C cayetanensis* for further details. Courtesy of Centers for Disease Control and Prevention/Alexander J. da Silva, PhD/Melanie Moser.

38

Cutaneous Larva Migrans

Clinical Manifestations

Nematode larvae produce pruritic, reddish papules at the site of skin entry, a condition referred to as creeping eruption. As the larvae migrate through skin, advancing several millimeters to a few centimeters a day, intensely pruritic serpiginous tracks or bullae are formed. This condition is most often caused by larvae of the dog and cat hookworm *Ancylostoma braziliense* but can be caused by other nematodes, including *Strongyloides* and human hookworm species. Larval activity can continue for several weeks or months, but the infection is self-limiting. Cutaneous larva migrans is a clinical diagnosis based on advancing serpiginous tracks in the skin with associated intense pruritus. Rarely, in infections with certain species of parasites, larvae may penetrate deeper tissues and cause pneumonitis (Löffler syndrome), which can be severe. Occasionally, the larvae of *Ancylostoma caninum* can reach the intestine and cause eosinophilic enteritis.

Etiology

Infective larvae of cat and dog hookworms (ie, *A braziliense* and *A caninum*) are the usual causes. Other skin-penetrating nematodes are occasional causes.

Epidemiology

Cutaneous larva migrans is a disease of children, utility workers, gardeners, sunbathers, and others who come in contact with soil contaminated with cat and dog feces. In the United States, the disease is most prevalent in the Southeast. Cases in the United States can also be imported by travelers returning from tropical and subtropical areas.

Diagnostic Tests

The diagnosis is made clinically, and biopsies typically are not indicated. Biopsy specimens typically demonstrate an eosinophilic inflammatory infiltrate, but the migrating parasite is not visualized. Eosinophilia and increased immunoglobulin E serum concentrations occur in some cases. Larvae have been detected in sputum and gastric washings in patients with pneumonitis. Enzyme immunoassay or Western blot analysis using antigens of *A caninum* have been developed in research laboratories, but these assays are not available for routine diagnostic use.

Treatment

The disease is usually self-limited, with spontaneous cure after several weeks or months. Orally administered albendazole or ivermectin is the recommended therapy.

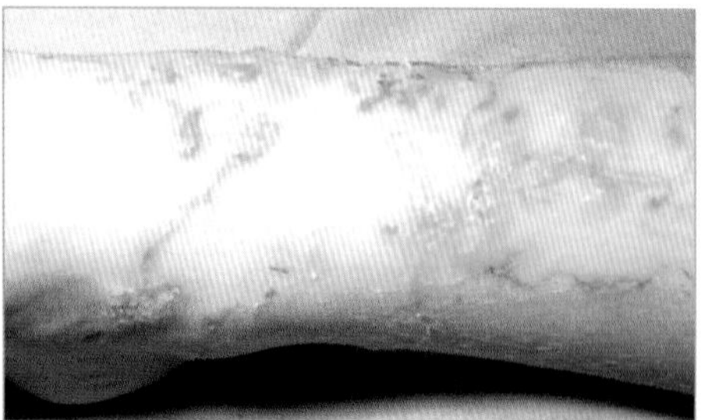

Image 38.1
Cutaneous larva migrans lesions on lower leg (caused by hookworm larvae of *Ancylostoma braziliense* and *Ancylostoma caninum*).

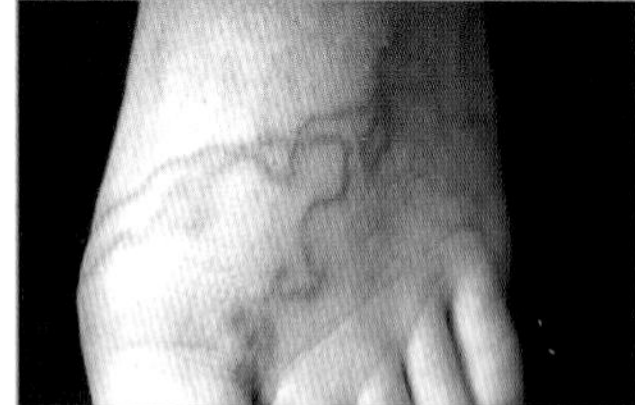

Image 38.2
Cutaneous larva migrans lesions of the foot of a 10-year-old girl. In the United States, this dog and cat hookworm infection is most commonly seen in the Southeast. These raised, serpiginous, pruritic, migrating eruptions may extend rapidly. Copyright Gary Williams, MD.

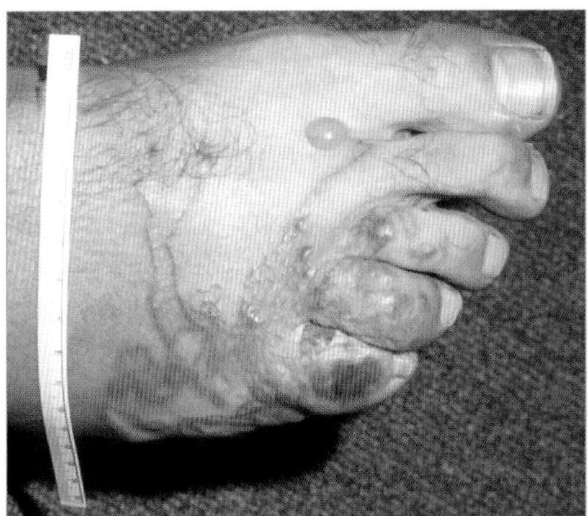

Image 38.3
Cutaneous larva migrans infection of the foot in an adolescent male. Courtesy of George Nankervis, MD.

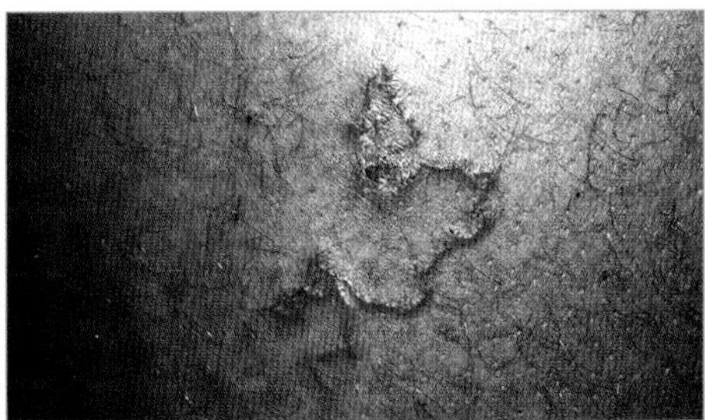

Image 38.4
Adult who noted a migrating skin lesion on left thigh for 2 weeks. Copyright Larry I. Corman.

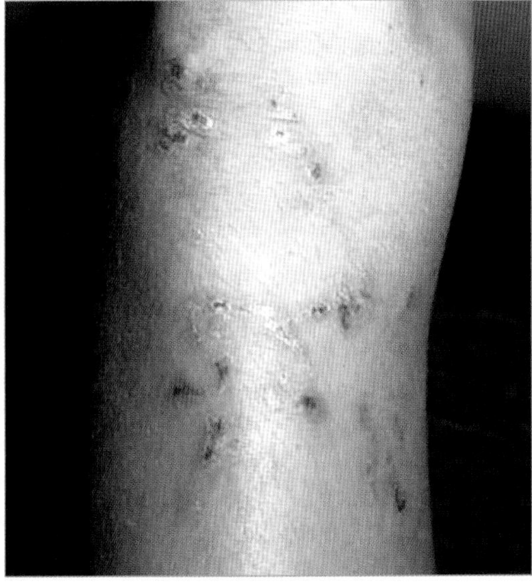

Image 38.5
Cutaneous larva migrans 48 hours after treatment. Orally administered albendazole or ivermectin is the recommended therapy.

39

Cyclosporiasis

Clinical Manifestations

Watery diarrhea is the most common symptom of cyclosporiasis; diarrhea can be profuse and protracted. Anorexia, nausea, vomiting, substantial weight loss, flatulence, abdominal cramping, myalgia, and prolonged fatigue can occur. Low-grade fever occurs in approximately 50% of patients. Biliary tract disease has been reported. Infection is usually self-limited, but untreated people may have remitting, relapsing symptoms for weeks to months. Asymptomatic infection has been most commonly documented in settings where cyclosporiasis is endemic.

Etiology

Cyclospora cayetanensis is a coccidian protozoan; oocysts (rather than cysts) are passed in stools.

Epidemiology

C cayetanensis is known to be endemic in many resource-limited countries and has been reported as a cause of traveler's diarrhea. Food- and waterborne outbreaks have been reported. Most outbreaks in the United States and Canada have been associated with consumption of imported fresh produce. Humans are the only known hosts for *C cayetanensis*. Direct person-to-person transmission is unlikely because excreted oocysts take days to weeks under favorable environmental conditions to sporulate and become infective. The oocysts are resistant to most disinfectants used in food and water processing and can remain viable for prolonged periods in cool, moist environments.

Incubation Period

Typically 1 week (range 2–14 days).

Diagnostic Tests

Diagnosis is made by identification of oocysts (8–10 µm in diameter) in stool, intestinal fluid/aspirate, or intestinal biopsy specimens. Oocysts may be shed at low levels, even by people with profuse diarrhea. This makes critical repeated stool examinations, sensitive recovery methods (eg, concentration procedures), and detection methods that highlight the organism. Oocysts are autofluorescent and are variably acid fast after modified acid fast staining of stool specimens.

Treatment

Trimethoprim-sulfamethoxazole, typically for 7 to 10 days, is the drug of choice. People infected with HIV may need long-term maintenance therapy.

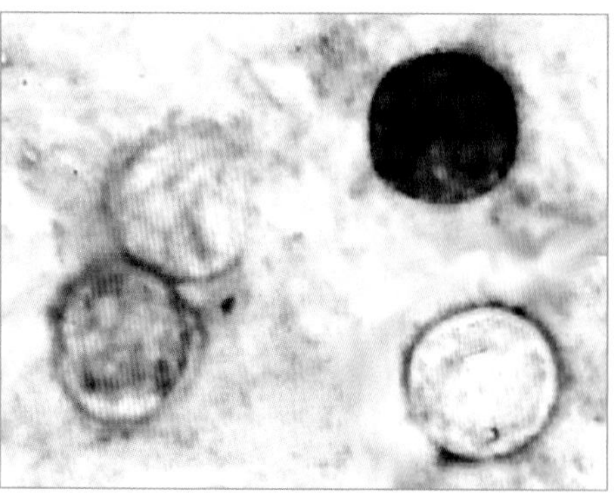

Image 39.1
Four *Cyclospora* oocysts from fresh stool fixed in 10% formalin (acid-fast stain). Compared with wet mount preparations, the oocysts are less perfectly round and have a wrinkled appearance. Most important, the staining is variable among the 4 oocysts. Courtesy of Centers for Disease Control and Prevention.

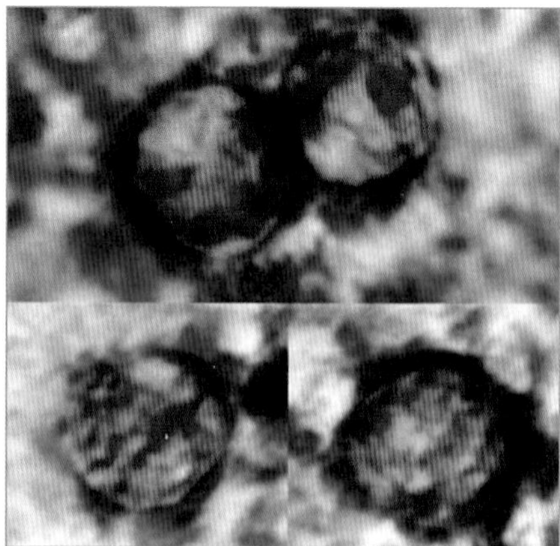

Image 39.2
Four *Cyclospora* oocysts from fresh stool fixed in 10% formalin and stained with safranin, showing the uniform staining of oocysts by this method. Courtesy of Centers for Disease Control and Prevention.

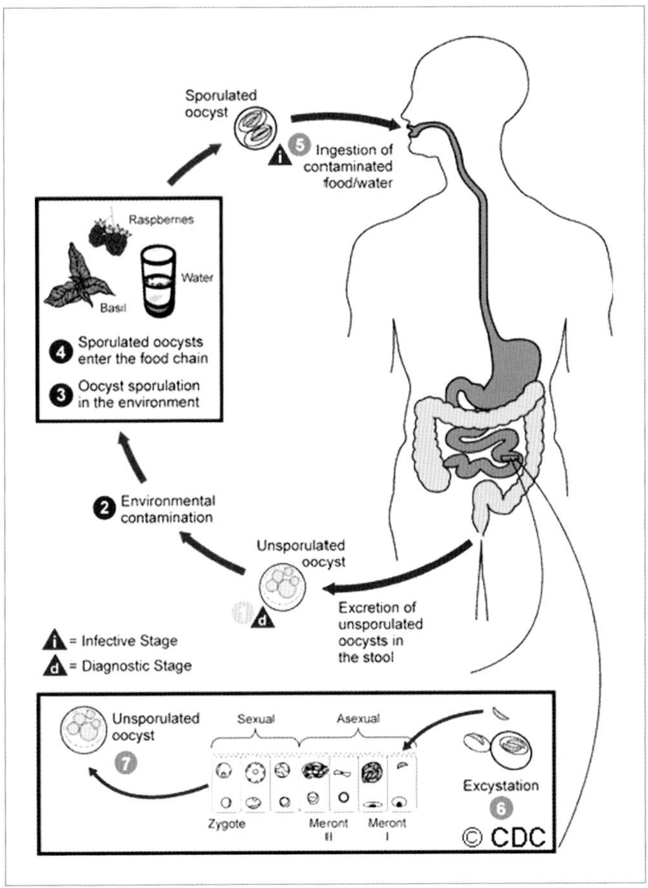

Image 39.3

Cyclospora cayetanensis. When freshly passed in stools, the oocyst is not infective (1) (thus, direct fecal-oral transmission cannot occur; this differentiates *Cyclospora* from another important coccidian parasite, *Cryptosporidium*). In the environment (2), sporulation occurs after days or weeks at temperatures between 22°C and 32°C (71.6°F–89.6°F), resulting in division of the sporont into 2 sporocysts, each containing 2 elongate sporozoites (3). Fresh produce and water can serve as vehicles for transmission (4) and the sporulated oocysts are ingested (in contaminated food or water) (5). The oocysts excyst in the gastrointestinal tract, freeing the sporozoites which invade the epithelial cells of the small intestine (6). Inside the cells, they undergo asexual multiplication and sexual development to mature into oocysts, which will be shed in stools (7). The potential mechanisms of contamination of food and water are still under investigation. Some of elements of this figure were created based on an illustration by Ortega YR, Sterling CR, Gilman RH. *Cyclospora cayetanensis. Adv Parasitol.* 1998;40:399–418. Courtesy of Centers for Disease Control and Prevention.

40

Cytomegalovirus Infection

Clinical Manifestations

Manifestations of acquired human cytomegalovirus (CMV) infection vary with age and host immunocompetence. Asymptomatic infections are the most common, particularly in children. An infectious mononucleosis-like syndrome with prolonged fever and mild hepatitis, occurring in the absence of heterophile antibody production ("monospot negative"), can occur in adolescents and adults. Pneumonia, colitis, retinitis, and a syndrome characterized by fever, thrombocytopenia, leukopenia, and mild hepatitis can occur in immunocompromised hosts, including people receiving treatment for malignant neoplasms, people infected with HIV, and people receiving immunosuppressive therapy for organ or hematopoietic stem cell transplantation. Less commonly, patients treated with biologic response can exhibit CMV end-organ disease, such as retinitis and hepatitis.

Congenital infection has a spectrum of clinical manifestations but usually is not evident at birth ("clinically silent" congenital CMV infection). Approximately 10% of neonates with congenital CMV infection exhibit clinical findings that are evident at birth (congenital CMV disease), with manifestations including intrauterine growth restriction, jaundice, purpura, hepatosplenomegaly, microcephaly, intracerebral (typically periventricular) calcifications, and retinitis; developmental delays are common among these neonates in later infancy and early childhood. Death attributable to congenital CMV is estimated to occur in 3% to 10% of neonates with congenital disease. Sensorineural hearing loss (SNHL) is the most common sequela following congenital CMV infection, with SNHL occurring in up to 50% of children with congenital disease at birth and up to 15% of those with clinically silent CMV infection. Congenital CMV infection is the leading nongenetic cause of SNHL in children in the United States. Progressive SNHL can occur following symptomatic or asymptomatic congenital CMV infection, with 50% of affected children continuing to have further deterioration (progression) of their hearing loss. Between 55% and 75% of clinically apparent and clinically silent newborns, respectively, who ultimately develop congenital CMV-associated SNHL will not have hearing loss detectable within the first month of life, illustrating the high frequency of late-onset SNHL in these children. For this reason, targeted CMV testing of neonates who fail their universal newborn hearing screen will not detect most neonates who are at risk of CMV-associated hearing loss. Approximately 20% of all hearing loss at birth and 25% of all hearing loss at 4 years of age are attributable to congenital CMV infection. As such, all children with congenital CMV infection should be regularly evaluated for early detection and intervention as appropriate.

Infection acquired from maternal cervical secretions during the intrapartum period, or in the postpartum period from human milk, is usually not associated with clinical illness in term neonates. In preterm neonates, however, postpartum infection resulting from human milk or from transfusion from CMV-seropositive donors has been associated with systemic infections, including hepatitis, interstitial pneumonia, and hematologic abnormalities, including thrombocytopenia and leukopenia, and a viral sepsis syndrome.

Etiology

Human CMV, also known as human herpesvirus 5, is a double-stranded DNA virus and a member of the herpesvirus family (Herpesviridae), β-herpesvirus subfamily (Betaherpesvirinae), and *Cytomegalovirus* genus.

Epidemiology

Cytomegalovirus is highly species specific, and only human CMV has been shown to infect humans and cause disease. The virus is ubiquitous and has numerous strain types (exhibits extensive genetic diversity). Transmission occurs horizontally (by direct person-to-person contact with virus-containing secretions), vertically (from mother to neonate before, during, or after birth), and via transfusions of blood, platelets, and white blood cells from infected donors. Cytomegalovirus can also be transmitted with organ or hematopoietic stem cell transplantation. Infections have no seasonal predilection. Cytomegalovirus persists in latent form after a primary infection, and intermittent virus shedding and symptomatic infection can occur throughout the lifetime of the infected person, particularly under conditions of immunosuppression. Reinfection with other strains of CMV can occur in seropositive hosts.

Horizontal transmission is probably the result of exposure to saliva and genital secretions from infected individuals, but contact with infected urine can also have a role. Spread of CMV in households and child care centers is well documented. Excretion rates from urine or saliva in children 1 to 3 years of age who attend child care centers usually range from 30% to 40% but can be as high as 70%. These children frequently excrete high quantities of virus. Young children can transmit CMV to their parents, including mothers who may be pregnant, and other caregivers, including child care staff. In adolescents and adults, sexual transmission occurs, as evidenced by detection of virus in seminal and cervical fluids. As such, CMV is considered to be a sexually transmitted infection.

Healthy cytomegalovirus-seropositive people have latent CMV in their leukocytes and tissues; hence, blood transfusions and organ transplantation can result in transmission. Severe CMV disease following transfusion or organ transplantation is more likely to occur if the recipient is immunosuppressed and CMV-seronegative or is a preterm neonate. In contrast, among nonautologous hematopoietic stem cell transplant recipients, CMV-seropositive recipients who receive transplants from seronegative donors are at greatest risk of disease when exposed to CMV after transplant, perhaps secondary to the failure of transplanted graft to provide immunity to the recipient. Latent CMV can reactivate in immunosuppressed people and result in disease if immunosuppression is severe (eg, patients with AIDS, solid organ or hematopoietic stem cell transplant recipients).

Vertical transmission of CMV to a neonate occurs in one of the following periods: in utero by transplacental passage of maternal bloodborne virus, at birth by passage through an infected maternal genital tract, or postnatally by ingestion of CMV-positive human milk or by transfusion. Between 0.5% and 1% of all liveborn neonates are infected in utero and excrete CMV at birth, making this the most common congenital viral infection in the United States. In utero fetal infection can occur in women with no preexisting CMV immunity (primary maternal infection) or in women with preexisting antibody to CMV (nonprimary maternal infection) by acquisition of a different viral strain during pregnancy or by reactivation of an existing maternal infection. Congenital infection and associated sequelae can occur irrespective of the trimester of pregnancy when the mother is infected, but severe sequelae are more commonly associated with primary maternal infection acquired during the first half of gestation. Damaging fetal infections following nonprimary maternal infection have been reported, and acquisition of a different viral strain during pregnancy in women with preexisting CMV antibody can cause clinically apparent congenital disease with sequelae. It is estimated that more than two-thirds of neonates with congenital CMV infection in the United States are born to women with nonprimary infection, and the contribution of nonprimary maternal infection as a cause of damaging congenital CMV infection is believed to be common in populations with higher maternal CMV seroprevalence than that of women in the United States. Thus, the definition of protective immunity in congenital CMV infection remains contentious.

Cervical excretion of CMV is common among seropositive women, resulting in exposure of many neonates to CMV at birth. Cervical excretion rates are higher among young mothers in lower socioeconomic groups. Similarly, although disease can occur in seronegative neonates fed CMV-infected human milk, most neonates who acquire CMV from ingestion of infected human milk do not develop clinical illness or sequelae, most likely because of the presence of passively transferred maternal antibody. Among neonates who acquire infection from maternal cervical secretions or human milk, preterm neonates born before 32 weeks' gestation are at greater risk of CMV disease than are full-term neonates.

Incubation Period

Horizontally transmitted CMV infections, unknown; 3 to 12 weeks and 1 to 4 months after blood transfusion and organ transplantation, respectively.

Diagnostic Tests

The diagnosis of CMV disease is confounded by the ubiquity of the virus, high rate of asymptomatic excretion, frequency of reactivated infections, development of serum immunoglobulin (Ig) M CMV-specific antibody in some episodes of reactivation, reinfection with different strains of CMV, and concurrent infection with other pathogens.

Virus can be isolated in cell culture from urine, oral fluids, peripheral blood leukocytes, human milk, semen, cervical secretions, and other tissues and body fluids. Recovery of virus from a target organ provides strong evidence that the disease is caused by CMV. Shell vial culture and immunofluorescence antibody stain for immediate early antigen provides results within days. A presumptive diagnosis of CMV infection beyond the neonatal period has been associated with a 4-fold antibody titer increase in paired serum specimens or by demonstration of virus excretion. Viral DNA can be detected by polymerase chain reaction (PCR) assay in tissues and some fluids, such as cerebrospinal fluid, urine, and saliva. Detection of CMV DNA by PCR assay in blood does not indicate acute infection or disease, especially in immunocompetent people. Detection of pp65 antigen or quantification of viral DNA (eg, by quantitative PCR assay) in white blood cells is often used to detect infection in immunocompromised hosts. Various serologic assays, including immunofluorescence, latex agglutination, and enzyme, are available for detecting CMV-specific antibodies.

Amniocentesis has been used in several small series of patients to establish the diagnosis of intrauterine infection. Following delivery, proof of congenital infection requires virologic detection of CMV in urine, oral fluids, respiratory tract secretions, blood, or cerebrospinal fluid obtained within 2 to 4 weeks of birth. The analytic sensitivity of CMV detection by PCR assay of dried blood spots is low, limiting use of this type of specimen for screening for congenital CMV infection. A positive PCR assay result from a neonatal dried blood spot confirms congenital infection, but a negative result does not exclude congenital infection. Differentiation between intrauterine and perinatal infection is difficult at later than 2 to 4 weeks of age unless clinical manifestations of the former are present. A strongly positive CMV-specific IgM during early infancy can be suggestive of congenital CMV infection; however, IgM serologic methods commonly have reduced specificity and frequently result in false-positive results.

Treatment

Intravenous ganciclovir is the drug of choice for induction and maintenance treatment of retinitis caused by acquired or recurrent CMV infection in immunocompromised adult patients, including HIV-infected patients, and for prophylaxis and treatment of CMV disease in adult transplant recipients. Valganciclovir, the oral prodrug of ganciclovir, is also approved for treatment (induction and maintenance) of CMV retinitis in immunocompromised adult patients, including HIV-infected patients, and for prevention of CMV disease in kidney, kidney-pancreas, or heart transplant recipients aged 4 months and older at high risk for CMV disease. Ganciclovir and valganciclovir are also used to treat CMV infections of other sites (esophagus, colon, lungs) and for preemptive treatment of immunosuppressed adults with CMV antigenemia or viremia. Oral valganciclovir is available in tablet and powder for oral solution formulations.

Neonates with symptomatic congenital CMV disease with or without central nervous system involvement have improved audiologic and neurodevelopmental outcomes at 2 years of age when treated with oral valganciclovir for 6 months. The dose should be adjusted each month to account for weight gain. Significant neutropenia occurs in one-fifth of neonates treated with oral valganciclovir and in two-thirds of neonates treated with parenteral ganciclovir. Absolute neutrophil counts should be performed weekly for 6 weeks, then at 8 weeks, then monthly for the duration of antiviral treatment; serum aminotransferase concentration should be measured monthly during treatment.

Preterm neonates with intrapartum-acquired CMV infection can have end-organ disease (eg, pneumonitis, hepatitis, thrombocytopenia). Antiviral treatment has not been studied in this population. In hematopoietic stem cell transplant recipients, the combination of intravenous immunoglobulin or CMV intravenous immunoglobulin and ganciclovir, administered intravenously, has been reported to be synergistic in treatment of CMV pneumonia. Valganciclovir and foscarnet can also be used for treatment and maintenance of CMV retinitis in adults with AIDS. Foscarnet is more toxic (with high rates of limiting nephrotoxicity) but may be advantageous for some patients with HIV infection, including people with disease caused by ganciclovir-resistant virus or who are unable to tolerate ganciclovir.

Cytomegalovirus establishes lifelong persistent infection, and as such, it is not eliminated from the body with antiviral treatment of CMV disease. Until immune reconstitution is achieved with antiretroviral therapy, chronic suppressive therapy should be administered to HIV-infected patients with a history of CMV end-organ disease (eg, retinitis, colitis, pneumonitis) to prevent recurrence. All patients who have had anti-CMV maintenance therapy discontinued should continue to undergo regular ophthalmologic monitoring at a minimum of 3- to 6-month intervals for early detection of CMV relapse as well as immune reconstitution uveitis.

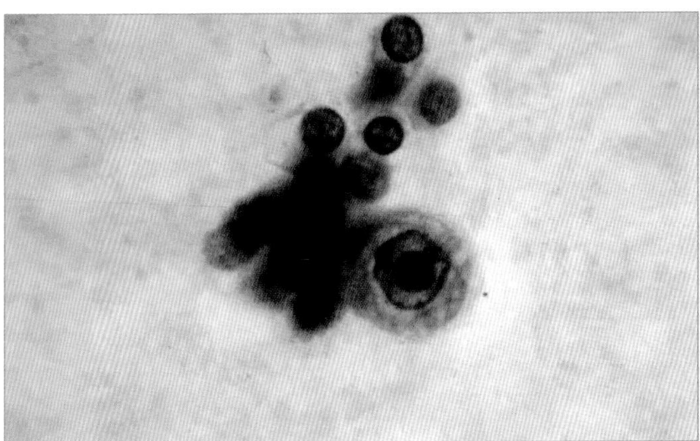

Image 40.1
Cells with intranuclear inclusions in the urine of infant with congenital cytomegalovirus disease.

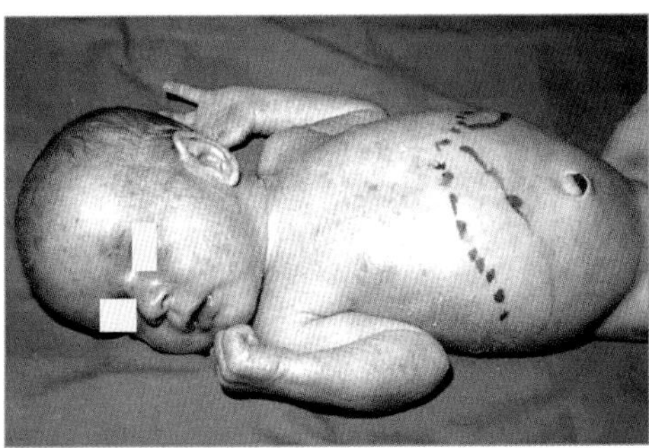

Image 40.2
A 3-week-old with congenital cytomegalovirus infection with purpuric skin lesions and hepatosplenomegaly. Courtesy of Edgar O. Ledbetter, MD, FAAP.

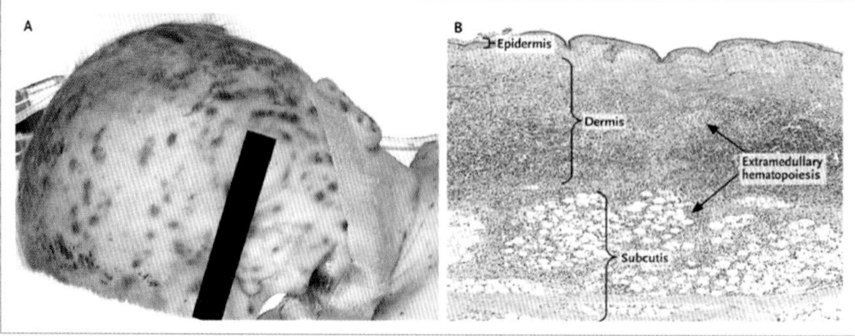

Image 40.3

A baby girl was delivered prematurely, at 30 weeks' gestation, by emergency cesarean delivery because of deceleration and no acceleration on fetal heart rate monitoring. In addition, she had severe intrauterine growth restriction, oligohydramnios, and increased peak systolic velocity of the middle cerebral artery on Doppler ultrasonography. The 39-year-old mother (gravida 7, para 5) had been well during pregnancy. On examination, the neonate was found to have respiratory distress, an extensive rash (A), and hepatomegaly. The rash consisted of purple-to-magenta, nonblanching macules that were 0.5 to 1.0 cm in diameter, as well as papules and petechiae covering her entire body. Laboratory investigation revealed anemia (hemoglobin level, 25 g/L [reference range, 121–191 g/L]) and thrombocytopenia (platelet count, 13,000/mm^3 [13 x 10^9/L [reference range, 195,000–450,000/mm^3 (195–434 x 10^9/L)]). Results of cytomegalovirus (CMV) IgM and IgG tests and serum and plasma DNA polymerase chain reaction assays were positive. Tests for parvovirus B19 and rubella IgM antibodies were negative. Despite aggressive care, the child did not survive. Postmortem examination confirmed disseminated CMV infection. Extramedullary hematopoiesis was present throughout the body, including the skin (B). Dermal hematopoiesis can occur in utero as a result of severe anemia, congenital rubella, parvovirus infection, or CMV infection. From *The New England Journal of Medicine,* Congenital Cytomegalovirus Infection, 362, 833. Copyright © 2010. Massachusetts Medical Society. Reprinted with permission from Massachusetts Medical Society.

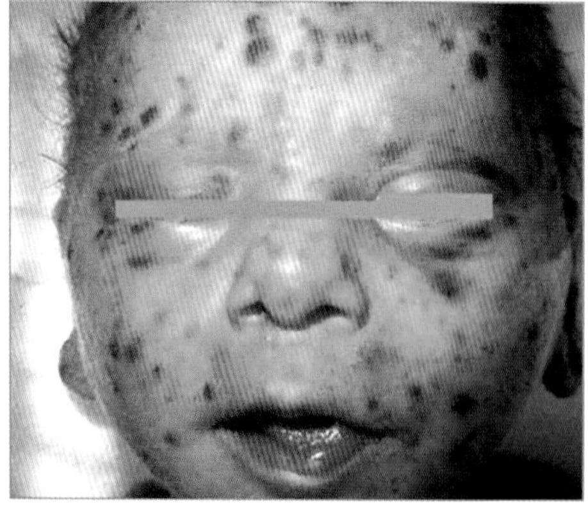

Image 40.4

Cytomegalovirus infection, congenital, with characteristic "blueberry muffin" lesions. Copyright David Clark.

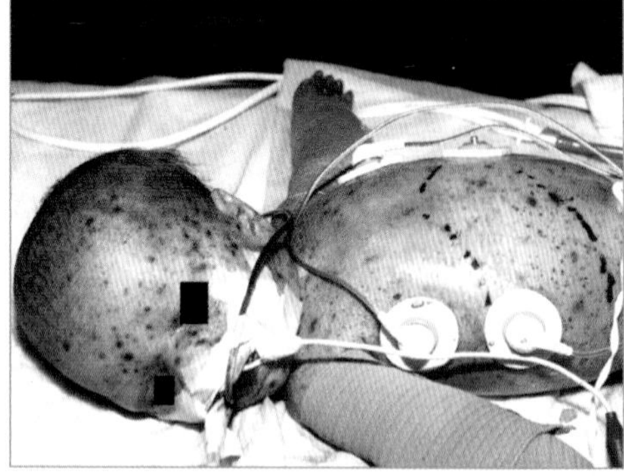

Image 40.5

This 1-day-old, who was small for gestational age, had microcephaly, hepatomegaly, jaundice, and a "blueberry muffin" rash. The neonate also developed thrombocytopenia and disseminated intravascular coagulation. The neonate died at 48 hours of age. Kidney and lung tissue culture tested positive for cytomegalovirus. Copyright Larry I. Corman.

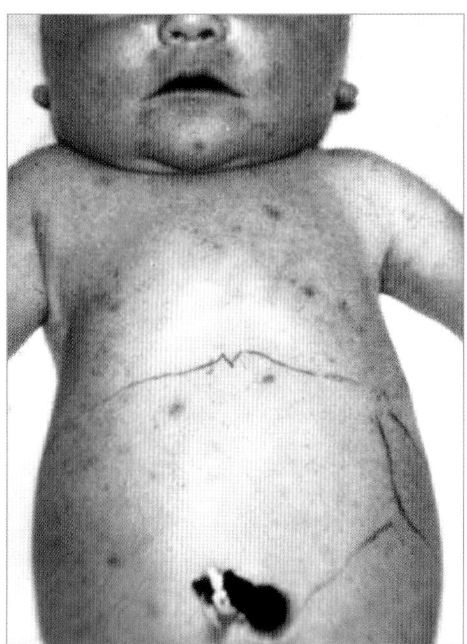

Image 40.6
Infant with lethal congenital cytomegalovirus disease with purpuric skin lesions and striking hepatosplenomegaly. Courtesy of Edgar O. Ledbetter, MD, FAAP.

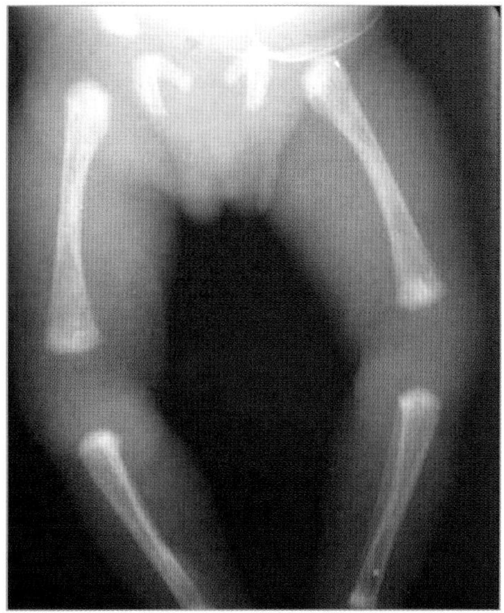

Image 40.7
Infant in Image 40.6 with lethal cytomegalovirus disease with radiographic changes in long bones of osteitis characterized by fine vertical metaphyseal striations. Courtesy of Edgar O. Ledbetter, MD, FAAP.

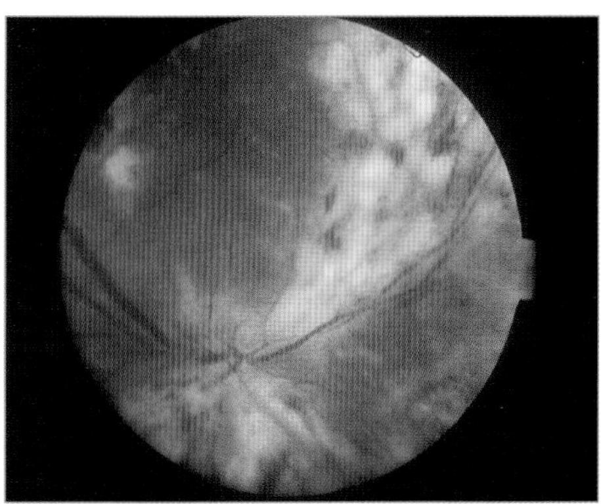

Image 40.8
Widespread "brushfire retinitis" in an infant with congenital cytomegalovirus infection. The perivascular infiltrates and diffuse hemorrhage may result in complete blindness whenever macular involvement occurs. Courtesy of George Nankervis, MD.

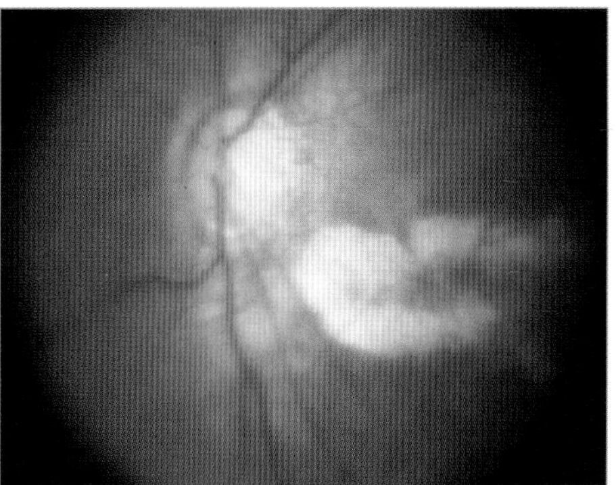

Image 40.9
Characteristic white perivascular infiltrates in the retina of an infant with congenital cytomegalovirus infection. Courtesy of George Nankervis, MD.

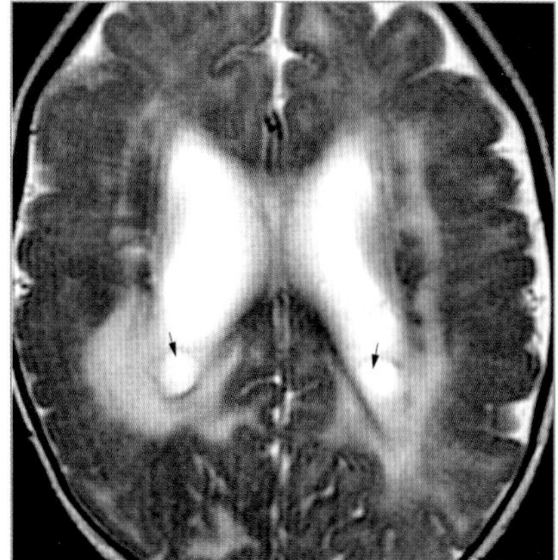

Image 40.10
Axial T2-weighted magnetic resonance image demonstrates periventricular germinolytic cysts (arrows). Also note the periventricular white matter hyperintensities that are representative of demyelination and gliosis.

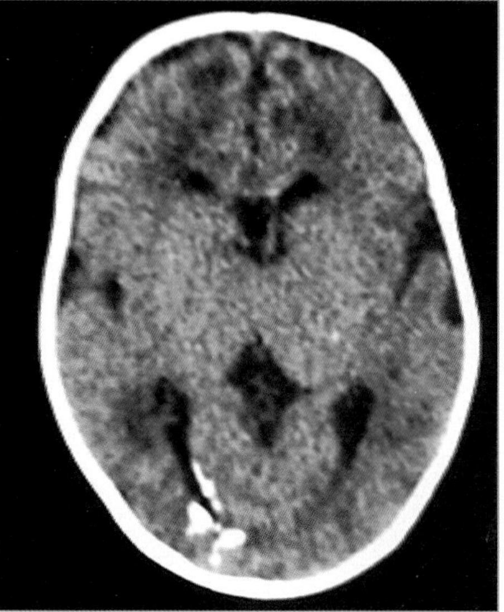

Image 40.11
Cytomegalovirus infection with periventricular calcification. Courtesy of Benjamin Estrada, MD.

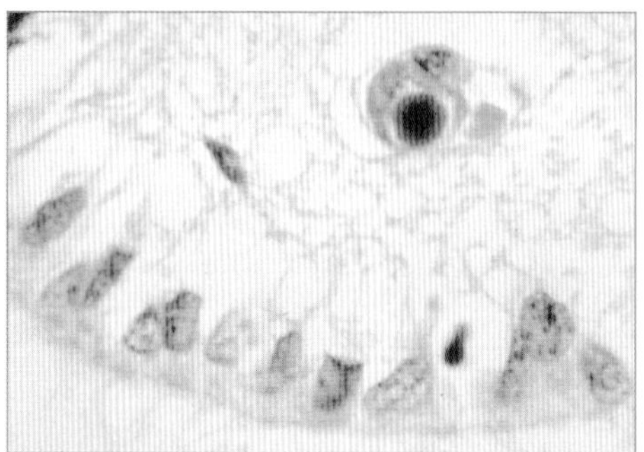

Image 40.12
Histopathology of cytomegalovirus infection of brain capillary endothelial cell. Courtesy of Centers for Disease Control and Prevention/Dr Haraszti.

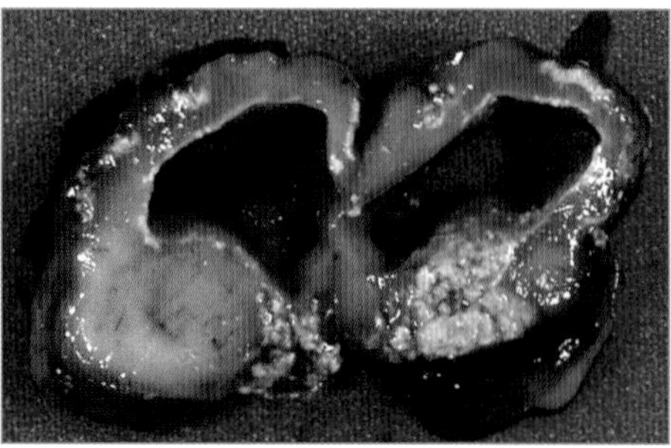

Image 40.13
Congenital cytomegalovirus encephalitis. Microcephaly and cerebral calcification. Courtesy of Dimitris P. Agamanolis, MD.

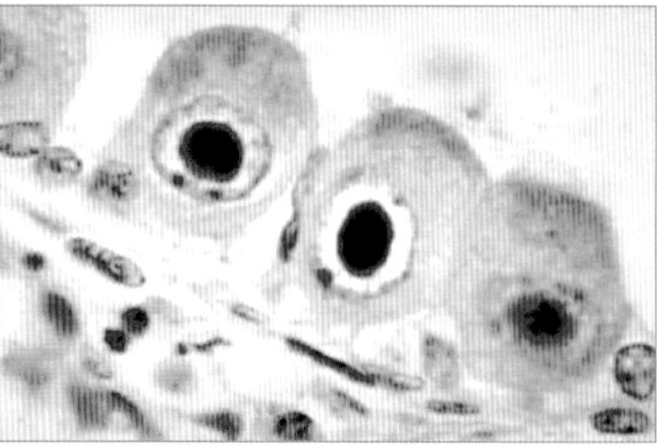

Image 40.14
Histopathologic features of cytomegalovirus infection of the kidney. Intranuclear inclusions are surrounded by a halo and the nuclear membrane, giving an "owl eye" appearance. Courtesy of Centers for Disease Control and Prevention/Dr Haraszti.

41

Dengue

Clinical Manifestations

Dengue has a wide range of clinical presentations, from asymptomatic infection to classic dengue fever and severe dengue (ie, dengue hemorrhagic fever or dengue shock syndrome). Approximately 5% of patients develop severe dengue, which is more common with second or other subsequent infections. Less common clinical syndromes include myocarditis, pancreatitis, hepatitis, and neuroinvasive disease.

Dengue begins with a nonspecific, acute febrile illness lasting 2 to 7 days (**febrile phase**), often accompanied by muscle, joint, or bone pain; headache; retro-orbital pain; facial erythema; injected oropharynx; macular or maculopapular rash; leukopenia; and petechiae or other minor bleeding manifestations. During fever defervescence, usually on days 3 through 7 of illness, an increase in vascular permeability in parallel with increasing hematocrit (hemoconcentration) may occur. The period of clinically significant plasma leakage usually lasts 24 to 48 hours (**critical phase**), followed by a **convalescent phase** with gradual improvement and stabilization of the hemodynamic status. Warning signs of progression to severe dengue occur in the late febrile phase and include persistent vomiting, severe abdominal pain, mucosal bleeding, difficulty breathing, early signs of shock, and a rapid decline in platelet count with an increase in hematocrit. Patients with nonsevere disease begin to improve during the critical phase, but people with clinically significant plasma leakage attributable to increased vascular permeability develop severe disease with pleural effusions or ascites, hypovolemic shock, and hemorrhage.

Etiology

Four related RNA viruses of the genus *Flavivirus*, dengue viruses (DENV) 1, 2, 3, and 4, cause symptomatic (~25%) and asymptomatic infections. Infection with one DENV type produces lifelong immunity against that type and a short period of cross-protection against infection with the other 3 types of DENV. After this short period, infection with a different strain may predispose to more severe disease. A person has a lifetime risk of up to 4 DENV infections.

Epidemiology

Dengue virus is primarily transmitted to humans through the bite of infected *Aedes aegypti* (and, less commonly, *Aedes albopictus* or *Aedes polynesiensis*) mosquitoes. Humans are the main amplifying host of DENV and the main source of virus for *Aedes* mosquitoes. A sylvatic nonhuman primate DENV transmission cycle exists in parts of Africa and Southeast Asia but rarely crosses to humans. During the approximately 7 days of viremia, DENV can be transmitted following receipt of blood products, donor organs, or tissue; percutaneous exposure to blood; and exposure in utero or at parturition.

Dengue is a major public health problem in the tropics and subtropics; an estimated 50 to 100 million dengue cases occur annually in more than 100 countries, and 40% of the world's population lives in areas with DENV transmission. In the United States, dengue is endemic in Puerto Rico, the Virgin Islands, and American Samoa. In addition, millions of US travelers, including children, are at risk because dengue is the leading cause of febrile illness among travelers returning from the Caribbean, Latin America, and South Asia. Outbreaks with local DENV transmission have occurred in Texas, Hawaii, and Florida in the last decade. However, although 16 states have *A aegypti* and 35 states have *A albopictus* mosquitoes, local dengue transmission is uncommon. Dengue occurs in children and adults; it is most likely to cause severe disease in young children, pregnant women, and patients with chronic diseases (eg, asthma, sickle cell anemia, diabetes mellitus).

Incubation Period

3 to 14 days before symptom onset. Infected people, symptomatic and asymptomatic, can transmit DENV to mosquitoes 1 to 2 days before symptoms develop and during viremia (approximately 7 days).

Diagnostic Tests

Laboratory confirmation of the clinical diagnosis of dengue can be made on a single serum specimen obtained during the febrile phase of the illness by testing for DENV by detection of DENV RNA by reverse transcriptase-polymerase chain reaction assay, detection of DENV nonstructural protein 1 antigen by immunoassay, or testing for anti-DENV immunoglobulin (Ig) M antibodies by enzyme immunoassay (EIA). Dengue virus is detectable by reverse transcriptase-polymerase chain reaction or nonstructural protein 1 antigen EIAs from the beginning of the febrile phase until day 7 to 10 after illness onset, but anti-DENV IgM antibodies are not detectable until at least 5 days after illness onset. Other tests, such as IgG anti-DENV EIA and hemagglutination inhibition assay, are not as specific. Anti-DENV IgG antibody remains elevated for life after DENV infection and is often falsely positive in people with prior infection with or immunization against other flaviviruses (eg, West Nile virus, Japanese encephalitis virus, yellow fever virus). A 4-fold or greater increase in anti-DENV IgG antibody titers between the acute (≤5 days after onset of symptoms) and convalescent (>15 days after onset of symptoms) samples confirms recent infection. A single anti-DENV IgG antibody titer of 1:1280 or greater is highly suggestive of a dengue diagnosis.

Treatment

No specific antiviral therapy exists for dengue. During the febrile phase, patients should stay well hydrated and avoid use of aspirin (acetylsalicylic acid), salicylate-containing drugs, and other nonsteroidal anti-inflammatory drugs (eg, ibuprofen) to minimize the potential for bleeding. Additional supportive care is required if the patient becomes dehydrated or develops signs of severe disease at the time of fever defervescence.

Early recognition of shock and intensive supportive therapy can reduce risk of death from approximately 10% to less than 1% in severe dengue. During the critical phase, maintenance of fluid volume and hemodynamic status is crucial to management of severe cases. Patients should be monitored for early signs of shock, occult bleeding, and resolution of plasma leak to avoid prolonged shock, end-organ damage, and fluid overload.

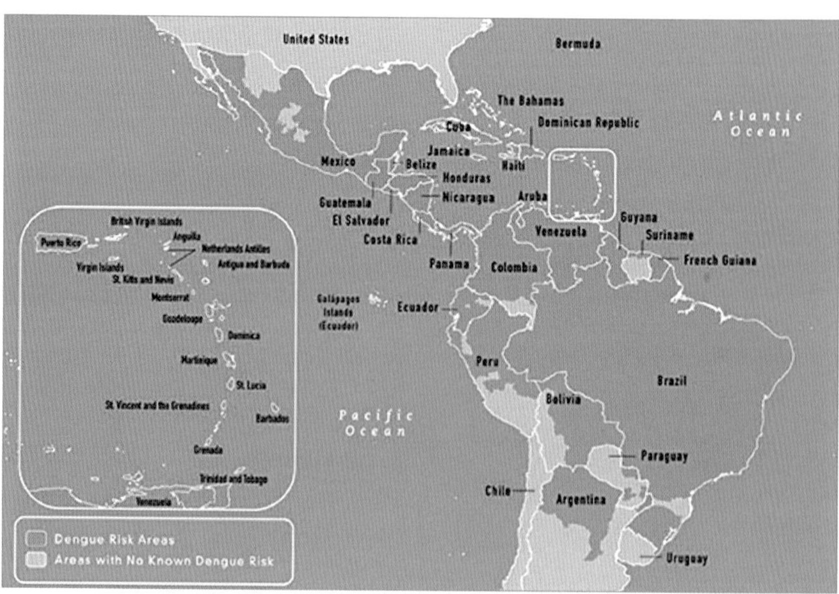

Image 41.1
Distribution of dengue, western hemisphere. Courtesy of Centers for Disease Control and Prevention.

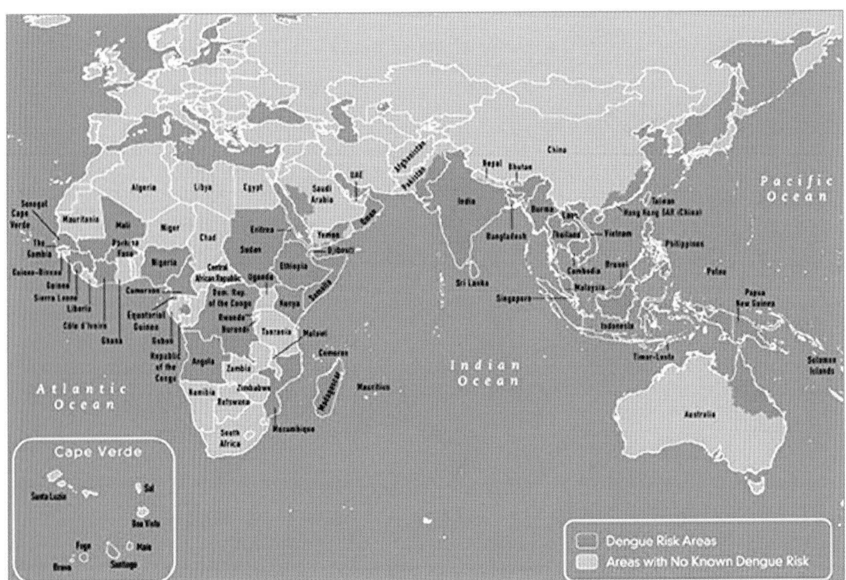

Image 41.2
Distribution of dengue, eastern hemisphere. Courtesy of Centers for Disease Control and Prevention.

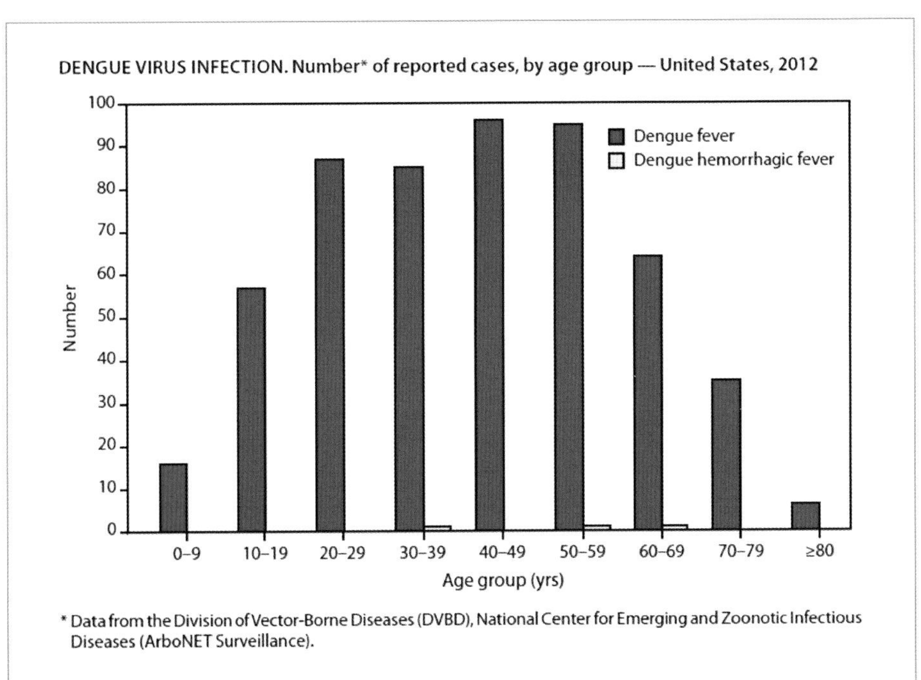

Image 41.3
Dengue virus infection. Number of reported cases, by age group—United States, 2012. Courtesy of *Morbidity and Mortality Weekly Report.*

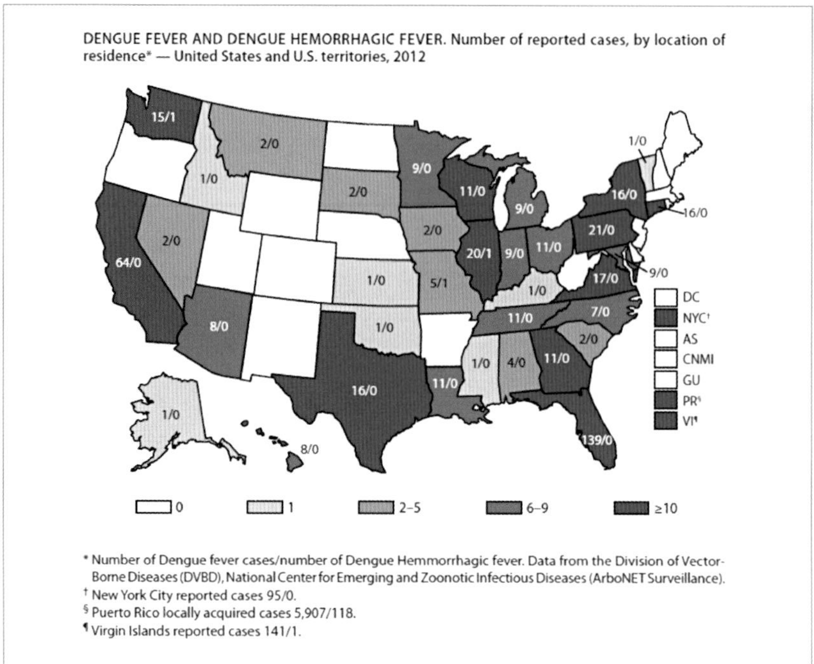

Image 41.4

Dengue and dengue hemorrhagic fever. Number of reported cases, by location of residence—United States and US territories, 2012. Courtesy of *Morbidity and Mortality Weekly Report.*

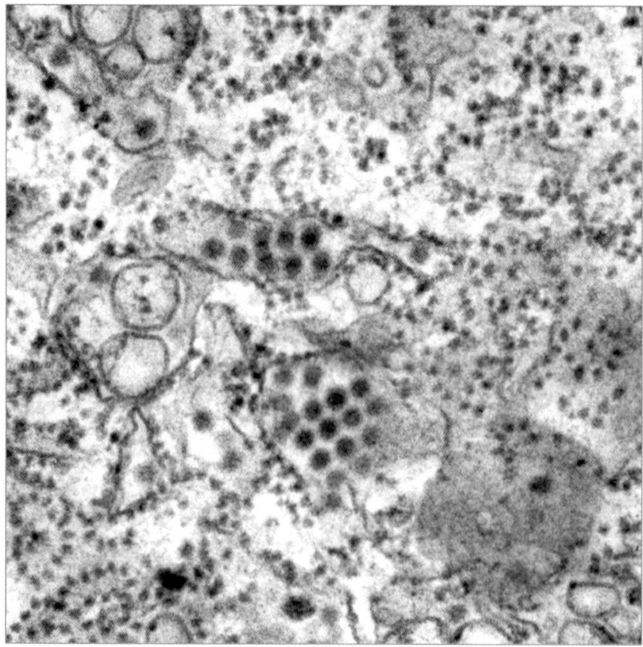

Image 41.5

This transmission electron micrograph depicts a number of round dengue virus particles that were revealed in this tissue specimen. Courtesy of Centers for Disease Control and Prevention/Frederick Murphy, Cynthia Goldsmith.

42

Diphtheria

Clinical Manifestations

Respiratory tract diphtheria usually occurs as membranous nasopharyngitis or obstructive laryngotracheitis. Membranous pharyngitis associated with a bloody nasal discharge should suggest diphtheria. Local infections are associated with a low-grade fever and gradual onset of manifestations over 1 to 2 days. Less commonly, diphtheria presents as cutaneous, vaginal, conjunctival, or otic infection. Cutaneous diphtheria is more common in tropical areas and among the urban homeless. Extensive neck swelling with cervical lymphadenitis (bull neck) is a sign of severe disease. Life-threatening complications of respiratory diphtheria include upper airway obstruction caused by extensive membrane formation; myocarditis, which is often associated with heart block; and cranial and peripheral neuropathies. Palatal palsy, characterized by nasal speech, frequently occurs in pharyngeal diphtheria.

Etiology

Diphtheria is caused by toxigenic strains of *Corynebacterium diphtheriae*. In industrialized countries, toxigenic strains of *Corynebacterium ulcerans* are emerging as an important cause of a diphtherialike illness. *C diphtheriae* is an irregularly staining, gram-positive, nonspore-forming, nonmotile, pleomorphic bacillus with 4 biotypes (*mitis, intermedius, gravis,* and *belfanti*). All biotypes of *C diphtheriae* may be toxigenic or nontoxigenic. The toxin inhibits protein synthesis in all cells, resulting in myocarditis, acute tubular necrosis, and delayed peripheral nerve conduction. Nontoxigenic strains of *C diphtheriae* can cause sore throat and, rarely, other invasive infections, including endocarditis and foreign body infections.

Epidemiology

Humans are the sole reservoir of *C diphtheriae*. Organisms are spread by respiratory tract droplets and by contact with discharges from skin lesions. In untreated people, organisms can be present in discharges from the nose and throat and from eye and skin lesions for 2 to 6 weeks after infection. Patients treated with an appropriate antimicrobial agent usually are not communicable 48 hours after treatment is initiated. Transmission results from intimate contact with patients or carriers. People who travel to areas where diphtheria is endemic or people who come into contact with infected travelers from such areas are at increased risk of being infected with the organism; rarely, fomites and raw milk or milk products can serve as vehicles of transmission. Severe disease occurs more often in people who are unimmunized or inadequately immunized. Fully immunized people may be asymptomatic carriers or have mild sore throat. The incidence of respiratory diphtheria is greatest during autumn and winter, but summer epidemics can occur in warm climates in which skin infections are prevalent. During the 1990s, epidemic diphtheria occurred throughout independent states of the former Soviet Union, with case-fatality rates ranging from 3% to 23%. Diphtheria remains endemic in these countries as well as in countries in Africa, Latin America, Asia, the Middle East, and parts of Europe, where childhood immunization coverage with diphtheria toxoid–containing vaccines is suboptimal. During 2012, one probable case of diphtheria was reported in the United States, representing the first case since 2003. Cases of cutaneous diphtheria likely still occur in the United States, but only respiratory tract cases are included for national notification.

Incubation Period

2 to 5 days (range, 1–10 days).

Diagnostic Tests

Specimens for culture should be obtained from the nose or throat and any mucosal or cutaneous lesion. Material should be obtained from beneath the membrane, or a portion of the membrane itself should be submitted for culture. Because special medium is required for isolation, laboratory personnel should be notified that *C diphtheriae* is suspected. Specimens collected for culture can be placed in any transport medium (eg, Amies, Stuart) or in a sterile container and transported at 4°C (39.2°F) or in silica gel packs to a reference laboratory for culture. All *C diphtheriae* isolates should be sent through the state health department to the Centers for Disease Control and Prevention.

Treatment

- **Antitoxin.** Because the condition of patients with diphtheria can deteriorate rapidly, a single dose of equine antitoxin should be administered on the basis of clinical diagnosis, even before culture results are available. Antitoxin and its indications for use and instructions for administration are available through the Centers for Disease Control and Prevention. To neutralize toxin from the organism as rapidly as possible, intravenous administration of the antitoxin is preferred. Before intravenous administration of antitoxin, tests for sensitivity to horse serum should be performed, initially with a scratch test. Allergic reactions of variable severity to horse serum can be expected in 5% to 20% of patients. The dose of antitoxin depends on the site and size of the diphtheria membrane, duration of illness, and degree of toxic effects; presence of soft, diffuse cervical lymphadenitis suggests moderate to severe toxin absorption. Antitoxin is probably of no value for cutaneous disease.
- **Antimicrobial therapy.** Erythromycin administered orally or parenterally for 14 days, aqueous penicillin G administered intravenously for 14 days, or penicillin G procaine administered intramuscularly for 14 days constitutes acceptable therapy. Antimicrobial therapy is required to stop toxin production, to eradicate the *C diphtheriae* organism, and to prevent transmission, but it is not a substitute for antitoxin, which is the primary therapy. Elimination of the organism should be documented 24 hours after completion of treatment by 2 consecutive negative cultures from specimens taken 24 hours apart.
- **Immunization.** Active immunization against diphtheria should be undertaken during convalescence from diphtheria; disease does not necessarily confer immunity.
- **Cutaneous diphtheria.** Thorough cleansing of the lesion with soap and water and administration of an appropriate antimicrobial agent for 10 days are recommended.

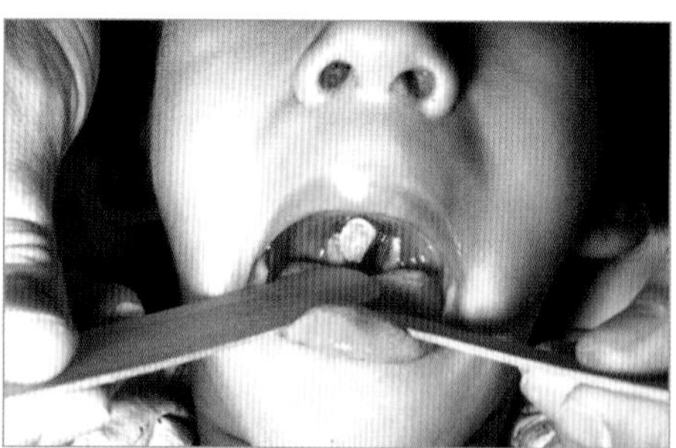

Image 42.1
Pharyngeal diphtheria with membranes covering the tonsils and uvula in a 15-year-old girl. Tonsillar and pharyngeal diphtheria may need to be differentiated from group A streptococcal pharyngitis, infectious mononucleosis, Vincent angina, acute toxoplasmosis, thrush, and leukemia, as well as other, less common entities, including tularemia and acute cytomegalovirus infection.

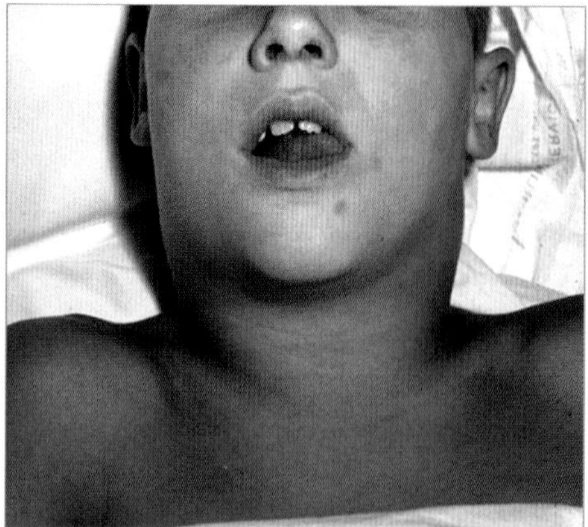

Image 42.2
Bull neck appearance of diphtheritic cervical lymphadenopathy in a 13-year-old boy.

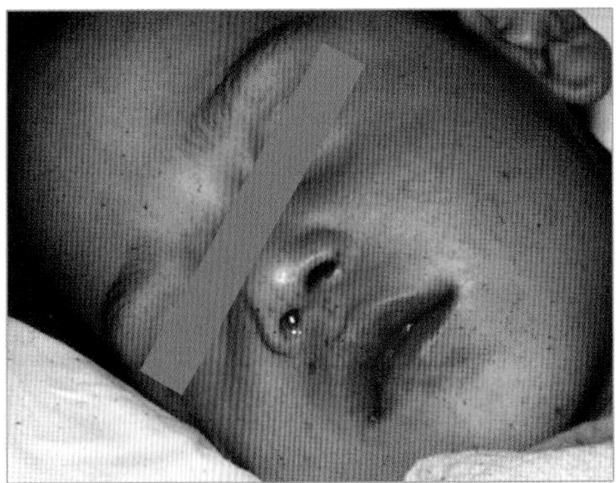

Image 42.3
A 5-year-old Latin American boy with nasal diphtheria. Courtesy of Paul Wehrle, MD.

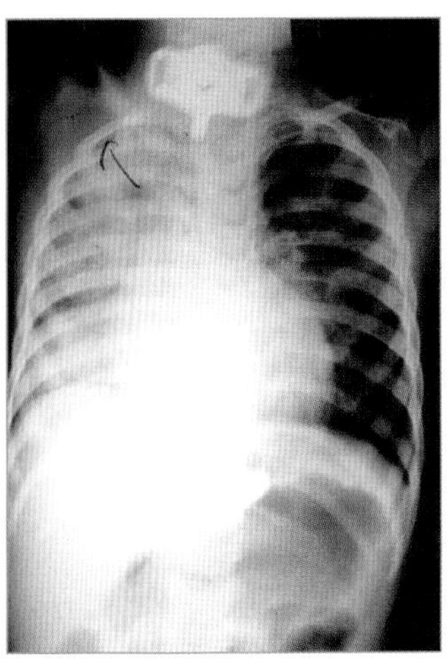

Image 42.5
Diphtheritic pneumonia 3 days after the admission radiograph in Image 42.4 following a tracheostomy complicated by early pneumothorax. Unfortunately, the tracheal membrane was not visualized at the time of tracheostomy and diphtheria antitoxin therapy was not prescribed. Courtesy of Edgar O. Ledbetter, MD, FAAP.

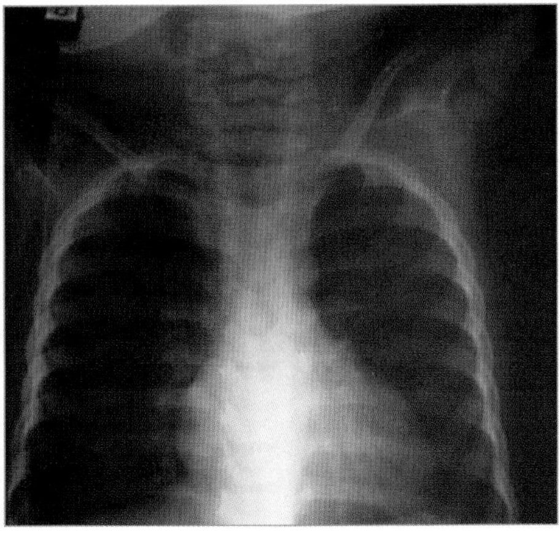

Image 42.4
Chest radiograph of a 2-year-old boy with laryngotracheal diphtheria. Diphtheritic pneumonia was obscured by hyperaeration on chest radiograph at time of admission to hospital due to laryngotracheal membranous obstruction. Courtesy of Edgar O. Ledbetter, MD, FAAP.

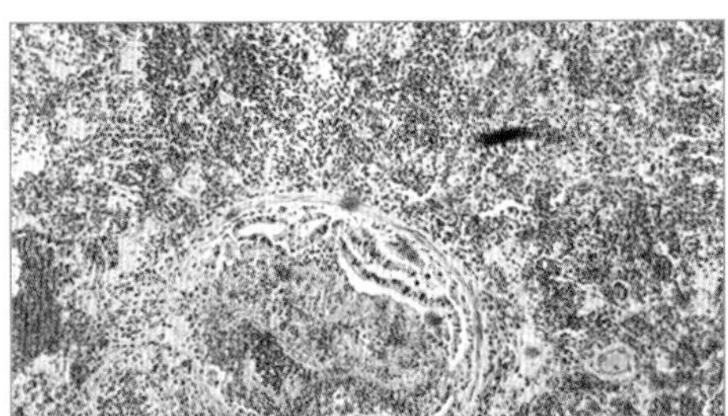

Image 42.6
Diphtheria pneumonia (hemorrhagic) with bronchiolar membranes (hematoxylin-eosin stain). From the patient in images 42.4 and 42.5. Courtesy of Edgar O. Ledbetter, MD, FAAP.

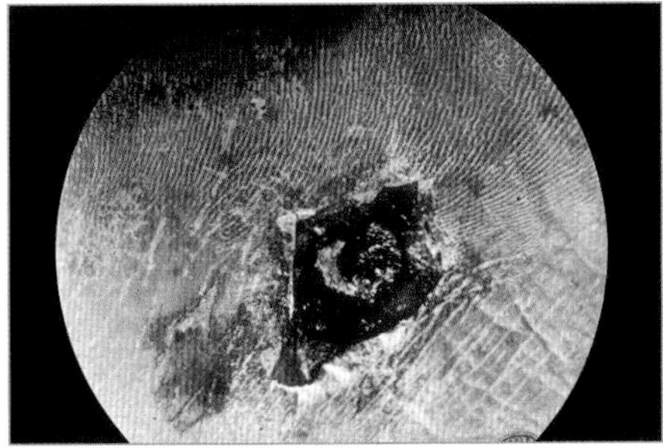

Image 42.7
This is a close-up of a diphtheria skin lesion caused by the organism *Corynebacterium diphtheriae.* Courtesy of Centers for Disease Control and Prevention/Dr Brodsky.

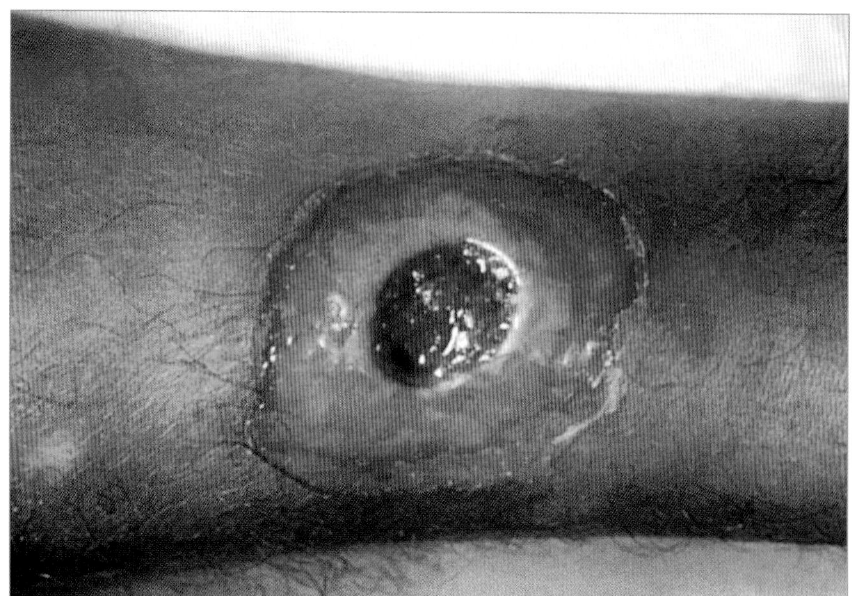

Image 42.8
A diphtheria skin lesion on the leg. *Corynebacterium diphtheriae* can not only affect the respiratory, cardiovascular, renal, and neurologic systems, but the cutaneous system as well, where it sometimes manifests as an open, isolated wound. Courtesy of Centers for Disease Control and Prevention.

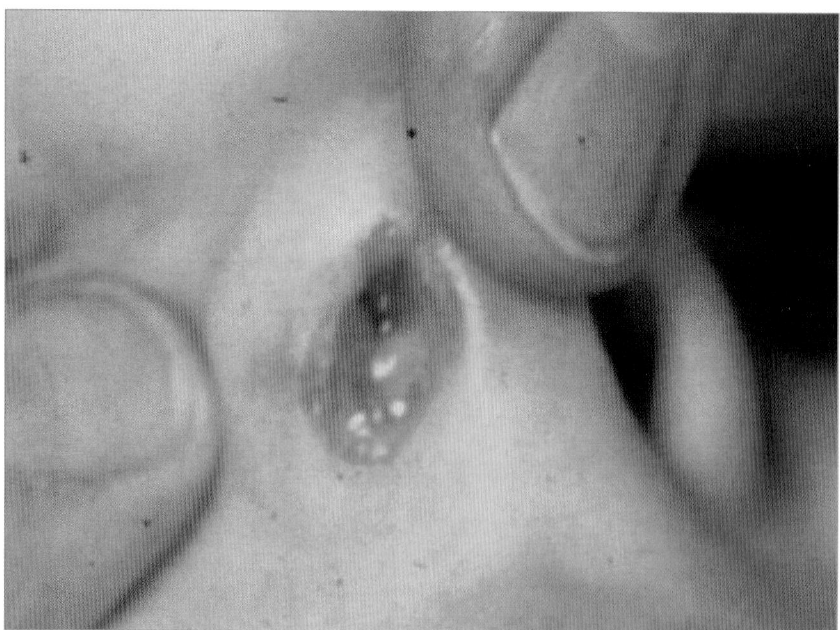

Image 42.9
Nasal membrane of diphtheria in a preschool-aged white boy. Courtesy of George Nankervis, MD.

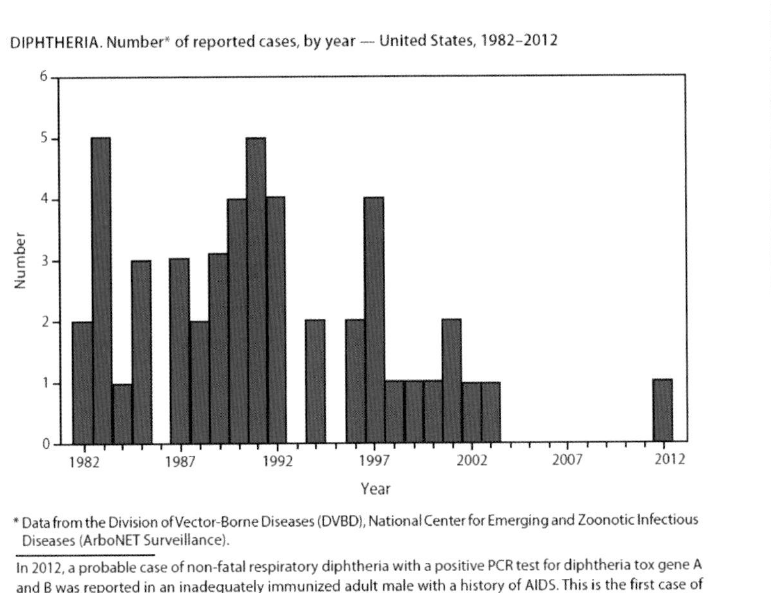

Image 42.10
Number of reported cases, by year—United States, 1982–2012. Courtesy of *Morbidity and Mortality Weekly Report.*

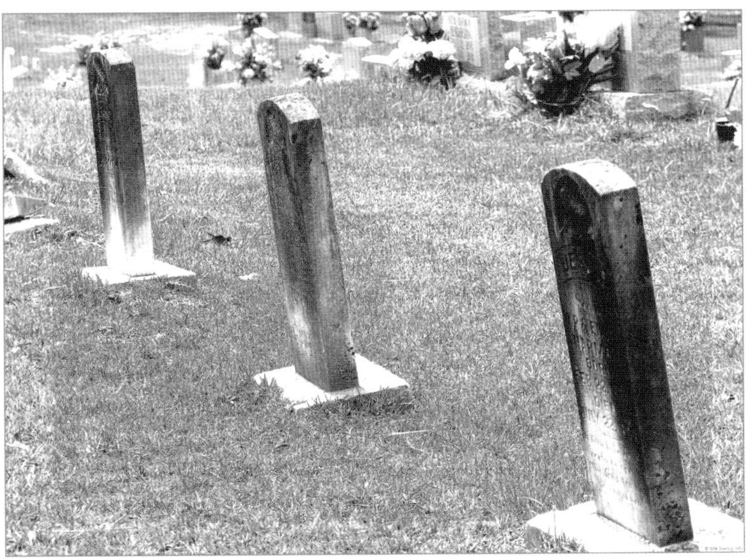

Image 42.11
Baby graves dating from the 1890s in a central Mississippi family cemetery. Diphtheria was a common cause of these infant deaths prior to the introduction of a toxoid vaccine around 1921. In the preantibiotic era, treatment was limited to comfort care or tracheotomy. Vaccination of children and adults has reduced the number of diphtheria cases in the United States. However, reluctance to immunize children sets the stage for another generation of rows of tiny memories. Courtesy of Will Sorey, MD.

43

Ehrlichia, Anaplasma, and Related Infections

(Human Ehrlichiosis, Anaplasmosis, and Related Infections)

Clinical Manifestations

Infections by members of the bacterial family Anaplasmataceae (genera *Anaplasma, Ehrlichia, Neorickettsia,* and the proposed genus *Neoehrlichia*) cause human illness with similar signs, symptoms, and clinical courses. All are acute, systemic, febrile illnesses, with common systemic manifestations, including fever, headache, chills, malaise, myalgia, and nausea. More variable symptoms include arthralgia, vomiting, diarrhea, cough, and confusion. Rash is more common in *Ehrlichia* infections than *Anaplasma* infections and is more common in children (up to 60% of cases). More severe manifestations of these diseases can include acute respiratory distress syndrome, encephalopathy, meningitis, disseminated intravascular coagulation, spontaneous hemorrhage, and renal failure. Significant laboratory findings in *Anaplasma* and *Ehrlichia* infections may include leukopenia, lymphopenia, thrombocytopenia, hyponatremia, and elevated serum hepatic transaminase concentrations. Cerebrospinal fluid abnormalities (ie, pleocytosis with a predominance of lymphocytes and increased total protein concentration) are common. Neorickettsiosis is characterized by lymphadenopathy, a sign that is not commonly seen with infections by other members of this bacterial family. As with ehrlichiosis and anaplasmosis, patients with neoehrlichiosis often have had leukocytosis and elevated C-reactive protein concentrations, but liver transaminase levels are usually within normal ranges. Most cases of neoehrlichiosis have been in people with underlying immunosuppressive conditions.

Without treatment, symptoms typically last 1 to 2 weeks, but prompt antimicrobial therapy will shorten the duration and reduce the risk of serious manifestations and sequelae. Following infection, fatigue may last several weeks; some reports suggest the occurrence of neurologic complications in some children after severe disease, and more commonly with *Ehrlichia* infections. Fatal infections have been reported more commonly for *Ehrlichia chaffeensis* infections (approximately 1%–3%) than for anaplasmosis (<1%). Typically, *E chaffeensis* presents with more severe disease than does *Anaplasma phagocytophilum*. People with underlying immunosuppression are at greater risk of severe disease.

Ehrlichia and *Anaplasma* species do not cause vasculitis or endothelial cell damage characteristic of some other rickettsial diseases. However, because of the nonspecific presenting symptoms, Rocky Mountain spotted fever should be considered. The recently discovered, tick-borne Heartland virus can also present similarly.

Etiology

In the United States, human ehrlichiosis and anaplasmosis are caused by at least 4 different species of obligate intracellular bacteria: *E chaffeensis, Ehrlichia ewingii, Ehrlichia muris*–like agent, and *A phagocytophilum* (Table 43.1). *Ehrlichia* and *Anaplasma* species are gram-negative cocci with tropisms for different white blood cell types. *E muris* is suspected to cause disease in Russia and Japan. *Neorickettsia sennetsu* may cause illness in Asia, while the organism designated as *Neoehrlichia mikurensis* has been found in various European and Asian countries.

Epidemiology

The reported incidences of *E chaffeensis* and *A phagocytophilum* infections during 2012 were 3.8 and 8.0 cases per million population, respectively. These diseases are underrecognized, and selected active surveillance programs have shown the incidence to be substantially higher in some areas with endemic infection. Most cases of *E chaffeensis* and *E ewingii* infection are reported from the south central and southeastern United States, as well as East Coast states. Ehrlichiosis caused by *E chaffeensis* and *E ewingii* are associated with the bite of the lone star tick (*Amblyomma americanum*). To date, cases attributable to the new *E muris*–like agent have been reported only from Minnesota and Wisconsin. Most cases of human anaplasmosis have been reported from the upper Midwest and northeast United States (eg, Wisconsin, Minnesota, Connecticut, New York) and northern California. In most of the United States, *A phagocytophilum* is transmitted by the black-legged tick (*Ixodes scapularis*), which is also the vector for Lyme disease (*Borrelia burgdorferi*) and babesiosis (*Babesia microti*). This tick is also suspected to be a vector for the *E muris*–like agent. In the western United States, the western black-legged tick (*Ixodes pacificus*) is the main vector for *A phagocytophilum*. Various mammalian wildlife reservoirs for the agents of human ehrlichiosis and anaplasmosis have been identified, including white-tailed deer and wild rodents. In other parts of the world, other bacterial species of this family are transmitted by the endemic tick vectors for that area. An exception is *N sennetsu*, which occurs in Asia and is transmitted through ingestion of infected trematodes residing in fish.

Reported cases of symptomatic ehrlichiosis and anaplasmosis are characteristically in older people, with age-specific incidences greatest in people older than 40 years. However, seroprevalence data indicate that exposure to *E chaffeensis* may be common in children. In the United States, most human infections occur between April and September, and the peak occurrence is from May through July. Coinfections of anaplasmosis with other tick-borne diseases, including babesiosis and Lyme disease, may cause illnesses that are more severe or of longer duration than a single infection.

Incubation Period

E chaffeensis, 5 to 14 days; *A phagocytophilum*, 5 to 21 days.

Diagnostic Tests

Detection of specific DNA in a clinical specimen by polymerase chain reaction assay is a sensitive and specific means for early diagnosis. Whole blood anticoagulated with ethylenediaminetetraacetic acid should be collected at the first presentation before antibiotic therapy has been initiated. Polymerase chain reaction assays for anaplasmosis and ehrlichiosis are available commercially. Sequence confirmation of the amplified product provides specific identification and is often necessary to identify infection with certain species (eg, *E ewingii*; *E muris*–like agent in the United States).

Identification of stained peripheral blood smears to look for classic clusters of organism known as **morulae** may occasionally indicate infection with Anaplasmataceae, but this method is generally insensitive and is not recommended as a first-line diagnostic tool. In many patients, serologic testing can be used to demonstrate evidence of a 4-fold change in immunoglobulin (Ig) G–specific antibody titer by indirect immunofluorescence antibody assay between paired serum specimens. Cross-reactivity between species can make it difficult to interpret the causative agent in areas where geographic distributions overlap. Detection of IgG antibodies in acute and convalescent sera is recommended when assessing acutely infected patients. *E ewingii* and *E muris*–like agent infections are best confirmed by molecular detection methods.

Treatment

Doxycycline is the drug of choice for treatment of human ehrlichiosis and anaplasmosis, regardless of patient age, and has also been shown to be effective for the other Anaplasmataceae infections. Ehrlichiosis and anaplasmosis can be severe or fatal in untreated patients or patients with predisposing conditions; initiation of therapy early in the course of disease helps minimize complications of illness. Most patients begin to respond within 48 hours of initiating doxycycline treatment. Treatment with trimethoprim-sulfamethoxazole has been linked to more severe outcome and is contraindicated. Treatment should continue for at least 3 days after defervescence; the standard course of treatment is 5 to 10 days. Unequivocal evidence of clinical improvement is generally within 7 days, although some symptoms (eg, headache, malaise) can persist for weeks.

Table 43.1
Human Ehrlichiosis, Anaplasmosis, and Related Infections

Disease	Causal Agent	Major Target Cell	Tick Vector	Geographic Distribution
Ehrlichiosis caused by *Ehrlichia chaffeensis* (also known as human monocytic ehrlichiosis, or HME)	*E chaffeensis*	Usually monocytes	Lone star tick (*Amblyomma americanum*)	US: Predominantly southeast, south central, and East Coast states; has been reported outside US
Anaplasmosis (also known as human granulocytic anaplasmosis, or HGA)	*Anaplasma phagocytophilum*	Usually granulocytes	Black-legged tick (*Ixodes scapularis*) or Western black-legged tick (*Ixodes pacificus*)	US: Northeastern and upper Midwestern states and northern California; Europe and Asia
Ehrlichiosis caused by *Ehrlichia ewingii*	*E ewingii*	Usually granulocytes	Lone star tick (*A americanum*)	US: Southeastern, south central, and Midwestern states; Africa, Asia
Ehrlichiosis caused by *Ehrlichia muris*–like agent	*E muris*–like agent	Unknown; suspected in monocytes	*I scapularis* is identified as a possible vector.	US: Minnesota, Wisconsin
Ehrlichiosis caused by *E muris*	*E muris sensu stricto*	Unknown; suspected in monocytes	*Ixodes persulcatus, Ixodes ovatus*	Asia
Thrombocytic anaplasmosis	*Anaplasma platys*	Platelets	*Rhipicephalus sanguineus* (suspected)	Venezuela
Ehrlichiosis caused by *Ehrlichia canis*	*E canis*	Monocytes	*R sanguineus* (suspected)	Venezuela
Neorickettsiosis, sennetsu fever, glandular fever	*Neorickettsia sennetsu*	Monocytes	Ingestion of infected trematodes residing in fish	Japan, Malaysia, Laos
Neoehrlichiosis	Candidatus *Neoehrlichia mikurensis*	Unknown	*Ixodes ricinus, Ixodes persulcatus, Haemaphysalis flava*	Europe and Asia

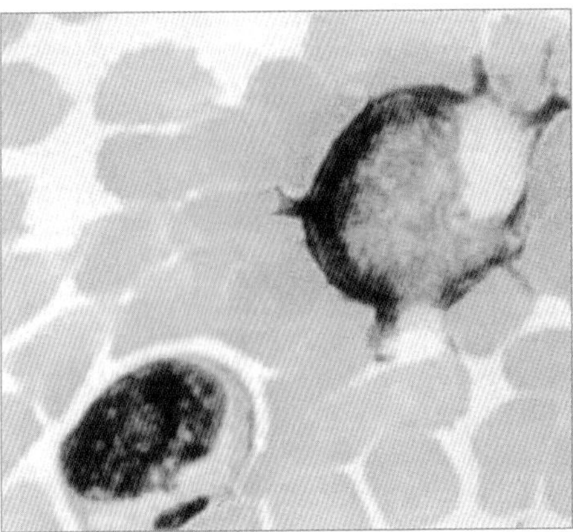

Image 43.1
The intracytoplasmic inclusion, or morula, of human monocytic ehrlichiosis in a cytocentrifuge preparation of cerebrospinal fluid from a patient with central nervous system involvement. Copyright Richard Jacobs, MD.

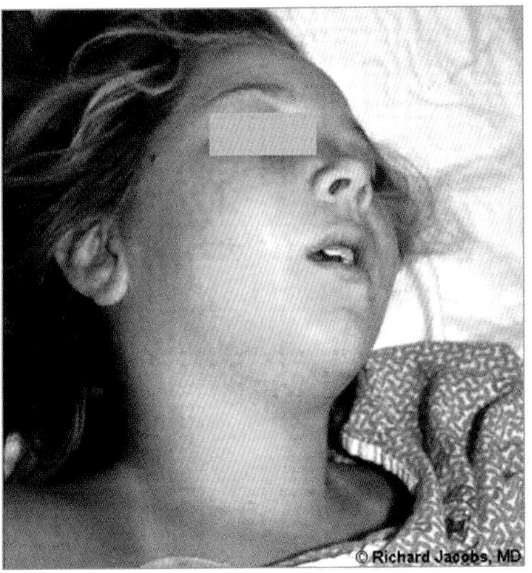

Image 43.3
Human monocytic ehrlichiosis (HME). A semicomatose 16-year-old girl with leukopenia, lymphopenia, thrombocytopenia, and elevated transaminase levels. The HME polymerase chain reaction and serologic test results were positive for HME. Copyright Richard Jacobs, MD.

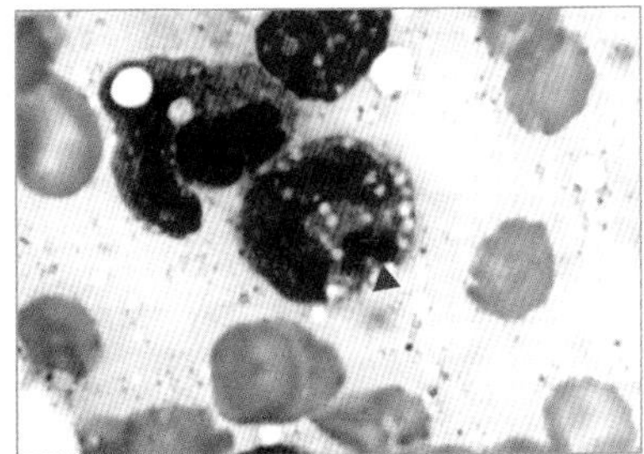

Image 43.2
Bone marrow examination (Wright stain, magnification x1,000). Intraleukocytic morulae of *Ehrlichia* can be seen (arrow) within monocytoid cells. Courtesy of *Emerging Infectious Diseases.*

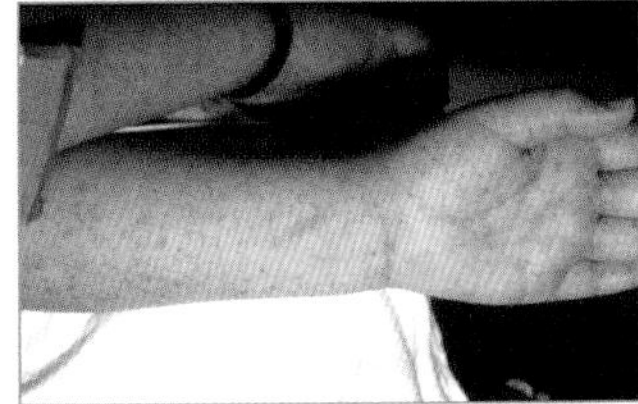

Image 43.4
The petechial and vasculitic rash of human monocytic ehrlichiosis in the patient in Image 43.3. Copyright Richard Jacobs, MD.

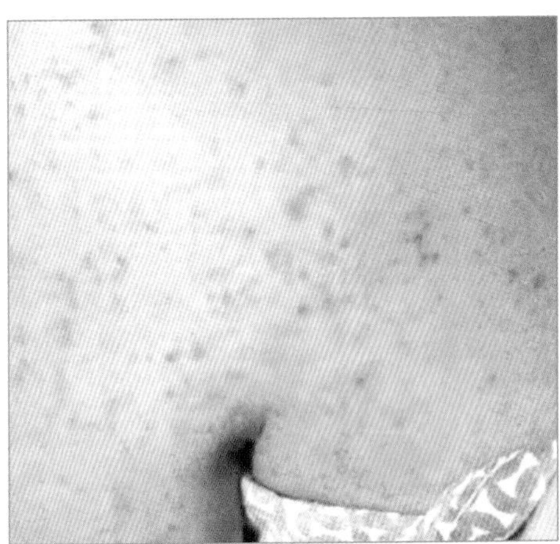

Image 43.5
The same characteristic rash of human monocytic ehrlichiosis in the patient in images 43.3 and 43.4. The differential diagnosis of this rash includes Rocky Mountain spotted fever, meningococcemia, and Stevens-Johnson syndrome. Other tick-borne diseases, such as Lyme disease, babesiosis, Colorado tick fever, relapsing fever, and tularemia, may need to be considered. Kawasaki disease has also caused some diagnostic confusion. Copyright Richard Jacobs, MD.

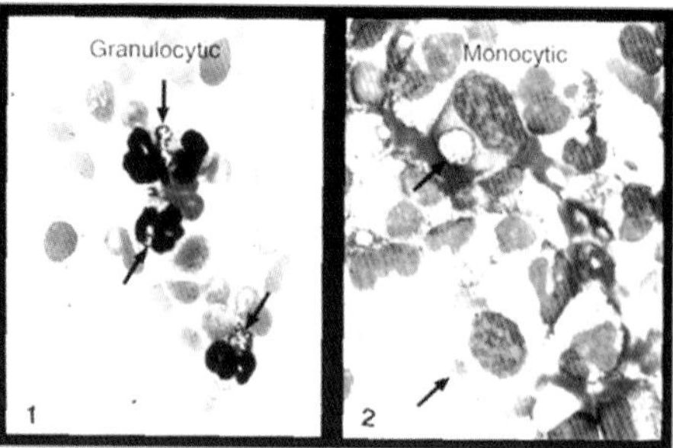

Image 43.6
Etiologic agents of ehrlichiosis. Photomicrographs of human white blood cells infected with the agent of human granulocytic ehrlichiosis (*Anaplasma phagocytophilum,* formerly *Ehrlichia phagocytophila*) and the agent of human monocytic ehrlichiosis (*Ehrlichia chaffeensis*). Courtesy of Centers for Disease Control and Prevention.

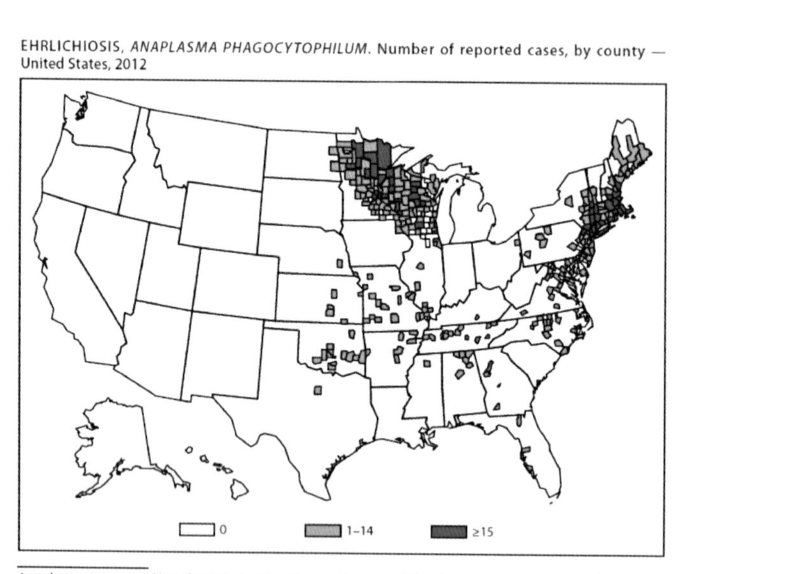

Image 43.7
Ehrlichiosis, *Anaplasma phagocytophilum.* Number of reported cases, by county—United States, 2012. Courtesy of *Morbidity and Mortality Weekly Report.*

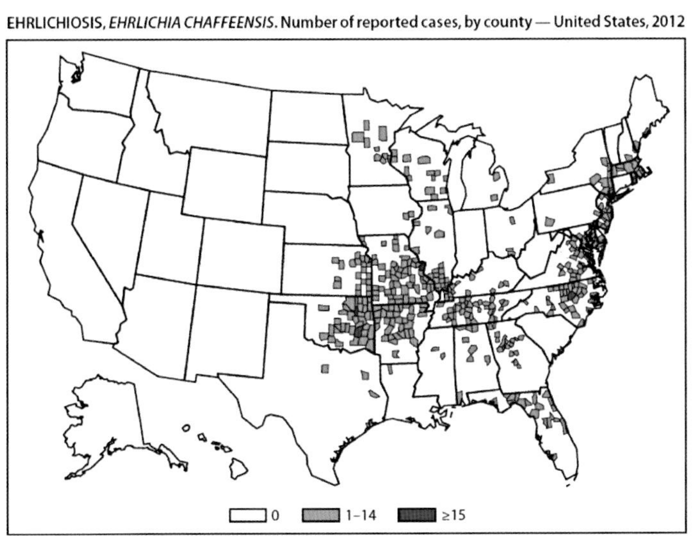

Ehrlichia chaffeensis is the most common type of ehrlichiosis infection in the United States. This tick-borne pathogen is transmitted by *Amblyomma americanum*, the lonestar tick. The majority of cases of *E. chaffeensis* are reported from the Midwest, South, and Northeast regions.

Image 43.8
Ehrlichiosis, *Ehrlichia chaffeensis.* Number of reported cases, by county—United States, 2012. Courtesy of *Morbidity and Mortality Weekly Report.*

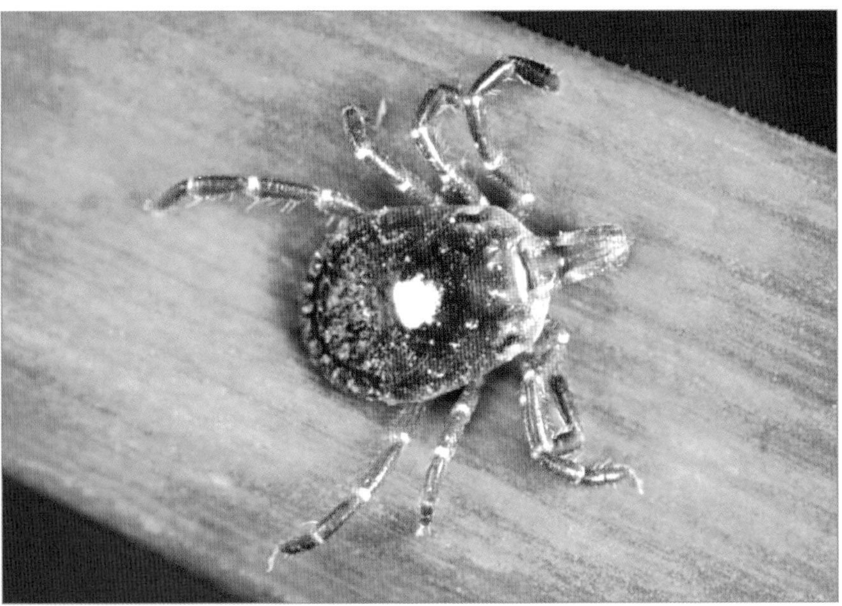

Image 43.9
This is a female lone star tick, *Amblyomma americanum,* and is found in the southeastern and mid-Atlantic United States. This tick is a vector of several zoonotic diseases, including human monocytic ehrlichiosis, southern tick-associated rash illness, tularemia, and Rocky Mountain spotted fever. Courtesy of Centers for Disease Control and Prevention/Michael L. Levin, PhD.

44

Enterovirus (Nonpoliovirus)

(Group A and B Coxsackieviruses, Echoviruses, Numbered Enteroviruses)

Clinical Manifestations

Nonpolio enteroviruses (EVs) are responsible for significant and frequent illnesses in infants and children and result in protean clinical manifestations. The most common manifestation is nonspecific febrile illness, which, in young infants, may lead to evaluation for bacterial sepsis. Other manifestations can include (1) respiratory: coryza, pharyngitis, herpangina, stomatitis, bronchiolitis, pneumonia, and pleurodynia; (2) skin: hand-foot-and-mouth disease, onychomadesis (periodic shedding of nails), and nonspecific exanthems; (3) neurologic: aseptic meningitis, encephalitis, and motor paralysis (acute flaccid paralysis); (4) gastrointestinal/genitourinary: vomiting, diarrhea, abdominal pain, hepatitis, pancreatitis, and orchitis; (5) eye: acute hemorrhagic conjunctivitis and uveitis; (6) heart: myopericarditis; and (7) muscle: pleurodynia and other skeletal myositis. Neonates, especially those who acquire infection in the absence of serotype-specific maternal antibody, are at risk of severe disease, including viral sepsis, meningoencephalitis, myocarditis, hepatitis, coagulopathy, and pneumonitis. Infection with EV 71 is associated with hand-foot-and-mouth disease, herpangina, and, in a small proportion of cases, severe neurologic disease, including brainstem encephalomyelitis, paralytic disease, and other neurologic manifestations; secondary pulmonary edema/hemorrhage and cardiopulmonary collapse can occur, occasionally resulting in fatalities and sequelae. Other noteworthy but not exclusive serotype associations include coxsackieviruses A6 and A16 with hand-foot-and-mouth disease, coxsackievirus A6 with atypical rashes, coxsackievirus A24 variant and EV 70 with acute hemorrhagic conjunctivitis, and coxsackieviruses B1 through B5 with pleurodynia and myopericarditis.

Enterovirus D68 (EV-D68) was first identified in California in 1962 and has been associated with mild to severe respiratory illness in infants, children, and teenagers. In August 2014, clusters of disease caused by EV-D68, prominently associated with exacerbation of asthma, were noted in Kansas City, MO, and Chicago, IL, with subsequent spread throughout the country. By the end of October 2014, EV-D68 had been detected in 48 states, with more than 1,100 patients. Almost all confirmed cases were among children, many of whom had asthma or a history of wheezing. Nine children died, although the contribution of EV-D68 to the fatal outcome is unknown. Additionally, a poliolike, acute neurologic syndrome was reported in a few children with a history of recent respiratory illnesses, some of which were caused by EV-D68. Illness consisted of spinal fluid pleocytosis and acute onset of limb weakness and changes on magnetic resonance imaging of the spinal cord demonstrating nonenhancing lesions restricted to the gray matter. As of December 2014, 94 children with acute flaccid myelitis have been reported in 33 states.

Patients with humoral and combined immune deficiencies can develop persistent central nervous system infections, a dermatomyositis-like syndrome, or disseminated infection. Severe neurologic or multisystem disease is reported in hematopoietic stem cell and solid organ transplant recipients, children with malignancies, and patients treated with anti-CD20 monoclonal antibody.

Etiology

The EVs comprise a genus in the Picornaviridae family of RNA viruses. The nonpolio EVs include more than 100 distinct serotypes formerly subclassified as group A coxsackieviruses, group B coxsackieviruses, echoviruses, and newer numbered EVs. A more recent classification system groups these nonpolio EVs into 4 species (EV-A, -B, -C, and -D) on the basis of genetic similarity; polioviruses are members of EV-C. Echoviruses 22 and 23 have been reclassified as human parechoviruses 1 and 2, respectively.

Epidemiology

Humans are the only known reservoir for human EVs, although some primates can become infected. Enterovirus infections are common and distributed worldwide. They are spread by fecal-oral and respiratory routes and from mother to newborn prenatally, in the peripartum period, and, possibly, via breast-feeding. Enteroviruses can survive on environmental surfaces for periods long enough to allow transmission from fomites. Hospital nursery and other institutional outbreaks can occur. Infection incidence, clinical attack rates, and disease severity are typically greatest in young children, and infections occur more frequently in tropical areas and where poor sanitation, poor hygiene, and overcrowding are present. Most EV infections in temperate climates occur in the summer and fall (June through October in the northern hemisphere), but seasonal patterns are less evident in the tropics. Epidemics of EV meningitis, EV 71–associated hand-foot-and-mouth disease with neurologic and cardiopulmonary complications (particularly in southeastern Asia), and EV 70– and coxsackievirus A24–associated acute hemorrhagic conjunctivitis (especially in tropical regions) occur. Fecal viral shedding can persist for several weeks or months after onset of infection, but respiratory tract shedding is usually limited to 1 to 3 weeks or less. Infection and viral shedding can occur without signs of clinical illness.

Incubation Period

3 to 6 days for all except acute hemorrhagic conjunctivitis, which is 24 to 72 hours.

Diagnostic Tests

Enteroviruses can be detected by reverse transcriptase-polymerase chain reaction (PCR) assay and culture from a variety of specimens, including stool, rectal, throat and conjunctival swabs, nasopharyngeal aspirates, tracheal aspirates, blood, urine, tissue biopsy specimens, and cerebrospinal fluid (CSF) when meningitis is present. Patients with EV 71 neurologic disease often have negative results of PCR assay and culture of CSF (even in the presence of CSF pleocytosis) and blood; PCR assay and culture of throat or rectal swab or vesicle fluid specimens are more frequently positive. Polymerase chain reaction assays for detection of EV RNA are available at many reference and commercial laboratories for CSF, blood, and other specimens. Polymerase chain reaction assay is more rapid and more sensitive than isolation of EVs in cell culture and can detect all EVs, including serotypes that are difficult to cultivate in viral culture. Sensitivity of culture ranges from 0% to 80% depending on serotype and cell lines used. Many group A coxsackieviruses grow poorly or not at all in vitro. Culture usually requires 3 to 8 days to detect growth. Acute infection with a known EV serotype can be determined at reference laboratories by demonstration of a change in neutralizing or other serotype-specific antibody titer between acute and convalescent serum specimens or detection of serotype-specific immunoglobulin M, but serologic assays are relatively insensitive and lack specificity.

Treatment

No specific antiviral therapy is available for EV infections. Intravenous immunoglobulin may be beneficial for chronic EV meningoencephalitis in patients who are immunodeficient. Intravenous immunoglobulin has also been used for life-threatening neonatal EV infections, severe EV infections in transplant recipients and people with malignancies, suspected viral myocarditis, and EV 71 neurologic disease, but proof of efficacy is lacking. Interferons occasionally have been used for treatment of EV-associated myocarditis, without definitive proof of efficacy. The antiviral drug, pleconaril, has activity against EVs (but likely not parechoviruses) but is not available commercially. Other agents with activity against EVs are in development (eg, pocapavir).

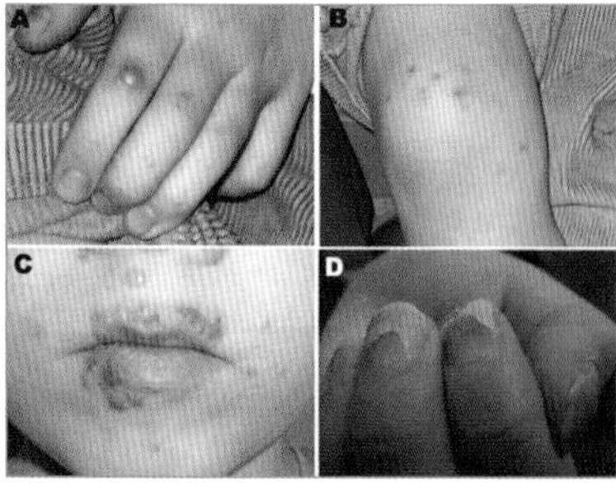

Image 44.1
Vesicular eruptions in hand (A), foot (B), and mouth (C) of a 6-year-old boy with coxsackievirus A6 infection. Several of his fingernails shed (D) 2 months after the pictures were taken. Courtesy of Centers for Disease Control and Prevention/ *Emerging Infectious Diseases.*

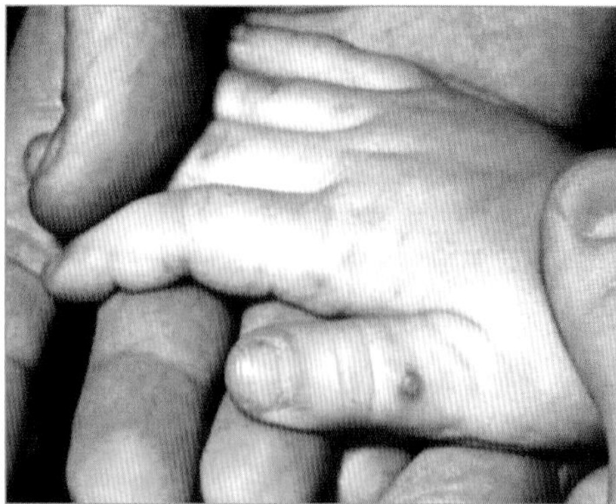

Image 44.2
Enterovirus infection in a preschool-aged girl. Hand-foot-and-mouth disease lesions are caused by coxsackievirus A16 and enterovirus 71.

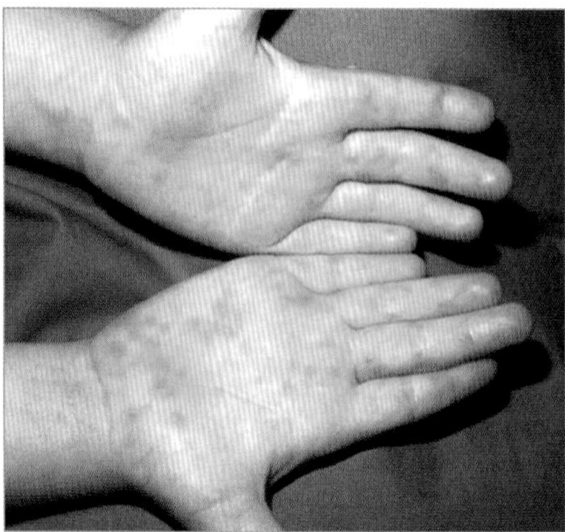

Image 44.3
Enterovirus infection (hand-foot-and-mouth disease) affecting the hands.

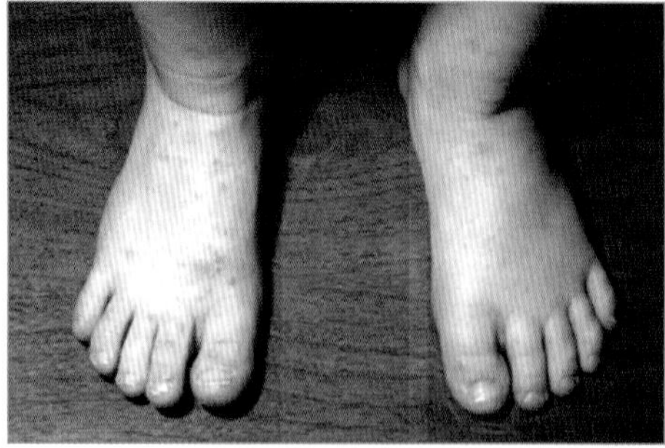

Image 44.4
Enterovirus infection (hand-foot-and-mouth disease) affecting the feet.

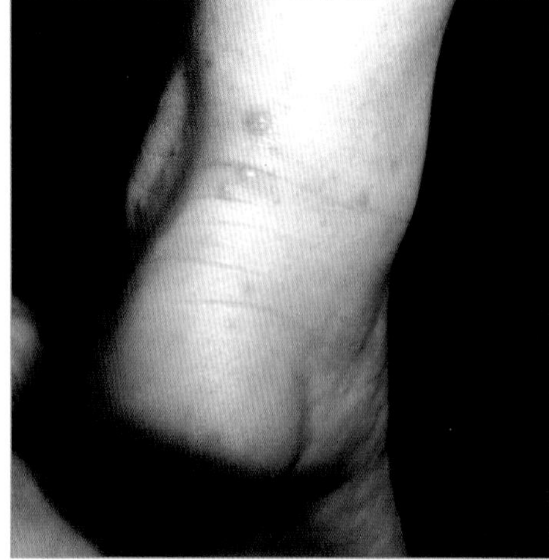

Image 44.5
Enterovirus infection (hand-foot-and-mouth disease) with typical papulovesicular lesions over the Achilles tendon area.

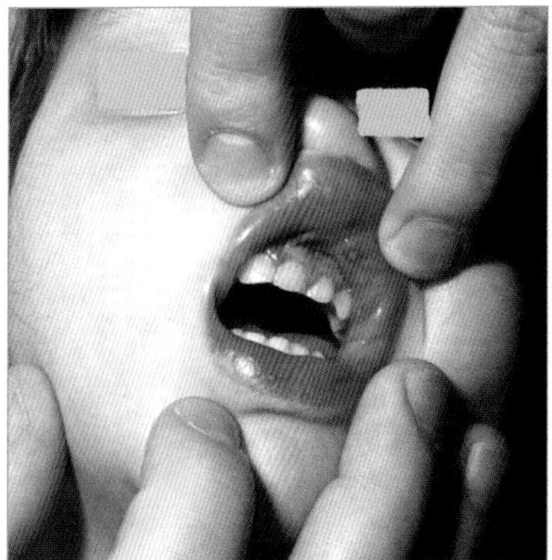

Image 44.6
Enterovirus infection (hand-foot-and-mouth disease) affecting the anterior buccal mucosa. These lesions are generally less painful than herpes simplex lesions.

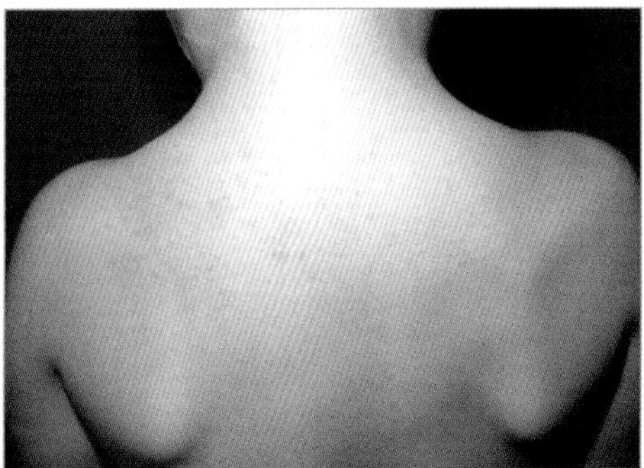

Image 44.8
Enterovirus infection (hand-foot-and-mouth disease). The rash may also be seen on the trunk.

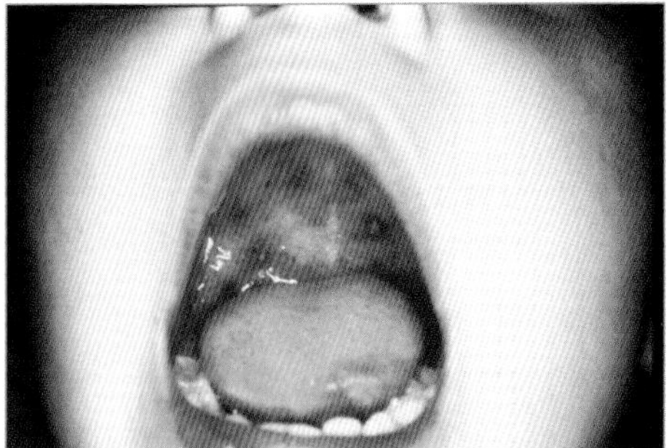

Image 44.10
Characteristic papulovesicular lesions of hand-foot-and-mouth disease in a 2-year-old boy. Courtesy of George Nankervis, MD.

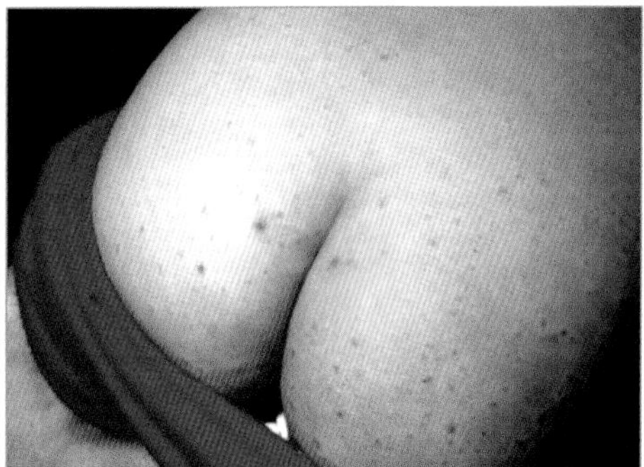

Image 44.7
Enterovirus infection (hand-foot-and-mouth disease). This rash, commonly seen over the buttocks, often appears macular, maculopapular, or papulovesicular and may be petechial.

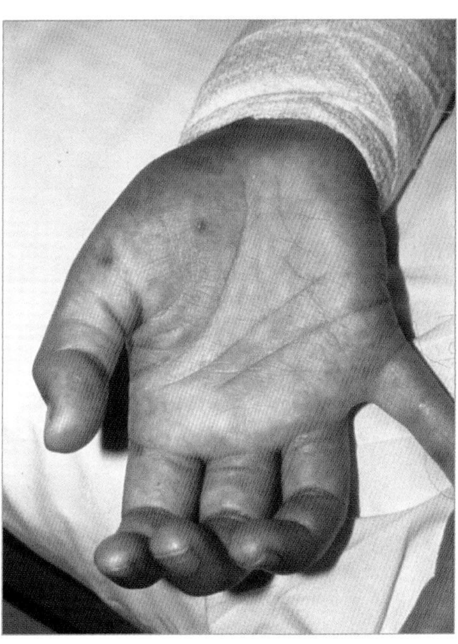

Image 44.9
Characteristic papulovesicular lesions on the palm of a 2-year-old boy with hand-foot-and-mouth disease, a coxsackievirus A infection, most often A16, or enterovirus 71. Courtesy of George Nankervis, MD.

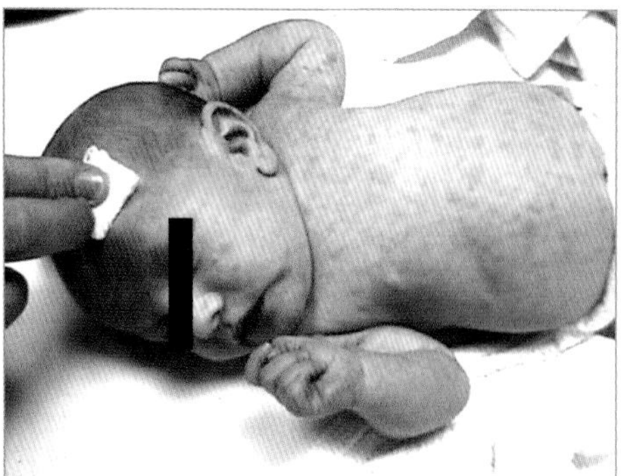

Image 44.11
Newborn with generalized enteroviral exanthem. Copyright Michael Rajnik, MD, FAAP.

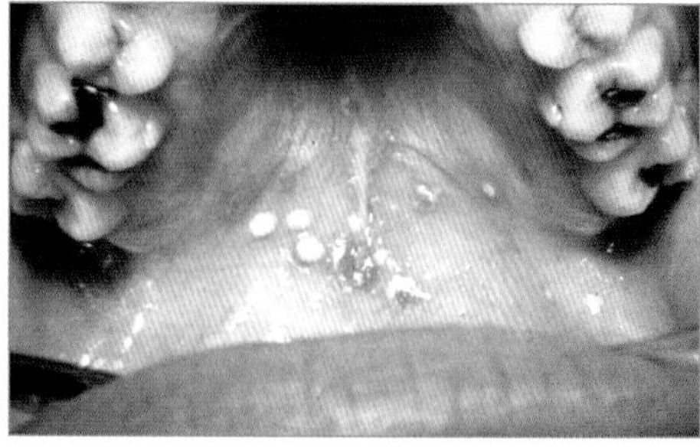

Image 44.12
Herpangina (coxsackievirus) lesions on the posterior palate of a young adult male. Coxsackievirus lesions are usually found in the posterior aspect of the oropharynx and may progress rapidly to painful ulceration.

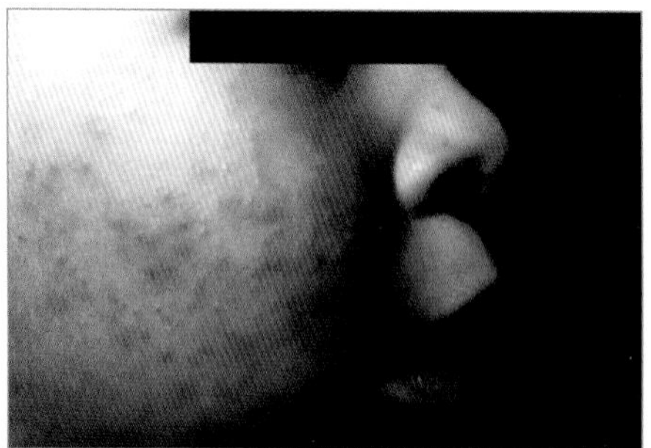

Image 44.13
Skin lesions on the side of a young girl's face due to echovirus 9. Courtesy of Centers for Disease Control and Prevention.

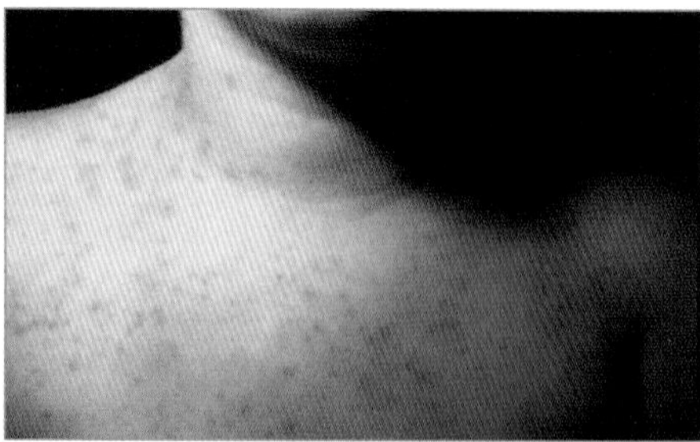

Image 44.14
Skin lesions on the neck and chest of a young girl due to echovirus 9. Echoviruses comprise 1 of 5 serotypes, which make up the genus *Enterovirus*, and are associated with illnesses, including aseptic meningitis, nonspecific rashes, encephalitides, and myositis. Courtesy of Centers for Disease Control and Prevention.

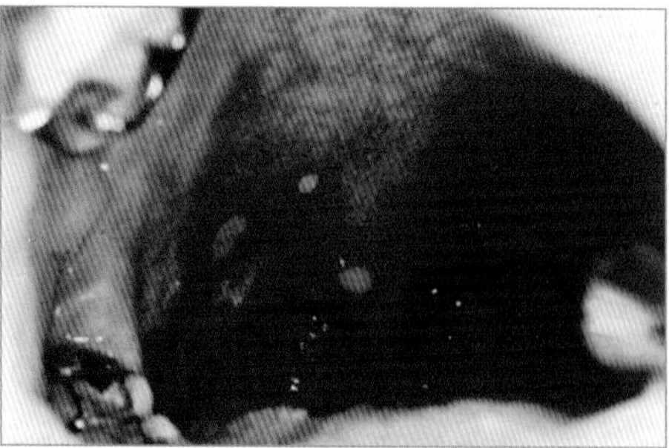

Image 44.15
A 4-year-old white girl with pharyngeal inflammation and palatal lesions of hand-foot-and-mouth disease, a coxsackievirus A infection. Copyright Larry Frenkel, MD.

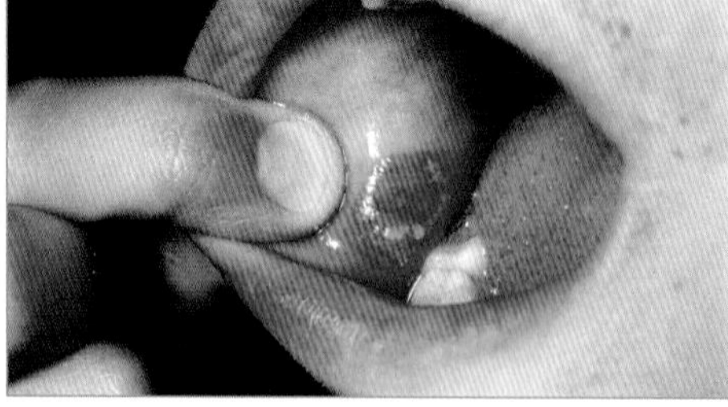

Image 44.16
This 7-year-old white girl presented with low-grade fever, malaise, sore throat, and these interesting, slightly raised oral lesions opposite the first molar. She also had approximately 10 maculopapular lesions on each buttock and a few on each foot. She had classic hand-foot-and-mouth disease. Coxsackievirus A16 was grown from throat and rectal swabs. Courtesy of Neal Halsey, MD.

45

Epstein-Barr Virus Infections

(Infectious Mononucleosis)

Clinical Manifestations

Infectious mononucleosis is the most common presentation of Epstein-Barr virus (EBV) infection. It typically manifests as fever, pharyngitis with petechiae, exudative pharyngitis, lymphadenopathy, hepatosplenomegaly, and atypical lymphocytosis. The spectrum of diseases is wide, ranging from asymptomatic to fatal infection. Infections are commonly unrecognized in infants and young children. Rash can occur and is more common in patients treated with ampicillin or amoxicillin, as well as with other penicillins. Central nervous system manifestations include aseptic meningitis, encephalitis, myelitis, optic neuritis, cranial nerve palsies, transverse myelitis, "Alice in Wonderland" syndrome, and Guillain-Barré syndrome. Hematologic complications include splenic rupture, thrombocytopenia, agranulocytosis, hemolytic anemia, and hemophagocytic lymphohistiocytosis (also called hemophagocytic syndrome). Pneumonia, orchitis, and myocarditis are infrequently observed. Early in the course of primary infection, up to 20% of circulating B lymphocytes are infected with EBV. Replication of EBV in B lymphocytes results in T lymphocyte proliferation and inhibition of B lymphocyte proliferation by T lymphocyte cytotoxic responses. Fatal disseminated infection or B or T lymphocyte lymphomas can occur in children with no detectable immunologic abnormality, as well as in children with congenital or acquired cellular immune deficiencies.

Epstein-Barr virus is associated with several other distinct disorders, including X-linked lymphoproliferative syndrome, posttransplantation lymphoproliferative disorders, Burkitt lymphoma, nasopharyngeal carcinoma, and undifferentiated B or T lymphocyte lymphomas. The syndrome is characterized by several phenotypic expressions, including occurrence of fatal infectious mononucleosis early in life among boys, nodular B lymphocyte lymphomas (often with central nervous system involvement), and profound hypogammaglobulinemia.

Epstein-Barr virus–associated lymphoproliferative disorders result in a number of complex syndromes in patients who are immunocompromised, such as transplant recipients or people infected with HIV. The highest incidence of these disorders occurs in liver and heart transplant recipients, in whom the proliferative states range from benign lymph node hypertrophy to monoclonal lymphomas. Other EBV syndromes are of greater importance outside the United States. Epstein-Barr virus is present in virtually 100% of people with endemic Burkitt lymphoma, found primarily in Central Africa, in contrast to 20% of people with sporadic Burkitt lymphoma (found in abdominal lymphoid tissue predominantly in North America and Europe). Epstein-Barr virus is found in nasopharyngeal carcinoma in Southeast Asia and the Inuit populations. Epstein-Barr virus has also been associated with Hodgkin disease (B lymphocyte tumor), non-Hodgkin lymphomas (B and T lymphocyte), gastric carcinoma "lymphoepitheliomas," and a variety of common epithelial malignancies.

Chronic fatigue syndrome is not related to EBV infection; however, fatigue lasting weeks to a few months may follow up to 10% of cases of classic infectious mononucleosis.

Etiology

Epstein-Barr virus (also known as human herpesvirus 4) is a gammaherpesvirus of the *Lymphocryptovirus* genus and is the most common cause of infectious mononucleosis (>90% of cases).

Epidemiology

Humans are the only known reservoir of EBV, and approximately 90% of US adults have been infected. Close personal contact is usually required for transmission. The virus is viable in saliva for several hours outside the body, but the role of fomites in transmission is unknown. Epstein-Barr virus can also be transmitted by blood transfusion or transplantation. Infection is commonly contracted early in life, particularly among members of lower socioeconomic groups, in which intrafamilial spread is common. Endemic infectious mononucleosis is common in group settings of adolescents, such as in educational institutions. No seasonal pattern has been documented. Intermittent excretion in saliva may occur throughout life after acute infection.

Incubation Period

30 to 50 days.

Diagnostic Tests

Routine diagnosis depends on serologic testing. Nonspecific tests for heterophile antibody, including the Paul-Bunnell test and slide agglutination reaction test, are available most commonly. The heterophile antibody response is primarily immunoglobulin (Ig) M, which appears during the first 2 weeks of illness and gradually disappears over a 6-month period. The results of heterophile antibody tests are often negative in children younger than 4 years, but heterophile antibody tests identify approximately 85% of cases of classic infectious mononucleosis in older children and adults. An absolute increase in atypical lymphocytes during the second week of illness with infectious mononucleosis is a characteristic but nonspecific finding. However, the finding of greater than 10% atypical lymphocytes together with a positive heterophile antibody test result in the classical illness pattern is considered diagnostic of acute infection.

Multiple specific serologic antibody tests for EBV infection are available. The most commonly performed test is for antibody against the viral capsid antigen (VCA). IgG antibodies against VCA occur in high titer early in infection and persist for life. Testing for presence of IgM anti-VCA antibody and the absence of antibodies to Epstein-Barr nuclear antigen (EBNA) identifies active and recent infections. Because serum antibody against EBNA is not present until several weeks to months after onset of infection, a positive anti-EBNA result excludes an active primary infection. Testing for antibodies against early antigen is not routinely performed. In selected cases, early antigen testing is useful. Epstein-Barr virus serologic tests are based on quantitative immunofluorescent antibody assays performed during various stages of mononucleosis and its resolution, although detection of antibodies by enzyme immunoassays is usually performed by clinical laboratories. Serologic testing for EBV is useful, particularly for evaluating patients who have heterophile-negative infectious mononucleosis and for cases in which the infectious mononucleosis syndrome is not completely present.

Isolation of EBV from oropharyngeal secretions by culture in cord blood cells is possible, but techniques for performing this procedure usually are not available in routine diagnostic laboratories, and viral isolation does not necessarily indicate acute infection. Polymerase chain reaction (PCR) assay for detection of EBV DNA in serum, plasma, and tissue and reverse transcriptase-polymerase chain reaction assay for detection of EBV RNA in lymphoid cells, tissue, or body fluids are available commercially and may be useful in evaluation of immunocompromised patients and in complex clinical problems.

Treatment

Patients suspected to have infectious mononucleosis should not be given ampicillin or amoxicillin, which cause nonallergic morbilliform rashes in a high proportion of patients. Although therapy with short-course corticosteroids may have a beneficial effect on acute symptoms, because of potential adverse effects, their use should be considered only for patients with marked tonsillar inflammation with impending airway obstruction, massive splenomegaly, myocarditis, hemolytic anemia, or hemophagocytic lymphohistiocytosis. Decreasing immunosuppressive therapy is beneficial for patients with EBV-induced posttransplant lymphoproliferative disorders.

Contact and collision sports should be avoided until the patient is recovered fully from infectious mononucleosis and the spleen is no longer palpable. In the setting of acute infectious mononucleosis, participation in strenuous and contact situations can result in splenic rupture. After 21 days, limited noncontact aerobic activity can be allowed if there are no symptoms and no overt splenomegaly. Clearance to participate in contact or collision sports is appropriate after 4 weeks after onset of symptoms if the athlete is asymptomatic and has no overt splenomegaly. Repeat monospot or EBV serologic testing is not recommended.

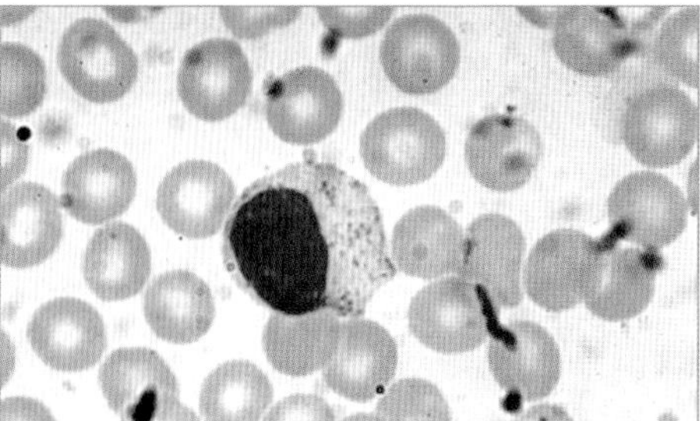

Image 45.1
Atypical lymphocyte in a peripheral blood smear of a patient with infectious mononucleosis. This lymphocyte is larger than normal lymphocytes, with a higher ratio of cytoplasm to nucleus. The cytoplasm is vacuolated and basophilic. This may also be present in cytomegalovirus infections.

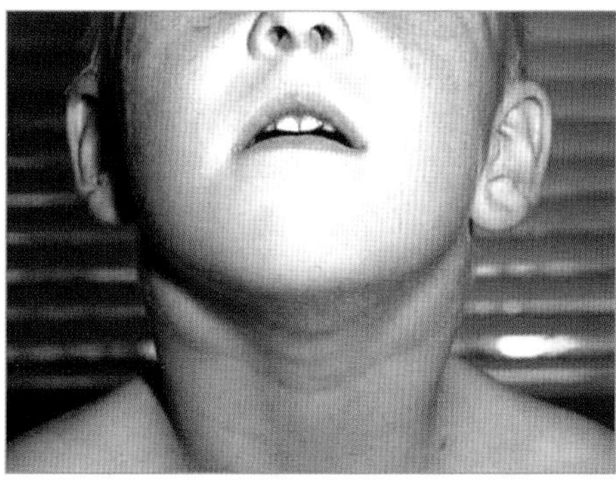

Image 45.2
Bilateral cervical lymphadenopathy in an 8-year-old boy with Epstein-Barr virus disease who remained relatively asymptomatic. Courtesy of Edgar O. Ledbetter, MD, FAAP.

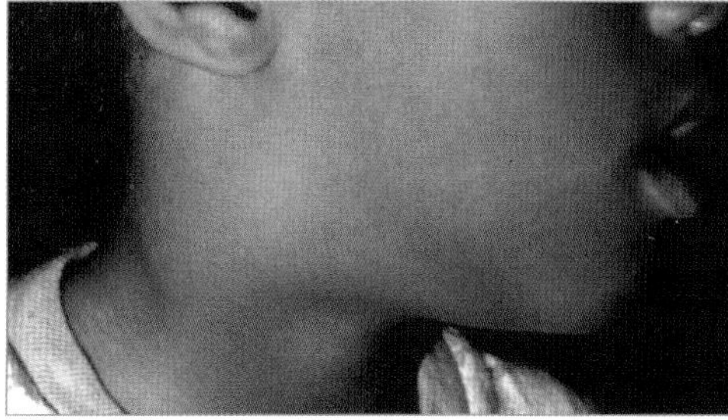

Image 45.3
Cervical lymphadenopathy in a 7-year-old girl with infectious mononucleosis.

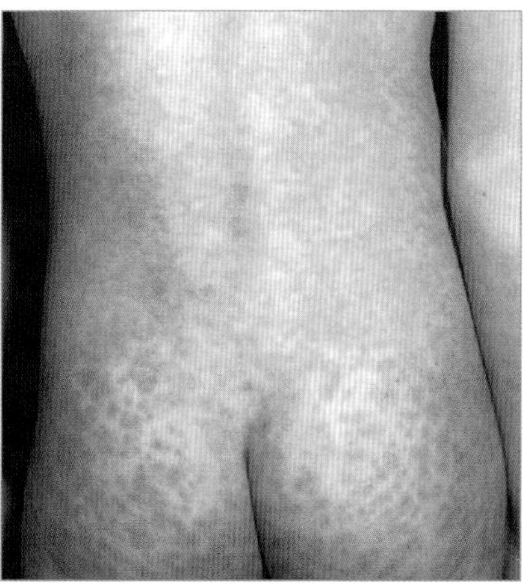

Image 45.4
This morbilliform rash arose in a patient with infectious mononucleosis after amoxicillin was prescribed. This is a nonallergic cutaneous eruption. Courtesy of Centers for Disease Control and Prevention/Dr Thomas F. Sellers, Emory University.

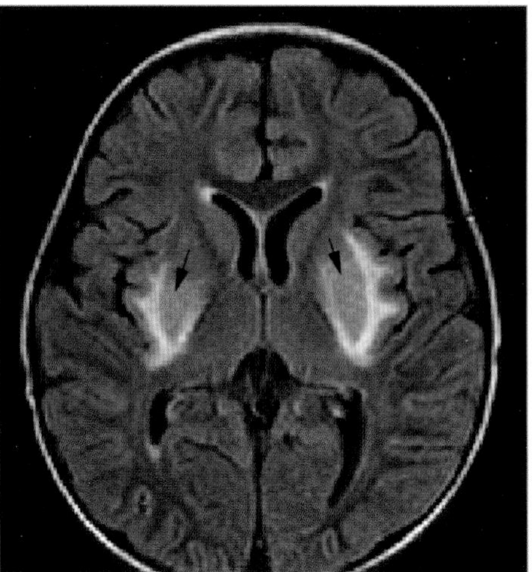

Image 45.5
Epstein-Barr virus encephalitis. Axial fluid attenuated inversion recovery magnetic resonance image shows basal ganglia hyperintensity (arrows).

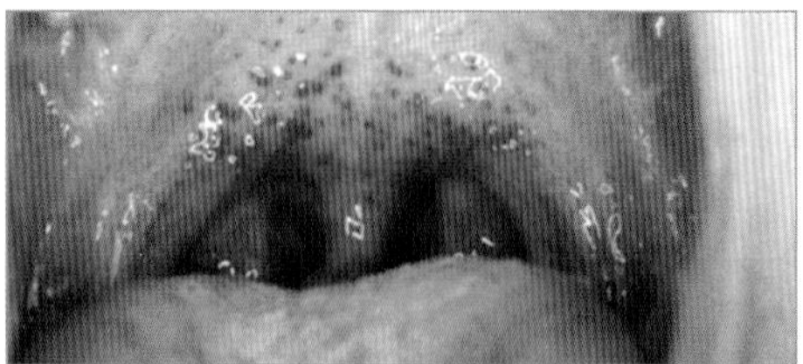

Image 45.6
A preadolescent child with infectious mononucleosis with petechiae on the soft palate and uvula without exudation.

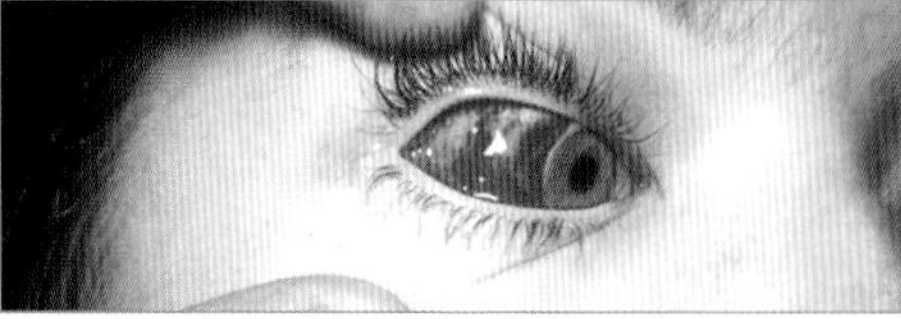

Image 45.7
A conjunctival hemorrhage of the right eye of a patient with infectious mononucleosis. At times, noninfectious conjunctivitis, as well as other corneal abnormalities, may manifest itself due to the body's systemic response to viral infections, such as infectious mononucleosis. Courtesy of Centers for Disease Control and Prevention/Dr Thomas F. Sellers, Emory University.

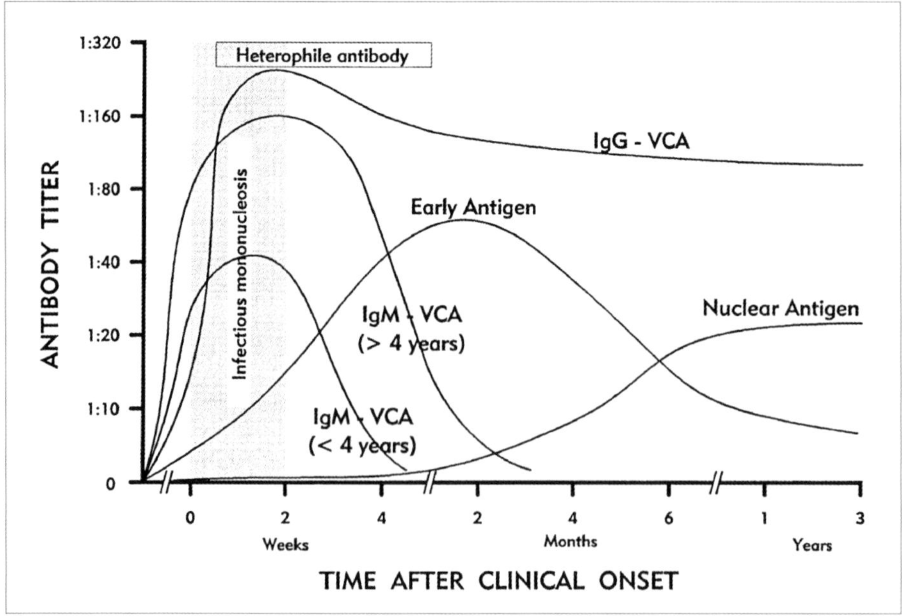

Image 45.8
Schematic representation of the evolution of antibodies to various Epstein-Barr virus antigens in patients with infectious mononucleosis. Reproduced with permission from American Society for Microbiology. Epstein-Barr virus. In: Rose NR, de Macario EC, Folds JD, eds. *Manual of Clinical Laboratory Immunology.* 5th ed. Washington, DC: American Society for Microbiology; 1997:634–643.

46

Escherichia coli and Other Gram-Negative Bacilli

(Septicemia and Meningitis in Neonates)

Clinical Manifestations

Neonatal septicemia or meningitis caused by *Escherichia coli* and other gram-negative bacilli cannot be differentiated clinically from septicemia or meningitis caused by other organisms. The early signs of sepsis can be subtle and similar to signs observed in noninfectious processes. Signs of septicemia include fever, temperature instability, heart rate abnormalities, grunting respirations, apnea, cyanosis, lethargy, irritability, anorexia, vomiting, jaundice, abdominal distention, cellulitis, and diarrhea. Meningitis, especially early in the course, can occur without overt signs suggesting central nervous system involvement. Some gram-negative bacilli, such as *Citrobacter koseri, Cronobacter* (formerly *Enterobacter*) *sakazakii, Serratia marcescens,* and *Salmonella* species, are associated with brain abscesses in neonates with meningitis caused by these organisms.

Etiology

E coli strains, often those with the K1 capsular polysaccharide antigen, are the most common cause of septicemia and meningitis in neonates. Other important gram-negative bacilli causing neonatal septicemia include *Klebsiella* species, *Enterobacter* species, *Proteus* species, *Citrobacter* species, *Salmonella* species, *Pseudomonas* species, *Acinetobacter* species, and *Serratia* species. Nonencapsulated strains of *Haemophilus influenzae* and anaerobic gram-negative bacilli are rare causes.

Epidemiology

The source of *E coli* and other gram-negative bacterial pathogens in neonatal infections during the first few days of life typically is the maternal genital tract. Reservoirs for gram-negative bacilli can also be present within the health care environment. Acquisition of gram-negative organisms can occur through person-to-person transmission from hospital nursery personnel and from nursery environmental sites, such as sinks, countertops, powdered infant formula, and respiratory therapy equipment, especially among very preterm neonates who require prolonged neonatal intensive care management. Predisposing factors in neonatal gram-negative bacterial infections include maternal intrapartum infection, gestation less than 37 weeks, low birth weight, and prolonged rupture of membranes. Metabolic abnormalities (eg, galactosemia), fetal hypoxia, and acidosis have been implicated as predisposing factors. Neonates with defects in the integrity of skin or mucosa (eg, myelomeningocele) or abnormalities of gastrointestinal or genitourinary tracts are at increased risk of gram-negative bacterial infections. In neonatal intensive care units, systems for respiratory and metabolic support, invasive or surgical procedures, indwelling vascular access catheters, and frequent use of broad-spectrum antimicrobial agents enable selection and proliferation of strains of gram-negative bacilli that are resistant to multiple antimicrobial agents.

Multiple mechanisms of resistance in gram-negative bacilli can be present simultaneously. Resistance resulting from production of chromosomally encoded or plasmid-derived AmpC β-lactamases or from plasmid-mediated extended-spectrum β-lactamases (ESBLs), occurring primarily in *E coli, Klebsiella* species, and *Enterobacter* species but reported in many other gram-negative species, has been associated with nursery outbreaks, especially in very low birth weight neonates. Organisms that produce ESBLs are typically resistant to penicillins, cephalosporins, and monobactams and can be resistant to aminoglycosides. Carbapenems-resistant strains have emerged among *Enterobacteriaceae,* especially *Klebsiella pneumoniae, Pseudomonas aeruginosa,* and *Acinetobacter* species. Extended-spectrum β-lactamase– and carbapenemase-producing bacteria often carry additional genes conferring resistance to aminoglycosides and sulfonamides, as well as fluoroquinolones.

Incubation Period

Variable, ranging from birth to several weeks after birth or longer in very low birth weight, preterm neonates with prolonged hospitalizations.

Diagnostic Tests

Diagnosis is established by growth of *E coli* or other gram-negative bacilli from blood, cerebrospinal fluid (CSF), or other, usually sterile sites. Special screening and confirmatory laboratory procedures are required to detect some multidrug-resistant gram-negative organisms. Molecular diagnostics are increasingly being used for identification of pathogens; specimens should be saved for resistance testing.

Treatment

Initial empiric treatment for suspected early-onset gram-negative septicemia in neonates is ampicillin and an aminoglycoside. An alternative regimen of ampicillin and an extended-spectrum cephalosporin (eg, cefotaxime) can be used, but rapid emergence of cephalosporin-resistant organisms, especially *Enterobacter* species, *Klebsiella* species, and *Serratia* species, and increased risk of colonization or infection with ESBL-producing *Enterobacteriaceae* can occur when use is routine in a neonatal unit. Hence, routine use of an extended-spectrum cephalosporin is not recommended unless gram-negative bacterial meningitis is suspected. The proportion of *E coli* bloodstream infections with onset within 72 hours of life that are resistant to ampicillin is high among very low birth weight neonates. These *E coli* infections are almost invariably susceptible to gentamicin, although monotherapy with an aminoglycoside is not recommended.

Once the causative agent and in vitro antimicrobial susceptibility pattern are known, nonmeningeal infections should be treated with ampicillin, an appropriate aminoglycoside, or an extended-spectrum cephalosporin (eg, cefotaxime). Many experts would treat nonmeningeal infections caused by *Enterobacter* species, *Serratia* species, or *Pseudomonas* species and some other, less commonly occurring gram-negative bacilli with a β-lactam antimicrobial agent and an aminoglycoside. For ampicillin-susceptible CSF isolates of *E coli,* meningitis can be treated with ampicillin or cefotaxime; meningitis caused by an ampicillin-resistant isolate is treated with cefotaxime with or without an aminoglycoside. Combination therapy with cefotaxime and an aminoglycoside antimicrobial agent is used for empirical therapy and until CSF is sterile. Some experts continue combination therapy for a longer duration. Expert advice from an infectious disease specialist can be helpful for management of meningitis.

The drug of choice for treatment of infections caused by ESBL-producing organisms is meropenem, which is active against gram-negative aerobic organisms with chromosomally mediated AmpC β-lactamases or ESBL-producing strains, except carbapenemase-producing strains, especially some *K pneumoniae* isolates. Of the aminoglycosides, amikacin retains the most activity against ESBL-producing strains. An aminoglycoside or cefepime can be used if the organism is susceptible. Expert advice from an infectious disease specialist can help in management of ESBL-producing gram-negative infections in neonates. The treatment of infections caused by carbapenemase-producing gram-negative organisms is guided by expert advice from an infectious disease specialist.

All neonates with gram-negative meningitis should undergo repeat lumbar puncture to ensure sterility of the CSF after 24 to 48 hours of therapy. If CSF remains culture positive, choice and doses of antimicrobial agents should be evaluated, and another lumbar puncture should be performed after another 48 to 72 hours. Duration of therapy is based on clinical and bacteriologic response of the patient and the site(s) of infection; the usual duration of therapy for uncomplicated bacteremia is 10 to 14 days, and for meningitis, minimum duration is 21 days. All neonates with gram-negative meningitis should undergo careful follow-up examinations, including testing for hearing loss, neurologic abnormalities, and developmental delay.

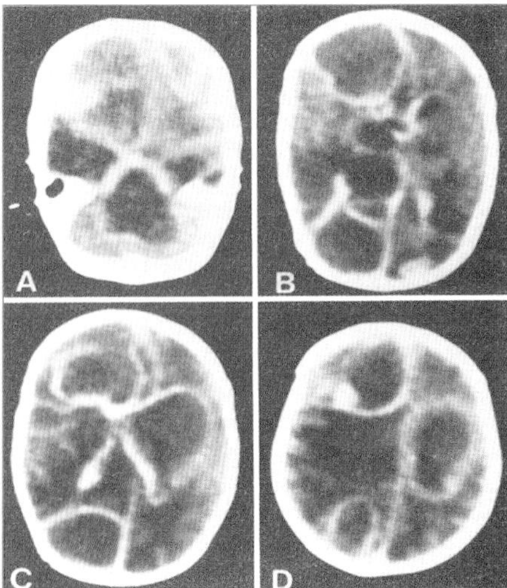

Image 46.1
Computed tomography scan of the head of a neonate 3 weeks after therapy for *Escherichia coli* meningitis demonstrating widespread destruction of cerebral cortex secondary to vascular thrombosis. Neonate was blind, deaf, and globally intellectually disabled and had diabetes insipidus. Courtesy of Carol J. Baker, MD, FAAP.

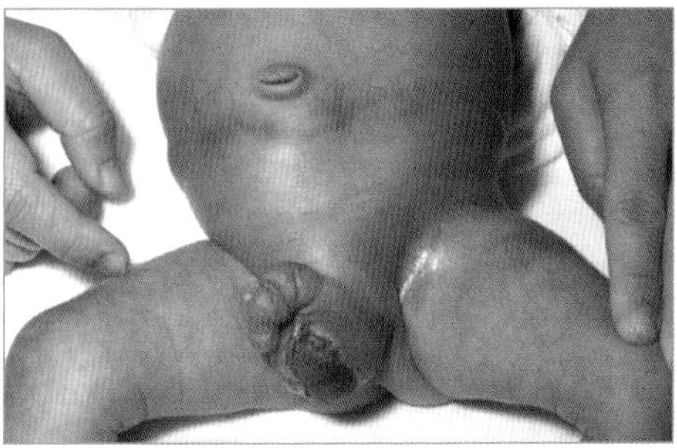

Image 46.3
Infant with *Escherichia coli* septicemia and perineal cellulitis, scrotal necrosis, and abdominal wall abscesses below the navel that required surgical drainage and antibiotics.

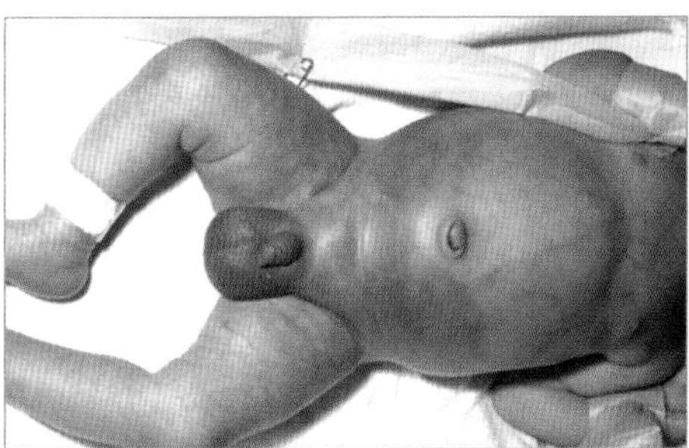

Image 46.2
Icteric premature neonate with septicemia and perineal and abdominal wall cellulitis due to *Escherichia coli*.

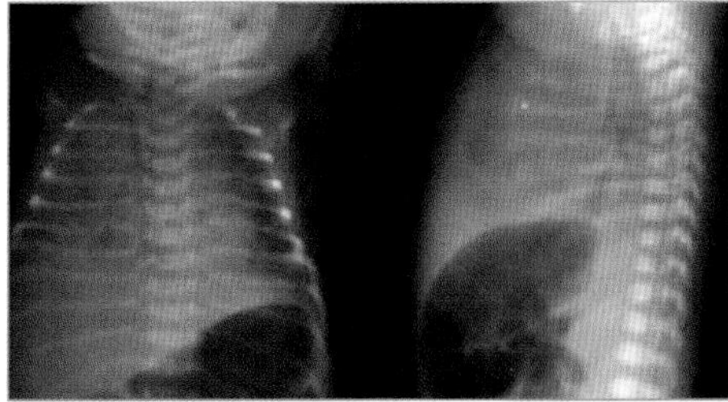

Image 46.4
Sepsis and pneumonia with empyema due to *Escherichia coli*. This newborn died at 12 hours of age.

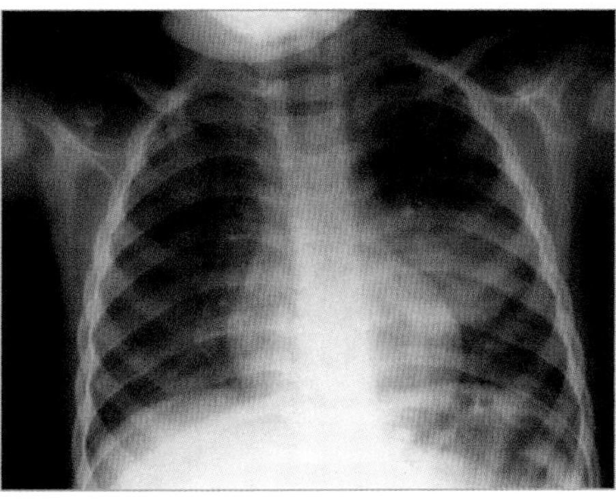

Image 46.5
Pneumonia due to *Klebsiella pneumoniae* with prebronchoscopy lung abscess. Courtesy of Edgar O. Ledbetter, MD, FAAP.

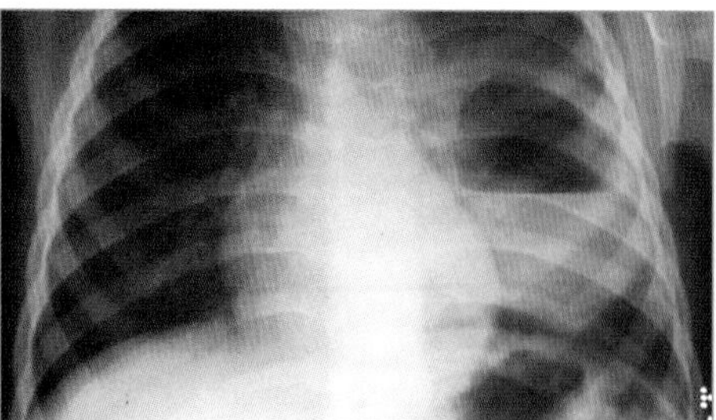

Image 46.6
Pneumonia due to *Klebsiella pneumoniae* with lung abscess. Cavitation with air-fluid level shown postbronchoscopy drainage. Repeat bronchoscopy was required for further drainage. Courtesy of Edgar O. Ledbetter, MD, FAAP.

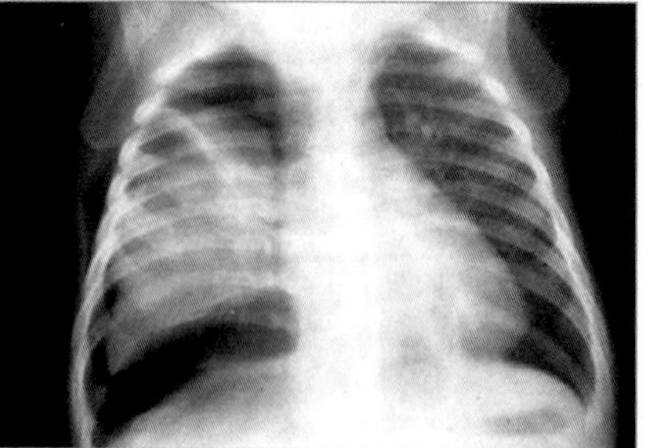

Image 46.7
Klebsiella pneumoniae pneumonia in a 4-month-old with spontaneous tension pneumothorax. Courtesy of Edgar O. Ledbetter, MD, FAAP.

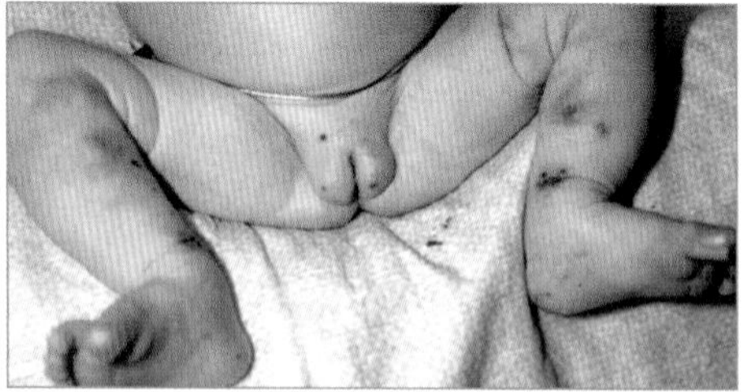

Image 46.8
A 5-week-old girl with *Klebsiella pneumoniae* sepsis and meningitis with bilateral saphenous vein thrombophlebitis (illness began with diarrhea). Copyright Martin G. Myers, MD.

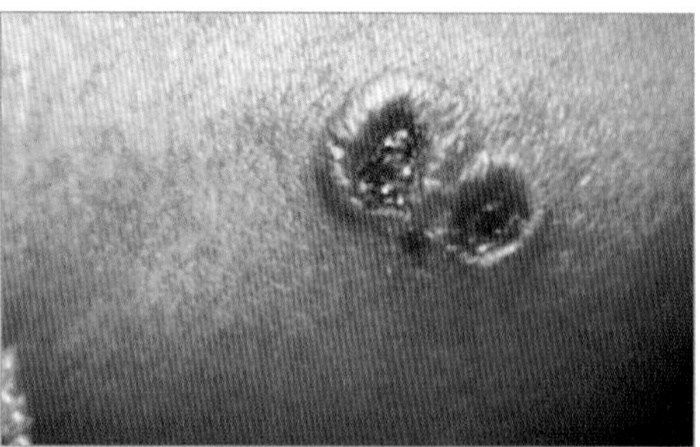

Image 46.9
Bullous, necrotic, umbilicated lesions in infant with septicemia due to *Pseudomonas aeruginosa*.

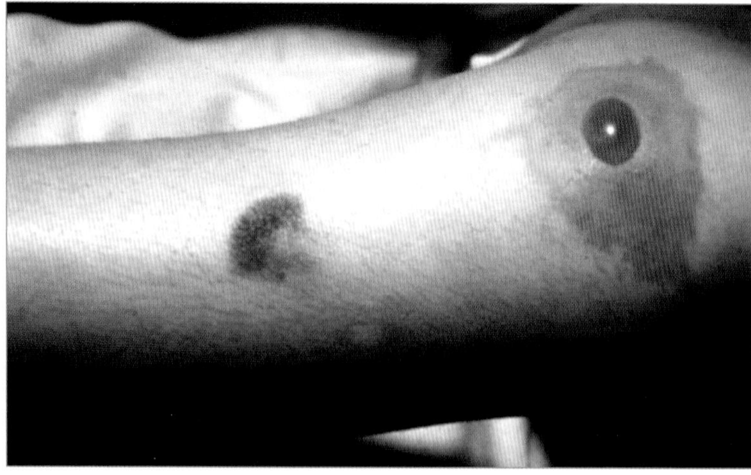

Image 46.10
Skin lesions due to *Pseudomonas aeruginosa* in child with neutropenia and septicemia.

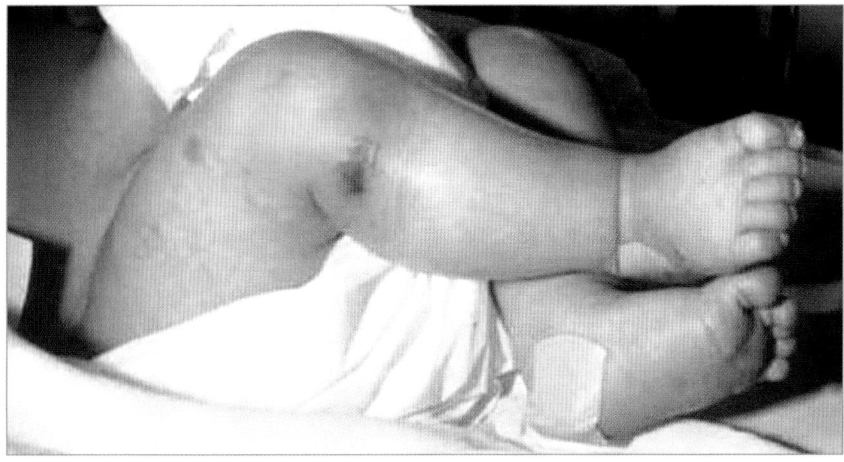

Image 46.11
Sepsis due to *Pseudomonas aeruginosa* with early ecthyma gangrenosum.

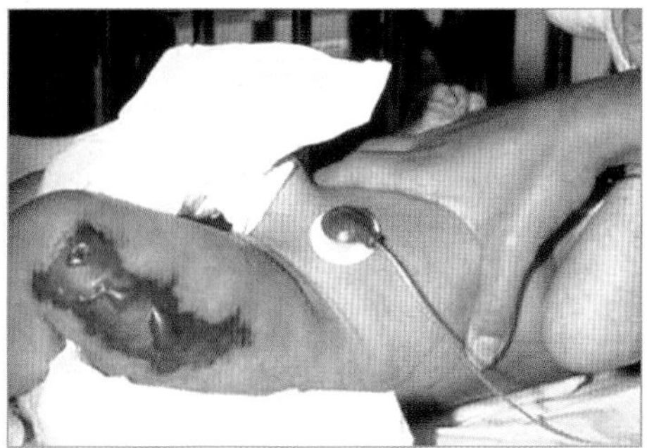

Image 46.12
Sepsis due to *Pseudomonas aeruginosa* with rapidly progressing ecthyma gangrenosum.

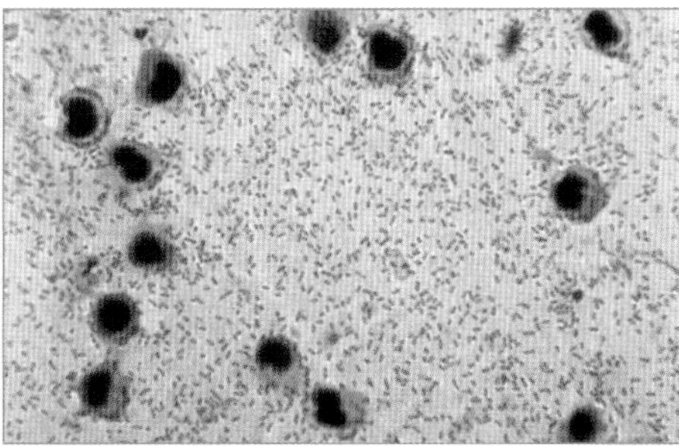

Image 46.13
Gram stain of *Escherichia coli* in the cerebrospinal fluid of a neonate with meningitis.

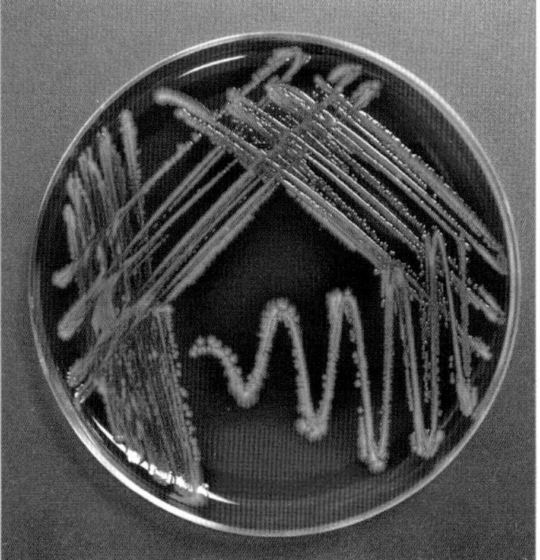

Image 46.14
Escherichia coli on sheep blood agar. Courtesy of Julia Rosebush, DO; Robert Jerris, PhD; and Theresa Stanley, M(ASCP).

47

Escherichia coli Diarrhea

(Including Hemolytic Uremic Syndrome)

Clinical Manifestations

At least 5 pathotypes of diarrhea-producing *Escherichia coli* strains have been identified. Clinical features of disease caused by each pathotype are summarized in Table 47.1.

- Shiga toxin-producing *E coli* (STEC) organisms are associated with diarrhea, hemorrhagic colitis, and hemolytic uremic syndrome (HUS). Shiga toxin-producing *E coli* O157:H7 is the serotype most often implicated in outbreaks and is consistently a virulent STEC serotype, but other serotypes can also cause illness. Shiga toxin-producing *E coli* illness typically begins with nonbloody diarrhea. Stools usually become bloody after 2 or 3 days, representing the onset of hemorrhagic colitis. Severe abdominal pain is typically short lived, and low-grade fever is present in approximately one-third of cases. In people with presumptive diagnoses of intussusception, appendicitis, inflammatory bowel disease, or ischemic colitis, disease caused by *E coli* O157:H7 and other STEC should be considered.
- Diarrhea caused by enteropathogenic *E coli* (EPEC) is watery. Although usually mild, diarrhea can result in dehydration and even death. Illness occurs almost exclusively in children younger than 2 years and predominantly in resource-limited countries, sporadically or in epidemics. In resource-limited countries, EPEC may be associated with high case fatality. Chronic EPEC diarrhea can be persistent and result in wasting or growth retardation. Enteropathogenic *E coli* infection is uncommon in breastfed infants.
- Diarrhea caused by enterotoxigenic *E coli* (ETEC) is a 1- to 5-day, self-limited illness of moderate severity, typically with watery stools and abdominal cramps. Enterotoxigenic *E coli* is common in infants in resource-limited countries and in travelers to those countries. Enterotoxigenic *E coli* infection is rarely diagnosed in the United States. However, outbreaks and studies with small numbers of patients have demonstrated that ETEC infection is occasionally acquired in the United States.
- Diarrhea caused by enteroinvasive *E coli* is clinically similar to diarrhea caused by *Shigella* species. Although dysentery can

Table 47.1
Classification of *Escherichia coli* Associated With Diarrhea

Pathotype	Epidemiology	Type of Diarrhea	Mechanism of Pathogenesis
Shiga toxin-producing *E coli* (STEC)	Hemorrhagic colitis and hemolytic uremic syndrome in all ages	Bloody or nonbloody	Shiga toxin production, large bowel attachment, coagulopathy
Enteropathogenic *E coli* (EPEC)	Acute and chronic endemic and epidemic diarrhea in infants	Watery	Small bowel adherence and effacement
Enterotoxigenic *E coli* (ETEC)	Infant diarrhea in resource-limited countries and traveler's diarrhea in all ages	Watery	Small bowel adherence, heat-stable/heat-labile enterotoxin production
Enteroinvasive *E coli* (EIEC)	Diarrhea with fever in all ages	Bloody or nonbloody; dysentery	Adherence, mucosal invasion and inflammation of large bowel
Enteroaggregative *E coli* (EAEC)	Acute and chronic diarrhea in all ages	Watery, occasionally bloody	Small and large bowel adherence, enterotoxin and cytotoxin production

occur, diarrhea is usually watery without blood or mucus. Patients are often febrile, and stools can contain leukocytes.

- Enteroaggregative *E coli* (EAEC) organisms cause watery diarrhea and are common in people of all ages in industrialized as well as resource-limited countries. Enteroaggregative *E coli* has been associated with prolonged diarrhea (≥14 days). Asymptomatic infection can be accompanied by subclinical inflammatory enteritis, which can cause growth disturbance.
- **Sequelae of STEC infection:** Hemolytic uremic syndrome is a serious sequela of STEC enteric infection. *E coli* O157:H7 is the STEC serotype most commonly associated with HUS, which is defined by the triad of microangiopathic hemolytic anemia, thrombocytopenia, and acute renal dysfunction. Children younger than 5 years are at highest risk of HUS, which occurs in approximately 15% of children infected with STEC. Hemolytic uremic syndrome typically develops 7 days (up to 2 weeks; rarely, 2–3 weeks) after onset of diarrhea. More than 50% of children with HUS require dialysis, and 3% to 5% die. Patients with HUS can develop neurologic complications (eg, seizures, coma, cerebral vessel thrombosis). Children presenting with an elevated white blood cell count (>20 x 10^9/mL) or oliguria or anuria are at higher risk of poor outcome, as are, seemingly paradoxically, children with hematocrit close to normal rather than low. Most who survive have a very good prognosis, which can be predicted by normal creatinine clearance and no proteinuria or hypertension 1 or more years after HUS.

Etiology

Five pathotypes of diarrhea-producing *E coli* have been distinguished by pathogenic and clinical characteristics. Each pathotype comprises characteristic serotypes, indicated by somatic (O) and flagellar (H) antigens.

Epidemiology

Transmission of most diarrhea-associated *E coli* strains is from food or water contaminated with human or animal feces or from infected symptomatic people. Shiga toxin-producing *E coli* is shed in feces of cattle and, to a lesser extent, sheep, deer, and other ruminants. Human infection is acquired via contaminated food or water or via direct contact with an infected person, a fomite, or a carrier animal or its environment. Many food vehicles have caused *E coli* O157 outbreaks, including undercooked ground beef (a major source), raw leafy greens, and unpasteurized milk and juice. Outbreak investigations have also implicated petting zoos, drinking water, and ingestion of recreational water. The infectious dose is low; thus, person-to-person transmission is common in households and has occurred in child care centers. Less is known about the epidemiology of STEC strains other than O157:H7. Among children younger than 5 years, the incidence of HUS is highest in 1-year-olds and lowest in infants. A severe outbreak of bloody diarrhea and HUS occurred in Europe in 2011; the outbreak was attributed to an EAEC strain of serotype O104:H4 that had acquired the Shiga toxin 2a-encoding phage. This experience highlights the importance of considering serotypes other than O157:H7 in outbreaks and cases of HUS.

With the exception of EAEC, non-STEC pathotypes are most commonly associated with disease in resource-limited countries, where food and water supplies commonly are contaminated and facilities and supplies for hand hygiene are suboptimal. For young children in resource-limited countries, transmission of ETEC, EPEC, and other diarrheal pathogens via contaminated weaning foods (sometimes by use of untreated drinking water in the foods) is also common. Enterotoxigenic *E coli* diarrhea occurs in people of all ages but is especially frequent and severe in infants in resource-limited countries. Enterotoxigenic *E coli* is a major cause of traveler's diarrhea. Enteroaggregative *E coli* is increasingly recognized as a cause of diarrhea in the United States.

Incubation Period

For most *E coli* strains, 10 hours to 6 days; for *E coli* O157:H7, 3 to 4 days (range, 1–8 days).

Diagnostic Tests

Diagnosis of infection caused by diarrhea-associated *E coli* other than STEC is difficult because tests are not widely available to distinguish these pathotypes from normal *E coli* strains present in stool flora. Culture-independent tests are necessary to detect non-O157:H7 STEC infections. Newly licensed multiplex polymerase chain reaction assays can detect a variety of enteric infections, including ETEC and STEC. Several commercially available, sensitive, specific, and rapid assays for Shiga toxins in stool or broth culture of stool, including enzyme immunoassays and immunochromatographic assays, have been approved by the US Food and Drug Administration. All stool specimens submitted for routine testing from patients with acute community-acquired diarrhea should be cultured simultaneously for *E coli* O157:H7 and tested with an assay that detects Shiga toxins. Most *E coli* O157:H7 isolates can be identified presumptively when grown on sorbitol-containing selective media.

Shiga toxin-producing *E coli* should also be sought in stool specimens from all patients diagnosed with postdiarrheal HUS. However, the absence of STEC does not preclude the diagnosis of probable STEC-associated HUS because HUS is typically diagnosed a week or more after onset of diarrhea, when the organism may not be detectable by conventional methods. Selective enrichment followed by immunomagnetic separation can markedly increase the sensitivity of STEC detection, so this testing is especially useful for patients who were not tested early in their diarrheal illness. The test is available at some state public health laboratories and at the Centers for Disease Control and Prevention. DNA probes are also available in reference and research laboratories. Serologic diagnosis using enzyme immunoassay to detect serum antibodies to *E coli* O157 and O111 lipopolysaccharides is available at the Centers for Disease Control and Prevention for outbreak investigations and for patients with HUS.

Treatment

Orally administered electrolyte-containing solutions are usually adequate to prevent or treat dehydration and electrolyte abnormalities. Antimotility agents should not be administered to children with inflammatory or bloody diarrhea. Patients with proven or suspected STEC infection should be fully but prudently rehydrated as soon as clinically feasible. Careful monitoring of patients with hemorrhagic colitis (including complete blood cell count with smear, blood urea nitrogen, and creatinine concentrations) is recommended to detect changes suggestive of HUS. If patients have no laboratory evidence of hemolysis, thrombocytopenia, or nephropathy 3 days after resolution of diarrhea, their risk of developing HUS is low. In resource-limited countries, nutritional rehabilitation should be provided as part of case management algorithms for diarrhea where feasible. Feeding, including breastfeeding, should be continued for young children with *E coli* enteric infection.

- **Antimicrobial therapy:** Most experts advise not prescribing antimicrobial therapy for children with *E coli* O157:H7 enteritis or a clinical or epidemiologic picture strongly suggestive of STEC infection. Empirical self-treatment of diarrhea for travelers to a resource-limited country is effective, and azithromycin or a fluoroquinolone has been the most reliable agent for therapy; the choice of therapy depends on the pathogen and local antibiotic resistance patterns. Rifaximin may be used for people 12 years and older.

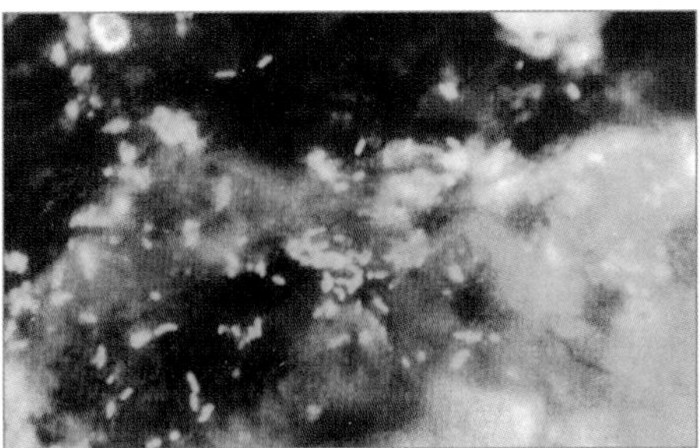

Image 47.1
Escherichia coli in the intestine of an 8-month-old suffering from chronic diarrhea (fluorescent antibody stain). In a small number of individuals (mostly children <5 years and the elderly), *E coli* can cause hemolytic uremic syndrome, in which the red blood cells are destroyed and the kidneys fail. Courtesy of Centers for Disease Control and Prevention.

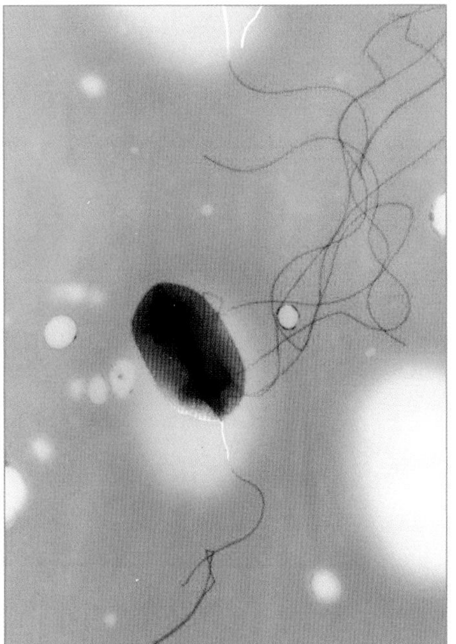

Image 47.2
Transmission electron micrograph of *Escherichia coli* O157:H7. Courtesy of Centers for Disease Control and Prevention/Peggy S. Hayes.

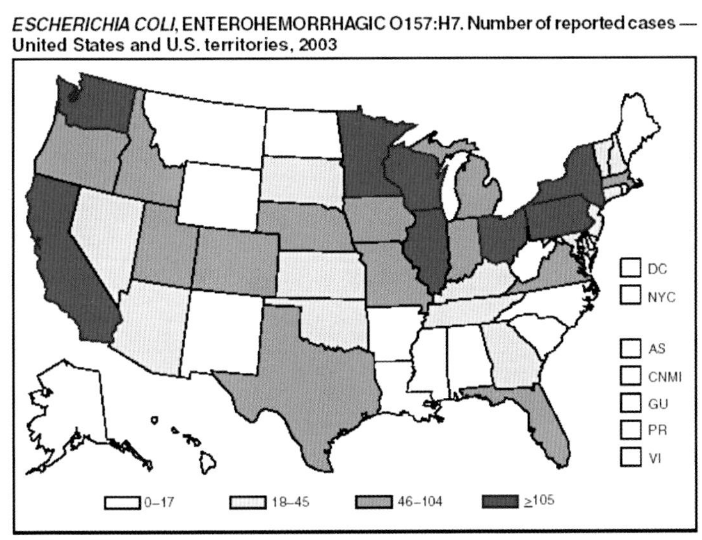

Image 47.3
Enterohemorrhagic *Escherichia coli* O157:H7. Number of reported cases in the United States and US territories, 2003. Courtesy of *Morbidity and Mortality Weekly Report.*

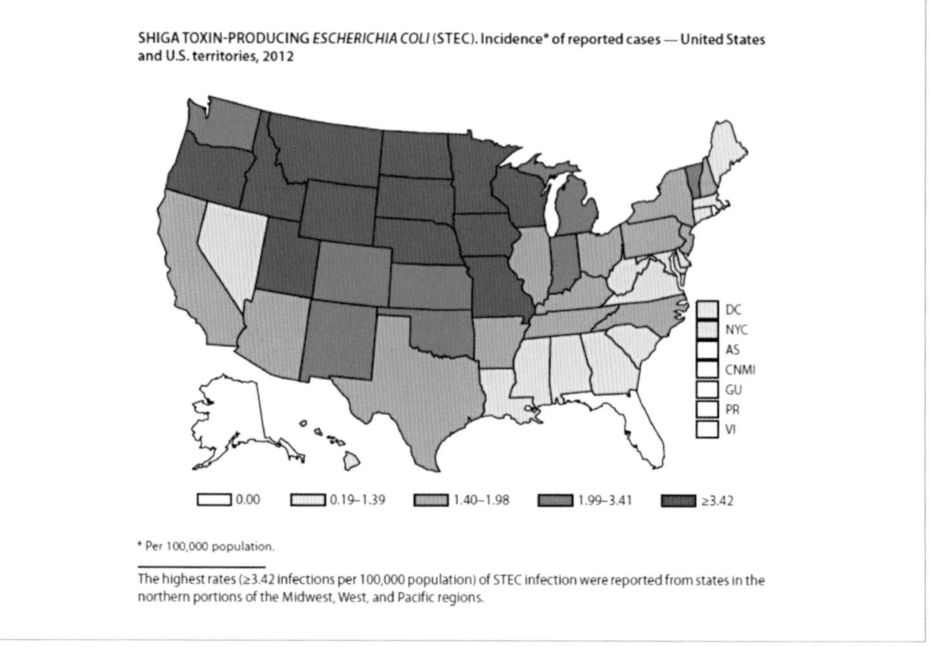

Image 47.4

Shiga toxin-producing *Escherichia coli.* Number of reported cases—United States and US territories, 2012. Courtesy of *Morbidity and Mortality Weekly Report.*

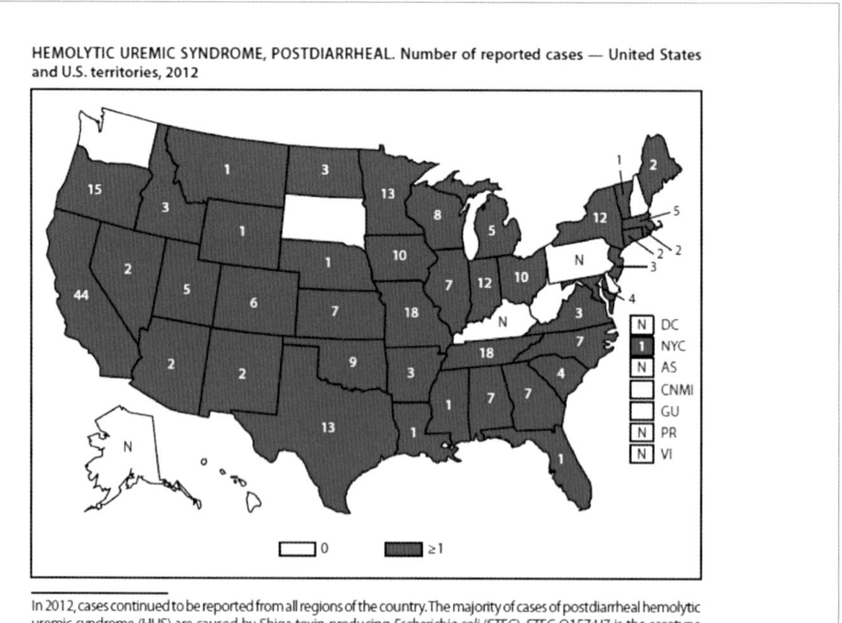

Image 47.5

Hemolytic uremic syndrome, postdiarrheal. Number of reported cases—United States and US territories, 2012. Courtesy of *Morbidity and Mortality Weekly Report.*

48

Fungal Diseases

In addition to the mycoses discussed in individual chapters (ie, aspergillosis, blastomycosis, candidiasis, coccidioidomycosis, cryptococcosis, histoplasmosis, paracoccidioidomycosis, sporotrichosis), uncommonly encountered fungi can cause infection in infants and children with immunosuppression or other underlying conditions. Children can acquire infection with these fungi through inhalation via the respiratory tract or through direct inoculation after traumatic disruption of cutaneous barriers. A list of these fungi and the pertinent underlying host conditions, reservoirs or routes of entry, clinical manifestations, diagnostic laboratory tests, and treatments can be found in Table 48.1. Taken as a group, few in vitro antifungal susceptibility data are available on which to base treatment recommendations for these uncommon invasive fungal infections, especially in children. Consultation with a pediatric infectious disease specialist experienced in the diagnosis and treatment of invasive fungal infections should be considered when caring for a child infected with one of these mycoses.

Table 48.1
Additional Fungal Diseases

Disease and Agent	Underlying Host Condition(s)	Reservoir(s) or Route(s) of Entry	Common Clinical Manifestations	Diagnostic Laboratory Test(s)	Treatment
Hyalohyphomycosis					
Fusarium species	Granulocytopenia; hematopoietic stem cell transplantation; severe immunocompromise	Respiratory tract; sinuses; skin	Pulmonary infiltrates; cutaneous lesions, sinusitis; disseminated infection	Culture of blood or tissue specimen	Voriconazole or L-AMB[a]
Malassezia species	Immunosuppression; preterm birth; exposure to parenteral nutrition that includes fat emulsions	Skin	Central line–associated bloodstream infection; interstitial pneumonitis; urinary tract infection; meningitis	Culture of blood, catheter tip, or tissue specimen (requires special laboratory handling)	Removal of catheters and temporary cessation of lipid infusion; L-AMB[a]
Penicilliosis					
Penicillium marneffei	HIV infection and exposure to southeast Asia	Respiratory tract	Pneumonitis; invasive dermatitis; disseminated infection	Culture of blood, bone marrow, or tissue; histopathologic examination of tissue	Itraconazole[b] or L-AMB
Phaeohyphomycosis					
Alternaria species	None or trauma or immunosuppression	Respiratory tract; skin	Sinusitis; cutaneous lesions	Culture and histopathologic examination of tissue	Voriconazole or high-dose L-AMB[a]
Bipolaris species	None, trauma, immunosuppression, or chronic sinusitis	Environment	Sinusitis; disseminated infection	Culture and histopathologic examination of tissue	Voriconazole, itraconazole,[b] or L-AMB[a]; surgical excision

Table 48.1
Additional Fungal Diseases (*continued*)

Disease and Agent	Under–lying Host Condition(s)	Reservoir(s) or Route(s) of Entry	Common Clinical Manifestations	Diagnostic Laboratory Test(s)	Treatment
Phaeohyphomycosis (*continued*)					
Curvularia species	Immunosuppression; altered skin integrity; asthma or nasal polyps; chronic sinusitis	Environment	Allergic fungal sinusitis; invasive dermatitis; disseminated infection	Culture and histopathologic examination of tissue	Allergic fungal sinusitis: surgery and corticosteroids Invasive disease: voriconazole, itraconazole,[b] or L-AMB[a]
Exophiala species, *Exserohilum* species	None or trauma or immunosuppression	Environment	Sinusitis; cutaneous lesions; disseminated infection; meningitis associated with contaminated steroid for epidural use	Culture and histopathologic examination of tissue	Voriconazole,[c] itraconazole,[b] L-AMB, or surgical excision
Pseudallescheria boydii (Scedosporium apiospermum) *Scedosporium* species	None or trauma or immunosuppression	Environment	Pneumonia; disseminated infection; osteomyelitis or septic arthritis; endocarditis	Culture and histopathologic examination of tissue	Voriconazole[d] or itraconazole
Trichosporonosis					
Trichosporon species	Immunosuppression; central venous catheter	Normal flora of gastrointestinal tract	Bloodstream infection; endocarditis; pneumonitis; disseminated infection	Blood culture; histopathologic examination of tissue; urine culture	Voriconazole
Mucormycosis (Formerly Zygomycosis)					
Rhizopus; Mucor; Lichtheimia (formerly *Absidia*) species; *Rhizomucor* species	Immunosuppression; hematologic malignant neoplasm; renal failure; diabetes mellitus; iron overload syndromes	Respiratory tract; skin	Rhinocerebral infection; pulmonary infection; disseminated infection; skin and gastrointestinal tract less commonly	Histopathologic examination of tissue and culture	High dose of L-AMB for initial therapy; surgical excision as feasible; posaconazole[e] for maintenance therapy (Voriconazole has no activity.)

Abbreviation: L-AMB, liposomal amphotericin B (if the patient is a neonate or young infant, or if L-AMP is not available, amphotericin B, D AMP, can be substituted).

[a] Consider use of a lipid-based formulation of amphotericin B.

[b] Itraconazole has been shown to be effective for cutaneous disease in adults, but safety and efficacy have not been established in children younger than 12 years.

[c] Voriconazole demonstrates activity in vitro, but limited clinical data are available for children.

[d] Itraconazole may be the treatment of choice, but data on safety and effectiveness in children are limited.

[e] Posaconazole demonstrates activity in vitro, but few clinical data are available for children.

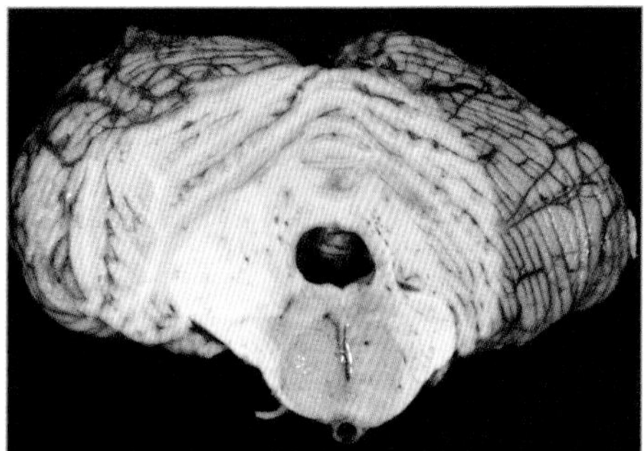

Image 48.1
Cerebral mucormycosis in a patient with acute lymphoblastic leukemia. Occlusion of the basilar artery and infarct of the pons. The patient had jaundice. Courtesy of Dimitris P. Agamanolis, MD.

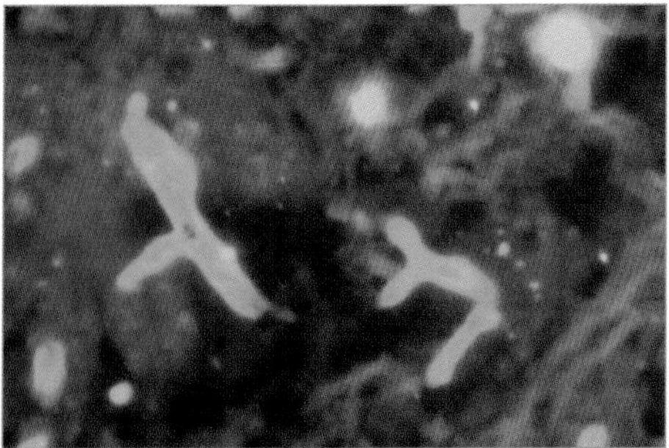

Image 48.3
This slide describes the histopathologic changes seen in zygomycosis due to *Rhizopus arrhizus* using fluorescent antibody stain technique. *R arrhizus*, the most common *Rhizopus* species, is known to be the cause of zygomycosis, an angiotropic disease, which means it tends to invade the blood vessels, thereby facilitating its systemic dissemination. Courtesy of Centers for Disease Control and Prevention/Dr William Kaplan.

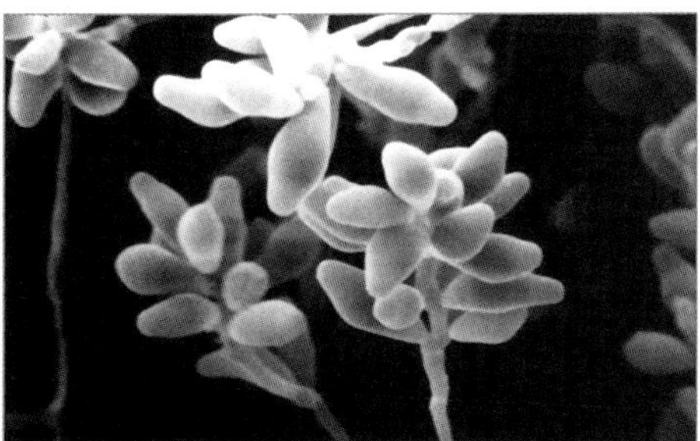

Image 48.5
Scanning electron micrograph of *Curvularia geniculata*. Courtesy of Centers for Disease Control and Prevention/Robert Simmons/Janice Haney Carr.

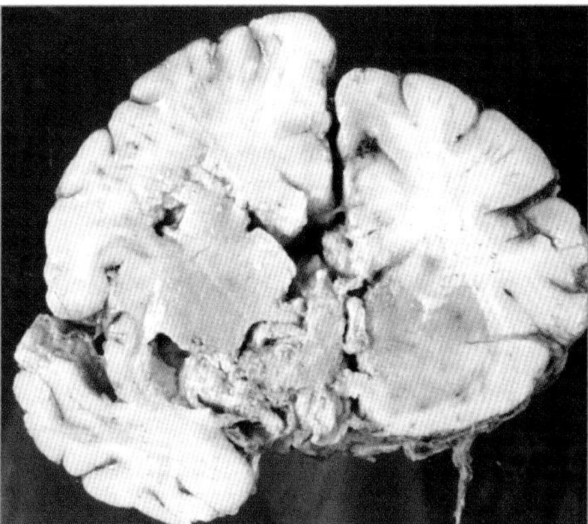

Image 48.2
Extensive cerebral necrosis in a patient with mucormycosis. Courtesy of Dimitris P. Agamanolis, MD.

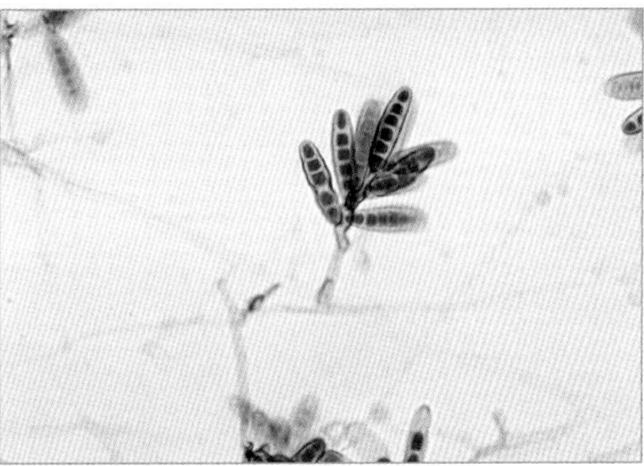

Image 48.4
This micrograph reveals a conidia-laden conidiophore of the fungus *Bipolaris hawaiiensis*. *Bipolaris* species are known to be one of the causative agents of the fungal illness phaeohyphomycosis, which can be superficially confined to the skin or systemically disseminated and involve the brain, lungs, and bones. Courtesy of Centers for Disease Control and Prevention.

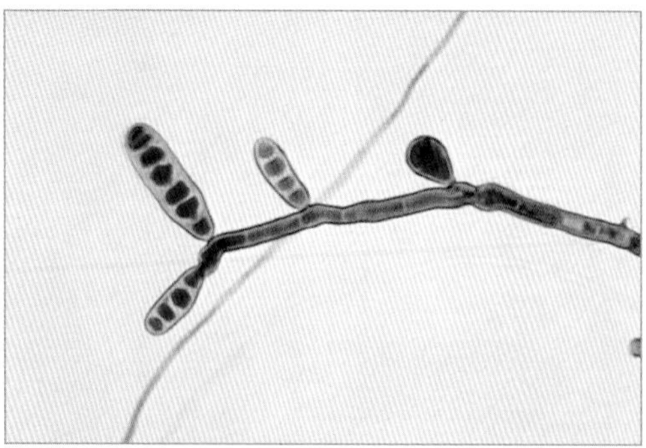

Image 48.6
Note the fine branching tubes of the fungus *Exserohilum rostratum,* which is the cause of phaeohyphomycosis. Phaeohyphomycosis is a fungal infection characterized by superficial and deep tissue involvement caused by dematiaceous, dark-walled fungi that form pigmented hyphae, or fine branching tubes, and yeastlike cells in the infected tissues. Courtesy of Centers for Disease Control and Prevention/Libero Ajello, MD.

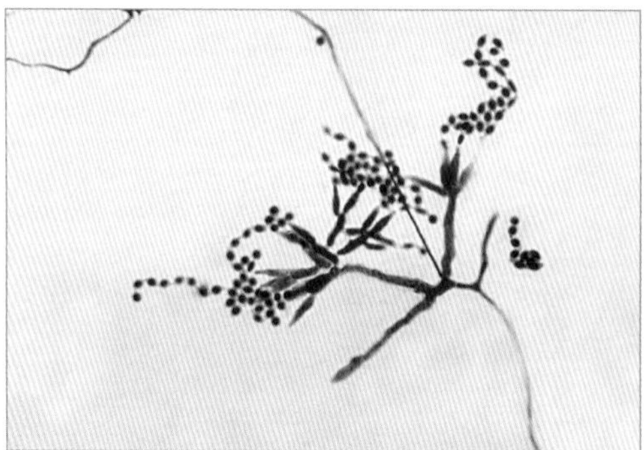

Image 48.7
This micrograph depicts multiple conidia-laden conidiophores and phialides of a *Penicillium marneffei* fungal organism. *Penicillium* species are known to cause penicilliosis, which usually affects immunocompromised individuals, such as those with AIDS or undergoing chemotherapy. *P marneffei* is normally acquired though inhalation of airborne spores. Courtesy of Centers for Disease Control and Prevention/Libero Ajello, MD.

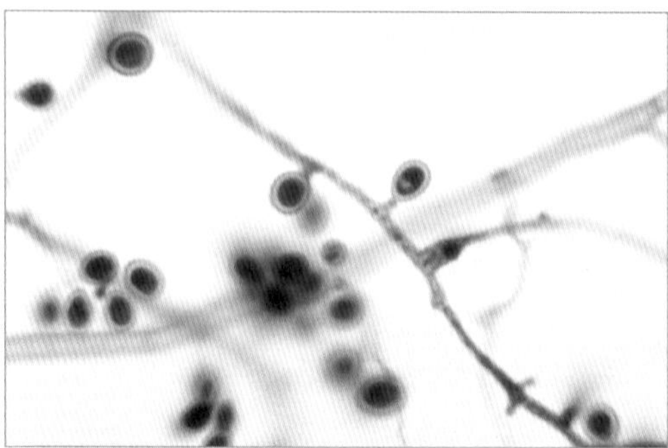

Image 48.8
This photomicrograph reveals the conidiophores with conidia of the fungus *Pseudallescheria boydii* from a slide culture. *P boydii* is pathogenic in humans, especially those who are immunocompromised, causing infections in almost all body regions, and which are classified under the broad heading of pseudallescheriasis. Courtesy of Centers for Disease Control and Prevention/Libero Ajello, MD.

49

Fusobacterium Infections

(Including Lemierre Disease)

Clinical Manifestations

Fusobacterium necrophorum and *Fusobacterium nucleatum* can be isolated from oropharyngeal specimens in healthy people, are frequent components of human dental plaque, and may lead to periodontal disease. Invasive disease attributable to *Fusobacterium* species has been associated with otitis media, tonsillitis, gingivitis, and oropharyngeal trauma, including dental surgery. Ten percent of cases of invasive *Fusobacterium* infections are associated with concomitant Epstein-Barr virus infection. Risk can be increased after macrolide use.

Invasive infection with *Fusobacterium* species can lead to life-threatening disease. Otogenic infection is the most frequent primary source in children and can be complicated by meningitis and thrombosis of dural venous sinuses. Invasive infection following tonsillitis was described early in the 20th century and was referred to as postanginal sepsis or Lemierre disease. Lemierre disease most often occurs in adolescents and young adults and is characterized by internal jugular vein septic thrombophlebitis or thrombosis (JVT), evidence of septic embolic lesions in lungs or other sterile sites, and isolation of *Fusobacterium* species from blood or other normally sterile sites. Lemierre-like syndromes have also been reported following infection with *Arcanobacterium haemolyticum*, *Bacteroides* species, anaerobic *Streptococcus* species, other anaerobic bacteria, and methicillin-susceptible and -resistant strains of *Staphylococcus aureus*. Fever and sore throat are followed by severe neck pain (anginal pain) that can be accompanied by unilateral neck swelling, trismus, and dysphagia. Patients with classic Lemierre disease have a sepsis syndrome with multiple organ dysfunction. Metastatic complications from septic embolic phenomena associated with suppurative JVT are common and may manifest as disseminated intravascular coagulation, pleural empyema, pyogenic arthritis, or osteomyelitis. Persistent headache or other neurologic signs may indicate the presence of cerebral venous sinus thrombosis (eg, cavernous sinus thrombosis), meningitis, or brain abscess.

Jugular vein septic thrombophlebitis or thrombosis can be completely vasoocclusive. Surgical debridement of necrotic tissue may be necessary for patients who do not respond to antimicrobial therapy. Some children with JVT associated with Lemierre disease have evidence of thrombophilia at diagnosis. These findings often resolve over several months and can indicate response to the inflammatory, prothrombotic process associated with infection rather than an underlying hypercoagulable state.

Etiology

Fusobacterium species are anaerobic, nonsporeforming, gram-negative bacilli. Human infection usually results from *F necrophorum* subsp *funduliforme*, but infections with other species, including *F nucleatum, Fusobacterium gonidiaformans, Fusobacterium naviforme, Fusobacterium mortiferum,* and *Fusobacterium varium,* have been reported. Infection with *Fusobacterium* species, alone or in combination with other oral anaerobic bacteria, may result in Lemierre disease.

Epidemiology

Fusobacterium species are commonly found in soil and the respiratory tracts of animals, including cattle, dogs, fowl, goats, sheep, and horses, and can be isolated from the oropharynx of healthy people. *Fusobacterium* infections are most common in adolescents and young adults, but infections, including fatal cases of Lemierre disease, have been reported in infants and young children. Those with sickle cell disease or diabetes mellitus may be at greater risk of infection.

Diagnostic Tests

Fusobacterium species can be isolated using conventional liquid anaerobic blood culture media. However, the organism grows best on semisolid media for fastidious anaerobic organisms or blood agar supplemented with vitamin K, hemin, menadione, and a reducing agent. Many strains fluoresce chartreuse green under ultraviolet light. Most *Fusobacterium* organisms are indole positive. The accurate identification of anaerobes to the species level has become important with the increasing incidence of microorganisms that are resistant to multiple drugs. Sequencing of the 16S rRNA gene and phylogenetic analysis can identify anaerobic bacteria to the genus or taxonomic group level and, frequently, to the species level.

The diagnosis of Lemierre disease should be considered in ill-appearing febrile children and adolescents with sore throat and exquisite neck pain over the angle of the jaw. Anaerobic blood culture in addition to aerobic blood culture should be performed to detect invasive *Fusobacterium* species infection. Computed tomography and magnetic resonance imaging are more sensitive than ultrasonography to document JVT early in the course of illness and to better identify thrombus extension.

Treatment

Fusobacterium species may be susceptible to metronidazole, clindamycin, chloramphenicol, carbapenems (meropenem or imipenem), cefoxitin, and ceftriaxone. Resistance to antimicrobial agents has increased in anaerobic bacteria during the last decade, and susceptibility is no longer predictable. Susceptibility testing is indicated for all clinically significant anaerobic isolates. Metronidazole is the treatment preferred by many experts but lacks activity against microaerophilic streptococci that can coinfect some patients. Clindamycin is generally an effective agent. *Fusobacterium* species are intrinsically resistant to gentamicin, fluoroquinolone agents, and, typically, macrolides. Tetracyclines have limited activity. Up to 50% of *F nucleatum* and 20% of *F necrophorum* isolates produce β-lactamases, rendering them resistant to penicillin, ampicillin, and some cephalosporins.

Because *Fusobacterium* infections are often polymicrobial, broad-spectrum therapy frequently is necessary. Therapy has been advocated with a penicillin-β-lactamase inhibitor combination (ampicillin-sulbactam or piperacillin-tazobactam) or a carbapenem (meropenem, imipenem, or ertapenem) or combination therapy with metronidazole or clindamycin in addition to other agents active against aerobic oral and respiratory tract pathogens (cefotaxime, ceftriaxone, or cefuroxime). Duration of antimicrobial therapy depends on the anatomic location and severity of infection but is usually several weeks. Surgical intervention involving debridement or incision and drainage of abscesses may be necessary. Anticoagulation therapy has been used in adults and children with JVT and cavernous sinus thrombosis. In cases with extensive thrombosis, anticoagulation therapy may decrease the risk of clot extension and shorten recovery time.

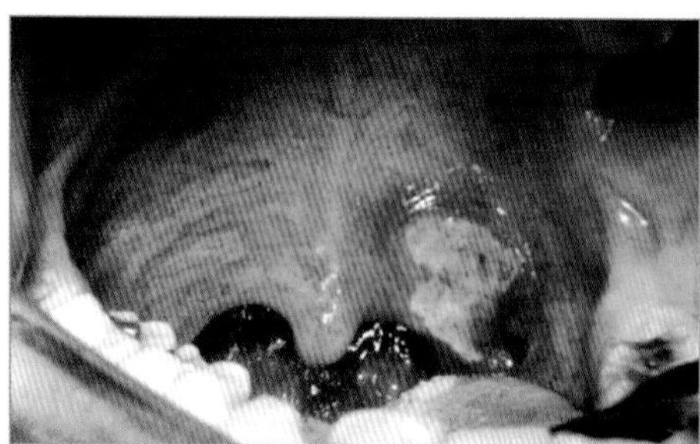

Image 49.1
Vincent stomatitis has been confused with diphtheria, although this infection is usually a mixed infection, including fusiform and spirochetal anaerobic bacteria including *Fusobacterium,* and is associated with severe pain and halitosis. Note ulceration of the soft palate with surrounding erythema. Courtesy of Edgar O. Ledbetter, MD, FAAP.

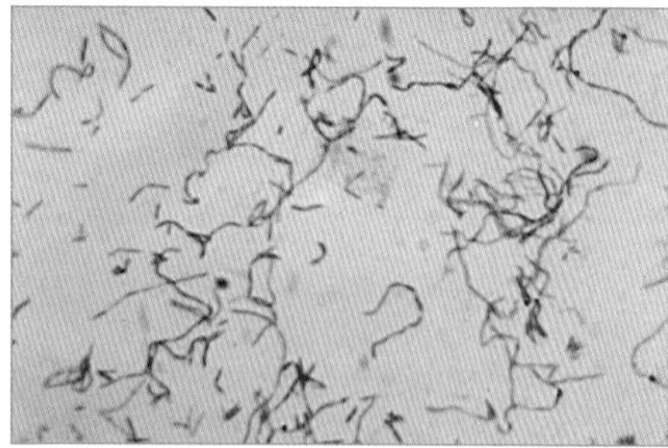

Image 49.2
This photomicrograph shows *Fusobacterium nucleatum* after being cultured in a thioglycollate medium for 48 hours. Courtesy of Centers for Disease Control and Prevention.

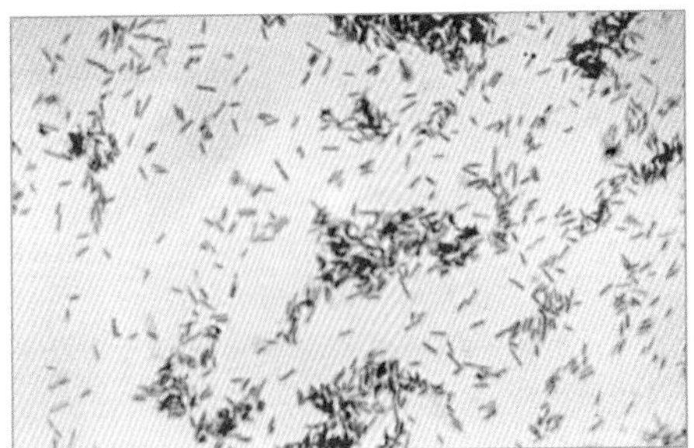

Image 49.3
This is a photomicrograph of *Fusobacterium russii* cultured in a thioglycollate medium for 48 hours. Like the genus *Bacteroides, Fusobacterium* species are anaerobic, gram-negative bacteria that are normal inhabiters of the oral cavity, intestine, and female genital tract. *Fusobacterium* species are most commonly associated with head and neck, pulmonary, and wound infections. Courtesy of Centers for Disease Control and Prevention/V. R. Dowell Jr, MD.

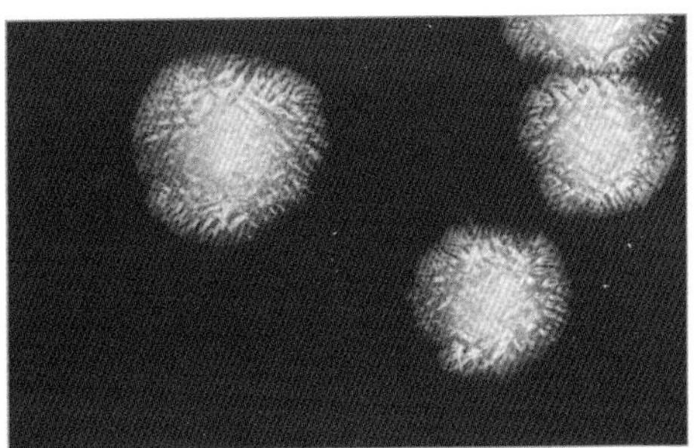

Image 49.4
This photograph demonstrates the morphology of 4 colonies of *Fusobacterium fusiforme* bacteria that were grown on blood agar medium for 48 hours. *Fusobacterium fusiforme* is a spindle-shaped gram-negative bacteria that colonizes the gingival sulcus of the human oral cavity and has also been isolated from infections of the upper respiratory tract. Courtesy of Centers for Disease Control and Prevention/V. R. Dowell Jr, MD.

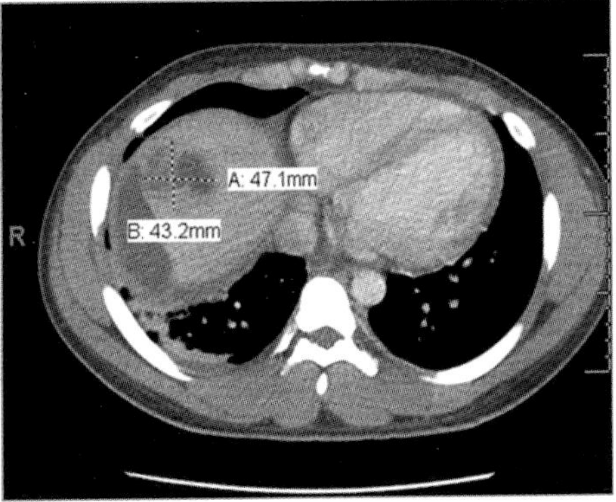

Image 49.5
An abdominal computed tomography scan of a 15-year-old football linebacker who presented with high fever, abdominal pain, and emesis for 5 days showing abscess collections in the liver. Aspiration of 3 discrete abscess areas grew only *Fusobacterium nucleatum*. Courtesy of Carol J. Baker, MD, FAAP.

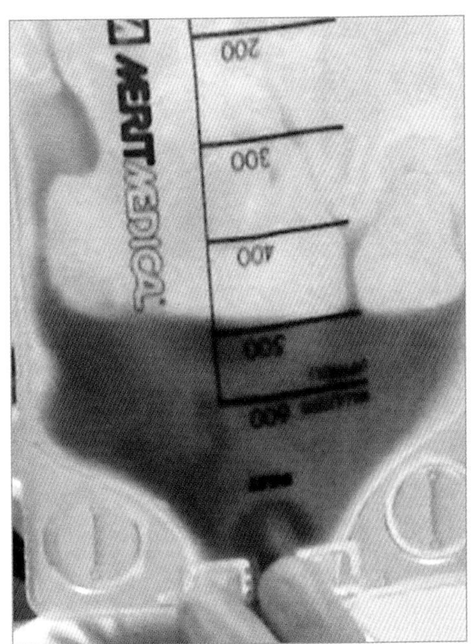

Image 49.6
80 mL of purulent material was aspirated from the liver abscess of the patient in Image 49.5. Courtesy of Carol J. Baker, MD, FAAP.

50

Giardia intestinalis (formerly *Giardia lamblia* and *Giardia duodenalis*) Infections

(Giardiasis)

Clinical Manifestations

Symptomatic infection with *Giardia intestinalis* causes a broad spectrum of clinical manifestations. Children can have occasional days of acute watery diarrhea with abdominal pain, or they may experience a protracted, intermittent, often debilitating disease characterized by passage of foul-smelling stools associated with anorexia, flatulence, and abdominal distention. Anorexia, combined with malabsorption, can lead to significant weight loss, failure to thrive, and anemia. Humoral immunodeficiencies predispose to chronic symptomatic *G intestinalis* infections. Asymptomatic infection is common; approximately 50% to 75% of people who acquired infection in outbreaks occurring in child care settings and in the community were asymptomatic.

Etiology

G intestinalis is a flagellate protozoan that exists in trophozoite and cyst forms; the infective form is the cyst. Infection is limited to the small intestine and biliary tract.

Epidemiology

Giardiasis is the most common intestinal parasitic infection of humans identified in the United States and globally with a worldwide distribution. Approximately 20,000 cases are reported in the United States each year, with highest incidence reported among children 1 to 9 years of age, adults 35 to 44 years of age, and residents of northern states. Peak onset of illness occurs annually during early summer through early fall. Humans are the principal reservoir of infection, but *Giardia* organisms can infect dogs, cats, beavers, rodents, sheep, cattle, nonhuman primates, and other animals. *G intestinalis* assemblages are quite species-specific, such that the organisms that affect nonhumans are usually not infectious to humans. People become infected directly from an infected person or through ingestion of fecally contaminated water or food. Most community-wide epidemics have resulted from a contaminated drinking water supply; outbreaks associated with recreational water have also been reported. Outbreaks resulting from person-to-person transmission occur in child care centers or institutional care settings, where staff and family members in contact with infected children or adults become infected themselves. Although less common, outbreaks associated with food or food handlers have also been reported. Surveys conducted in the United States have identified overall prevalence rates of *Giardia* organisms in stool specimens that range from 5% to 7%, with variations depending on age, geographic location, and seasonality. Duration of cyst excretion is variable but can range from weeks to months. Giardiasis is communicable for as long as the infected person excretes cysts.

Incubation Period

1 to 3 weeks.

Diagnostic Tests

Commercially available, sensitive, and specific enzyme immunoassay and direct fluorescence antibody assays are the standard tests used for diagnosis of giardiasis in the United States. Enzyme immunoassay has a sensitivity of up to 95% and a specificity of 98% to 100% when compared with microscopy. Direct fluorescence antibody assay has the advantage that organisms are visualized. Diagnosis has traditionally been based on the microscopic identification of trophozoites or cysts in stool specimens; this requires an experienced microscopist, and sensitivity can be suboptimal. Stool needs to be examined as soon as possible or placed immediately in a preservative, such as neutral-buffered 10% formalin or polyvinyl alcohol. A single direct smear examination of stool has a sensitivity of 75% to 95%. Sensitivity is higher for diarrheal stool specimens because they contain higher concentrations of organisms. Sensitivity of microscopy is increased by examining 3 or more specimens collected every other day. Commercially available stool collection kits in child-proof containers are convenient for preserving stool specimens collected at home. When giardiasis is suspected clinically but the organism is not found on repeated stool examination, inspection of duodenal contents obtained by direct aspiration or by using a commercially available string test (eg, Entero-Test) may be diagnostic. Rarely, duodenal biopsy is required for diagnosis.

Treatment

Some infections are self-limited, and treatment is not required. Dehydration and electrolyte abnormalities can occur and should be corrected. Metronidazole, nitazoxanide, and tinidazole are the drugs of choice. Metronidazole (if used for a 5-day course) is the least expensive of these therapies. A 5- to 10-day course of metronidazole has an efficacy of 80% to 100% in pediatric patients, but poor palatability has been noted for metronidazole suspension. A 1-time dose of tinidazole, for children 3 years and older, has a similar efficacy in pediatric patients and has fewer adverse effects than does metronidazole. A 3-day course of nitazoxanide oral suspension also has similar efficacy to metronidazole and has the advantage(s) of treating other intestinal parasites and is approved for use in children 1 year and older.

Symptom recurrence after completing antimicrobial treatment can be attributable to reinfection, post-*Giardia* lactose intolerance (occurs in 20%–40% of patients), immune suppression, insufficient treatment, or drug resistance. If reinfection is suspected, a second course of the same drug should be effective. Treatment with a different class of drug is recommended for resistant giardiasis. Other treatment options include combination of a nitroimidazole plus quinacrine for at least 2 weeks or high-dose courses of the original agent.

Patients who are immunocompromised because of hypogammaglobulinemia or lymphoproliferative disease are at higher risk of giardiasis, and it is more difficult to treat in these patients. Among HIV-infected children without AIDS, effective combination and antiparasitic therapy are the major initial treatments for these infections. Especially in HIV-infected children without AIDS, combination antiretroviral therapy should be part of the primary initial treatment for giardiasis. Patients with AIDS often respond to standard therapy; however, in some cases, additional treatment is required. If giardiasis is refractory to standard treatment among patients with AIDS, high doses, longer treatment duration, or combination therapy may be appropriate.

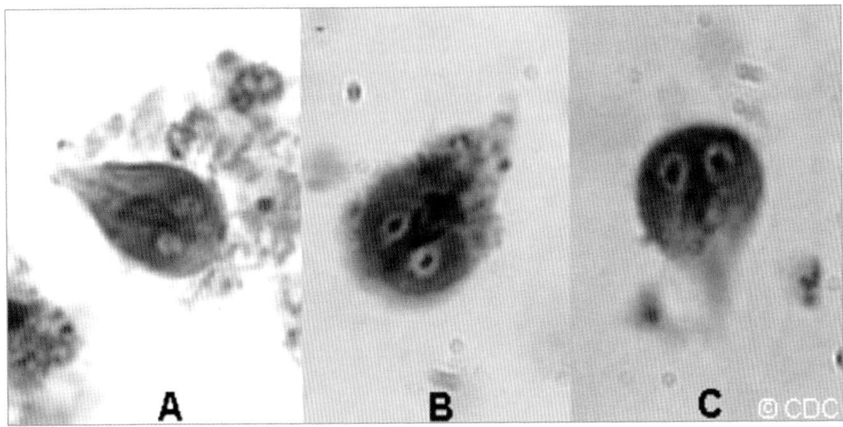

Image 50.1
Three trophozoites of *Giardia intestinalis* (A, trichrome stain; B and C, iron hematoxylin stain). Each cell has 2 nuclei with a large, central karyosome. Cell length is 9 to 21 µm. Trophozoites are usually seen in fresh diarrheal stool or in duodenal mucus. Courtesy of Centers for Disease Control and Prevention.

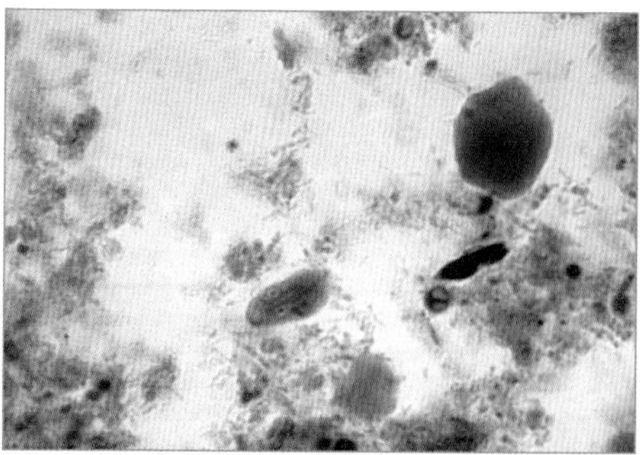

Image 50.2
Photomicrograph of a *Giardia intestinalis* cyst seen using a trichrome stain. *G intestinalis* is the protozoan organism that causes the disease giardiasis, a diarrheal disorder directly affecting the small intestine. Courtesy of Centers for Disease Control and Prevention.

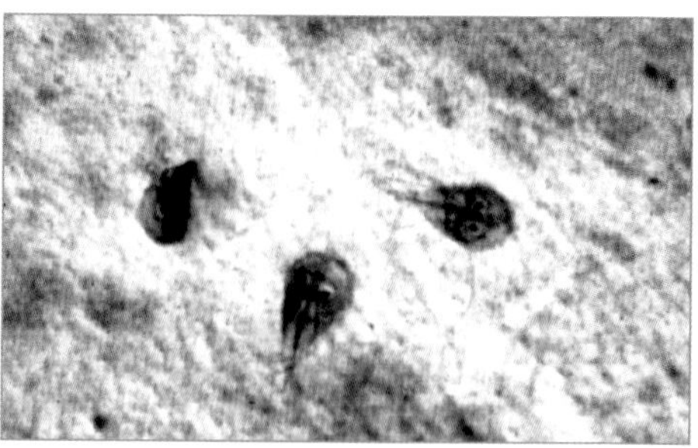

Image 50.3
Giardia intestinalis cysts (trichrome stain). Person-to-person transmission is the most common mode of transmission of giardiasis.

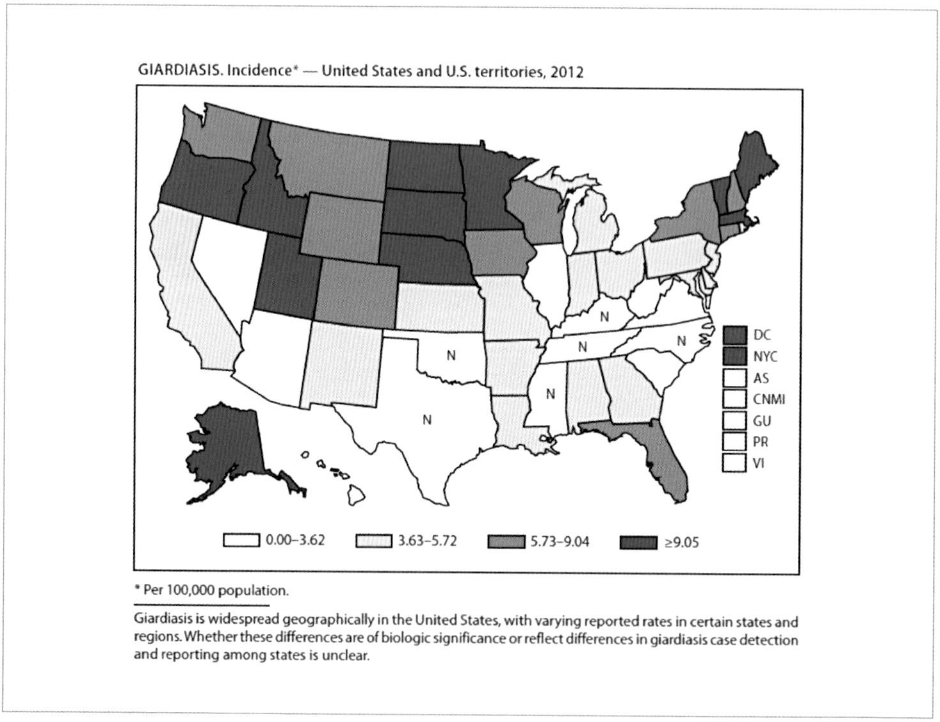

GIARDIASIS. Incidence* — United States and U.S. territories, 2012

N
N
N
N
N
N
DC
NYC
AS
CNMI
GU
PR
VI
0.00–3.62
3.63–5.72
5.73–9.04
≥9.05

* Per 100,000 population.

Giardiasis is widespread geographically in the United States, with varying reported rates in certain states and regions. Whether these differences are of biologic significance or reflect differences in giardiasis case detection and reporting among states is unclear.

Image 50.4
Giardiasis. Incidence—United States and US territories, 2012. Courtesy of *Morbidity and Mortality Weekly Report.*

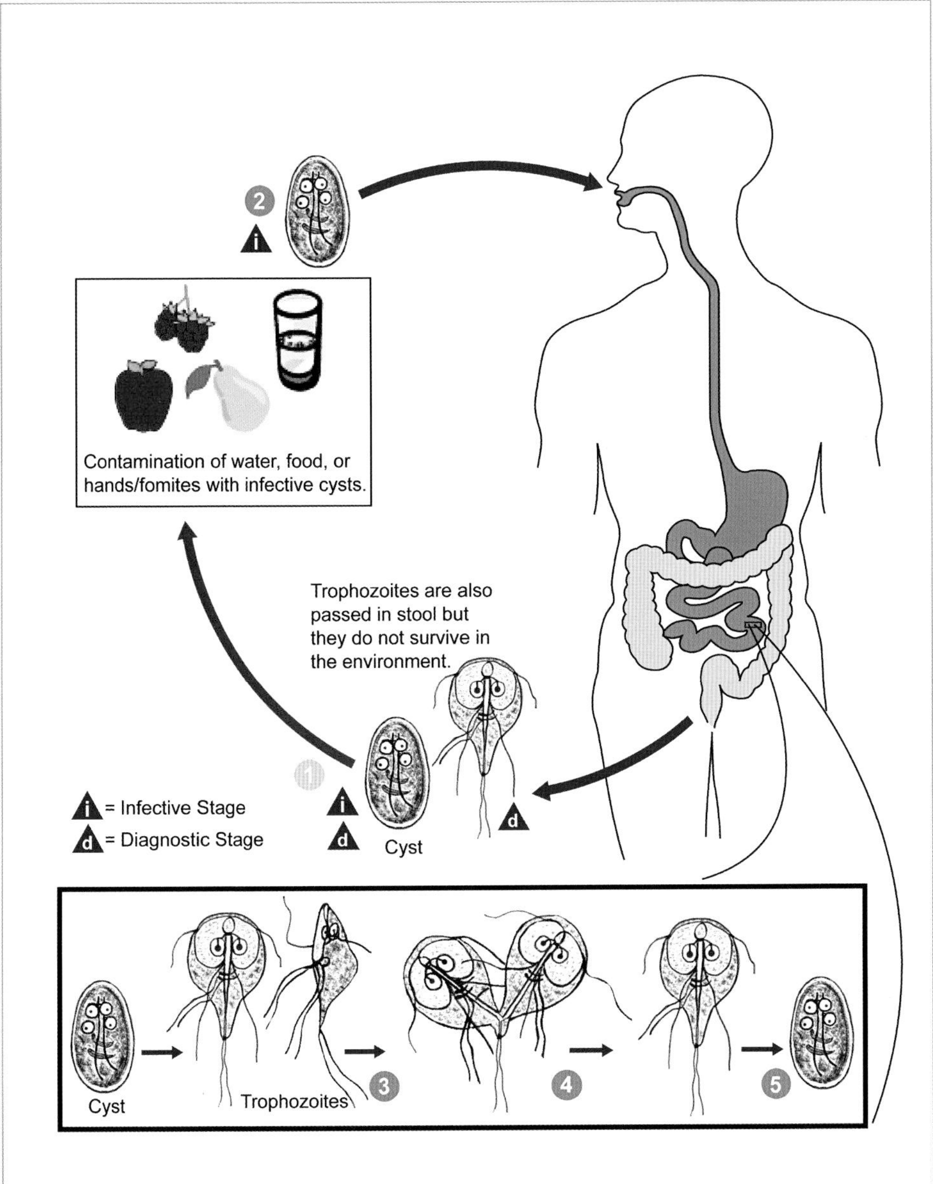

Image 50.5

Cysts are resistant forms and responsible for transmission of giardiasis. Cysts and trophozoites can be found in the feces (diagnostic stages) (1). The cysts are hardy and can survive several months in cold water. Infection occurs by the ingestion of cysts in contaminated water or food or by the fecal-oral route (hands or fomites) (2). In the small intestine, excystation releases trophozoites (each cyst produces 2 trophozoites) (3). Trophozoites multiply by longitudinal binary fission, remaining in the lumen of the proximal small bowel, where they can be free or attached to the mucosa by a ventral sucking disk (4). Encystation occurs as the parasites transit toward the colon. The cyst is the stage found most commonly in nondiarrheal feces (5). Because the cysts are infectious when passed in the stool or shortly afterward, person-to-person transmission is possible. While animals are infected with *Giardia,* their importance as a reservoir is unclear. Courtesy of Centers for Disease Control and Prevention/Alexander J. da Silva, PhD/Melanie Moser.

51

Gonococcal Infections

Clinical Manifestations

Gonococcal infections in newborns, infants, children, and adolescents occur in 3 distinct age groups.

- Infection in the **newborn** usually involves the eyes. Other possible manifestations of neonatal gonococcal infection include scalp abscess (which can be associated with fetal scalp monitoring) and disseminated disease with bacteremia, arthritis, or meningitis. Vaginitis and urethritis may occur as well.
- In children beyond the newborn period, including **prepubertal children,** gonococcal infection may occur in the genital tract and is almost always transmitted sexually. Vaginitis is the most common manifestation in prepubertal females. Progression to pelvic inflammatory disease (PID) appears to be less common in this age group than in older adolescents. Gonococcal urethritis is possible but uncommon in prepubertal males. Anorectal and tonsillopharyngeal infection can also occur in prepubertal children and is often asymptomatic.
- In **sexually active adolescent and young adult females,** gonococcal infection of the genital tract is often asymptomatic. Common clinical syndromes include urethritis, endocervicitis, and salpingitis. In males, infection is often symptomatic, and the primary site is the urethra. Infection of the rectum and pharynx can occur alone or with genitourinary tract infection in either gender. Rectal and pharyngeal infections are often asymptomatic. Extension from primary genital mucosal sites in males can lead to epididymitis; in females, it can lead to bartholinitis, PID with resultant tubal scarring, and perihepatitis (Fitz-Hugh–Curtis syndrome). Even asymptomatic infection in females can progress to PID, with tubal scarring that can result in ectopic pregnancy, infertility, or chronic pelvic pain. Infection involving other mucous membranes can produce conjunctivitis, pharyngitis, or proctitis. Hematogenous spread from mucosal sites can involve skin and joints (arthritis-dermatitis syndrome; disseminated gonococcal infection) and occurs in up to 3% of untreated people with mucosal gonorrhea. Bacteremia can result in a maculopapular rash with necrosis, tenosynovitis, and migratory arthritis. Arthritis may be reactive (sterile) or septic in nature. Meningitis and endocarditis occur rarely.

Etiology

Neisseria gonorrhoeae is a gram-negative, oxidase-positive diplococcus.

Epidemiology

Gonococcal infections only occur in humans. The source of the organism is exudate and secretions from infected mucosal surfaces; *N gonorrhoeae* is communicable as long as a person harbors the organism. Transmission results from intimate contact, such as sexual acts, parturition, and, very rarely, household exposure in prepubertal children. Sexual abuse should be strongly considered when genital, rectal, or pharyngeal colonization or infection is diagnosed in prepubertal children beyond the newborn period. *N gonorrhoeae* infection is the second most commonly reported sexually transmitted infection in the United States, following *Chlamydia trachomatis* infection. In 2012, a total of 334,826 cases of gonorrhea were reported in the United States, a rate of 108 cases per 100,000 population. The reported rate of diagnosis is highest in females 15 through 24 years of age. Among males, the rate is highest in those 20 through 24 years of age. In 2012, the rate of gonorrhea among black people was 15 times the rate among white people. Rates were 4 times higher among American Indian/Alaska Native people, 3 times higher among Native Hawaiian/Pacific Islander people, and 2 times higher among Hispanic people than among whites. Disparities in gonorrhea rates are observed by sexual behavior. Among males who have sex with males, very high proportions of positive gonorrhea pharyngeal, urethral, and rectal test results, as well as coinfection with other sexually transmitted infections and HIV, have been found.

Incubation Period

2 to 7 days.

Diagnostic Tests

Microscopic examination of Gram-stained smears of exudate from the conjunctivae, vagina of prepubertal girls, male urethra, skin lesions, synovial fluid, and, when clinically warranted, cerebrospinal fluid (CSF) can be useful in the initial evaluation. Identification of gram-negative intracellular diplococci in these smears can be helpful, particularly if the organism is not recovered in culture. However, because of low sensitivity, a negative smear result should not be considered sufficient for ruling out infection. *N gonorrhoeae* can be isolated from normally sterile sites, such as blood, CSF, or synovial fluid, using nonselective chocolate agar with incubation in 5% to 10% carbon dioxide. Selective media that inhibit normal flora and nonpathogenic *Neisseria* organisms are used for cultures from nonsterile sites, such as the cervix, vagina, rectum, urethra, and pharynx. Specimens for *N gonorrhoeae* culture from mucosal sites should be inoculated immediately onto appropriate agar because the organism is extremely sensitive to drying and temperature changes.

Caution should be exercised when interpreting the significance of isolation of *Neisseria* organisms because *N gonorrhoeae* can be confused with other *Neisseria* species that colonize the genitourinary tract or pharynx. At least 2 confirmatory bacteriologic tests involving different biochemical principles should be performed by the laboratory. Interpretation of culture of *N gonorrhoeae* from the pharynx of young children necessitates particular caution because of the high carriage rate of nonpathogenic *Neisseria* species and the serious implications of such a culture result.

Nucleic acid amplification tests (NAATs) are far superior in overall performance compared with other *N gonorrhoeae* culture and nonculture diagnostic methods to test genital and nongenital specimens, but performance varies by NAAT type. These tests include polymerase chain reaction, transcription-mediated amplification, and strand-displacement amplification. Most commercially available products are now approved for testing male urethral swab specimens, female endocervical or vaginal swab specimens, male or female urine specimens, or liquid cytology specimens. Use of less-invasive specimens, such as urine or vaginal swab specimens, increases feasibility of routine testing of sexually active adolescents by their primary care physicians and in other clinical settings. Nucleic acid amplification tests also permit dual testing of specimens for *C trachomatis* and *N gonorrhoeae*. The Centers for Disease Control and Prevention (CDC) recommends the vaginal swab specimen as the preferred means of screening females and urine as the preferred means for screening males for *N gonorrhoeae* infection.

For identifying *N gonorrhoeae* from nongenital sites, culture is the most widely used test and allows for antimicrobial susceptibility testing to aid in management should infection persist following initial therapy. Nucleic acid amplification tests are not cleared by the US Food and Drug Administration for *N gonorrhoeae* testing on rectal or pharyngeal swabs. Many commercial laboratories have validated gonorrhea NAAT performance on rectal or pharyngeal swab specimens. Some NAATs have the potential to cross-react with nongonococcal *Neisseria* species that are commonly found in the throat, leading to false-positive test results. A limited number of nonculture tests are approved by the Food and Drug Administration for conjunctival specimens.

- **Sexual abuse.** In all prepubertal children beyond the newborn period and in adolescents who have gonococcal infection but report no prior sexual activity, sexual abuse must be considered to have occurred until proven otherwise. Health care professionals have a responsibility to report suspected sexual abuse to the state child protective services agency if there is "reasonable cause to suspect abuse." Cultures should be performed on genital, rectal, and pharyngeal swab specimens for all patients before antimicrobial treatment is given. All gonococcal isolates from such patients should be preserved. Nonculture gonococcal tests, including Gram stain, DNA probes, enzyme immunoassays, or NAATs of oropharyngeal, rectal, or genital tract swab specimens in children, cannot be relied on as the sole method for diagnosis of gonococcal infection for this purpose because false-positive results can occur. Culture remains the preferred method for urethral specimens from boys and extragenital specimens (pharynx and rectum) in boys and girls.

Treatment

The rapid emergence of antimicrobial resistance has led to a limited number of approved therapies for gonococcal infections. Resistance to penicillin and tetracycline is widespread, and as of 2007, the CDC no longer recommends the use of fluoroquinolones for gonorrhea because of the increased prevalence of quinolone-resistant *N gonorrhoeae* in the United States. This leaves cephalosporins as the only recommended antimicrobial class for the treatment of gonococcal infections. Over the past decade, the minimum inhibitory concentrations for oral cefixime activity against *N gonorrhoeae* strains circulating in the United States and other countries has increased, suggesting that resistance to this drug is emerging. As of 2012, the CDC no longer recommends the use of cefixime as a first-line treatment for gonococcal infection. Ceftriaxone, intramuscularly, once, with azithromycin, once, or doxycycline, twice daily for 7 days, is the recommended treatment for all gonococcal infections, regardless of age. Azithromycin is preferred to doxycycline because of the convenience of single-dose therapy and because gonococcal resistance to tetracycline appears to be greater than resistance to azithromycin.

Test-of-cure samples are not required in adolescents or adults with uncomplicated gonorrhea who are asymptomatic after being treated with a recommended antimicrobial regimen that includes ceftriaxone alone. If an alternative regimen is used for treatment of pharyngeal gonorrhea infection, the CDC recommends a test of cure 14 days after treatment is completed, ideally using culture so that antimicrobial susceptibility testing may be performed. If culture is not available, the CDC recommends testing with a NAAT. If the NAAT result remains positive, every effort should be made to obtain a culture for susceptibility testing. Patients who have symptoms that persist after treatment or whose symptoms recur shortly after treatment should be reevaluated by culture for *N gonorrhoeae,* and any gonococci isolated should be tested for antimicrobial susceptibility.

Because patients may be reinfected by a new or untreated partner within a few months after diagnosis and treatment, practitioners should advise all adolescents and adults diagnosed with gonorrhea to be retested approximately 3 months after treatment. Patients who do not receive a test of reinfection at 3 months should be tested whenever they are seen for care within the next 12 months. All patients with presumed or proven gonorrhea should be evaluated for concurrent syphilis, HIV, and *C trachomatis* infections.

Specific recommendations for management and antimicrobial therapy are as follows:

- **Neonatal disease.** Infants with clinical evidence of ophthalmia neonatorum, scalp abscess, or disseminated infections attributable to *N gonorrhoeae* should be hospitalized. Cultures of blood, eye discharge, and other potential sites of infection, such as CSF, should be performed on specimens from infants to confirm the diagnosis and to determine antimicrobial susceptibility. Tests for concomitant infection with *C trachomatis,* congenital syphilis, and HIV infection should be performed. Results of the maternal test for hepatitis B surface antigen should be confirmed. The mother and her partner(s) also need appropriate examination and treatment for *N gonorrhoeae.*
- **Nondisseminated neonatal infections.** Recommended antimicrobial therapy for ophthalmia neonatorum caused by *N gonorrhoeae* is a single one-time dose of ceftriaxone, intravenously or intramuscularly. Infants with gonococcal ophthalmia should receive eye irrigations with saline solution immediately and at frequent intervals until discharge is eliminated. Topical antimicrobial treatment alone is inadequate and unnecessary when recommended systemic antimicrobial treatment is given.

Infants with gonococcal ophthalmia should be hospitalized and evaluated for disseminated infection (sepsis, arthritis, meningitis).

- **Disseminated neonatal infections and scalp abscesses.** Recommended therapy for arthritis, septicemia, or abscess is ceftriaxone, intravenously or intramuscularly, for 7 days. Cefotaxime, intravenously every 12 hours, is recommended for infants with hyperbilirubinemia. If meningitis is documented, treatment should be continued for a total of 10 to 14 days.
- **Gonococcal infections in children beyond the neonatal period and adolescents.** Patients with uncomplicated infections of the vagina, endocervix, urethra, or anorectum and a history of severe adverse reactions to cephalosporins (eg, anaphylaxis, ceftriaxone-induced hemolysis, Stevens-Johnson syndrome, toxic epidermal necrolysis) should consult an expert in infectious diseases. In adults, dual treatment with a single dose of gemifloxacin, plus oral azithromycin, or dual treatment with a single dose of intramuscular gentamicin plus oral azithromycin, are potential therapeutic options. However, there are no data on the efficacy of these regimens in children or adolescents. Because data are limited on alternative regimens for treating gonorrhea among people who have documented severe cephalosporin allergy, consultation with an expert in infectious diseases may be warranted.
- **Pharyngeal infection** is generally more difficult to treat than anogenital infection; therefore, single-dose ceftriaxone and azithromycin are recommended. Children or adolescents with HIV infection should receive the same treatment for gonococcal infection as children without HIV infection.
- **Acute PID.** *N gonorrhoeae* and *C trachomatis* are implicated in many cases of PID; most cases have a polymicrobial etiology. No reliable clinical criteria distinguish gonococcal from nongonococcal-associated PID. Hence, broad-spectrum treatment regimens are recommended.
- **Acute epididymitis.** Sexually transmitted organisms, such as *N gonorrhoeae* or *C trachomatis*, can cause acute epididymitis in sexually active adolescents and young adults but rarely, if ever, cause acute epididymitis in prepubertal children. The recommended regimen for epididymitis is single-dose ceftriaxone plus doxycycline, for 14 days.

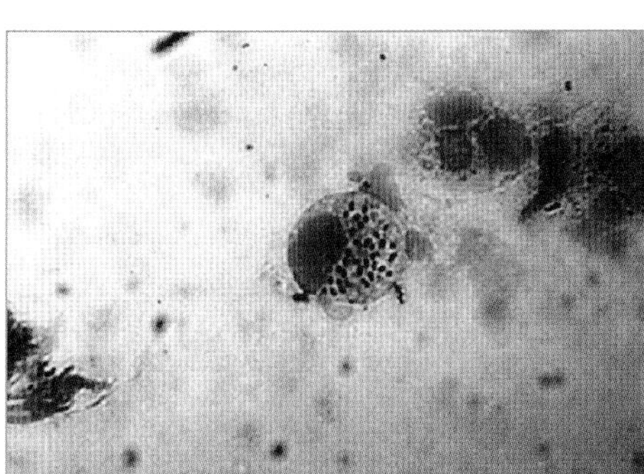

Image 51.1
Gram stain of cervical discharge in an adolescent who has gonococcal cervicitis. Note multiple intracellular diplococci. In children with suspected abuse, it is imperative the gonococcus be cultured and identified to distinguish pathogens from normal flora.

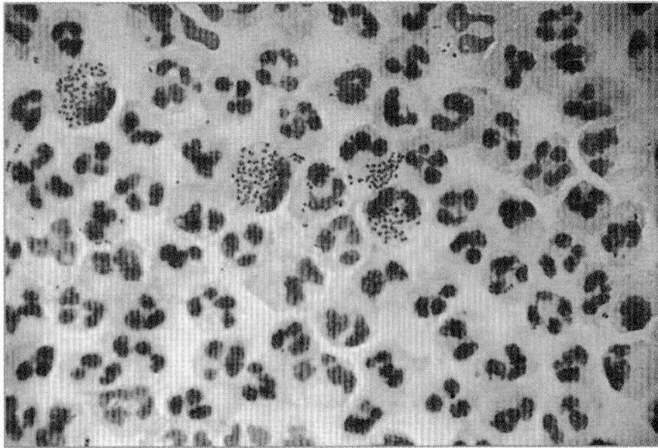

Image 51.2
This photomicrograph reveals the histopathology in an acute case of gonococcal urethritis (Gram stain). This image demonstrates the nonrandom distribution of gonococci among polymorphonuclear neutrophils. Note there are intracellular and extracellular bacteria in the field of view. Courtesy of Centers for Disease Control and Prevention/Joe Miller.

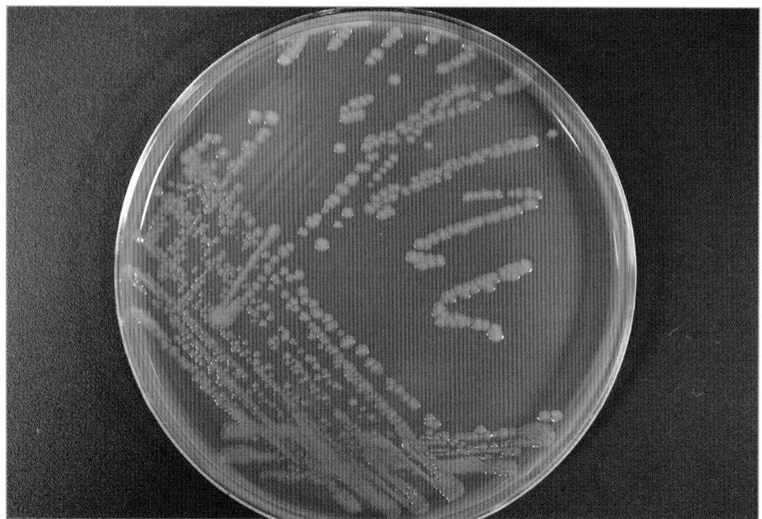

Image 51.3
Neisseria gonorrhoeae on chocolate agar. Colonies appear off-white with no discoloration of the agar. Courtesy of Julia Rosebush, DO; Robert Jerris, PhD; and Theresa Stanley, M(ASCP).

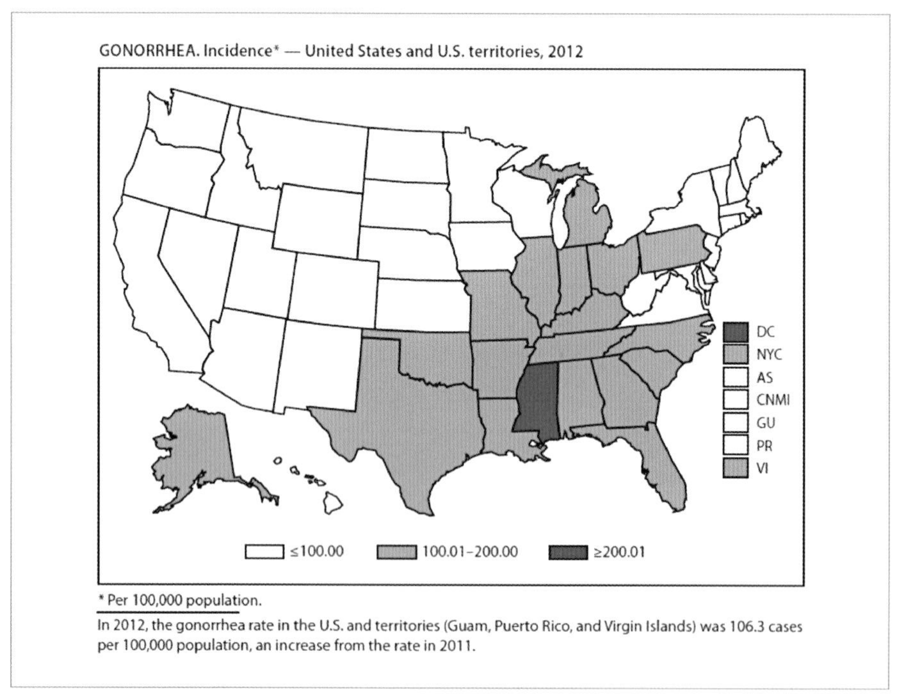

Image 51.4
Gonorrhea. Incidence—United States and US territories, 2012. Courtesy of *Morbidity and Mortality Weekly Report.*

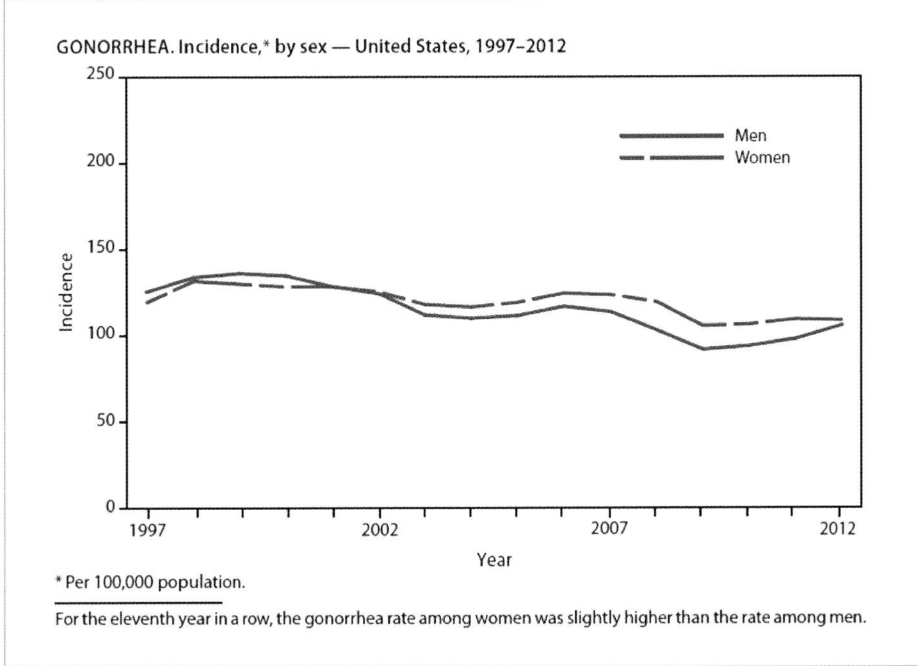

Image 51.5
Gonorrhea. Incidence, by sex—United States, 1997–2012. Courtesy of *Morbidity and Mortality Weekly Report.*

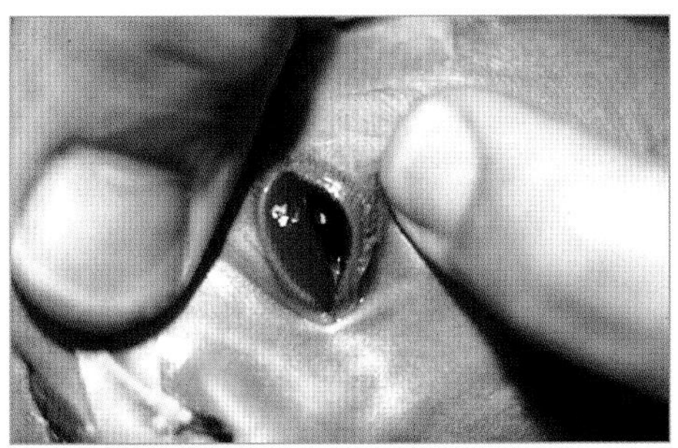

Image 51.6
An infant with gonococcal ophthalmia. In-hospital evaluation and treatment is recommended for infants with gonococcal ophthalmia. Copyright Martin G. Myers, MD.

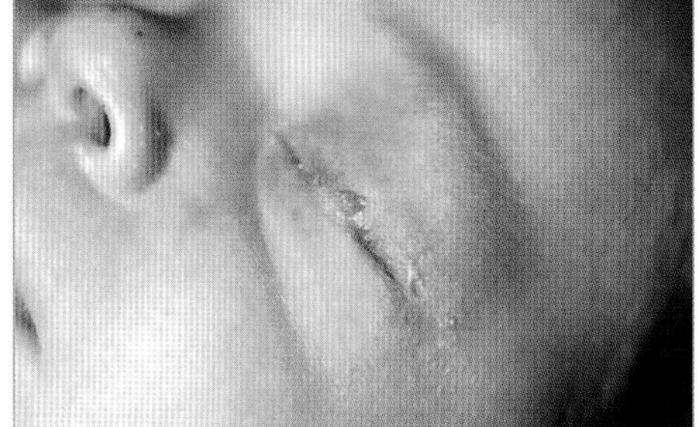

Image 51.7
An 8-day-old with gonococcal ophthalmia. Therapy for *Chlamydia trachomatis* is recommended, as concomitant infection may occur. Copyright Martin G. Myers, MD.

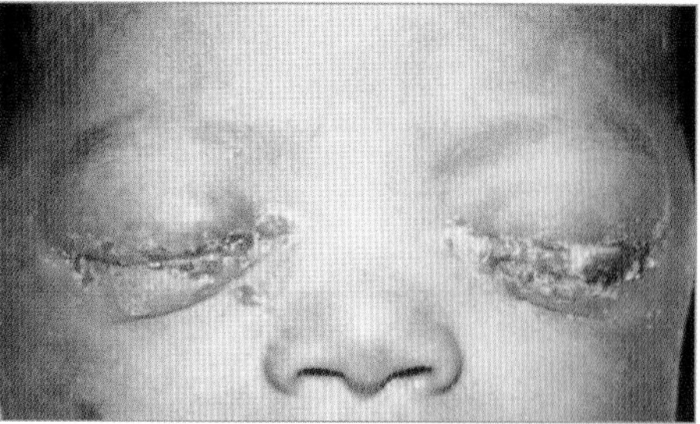

Image 51.8
This newborn has gonococcal ophthalmia neonatorum caused by a maternally transmitted gonococcal infection. Unless preventive measures are taken, it is estimated that gonococcal ophthalmia neonatorum will develop in 28% of neonates born to women with gonorrhea. It affects the corneal epithelium, causing microbial keratitis, ulceration, and perforation. Courtesy of Centers for Disease Control and Prevention/J. Pledger.

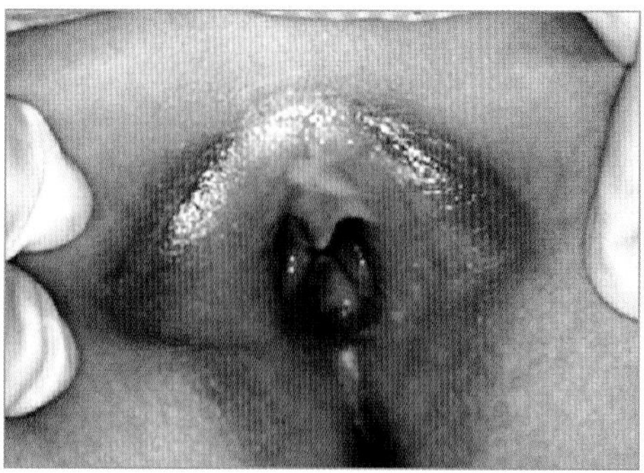

Image 51.9
Profuse, purulent vaginal discharge in an 18-month-old girl who has gonococcal vulvovaginitis. In preadolescent children, this infection is almost always associated with sexual abuse. Identification of the species of cultured gonococci is imperative in suspected cases of sexual abuse.

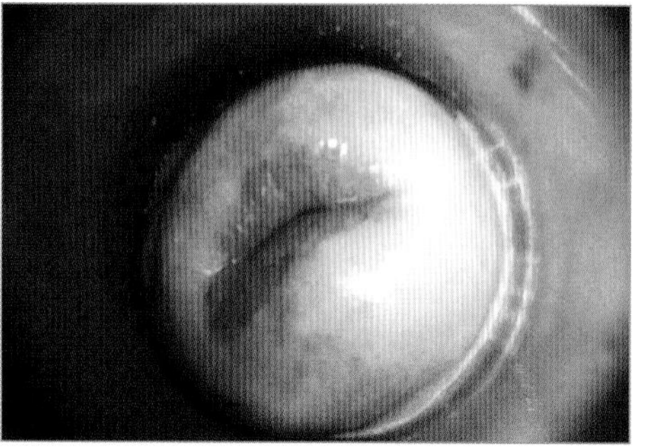

Image 51.10
This colposcopic view of this patient's cervix revealed an eroded ostium due to *Neisseria gonorrhoeae* infection. A chronic *N gonorrhoeae* infection can lead to complications that can be apparent, such as this cervical inflammation, and some can be quite insipid, giving the impression that the infection has subsided while treatment is still needed. Courtesy of Centers for Disease Control and Prevention.

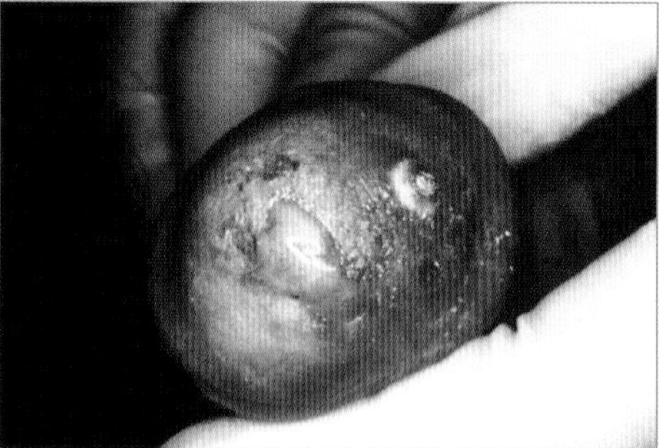

Image 51.11
This male presented with purulent penile discharge due to gonorrhea with an overlying penile pyoderma lesion. Pyoderma involves the formation of a purulent skin lesion, as in this case, located on the glans penis and overlying the sexually transmitted infection gonorrhea. Courtesy of Centers for Disease Control and Prevention/Joe Miller.

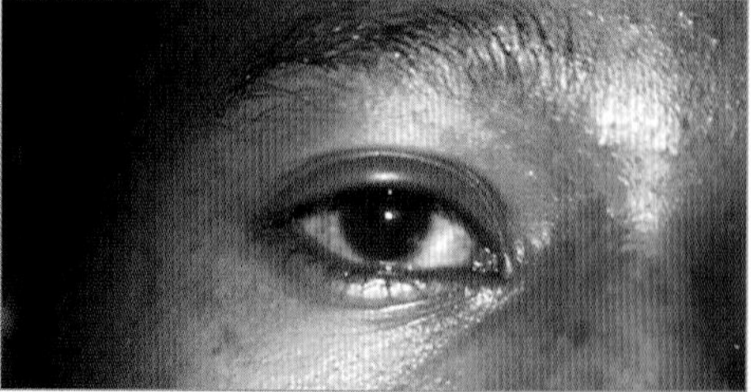

Image 51.12
This patient presented with gonococcal urethritis and gonococcal conjunctivitis of the right eye. If untreated, *Neisseria gonorrhoeae* may spread to the bloodstream and throughout the body. Courtesy of Centers for Disease Control and Prevention/Joe Miller.

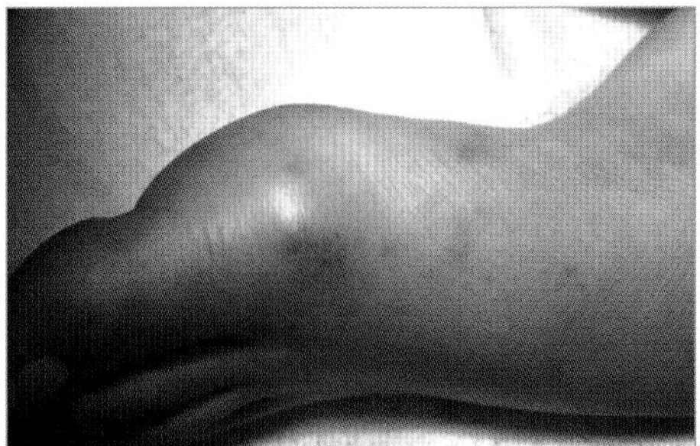

Image 51.13
Gonococcemia with maculopapular and petechial skin lesions, most commonly seen on the hands and feet.

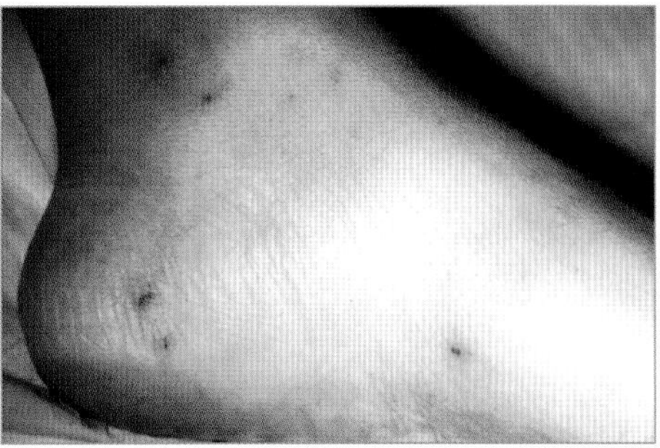

Image 51.14
Adolescent with septic arthritis of left ankle with petechial and necrotic skin lesions on the feet. Blood culture results were positive for *Neisseria gonorrhoeae*.

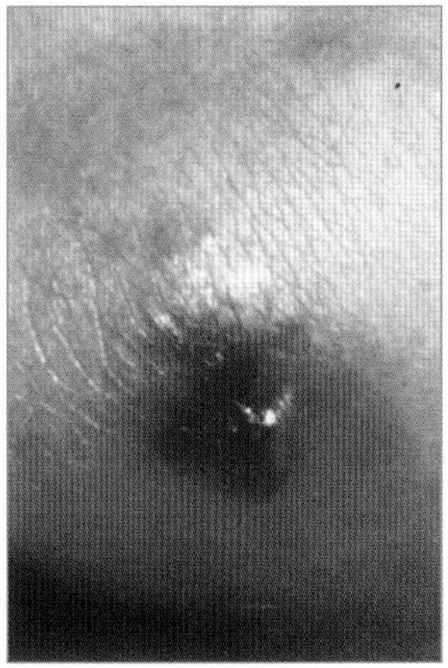

Image 51.15
An acute gonococcal skin lesion with cutaneous necrosis over the elbow of a 19-year-old male with gonococcal septicemia. Courtesy of George Nankervis, MD.

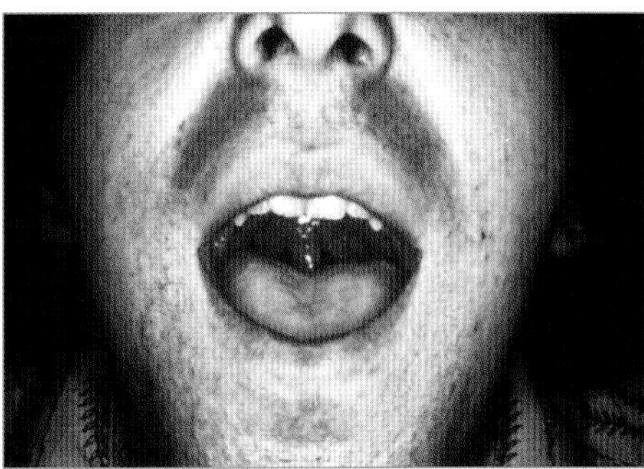

Image 51.16
This patient presented with symptoms later diagnosed as due to gonococcal pharyngitis. Gonococcal pharyngitis is a sexually transmitted infection acquired through oral sex with an infected partner. Most throat infections caused by gonococci have no symptoms, but some can suffer from mild to severe sore throat. Courtesy of Centers for Disease Control and Prevention/ Dr N. J. Flumara, Dr Gavin Hart.

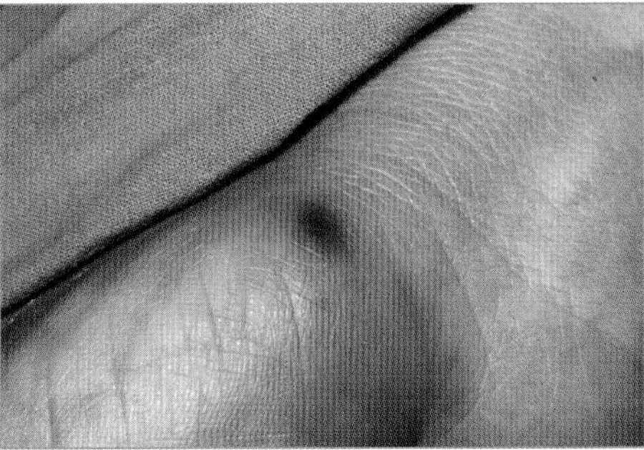

Image 51.17
Disseminated gonococcal infection. Courtesy of Gary Overturf, MD.

52

Granuloma Inguinale

(Donovanosis)

Clinical Manifestations

Initial lesions of this sexually transmitted infection are single or multiple subcutaneous nodules that gradually ulcerate. These nontender, granulomatous ulcers are beefy red and highly vascular and bleed readily on contact. Lesions usually involve the genitalia without regional adenopathy, but anal infections occur in 5% to 10% of patients; lesions at distant sites (eg, face, mouth, liver) are rare. Subcutaneous extension into the inguinal area results in induration that can mimic inguinal adenopathy (ie, "pseudobubo"). Verrucous, necrotic, and fibrous lesions may occur as well. Fibrosis manifests as sinus tracts, adhesions, and lymphedema, resulting in extreme genital deformity. Urethral obstruction can occur.

Etiology

Granuloma inguinale, also called donovanosis, is caused by *Klebsiella granulomatis* (formerly known as *Calymmatobacterium granulomatis*), an intracellular gram-negative bacillus.

Epidemiology

Indigenous granuloma inguinale occurs very rarely in the United States and most industrialized nations. The disease is endemic in some tropical and developing areas, including India, Papua New Guinea, the Caribbean, central Australia, and southern Africa. The incidence of infection seems to correlate with sustained high temperatures and high relative humidity. Infection is usually acquired by sexual intercourse, most commonly with a person with active infection but possibly also from a person with asymptomatic rectal infection. Young children can acquire infection by contact with infected secretions. The period of communicability extends throughout the duration of active lesions or rectal colonization.

Incubation Period

8 to 80 days.

Diagnostic Tests

The causative organism is difficult to culture, and diagnosis requires microscopic demonstration of dark-staining intracytoplasmic *K granulomatis* (also called Donovan bodies) on Wright or Giemsa staining of a crush preparation from subsurface scrapings of a lesion or tissue. The microorganism can also be detected by histologic examination of biopsy specimens. Lesions should be cultured for *Haemophilus ducreyi* to exclude chancroid. Granuloma inguinale is often misdiagnosed as carcinoma, which can be excluded by histologic examination of tissue or by response of the lesion to antimicrobial agents.

Treatment

Doxycycline for at least 21 days and until the lesions are completely healed is the treatment of choice. Azithromycin orally, once per week for at least 3 weeks and until all lesions have completely healed, is an alternative regimen. Trimethoprim-sulfamethoxazole, ciprofloxacin, and erythromycin may be used in appropriate patients. Gentamicin can be added if no improvement is evident after several days of therapy. Partial healing is usually noted within 7 days of initiation of therapy. Relapse can occur, especially if the antimicrobial agent is stopped before the primary lesion has healed completely. Complicated or long-standing infection can require surgical intervention.

Patients should be evaluated for other sexually transmitted infections, such as gonorrhea, syphilis, chancroid, chlamydia, hepatitis B virus, and HIV infections. Initiation or completion of the series of vaccines for hepatitis B and human papillomavirus should be given, if appropriate for the age group.

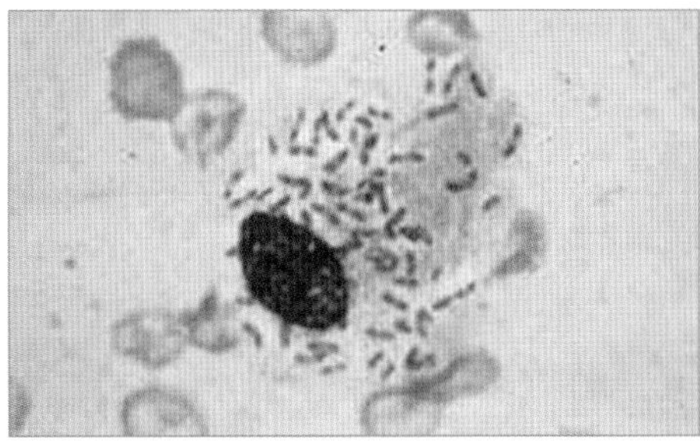

Image 52.1
Giemsa-stained *Klebsiella granulomatis* (Donovan bodies) of granuloma inguinale. Courtesy of Robert Jerris, MD.

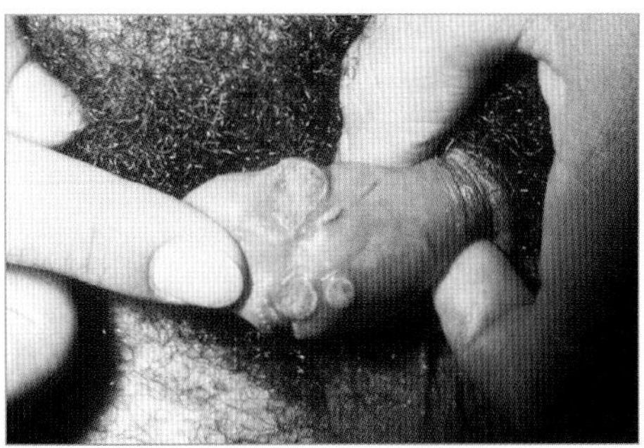

Image 52.2
This patient's penile lesions were due to gram-negative *Klebsiella granulomatis,* formerly known as *Calymmatobacterium granulomatis. K granulomatis* cause granuloma inguinale, or donovanosis, a sexually transmitted infection that is a slowly progressive, ulcerative condition of the skin and lymphatics of the genital and perianal area. A definitive diagnosis is achieved when a tissue smear test result is positive for the presence of *K granulomatis* (Donovan bodies). Courtesy of Centers for Disease Control and Prevention/Joe Miller; Source: Dr Cornelio Arevalo, Venezuela.

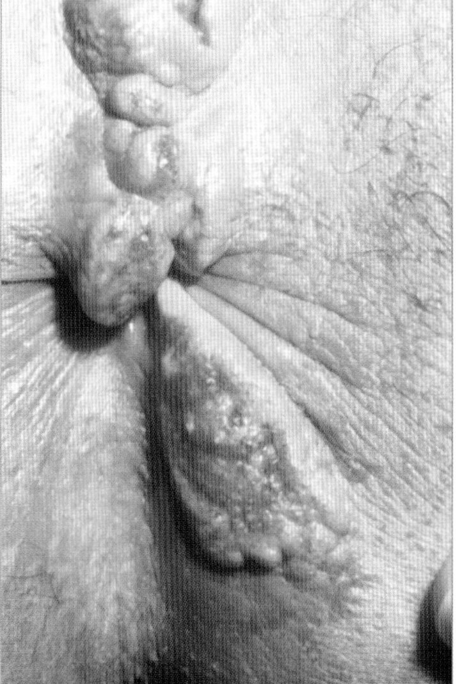

Image 52.3
Granuloma inguinale accompanied by perianal skin ulceration due to the bacterium *Klebsiella granulomatis* (formerly *Calymmatobacterium granulomatis*). The ulcerations are, for the most part, painless and granulomatous in nature (ie, chronic inflammation). Courtesy of the Centers for Disease Control and Prevention/Joe Miller; Source: Dr Cornelio Arevalo, Venezuela.

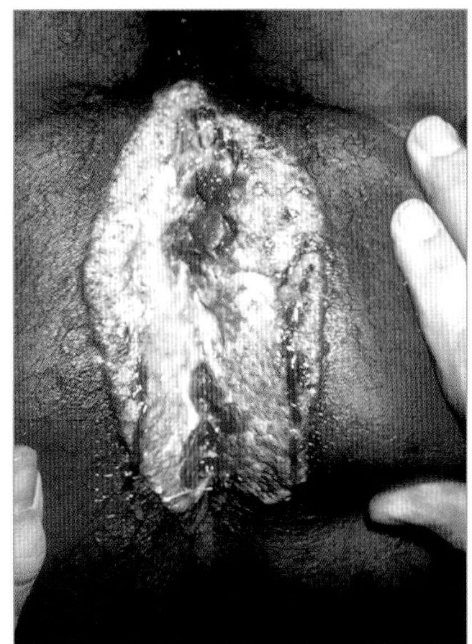

Image 52.4
Granuloma inguinale accompanied by perianal skin ulceration due to the bacterium *Klebsiella granulomatis* (formerly *Calymmatobacterium granulomatis*). The ulcerations are, for the most part, painless and granulomatous in nature (ie, chronic inflammation). Courtesy of Centers for Disease Control and Prevention/Dr Thomas F. Sellers/Emory University.

53

Haemophilus influenzae Infections

Clinical Manifestations

Haemophilus influenzae type b (Hib) causes pneumonia, bacteremia, meningitis, epiglottitis, septic arthritis, cellulitis, otitis media, purulent pericarditis, and, less commonly, endocarditis, endophthalmitis, osteomyelitis, peritonitis, and gangrene. Nontype b–encapsulated strains present in a similar manner to type b infections. Nontypable strains more commonly cause infections of the respiratory tract (eg, otitis media, sinusitis, pneumonia, conjunctivitis) and, less often, bacteremia, meningitis, chorioamnionitis, and neonatal septicemia.

Etiology

H influenzae is a pleomorphic gram-negative coccobacillus. Encapsulated strains express 1 of 6 antigenically distinct capsular polysaccharides (a–f); nonencapsulated strains lack capsule genes and are designated nontypable.

Epidemiology

The mode of transmission is person to person by inhalation of respiratory tract droplets or by direct contact with respiratory tract secretions. In neonates, infection is acquired intrapartum by aspiration of amniotic fluid or by contact with genital tract secretions containing the organism. Pharyngeal colonization by *H influenzae* is relatively common, especially with nontypable and nontype b capsular-type strains. Similar to findings in the pre-Hib vaccine era, in resource-limited countries where Hib vaccine has not been routinely implemented, the major reservoir of Hib is young infants and toddlers, who carry the organism in the upper respiratory tract. Before introduction of effective Hib conjugate vaccines, Hib was the most common cause of bacterial meningitis in children in the United States. The peak incidence of invasive Hib infections occurred between 6 and 18 months of age. In contrast, the peak age for Hib epiglottitis was 2 to 4 years of age.

Unimmunized children younger than 4 years are at increased risk of invasive Hib disease. Factors that predispose to invasive disease include sickle cell disease, asplenia, HIV infection, certain immunodeficiency syndromes, and malignant neoplasms. Historically, invasive Hib was more common in black, Alaska Native, Apache, and Navajo children; boys; child care attendees; children living in crowded conditions; and children who were not breastfed.

Since introduction of Hib conjugate vaccines in the United States, the incidence of invasive Hib disease has decreased by 99% to fewer than 1 cases per 100,000 children younger than 5 years. In 2012, 30 cases of invasive type b disease were reported in children younger than 5 years. In the United States, invasive Hib disease occurs primarily in unimmunized or under-immunized children and among infants too young to have completed the primary immunization series. *H influenzae* type b remains an important pathogen in many resource-limited countries where Hib vaccines are not routinely available. The epidemiology of invasive *H influenzae* disease in the United States has shifted in the postvaccination era. Nontypable *H influenzae* now causes most invasive *H influenzae* disease in all age groups. From 1999 through 2008, the annual incidence of invasive nontypable *H influenzae* disease was 1.73 per 100,000 children younger than 5 years. Nontypable *H influenzae* causes approximately 50% of episodes of acute otitis media and sinusitis in children and is a common cause of recurrent otitis media. The rate of nontypable *H influenzae* infections in boys is twice that in girls and peaks in the late fall.

In some North American indigenous populations, *H influenzae* type a (Hia) has emerged as a significant cause of invasive disease. The 2002–2012 incidence of Hia in Alaska Native children younger than 5 years was 18 per 100,000 per year (vs 0.5/100,000 in nonnative children). The incidence was highest in southwestern Alaska Native children younger than 5 years (72/100,000/y). Similarly, Hia has emerged among northern Canadian indigenous children, who experienced an incidence of 102 per 100,000 per year in children younger than 2 years. There has been an ongoing lower level of Hia disease in Navajo children younger than 5 years (20/100,000/y, 1988–2003). Invasive disease has also been caused by other encapsulated nontype b strains.

Incubation Period

Unknown.

Diagnostic Tests

The diagnosis of invasive disease is established by growth of *H influenzae* from cerebrospinal fluid, blood, synovial fluid, pleural fluid, or pericardial fluid. Gram stain of an infected body fluid specimen can facilitate presumptive diagnosis. All *H influenzae* isolates associated with invasive infection should be serotyped. Although the potential for suboptimal sensitivity and specificity exists with slide agglutination serotyping depending on reagents used, slide agglutination serotyping and genotyping by polymerase chain reaction are acceptable methods for capsule typing. If polymerase chain reaction capsular typing is not available locally, isolates should be submitted to the state health department or to a reference laboratory for testing.

Otitis media attributable to *H influenzae* is diagnosed by culture of tympanocentesis fluid; organisms isolated from other respiratory tract swab specimens (eg, throat, ear drainage) may not be the same as those from middle-ear culture.

Treatment

Initial therapy for children with *H influenzae* meningitis is intravenous cefotaxime or ceftriaxone. Ampicillin should be substituted if the Hib isolate is susceptible. Treatment of other invasive *H influenzae* infections is similar. Therapy is continued for 7 to 10 days and longer in complicated infections. Dexamethasone is beneficial for treatment of infants and children with Hib meningitis to diminish the risk of hearing loss, if given before or concurrently with the first dose of antimicrobial agent(s). Epiglottitis is a medical emergency. An airway must be established promptly via controlled intubation. Infected pleural or pericardial fluid should be drained.

For empiric treatment of acute otitis media in children younger than 2 years or in children 2 years or older with severe disease, oral amoxicillin is recommended for 10 days. A 7-day course is considered for children 2 through 5 years of age, and a 5-day course can be used for older children. In the United States, approximately 30% to 40% of *H influenzae* isolates produce β-lactamase, so amoxicillin may fail, necessitating use of a β-lactamase–resistant agent, such as amoxicillin-clavulanate, or an oral cephalosporin, such as cefdinir, cefuroxime, or cefpodoxime. Azithromycin is recommended for children with an allergy to β-lactam antibiotics. In vitro susceptibility testing of isolates from middle-ear fluid specimens helps guide therapy in complicated or persistent cases.

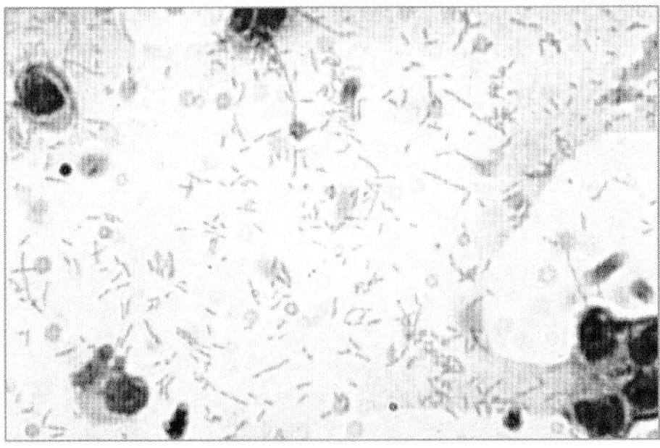

Image 53.1
Gram stain of cerebrospinal fluid (culture positive for *Haemophilus influenzae* type b).

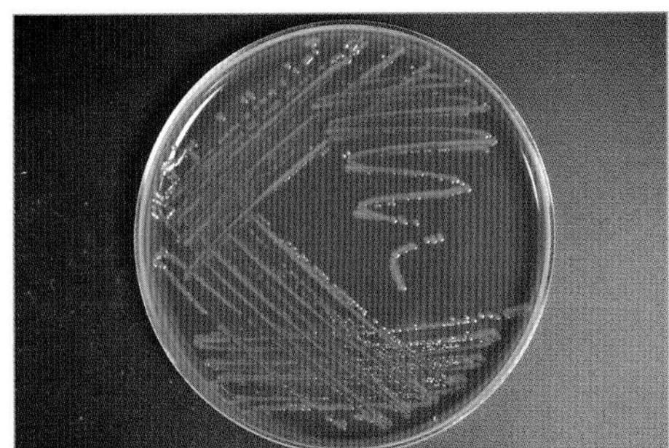

Image 53.2
Haemophilus influenzae on chocolate agar. This organism thrives on chocolate agar because of the supplication of factors X and V required for its growth. Individual colonies appear gray in color and sometimes mucoid or glistening in quality. Courtesy of Julia Rosebush, DO; Robert Jerris, PhD; and Theresa Stanley, M(ASCP).

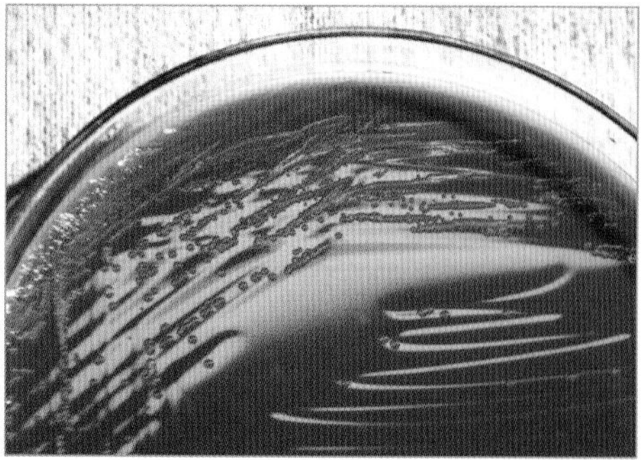

Image 53.3
This photograph depicts the colonial morphology displayed by gram-negative *Haemophilus influenzae* bacteria, which was grown on a medium of chocolate agar for a 24-hour period at a temperature of 37°C (98.6°F). Invasive disease caused by *H influenzae* type b can affect many organ systems. The most common types of invasive disease are pneumonia, occult febrile bacteremia, meningitis, epiglottitis, septic arthritis, cellulitis, otitis media, purulent pericarditis, and other, less common infections, such as endocarditis and osteomyelitis. Courtesy of Centers for Disease Control and Prevention/Amanda Moore, MT; Todd Parker, PhD; Audra Marsh.

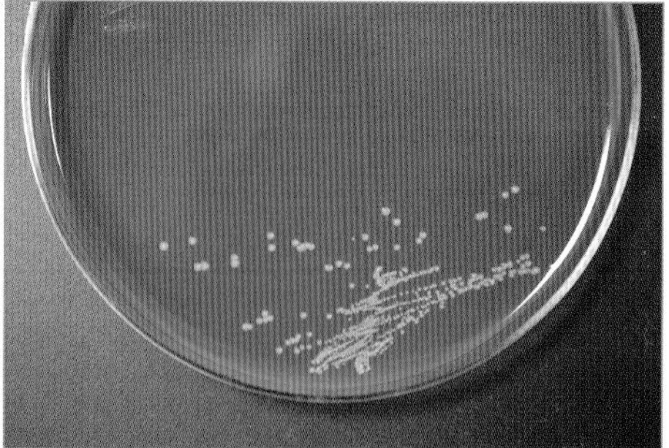

Image 53.4
Aggregatibacter (formerly *Haemophilus*) *aphrophilus* on chocolate agar. Colonies appear to grow down into the plate. This organism, a member of the *A (H) aphrophilus, Actinobacillus actinomycetemcomitans, Cardiobacterium hominis, Eikenella corrodens*, and *Kingella* species (HACEK) group, is associated with brain abscesses and endocarditis. Courtesy of Julia Rosebush, DO; Robert Jerris, PhD; and Theresa Stanley, M(ASCP).

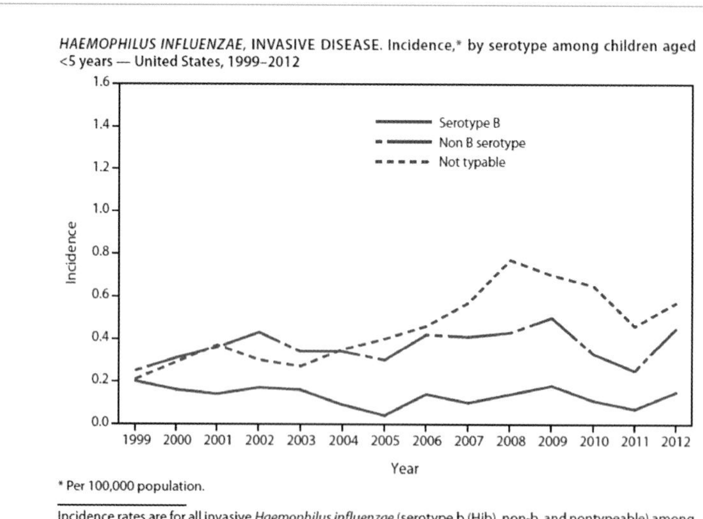

Incidence rates are for all invasive *Haemophilus influenzae* (serotype b (Hib), non-b, and nontypeable) among children aged <5 years. The epidemiology of invasive *Haemophilus influenzae* disease has changed in the United States in the post vaccine era. Since the introduction of conjugate Hib vaccines in 1987, the incidence of invasive Hib disease among children aged <5 years decreased by 99% to <1 case per 100,000 children. Nontypeable *Haemophilus influenzae* now causes the majority of invasive disease in all age groups. To ensure appropriate chemophrophylaxis measures for contacts of invasive Hib disease and to detect emergence of invasive non-Hib disease, serotyping of all *Haemophilus influenzae* isolates in children <5 years, and thorough and timely investigation of all cases of Hib disease are essential.

Image 53.5
Haemophilus influenzae, invasive disease. Incidence by serotype among persons younger than 5 years—United States, 1999–2012. Courtesy of *Morbidity and Mortality Weekly Report.*

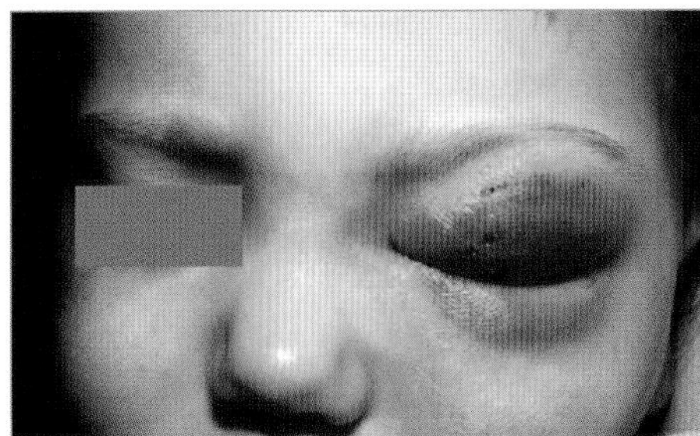

Image 53.6
Haemophilus influenzae type b periorbital cellulitis. Courtesy of Neal Halsey, MD.

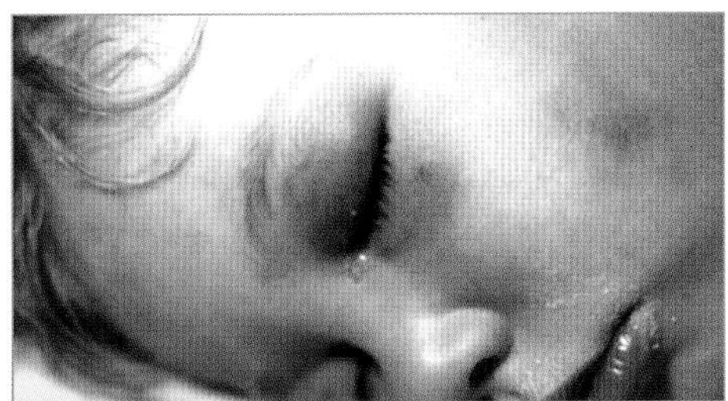

Image 53.7
A 16-month-old girl with periorbital and facial cellulitis caused by *Haemophilus influenzae* type b. The patient had no history of trauma. Copyright Martin G. Myers, MD.

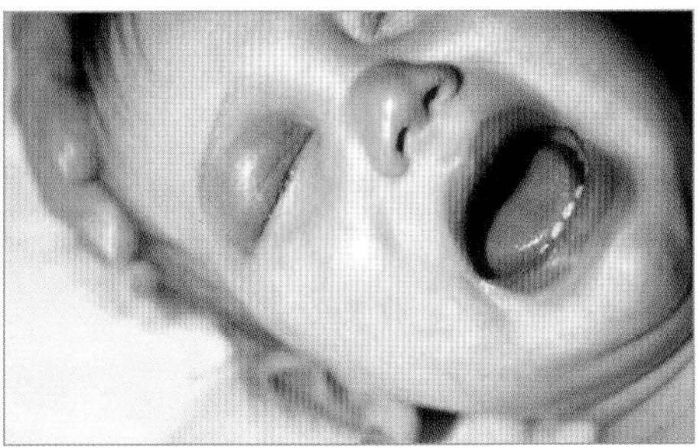

Image 53.8
A 10-month-old white boy with periorbital cellulitis due to *Haemophilus influenzae* type b. Copyright Martin G. Myers, MD.

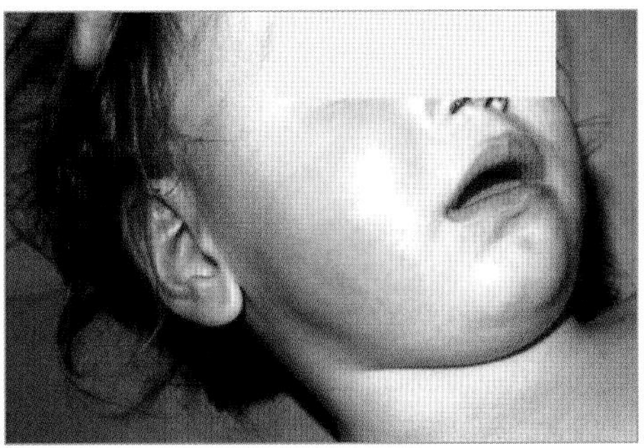

Image 53.9
Haemophilus influenzae type b cellulitis of the face proved by positive subcutaneous aspirate cultures and blood cultures. The cerebrospinal fluid culture was negative. (This is the first of 3 preschool boys from the same child care center who were examined within a period of 72 hours.)

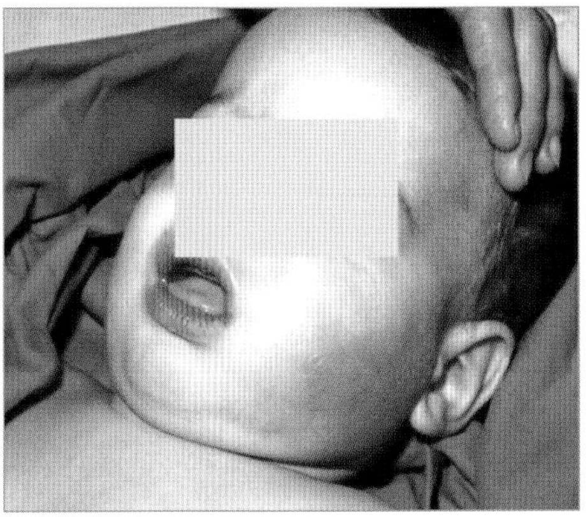

Image 53.10
The second of 3 preschool-aged boys with *Haemophilus influenzae* type b cellulitis of the face proved by positive subcutaneous aspirate cultures and blood cultures.

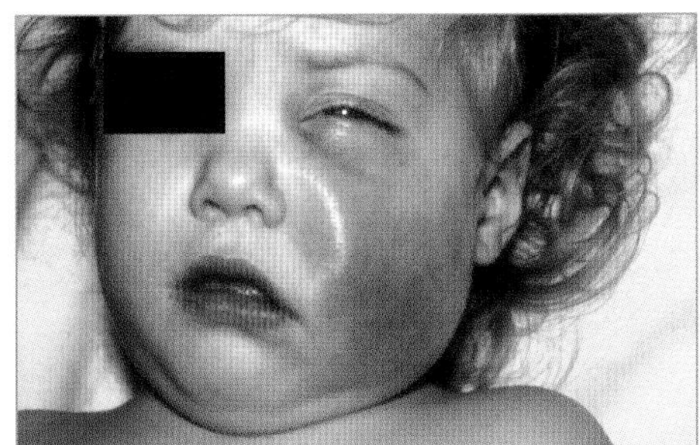

Image 53.11
A classic presentation of *Haemophilus influenzae* type b (Hib) facial cellulitis in a 10-month-old white girl. This once-common infection has been nearly eliminated among children who have been immunized with the Hib vaccine. Courtesy of George Nankervis, MD.

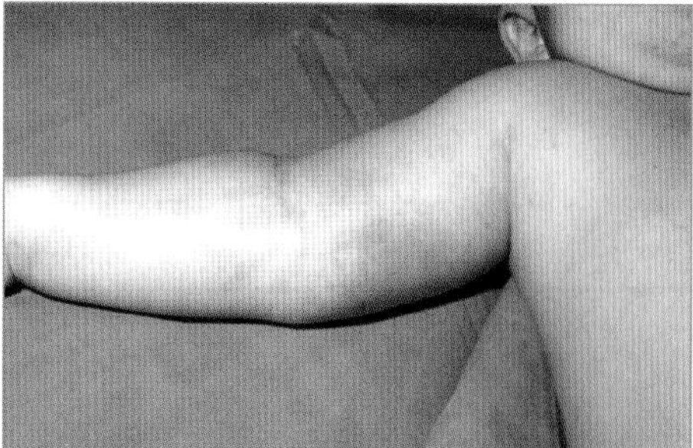

Image 53.12
Haemophilus influenzae type b cellulitis of the arm proved by positive blood culture.

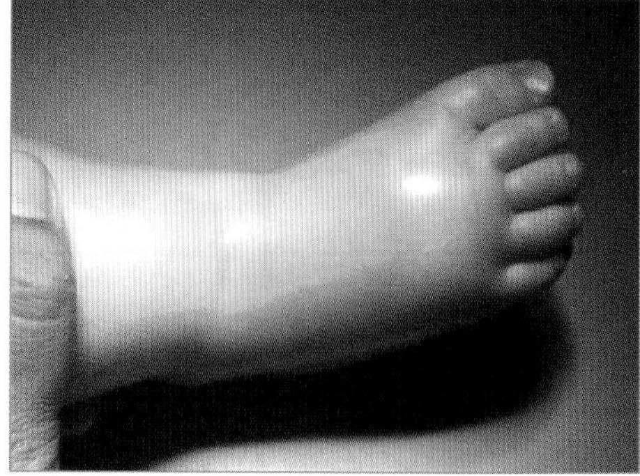

Image 53.13
Haemophilus influenzae type b cellulitis of the foot proved by positive blood culture.

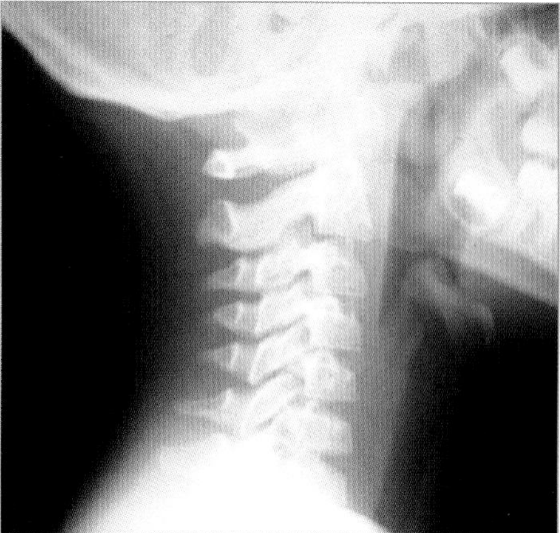

Image 53.14
Acute epiglottitis due to *Haemophilus influenzae* type b proved by blood culture. The swollen inflamed epiglottis looks like the shadow of a thumb on the lateral neck radiograph.

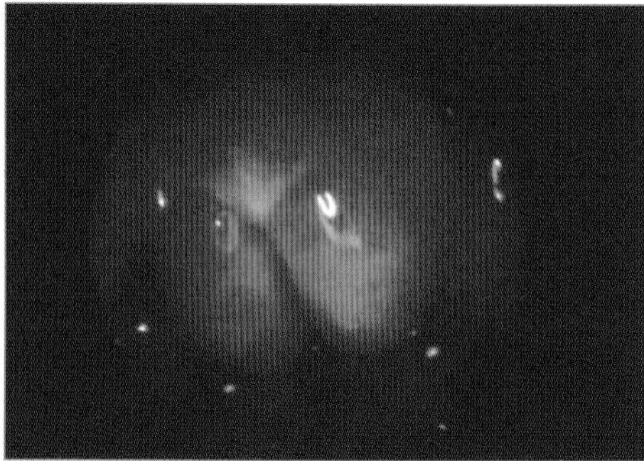

Image 53.15
Acute *Haemophilus influenzae* type b epiglottitis with striking erythema and swelling of the epiglottis. Courtesy of Edgar O. Ledbetter, MD, FAAP.

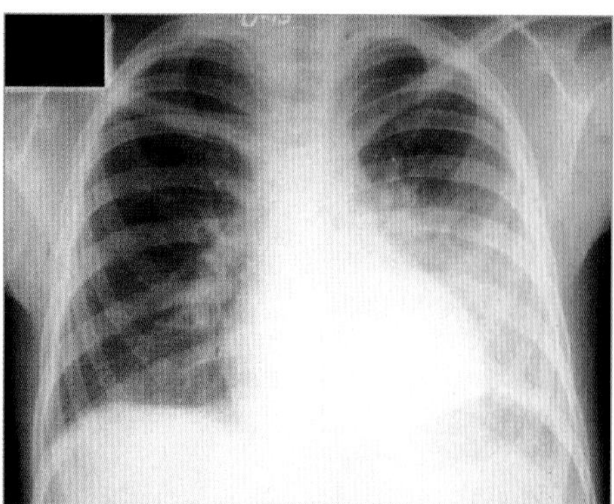

Image 53.16
Haemophilus influenzae type b pneumonia, bilateral, in a patient with acute epiglottitis (proved by blood culture). This is the same patient as in Image 53.15.

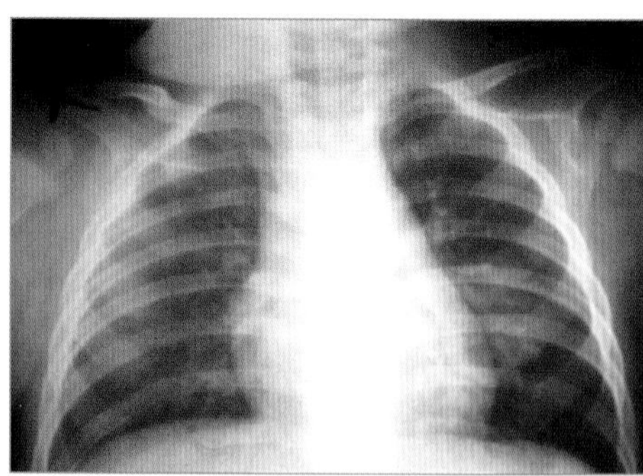

Image 53.17
Retrocardiac *Haemophilus influenzae* type b pneumonia proved by blood culture. Note the air bronchogram.

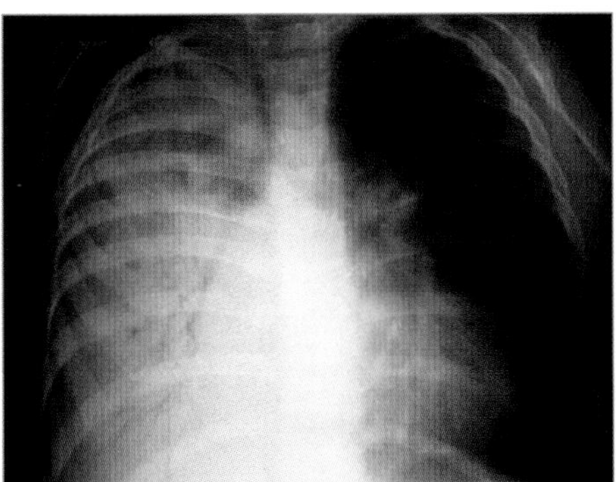

Image 53.18
Air bronchogram of fulminant *Haemophilus influenzae* type b pneumonia of the right lung in a child with congenital heart disease. Blood culture was positive. Courtesy of Edgar O. Ledbetter, MD, FAAP.

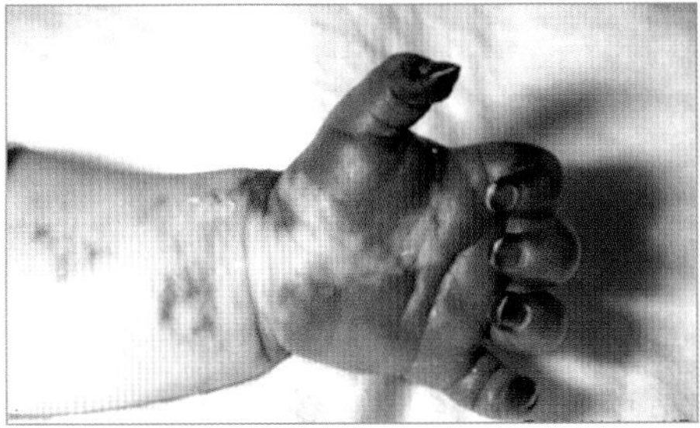

Image 53.20
Haemophilus influenzae type b sepsis with gangrene of the hand. Courtesy of Neal Halsey, MD.

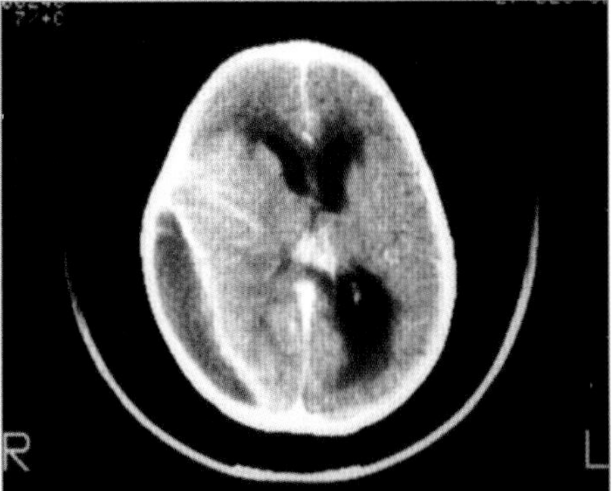

Image 53.22
Magnetic resonance image showing subdural empyema that developed in a patient with *Haemophilus influenzae* type b meningitis.

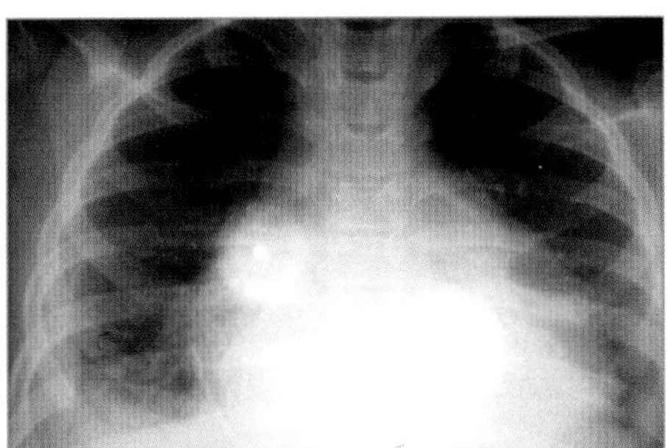

Image 53.19
Haemophilus influenzae type b bilateral pneumonia, empyema, and purulent pericarditis. Pericardiostomy drainage is important in preventing cardiac restriction.

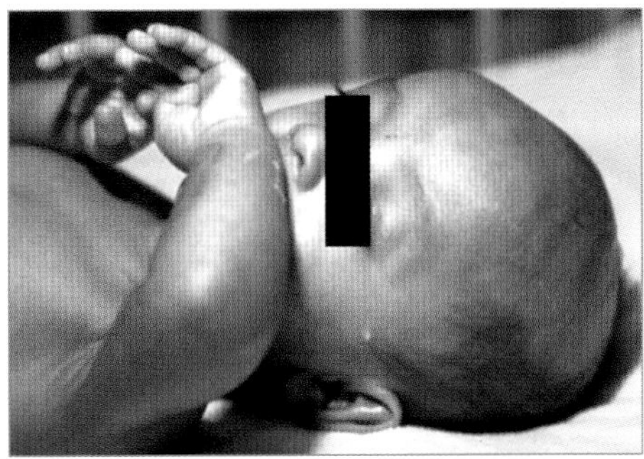

Image 53.21
A 2-year-old boy with *Haemophilus influenzae* type b meningitis and subdural empyema. Note the prominent anterior fontanelle secondary to increased intracranial pressure. Copyright Martin G. Myers, MD.

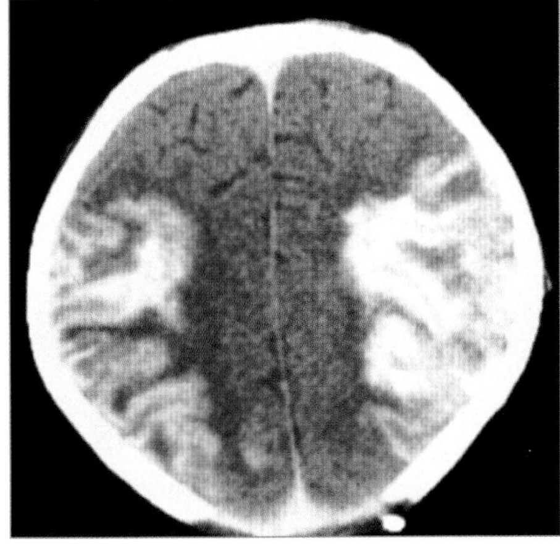

Image 53.23
Magnetic resonance image showing localized cerebritis and vasculitis in a patient with *Haemophilus influenzae* type b meningitis.

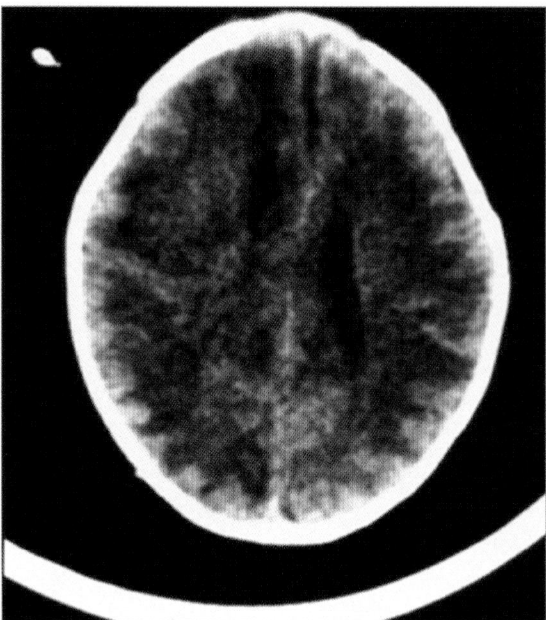

Image 53.24
Magnetic resonance image showing cerebral infarction in a patient who had *Haemophilus influenzae* type b (Hib) meningitis. The routine administration of Hib vaccine has virtually eliminated this type of devastating illness in the United States.

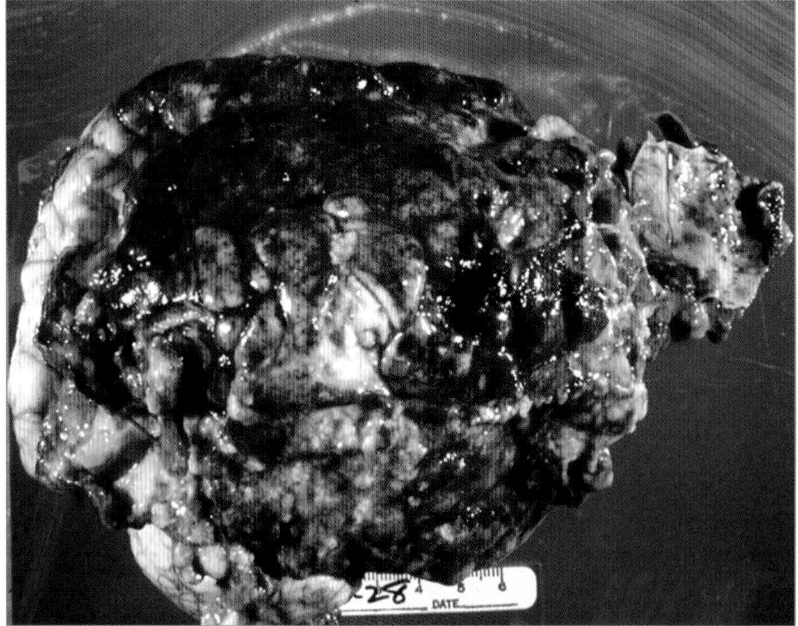

Image 53.25
Haemophilus influenzae meningitis in a 4-month-old who was evaluated in the morning for a well-child visit with normal clinical findings. By afternoon, the child had necrosis of the hands and feet and died 12 hours later. This is the brain of the infant 24 hours after the well-child visit. No immunologic deficit was diagnosed. Copyright Jerri Ann Jenista, MD.

54

Hantavirus Pulmonary Syndrome

Clinical Manifestations

Hantaviruses cause 2 distinct clinical syndromes: hantavirus pulmonary syndrome (HPS), a noncardiogenic pulmonary edema observed in the western hemisphere; and hemorrhagic fever with renal syndrome, which occurs worldwide. The prodromal illness of HPS is 3 to 7 days and is characterized by fever; chills; headache; myalgia of the shoulders, lower back, and thighs; nausea; vomiting; diarrhea; dizziness; and, sometimes, cough. Respiratory tract symptoms or signs usually do not occur during the prodrome, but pulmonary edema and severe hypoxemia appear abruptly after the onset of cough and dyspnea. The disease then progresses over a number of hours. In severe cases, persistent hypotension caused by myocardial dysfunction is present. In fatal cases, death occurs in 1 to 2 days following hospitalization.

Extensive bilateral interstitial and alveolar pulmonary edema and pleural effusions are the result of a diffuse pulmonary capillary leak and appear to be immune mediated in the endothelial cells of the microvasculature. Endotracheal intubation and assisted ventilation are usually required for only 2 to 4 days, with resolution heralded by onset of diuresis and rapid clinical improvement.

The severe myocardial depression is different from that of septic shock, with low cardiac indices and stroke volume index, normal pulmonary wedge pressure, and increased systemic vascular resistance. Poor prognostic indicators include persistent hypotension, marked hemoconcentration, a cardiac index of less than 2, and abrupt onset of lactic acidosis with a serum lactate concentration of greater than 4 mmol/L (36 mg/dL).

The mortality rate for patients with HPS is between 30% and 40%. Asymptomatic and milder forms of disease are rare. Limited information suggests clinical manifestations and prognosis are similar in adults and children. Serious sequelae are uncommon.

Etiology

Hantaviruses are RNA viruses of the Bunyaviridae family. Sin Nombre virus is the major cause of HPS in the western and central regions of the United States. Bayou virus, Black Creek Canal virus, Monongahela virus, and New York virus are responsible for sporadic cases in Louisiana, Texas, Florida, New York, and other areas of the eastern United States. Hantavirus serotypes associated with HPS in South and Central America include Andes virus, Oran virus, Laguna Negra virus, and Choclo virus. During the past decade, Brazil, Chile, and Argentina have reported most of the HPS cases in the Americas.

Epidemiology

Rodents, the natural hosts for hantaviruses, acquire lifelong, asymptomatic, chronic infection with prolonged viruria and virus in saliva, urine, and feces. Humans acquire infection through direct contact with infected rodents, rodent droppings, or rodent nests or through the inhalation of aerosolized virus particles from rodent urine, droppings, or saliva. Rarely, infection may be acquired from rodent bites or contamination of broken skin with excreta. Person-to-person transmission of hantaviruses has not been demonstrated in the United States but has been reported in Chile and Argentina. At-risk activities include handling or trapping rodents, cleaning or entering closed or rarely used rodent-infested structures, cleaning feed storage or animal shelter areas, hand plowing, and living in a home with an increased density of mice. For backpackers or campers, sleeping in a structure also inhabited by rodents has been associated with HPS. Weather conditions resulting in exceptionally heavy rainfall and improved rodent food supplies can result in a large increase in the rodent population with more frequent contact between humans and infected mice, resulting in an increase in human disease. Most cases occur during the spring and summer, with the geographic location determined by the habitat of the rodent carrier.

Sin Nombre virus is transmitted by the deer mouse, *Peromyscus maniculatus;* Black Creek Canal virus is transmitted by the cotton rat, *Sigmodon hispidus;* Bayou virus is transmitted by the rice rat, *Oryzomys palustris;* and New York virus is transmitted by the white-footed mouse, *Peromyscus leucopus.*

Incubation Period

1 to 6 weeks.

Diagnostic Tests

Characteristic laboratory findings include neutrophilic leukocytosis with immature granulocytes, including more than 10% immunoblasts, thrombocytopenia, and increased hematocrit. Sin Nombre virus RNA has been detected by reverse transcriptase-polymerase chain reaction assay of peripheral blood mononuclear cells and other clinical specimens from the early phase of the disease, frequently before the hospitalization. Viral RNA is not readily detected in bronchoalveolar lavage fluids.

Hantavirus-specific immunoglobulin (Ig) M and IgG antibodies are often present at the onset of clinical disease, and serologic testing is the method of choice for diagnosis. IgG can be negative in rapidly fatal cases. Rapid diagnosis can facilitate immediate appropriate supportive therapy and early transfer to a tertiary care facility. Enzyme immunoassay (available through many state health departments and the Centers for Disease Control and Prevention) and Western blot assays use recombinant antigens and have a high degree of specificity for detection of IgG and IgM antibody. Finally, immunohistochemistry in tissues (staining of capillary endothelial cells of the lungs and almost every organ in the body) obtained from autopsy can also establish the diagnosis retrospectively.

Treatment

Patients with suspected HPS should be transferred immediately to a tertiary care facility where supportive management of pulmonary edema, severe hypoxemia, and hypotension can occur during the first critical 24 to 48 hours. In severe forms, early mechanical ventilation and inotropic and pressor support are necessary. Extracorporeal membrane oxygenation should be considered when pulmonary wedge pressure and cardiac indices have deteriorated and may provide short-term support for the severe capillary leak syndrome in the lungs. Ribavirin is active in vitro against hantaviruses, including Sin Nombre virus. However, 2 clinical studies of intravenous ribavirin failed to show benefit in treatment of HPS in the cardiopulmonary stage.

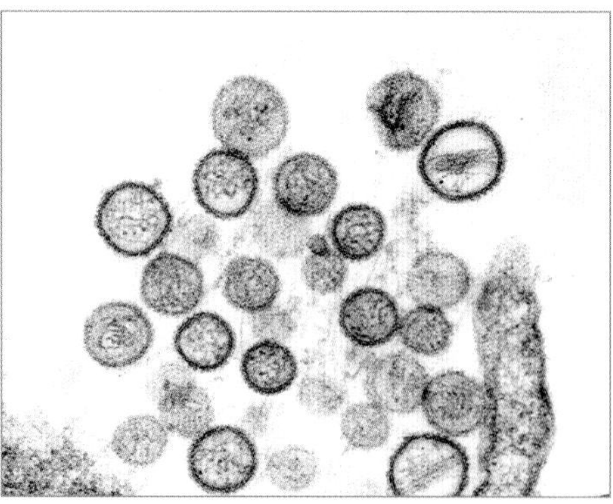

Image 54.1
Transmission electron micrograph of Sin Nombre virus, a frequent cause of hantavirus pulmonary syndrome. Courtesy of Centers for Disease Control and Prevention/Photo credit: Cynthia Goldsmith.

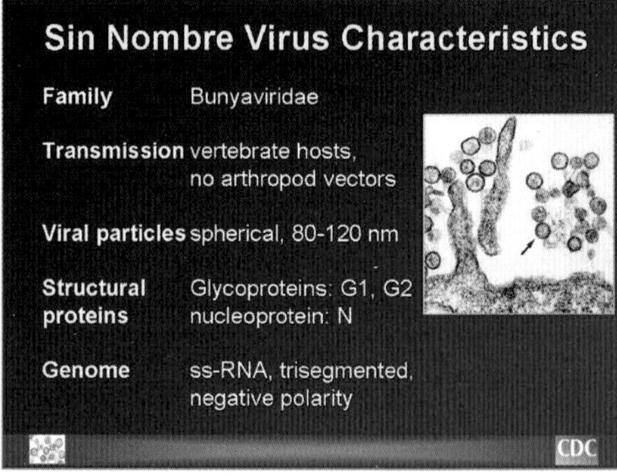

Image 54.2
Characteristics of Sin Nombre virus. Sin Nombre virus belongs to the family Bunyaviridae and contains 3 genomic RNA segments of negative polarity. The virion of Sin Nombre virus is spherical and is 80 to 120 nm in diameter. The virion contains 2 glycoproteins, G1 and G2, located on the outer surface, which are the nucleoprotein and the viral polymerase. Courtesy of Centers for Disease Control and Prevention.

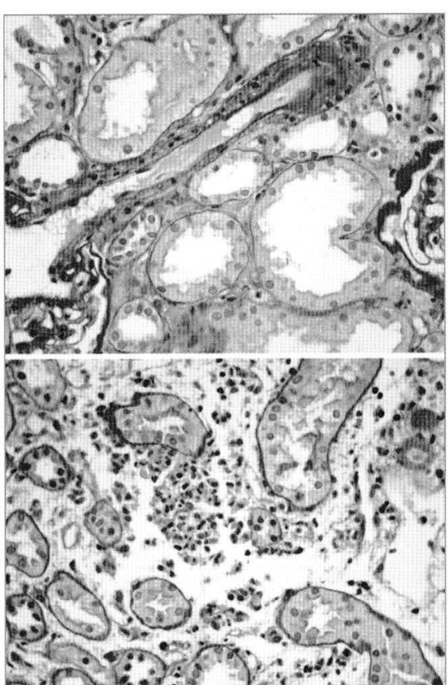

Image 54.3
Rodentborne hantavirus infections causing hemorrhagic fever with renal syndrome (HFRS) occur throughout most of Europe and Russia. The clinical manifestations of hantavirus infection vary and depend largely on the strain of the infecting virus. Classic HFRS is characterized by fever, acute renal failure, hypotension, hemorrhage, and vascular leakage. Acute tubular necrosis in a renal biopsy specimen is shown in this photograph. Courtesy of Centers for Disease Control and Prevention/*Emerging Infectious Diseases.*

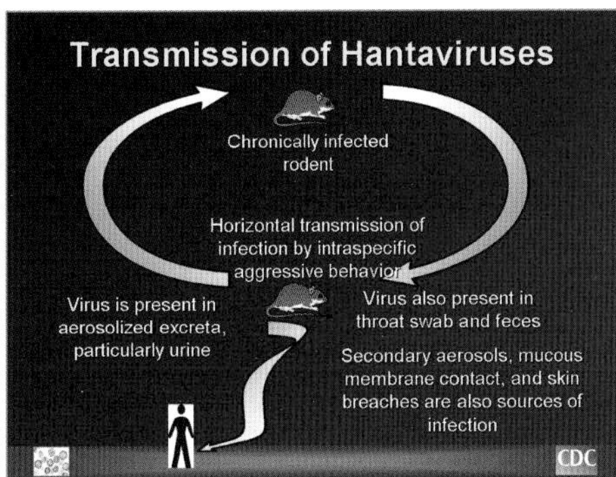

Image 54.4
Transmission of hantaviruses. The virus is horizontally transmitted between rodents through intraspecific aggressive behaviors, such as biting. The virus is transmitted to humans from aerosolized rodent excreta, particularly urine. Transmission to humans can also occur from inhalation of secondary aerosols and from rodent bites or other direct contact of infectious material with mucous membranes or broken skin. Courtesy of Centers for Disease Control and Prevention.

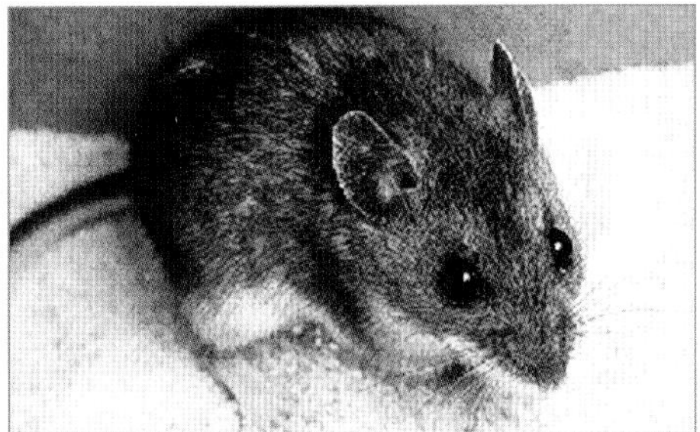

Image 54.5
Deer mouse (*Peromyscus maniculatus*). The deer mouse is a carrier of Sin Nombre virus, an etiologic agent of hantavirus pulmonary syndrome. Courtesy of Centers for Disease Control and Prevention.

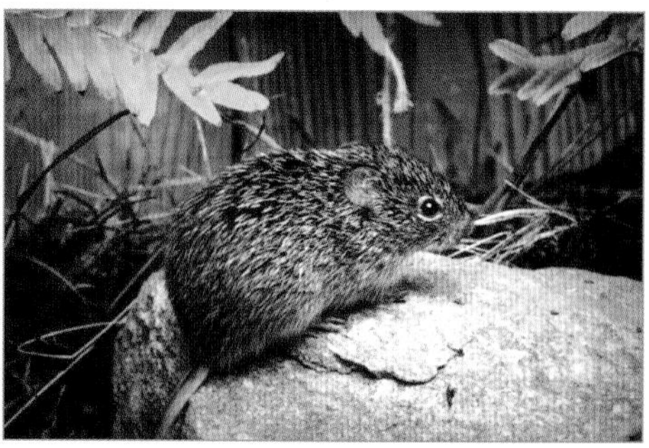

Image 54.6

This photograph depicts a cotton rat, *Sigmodon hispidus*, whose habitat includes the southeastern United States and way down into Central and South America. Its body is larger than the deer mouse, *Peromyscus maniculatus*, and measures about 5 to 7 inches, which includes the head and body; the tail measures an additional 3 to 4 inches. Its hair is longer and coarser than *P maniculatus* and is a grayish-brown color, sometimes grayish-black. The cotton rat prefers overgrown areas with shrubs and tall grasses. The cotton rat is a hantavirus carrier that becomes a threat when it enters human habitation in rural and suburban areas. Hantavirus pulmonary syndrome (HPS) is a deadly disease transmitted by infected rodents through urine, droppings, or saliva. Humans can contract the disease when they breathe in aerosolized virus. All hantaviruses known to cause HPS are carried by western hemisphere rats and mice of the family Muridae, subfamily Sigmodontinae. Courtesy of Centers for Disease Control and Prevention/James Gathany.

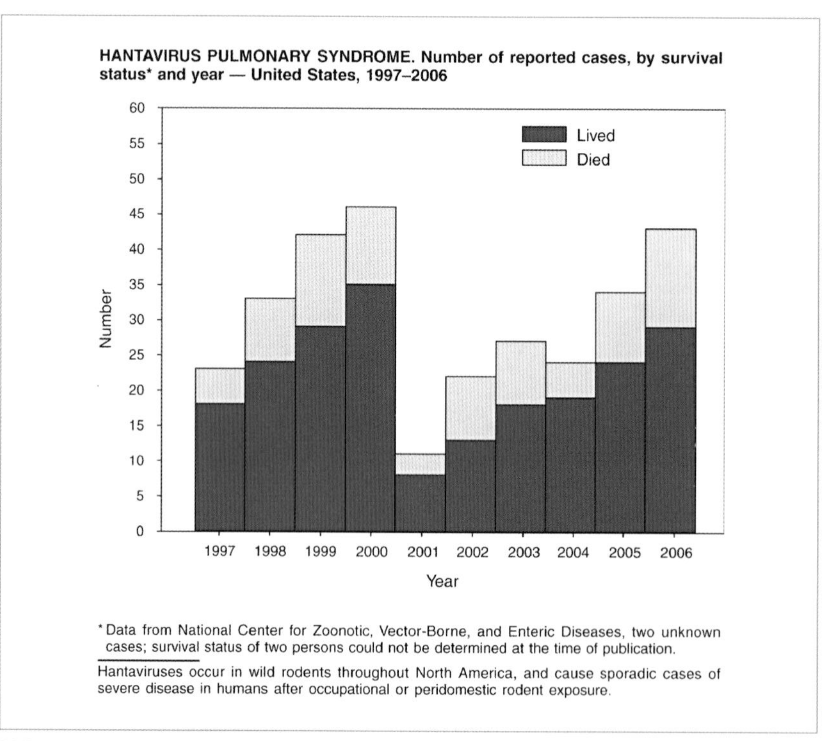

Image 54.7

Hantavirus pulmonary syndrome. Number of reported cases by survival status and year in the United States, 1997–2006. Courtesy of *Morbidity and Mortality Weekly Report.*

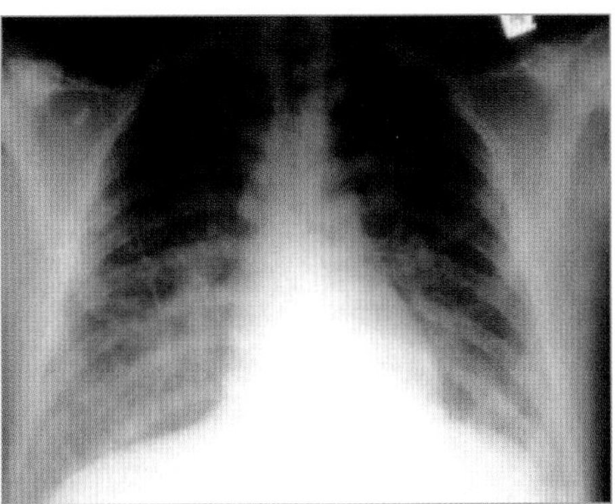

Image 54.8
Hantavirus pulmonary syndrome in a 16-year-old boy with a 36-hour history of fever, myalgia, and shortness of breath. Diffuse interstitial infiltrates with Kerley B lines. Diffuse nodular confluent alveolar opacities with some consolidation consistent with adult respiratory distress syndrome. Hantavirus serology confirmatory by immunoglobulin M at 1:6,400. Patient recovered with supportive care including inhaled nitric oxide. Copyright David Waagner.

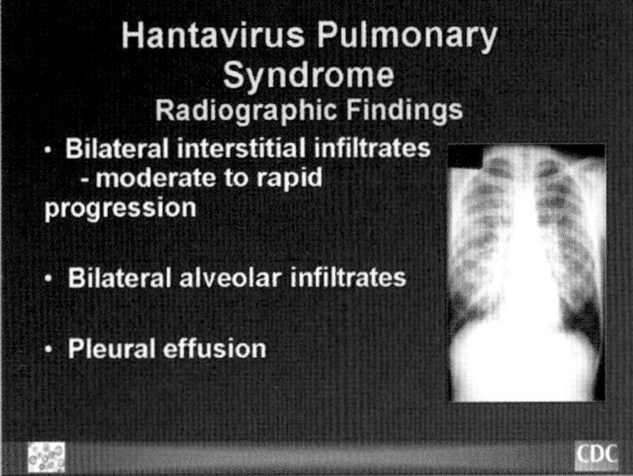

Image 54.10
Radiographic findings of hantavirus pulmonary syndrome. Findings usually include interstitial edema, Kerley B lines, hilar indistinctness, and peribronchial cuffing with normal cardiothoracic ratios. Hantavirus pulmonary syndrome begins with minimal changes of interstitial pulmonary edema and rapidly progresses to alveolar edema with severe bilateral involvement. Pleural effusions are common and are often large enough to be evident radiographically. Courtesy of Centers for Disease Control and Prevention.

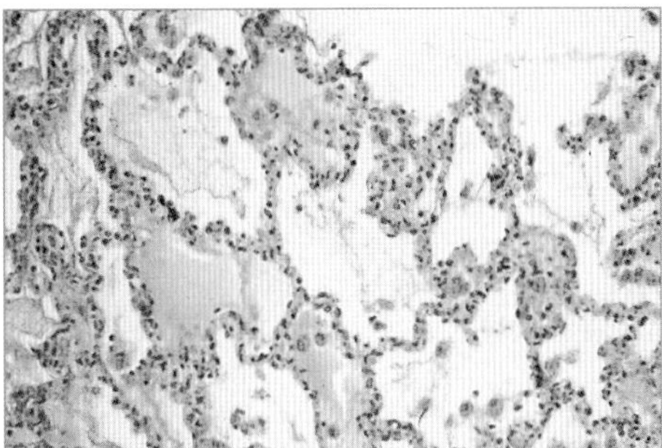

Image 54.9
Histopathologic features of lung in hantavirus pulmonary syndrome include interstitial pneumonitis and intra-alveolar edema. Courtesy of Centers for Disease Control and Prevention/Dr Sherif R. Zaki.

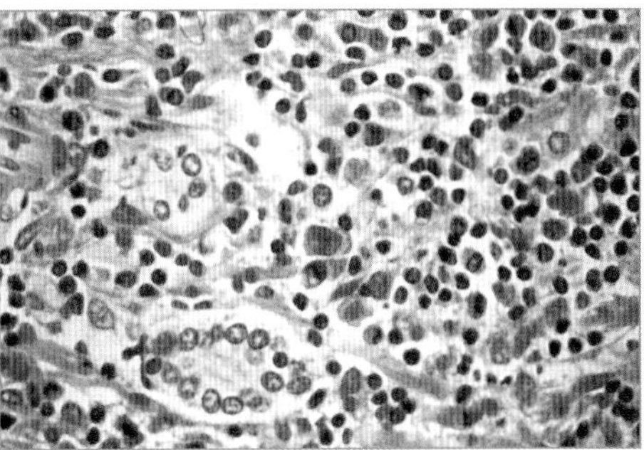

Image 54.11
This photograph shows liver tissue from a patient with hantavirus pulmonary syndrome. Courtesy of Centers for Disease Control and Prevention.

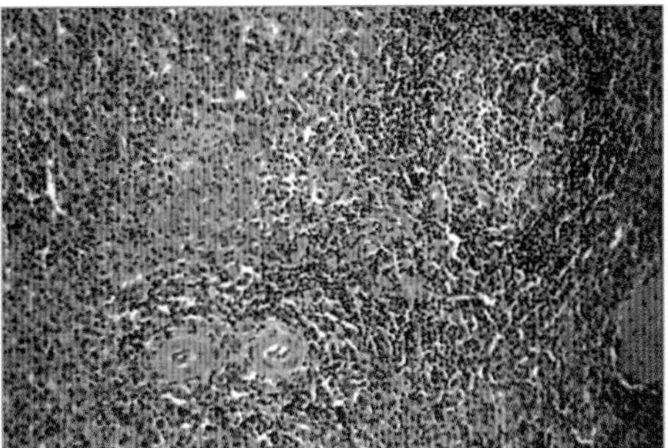

Image 54.12
This photograph shows splenic tissue from a patient with hantavirus pulmonary syndrome (HPS). In HPS splenic histopathology, one will note a lymphohistiocytic infiltrate throughout the red pulp region and concentrated to some extent in the periarteriolar white pulp area as well. Courtesy of Centers for Disease Control and Prevention.

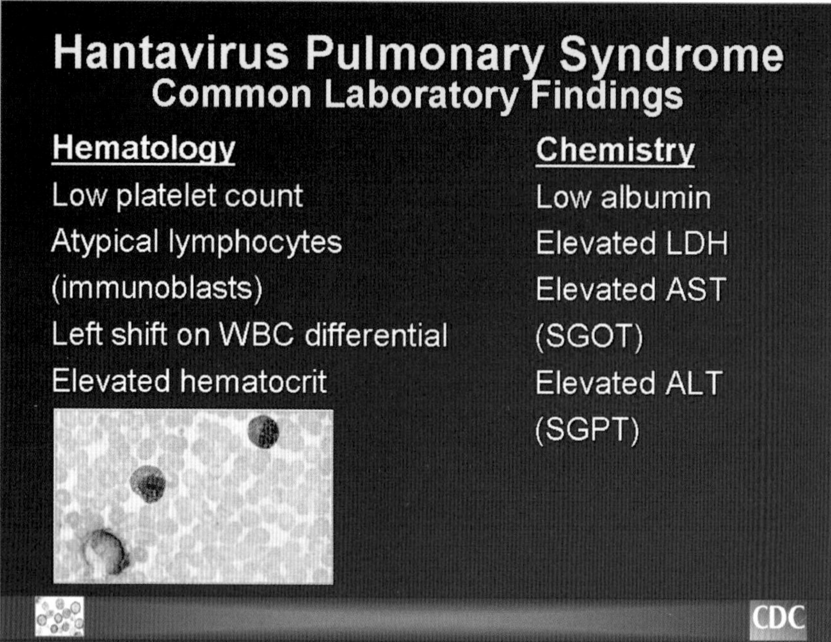

Image 54.13
Common laboratory findings. Notable hematologic findings include low platelet count, immunoblasts, left shift on white blood cell count differential, elevated white blood cell count, and elevated hematocrit. The large atypical lymphocyte shown here is an example of one of the laboratory findings that, when combined with a bandemia and dropping platelet count, are characteristic of hantavirus pulmonary syndrome. Notable blood chemistry findings include low albumin, elevated lactate dehydrogenase, elevated aspartate aminotransferase, and elevated alanine aminotransferase. Courtesy of Centers for Disease Control and Prevention.

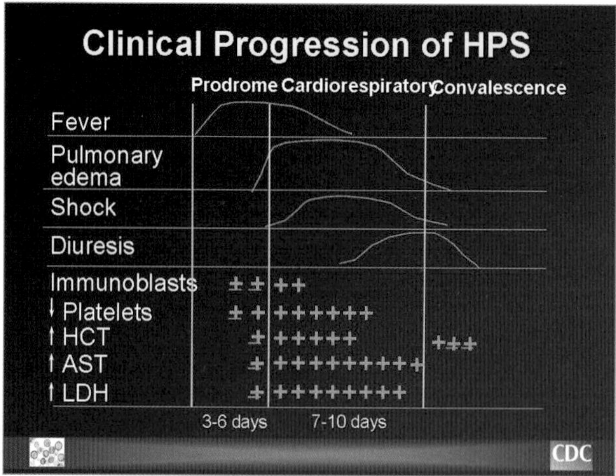

Image 54.14
Clinical course of hantavirus pulmonary syndrome starts with a febrile prodrome that may ultimately lead to hypotension and end-organ failure. The onset of the immune response precedes severe organ failure, which is thought to be immunopathologic in nature. Hypotension does not result in shock until the onset of respiratory failure, but this may reflect the severe physiological effect of lung edema. Courtesy of Centers for Disease Control and Prevention.

55

Helicobacter pylori Infections

Clinical Manifestations

Helicobacter pylori causes chronic active gastritis and can result in duodenal and, to a lesser extent, gastric ulcers. Persistent infection with *H pylori* increases the risk of gastric cancer. In children, *H pylori* infection can result in gastroduodenal inflammation that can manifest as epigastric pain, nausea, vomiting, hematemesis, and guaiac-positive stools. Symptoms can resolve within a few days or can wax and wane. Extraintestinal conditions in children that have been associated with *H pylori* infection can include iron deficiency anemia and short stature. However, most infections are thought to be asymptomatic. Moreover, there is no clear association between infection and recurrent abdominal pain, in the absence of peptic ulcer disease. The organism can persist in the stomach for years or for life. *H pylori* infection is not associated with secondary gastritis (eg, autoimmune, associated with nonsteroidal anti-inflammatory agents).

Etiology

H pylori is a gram-negative, spiral, curved, or U-shaped microaerophilic bacillus that has single or multiple flagella at one end. The organism is catalase, oxidase, and urease positive.

Epidemiology

H pylori organisms have been isolated from humans and other primates. An animal reservoir for human transmission has not been demonstrated. Organisms are thought to be transmitted from infected humans by the fecal-oral, gastro-oral, and oral-oral routes. Nearly half of the world's population is infected with *H pylori*, with a disproportionally high prevalence rate in resource-limited countries. Infection rates are low in children in resource-rich, industrialized countries, except in children from lower socioeconomic groups. Most infections are acquired in the first 5 years of life and can reach prevalence rates of up to 80% in resource-limited countries. Approximately 70% of infected people are asymptomatic, 20% of people have macroscopic (ie, visual) and microscopic findings of ulceration, and an estimated 1% have features of neoplasia.

Incubation Period

Unknown.

Diagnostic Tests

H pylori infection can be diagnosed by culture of gastric biopsy tissue on nonselective or selective media at 37°C (98.6°F) under microaerobic conditions for 3 to 7 days. The organism can also be identified by polymerase chain reaction or fluorescence in situ hybridization of gastric biopsy tissue. Organisms can usually be visualized on histologic sections with Warthin-Starry silver, Steiner, Giemsa, or Genta staining. Because of production of urease by organisms, urease testing of a gastric specimen can give a rapid and specific microbiologic diagnosis. Each of these tests requires endoscopy and biopsy. The first *H pylori* breath test for children 3 to 17 years of age became available in 2012. A stool antigen test (by enzyme immunoassay) is also available and can be used for children of any age, especially before and after treatment. Each of these commercially available tests for active infection (ie, breath or stool tests) has a high sensitivity and specificity.

Treatment

Treatment is recommended for infected patients who have peptic ulcer disease (currently or in the past 1–5 years), gastric mucosa–associated lymphoid tissue-type lymphoma, or early gastric cancer. Screening for and treatment of infection, if found, can be considered for children with one or more primary relatives with gastric cancer, children who are in a high-risk group for gastric cancer (eg, immigrants from resource-limited countries or countries with high rates of gastric cancer), or children who have unexplained iron deficiency anemia. Treatment may also be considered if infection is found at the time of diagnostic endoscopy.

A number of treatment regimens have been evaluated and are approved for use in adults; the safety and efficacy of these regimens in pediatric patients have not been established. First-line eradication regimens include triple therapy with a proton pump inhibitor (PPI) plus amoxicillin plus clarithromycin or metronidazole, or bismuth salts plus amoxicillin plus metronidazole. An alternative sequential regimen that may be more effective includes dual therapy with amoxicillin and a PPI for 5 days, followed by 5 days of triple therapy (a PPI plus clarithromycin and metronidazole). These regimens are effective in eliminating the organism, healing the ulcer, and preventing recurrence. Alternate therapies in people 8 years and older include bismuth subsalicylate plus metronidazole plus tetracycline plus either a PPI or an H_2-receptor antagonist (eg, cimetidine, famotidine, nizatidine, ranitidine), or bismuth subcitrate potassium plus metronidazole plus tetracycline plus omeprazole. A breath or stool test may be performed as follow-up to document organism eradication 4 to 8 weeks after completion of therapy, although the stool antigen test result can remain positive for up to 90 days after treatment.

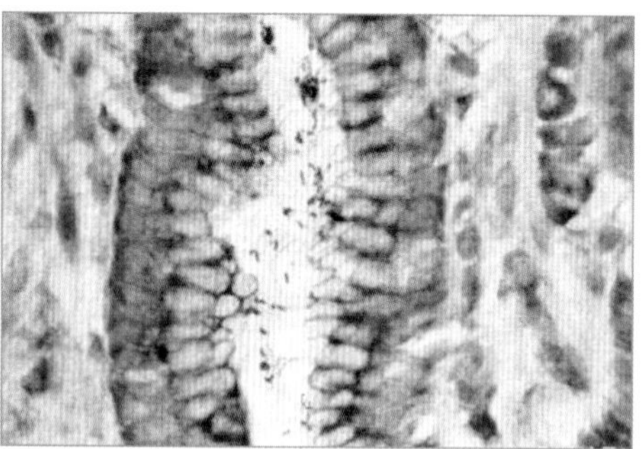

Image 55.1
Histology of the gastric mucosa demonstrates the characteristic curved organisms in the gastric glands. Courtesy of H. Cody Meissner, MD, FAAP.

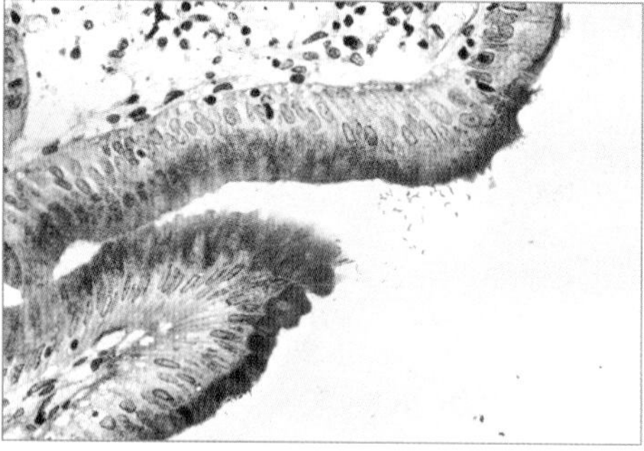

Image 55.2
A biopsy of gastric mucosa stained with Warthin-Starry silver stain showing *Helicobacter pylori* organisms. Courtesy of Brian Oliver, MD.

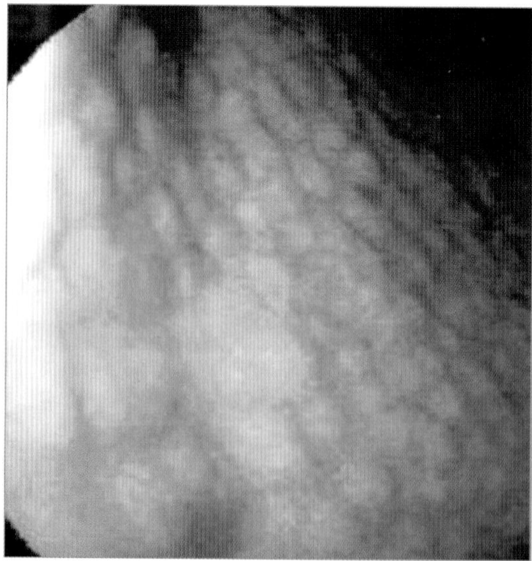

Image 55.3
Helicobacter pylori infection is a known risk factor for gastritis and duodenal ulcers in children and adults. Rarely, and primarily in older adulthood, *H pylori* is also associated with a gastric lymphoma of the mucosal-associated lymphoid tissue. The gold standard for the diagnosis of *H pylori* infection of the stomach is endoscopy with biopsy. Endoscopy may show a nodular gastritis of the antrum. Courtesy of H. Cody Meissner, MD, FAAP.

56

Hemorrhagic Fevers Caused by Arenaviruses

Clinical Manifestations

Arenaviruses are responsible for several hemorrhagic fevers (HFs): LCMV-LASV complex (formerly Old World) arenavirus HFs include Lassa fever and the recently described Lujo virus infections; Tacaribe complex (formerly New World) arenavirus HFs include Argentine, Bolivian, Brazilian, Venezuelan, and Chapare virus infection. Lymphocytic choriomeningitis virus is an arenavirus that generally induces less severe disease, although it can cause HFs in immunosuppressed patients; it is discussed in a separate chapter. Disease associated with arenaviruses ranges in severity from mild, acute, febrile infections to severe illnesses in which vascular leak, shock, and multiorgan dysfunction are prominent features. Fever, headache, myalgia, conjunctival suffusion, retro-orbital pain, facial flushing, bleeding, and abdominal pain are common early symptoms in all infections. Thrombocytopenia, leukopenia, axillary petechiae, generalized lymphadenopathy, and encephalopathy are usually present in Argentine HF, Bolivian HF, and Venezuelan HF, and exudative pharyngitis often occurs in Lassa fever. Mucosal bleeding occurs in severe cases as a consequence of vascular damage, thrombocytopenia, and platelet dysfunction. Proteinuria is common, but renal failure is unusual. Increased serum concentrations of aspartate transaminase can portend a severe or possibly fatal outcome of Lassa fever. Shock develops 7 to 9 days after onset of illness in more severely ill patients with these infections. Upper and lower respiratory tract symptoms can develop in people with Lassa fever. Encephalopathic signs, such as tremor, alterations in consciousness, and seizures, can occur in South American HFs and in severe cases of Lassa fever. Transitory deafness is reported in 30% of early convalescents of Lassa fever. The mortality rate in South American HFs is 15% to 30%.

Etiology

Arenaviruses are single-stranded RNA viruses. The major arenavirus HFs occurring in the western hemisphere are caused by the Tacaribe serocomplex of arenaviruses: Argentine HF caused by Junin virus, Bolivian HF caused by Machupo virus, and Venezuelan HF caused by Guanarito virus. A fourth arenavirus, Sabia virus, has been recognized to cause 2 unrelated cases of naturally occurring HF in Brazil and 2 laboratory-acquired cases. Chapare virus has been isolated from a fatal human case in Bolivia. The LCMV-LASV complex of arenaviruses includes Lassa virus, which causes Lassa fever in West Africa, as well as Lujo virus, which was described in southern Africa during an outbreak characterized by fatal human-to-human transmission. Several other arenaviruses are known only from their rodent reservoirs in both hemispheres.

Epidemiology

Arenaviruses are maintained in nature by association with specific rodent hosts, in which they produce chronic viremia and viruria. The principal routes of infection are inhalation and contact of mucous membranes and skin (ie, through cuts, scratches, or abrasions) with urine and salivary secretions from these persistently infected rodents. Ingestion of food contaminated by rodent excrement may also cause disease transmission. All arenaviruses are infectious as aerosols, and arenaviruses causing HF should be considered highly hazardous to people working with any of these viruses in the laboratory. Laboratory-acquired infections have been documented with Lassa, Machupo, Junin, and Sabia viruses. The geographic distribution and habitats of the specific rodents that serve as reservoir hosts largely determine the areas with endemic infection and the populations at risk. Before a vaccine became available in Argentina, several hundred cases of Argentine HF occurred annually in agricultural workers and inhabitants of the Argentine pampas. The Argentine HF vaccine is not licensed in the United States. Epidemics of Bolivian HF occurred in small towns between 1962 and 1964; sporadic disease activity in the countryside has continued since then.

Venezuelan HF was first identified in 1989 and occurs in rural north-central Venezuela. Lassa fever is endemic in most of West Africa, where rodent hosts live in proximity with humans, causing thousands of infections annually. Lassa fever has been reported in the United States and Western Europe in people who have traveled to West Africa.

Incubation Period

6 to 17 days.

Diagnostic Tests

Viral nucleic acid can be detected in acute disease by reverse transcriptase-polymerase chain reaction assay. These viruses can be isolated from blood of acutely ill patients as well as from various tissues obtained postmortem, but isolation should be attempted only under Biosafety level 4 conditions. Virus antigen is detectable by enzyme immunoassay in acute specimens and postmortem tissues. Virus-specific immunoglobulin (Ig) M antibodies are present in the serum during acute stages of illness but may be undetectable in rapidly fatal cases. The IgG antibody response is delayed. Diagnosis can be made retrospectively by immunohistochemistry in formalin-fixed tissues obtained from autopsy.

Treatment

Intravenous ribavirin substantially decreases the mortality rate in patients with severe Lassa fever, particularly if they are treated during the first week of illness. For Argentine HF, transfusion of immune plasma in defined doses of neutralizing antibodies is the standard specific treatment when administered during the first 8 days from onset of symptoms. Intravenous ribavirin has been used with success to abort a Sabia laboratory infection and to treat Bolivian HF patients and the only Lujo infection survivor. Ribavirin did not reduce mortality when initiated 8 days or more after onset of Argentine HF symptoms. Whether ribavirin treatment initiated early in the course of the disease has a role in the treatment of Argentine HF remains unknown. Meticulous fluid balance is an important aspect of supportive care in each of the HFs.

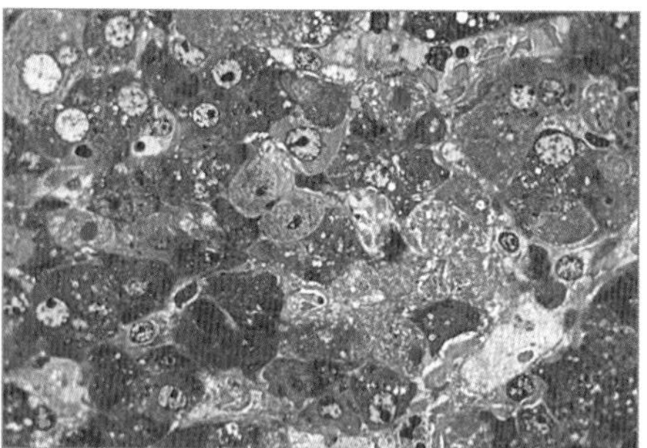

Image 56.1
This photomicrograph shows hepatitis caused by the Lassa virus (toluidine-blue azure II stain). The Lassa virus, which can cause altered liver morphology with hemorrhagic necrosis and inflammation, is a member of the family Arenaviridae and is a single-stranded RNA, zoonotic, or animal-borne pathogen. Courtesy of Centers for Disease Control and Prevention/ Dr Fred Murphy; Sylvia Whitfield.

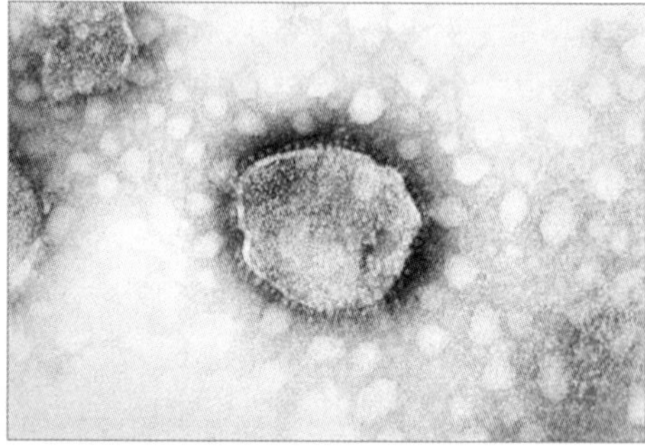

Image 56.2
Electron micrograph of *Arenaviridae* Tacaribe complex arenaviruses. *Arenaviridae* are RNA viruses whose particles are spherical and have an average diameter of 110 to 130 nm. *Arenaviridae* members are zoonotic, which means in nature, they are found in reservoir animal hosts—primarily rodents. Courtesy of Centers for Disease Control and Prevention/ E. L. Palmer.

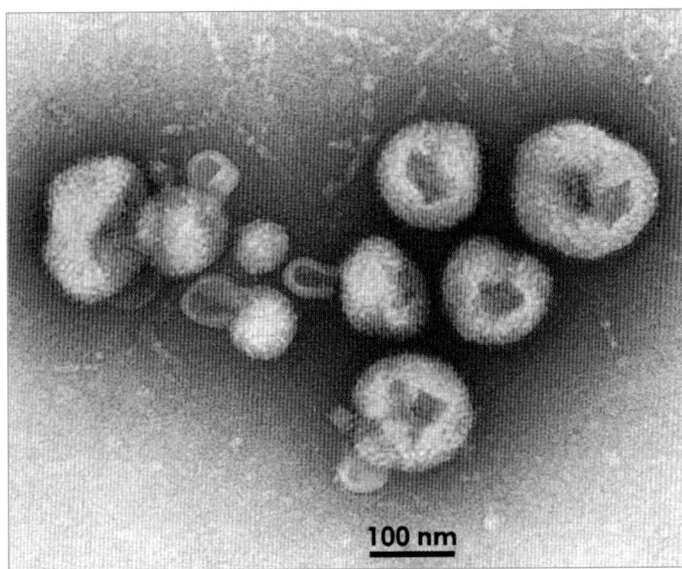

Image 56.3
This transmission electron micrograph depicts virions (viral particles) that are members of the genus *Arenavirus*. Arenaviruses include lymphocytic choriomeningitis virus and the agents of 5 hemorrhagic fevers, including West African Lassa fever virus and Bolivian hemorrhagic fever, also known as Machupo virus. Spread to humans occurs through inhalation of airborne particulates originating from rodent excrement, which can occur during the simple act of sweeping a floor. Courtesy of Centers for Disease Control and Prevention/Charles Humphrey.

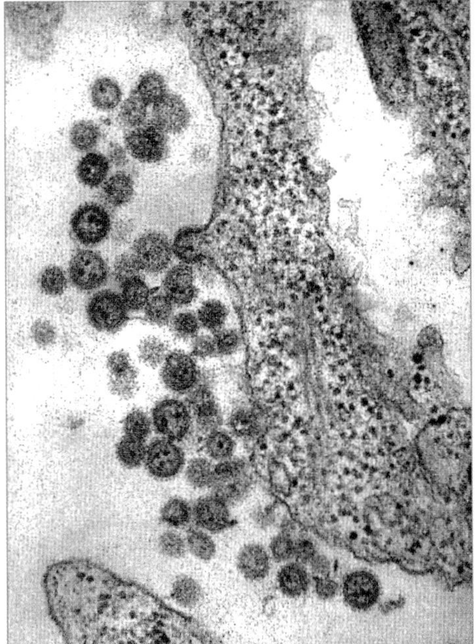

Image 56.4
Electron photomicrograph of the Machupo virus. Machupo virus is a member of the arenavirus family, isolated in the Beni province of Bolivia in 1963; viral hemorrhagic fever. Courtesy of Centers for Disease Control and Prevention/Dr W. Winn.

57

Hemorrhagic Fevers Caused by Bunyaviruses

Clinical Manifestations

Bunyaviruses are vectorborne infections (except for hantavirus) that often result in severe febrile disease with multisystem involvement. Human infection by bunyaviruses can be associated with high rates of morbidity and mortality. In the United States, disease attributable to a bunyavirus is most likely caused by hantavirus or members of the California serogroup.

Hemorrhagic fever with renal syndrome (HFRS) is a complex, multiphasic disease characterized by vascular instability and varying degrees of renal insufficiency. Fever, flushing, conjunctival injection, headache, blurred vision, abdominal pain, and lumbar pain are followed by hypotension, oliguria, and, subsequently, polyuria. Petechiae are frequent, but more serious bleeding manifestations are rare. Shock and acute renal insufficiency may occur. Nephropathia epidemica (attributable to Puumala virus) occurs in Europe and presents as a milder disease with acute influenza-like illness, abdominal pain, and proteinuria. Acute renal dysfunction also occurs, but hypotensive shock or requirement for dialysis is rare. However, more severe forms of HFRS (ie, attributable to Dobrava-Belgrade virus) also occur in Europe.

Crimean-Congo hemorrhagic fever (CCHF) is a multisystem disease characterized by hepatitis and profuse bleeding. Fever, headache, and myalgia are followed by signs of a diffuse capillary leak syndrome with facial suffusion, conjunctivitis, icteric hepatitis, proteinuria, and disseminated intravascular coagulation associated with petechiae and purpura on the skin and mucous membranes. A hypotensive crisis often occurs after the appearance of frank hemorrhage from the gastrointestinal tract, nose, mouth, or uterus. Mortality rates range from 20% to 35%.

Rift Valley fever (RVF), in most cases, is a self-limited, undifferentiated febrile illness. Occasionally, hemorrhagic fever with shock and icteric hepatitis, encephalitis, or retinitis develops.

Etiology

Bunyaviridae are single-stranded RNA viruses with different geographic distributions depending on their vector or reservoir. Hemorrhagic fever syndromes are associated with viruses from 3 genera: hantaviruses, *Nairovirus* (CCHF virus), and *Phlebovirus* (RVF, Heartland virus in the United States, sandfly fever viruses in Europe, and severe fever with thrombocytopenia syndrome virus in China). Old World hantaviruses (Hantaan, Seoul, Dobrava, and Puumala viruses) cause HFRS, and New World hantaviruses (Sin Nombre and related viruses) cause hantavirus pulmonary syndrome.

Epidemiology

The epidemiology of these diseases is mainly a function of the distribution and behavior of their reservoirs and vectors. All genera except hantaviruses are associated with arthropod vectors, and hantavirus infections are associated with airborne exposure to infected wild rodents, primarily via inhalation of virus-contaminated urine, droppings, or nesting materials.

Classic HFRS occurs throughout much of Asia and Eastern and Western Europe, with up to 100,000 cases per year. The most severe form of the disease is caused by the prototype Hantaan virus and Dobrava-Belgrade viruses in rural Asia and Europe, respectively; Puumala virus is associated with milder disease (nephropathia epidemica) in Western Europe. Seoul virus is distributed worldwide in association with *Rattus* species and can cause a disease of variable severity. Person-to-person transmission never has been reported with HFRS.

Crimean-Congo hemorrhagic fever occurs in much of sub-Saharan Africa, the Middle East, areas in West and Central Asia, and the Balkans. Crimean-Congo hemorrhagic fever virus is transmitted by ticks and occasionally by contact with viremic livestock and wild animals at slaughter. Health care–associated transmission of CCHF is a frequent and serious hazard.

Rift Valley fever occurs throughout sub-Saharan Africa and has caused large epidemics in Egypt in 1977 and 1993–1995, Mauritania in 1987, Saudi Arabia and Yemen in 2000, Kenya in 1997 and 2006–2007, Madagascar in 1990 and 2008, and South Africa in 2010. The virus is arthropodborne and is transmitted from domestic livestock to humans by mosquitoes. The virus can also be transmitted by aerosol and by direct contact with infected aborted tissues or freshly slaughtered infected animal carcasses. Person-to-person transmission has not been reported.

Incubation Period

Crimean-Congo hemorrhagic fever and RVF, 2 to 10 days; HFRS, 7 to 42 days.

Diagnostic Tests

Crimean-Congo hemorrhagic fever and RVF viruses can be cultivated readily (in a Biosafety level 4 laboratory) from blood and tissue specimens of infected patients. Polymerase chain reaction assays performed with appropriate safety precautions are usually sensitive on samples obtained during the acute phase of CCHF and RVF but less for HFRS. Detection of viral antigen by enzyme immunoassay is a useful alternative for CCHF and RVF. Serum immunoglobulin (Ig) M and IgG virus-specific antibodies typically develop early in convalescence in CCHF and RVF but could be absent in rapidly fatal cases of CCHF. In HFRS, IgM and IgG antibodies are usually detectable at the time of onset of illness or within 48 hours, when it is too late for virus isolation and polymerase chain reaction assay. IgM antibodies or rising IgG titers in paired serum specimens, as demonstrated by enzyme immunoassay, are diagnostic; neutralizing antibody tests provide greater virus-strain specificity but are rarely utilized. Diagnosis can be made retrospectively by immunohistochemistry assay of formalin-fixed tissues obtained from necropsy.

Treatment

Ribavirin administered intravenously to patients with HFRS within the first 4 days of illness may be effective in decreasing renal dysfunction, vascular instability, and mortality. However, intravenous ribavirin is not available commercially in the United States. Health care professionals who need to obtain intravenous ribavirin should contact the manufacture. Supportive therapy for HFRS should include treatment of shock, monitoring of fluid balance, dialysis for complications of renal failure, control of hypertension during the oliguric phase, and early recognition of possible myocardial failure with appropriate therapy.

Oral and intravenous ribavirin given to patients with CCHF has been associated with milder disease, although no controlled studies have been performed.

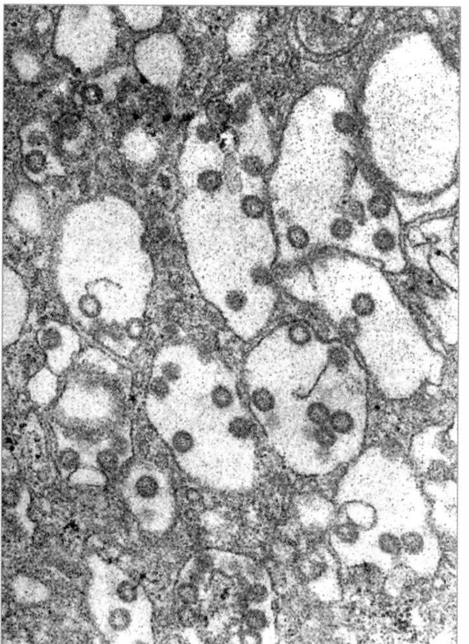

Image 57.1
Electron micrograph of the Rift Valley fever virus, which is a member of the genus *Phlebovirus* in the family Bunyaviridae, first reported in livestock in Kenya around 1900. Courtesy of Centers for Disease Control and Prevention/Dr Fred Murphy.

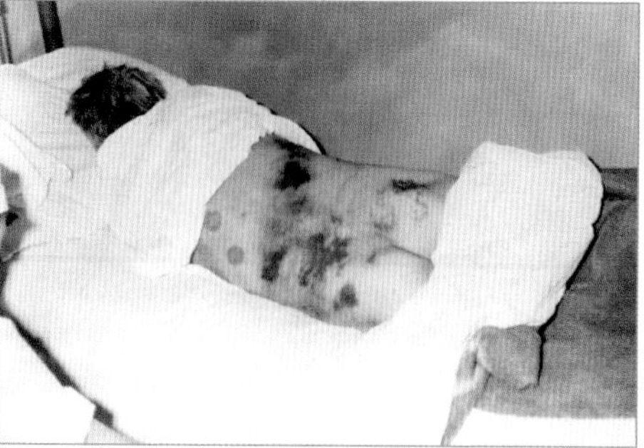

Image 57.2
Isolated male patient diagnosed with Crimean-Congo hemorrhagic fever, a tick-borne hemorrhagic fever with documented person-to-person transmission and a case-fatality rate of approximately 30%. This widespread virus has been found in Africa, Asia, the Middle East, and eastern Europe. Courtesy of Centers for Disease Control and Prevention/Dr B.E. Henderson.

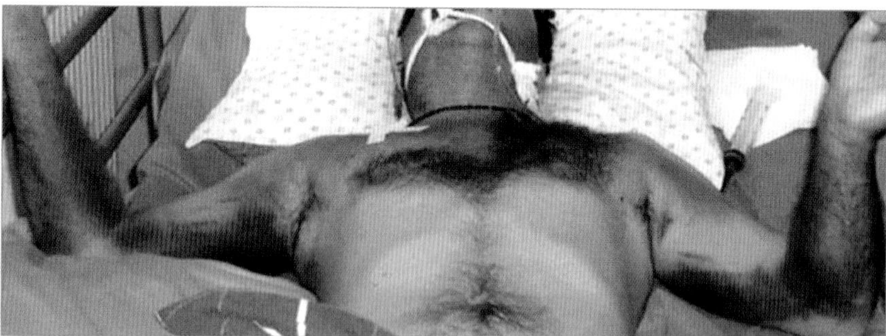

Image 57.3
Intubated patient with Crimean-Congo hemorrhagic fever, Republic of Georgia, 2009, showing massive ecchymoses on the upper extremities that extend to the chest. Courtesy of *Emerging Infectious Diseases.*

58

Hemorrhagic Fevers Caused by Filoviruses: Ebola and Marburg

Clinical Manifestations

Information on Ebola and Marburg virus infections is primarily derived from adult populations. More is known about Ebola virus disease than Marburg virus disease, although the same principles apply generally to all filoviruses that cause human disease. Asymptomatic cases of human filovirus infections have been reported, and symptomatic disease ranges from mild to severe; case fatality rates for severely affected people range from 25% to 90% (approximately 70% in the 2014 outbreak). Onset in children and adults begins with nonspecific signs and symptoms, including fever, headache, myalgia, abdominal pain, and weakness, followed several days later by vomiting, diarrhea, and unexplained bleeding or bruising. Respiratory symptoms are more common in children, and central nervous system manifestations are more common in adults. A fleeting maculopapular rash on the torso or face after approximately 4 to 5 days of illness can occur. Conjunctival injection or subconjunctival hemorrhage can be present. Hepatic dysfunction, with elevations in aspartate transaminase markedly higher than alanine transaminase, and metabolic derangements, including hypokalemia, hyponatremia, hypocalcemia, and hypomagnesemia, are common. In the most severe cases, microvascular instability ensues around the end of the first week of disease. Although hemostasis is impaired, hemorrhagic manifestations develop in a minority of patients. In the 2001 Uganda Sudan Ebola virus outbreak, all children with laboratory-confirmed Ebola virus disease were febrile, and only 16% had hemorrhage. The most common hemorrhagic manifestations consist of bleeding from the gastrointestinal tract, sometimes with oozing from the mucous membranes or venipuncture sites in the late stages. Central nervous system manifestations and renal failure are frequent in end-stage disease. In fatal cases, death typically occurs around 10 to 12 days after symptom onset, usually resulting from viral- or bacterial-induced septic shock and multiorgan system failure. Approximately 30% of pregnant women with Ebola virus disease present with spontaneous abortion and vaginal bleeding. Maternal mortality approaches 90% when infection occurs during the third trimester. All neonates born to mothers with active Ebola virus disease to date have died. The exact cause of the neonatal deaths is unknown, but high viral loads of Ebola virus have been documented in amniotic fluid, placental tissue, and fetal tissues of stillborn neonates.

Etiology

The Filoviridae (from the Latin *filo* meaning thread, referring to their filamentous shape) are single-stranded, negative-sense RNA viruses. Four of the 5 species of virus in the Ebola virus genus and both of the known species of virus in the Marburg virus genus are associated with human disease. All of the known human pathogenic filoviruses are endemic only in sub-Saharan Africa.

Epidemiology

Fruit bats are believed to be the animal reservoir for Ebola virus. Human infection is believed to occur from inadvertent exposure to infected bat excreta or saliva following entry into roosting areas in caves, mines, and forests. Nonhuman primates, especially gorillas and chimpanzees, and other wild animals can also become infected from bat contact and serve as intermediate hosts that transmit filoviruses to humans through contact with their blood and body fluids, usually associated with hunting and medical work. For unclear reasons, filovirus outbreaks tend to occur after prolonged dry seasons.

Although filoviruses are the most transmissible of all hemorrhagic fever viruses, secondary attack rates in households are generally still only 15% to 20% in African communities and are lower if proper universal and contact precautions are maintained. Human-to-human transmission usually occurs through oral, mucous membrane, or nonintact skin exposure to body fluids of a symptomatic person with filovirus disease, most often in the context of providing care to a sick family or community member (community transmission) or patient (health care–associated transmission). Funeral rituals that entail touching of the corpse have also been implicated, as has transmission through breastfeeding from infected mothers. Health care–associated transmission is highly unlikely if rigorous infection control practices are in place in health care facilities. Ebola is not spread through the air, by water, or, in general, by food. Respiratory spread of virus does not occur.

The degree of viremia appears to correlate with the clinical state. People are most infectious late in the course of severe disease, especially when copious vomiting, diarrhea, or bleeding is present. Transmission during the incubation period, when the person is asymptomatic, is not believed to occur. Virus may persist in a few immunologically protected sites for several weeks after clinical recovery, including in testicles/semen, human milk, and chambers of the eye (resulting in transient uveitis and other ocular problems). Because of the risk of sexual transmission, abstinence or use of condoms is recommended for 3 months after recovery.

The 2014 West Africa Ebola outbreak is the largest since the virus was first identified in 1976 and the first in that region of the continent. A simultaneous outbreak of Ebola occurred in the Democratic Republic of the Congo (formerly Zaire), but this outbreak was caused by a different species than the species causing the outbreak in West Africa.

Incubation Period

8 to 10 days (range, 2–21 days).

Diagnostic Tests

The diagnosis of Ebola virus infection should be considered in a person who develops a fever within 21 days of travel to an endemic area. Because initial clinical manifestations are difficult to distinguish from those of more common febrile diseases, prompt laboratory testing is imperative in a suspected case. Filovirus disease can be diagnosed by testing of blood by reverse transcriptase-polymerase chain reaction assay, enzyme-linked immunosorbent assay for viral antigens or immunoglobulin (Ig) M, and cell culture, with the latter being attempted only under Biosafety level 4 conditions. Viral RNA is generally detectable by reverse transcriptase-polymerase chain reaction assay within 3 to 10 days after the onset of symptoms. Postmortem diagnosis can be made via immunohistochemistry testing of skin, liver, or spleen. Local or state public health department officials must be contacted and can facilitate testing at a regional certified laboratory or at the Centers for Disease Control and Prevention.

Treatment

People suspected of having Ebola or Marburg virus infection should immediately be placed in isolation, and public health officials should be notified. Management of patients with filovirus disease is primarily supportive, including oral or intravenous fluids with electrolyte repletion, vasopressors, blood products, total parenteral nutrition, and antimalarial and antibiotic medications when coinfections are suspected or confirmed. Volume losses can be enormous (10 L/d in adults), and some centers report better results with repletion using lactated Ringer injection rather than normal saline solution in management of adult patients in the United States. When antibiotics are used to empirically treat sepsis, these should be active against intestinal microbiota that can be translocated from the gut into the blood of patients with filovirus disease. Nonsteroidal anti-inflammatory drugs, aspirin, and intramuscular injections should be avoided because of the risk of bleeding.

Ribavirin has no efficacy against filoviruses and should not be used. Corticosteroids should not be administered except for replacement in suspected or confirmed adrenal insufficiency or refractory septic shock.

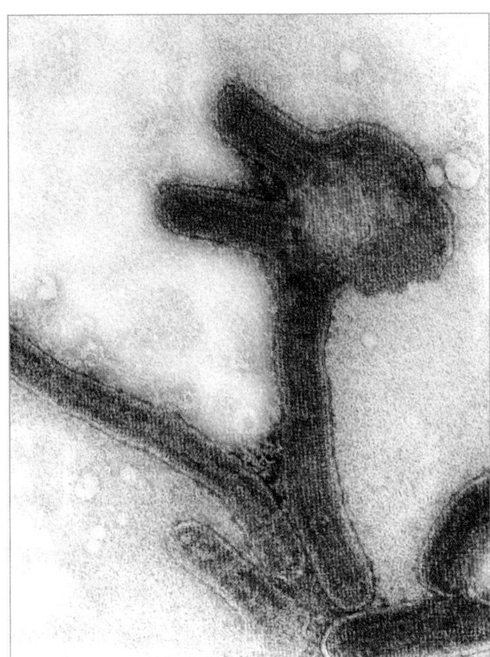

Image 58.1

This colorized negative stained transmission electron micrograph, captured by F.A. Murphy in 1968, depicts a number of Marburg virus virions, which had been grown in an environment of tissue culture cells. Marburg hemorrhagic fever is a rare, severe type of hemorrhagic fever that affects humans and nonhuman primates. Caused by a genetically unique zoonotic (ie, animalborne) RNA virus of the *Filovirus* family, its recognition led to the creation of this virus family. The 4 species of Ebola virus are the only other known members of the *Filovirus* family. After an incubation period of 5 to 10 days, onset of the disease is sudden and is marked by fever, chills, headache, and myalgia. Around the fifth day after the onset of symptoms, a maculopapular rash, most prominent on the trunk (ie, chest, back, stomach), may occur. Nausea, vomiting, chest pain, a sore throat, abdominal pain, and diarrhea may then appear. Symptoms become increasingly severe and may include jaundice, inflammation of the pancreas, severe weight loss, delirium, shock, liver failure, and multiorgan dysfunction. Because many of the signs and symptoms of Marburg hemorrhagic fever are similar to those of other infectious diseases, such as malaria or typhoid fever, diagnosis of the disease can be difficult, especially if only a single case is involved. Courtesy of Centers for Disease Control and Prevention/Frederick Murphy, MD.

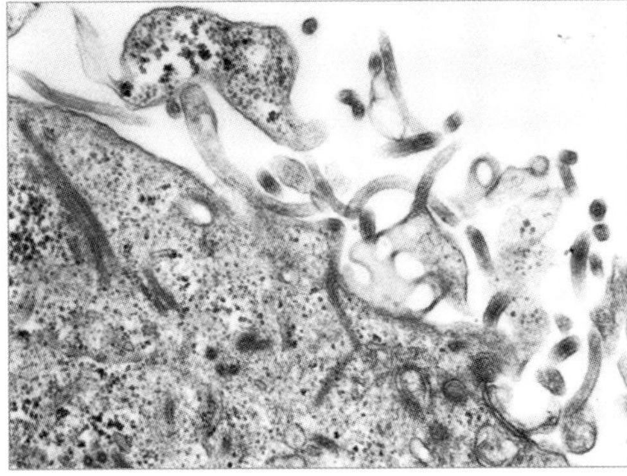

Image 58.2

This electron micrograph shows a thin section containing the Ebola virus, the causative agent for African hemorrhagic fever. Courtesy of Centers for Disease Control and Prevention/Frederick Murphy, MD.

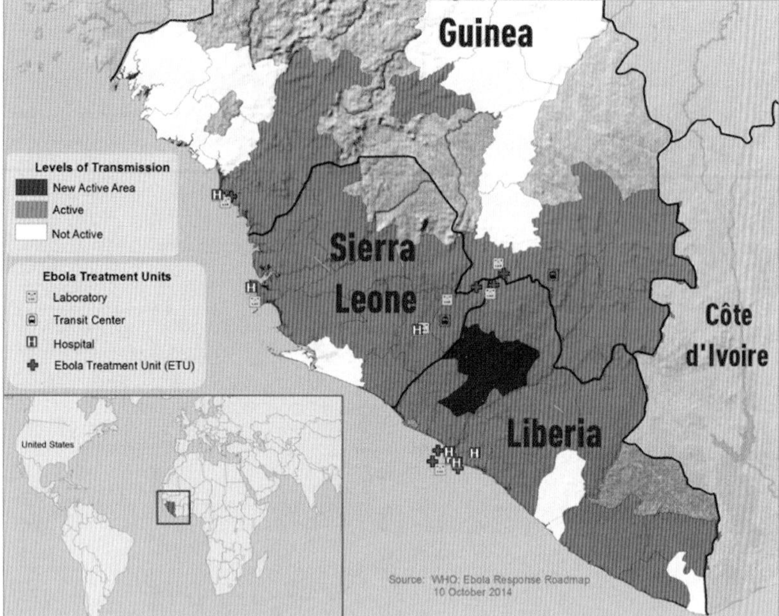

Image 58.3
This map illustrates the geographic distribution, as of October 10, 2014, of the West African Ebola outbreak and demarcates some of the salient focal points involved in the epidemiologic investigation of what became an international epidemic, including the location of Ebola treatment units, field laboratories, transit centers, and hospitals. Also indicated were the regions where there were newly active and previously active cases and areas where there were no suspected cases. The 2014 Ebola outbreak is one of the largest Ebola outbreaks in history and the first in West Africa. At the time of this map's creation, countries classified as sustaining "widespread transmission" included Guinea, Liberia, and Sierra Leone. Countries exhibiting "localized transmission" included Nigeria (Port Harcourt and Lagos), Spain (Madrid), and the United States (Dallas, TX). Finally, Senegal exhibited a single case in its capital city of Dakar. Courtesy of World Health Organization.

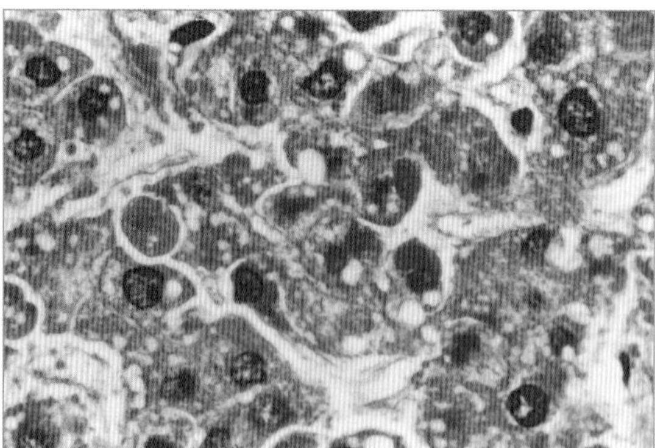

Image 58.4
Under a high magnification of x400, this hematoxylin-eosin–stained photomicrograph depicts the cytoarchitectural changes found in a liver tissue specimen extracted from a patient with Ebola virus infection in the Democratic Republic of the Congo. This particular view reveals an acidophilic necrosis leading to the formation of a Councilman body and cytoplasmic inclusions. A steatotic (fatty change) vesicle was caught in the process of formation. Courtesy of Centers for Disease Control and Prevention/ Dr Yves Robin and Dr Jean Renaudet, Arbovirus Laboratory at the Pasteur Institute in Dakar, Senegal; World Health Organization.

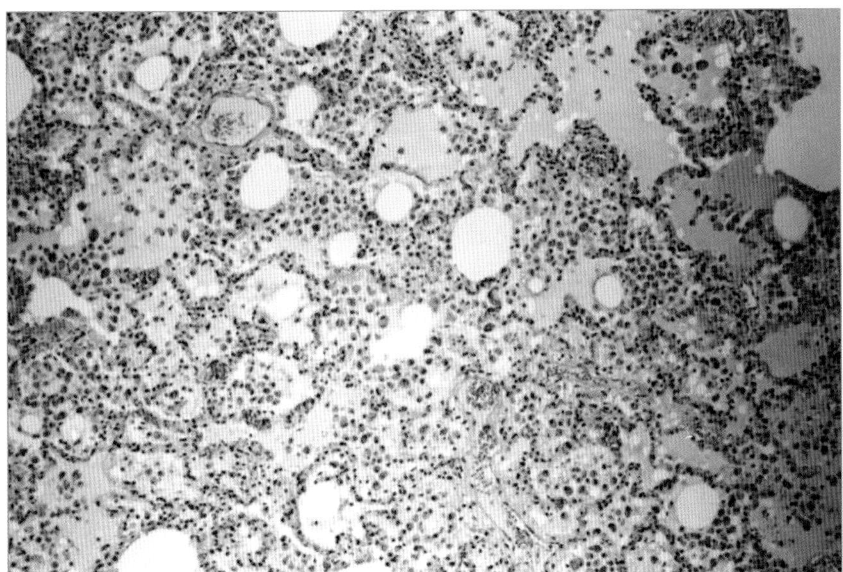

Image 58.5
This photomicrograph revealed the cytoarchitectural histopathologic changes detected in a lung biopsy tissue section from a patient with Marburg virus infection who was treated in Johannesburg, South Africa. Note the necrotic changes indicated by the breakdown of the alveolar walls resulting in pulmonary edema. There is also the presence of numerous alveolar macrophages due to the *Filovirus* infiltrate. Courtesy of Centers for Disease Control and Prevention/Dr J. Lyle Conrad.

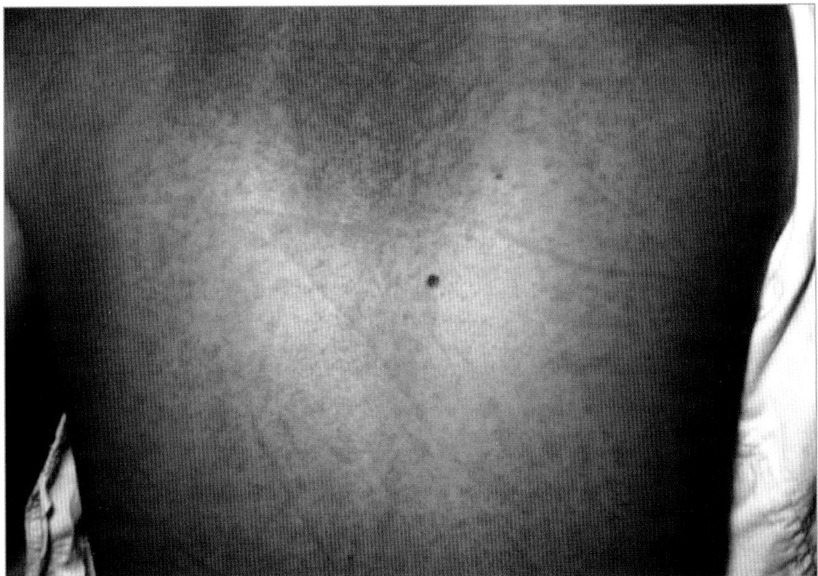

Image 58.6
This patient with Marburg virus infection presented with a measleslike rash located on her back and was hospitalized in Johannesburg, South Africa, in 1975. This type of maculopapular rash, which can appear on patient with Marburg virus infection around the fifth day after the onset of symptoms, may usually be found on the patient's chest, back, and stomach. This patient's skin blanched under pressure, which is a common characteristic of a Marburg virus rash. Courtesy of Centers for Disease Control and Prevention/Dr J. Lyle Conrad.

59

Hepatitis A

Clinical Manifestations

Hepatitis A characteristically is an acute, self-limited illness associated with fever, malaise, jaundice, anorexia, and nausea. Symptomatic hepatitis A virus (HAV) infection occurs in approximately 30% of infected children younger than 6 years; few of these children will have jaundice. Among older children and adults, infection is usually symptomatic and typically lasts several weeks, with jaundice occurring in 70% or more. Signs and symptoms typically last less than 2 months, although 10% to 15% of symptomatic people have prolonged or relapsing disease lasting as long as 6 months. Fulminant hepatitis is rare but is more common in people with underlying liver disease. Chronic infection does not occur.

Etiology

Hepatitis A virus is an RNA virus classified as a member of the Picornaviridae family, genus *Hepatovirus*.

Epidemiology

The most common mode of transmission is person to person, resulting from fecal contamination and oral ingestion (ie, the fecal-oral route). In resource-limited countries where infection is endemic, most people are infected during the first decade of life. In the United States, hepatitis A was one of the most frequently reported vaccine-preventable diseases in the prevaccine era, but incidence of disease attributable to HAV has declined significantly since hepatitis A vaccine was licensed in 1995. These declining rates have been accompanied by a shift in age-specific rates. Historically, the highest rates occurred among children 5 to 14 years of age and the lowest rates occurred among adults older than 40 years. Beginning in the late 1990s, national age-specific rates declined more rapidly among children than among adults; as a result, in recent years, rates have been similar among all age groups. In addition, the previously observed unequal geographic distribution of hepatitis A incidence in the United States, with the highest rates of disease occurring in a limited number of states and communities, disappeared after introduction of targeted immunization in 1999. Rates in the United States were 1.0 per 100,000 population in 2007, which was the year hepatitis A vaccine was recommended for routine use in all US children 12 through 23 months of age, and declined to 0.4 per 100,000 in 2011. The 1,398 HAV cases in 2011 represented the lowest number ever recorded; rates have plateaued since then. An increasing proportion of adults in the United States are susceptible to hepatitis A because of reduced exposure to HAV earlier in life. The mean age of people hospitalized for HAV infection has increased significantly between 2002 and 2011 (mean age of 37.6 years in 2002–2003, compared with 45.5 years in 2010–2011).

Among reported cases of hepatitis A, recognized risk factors include close personal contact with a person infected with HAV, international travel, household or personal contact with a child who attends a child care center, household or personal contact with a newly arriving international adoptee, a recognized foodborne outbreak, men who have sex with men, and use of illegal drugs. In approximately two-thirds of reported cases, the source cannot be determined. Fecal-oral spread from people with asymptomatic infections, particularly young children, likely accounts for many of these cases with an unknown source. Transmission by blood transfusion or from mother to newborn (ie, vertical transmission) seldom occurs.

Before availability of vaccine, most HAV infection and illness occurred in the context of community-wide epidemics, in which infection was primarily transmitted in households and extended-family settings. Community-wide epidemics have not been observed in recent years. Common-source foodborne outbreaks occur; waterborne outbreaks are rare. Waterborne outbreaks are usually associated with sewage-contaminated or inadequately treated water. Health care–associated transmission is unusual, but, very rarely, outbreaks have occurred in neonatal intensive care units from neonates infected through transfused blood who subsequently transmitted HAV to other neonates and staff.

In child care centers, recognized symptomatic (icteric) illness occurs primarily among adult contacts of children. Most infected children younger than 6 years are asymptomatic or have nonspecific manifestations. Hence, spread of HAV infection within and outside a child care center often occurs before recognition of the index case(s). Outbreaks have occurred most commonly in large child care centers and specifically in facilities that enroll children in diapers.

Patients infected with HAV are most infectious during the 1 to 2 weeks before onset of jaundice or elevation of liver enzymes, when concentration of virus in the stool is highest. The risk of transmission subsequently diminishes and is minimal by 1 week after onset of jaundice. However, HAV can be detected in stool for longer periods, especially in neonates and young children.

Incubation Period

Average 28 days (range, 15–50 days).

Diagnostic Tests

Serologic tests for HAV-specific total (ie, immunoglobulin [Ig] G and IgM) anti-HAV are available commercially. The presence of serum IgM anti-HAV indicates current or recent infection, although false-positive results can occur. IgM anti-HAV is detectable in up to 20% of vaccinees when measured 2 weeks after hepatitis A immunization. In most infected people, serum IgM anti-HAV becomes detectable 5 to 10 days before onset of symptoms and declines to undetectable concentrations within 6 months after infection. People who test positive for IgM anti-HAV more than 1 year after infection have been reported. IgG anti-HAV is detectable shortly after appearance of IgM. A positive total anti-HAV (ie, IgM and IgG) test result with a negative IgM anti-HAV test result indicates immunity from past infection or vaccination. Polymerase chain reaction assays for hepatitis A are available.

Treatment

Supportive.

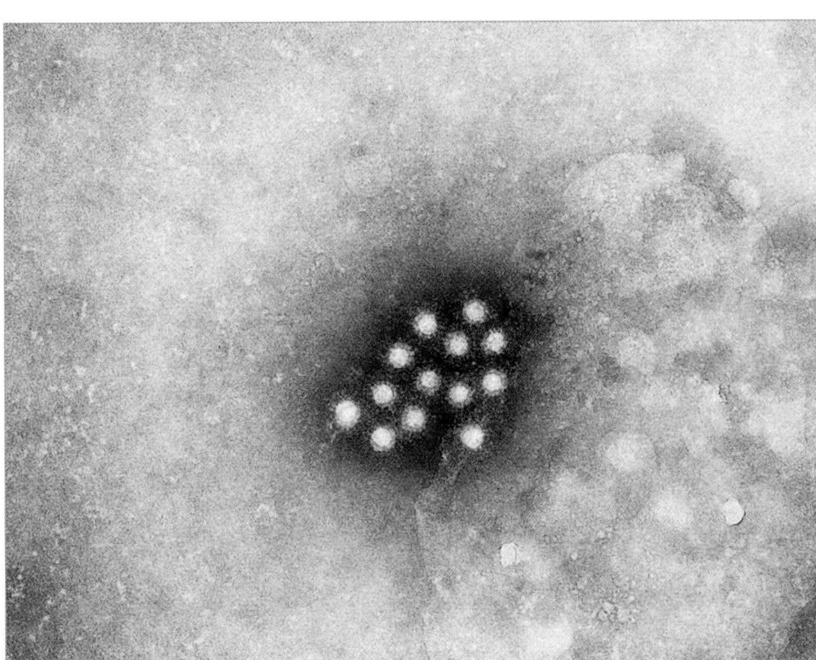

Image 59.1

An electron micrograph of the hepatitis A virus, an RNA virus classified as a member of the picornavirus group. Courtesy of Centers for Disease Control and Prevention/Betty Partin.

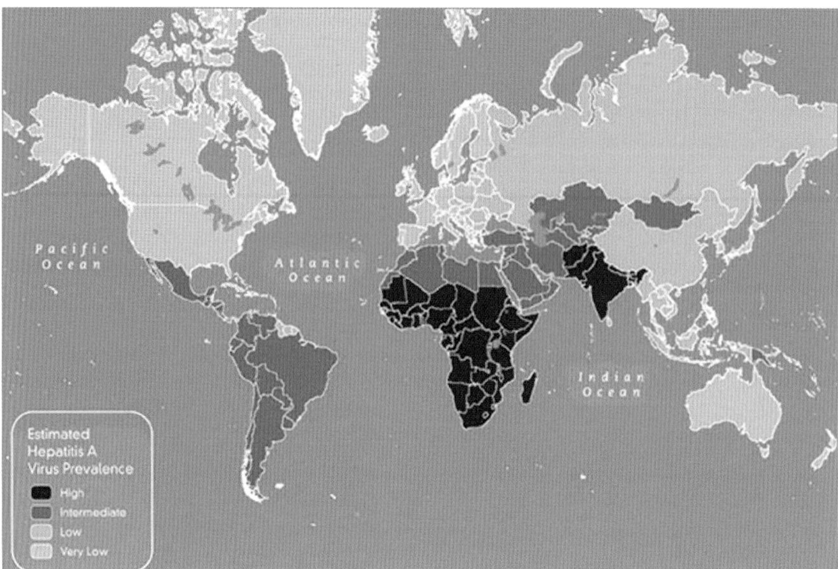

Image 59.2
Estimated prevalence of hepatitis A virus. Centers for Disease Control and Prevention National Center for Emerging and Zoonotic Infectious Diseases (NCEZID) Division of Global Migration and Quarantine (DGMQ).

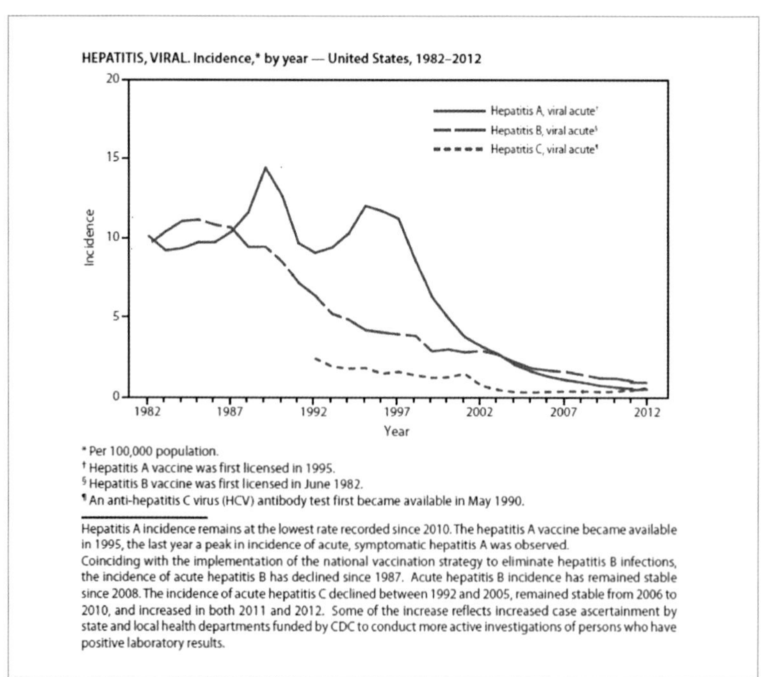

Image 59.3
Hepatitis, viral. Incidence, by year—United States, 1982–2012. Courtesy of *Morbidity and Mortality Weekly Report.*

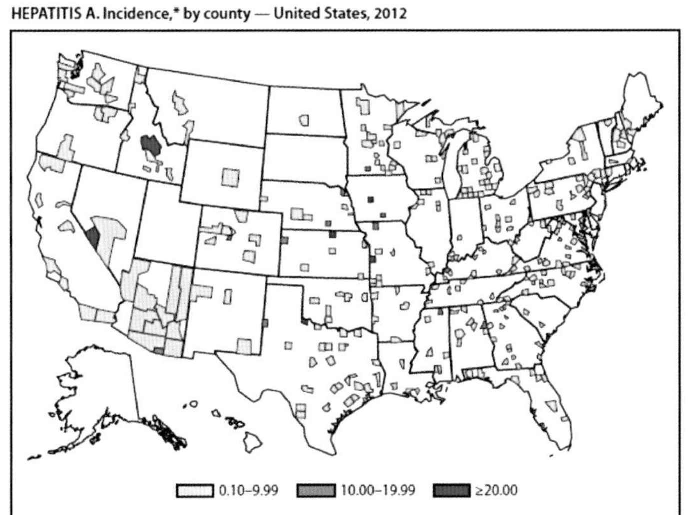

Image 59.4
Hepatitis A. Incidence, by county—United States, 2012. Courtesy of *Morbidity and Mortality Weekly Report.*

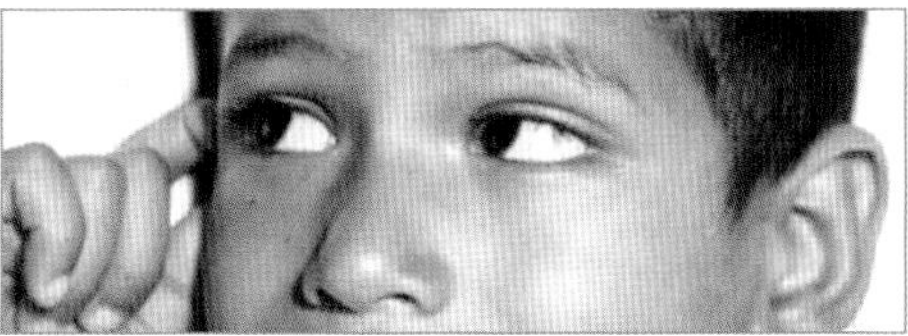

Image 59.5
Acute hepatitis A infection with scleral icterus in a 10-year-old boy. Courtesy of Edgar O. Ledbetter, MD, FAAP.

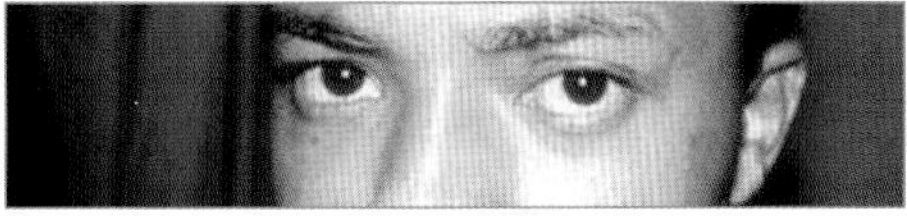

Image 59.6
Hepatitis A infection has caused this man's skin and the whites of his eyes to turn yellow. Other symptoms of hepatitis A can include loss of appetite, abdominal pain, nausea or vomiting, fever, headaches, and dark urine. Courtesy of Centers for Disease Control and Prevention/ Dr Thomas F. Sellers; Emory University.

60

Hepatitis B

Clinical Manifestations

People acutely infected with hepatitis B virus (HBV) may be asymptomatic or symptomatic. The likelihood of developing symptoms of acute hepatitis is age dependent: less than 1% of infants younger than 1 year, 5% to 15% of children 1 through 5 years of age, and 30% to 50% of people older than 5 years are symptomatic, although few data are available for adults older than 30 years. The spectrum of signs and symptoms is varied and includes subacute illness with nonspecific symptoms (eg, anorexia, nausea, malaise), clinical hepatitis with jaundice, or fulminant hepatitis. Extrahepatic manifestations, such as arthralgia, arthritis, macular rashes, thrombocytopenia, polyarteritis nodosa, glomerulonephritis, or papular acrodermatitis (Gianotti-Crosti syndrome), can occur early in the course of illness and can precede jaundice. Acute HBV infection cannot be distinguished from other forms of acute viral hepatitis on the basis of clinical signs and symptoms or nonspecific laboratory findings.

Chronic HBV infection is defined as presence of any one of hepatitis B surface antigen (HBsAg), HBV DNA, or hepatitis B e antigen (HBeAg) in serum for at least 6 months. Chronic HBV infection is likely in the presence of HBsAg, nucleic acid, HBV DNA, or HBeAg in serum from a person who tests negative for antibody of the immunoglobulin (Ig) M subclass to hepatitis B core antigen (anti-HBc).

Age at the time of infection is the primary determinant of risk of progressing to chronic infection. Up to 90% of infants infected perinatally or in the first year of life will develop chronic HBV infection. Between 25% and 50% of children infected between 1 and 5 years of age become chronically infected, whereas 5% to 10% of infected older children and adults develop chronic HBV infection. Patients who become HBV infected while immunosuppressed or with an underlying chronic illness (eg, end-stage renal disease) have an increased risk of developing chronic infection. In the absence of treatment, up to 25% of infants and children who acquire chronic HBV infection will die prematurely from HBV-related hepatocellular carcinoma (HCC) or cirrhosis. Risk factors for developing HCC include long duration of infection, male gender, elevation of serum alanine aminotransferase (ALT), HBeAg positivity, degree of histologic injury of the liver, replicative state of the virus (HBV DNA levels), presence of cirrhosis, and concomitant infection with hepatitis C virus or HIV.

The clinical course of untreated chronic HBV infection varies according to the population studied, reflecting differences in age at acquisition, rate of loss of HBeAg, and, possibly, HBV genotype. Most children have asymptomatic infection. Perinatally infected children usually have normal ALT concentrations and minimal or mild liver histologic abnormalities, with detectable HBeAg and high HBV DNA concentrations (≥20,000 IU/mL) for years to decades after initial infection ("immune tolerant phase"). Children with chronic HBV may exhibit growth impairment. Chronic HBV infection acquired during later childhood or adolescence is usually accompanied by more active liver disease and increased serum aminotransferase concentrations. Patients with detectable HBeAg (HBeAg-positive chronic hepatitis B) usually have high concentrations of HBV DNA and HBsAg in serum and are more likely to transmit infection. Because HBV-associated liver injury is thought to be immune mediated, in people coinfected with HIV and HBV, the return of immune competence with antiretroviral treatment of HIV infection may lead to a reactivation of HBV-related liver inflammation and damage. Over time (years to decades), HBeAg becomes undetectable in many chronically infected people. This transition is often accompanied by development of antibody to HBeAg (anti-HBe) and decreases in serum HBV DNA and serum aminotransferase concentrations and may be preceded by a temporary exacerbation of liver disease. These patients have **inactive chronic infection** but still may have exacerbations of hepatitis. Serologic reversion (reappearance of HBeAg) is more common if loss of HBeAg is not accompanied by development of anti-HBe; reversion with loss of anti-HBe can also occur.

Some patients who lose HBeAg may continue to have ongoing histologic evidence of liver damage and moderate to high concentrations of HBV DNA (HBeAg-negative chronic hepatitis B). Patients with histologic evidence of chronic HBV infection, regardless of HBeAg status, remain at higher risk of death attributable to liver failure compared with HBV-infected people with no histologic evidence of liver inflammation and fibrosis. Other factors that may adversely influence the natural history of chronic infection include male gender, high HBV DNA level, elevation of serum aminotransferase concentrations, HBeAg positivity, race, alcohol use, and coinfection with hepatitis C virus, hepatitis D virus, or HIV.

Resolved hepatitis B is defined as clearance of HBsAg, normalization of serum aminotransferase concentrations, and development of antibody to HBsAg (anti-HBs). Chronically infected adults clear HBsAg and develop anti-HBs at the rate of 1% to 2% annually; during childhood, the annual clearance rate is less than 1%. Reactivation of resolved chronic infection is possible if these patients become immunosuppressed and is also well reported among HBsAg-positive patients receiving antitumor necrosis factor agents or disease-modifying antirheumatic drugs (12% of patients).

Etiology

Hepatitis B virus is a DNA-containing, 42-nm-diameter hepadnavirus. Important components of the viral particle include an outer lipoprotein envelope containing HBsAg and an inner nucleocapsid consisting of anti-HBc. Viral polymerase activity can be detected in preparations of plasma containing HBV.

Epidemiology

Hepatitis B virus is transmitted through infected blood or body fluids. Although HBsAg has been detected in multiple body fluids, including human milk, saliva, and tears, only blood, serum, semen, vaginal secretions, and cerebrospinal, synovial, pleural, pericardial, peritoneal, and amniotic fluids are considered the most potentially infectious. People with chronic HBV infection are the primary reservoirs for infection. Common modes of transmission include percutaneous and mucosal exposure to infectious body fluids; sharing or using nonsterilized needles, syringes, or glucose monitoring equipment or devices; sexual contact with an infected person; perinatal exposure to an infected mother; and household exposure to a person with chronic HBV infection. The risk of HBV acquisition when a susceptible child bites a child who has chronic HBV infection is unknown. A theoretic risk exists if HBsAg-positive blood enters the oral cavity of the biter, but transmission by this route has not been reported. Transmission by transfusion of contaminated blood or blood products is rare in the United States because of routine screening of blood donors and viral inactivation of certain blood products before administration.

Perinatal transmission of HBV is highly efficient and usually occurs from blood exposures during labor and delivery. In utero transmission accounts for less than 2% of all vertically transmitted HBV infections in most studies. Without postexposure prophylaxis, the risk of a neonate acquiring HBV from an infected mother as a result of perinatal exposure is 70% to 90% for neonates born to mothers who are HBsAg and HBeAg positive; the risk is 5% to 20% for neonates born to HBsAg-positive but HBeAg-negative mothers.

Person-to-person spread of HBV can occur in settings involving interpersonal contact over extended periods, such as in a household with a person with chronic HBV infection. In regions of the world with a high prevalence of chronic HBV infection, transmission between children in household settings may account for a substantial amount of transmission. The precise mechanisms of transmission from child to child are unknown; however, frequent interpersonal contact of nonintact skin or mucous membranes with blood-containing secretions, open skin lesions, or blood-containing saliva are potential means of transmission. Transmission from sharing inanimate objects, such as razors or toothbrushes, can also occur. Hepatitis B virus can survive in the environment for 7 or more days but is inactivated by commonly used disinfectants, including household bleach diluted 1:10 with water. Hepatitis B virus is not transmitted by the fecal-oral route.

Transmission among children born in the United States is unusual because of high coverage with hepatitis B vaccine starting at birth. The risk of HBV transmission is higher in children who have not completed a vaccine series, children undergoing hemodialysis, institutionalized children with developmental disabilities, and children emigrating from countries with endemic HBV (eg, Southeast Asia, China, Africa). Person-to-person transmission has been reported in child care settings, but risk of transmission in child care facilities in the United States has become negligible as a result of high infant hepatitis B immunization rates.

Acute HBV infection is most commonly reported among adults 30 through 49 years of age in the United States. Since 1990, the incidence of acute HBV infection has declined in all age categories, with a 98% decline in children younger than 19 years and a 93% decline in young adults 20 through 29 years of age, with most of the decline among people 20 through 24 years of age. Among patients with acute hepatitis B interviewed in 2010, groups constituting the largest proportion of acute hepatitis B cases included users of injection drugs, people with multiple heterosexual partners, men who have sex with men, and people who reported surgery during the 6 weeks to 6 months before onset of symptoms. Others at increased risk include people with occupational exposure to blood or body fluids, staff of institutions and nonresidential child care programs for children with developmental disabilities, patients undergoing hemodialysis, and sexual or household contacts of people with an acute or chronic infection. Approximately 68% of infected people who were interviewed in 2010 did not have a readily identifiable risk characteristic. Hepatitis B virus infection in adolescents and adults is associated with other sexually transmitted infections. Outbreaks in nonhospital health care settings, including assisted-living facilities and nursing homes, highlight the increased risk among people with diabetes mellitus undergoing assisted blood glucose monitoring.

The prevalence of HBV infection and patterns of transmission vary markedly throughout the world (Table 60.1). Approximately 45% of people worldwide live in regions of high HBV endemicity, where the prevalence of chronic HBV infection is 8% or greater. Historically, in these regions, most new infections occurred as a result of perinatal or early childhood infections. In regions of intermediate HBV endemicity, where the prevalence of HBV infection is 2% to 7%, multiple modes of transmission (ie, perinatal, household, sexual, injection drug use, and health care–associated) contribute to the burden of infection. In countries of low endemicity, where chronic HBV infection prevalence is less than 2% (including the United States) and where routine immunization has been adopted, new infections are increasingly among unimmunized age groups. Many people born in countries with high endemicity live in the United States. Infant immunization programs in some of these countries have, in recent years, greatly reduced the seroprevalence of HBsAg, but many other countries with endemic HBV have yet to implement widespread routine childhood hepatitis B immunization programs.

Incubation Period

Acute infection, 90 days (range, 45–160 days).

Diagnostic Tests

Serologic antigen tests are available commercially to detect HBsAg and HBeAg. Serologic assays are also available for detection of anti-HBs, anti-HBc (total), IgM anti-HBc, and anti-HBe. In addition, nucleic acid amplification testing, gene-amplification techniques (eg, polymerase chain reaction assay, branched DNA methods), and hybridization assays are available to detect and quantify HBV DNA. Tests to quantify HBsAg and HBeAg are currently being developed but are not yet commercially available. Hepatitis B surface antigen is detectable during acute infection. If HBV infection is self-limited, HBsAg disappears in most patients within a few weeks to several months after infection, followed by appearance of anti-HBs. The time between disappearance of HBsAg and appearance of anti-HBs is termed the **window period** of infection. During the window period, the only marker of acute infection is IgM anti-HBc, which is highly specific for establishing the diagnosis of acute infection. However, IgM anti-HBc is not usually present in neonates infected perinatally. People with chronic HBV infection have circulating HBsAg and circulating total anti-HBc; on rare occasions, anti-HBs is also present. Anti-HBs and total anti-HBc are present in people with resolved infection, whereas anti-HBs alone is present in people immunized with hepatitis B vaccine. Transient HBsAg antigenemia can occur following receipt of hepatitis B vaccine, with HBsAg being detected as early as 24 hours after and up to 2 to 3 weeks following administration of the vaccine. The presence of HBeAg in serum correlates with higher concentrations of HBV and greater infectivity. Tests for HBeAg and HBV DNA are useful in selection of candidates to receive antiviral therapy and to monitor response to therapy.

Treatment

No specific therapy for acute HBV infection is available, and acute HBV infection usually does not warrant referral to a hepatitis specialist. However, acute HBV infection may be difficult to distinguish from reactivation of HBV, so if reactivation is a possibility, referral to a hepatitis specialist would be warranted.

Children and adolescents who have chronic HBV infection are at risk of developing serious liver disease, including primary HCC, with advancing age and, therefore, should receive hepatitis A vaccine. Although the peak incidence of primary HCC attributable to HBV infection is in the fifth decade of life, HCC occurs in children as young as 6 years who become infected perinatally or in early childhood. Several algorithms have been published describing the initial evaluation, monitoring, and criteria for treatment. Children with chronic HBV infection should be screened periodically for hepatic complications using serum aminotransferase tests, α-fetoprotein concentration, and abdominal ultrasonography. Definitive recommendations on the frequency and indications for specific tests are not yet available because of lack of data on their reliability in predicting sequelae. Patients with serum ALT concentrations persistently exceeding the upper limit of normal and patients with an increased serum α-fetoprotein concentration or abnormal findings on abdominal ultrasonography should be referred to a specialist in management of chronic HBV infection for further management and treatment.

The goal of treatment in chronic HBV infection is to prevent progression to cirrhosis, hepatic failure, and HCC. Current indications for treatment of chronic HBV infection include evidence of ongoing hepatitis B viral replication, as indicated by the presence for longer than 6 months of serum HBV DNA greater than 20,000 IU/mL without HBeAg positivity, greater than 2,000 IU/mL with HBeAg positivity, and elevated serum ALT concentrations for longer than 6 months or evidence of chronic hepatitis on liver biopsy. Children without necroinflammatory liver disease and children with immunotolerant chronic HBV infection (ie, normal ALT concentrations despite presence of HBV DNA) usually do not warrant antiviral therapy. Treatment response is measured by biochemical, virologic, and histologic response. An important consideration in the choice of treatment is to avoid selection of antiviral-resistant mutations.

The US Food and Drug Administration has approved 3 nucleoside analogues (entecavir, lamivudine, and telbivudine), 2 nucleotide analogues (tenofovir and adefovir), and 2 interferon alfa drugs (interferon alfa-2b and pegylated interferon alfa-2a) for treatment of chronic HBV infection in adults. Tenofovir, entecavir, and pegylated interferon alfa-2a are preferred in adults as first-line therapy because of the lower likelihood of developing antiviral resistance mutations over long-term therapy. Of these, Food and Drug Administration licensure in the pediatric population is as follows: interferon, 1 year and older; lamivudine, 3 months and older; adefovir, 12 years and older; telbivudine, 16 years and older; and entecavir, 16 years and older. Pediatric trials of telbivudine, tenofovir, pegylated interferon, and entecavir are currently underway. The optimal agent(s) and duration of therapy for chronic HBV infection in children remain unclear. There are few large randomized, controlled trials of antiviral therapies for chronic hepatitis B in childhood. Studies indicate approximately 17% to 58% of children with increased serum aminotransferase concentrations who are treated with interferon alfa-2b for 6 months lose HBeAg, compared with approximately 8% to 17% of untreated controls. Response to interferon alfa is better for children from Western countries (20%–58%) as compared with Asian countries (17%). Children from Asian countries with HBV infection are more likely to have acquired infection perinatally, have a prolonged immune tolerant phase of infection, and be infected with HBV genotype C. All 3 of these factors are associated with lower response rates to interferon alfa, which is less effective for chronic infections acquired during early childhood, especially if serum aminotransferase concentrations are normal. Children with chronic HBV infection who were treated with lamivudine had higher rates of virologic response (loss of detectable HBV DNA and loss of HBeAg) after 1 year of treatment than did children who received placebo (23% vs 13%). Resistance to lamivudine can develop while on treatment and may occur early. The optimal duration of lamivudine therapy is not known, but a minimum of 1 year is required. For those who have not yet seroreverted but do not have resistant virus, therapy beyond 1 year may be beneficial (ie, continued seroreversions). However, the high rates of lamivudine resistance (~70% after 3 years of therapy) have decreased enthusiasm for the use of this drug. Combination therapy with lamivudine and interferon alfa has been studied with mixed results, as compared with monotherapy with interferon alfa. Children coinfected with HIV and HBV should receive the lamivudine dose approved for treatment of HIV. Consultation with health care professionals with expertise in treating chronic hepatitis B in children is recommended.

Table 60.1

Estimated International Hepatitis B Surface Antigen Prevalence[a]

Region	Estimated HBsAg Prevalence[b]
North America	0.1%
Mexico and Central America	0.3%
South America	0.7%
Western Europe	0.7%
Australia and New Zealand	0.9%
Caribbean (except Haiti)	1.0%
Eastern Europe and North Asia	2.8%
South Asia	2.8%
Middle East	3.2%
Haiti	5.6%
East Asia	7.4%
Southeast Asia	9.1%
Africa	9.3%
Pacific Islands	12.0%

Abbreviation: HBsAg, hepatitis B surface antigen.

[a] Centers for Disease Control and Prevention. A comprehensive immunization strategy to eliminate transmission of hepatitis B virus infection in the United States: recommendations of the Advisory Committee on Immunization Practices (ACIP) part II: immunization of adults. *MMWR Recomm Rep*. 2006;55(RR-16):1–33.

[b] Level of hepatitis B virus endemicity defined as high (≥8%), intermediate (2%–7%), and low (<2%).

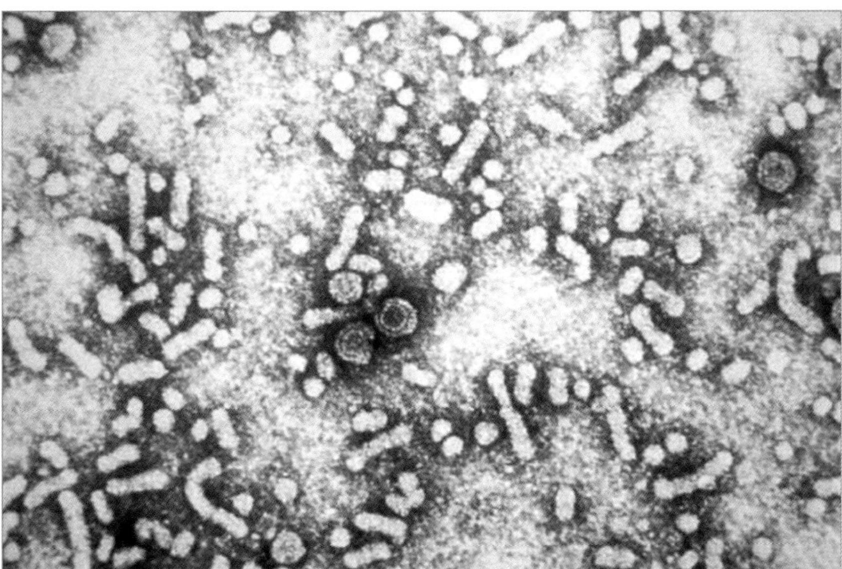

Image 60.1
This electron micrograph reveals the presence of hepatitis B virus (HBV). Infectious HBV virions are also known as Dane particles. These particles measure 42 nm in their overall diameter and contain a DNA-based core that is 27 nm in diameter. Courtesy of Centers for Disease Control and Prevention.

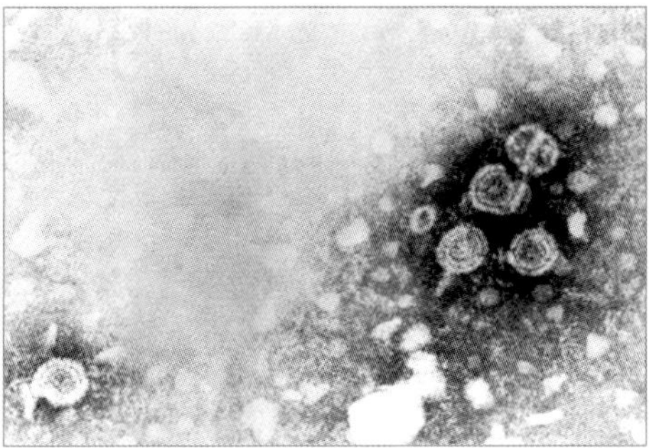

Image 60.2
Transmission electron micrograph of hepatitis B virions, also known as Dane particles. Courtesy of Centers for Disease Control and Prevention/Erskine Palmer, MD.

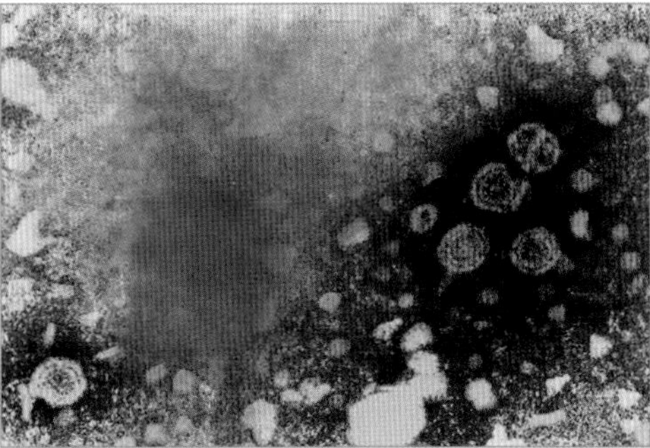

Image 60.3
This transmission electron micrograph revealed the presence of hepatitis B virions. Courtesy of Centers for Disease Control and Prevention/Erskine Palmer, MD.

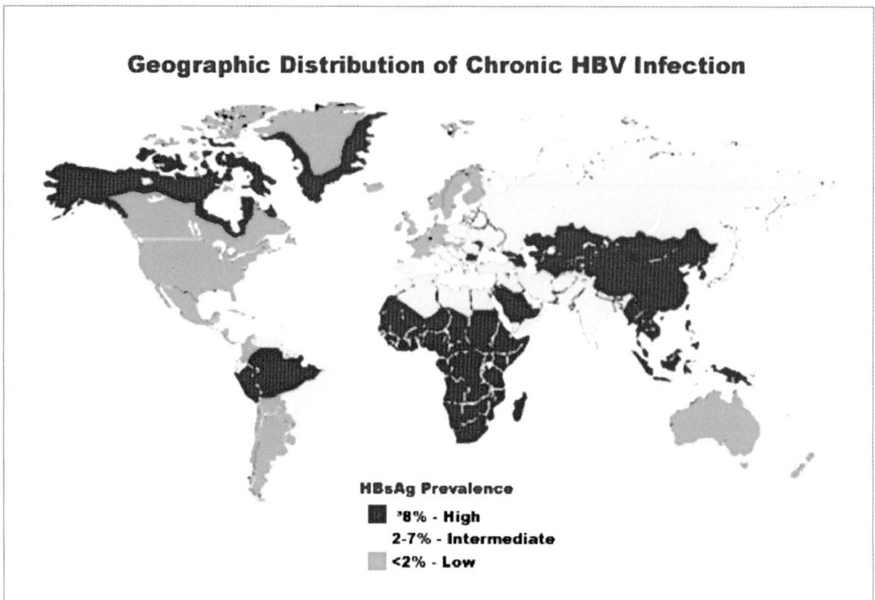

Image 60.4
World map for hepatitis B endemicity. Courtesy of Centers for Disease Control and Prevention.

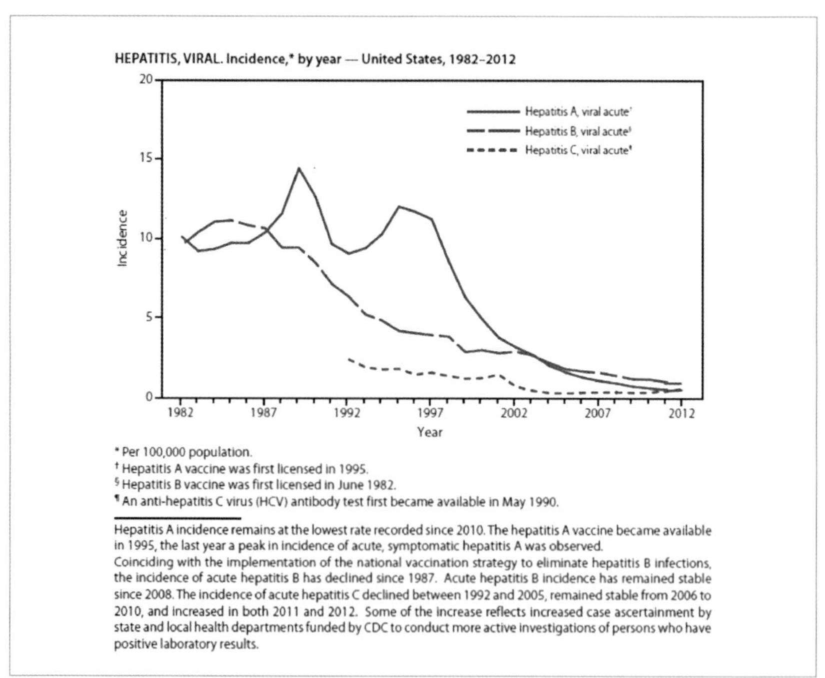

Image 60.5
Hepatitis, viral. Incidence, by year—United States, 1982–2012. Courtesy of *Morbidity and Mortality Weekly Report.*

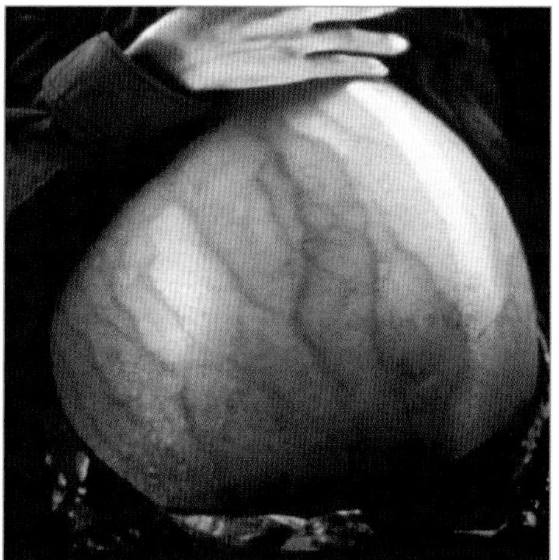

Image 60.6
This female Cambodian patient presented with a distended abdomen due to a hepatoma resulting from chronic hepatitis B infection. Courtesy of Centers for Disease Control and Prevention/ Patricia Walker, MD, Regions Hospital, MN.

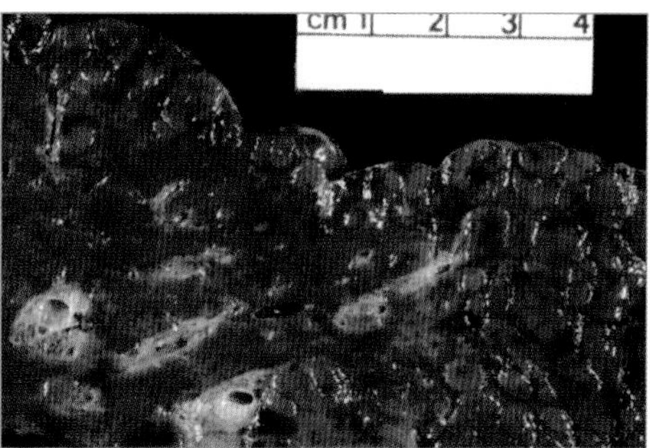

Image 60.7
Section of liver damaged by hepatitis B virus. Note the enlarged cells and blistering of the capsular surface. Copyright Anthony Demetris, MD, Director, Division of Transplantation Pathology, University of Pittsburgh Medical Center.

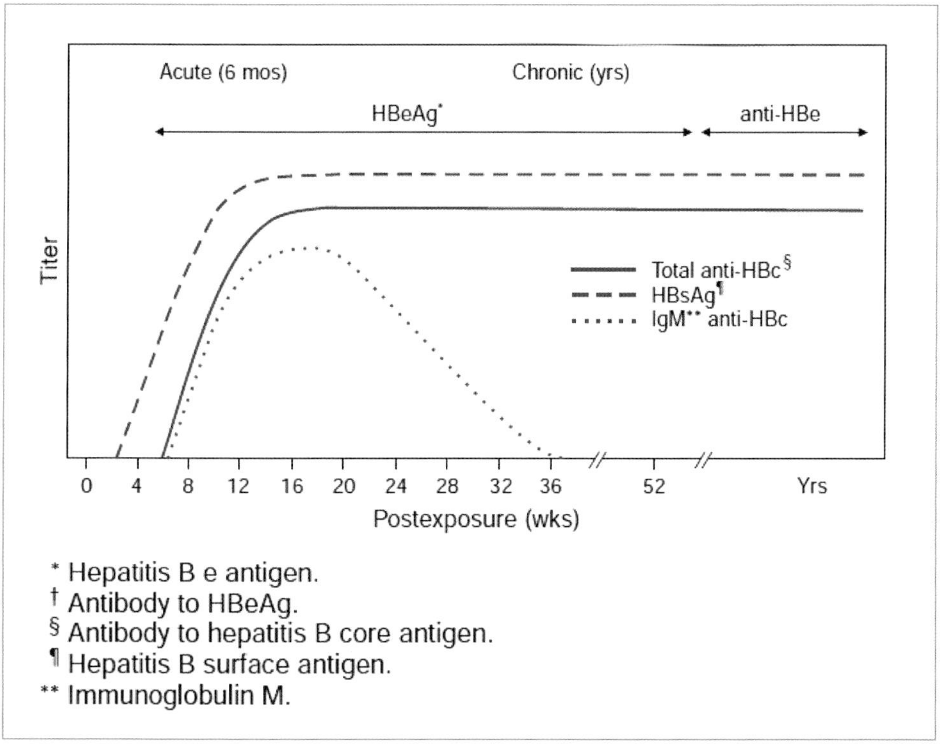

Acute (6 mos)
Chronic (yrs)
HBeAg*
anti-HBe†
Titer
Total anti-HBc§
HBsAg¶
IgM** anti-HBc
0 4 8 12 16 20 24 28 32 36 52 Yrs
Postexposure (wks)

* Hepatitis B e antigen.
† Antibody to HBeAg.
§ Antibody to hepatitis B core antigen.
¶ Hepatitis B surface antigen.
** Immunoglobulin M.

Image 60.8
Typical serologic course of acute hepatitis B virus (HBV) infection with progression to chronic HBV infection. From Centers for Disease Control and Prevention. Recommendations for identification and public health management of persons with chronic hepatitis B virus infection. *MMWR Recomm Rep.* 2008;57(RR-8):1–20.

61

Hepatitis C

Clinical Manifestations

Signs and symptoms of hepatitis C virus (HCV) infection are indistinguishable from those of hepatitis A or hepatitis B virus infections. Acute disease tends to be mild and insidious in onset, and most infections are asymptomatic. Jaundice occurs in fewer than 20% of patients, and abnormalities in serum aminotransferase concentrations are generally less pronounced than abnormalities in patients with hepatitis B virus infection. Persistent infection with HCV occurs in up to 80% of infected children, even in the absence of biochemical evidence of liver disease. Most children with chronic infection are asymptomatic. Although chronic hepatitis develops in approximately 70% to 80% of infected adults, limited data indicate chronic hepatitis and cirrhosis occur less commonly in children, in part because of the usually indolent nature of infection in pediatric patients. Liver failure secondary to HCV infection is the leading indication for liver transplantation among adults in the United States.

Etiology

Hepatitis C virus is a small, single-stranded RNA virus and is a member of the *Flavivirus* family. At least 6 HCV genotypes exist with multiple subtypes.

Epidemiology

The incidence of acute symptomatic HCV infection in the United States was 0.2 per 100,000 population in 2005; after asymptomatic infection and underreporting were considered, approximately 20,000 new cases were estimated to have occurred. For all age groups, the incidence of HCV infection has markedly decreased in the United States since the 1990s and has remained low since 2006. However, there was a 45% increase in reported cases of acute HCV in the United States in 2011 compared with 2004 through 2010. This increase was mostly seen in white, nonurban young people with a history of using injection drugs and opioid agonists such as oxycodone. A substantial burden of disease still exists in the United States because of the propensity of HCV to establish chronic infection and the high incidence of acute HCV infection through the 1980s. The prevalence of HCV infection in the general population of the United States is estimated at 1.3%, equating to an estimated 3.2 million people in the United States who have chronic HCV infection. The seroprevalence of HCV in children was approximately 0.1%, although the numbers of HCV infections in the younger age groups were too small for reliable estimates. Worldwide, the prevalence of chronic HCV infection is highest in Africa, especially Egypt.

Hepatitis C virus is primarily spread by parenteral exposure to blood of HCV-infected people. The most common risk factors for adults to acquire infection are injection drug use, multiple sexual partners, or receipt of blood products before 1992. The current risk of HCV infection after blood transfusion in the United States is estimated to be 1 per 2 million units transfused because of exclusion of high-risk donors since 1992 and of HCV-positive units after antibody testing as well as screening of pools of blood units. The most common route of infection in children is maternal-fetal transmission.

Approximately 60% of chronic HCV cases are in injection drug users who have shared needles or injection paraphernalia; almost all infected people are outside the pediatric age range. Data from recent multicenter, population-based cohort studies indicate approximately one-third of young injection drug users 18 to 30 years of age are infected with HCV. Approximately half of the 18,000 people with hemophilia who received transfusions before adoption of heat treatment of clotting factors in 1987 are HCV seropositive. Also, more recently appreciated has been the number of infections acquired in the health care setting, especially nonhospital clinics where infection control and needle and intravenous hygienic procedures have not been practiced strictly. Prevalence is high among people with frequent but smaller direct percutaneous exposures, such as patients receiving hemodialysis (10%–20%). Transmission among family contacts is uncommon but can occur from direct or inapparent percutaneous or mucosal exposure to blood.

Seroprevalence among pregnant women in the United States has been estimated at 1% to 2%. The risk of perinatal transmission averages 5% to 6% and transmission occurs only from women who are HCV RNA positive at the time of delivery. Maternal coinfection with HIV has been associated with increased risk of perinatal transmission of HCV, with transmission rates between 10% and 20%; transmission depends in part on the amount of HCV RNA in the mother's blood. Although HCV RNA has been detected in colostrum, the risk of HCV transmission is similar in breastfed and formula-fed neonates and infants.

Incubation Period

Average, 6 to 7 weeks (range, 2 weeks–6 months); time from exposure to development of viremia, 1 to 2 weeks.

Diagnostic Tests

The 2 types of tests available for laboratory diagnosis of HCV infections are immunoglobulin (Ig) G antibody enzyme immunoassays for HCV and nucleic acid amplification tests to detect HCV RNA. Assays for IgM to detect early or acute infection are not available. Third-generation enzyme immunoassays are at least 97% sensitive and more than 99% specific. In June 2010, the US Food and Drug Administration approved for use in people 15 years and older the OraQuick rapid blood test, which uses a test strip that produces a blue line within 20 minutes if anti-HCV antibodies are present. False-negative results early in the course of acute infection can result from any of the HCV serologic tests because of the prolonged interval between exposure and onset of illness and seroconversion. Within 15 weeks after exposure and within 5 to 6 weeks after onset of hepatitis, 80% of patients will have positive test results for serum anti-HCV antibody. Among neonates born to anti-HCV–positive mothers, passively acquired maternal antibody may persist for up to 18 months.

Nucleic acid amplification tests for qualitative detection of HCV RNA are available. Hepatitis C virus RNA can be detected in serum or plasma within 1 to 2 weeks after exposure to the virus and weeks before onset of liver enzyme abnormalities or appearance of anti-HCV. Assays for detection of HCV RNA are commonly used in clinical practice to identify anti-HCV–positive patients who are viremic, for identifying infection in neonates/infants early in life (ie, perinatal transmission) when maternal antibody interferes with ability to detect antibody produced by the neonate/infant, and for monitoring patients receiving antiviral therapy. However, false-positive and false-negative results of nucleic acid amplification tests can occur from improper handling, storage, and contamination of test specimens. Viral RNA may be detected intermittently in acute infection (ie, in the first 6 or 12 months following infection); thus, a single negative assay result is not conclusive if performed during this acute infection period. Highly sensitive quantitative assays for measuring the concentration of HCV RNA have largely replaced qualitative assays. The clinical value of these quantitative assays appears to be primarily as a prognostic indicator for patients undergoing or about to undergo antiviral therapy.

Treatment

Patients diagnosed with HCV infection should be referred to a pediatric hepatitis specialist for clinical monitoring and consideration of antiviral treatment. Therapy is aimed at inhibiting HCV replication, eradicating infection, and improving the natural history of disease. Therapies are expensive and can have significant adverse reactions. Response to treatment varies depending on the genotype with which the person is infected. Genotype 1 is the most common genotype in North America. Genotypes 1 and 4 respond less well than genotypes 2 and 3 to antiviral therapy. Currently, the only Food and Drug Administration–approved treatment for HCV in children 3 to 17 years of age consists of a combination of peginterferon and ribavirin. The few studies of peginterferon and ribavirin combination therapy in children suggest that children have fewer adverse events compared with adults; however, all treatment regimens are associated with adverse events. Major adverse effects of combination therapy in pediatric patients include influenza-like symptoms, hematologic abnormalities, neuropsychiatric symptoms, thyroid abnormalities, ocular abnormalities including ischemic retinopathy and uveitis, and growth disturbances. The recent data for combination antivirals without significant adverse effects in adults suggest that, ultimately, pediatric patients with HCV infection will also have effective therapies.

All patients with chronic HCV infection should be immunized against hepatitis A and hepatitis B. Among children, progression of liver disease appears to be accelerated when comorbid conditions, including childhood cancer, iron overload, or thalassemia, are present. Pediatricians need to be alert to concomitant infections, alcohol abuse, and concomitant use of drugs, such as acetaminophen and some antiretroviral agents (eg, stavudine), in patients with HCV infection. Children with chronic infection should be followed closely, including sequential monitoring of serum aminotransferase concentrations, because of the potential for chronic liver disease.

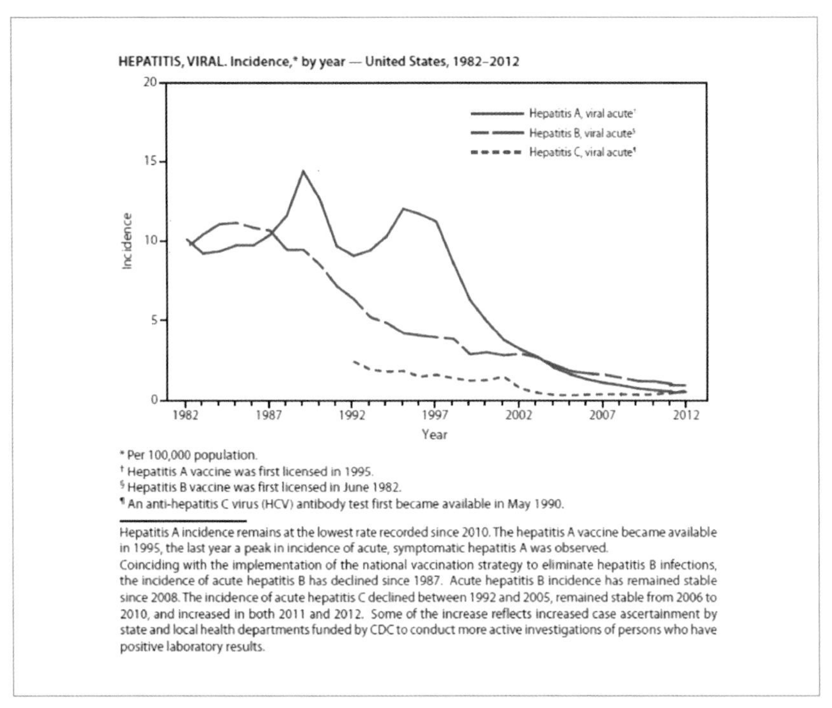

Image 61.1

Hepatitis, viral. Incidence, by year—United States, 1982–2012. Courtesy of *Morbidity and Mortality Weekly Report.*

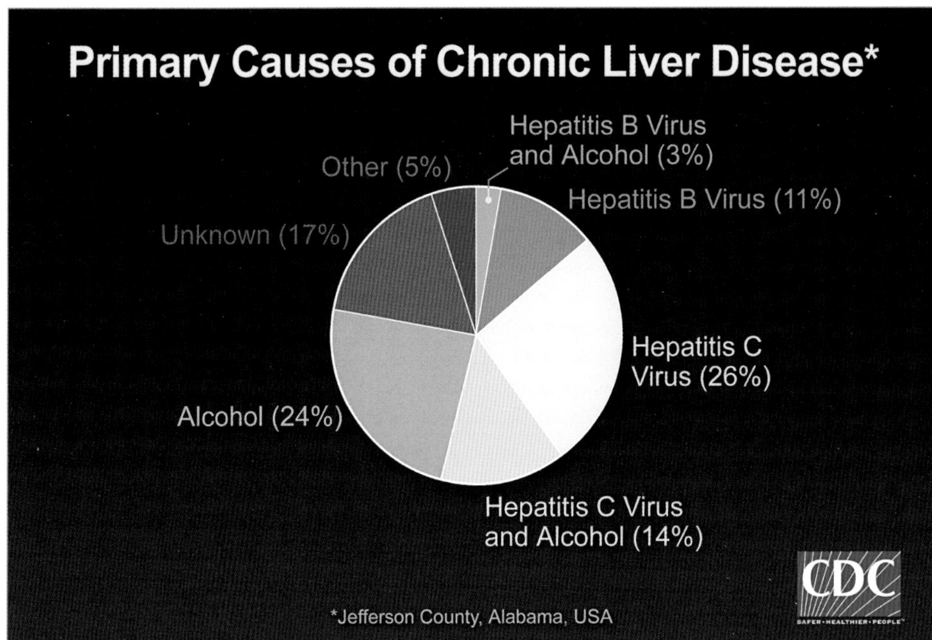

Image 61.2
Pie chart showing causes of chronic liver disease in residents of Jefferson County, AL. Hepatitis B and hepatitis C viruses contributed to most cases of chronic liver disease in this population. Courtesy of Centers for Disease Control and Prevention.

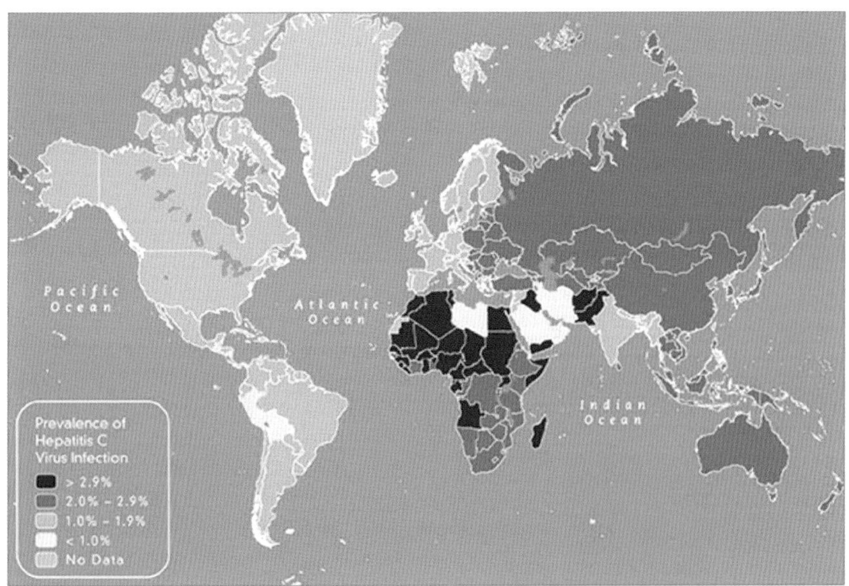

Image 61.3
Prevalence of chronic hepatitis C infection. Centers for Disease Control and Prevention National Center for Emerging and Zoonotic Infectious Diseases (NCEZID) Division of Global Migration and Quarantine (DGMQ).

62

Hepatitis D

Clinical Manifestations

Hepatitis D virus (HDV) causes infection only in people with acute or chronic hepatitis B virus (HBV) infection. Hepatitis D virus requires HBV as a helper virus for replication and cannot produce infection in the absence of HBV. The importance of HDV infection lies in its ability to convert an asymptomatic or mild chronic HBV infection into fulminant or more severe or rapidly progressive disease. Acute coinfection with HBV and HDV usually causes an acute illness indistinguishable from acute HBV infection alone, except that the likelihood of fulminant hepatitis can be as high as 5%.

Etiology

Hepatitis D virus measures 36 to 43 nm in diameter and consists of an RNA genome and a delta protein antigen, both of which are coated with hepatitis B surface antigen.

Epidemiology

Hepatitis D virus infection is present worldwide, in all age groups, and an estimated 18 million people are infected with the virus. Over the past 20 years, HDV prevalence has decreased significantly in Western and Southern Europe because of long-standing hepatitis B immunization programs, although HDV remains a significant health problem in resource-limited countries. At least 8 genotypes of HDV have been described, each with a typical geographic pattern, with genotype 1 being the predominant type in Europe and North America. Hepatitis D virus can cause an infection at the same time as the initial HBV infection (coinfection), or it can infect a person already chronically infected with HBV (superinfection). Acquisition of HDV is by parenteral, percutaneous, or mucous membrane inoculation. Hepatitis D virus can be acquired from blood or blood products, through injection drug use, or by sexual contact, but only if HBV is also present. Transmission from mother to newborn is uncommon. Intrafamilial spread can occur among people with chronic HBV infection. High-prevalence areas include parts of Eastern Europe, South America, Africa, Central Asia (particularly Pakistan), and the Middle East. In the United States, HDV infection is most commonly found in people who abuse injection drugs, people with hemophilia, and people who have emigrated from areas with endemic HDV infection.

Incubation Period

Approximately 2 to 8 weeks; when HBV and HDV viruses infect simultaneously, average 90 days (range, 45–160).

Diagnostic Tests

People with chronic HBV infection are at risk of HDV coinfection. Accordingly, their care should be supervised by an expert in hepatitis treatment, and consideration should be given to testing for anti-HDV immunoglobulin (Ig) G antibodies using a commercially available test if they have increased transaminase concentrations, particularly if they recently came from a country with high prevalence of HDV. Anti-HDV may not be present until several weeks after onset of illness, and acute and convalescent sera can be required to confirm the diagnosis. In a person with anti-HDV, the absence of IgM hepatitis B core antibody, which is indicative of chronic HBV infection, suggests the person has chronic HBV infection and superinfection with HDV. Presence of anti-HDV IgG antibodies does not prove active infection; thus, HDV RNA testing should be performed for diagnostic and therapeutic considerations. Patients with circulating HDV RNA should be staged for severity of liver disease, have surveillance for development of hepatocellular carcinoma, and be considered for treatment. Presence of anti-HDV IgM is of lesser utility because it is present in acute and chronic HDV infections.

Treatment

Hepatitis D virus has proven difficult to treat. However, data suggest pegylated interferon alfa may result in up to 40% of patients having a sustained response to treatment. Clinical trials suggest at least a year of therapy may be associated with sustained responses, and longer courses may be warranted if the patient is able to tolerate therapy. Further study of pegylated interferon monotherapy or as combination therapy with a direct-acting antiviral agent needs to be performed before treatment of HDV can be routinely advised.

63

Hepatitis E

Clinical Manifestations

Hepatitis E virus (HEV) infection causes an acute illness with symptoms including jaundice, malaise, anorexia, fever, abdominal pain, and arthralgia. Disease is more common among adults than among children and is more severe in pregnant women, in whom mortality rates can reach 10% to 25% during the third trimester. Chronic HEV infection is rare and has been reported only in recipients of solid organ transplants and people with severe immunodeficiency.

Etiology

Hepatitis E virus is a spherical, nonenveloped, positive-sense RNA virus. It is classified in the genus *Hepevirus* of the family Hepeviridae. There are 4 major recognized genotypes with a single known serotype.

Epidemiology

Hepatitis E virus is the most common cause of viral hepatitis in the world. Globally, an estimated 20 million HEV infections occur annually, resulting in 3.4 million cases of acute hepatitis and 70,000 deaths. In developing countries, ingestion of fecally contaminated water is the most common route of HEV transmission, and large waterborne outbreaks occur frequently. Sporadic HEV infection has been reported throughout the world and is common in Africa and the Indian subcontinent. Unlike the other agents of viral hepatitis, certain HEV genotypes (genotypes 3 and 4) also have zoonotic hosts, such as swine, and can be transmitted by eating undercooked pork. Hepatitis E virus genotypes 1 and 2 exclusively infect humans. Person-to-person transmission appears to be much less efficient than with hepatitis A virus but occurs in sporadic and outbreak settings. Mother-to-newborn transmission of HEV occurs frequently and accounts for a significant proportion of fetal loss and perinatal mortality. Hepatitis E is also transmitted through blood product transfusion. Transfusion-transmitted hepatitis E occurs primarily in countries with endemic disease and is rarely reported in areas without endemic infection. In the United States, serologic studies have demonstrated that approximately 20% of the population has immunoglobulin (Ig) G against HEV. However, symptomatic HEV infection in the United States is uncommon and generally occurs in people who acquire HEV genotype 1 infection after traveling to countries with endemic HEV. Nonetheless, a number of people without a travel history have been diagnosed with acute HEV, and evidence for the infection should be sought in cases of acute hepatitis without an etiology. Acute HEV can masquerade as drug-induced liver injury.

Diagnostic Tests

Testing for IgM and IgG anti-HEV is available through some research and commercial reference laboratories. Because anti-HEV assays are not approved by the US Food and Drug Administration and their performance characteristics are not well defined, results should be interpreted with caution, particularly in cases lacking a discrete onset of illness associated with jaundice or with no recent history of travel to a country with endemic infection. Definitive diagnosis may be made by demonstrating viral RNA in serum or stool by means of reverse transcriptase-polymerase chain reaction assay, which is available only in research settings (with prior approval through the Centers for Disease Control and Prevention). Because virus circulates in the body for a relatively short period, the inability to detect HEV in serum or stool does not eliminate the possibility that the person was infected with HEV.

Treatment

Supportive care.

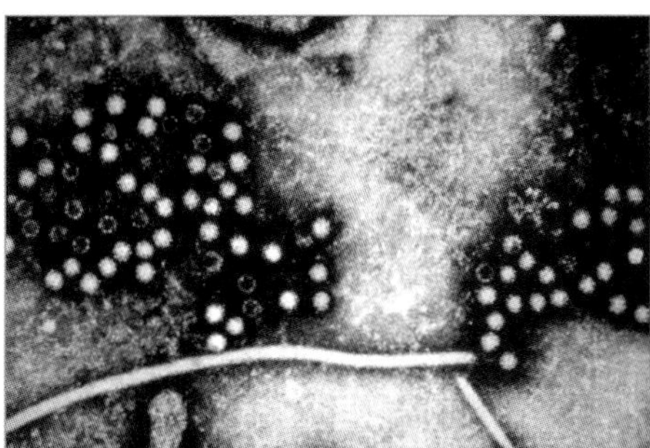

Image 63.1
This electron micrograph depicts hepatitis E viruses. Hepatitis E virus was classified as a member of the Caliciviridae family but has been reclassified in the genus *Hepevirus* of the family Hepeviridae. There are 4 major recognized genotypes with a single known serotype. Hepatitis E virus, the major etiologic agent of enterically transmitted non-A, non-B hepatitis worldwide, is a spherical, nonenveloped, single-stranded RNA virus that is approximately 32 to 34 nm in diameter. Courtesy of Centers for Disease Control and Prevention.

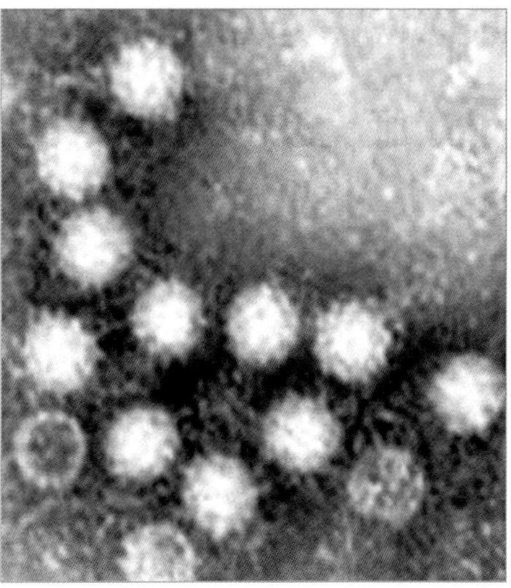

Image 63.2
Electron micrograph of nonhuman primate (marmoset) passaged hepatitis E virus (HEV) (Nepal isolate). Virus is aggregated with convalescent antisera to HEV and negatively stained in phosphotungstic acid. Particle size ranges from 27 to 30 nm. Courtesy of Centers for Disease Control and Prevention.

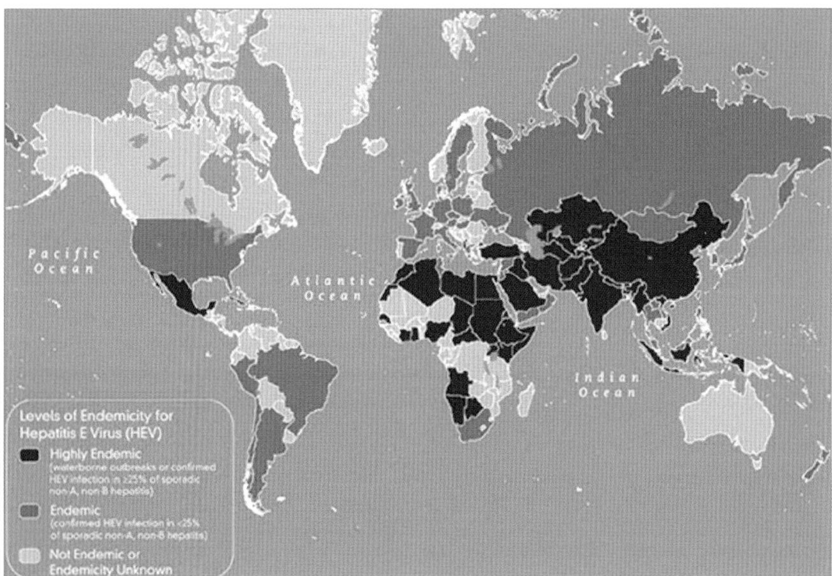

Image 63.3
Distribution of hepatitis E infection, 2010. Centers for Disease Control and Prevention National Center for Emerging and Zoonotic Infectious Diseases (NCEZID) Division of Global Migration and Quarantine (DGMQ).

64

Herpes Simplex

Clinical Manifestations

Neonatal. In newborns, herpes simplex infection can manifest as 3 syndromes: (1) **disseminated disease** involving multiple organs, most prominently liver and lungs, and, in 60% to 75% of cases, also involving the central nervous system (CNS); (2) **CNS disease,** with or without skin involvement; or (3) disease **localized to the skin, eyes, or mouth (SEM disease).** Approximately 25% of cases of neonatal herpes simplex manifest as disseminated disease, 30% of cases manifest as CNS disease, and 45% of cases manifest as SEM disease. More than 80% of neonates with SEM disease have skin vesicles; those without have infection limited to the eyes or oral mucosa. Approximately two-thirds of neonates with disseminated or CNS disease have skin lesions, but these lesions may not be present at the time of onset of symptoms. Disseminated infection should be considered in neonates with sepsis syndrome, negative bacteriologic culture results, severe liver dysfunction, or consumptive coagulopathy. Herpes simplex should also be considered as a causative agent in neonates with fever, a vesicular rash, or abnormal cerebrospinal fluid (CSF) findings, especially in the presence of seizures or during a time of year when enteroviruses are not circulating in the community. Although asymptomatic herpes simplex infection is common in older children, it rarely, if ever, occurs in neonates.

Neonatal herpetic infections are often severe, with attendant high mortality and morbidity rates, even when antiviral therapy is promptly administered. Recurrent skin lesions are common in surviving neonates, occurring in approximately 50% of survivors, often within 1 to 2 weeks of discontinuing the initial treatment course.

Initial signs of herpes simplex infection most often develop within the first month of life. Neonates with disseminated disease and SEM disease have an earlier age of onset, typically presenting between the first and second weeks of life; neonates with CNS disease usually present with illness between the second and third weeks of life.

Children beyond the neonatal period and adolescents. Most primary herpes simplex childhood infections beyond the neonatal period are asymptomatic.

Gingivostomatitis, which is the most common clinical manifestation of herpes simplex during childhood, is caused by herpes simplex virus type 1 (HSV-1) and is characterized by fever, irritability, tender submandibular adenopathy, and an ulcerative enanthem involving the gingiva and mucous membranes of the mouth, often with perioral vesicular lesions.

Genital herpes, which is the most common manifestation of primary herpes simplex infection in adolescents and adults, is characterized by vesicular or ulcerative lesions of the male or female genital organs, perineum, or both. Until recent years, genital herpes was most often caused by herpes simplex virus type 2 (HSV-2), but HSV-1 now accounts for more than half of all cases of genital herpes in the United States. Most cases of primary genital herpes infection in males and females are asymptomatic and are not recognized by the infected person or diagnosed by a health care professional.

Eczema herpeticum can develop in patients with atopic dermatitis who are infected with herpes simplex. Examination may reveal skin with punched-out erosions, hemorrhagic crusts, or vesicular lesions.

In patients who are immunocompromised, severe local lesions and, less commonly, disseminated herpes simplex infection with generalized vesicular skin lesions and visceral involvement can occur.

After primary infection, herpes simplex persists for life in a latent form. The site of latency for the virus causing herpes labialis is the trigeminal ganglion, and the usual site of latency for genital herpes is the sacral dorsal root ganglia, although any of the sensory ganglia can be involved depending on the site of primary infection. Reactivation of latent virus most commonly is asymptomatic. When symptomatic, recurrent HSV-1 herpes labialis manifests as single or grouped vesicles in the perioral region, usually on the vermilion border of the lips (typically called "cold sores" or "fever blisters"). Symptomatic recurrent genital herpes manifests as vesicular lesions on the penis, scrotum, vulva, cervix, buttocks, perianal areas, thighs, or back. Among immunocompromised patients, genital HSV-2 recurrences are more frequent and of longer duration. Recurrences may be heralded by a prodrome of burning or itching at the site of an incipient recurrence, identification of which can be useful in instituting antiviral therapy early.

Conjunctivitis and **keratitis** can result from primary or recurrent herpes simplex infection. **Herpetic whitlow** consists of single or multiple vesicular lesions on the distal fingers. Herpes simplex infection can be a precipitating factor in erythema multiforme, and recurrent erythema multiforme is often caused by symptomatic or asymptomatic herpes simplex recurrences. Wrestlers can develop **herpes gladiatorum** if they become infected with herpes simplex.

Herpes simplex encephalitis (HSE) occurs in children beyond the neonatal period or in adolescents and adults and can result from primary or recurrent HSV-1 infection. One-fifth of HSE cases occur in the pediatric age group. Symptoms and signs usually include fever, alterations in the state of consciousness, personality changes, seizures, and focal neurologic findings. Encephalitis commonly has an acute onset with a fulminant course, leading to coma and death in untreated patients. Herpes simplex encephalitis usually involves the temporal lobe; thus, temporal lobe abnormalities on imaging studies or electroencephalography in the context of a consistent clinical picture should increase the suspicion of HSE. Magnetic resonance imaging is the most sensitive neuroimaging modality to demonstrate temporal lobe involvement. Cerebrospinal fluid pleocytosis with a predominance of lymphocytes is typical.

Herpes simplex infection can also cause **aseptic meningitis** with nonspecific clinical manifestations that are usually mild and self-limited. Such episodes of meningitis are usually associated with genital HSV-2 infection. A number of unusual CNS manifestations of herpes simplex have been described, including Bell palsy, atypical pain syndromes, trigeminal neuralgia, ascending myelitis, transverse myelitis, postinfectious encephalomyelitis, and recurrent (Mollaret) meningitis.

Etiology

Herpes simplex viruses are enveloped, double-stranded, DNA viruses. At least 9 herpesvirus species, including HSV, infect humans. Two distinct types exist: HSV-1 and HSV-2. Infections with HSV-1 usually involve the face and skin above the waist; however, an increasing number of genital herpes cases are attributable to HSV-1. Infections with HSV-2 usually involve the genitalia and skin below the waist in sexually active adolescents and adults. However, HSV-1 and HSV-2 can be found in either area and both cause herpes disease in neonates. As with all human herpesviruses, HSV-1 and HSV-2 establish latency following primary infection, with periodic reactivation to cause recurrent symptomatic disease or asymptomatic viral shedding.

Epidemiology

Herpes simplex infections are ubiquitous and can be transmitted from people who are symptomatic or asymptomatic with primary or recurrent infections.

Neonatal. The incidence of neonatal herpes simplex infection is estimated to range from 1 in 3,000 to 1 in 20,000 live births. Herpes simplex virus is transmitted to a neonate most often during birth through an infected maternal genital tract but can be caused by an ascending infection through ruptured or apparently intact amniotic membranes. Intrauterine infections causing congenital malformations have been implicated in rare cases. Other, less common sources of neonatal infection include postnatal transmission from a parent or other caregiver, most often from a nongenital infection (eg, mouth, hands).

The risk of HSV transmission to a neonate born to a mother who acquires primary genital infection near the time of delivery is estimated to be 25% to 60%. In contrast, the risk to a neonate born to a mother shedding HSV as a result of reactivation of infection acquired during the first half of pregnancy or earlier is less than 2%. Distinguishing between primary and recurrent herpes simplex infections in women by history or physical examination alone may be impossible because primary and recurrent genital infections may be asymptomatic or associated with nonspecific findings (eg, vaginal discharge, genital pain, shallow ulcers). History of maternal genital herpes simplex infection is not helpful in diagnosing neonatal herpes simplex disease because more than three-quarters of neonates who contract herpes simplex infection are born to women with no history or clinical findings suggestive of genital herpes simplex infection during or preceding pregnancy.

Children beyond the neonatal period and adolescents. Twenty-six percent of US children have serologic evidence of HSV-1 infection by 7 years of age. Patients with primary gingivostomatitis or genital herpes usually shed virus for at least 1 week and, occasionally, for several weeks. Patients with symptomatic recurrences shed virus for a shorter period, typically 3 to 4 days. Intermittent asymptomatic reactivation of oral and genital herpes is common and likely occurs throughout the remainder of a person's life. The greatest concentration of virus is shed during symptomatic primary infections and the lowest concentration of virus is shed during asymptomatic reactivation.

Infections with HSV-1 usually result from direct contact with virus shed from visible or microscopic orolabial lesions or in infected oral secretions. Infections with HSV-2 usually result from direct contact with virus shed from visible or microscopic genital lesions or in genital secretions during sexual activity. Genital herpes simplex infections increase the risk of acquisition of HIV. Genital infections caused by HSV-1 in children can result from autoinoculation of virus from the mouth. Sexual abuse should always be considered in prepubertal children with genital HSV-2 infections. Therefore, genital HSV isolates from children should be typed to differentiate between HSV-1 and HSV-2.

The incidence of HSV-2 infection correlates with the number of sexual partners and with acquisition of other sexually transmitted infections. After primary genital infection, which is often asymptomatic, some people experience frequent clinical recurrences, and others have no clinically apparent recurrences. Genital HSV-2 infection is more likely to recur than is genital HSV-1 infection.

Inoculation of abraded skin occurs from direct contact with herpes simplex virus shed from oral, genital, or other skin sites. This contact can result in herpes gladiatorum among wrestlers, herpes rugbiaforum among rugby players, or herpetic whitlow of the fingers in any exposed person.

Incubation Period

For infection beyond the neonatal period, range from 2 days to 2 weeks.

Diagnostic Tests

Herpes simplex grows readily in cell culture. Special transport media are available that allow transport to local or regional laboratories for culture. Cytopathogenic effects typical of herpes simplex infection are usually observed 1 to 3 days after inoculation. Methods of culture confirmation include fluorescent antibody staining, enzyme immunoassays, and monolayer culture with typing. Cultures that remain negative by day 5 likely will continue to remain negative. Polymerase chain reaction (PCR) assay can often detect herpes simplex DNA in CSF from neonates with CNS infection (neonatal herpes simplex CNS disease) and from older children and adults with HSE and is the diagnostic method of choice for CNS herpes simplex involvement. Polymerase chain reaction assay of CSF can yield negative results in cases of HSE, especially early in the disease course. In difficult cases in which repeated CSF PCR assay results are negative, histologic examination and viral culture of a brain tissue biopsy specimen is the most definitive method of confirming the diagnosis of HSE. Detection of intrathecal antibody against herpes simplex can also assist in the diagnosis. Viral cultures of CSF from a patient with HSE are usually negative.

For diagnosis of neonatal herpes simplex infection, the following specimens should be obtained: swab specimens from the mouth, nasopharynx, conjunctivae, and anus ("surface cultures") for herpes simplex culture (a single swab can be used) and, if desired, for herpes simplex PCR assay; specimens of skin vesicles for herpes simplex culture and, if desired, for PCR assay; CSF sample for herpes simplex PCR assay; whole blood sample for herpes simplex PCR assay; and whole blood sample for measuring alanine aminotransferase. The performance of PCR assay on skin and mucosal specimens from neonates has not been studied; if used, surface or skin PCR assays should be performed in addition to surface cultures. Positive culture results obtained from any of the surface sites **more than 12 to 24 hours after birth** indicate viral replication and are suggestive of neonatal infection rather than contamination after intrapartum exposure. As with any PCR assay, false-negative and false-positive results can occur. Whole blood PCR assay may be of benefit in diagnosis of neonatal herpes simplex disease, but its use should not supplant standard diagnostic studies (ie, surface cultures and CSF PCR assay). Any of the 3 syndromes of neonatal herpes simplex can have associated viremia, so a positive whole blood PCR assay should not be used to determine extent of disease; similarly, no data exist to support use of serial blood PCR assay to monitor response to therapy. Rapid diagnostic techniques are also available, such as direct fluorescent antibody staining of vesicle scrapings or enzyme immunoassay detection of herpes simplex antigens. These techniques are as specific but slightly less sensitive than culture. Typing herpes simplex strains differentiates between HSV-1 and HSV-2 isolates. Radiographs and clinical manifestations can suggest herpes simplex pneumonitis, and elevated transaminase values can suggest herpes simplex hepatitis; both occur commonly in neonatal herpes simplex disseminated disease. Histologic examination of lesions for presence of multinucleated giant cells and eosinophilic intranuclear inclusions typical of herpes simplex (eg, with Tzanck test) has low sensitivity and should not be performed.

Herpes simplex PCR assay and cell culture are the preferred tests for detecting herpes simplex in genital ulcers or other mucocutaneous lesions consistent with genital herpes. The sensitivity of viral culture is low and declines rapidly as lesions begin to heal. Polymerase chain reaction assays for herpes simplex DNA are more sensitive and are increasingly used in many settings. Failure to detect herpes simplex in genital lesions by culture or PCR assay does not indicate an absence of herpes simplex infection because viral shedding is intermittent.

Type-specific and type-common antibodies to herpes simplex develop during the first several weeks after infection and persist indefinitely. The median time to seroconversion is 21 days with the Focus type-specific enzyme-linked immunosorbent assay, and more than 95% of people seroconvert by 12 weeks following infection. Although type-specific HSV-2 antibody usually indicates previous anogenital infection, the presence of HSV-1 antibody does not reliably distinguish anogenital from orolabial infection because a substantial proportion of initial genital infections are caused by HSV-1. Type-specific serologic tests can be useful in confirming a clinical diagnosis of genital herpes caused by HSV-2. There is growing evidence that type-specific antibody avidity testing may prove useful for evaluating risk of maternal transmission of herpes simplex to neonates. Serologic testing is not useful in neonates.

Several glycoprotein G–based type-specific assays including at least one that can be used as a point-of-care test. The sensitivities and specificities of these tests for detection of HSV-2 IgG antibody vary from 90% to 100%; false-negative results may occur, especially early after infection, and false-positive results can occur, especially in patients with low likelihood of herpes simplex infection.

Treatment

Acyclovir is the drug of choice for many herpes simplex infections (Table 64.1). Valacyclovir is an L-valyl ester of acyclovir that is metabolized to acyclovir after oral administration, resulting in higher serum concentrations than are achieved with oral acyclovir and similar serum concentrations as are achieved with intravenous administration of acyclovir. Famciclovir is converted rapidly to penciclovir after oral administration.

Neonatal. Parenteral acyclovir is the recommended treatment for neonatal herpes simplex infections, regardless of manifestations and clinical findings. The duration of therapy is 14 days in SEM disease and a minimum of 21 days in CNS disease or disseminated disease. The best outcomes in terms of morbidity and mortality are observed among neonates with SEM disease. Approximately 50% of neonates surviving neonatal herpes simplex experience cutaneous recurrences, with the first skin recurrence often occurring within 1 to 2 weeks of stopping intravenous acyclovir treatment.

All neonates with neonatal herpes simplex disease, regardless of syndrome, should have an ophthalmologic examination and neuroimaging to establish baseline brain anatomy. All neonates with CNS involvement should have a repeat lumbar puncture performed near the end of therapy to document that the CSF is negative for herpes simplex DNA on PCR assay; if this remains positive, consultation with an infectious diseases specialist is warranted.

Oral acyclovir suppressive therapy for the 6 months following treatment of acute neonatal herpes simplex infection improves neurodevelopmental outcomes in infants with herpes simplex CNS disease and prevents skin recurrences in infants with any disease classification of neonatal herpes simplex. Infants with ocular involvement attributable to herpes simplex infection should receive a topical ophthalmic antiviral drug. An ophthalmologist should be involved in the management and treatment of acute neonatal ocular herpes simplex infection.

Table 64.1
Recommended Therapy for Herpes Simplex Infections[a]

Infection	Drug[b]
Neonatal	Parenteral acyclovir
Keratoconjunctivitis	Trifluridine[c] **OR** Iododeoxyuridine **OR** Topical ganciclovir
Genital	Acyclovir **OR** Famciclovir **OR** Valacyclovir
Mucocutaneous (immunocompromised or primary gingivostomatitis)	Acyclovir **OR** Famciclovir **OR** Valacyclovir
Acyclovir-resistant (severe infections, immunocompromised)	Parenteral foscarnet
Encephalitis	Parenteral acyclovir

[a] See text for details.
[b] Famciclovir and valacyclovir are approved by the US Food and Drug Administration for treatment of adults.
[c] Treatment of herpes simplex ocular infection should involve an ophthalmologist.

Genital infection

- **Primary.** Many patients with first-episode genital herpes initially have mild clinical manifestations but may go on to develop severe or prolonged symptoms with viral reactivation. Therefore, most patients with initial genital herpes should receive antiviral therapy. In adults, acyclovir and valacyclovir decrease the duration of symptoms and viral shedding in primary genital herpes. Oral acyclovir therapy, initiated within 6 days of onset of disease, shortens the duration of illness and viral shedding by 3 to 5 days. Valacyclovir and famciclovir do not seem to be more effective than acyclovir but offer the advantage of less frequent dosing. Intravenous acyclovir is indicated for patients with a severe or complicated primary infection that requires hospitalization followed by oral antiviral therapy to complete at least 10 days of total therapy.
- **Recurrent.** Antiviral therapy for recurrent genital herpes can be administered episodically to ameliorate or shorten the duration of lesions or continuously as suppressive therapy to decrease the frequency of recurrences. Many people prefer suppressive therapy, which has the additional advantage of decreasing the risk of genital HSV-2 transmission to susceptible partners.

In adults with frequent genital herpes simplex recurrences, daily oral acyclovir suppressive therapy is effective for decreasing the frequency of symptomatic recurrences and improving quality of life. After approximately 1 year of continuous daily therapy, acyclovir should be discontinued, and the recurrence rate should be assessed. If frequent recurrences are observed, additional suppressive therapy should be considered. Acyclovir appears to be safe for adults receiving the drug for more than 15 years, but longer-term effects are unknown.

Acyclovir or valacyclovir may be administered orally to pregnant women with first-episode genital herpes or severe recurrent herpes, and acyclovir should be given intravenously to pregnant women with severe herpes simplex infection. Pregnant women or women of childbearing age with genital herpes should be encouraged to inform their health care professionals and those who will care for the newborn (Table 64.2).

Table 64.2

Maternal Infection Classification by Genital Herpes Simplex Viral Type and Maternal Serologic Test Results[a]

Classification of Maternal Infection	PCR/Culture From Genital Lesion	Maternal HSV-1 and HSV-2 IgG Antibody Status
Documented first-episode primary infection	Positive, either virus	Both negative
Documented first-episode nonprimary infection	Positive for HSV-1	Positive for HSV-2 **AND** negative for HSV-1
	Positive for HSV-2	Positive for HSV-1 **AND** negative for HSV-2
Assumed first-episode (primary or nonprimary) infection	Positive for HSV-1 **OR** HSV-2	Not available
	Negative **OR** not available[b]	Negative for HSV-1 and/or HSV-2, **OR** not available
Recurrent infection	Positive for HSV-1	Positive for HSV-1
	Positive for HSV-2	Positive for HSV-2

Abbreviations: HSV, herpes simplex virus; IgG, immunoglobulin G; PCR, polymerase chain reaction (assay).

[a] To be used for women without a clinical history of genital herpes.

[b] When a genital lesion is strongly suspicious for HSV, clinical judgment should supersede the virologic test results for the conservative purposes of this neonatal management algorithm. Conversely, if, in retrospect, the genital lesion was not likely to be caused by HSV and the PCR assay culture result is negative, departure from the evaluation and management in this conservative algorithm may be warranted.

Mucocutaneous

- **Immunocompromised hosts.** Intravenous acyclovir is effective for treatment of mucocutaneous herpes simplex infection. Acyclovir-resistant strains of HSV have been isolated from immunocompromised people receiving prolonged treatment with acyclovir. Under these circumstances, progressive disease may be observed despite acyclovir therapy. Foscarnet is the drug of choice for disease caused by acyclovir-resistant HSV isolates.
- **Immunocompetent hosts.** Limited data are available on effects of acyclovir on the course of primary or recurrent nongenital mucocutaneous herpes simplex infection in immunocompetent hosts. Therapeutic benefit has been noted in a limited number of children with primary gingivostomatitis treated with oral acyclovir. Slight therapeutic benefit of oral acyclovir therapy has been demonstrated among adults with recurrent herpes labialis.

Other herpes simplex infections

- **Central nervous system.** Patients with HSE should be treated for 21 days with intravenous acyclovir. Patients who are comatose or semicomatose at initiation of therapy have a poorer outcome. For people with Bell palsy, the combination of acyclovir and prednisone may be considered.
- **Ocular.** Treatment of eye lesions should be undertaken in consultation with an ophthalmologist. Several topical drugs, such as 1% trifluridine, 0.1% iododeoxyuridine, and 0.15% ganciclovir, have proven efficacy for superficial keratitis. Topical corticosteroids, by themselves, are contraindicated in suspected herpes simplex conjunctivitis; however, ophthalmologists may choose to use corticosteroids in conjunction with antiviral drugs to treat locally invasive infections.

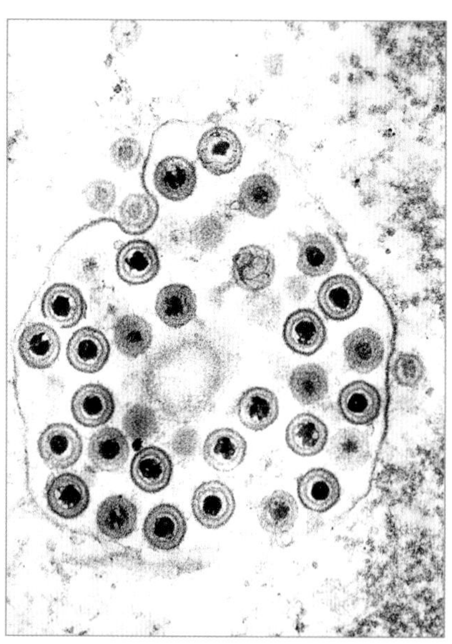

Image 64.1
This negatively stained transmission electron micrograph reveals the presence of numerous herpesvirus virions, members of the Herpesviridae virus family. Courtesy of Centers for Disease Control and Prevention/Dr Fred Murphy; Sylvia Whitfield.

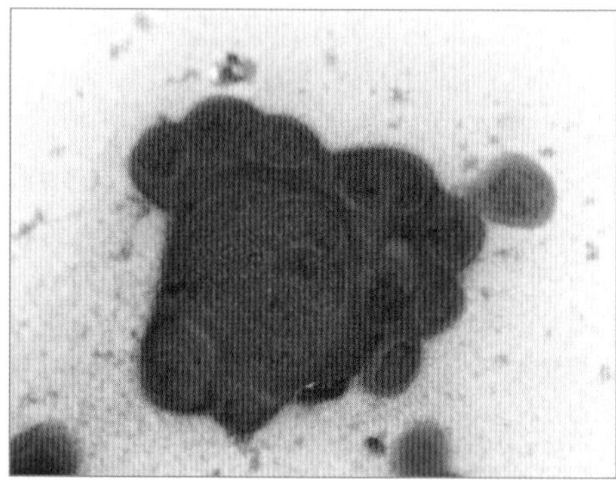

Image 64.2
Tzanck test showing multinucleated giant cells (magnification x100). Courtesy of Robert Jerris, MD.

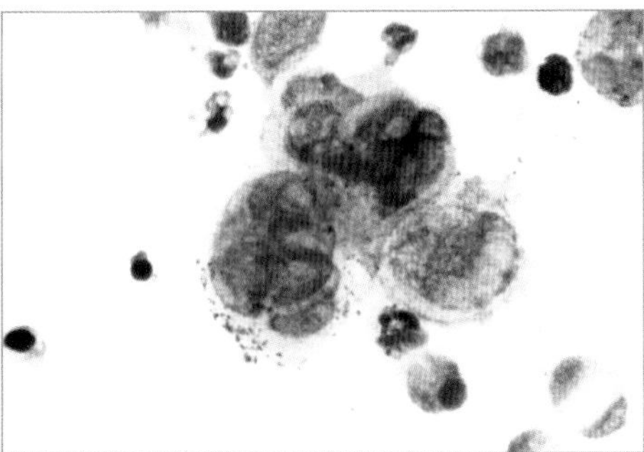

Image 64.3
This micrograph depicts results indicating the presence of herpes simplex virus in a Tzanck test specimen from a penile lesion. A Tzanck test involves extracting a sample of tissue from the base of a vesicle to look for multinucleated giant cells. Courtesy of Centers for Disease Control and Prevention/Joe Miller.

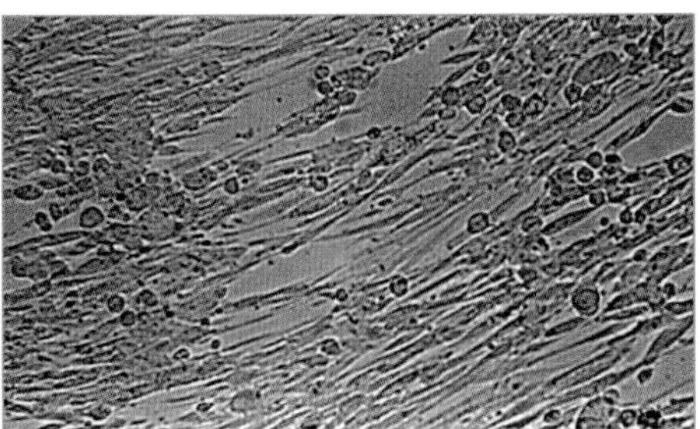

Image 64.5
The cytopathic effect of herpes simplex virus develops rapidly in cell culture. Cytopathogenic effects can usually be seen in 1 to 3 days after tissue-culture inoculation.

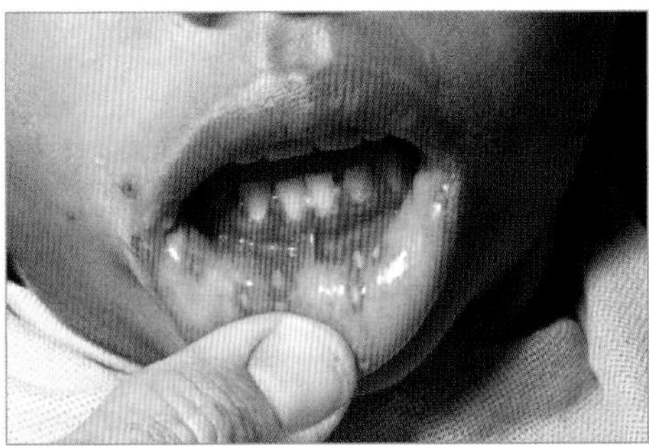

Image 64.7
Herpes simplex stomatitis, primary infection of the anterior oral mucous membranes. Tongue lesions are also common with primary herpes simplex infections.

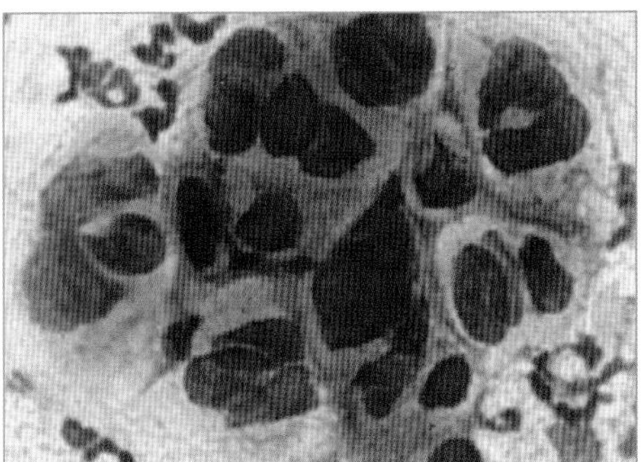

Image 64.4
Multinucleated giant cells formed by the fusion of keratinocytes are often present in association with herpes simplex infection. Courtesy of Daniel P. Krowchuk, MD, FAAP.

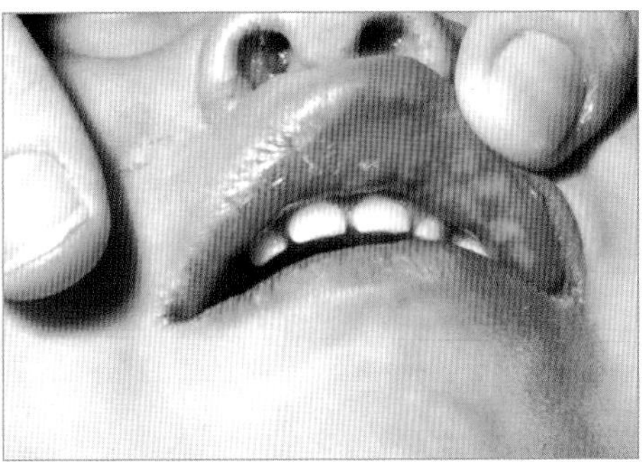

Image 64.6
Herpes simplex stomatitis, primary infection.

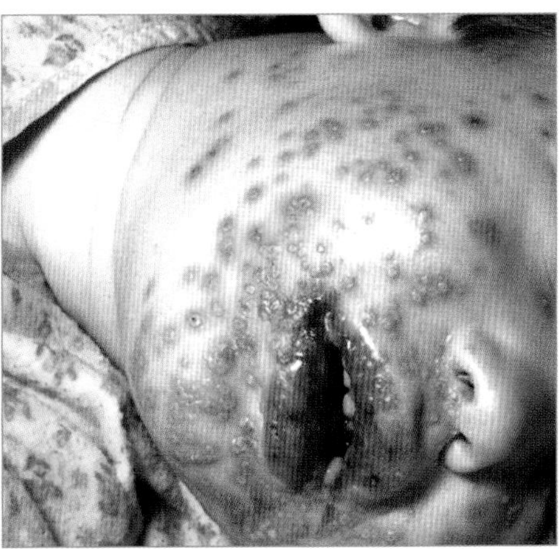

Image 64.8
Herpes simplex stomatitis, primary infection with extension to the face.

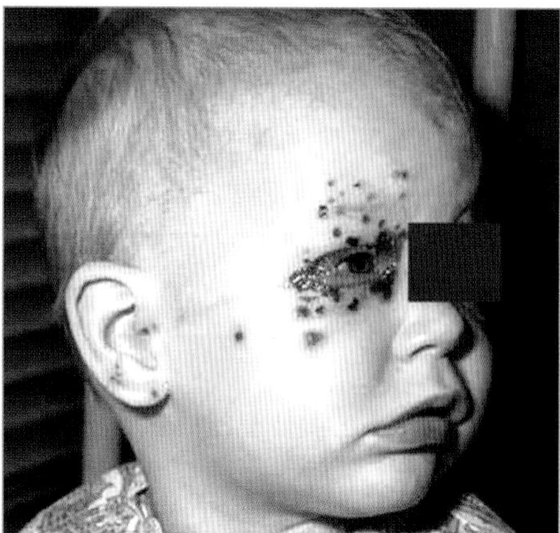

Image 64.9
Recurrent herpes simplex periorbital, ear, and facial vesicles. Copyright Martha Lepow.

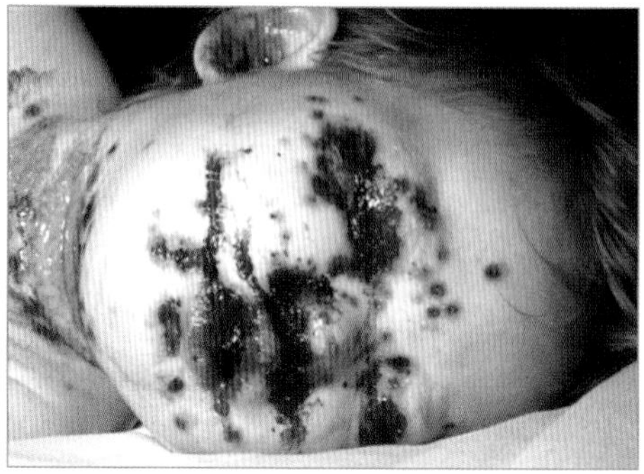

Image 64.11
Herpes simplex infection in a child with eczema with Kaposi varicelliform eruption and Stevens-Johnson syndrome.

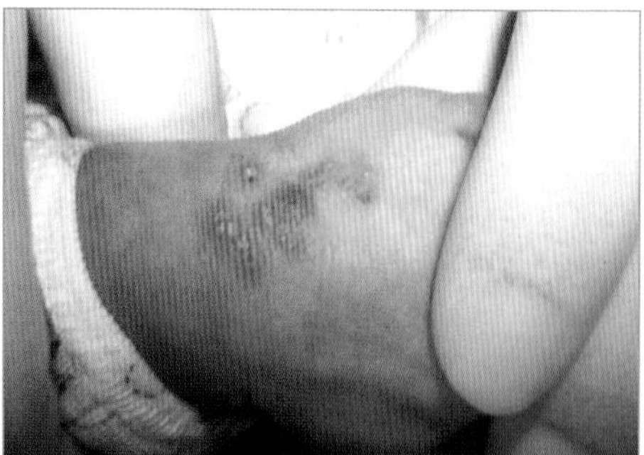

Image 64.13
A neonate born with "sucking blisters" on hand who developed neonatal herpes simplex lesions at the site. The patient responded well while receiving treatment with acyclovir. Copyright Jerri Ann Jenista, MD.

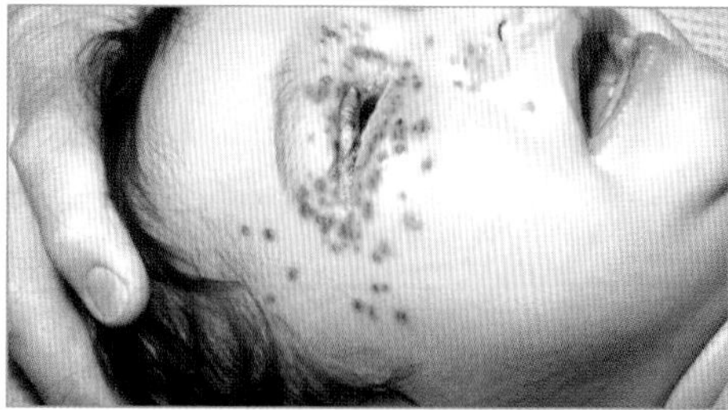

Image 64.10
Recurrent herpes simplex infection of the face, most pronounced in the periorbital area.

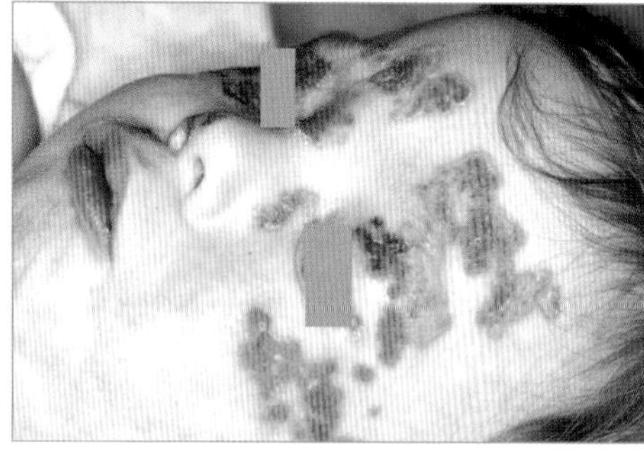

Image 64.12
Eczema herpeticum on the face of a boy with eczema and primary herpetic gingivostomatitis, day 3 to 4 of the onset. The herpetic lesions spread over a period of 2 to 3 days to extensive covering of the skin, and systemic therapy with acyclovir was provided. The patient recovered after a prolonged hospital stay for secondary nosocomial bacterial infections. Copyright Jerri Ann Jenista, MD.

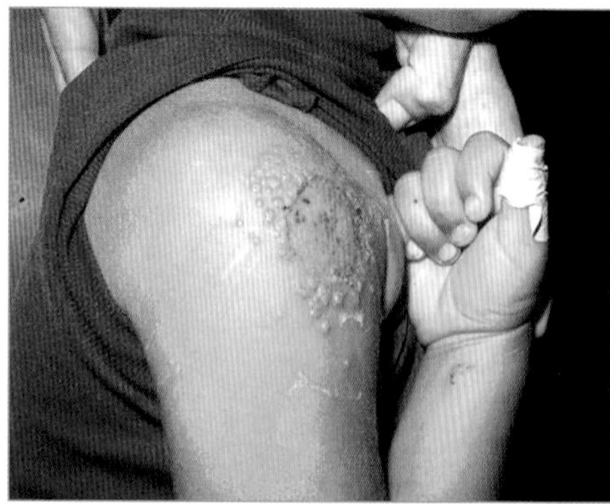

Image 64.14
Herpes simplex infection at a diphtheria, tetanus, and pertussis vaccine injection site reflecting self-inoculation. Courtesy of Edgar O. Ledbetter, MD, FAAP.

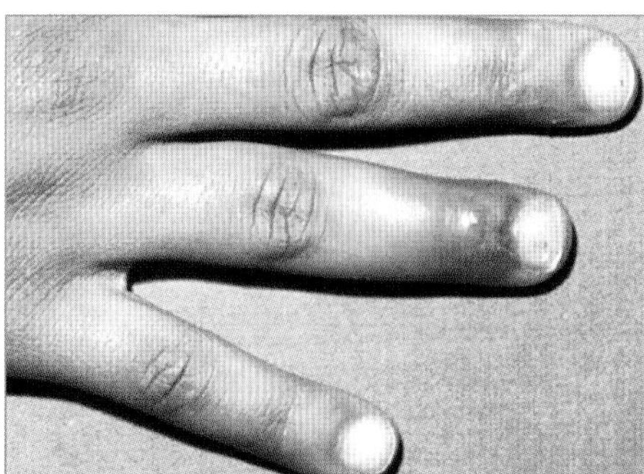

Image 64.15
Herpetic whitlow in a 10-year-old boy with recurrent herpes simplex infection.

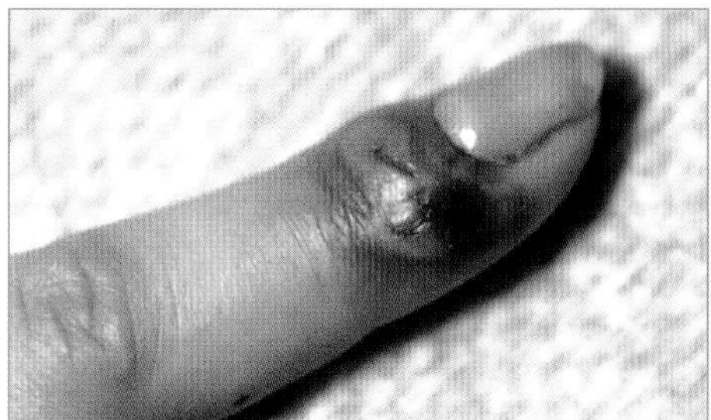

Image 64.16
An adolescent girl with herpetic whitlow secondary to orolabial lesions with self-inoculation. Copyright Martin G. Myers, MD.

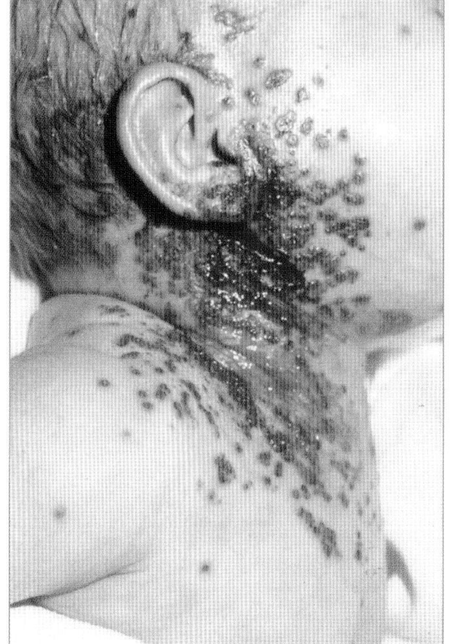

Image 64.17
A 7-month-old boy with eczema and suppurative drainage from otitis media complicated by herpes simplex infection (Kaposi varicelliform eruption). Courtesy of George Nankervis, MD.

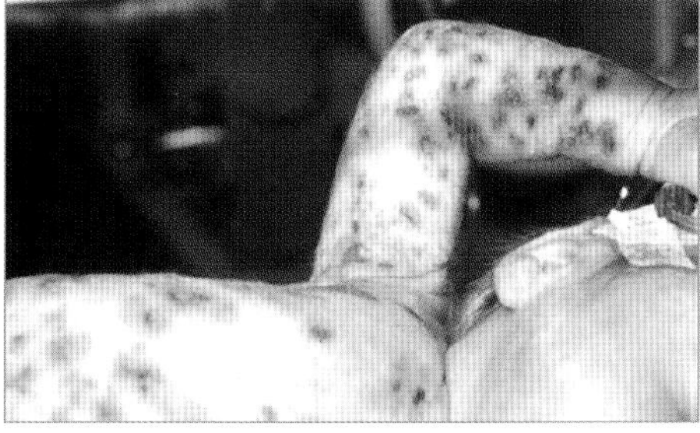

Image 64.18
Neonatal herpes simplex infection with disseminated vesicular lesions.

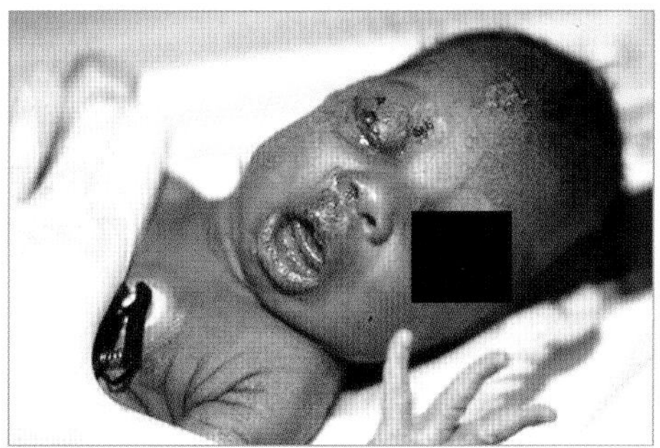

Image 64.19
Neonatal herpes skin lesions of the face. A premature 14-day-old developed vesicular lesions over the right eye and face on days 11 to 14 of life. Herpes simplex virus type 2 was recovered from viral culture of the vesicular fluid. Keratoconjunctivitis was diagnosed by ophthalmology and the neonate was treated with topical antiviral eyedrops in addition to intravenous acyclovir. The neonate was born via a spontaneous vaginal delivery with a vertex presentation. Membranes had ruptured 8 hours prior to delivery. There was no history of genital herpes or fever blisters in either parent. The lesions were concentrated on the face and head, the presenting body parts in delivery. Copyright Barbara Jantausch, MD, FAAP.

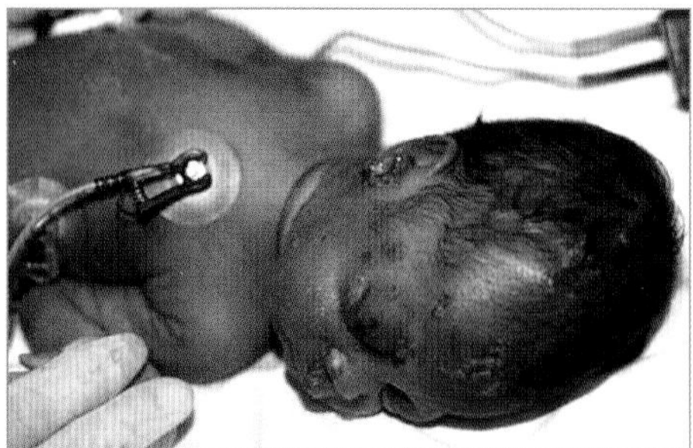

Image 64.20
Neonatal herpes skin lesions of the head and face. This is the same patient as shown in Image 64.19. Copyright Barbara Jantausch, MD, FAAP.

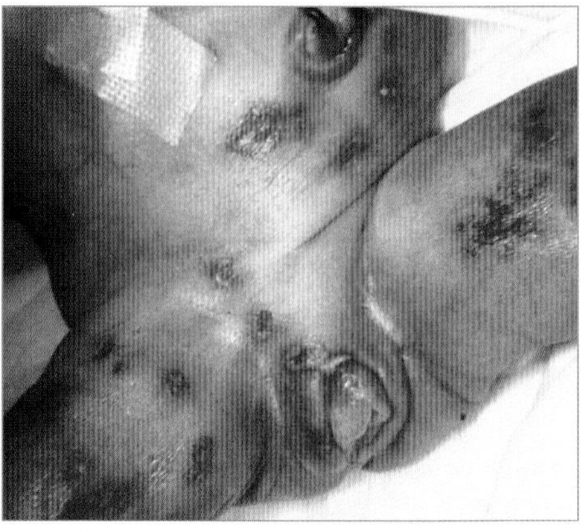

Image 64.21
A 2-hour-old girl with characteristic vesicular and ulcerative lesions below the umbilicus and over the genital area that grew herpes simplex type 1. Courtesy of Neal Halsey, MD.

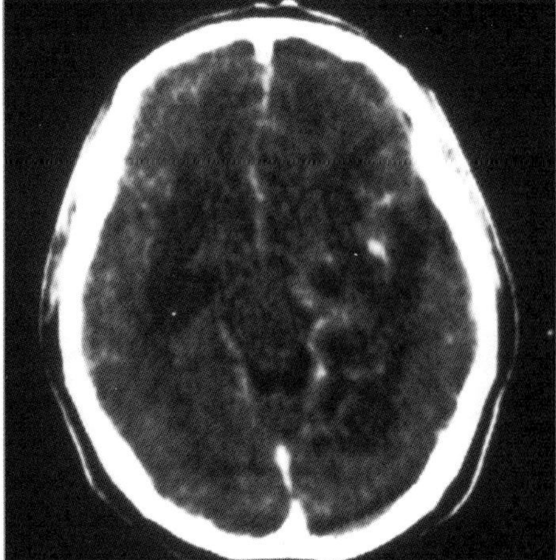

Image 64.22
Computed tomography scan of a patient with herpes simplex encephalitis with temporal lobe changes.

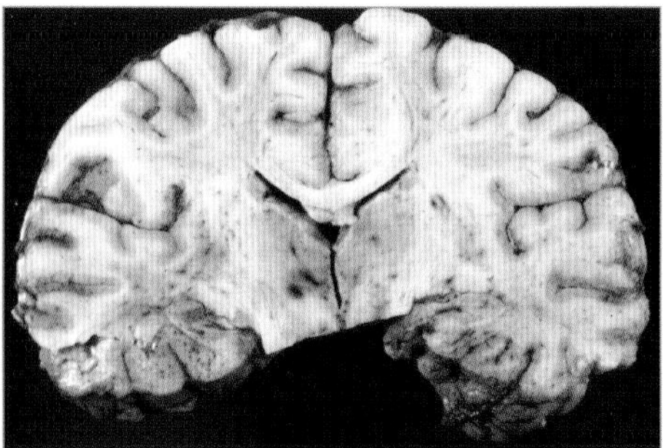

Image 64.23
Postneonatal herpes simplex encephalitis. Hemorrhagic necrosis of the temporal lobes. Courtesy of Dimitris P. Agamanolis, MD.

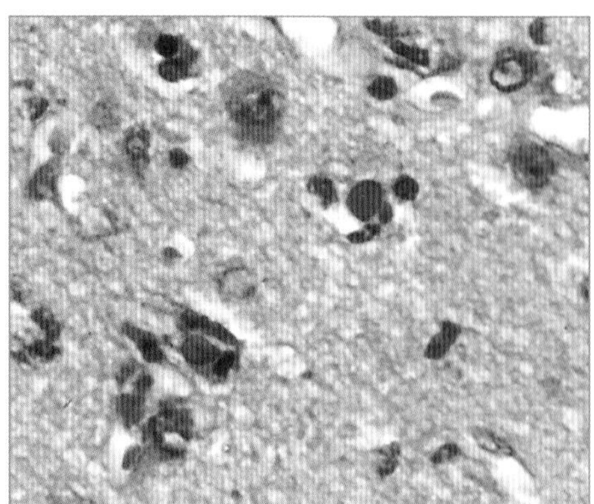

Image 64.24
Herpes simplex encephalitis. Viral intranuclear inclusions. Courtesy of Dimitris P. Agamanolis, MD.

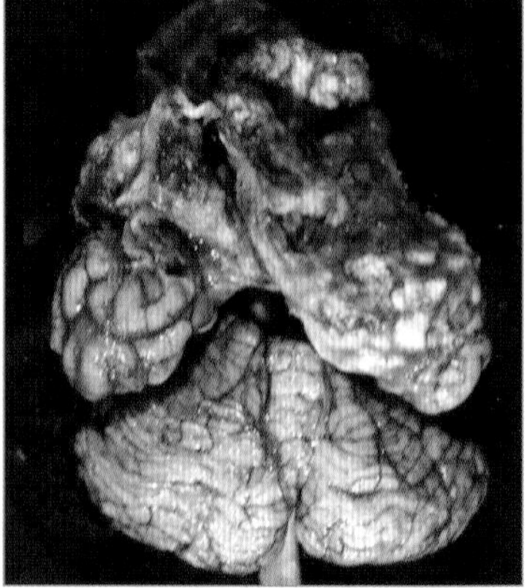

Image 64.25
Burned out neonatal herpes simplex encephalitis. Severe atrophy and distortion of the cerebral hemispheres. Courtesy of Dimitris P. Agamanolis, MD.

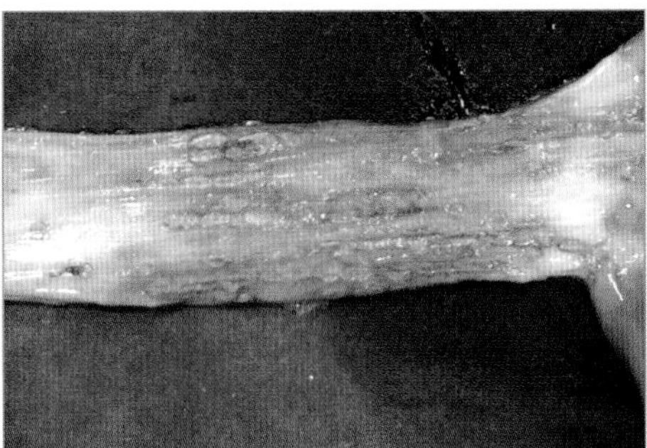

Image 64.26
Herpes simplex esophagitis. Courtesy of Dimitris P. Agamanolis, MD.

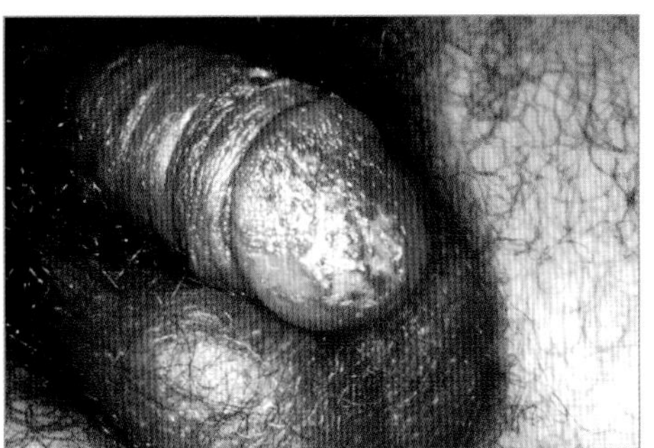

Image 64.27
This male presented with primary vesiculopapular herpes genitalis lesions on his glans penis and penile shaft. When signs of herpes genitalis occur, they typically appear as one or more blisters on or around the genitals or rectum. The blisters break, leaving tender ulcers (sores) that may take 2 to 4 weeks to heal the first time they occur. Courtesy of Centers for Disease Control and Prevention/Dr N. J. Flumara; Dr Gavin Hart.

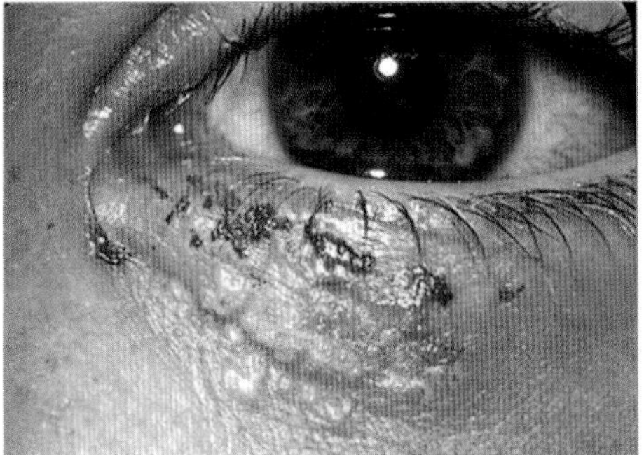

Image 64.28
A 15-year-old white girl with recurrent facial and ocular herpes simplex infection. Courtesy of Larry Frenkel, MD.

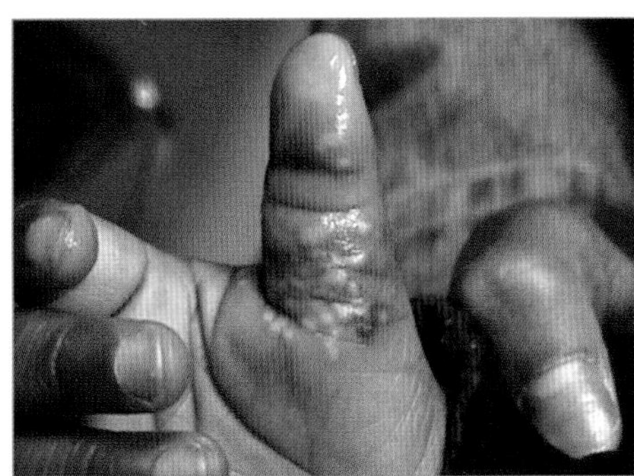

Image 64.29
Herpetic whitlow in a 6-year-old boy with a history of herpes labialis. Courtesy of Benjamin Estrada, MD.

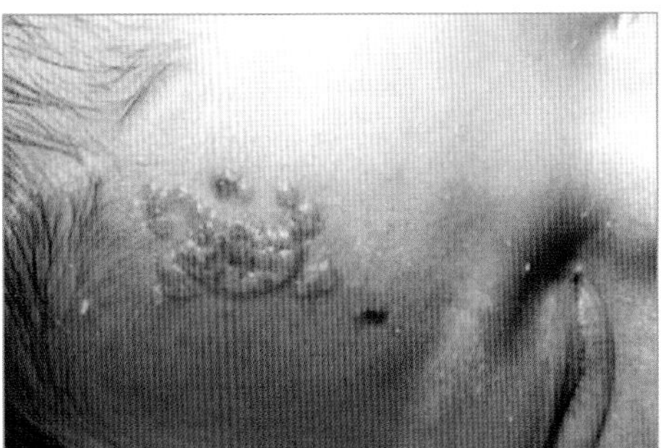

Image 64.30
Herpes simplex infection is characterized by clustered vesicles on an erythematous base. Courtesy of Daniel P. Krowchuk, MD, FAAP.

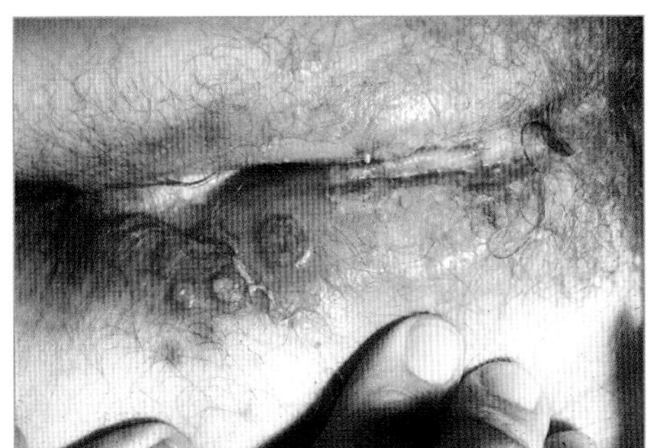

Image 64.31
A 15-year-old girl with a primary herpes simplex infection of the genital area. Courtesy of Larry Frenkel, MD.

65

Histoplasmosis

Clinical Manifestations

Histoplasma capsulatum causes symptoms in fewer than 5% of infected people. Clinical manifestations are classified according to site (pulmonary or disseminated), duration (acute, subacute, or chronic), and pattern (primary or reactivation) of infection. Most symptomatic patients have acute pulmonary histoplasmosis, a self-limited illness characterized by fever, chills, nonproductive cough, and malaise. Typical radiographic finding in mild infections is an area of focal pneumonitis associated with hilar or mediastinal adenopathy; high inoculum exposure can result in diffuse interstitial or reticulonodular pulmonary infiltrates. Most patients recover without treatment 2 to 3 weeks after onset of symptoms. Exposure to a large inoculum of conidia can cause severe pulmonary infection associated with high fevers, hypoxemia, diffuse reticulonodular infiltrates, and acute respiratory distress syndrome. Mediastinal involvement, usually a complication of pulmonary histoplasmosis, includes mediastinal lymphadenitis, which can cause airway encroachment in young children. Inflammatory syndromes (pericarditis and rheumatologic syndromes) can also develop; erythema nodosum can occur in adolescents and adults. Primary cutaneous infections after trauma are rare. Chronic cavitary pulmonary histoplasmosis is extremely rare in children.

Disseminated histoplasmosis can be self-limited or progressive. Progressive disseminated histoplasmosis (PDH) can occur in otherwise healthy infants and children younger than 2 years or in older children with primary or acquired cellular immune dysfunction. Progressive disseminated histoplasmosis can be a rapidly progressive illness following acute infection or can be a more chronic, slowly progressive disease. Progressive disseminated histoplasmosis in adults occurs most often in people with underlying immune deficiency (eg, HIV/AIDS, solid organ transplant, hematologic malignancy, biologic response modifiers including tumor necrosis factor antagonists) or in people older than 65 years. Early manifestations of PDH in children include prolonged fever, failure to thrive, and hepatosplenomegaly; if untreated, malnutrition, diffuse adenopathy, pneumonitis, mucosal ulceration, pancytopenia, disseminated intravascular coagulopathy, and gastrointestinal tract bleeding can ensue. Central nervous system involvement is common. Chronic PDH generally occurs in adults with immune suppression and is characterized by prolonger fever, night sweats, weight loss, and fatigue; signs include hepatosplenomegaly, mucosal ulcerations, adrenal insufficiency, and pancytopenia. Clinicians should be alert to the risk of disseminated endemic mycoses in patients receiving tumor necrosis factor-α antagonists and disease-modifying antirheumatic drugs.

Etiology

H capsulatum var *capsulatum* is a thermally dimorphic, endemic fungus that grows in the environment as a microconidia-bearing mold but converts to its yeast phase at 37°C (98.6°F). *H capsulatum* var *duboisii* is the cause of African histoplasmosis and is found only in central and western Africa.

Epidemiology

H capsulatum is encountered in most parts of the world (including Africa, the Americas, Asia, and Europe) and is highly endemic in the central United States, particularly the Mississippi, Ohio, and Missouri river valleys. Infection is acquired following inhalation of conidia that are aerosolized by disturbance of soil or abandoned structures contaminated with bat guano or bird droppings. The inoculum size, strain virulence, and immune status of the host affect the severity of the ensuing illness. Infections occur sporadically, in outbreaks when weather conditions (dry and windy) predispose to spread of conidia, or in point-source epidemics after exposure to activities that disturb contaminated sites. In regions with endemic disease, recreational and occupational activities, such as playing in hollow trees, caving, construction, excavation, demolition, farming, and cleaning of contaminated buildings, have been associated with outbreaks. Person-to-person transmission does not occur. Prior infection confers partial immunity; reinfection can occur but requires a larger inoculum.

Incubation Period

Variable; usually 1 to 3 weeks.

Diagnostic Tests

Culture is the definitive method of diagnosis. *H capsulatum* organisms from bone marrow, blood, sputum, and tissue specimens grow on standard mycologic media in 1 to 6 weeks. The lysis-centrifugation method is preferred for blood cultures. A DNA probe for *H capsulatum* permits rapid identification of cultured isolates. Demonstration of typical intracellular yeast forms by examination with Gomori methenamine silver or other stains of tissue, blood, bone marrow, or bronchoalveolar lavage specimens strongly supports the diagnosis of histoplasmosis when clinical, epidemiologic, and other laboratory studies are compatible.

Detection of *H capsulatum* antigen in serum, urine, bronchoalveolar lavage fluid, or cerebrospinal fluid using a quantitative immunoassay is possible with a rapid, commercially available diagnostic test. Antigen detection in blood and urine specimens is most sensitive for severe, acute pulmonary infections and for progressive disseminated infections. Results are often transiently positive early in the course of acute, self-limited pulmonary infections. A negative test result does not exclude infection. If the result is initially positive, the antigen test is also useful for monitoring treatment response and, thereafter, promptly identifying relapse or reexposure to *H capsulatum* conidia. Cross-reactions occur in patients with blastomycosis, coccidioidomycosis, paracoccidioidomycosis, and penicilliosis; clinical and epidemiologic distinctions aid in differentiating these entities.

Serologic testing is available and is most useful in patients with subacute or chronic pulmonary disease. A 4-fold increase in yeast-phase or mycelial-phase complement fixation titers or a single titer of 1:32 or greater in either test is strong presumptive evidence of active or recent infection in patients exposed to or residing within regions of endemicity. Cross-reacting antibodies can result from *Aspergillus* species, *Blastomyces dermatitidis*, and *Coccidioides* species infections. The immunodiffusion test is more specific than the complement fixation test, but the complement fixation test is more sensitive.

Treatment

Immunocompetent children with uncomplicated or mild-to-moderate acute pulmonary histoplasmosis may not require antifungal therapy because infection is usually self-limited. However, if the patient does not improve within 4 weeks, itraconazole should be given for 6 to 12 weeks.

For severe or disseminated infections, a lipid formulation of amphotericin B followed by itraconazole is recommended. Itraconazole is preferred over other azoles by most experts. Although safety and efficacy of itraconazole for use in children have not been established, anecdotal experience has found it to be well tolerated and effective. Serum trough concentrations of itraconazole should be 1 or greater but less than 10 mcg/mL. Concentrations should be checked after 2 weeks of therapy to ensure adequate drug exposure.

For severe, acute pulmonary infections, treatment with a lipid formulation of amphotericin B is recommended for 1 to 2 weeks. After clinical improvement occurs, itraconazole is recommended for an additional 12 weeks. Methylprednisolone during the first 1 to 2 weeks of therapy may be considered if severe respiratory complications develop.

All patients with chronic pulmonary histoplasmosis should be treated. Mild to moderate cases should be treated with itraconazole for 1 to 2 years. Severe cases should be treated initially with a lipid formulation amphotericin B followed by itraconazole for the same duration.

Mediastinal and inflammatory manifestations of infection generally do not need to be treated with antifungal agents. However, mediastinal adenitis that causes obstruction of a bronchus, the esophagus, or another mediastinal structure may improve with a brief course of corticosteroids. In these instances, itraconazole should be used concurrently and continued for 6 to 12 weeks. Dense fibrosis of mediastinal structures without an associated granulomatous inflammatory component does not respond to antifungal therapy, and surgical intervention may be necessary for severe cases. Pericarditis and rheumatologic syndromes may respond to treatment with nonsteroidal anti-inflammatory agents.

For treatment of moderately severe to severe PDH in an infant or child, a lipid formulation of amphotericin B is the drug of choice and is usually given for a minimum of 2 weeks. When the child has demonstrated substantial clinical improvement and a decline in the serum concentration of *Histoplasma* antigen, oral itraconazole is administered for 12 weeks. Prolonged therapy for up to 12 months may be required for patients with severe disease, primary immunodeficiency syndromes, or acquired immunodeficiency that cannot be reversed, or patients who experience relapse despite appropriate therapy.

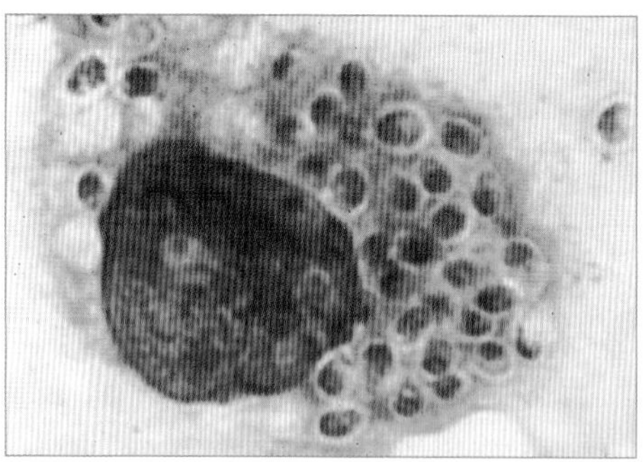

Image 65.1
Pulmonary histiocyte containing numerous yeast cells of *Histoplasma capsulatum*. Courtesy of Centers for Disease Control and Prevention/ Dr J.T. McClellan, Lexington, KY.

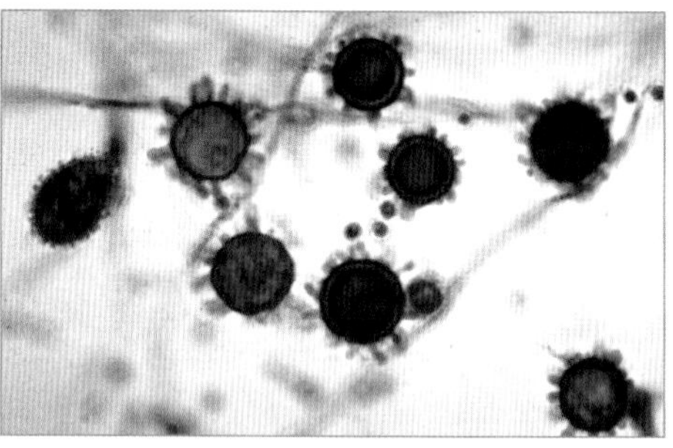

Image 65.2
Asexual spores (conidia). Tuberculate macroconidia of *Histoplasma capsulatum* (toluidine blue stain). Microconidia are also present. Courtesy of Centers for Disease Control and Prevention.

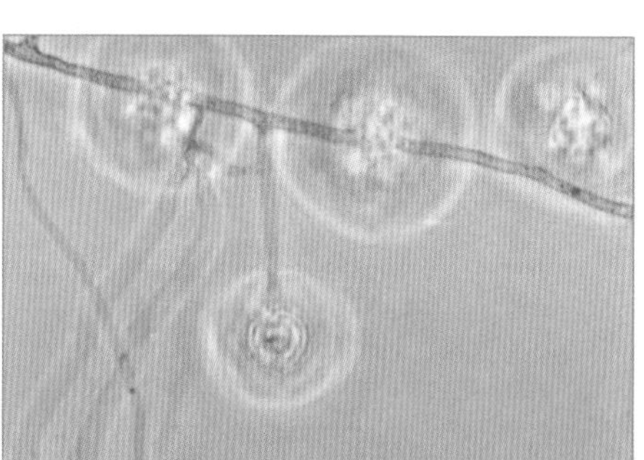

Image 65.3
This photomicrograph reveals a conidiophore of the fungus *Histoplasma capsulatum*. *H capsulatum* grows in soil and material contaminated with bat or bird droppings. Spores become airborne when contaminated soil is disturbed. Breathing the spores causes pulmonary histoplasmosis. Courtesy of Centers for Disease Control and Prevention/Libero Ajello, MD.

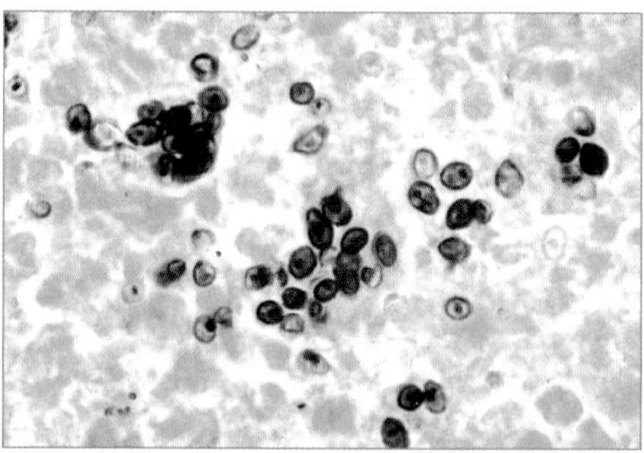

Image 65.4
Methenamine silver stain reveals *Histoplasma capsulatum* fungi. Courtesy of Centers for Disease Control and Prevention.

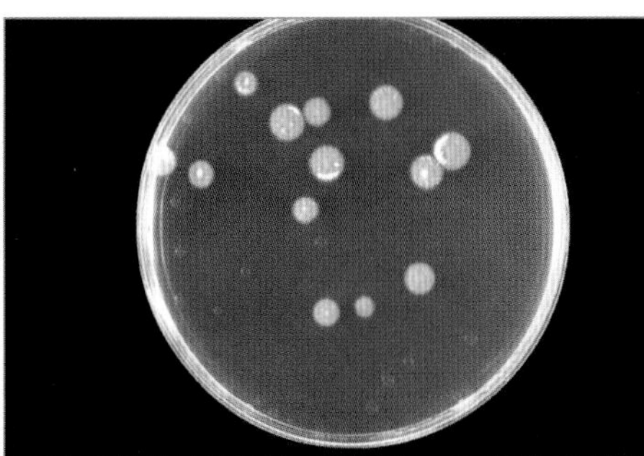

Image 65.5
Pictured is a Sabhi agar plate culture of the fungus *Histoplasma capsulatum* grown at 20°C (68°F). Positive histoplasmin skin tests occur in as many as 80% of the people living in areas where *H capsulatum* is common, such as the eastern and central United States. Courtesy of Centers for Disease Control and Prevention/Dr William Kaplan.

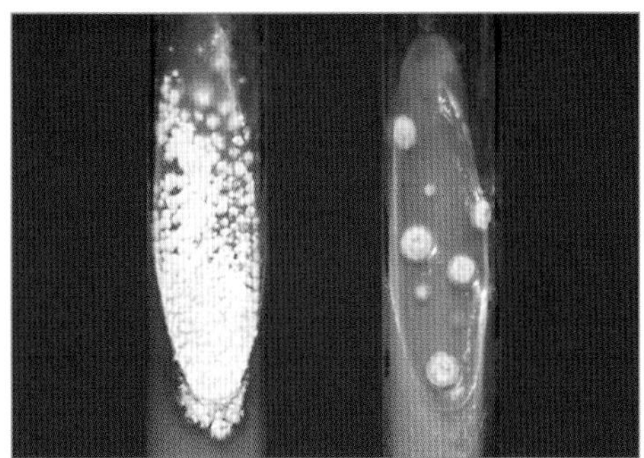

Image 65.6
These 2 slant cultures grew *Histoplasma capsulatum* colonies (left tube: Sabouraud agar; right tube: Sabhi agar). *H capsulatum* is the most common cause of fungal respiratory infections globally. While most infections are mild, 10% of cases can be life-threatening, such as inflammation of the pericardium and fibrosis of major blood vessels. Courtesy of Centers for Disease Control and Prevention.

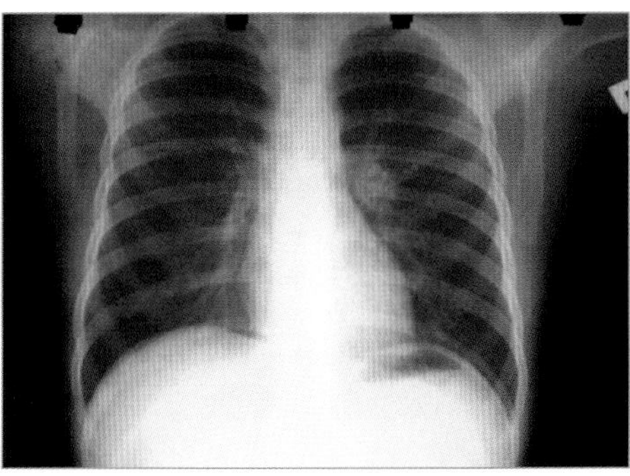

Image 65.7
A 10-year-old boy with calcified left hilar lymph nodes secondary to histoplasmosis.

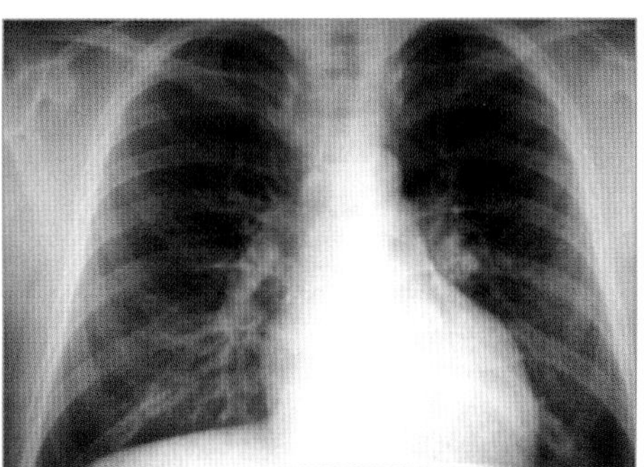

Image 65.8
A preadolescent with calcified left hilar lymph nodes bilaterally secondary to histoplasmosis.

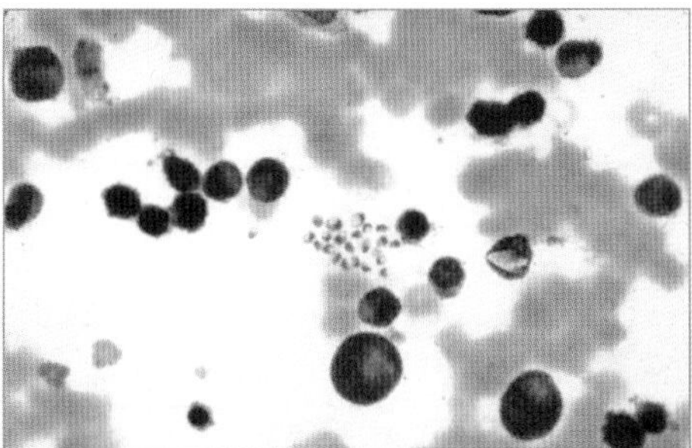

Image 65.9
Histoplasma capsulatum in peripheral blood smear. Copyright Martha Lepow.

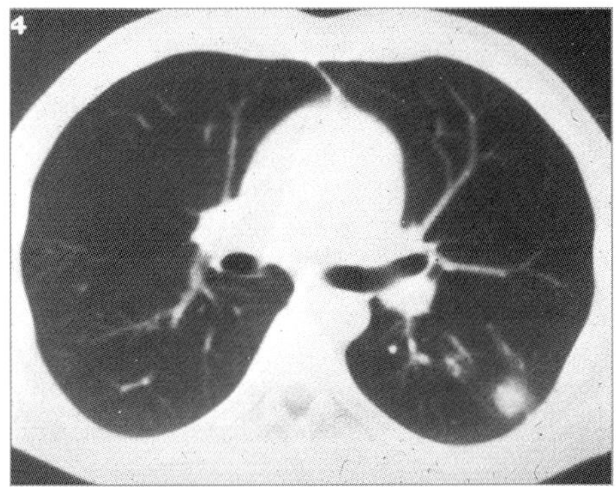

Image 65.10
Computed tomography scan showing single pulmonary nodule of histoplasmosis. Courtesy of Centers for Disease Control and Prevention.

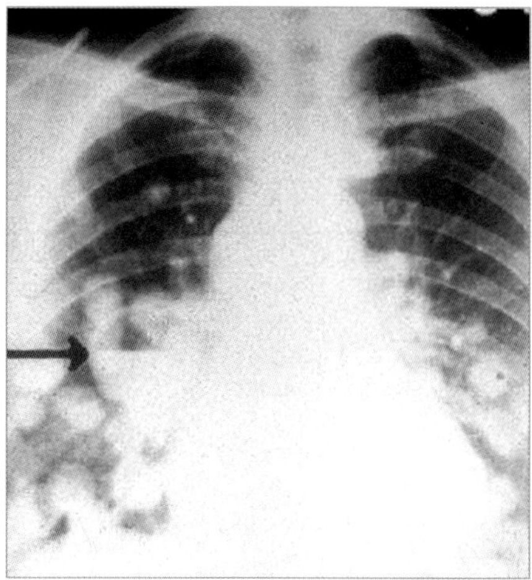

Image 65.11
Chest radiograph showing miliary densities in both lung fields plus a thin-walled cavity with a fluid level. Copyright American Society for Clinical Pathology.

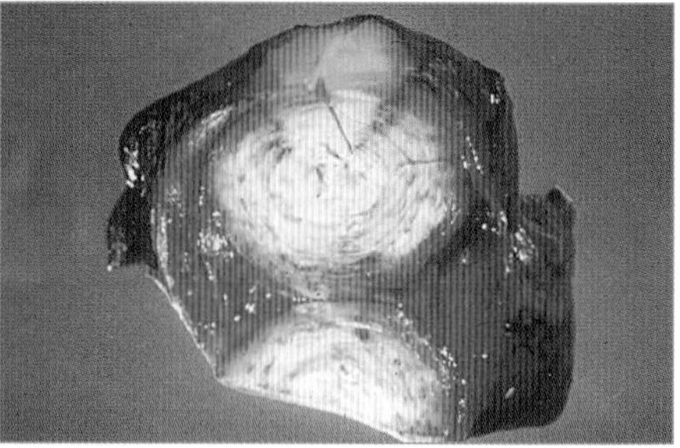

Image 65.12
Gross pathology specimen of lung showing cut surface of fibrocaseous nodule due to *Histoplasma capsulatum*. Copyright American Society for Clinical Pathology.

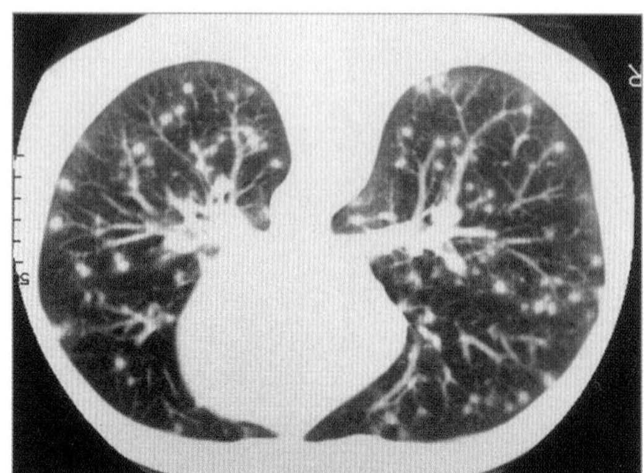

Image 65.13
Computed tomography scan of lungs showing classic snowstorm appearance of acute histoplasmosis. Courtesy of Centers for Disease Control and Prevention.

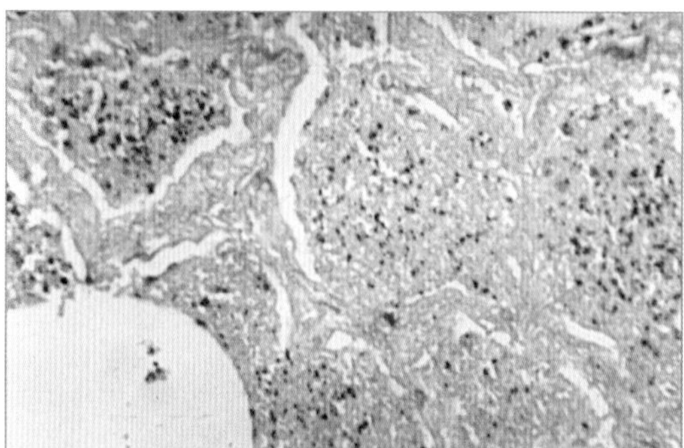

Image 65.14
This partially calcified fibrocaseous nodule depicts the histopathologic changes associated with histoplasmosis of the lung. Courtesy of Centers for Disease Control and Prevention/Martin Hicklin, MD.

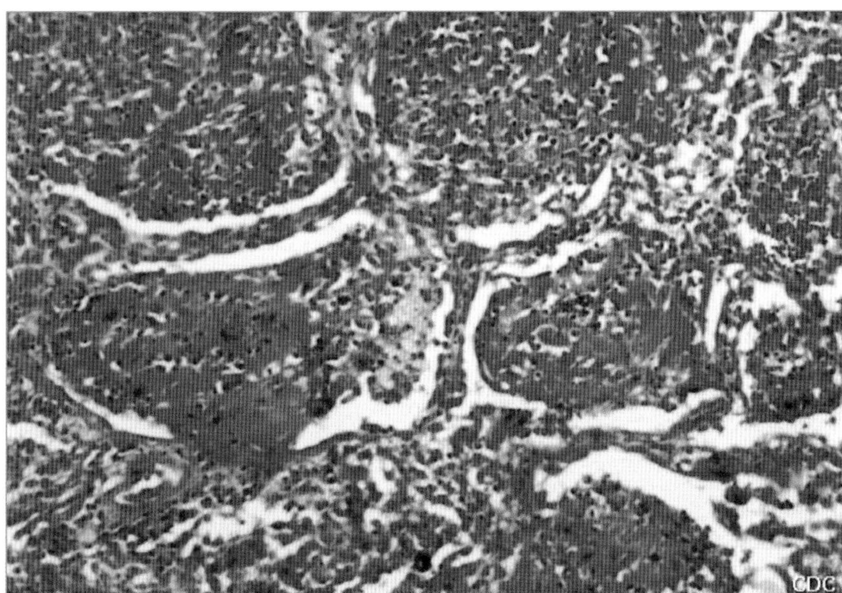

Image 65.15
This micrograph depicts the histopathologic changes associated with histoplasmosis of the lung. Courtesy of Centers for Disease Control and Prevention/Martin Hicklin, MD.

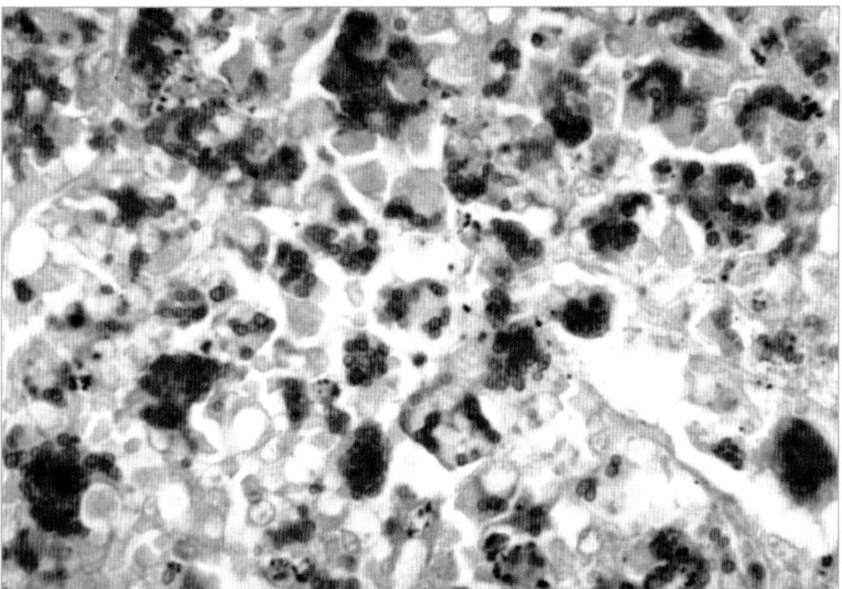

Image 65.16
This micrograph depicts the histopathologic changes associated with histoplasmosis of the spleen (Gridley stain). Courtesy of Centers for Disease Control and Prevention/Martin Hicklin, MD.

66

Hookworm Infections

(*Ancylostoma duodenale* and *Necator americanus*)

Clinical Manifestations

Patients with hookworm infection are often asymptomatic; however, chronic hookworm infection is a common cause of moderate to severe hypochromic, microcytic anemia in people living in tropical developing countries, and heavy infestation can cause hypoproteinemia with edema. Chronic hookworm infection in children can lead to physical growth delay, deficits in cognition, and developmental delay. After contact with contaminated soil, initial skin penetration of larvae, often involving the feet, can cause a stinging or burning sensation followed by pruritus and a papulovesicular rash that may persist for 1 to 2 weeks. Pneumonitis associated with migrating larvae (Löffler-like syndrome) is uncommon and usually mild, except in heavy infections. Colicky abdominal pain, nausea, diarrhea, and marked eosinophilia can develop 4 to 6 weeks after exposure. Blood loss secondary to hookworm infection develops 10 to 12 weeks after initial infection, and symptoms related to serious iron deficiency anemia can develop in long-standing moderate or heavy hookworm infections. Pharyngeal itching, hoarseness, nausea, and vomiting can develop shortly after oral ingestion of infectious *Ancylostoma duodenale* larvae.

Etiology

Necator americanus is the major cause of hookworm infection worldwide, although *A duodenale* is also an important hookworm in some regions. Mixed infections can also occur. Both are roundworms (nematodes) with similar life cycles.

Epidemiology

Humans are the only reservoir. Hookworms are prominent in rural, tropical, and subtropical areas where soil contamination with human feces is common. Although the prevalence of both hookworm species is equal in many areas, *A duodenale* is the predominant species in the Mediterranean region, northern Asia, and selected foci of South America. *N americanus* is predominant in the western hemisphere, sub-Saharan Africa, Southeast Asia, and a number of Pacific islands. Larvae and eggs survive in loose, sandy, moist, shady, well-aerated, warm soil (optimal temperature 23°C–33°C [73°F–91°F]). Hookworm eggs from stool hatch in soil in 1 to 2 days as rhabditiform larvae. These larvae develop into infective filariform larvae in soil within 5 to 7 days and can persist for 3 to 4 weeks. Percutaneous infection occurs after exposure to infectious larvae. *A duodenale* transmission can occur by oral ingestion and, possibly, through human milk. Untreated infected patients can harbor worms for 5 years or longer.

Incubation Period

The time from exposure to development of noncutaneous symptoms is 4 to 12 weeks.

Diagnostic Tests

Microscopic demonstration of hookworm eggs in feces is diagnostic. Adult worms or larvae are rarely seen. Approximately 5 to 8 weeks are required after infection for eggs to appear in feces. A direct stool smear with saline solution or potassium iodide saturated with iodine is adequate for diagnosis of heavy hookworm infection; light infections require concentration techniques. Quantification techniques (eg, Kato test, Beaver direct smear, or Stoll egg-counting techniques) to determine the clinical significance of infection and the response to treatment may be available from state or reference laboratories.

Treatment

Albendazole, mebendazole, and pyrantel pamoate are all effective treatments. In 1-year-olds, the World Health Organization recommends reducing the albendazole dose to half of that given to older children and adults. Reexamination of stool specimens 2 weeks after therapy to determine whether worms have been eliminated is helpful for assessing response to therapy. Retreatment is indicated for persistent infection. Nutritional supplementation, including iron, is important when severe anemia is present. Severely affected children may also require blood transfusion.

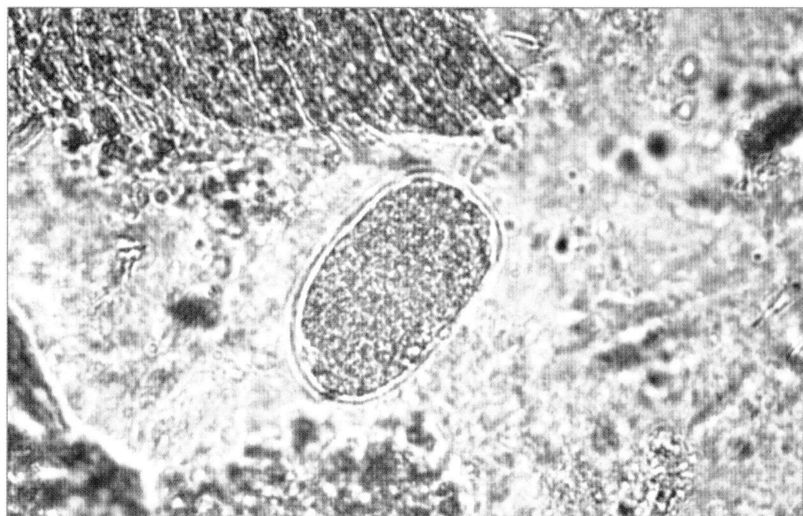

Image 66.1
Hookworm (*Necator americanus*) ova in stool preparation.

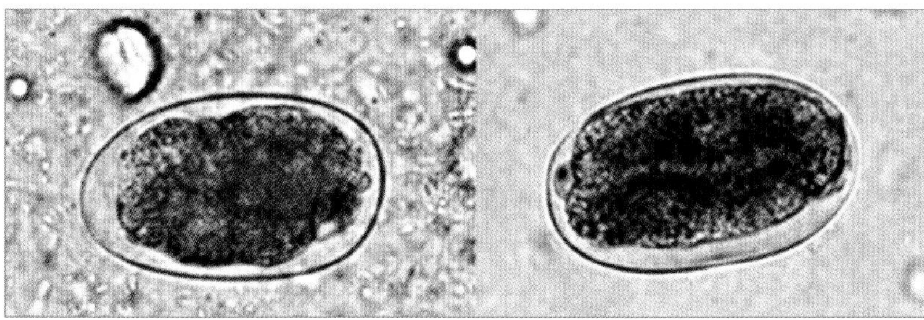

Image 66.2
Hookworm eggs examined on wet mount (eggs of *Ancylostoma duodenale* and *Necator americanus* cannot be distinguished morphologically). Diagnostic characteristics: 57 to 76 μm by 35 to 47 μm, oval or ellipsoidal, thin shell. The embryo (right) has begun cellular division and is at an early developmental stage (gastrula). Courtesy of Centers for Disease Control and Prevention.

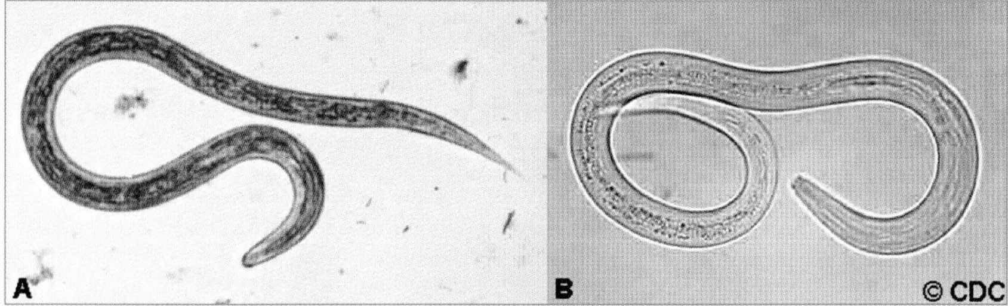

Image 66.3
Hookworm filariform larva (wet preparation). Courtesy of Centers for Disease Control and Prevention/ Dr Mae Melvin.

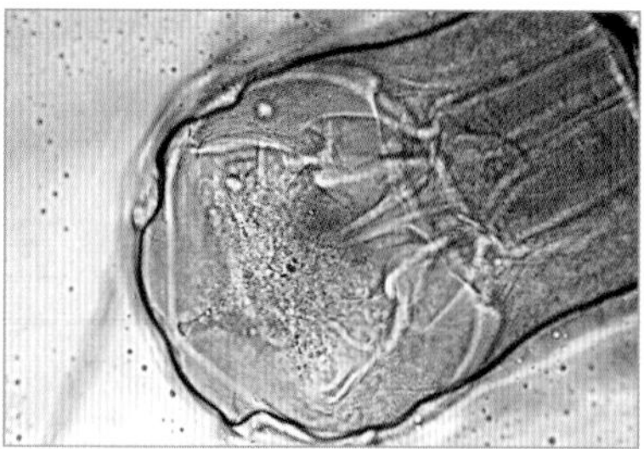

Image 66.4
This micrograph reveals the head of the hookworm *Necator americanus* and its mouth's cutting plates (magnification x400). The hookworm uses these sharp cutting teeth to grasp firmly to the intestinal wall and, while remaining fastened in place, ingests the host's blood, obtaining its nutrients in this fashion. Courtesy of Centers for Disease Control and Prevention/ Dr Mae Melvin.

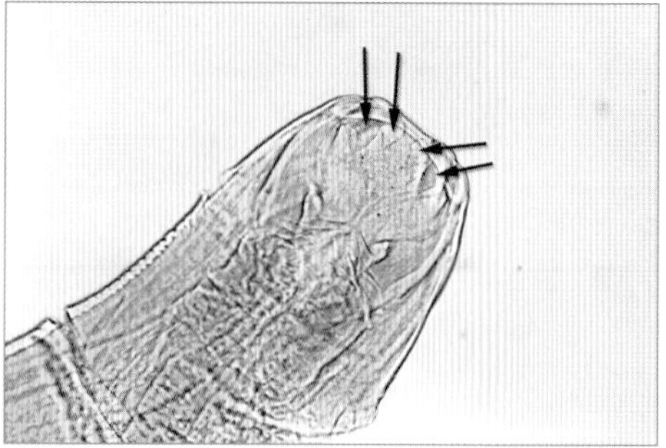

Image 66.5
This unstained micrograph reveals the *Ancylostoma duodenale* hookworm's mouth parts (magnification x125). Courtesy of Centers for Disease Control and Prevention/Dr Mae Melvin.

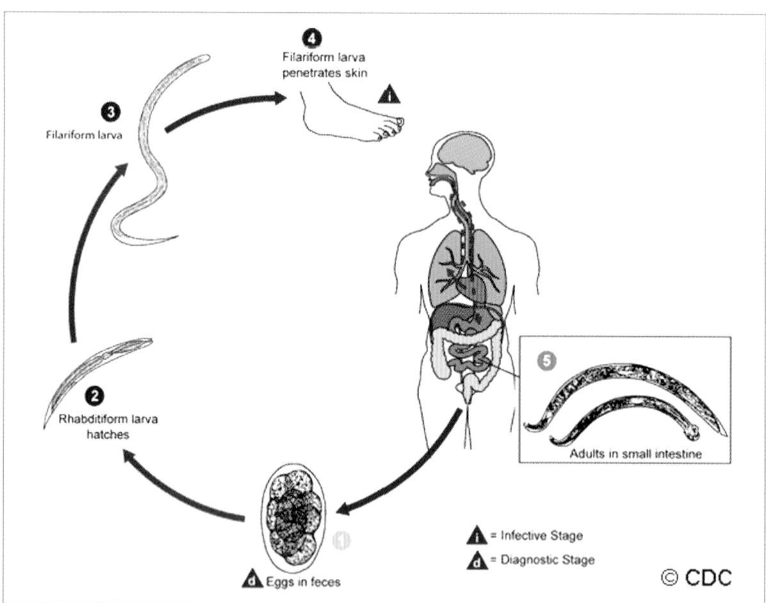

Image 66.6
Eggs are passed in the stool (1) and, under favorable conditions (moisture, warmth, shade), larvae hatch in 1 to 2 days. The released rhabditiform larvae grow in the feces or the soil (2), and, after 5 to 10 days (and 2 molts), they become filariform (third-stage) larvae that are infective (3). These infective larvae can survive 3 to 4 weeks in favorable environmental conditions. On contact with the human host, the larvae penetrate the skin and are carried through the veins to the heart and then to the lungs. They penetrate into the pulmonary alveoli, ascend the bronchial tree to the pharynx, and are swallowed (4). The larvae reach the small intestine, where they reside and mature into adults. Adult worms live in the lumen of the small intestine, where they attach to the intestinal wall with resultant blood loss by the host (5). Most adult worms are eliminated in 1 to 2 years, but longevity records can reach several years. Some *Ancylostoma duodenale* larvae, following penetration of the host skin, can become dormant (in the intestine or muscle). In addition, infection by *A duodenale* may also occur by the oral and transmammary route. *Necator americanus,* however, requires a transpulmonary migration phase. Courtesy of Centers for Disease Control and Prevention.

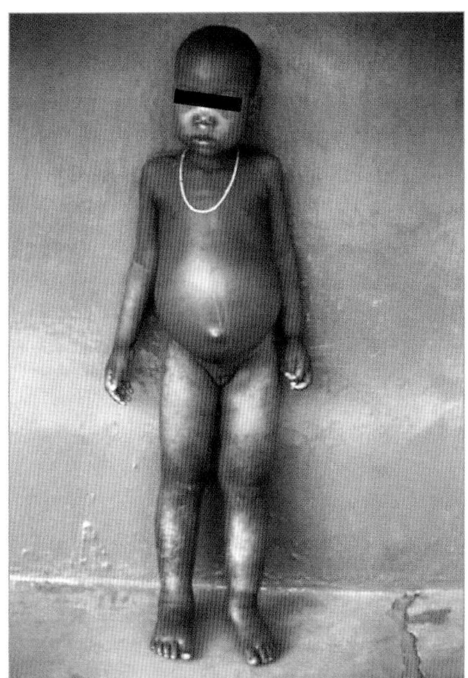

Image 66.7
This child with hookworm shows visible signs of edema and was diagnosed with anemia as well. Courtesy of Centers for Disease Control and Prevention/Dr Myron Schultz.

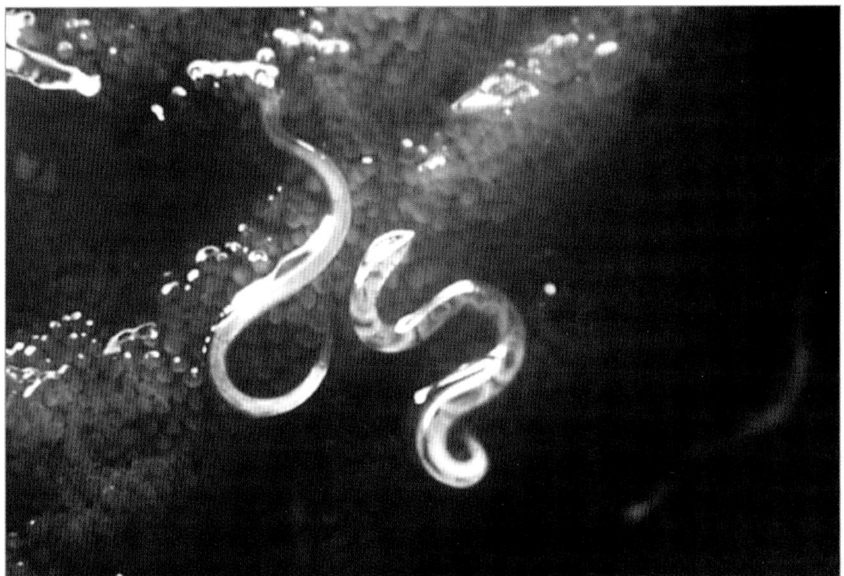

Image 66.8
This enlargement shows hookworms, *Ancylostoma caninum,* attached to the intestinal mucosa. Barely visible larvae penetrate the skin (often through bare feet), are carried to the lungs, go through the respiratory tract to the mouth, are swallowed, and eventually reach the small intestine. This journey takes about a week. Courtesy of Centers for Disease Control and Prevention.

67

Human Herpesvirus 6 (Including Roseola) and 7

Clinical Manifestations

Clinical manifestations of primary infection with human herpesvirus 6 (HHV-6) include roseola (exanthem subitum) in approximately 20% of infected children, with the other 80% having an undifferentiated febrile illness without rash or localizing signs. Human herpesvirus 6 infection is often accompanied by cervical and characteristic occipital lymphadenopathy, gastrointestinal tract or respiratory tract signs, and inflamed tympanic membranes. Fever is usually high (temperature >39.5°C [103.0°F]) and persists for 3 to 7 days. Approximately 20% of all emergency department visits for febrile children 6 through 12 months of age are attributable to HHV-6. Roseola is distinguished by the erythematous maculopapular rash that appears once fever resolves and can last hours to days. Febrile seizures, sometimes leading to status epilepticus, are the most common complication and reason for hospitalization among children with primary HHV-6 infection. Approximately 10% to 15% of children develop febrile seizures, predominantly between the ages of 6 and 18 months. Other neurologic manifestations that can accompany primary infection include a bulging fontanelle and encephalopathy or encephalitis. Hepatitis is a rare manifestation. Approximately 5% of mononucleosis cases are attributable to HHV-6. Congenital HHV-6 infection, which occurs in approximately 1% of newborns, has not been linked to any clinical disease.

The clinical manifestations occurring with human herpesvirus 7 (HHV-7) infections are indistinct. Most primary infections are asymptomatic or mild. Some initial infections can present as typical roseola and may account for second or recurrent cases of roseola. Febrile illnesses associated with seizures have also been documented to occur during primary HHV-7 infection. Some investigators suggest the association of HHV-7 with these clinical manifestations results from the ability of HHV-7 to reactivate latent HHV-6.

Following primary infection, HHV-6 and HHV-7 remain latent and can reactivate. The clinical circumstances and manifestations of reactivation in healthy people are unclear. Illness associated with HHV-6 reactivation has been described primarily among recipients of solid organ and hematopoietic stem cell transplants. Among the clinical findings associated with HHV-6 reactivation in these patients are fever, rash, hepatitis, bone marrow suppression, graft rejection, pneumonia, and encephalitis. A few cases with central nervous system symptoms have been reported in association with HHV-7 reactivation in immunocompromised hosts, but clinical findings are less frequently with HHV-7 than with HHV-6 reactivation.

Etiology

Human herpesviruses 6 and 7 are lymphotropic agents that are closely related members of the Herpesviridae family, subfamily Betaherpesvirinae. Among the human herpesviruses, HHV-6 and HHV-7 are most closely related to cytomegalovirus. Human herpesviruses 6 and 7 establish lifelong infection after initial exposure. There are 2 species of HHV-6, HHV-6A and HHV-6B. Essentially all primary infections in children are caused by HHV-6B, except infections in some parts of Africa. Among congenital HHV-6 infections, however, as many as one-third may be caused by HHV-6A.

Epidemiology

Human herpesviruses 6 and 7 cause ubiquitous infections in children worldwide. Humans are the only natural host. Nearly all children acquire HHV-6 infection within the first 2 years of life, probably resulting from asymptomatic shedding of infectious virus in secretions of a healthy family member or other close contact. During the acute phase of primary infection, HHV-6 and HHV-7 can be isolated from peripheral blood mononuclear cells and from saliva of some children. Viral DNA subsequently can be detected throughout life by polymerase chain reaction assay in multiple body sites. Although HHV-6 and HHV-7 can be detected in blood mononuclear cells, salivary glands, lung, and skin, only HHV-6 is found in brain and only HHV-7 is found in mammary glands. Virus-specific maternal antibody, which is uniformly present in the sera of neonates at birth, provides transient partial protection. As maternal antibody concentration decreases during the first year of life, the infection rate increases rapidly, peaking between 6 and 24 months of age. Essentially all children are seropositive for HHV-6 by 4 years of age. Infections occur throughout the year. Occasional outbreaks of roseola occur.

Human herpesvirus 7 infection usually occurs later in childhood than HHV-6 infection. The seroprevalence of HHV-7 is approximately 85% in adults. Contact with infected respiratory tract secretions of healthy people is the probable mode of transmission of HHV-7 to young children. Human herpesvirus 7 has been detected in human milk, peripheral blood mononuclear cells, cervical secretions, and other body sites. Congenital HHV-7 infection has not been demonstrated by the examination of large numbers of cord blood samples for HHV-7 DNA.

Incubation Period

For HHV-6, 9 to 10 days; for HHV-7, unknown.

Diagnostic Tests

Multiple assays for detection of HHV-6 and HHV-7 have been developed, but few are available commercially, and many do not differentiate between new, past, and reactivated infection. These tests have limited utility in clinical practice.

Serologic tests include immunofluorescent antibody, neutralization, immunoblot, and enzyme immunoassays. A 4-fold increase in serum antibody concentration alone does not necessarily indicate new infection because an increase in titer may also occur with reactivation and in association with other infections, especially other Betaherpesvirinae infections. Detection of specific immunoglobulin (Ig) M antibody is not reliable for diagnosing new infection. These antibody assays do not differentiate HHV-6A from HHV-6B infections. Reference laboratories offer diagnostic testing for HHV-6 and HHV-7 infections by detection of viral DNA in blood and cerebrospinal fluid specimens. However, detection of HHV-6 DNA or HHV-7 DNA in peripheral blood mononuclear cells, other body fluids, and tissues generally does not differentiate between new infection and persistence of virus from past infection.

Treatment

Supportive.

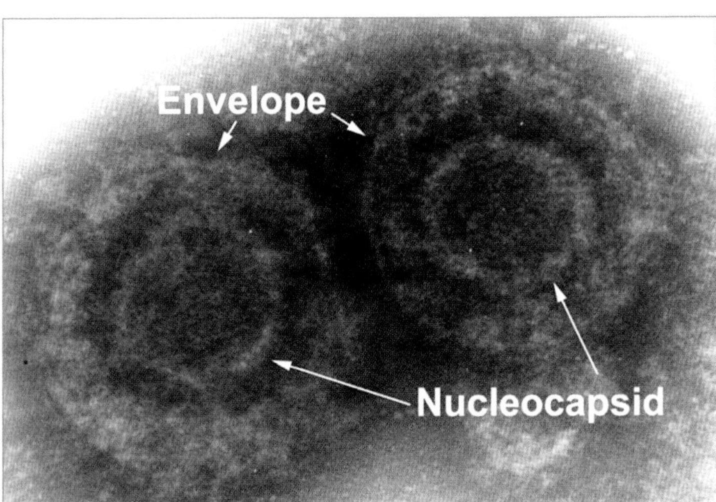

Image 67.1
Thin-section electron micrograph image of human herpesvirus 7, which, like human herpesvirus 6, can cause roseola. Virions consist of a darkly staining core within the capsid that is surrounded by a proteinaceous tegument layer and enclosed within the viral envelope. Courtesy of Centers for Disease Control and Prevention.

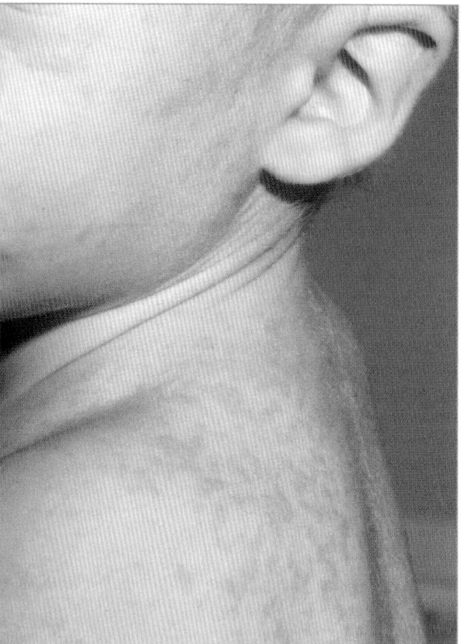

Image 67.2
A 13-month-old white boy developed high fever that persisted for 4 days without recognized cause. The child appeared relatively well and the fever subsided to be followed by a maculopapular rash that began on the trunk and spread to involve the face and extremities. The course was typical for roseola infantum. Courtesy of George Nankervis, MD.

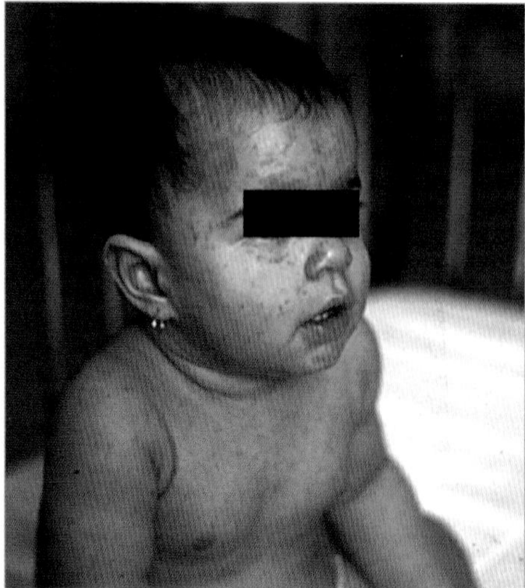

Image 67.4
A Hispanic female toddler with the exanthem of roseola following several days of high fever. Courtesy of Larry Frenkel, MD.

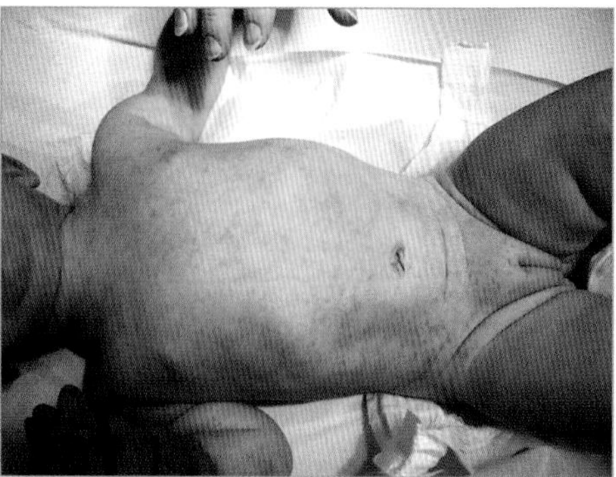

Image 67.3
An 8-month-old with a temperature between 38°C and 39°C (101°F and 103°F) for 3 consecutive days. The child appeared well, with no additional symptoms aside from mild irritability and decreased appetite. After cessation of the fever, the patient developed a maculopapular rash heavy on the trunk, but, aside from this, the patient still appeared well. The rash resolved in the next 48 hours. The clinical course and rash are compatible with roseola. Copyright Stan Block, MD, FAAP.

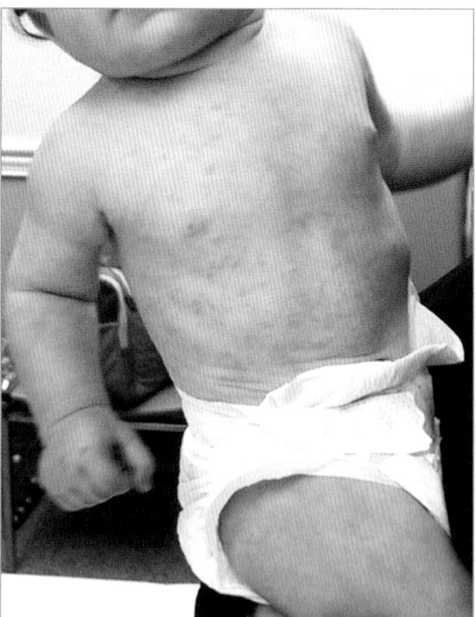

Image 67.5
Clinical course and rash compatible with roseola. Copyright Stan Block, MD, FAAP.

68

Human Herpesvirus 8

Clinical Manifestations

Human herpesvirus 8 (HHV-8) is the etiologic agent associated with Kaposi sarcoma (KS), primary effusion lymphoma, and multicentric Castleman disease. More recently, a syndrome termed KS herpesvirus-associated inflammatory cytokine syndrome, which presents as a systemic inflammatory illness, has been described in adults with HHV-8 infection in the United States. Human herpesvirus 8 is one of the triggers of hemophagocytic lymphohistiocytosis. In regions with endemic HHV-8, the following primary infection syndrome in immunocompetent children has been described: fever and a maculopapular rash, often accompanied by upper respiratory tract signs. Primary infection among immunocompromised people and men who have sex with men tends to have more severe manifestations that include pancytopenia, fever, rash, lymphadenopathy, splenomegaly, diarrhea, arthralgia, disseminated disease, and KS. In parts of Africa, among children with and without HIV infection, KS is a frequent, aggressive malignancy. In the United States, KS is rare in children but occurs commonly in those severely immunocompromised by HIV. Among organ transplant recipients and other immunosuppressed patients, KS is an important cause of cancer-related deaths. Primary effusion lymphoma is rare among children. Multicentric Castleman disease has been described in immunosuppressed and immunocompetent children, but the proportion of cases attributable to infection with HHV-8 is unknown.

Etiology

Human herpesvirus 8 is a member of the family Herpesviridae, the Gammaherpesvirinae subfamily, and the *Rhadinovirus* genus and is related closely to herpesvirus saimiri of monkeys and Epstein-Barr virus.

Epidemiology

In areas of Africa, the Amazon basin, the Mediterranean, and the Middle East, HHV-8 is endemic and seroprevalence ranges from approximately 30% to 80%. Low rates of seroprevalence, generally less than 5%, have been reported in the United States, Northern and Central Europe, and most areas of Asia. Higher rates, however, occur in specific geographic regions, among adolescents and adults with or at high risk of acquiring HIV infection, injection drug users, and internationally adopted children coming from some Eastern European countries.

Acquisition of HHV-8 in areas with endemic infection frequently occurs before puberty, likely by oral inoculation of saliva of close contacts, especially secretions of mothers and siblings. Virus is shed frequently in saliva of infected people and becomes latent for life in peripheral blood mononuclear cells, primarily $CD19^+$ B lymphocytes, and lymphoid tissue. In areas where infection is not endemic, sexual transmission appears to be the major route of infection, especially among men who have sex with men. Studies from areas with endemic infection have suggested transmission can occur by blood transfusion, but in the United States, such evidence is lacking. Transplantation of infected donor organs has been documented to result in HHV-8 infection in the recipient. Human herpesvirus 8 DNA has been detected in blood drawn at birth from neonates born to HHV-8 seropositive mothers, but vertical transmission is rare.

Incubation Period

Unknown.

Diagnostic Tests

Nucleic acid amplification testing and serologic assays for HHV-8 are available, and new assays with greater clinical utility are being developed. Polymerase chain reaction assays can be used on peripheral blood and tissue biopsy specimens of patients with HHV-8–associated disease, such as KS. Detection of HHV-8 in peripheral blood specimens by polymerase chain reaction assay has been used to support the diagnosis of KS and to identify exacerbations of HHV-8–associated diseases, primarily multicentric Castleman disease and KS herpesvirus-associated inflammatory cytokine syndrome. However, HHV-8 DNA detection in the peripheral blood does not differentiate between latent and active replicating infection.

Currently available serologic assays measuring antibodies to HHV-8 include immunofluorescence assay, enzyme immunoassays, and Western blot assays using recombinant HHV-8 proteins. These serologic assays can detect latent and lytic infection, but each has challenges with accuracy or convenience, thereby limiting use in the diagnosis and management of acute disease.

Treatment

No antiviral treatment is approved for HHV-8 disease. Ganciclovir has been shown to inhibit HHV-8 replication in the only randomized trial of an antiviral drug for this infection. Valacyclovir and famciclovir more modestly reduce HHV-8 replication. Retrospective cohort studies suggest antiretroviral therapy (particularly zidovudine and nelfinavir) may inhibit HHV-8 replication in patients infected with HIV.

69

Human Immunodeficiency Virus Infection

Clinical Manifestations

HIV infection results in a wide array of clinical manifestations and varied natural history. HIV type 1 (HIV-1) is much more common in the United States than is HIV type 2 (HIV-2). Unless otherwise specified, this chapter addresses HIV-1 infection.

AIDS is the name given to an advanced stage of HIV infection. The Centers for Disease Control and Prevention (CDC) uses a case definition that comprises AIDS-defining conditions for surveillance (Box 69.1). The CDC classifies all HIV-infected children younger than 13 years according to clinical stage of disease (Box 69.2) and immunologic status (Table 69.1). For purposes of surveillance of HIV disease, the CDC has updated the immunologic classification system; however, some clinical guidelines continue to make use of the 1994 CDC immunologic classification. This pediatric classification system emphasizes the importance of the $CD4^+$ T-lymphocyte count and percentage as critical immunologic parameters and as markers of prognosis. Data on plasma HIV-1 RNA concentration (viral load) are not included in this classification.

With timely diagnostic testing and appropriate treatment, clinical manifestations of HIV-1 infection and occurrence of AIDS-defining

Box 69.1
1993 Revised Case Definition of AIDS-Defining Conditions for Adults and Adolescents 13 Years and Older

- Candidiasis of bronchi, trachea, or lungs
- Candidiasis, esophageal
- Cervical cancer, invasive
- Coccidioidomycosis, disseminated or extrapulmonary
- Cryptococcosis, extrapulmonary
- Cryptosporidiosis, chronic intestinal (>1 mo duration)
- Cystoisosporiasis (isosporiasis), chronic intestinal (>1 mo duration)
- Cytomegalovirus disease (other than liver, spleen, or nodes)
- Cytomegalovirus retinitis (with loss of vision)
- Encephalopathy, HIV related
- Herpes simplex: chronic ulcer(s) (>1 mo duration) or bronchitis, pneumonitis, or esophagitis
- Histoplasmosis, disseminated or extrapulmonary
- Kaposi sarcoma
- Lymphoma, Burkitt (or equivalent term)
- Lymphoma, immunoblastic (or equivalent term)
- Lymphoma, primary or brain
- *Mycobacterium avium* complex or *Mycobacterium kansasii* infection, disseminated or extrapulmonary
- *Mycobacterium tuberculosis* infection, any site, pulmonary or extrapulmonary
- *Mycobacterium,* other species or unidentified species infection, disseminated or extrapulmonary
- *Pneumocystis jiroveci* pneumonia
- Pneumonia, recurrent
- Progressive multifocal leukoencephalopathy
- *Salmonella* septicemia, recurrent
- Toxoplasmosis of brain
- Wasting syndrome attributable to HIV
- $CD4^+$ T-lymphocyte count <200/µL (0.20×10^9/L) or $CD4^+$ T-lymphocyte percentage <15%

Abbreviations: AIDS, acquired immunodeficiency syndrome; HIV, human immunodeficiency virus.
Modified from Centers for Disease Control and Prevention. 1993 revised classification system for HIV infection and expanded surveillance case definition for AIDS among adolescents and adults. *MMWR Recomm Rep.* 1992;41(RR-17):1–19.

Box 69.2

Clinical Categories for Children Younger Than 13 Years With HIV Infection

Category N: Not Symptomatic

Children who have no signs or symptoms considered to be the result of HIV infection or have only 1 of the conditions listed in Category A.

Category A: Mildly Symptomatic

- Children with 2 or more of the conditions listed but none of the conditions listed in categories B and C
- Lymphadenopathy (≥0.5 cm at more than 2 sites; bilateral at 1 site)
- Hepatomegaly
- Splenomegaly
- Dermatitis
- Parotitis
- Recurrent or persistent upper respiratory tract infection, sinusitis, or otitis media

Category B: Moderately Symptomatic

- Children who have symptomatic conditions other than those listed for category A or C that are attributed to HIV infection
- Anemia (hemoglobin <8 g/dL [<80 g/L]), neutropenia (white blood cell count <1,000/µL [<1.0 x 10^9/L]), and/or thrombocytopenia (platelet count <100 x 10^3/µL [<100 x 10^9/L]) persisting for ≥30 d
- Bacterial meningitis, pneumonia, or sepsis (single episode)
- Candidiasis, oropharyngeal (thrush), persisting (>2 mo) in children older than 6 mo
- Cardiomyopathy
- Cytomegalovirus infection, with onset before 1 mo of age
- Diarrhea, recurrent or chronic
- Hepatitis
- Herpes simplex stomatitis, recurrent (>2 episodes within 1 y)
- Herpes simplex bronchitis, pneumonitis, or esophagitis with onset before 1 mo of age
- Herpes zoster (shingles) involving at least 2 distinct episodes or more than 1 dermatome
- Leiomyosarcoma
- Lymphoid interstitial pneumonia or pulmonary lymphoid hyperplasia complex
- Nephropathy
- Nocardiosis
- Persistent fever (lasting >1 mo)
- Toxoplasmosis, onset before 1 mo of age
- Varicella, disseminated (complicated chickenpox)

Box 69.2
Clinical Categories for Children Younger Than 13 Years With HIV Infection, continued

Category C: Severely Symptomatic

- Serious bacterial infections, multiple or recurrent (ie, any combination of at least 2 culture-confirmed infections within a 2-y period), of the following types: septicemia, pneumonia, meningitis, bone or joint infection, or abscess of an internal organ or body cavity (excluding otitis media, superficial skin or mucosal abscesses, and indwelling catheter-related infections)
- Candidiasis, esophageal or pulmonary (bronchi, trachea, lungs)
- Coccidioidomycosis, disseminated (at site other than or in addition to lungs or cervical or hilar lymph nodes)
- Cryptococcosis, extrapulmonary
- Cryptosporidiosis or cystoisosporiasis with diarrhea persisting >1 mo
- Cytomegalovirus disease with onset of symptoms after 1 mo of age (at a site other than liver, spleen, or lymph nodes)
- Encephalopathy (at least 1 of the following progressive findings present for at least 2 mo in the absence of a concurrent illness other than HIV infection that could explain the findings): (1) failure to attain or loss of developmental milestones or loss of intellectual ability, verified by standard developmental scale or neuropsychologic tests; (2) impaired brain growth or acquired microcephaly demonstrated by head circumference measurements or brain atrophy demonstrated by computed tomography or magnetic resonance imaging (serial imaging required for children <2 y); (3) acquired symmetric motor deficit manifested by 2 or more of the following: paresis, pathologic reflexes, ataxia, or gait disturbance
- Herpes simplex infection causing a mucocutaneous ulcer that persists for greater than 1 mo or bronchitis, pneumonitis, or esophagitis for any duration affecting a child older than 1 mo
- Histoplasmosis, disseminated (at a site other than or in addition to lungs or cervical or hilar lymph nodes)
- Kaposi sarcoma
- Lymphoma, primary, in brain
- Lymphoma, small, noncleaved cell (Burkitt), or immunoblastic; or large-cell lymphoma of B-lymphocyte or unknown immunologic phenotype
- *Mycobacterium tuberculosis,* disseminated or extrapulmonary
- *Mycobacterium,* other species or unidentified species infection, disseminated (at a site other than or in addition to lungs, skin, or cervical or hilar lymph nodes)
- *Pneumocystis jiroveci* pneumonia
- Progressive multifocal leukoencephalopathy
- *Salmonella* (nontyphoid) septicemia, recurrent
- Toxoplasmosis of the brain with onset at or after 1 mo of age
- Wasting syndrome in the absence of a concurrent illness other than HIV infection that could explain the following findings: (1) persistent weight loss >10% of baseline; (2) downward crossing of at least 2 of the following percentile lines on the weight-for-age chart (eg, 95th, 75th, 50th, 25th, 5th) in a child 1 y or older; OR (3) <5th percentile on weight-for-height chart on 2 consecutive measurements, ≥30 days apart; PLUS
  (1) chronic diarrhea (ie, at least 2 loose stools per day for >30 d);
  OR
  (2) documented fever (for >30 d, intermittent or constant)

Modified from Centers for Disease Control and Prevention. 1994 revised classification system for human immunodeficiency virus infection in children less than 13 years of age. Official authorized addenda: human immunodeficiency virus infection codes and official guidelines for coding and reporting ICD-9-CM. *MMWR Recomm Rep.* 1994;43(RR-12):1–19.

Table 69.1

HIV Infection Stage, Based on Age-Specific CD4$^+$ T-Lymphocyte Count or CD4$^+$ T-Lymphocyte Percentage of Total Lymphocytes[a]

	Age on Date of CD4 T-Lymphocyte Test					
	<1 y		1–5 y		6 y–Adult	
Stage[a]	Cells/μL	%	Cells/μL	%	Cells/μL	%
1	≥1,500	≥30	≥1,000	≥26	≥500	≥26[b]
2	750–1,499	20–29	500–999	14–25	200–499	14–25
3	<750	<20	<500	<14	<200	<14

[a] The stage is based primarily on the CD4$^+$ T-lymphocyte count; it is based on the CD4$^+$ T-lymphocyte percentage only if the count is missing. There are 3 situations in which the stage is not based on this table: (1) if the criteria for stage 0 are met, the stage is 0 regardless of criteria for other stages (CD4$^+$ T-lymphocyte test results and opportunistic illness diagnoses); (2) if the criteria for stage 0 are not met and a stage-3–defining opportunistic illness has been diagnosed, the stage is 3 regardless of CD4$^+$ T-lymphocyte test results; and (3) if the criteria for stage 0 are not met and information on the above criteria for other stages is missing, the stage is U (unknown).

[b] The change in the upper CD4$^+$ T-lymphocyte percentage threshold from 29% (as in the case definition of 2008) to 26% (as in the revision above) is contingent on data being published that support it, to corroborate unpublished analyses of surveillance data.

illnesses are now rare among children in the United States and other industrialized countries. Early clinical manifestations of pediatric HIV infection include unexplained fevers, generalized lymphadenopathy, hepatomegaly, splenomegaly, failure to thrive, persistent or recurrent oral and diaper candidiasis, recurrent diarrhea, parotitis, hepatitis, central nervous system disease (eg, hyperreflexia, hypertonia, floppiness, developmental delay), lymphoid interstitial pneumonia, recurrent invasive bacterial infections, and other opportunistic infections (OIs) (eg, viral, fungal).

In the era of combination antiretroviral therapy (cART), there has been a substantial decrease in frequency of all OIs. Frequency of different OIs in the pre-cART era varied by age, pathogen, previous infection history, and immunologic status. In the pre-cART era, the most common OIs observed among children in the United States were infections caused by invasive encapsulated bacteria, *Pneumocystis jiroveci*, varicella-zoster virus, cytomegalovirus (CMV), human herpesvirus (herpes simplex), *Mycobacterium avium* complex, and *Candida* species. Less commonly observed opportunistic pathogens included Epstein-Barr virus, *Mycobacterium tuberculosis, Cryptosporidium* species, *Cystoisospora* (formerly *Isospora*) species, other enteric pathogens, *Aspergillus* species, and *Toxoplasma gondii.*

Immune reconstitution inflammatory syndrome is a paradoxical clinical deterioration often seen in severely immunosuppressed people that occurs shortly after the initiation of cART. Local or systemic symptoms develop secondary to an inflammatory response as cell-mediated immunity is restored. Underlying infection with mycobacteria (including *M tuberculosis*), herpesviruses, and fungi (including *Cryptococcus* species) predispose to immune reconstitution inflammatory syndrome.

Malignant neoplasms in children with HIV-1 infection are relatively uncommon, but leiomyosarcomas and non-Hodgkin B-cell lymphomas of the Burkitt type (including some that occur in the central nervous system) occur more commonly in children with HIV infection than in immunocompetent children. Kaposi sarcoma is rare in children in the United States but has been documented in HIV-infected children who have emigrated from sub-Saharan African countries. The incidence of malignant neoplasms in HIV-infected children has decreased during the cART era.

The incidence of HIV encephalopathy is high among untreated HIV-infected infants and young children. In the United States, pediatric HIV encephalopathy has decreased substantially in the cART era, although other neurologic signs and symptoms have been appreciated, such as myelopathy or peripheral neuropathies, sometimes associated with antiretroviral therapy (ART).

Prognosis for survival is poor for untreated neonates who acquired HIV infection through mother-to-child transmission and who have high viral loads (ie, >100,000 copies/mL) and severe suppression of $CD4^+$ T-lymphocyte counts (Table 69.2). In these infants, AIDS-defining conditions developing during the first 6 months of life, including *P jiroveci* pneumonia (PCP), progressive neurologic disease, and severe wasting, are predictors of a poor outcome. When cART regimens are begun early, prognosis and survival rates improve dramatically. Although deaths attributable to OIs have declined, non–AIDS-defining infections and multiorgan failure remain major causes of death. In the United States, mortality in a longitudinal cohort of HIV-infected children whose age at enrollment ranged from birth to 21 years declined from 7.2 per 100 person years in 1993 to 0.8 per 100 person years in 2006. The HIV mortality rate in 2006 was equivalent to that of the general US pediatric population younger than 5 years (0.8/100) in 2011.

Although B-lymphocyte counts remain normal or are somewhat increased, humoral immune dysfunction may precede or accompany cellular dysfunction. Polyclonal B-lymphocyte hyperactivation occurs as part of a spectrum of chronic immune activation, leading to production of immunoglobulins that are not directed against specific pathogens encountered by the child. With advancing immunosuppression, recall antibody responses, including responses to vaccine-associated antigens, are slow and diminish in magnitude. A small proportion (<10%) of patients will develop panhypogammaglobulinemia. In the absence of treatment with cART, such patients have a particularly poor prognosis.

Etiology

As noted previously, 2 types of HIV cause disease in humans: HIV-1 and HIV-2. These viruses are cytopathic lentiviruses belonging to the family Retroviridae, and they are related closely to simian immunodeficiency viruses (SIVs), agents found in a variety of nonhuman primate species in sub-Saharan Africa. HIV-1 species infecting humans have evolved from SIVs found in chimpanzees and gorillas, whereas HIV-2 evolved from an SIV in sooty mangabeys. Three distinct genetic groups of HIV-1 exist worldwide: M (major), O (outlier), and N (new). Group M viruses are the most prevalent worldwide and comprise 8 genetic subtypes, or clades, known as A through H, which each have distinct geographic distribution. The HIV-1 genome is 10 kb in length and has conserved and highly variable domains. Three principal genes (*gag, pol,* and *env*) encode the major structural and enzymatic proteins, and 6 accessory genes regulate gene expression and aid in assembly and release of

Table 69.2
Laboratory Diagnosis of HIV Infection[a]

Test	Comment
HIV DNA PCR	Preferred test to diagnose HIV-1 subtype B infection in infants and children younger than 18 mo; highly sensitive and specific by 2 wk of age and available; performed on peripheral blood mononuclear cells. False-negative results can occur in non-B subtype HIV-1 infections.
HIV p24 Ag	Less sensitive, false-positive results during first month of life, variable results; not recommended.
ICD p24 Ag	Negative test result does not rule out infection; not recommended.
HIV culture	Expensive, not easily available, requires up to 4 wk for results; not recommended.
HIV RNA PCR	Preferred test to identify non-B subtype HIV-1 infections. Similar sensitivity and specificity to HIV DNA PCR in infants and children younger than 18 mo, but DNA PCR is generally preferred because of greater clinical experience with that assay.

Abbreviations: Ag, antigen; HIV, human immunodeficiency virus; ICD, immune complex dissociated; PCR, polymerase chain reaction.

[a] Read JS; American Academy of Pediatrics Committee on Pediatric AIDS. Diagnosis of HIV-1 infection in children younger than 18 months in the United States, *Pediatrics.* 2007;120(6):e1547–e1562. Reaffirmed April 2010. http://pediatrics.aappublications.org/cgi/content/full/120/6/e1547. Accessed May 23, 2016.

infectious virions. The envelope glycoprotein interacts with the $CD4^+$ receptor and with 1 of 2 major coreceptors (CCR5 or CXCR4) on the host cell membrane. HIV-1 is a single-stranded RNA virus that requires the activity of a viral enzyme, reverse transcriptase, to convert to double-stranded DNA. A double-stranded DNA copy of the viral genome then randomly integrates into the host cell genome, where it persists as a provirus.

HIV-2, the second AIDS-causing virus, is predominantly found in West Africa, with the highest rates of infection in Guinea-Bissau. The prevalence of HIV-2 in the United States is extremely low. HIV-2 is thought to have a milder disease course with a longer time to development of AIDS than HIV-1. Nonnucleoside reverse transcriptase inhibitors and at least 1 fusion inhibitor (enfuvirtide) are not effective against HIV-2, whereas nucleoside reverse transcriptase inhibitors and protease inhibitors have varying efficacy against HIV-2.

Epidemiology

Humans are the only known reservoir for HIV-1 and HIV-2. Latent virus persists in peripheral blood mononuclear cells and in cells of the brain, bone marrow, and genital tract even when plasma viral load is undetectable. Only blood, semen, cervicovaginal secretions, and human milk have been implicated epidemiologically in transmission of infection.

Established modes of HIV transmission include sexual contact (vaginal, anal, or orogenital); percutaneous blood exposure (from contaminated needles or other sharp instruments); mucous membrane exposure to contaminated blood or other body fluids; mother-to-child transmission in utero, around the time of labor and delivery, and postnatally through breastfeeding; and transfusion with contaminated blood products. Cases of probable HIV transmission from an HIV-infected caregiver to an infant through feeding blood-tinged premasticated food have been reported in the United States. As a result of highly effective screening methods, transfusion of blood, blood components, and clotting factors has virtually been eliminated as a cause of HIV transmission in the United States since 1985. Also, transmission of HIV has not been documented with normal activities in households; transmission has been documented after contact of nonintact skin with blood-containing body fluids. Moreover, transmission of HIV has not been documented in schools or child care settings in the United States.

Children younger than 13 years accounted for 0.3% of all estimated HIV diagnoses in the United States in 2011. Since the mid-1990s, the number of reported pediatric AIDS cases has decreased significantly, primarily because of prevention of mother-to-child transmission of HIV. This decrease in rate of mother-to-child transmission of HIV in the United States was attributable to the development and implementation of antenatal HIV testing programs and other interventions to prevent transmission, including antiretroviral prophylaxis during the antepartum, intrapartum, and postnatal periods; cesarean delivery before labor and before rupture of membranes; and complete avoidance of breastfeeding. Combination antiretroviral regimens during pregnancy have been associated with lower rates of mother-to-child transmission than zidovudine monotherapy taken antenatally. Currently, in the United States, most HIV-infected pregnant women receive 3-drug combination antiretroviral regimens for treatment of their own HIV infection or, if criteria for treatment are not yet met, for prevention of mother-to-child transmission of HIV (in which case the drugs can be stopped after delivery). The CDC estimates perinatally transmitted HIV cases in the United States have decreased from a peak of 1,650 in 1991 to 57 in 2010.

The risk of infection for a neonate born to an HIV-seropositive mother who did not receive interventions to prevent transmission is estimated to range from 22.6% to 25.5% in the United States. Most mother-to-child transmission occurs during the intrapartum period, with fewer transmission events occurring in utero and postnatally through breastfeeding. Risk factors for mother-to-child transmission of HIV can be categorized as follows: the amount of virus to which the child is exposed (a higher maternal viral load is associated with a lower maternal $CD4^+$ T-lymphocyte count and with more advanced maternal clinical disease or with recent seroconversion); the duration of exposure (eg, duration of ruptured membranes or of breastfeeding, vaginal versus cesarean delivery before labor and before rupture of membranes); and factors that facilitate the transfer of virus from mother to child (eg, maternal breast pathologic lesions, infant oral candidiasis). In addition to these factors, characteristics of the virus and the child's susceptibility to infection are important. Of note, although maternal viral load is a critical determinant affecting the likelihood of mother-to-child transmission of HIV, transmissions have been observed across the entire range of maternal viral loads. The risk of mother-to-child transmission increases with each hour increase in the duration of rupture of membranes, and the duration of ruptured membranes should be considered when evaluating the need for obstetric interventions. Cesarean delivery performed before onset of labor and before rupture of membranes has been shown to reduce mother-to-child intrapartum transmission. Current US guidelines recommend cesarean delivery at 38 weeks' gestation, before onset of labor and before rupture of membranes, for HIV-infected women with a viral load greater than 1,000 copies/mL (irrespective of use of ART during pregnancy) and for women with unknown viral load near the time of delivery. Cesarean delivery for women with an undetectable viral load is not routinely recommended.

Postnatal transmission to neonates and young infants occurs mainly through breastfeeding. Worldwide, an estimated one-third to one-half of cases of mother-to-child transmission of HIV occurs as a result of breastfeeding. HIV genomes have been detected in cell-associated and cell-free fractions of human milk. In the United States, HIV-infected mothers are advised not to breastfeed because safe alternatives to human milk are available. Because human milk cell-associated HIV can be detected even in women receiving cART and perinatal transmission still occurs among a small percentage of cART-receiving virologically suppressed women, replacement (formula) feeding continues to be recommended for US mothers receiving cART. In resource-limited locations, women whose HIV infection status is unknown are encouraged to breastfeed their infants exclusively for the first 6 months of life because the morbidity associated with formula feeding is unacceptably high. In addition, these women should be offered HIV testing. The World Health Organization recommended in 2010 that HIV-infected mothers exclusively breastfeed their infants for the first 6 months of life. Introduction of complementary foods should occur after 6 months of life, and breastfeeding should continue through 12 months of life. Breastfeeding should be replaced only when a nutritionally adequate and safe diet can be maintained without human milk. In areas where ART is available, infants should receive daily nevirapine prophylaxis until 1 week after human milk consumption stops, and mothers should receive ART (consisting of an effective cART regimen) for the first 6 months of their infants' lives. For infants known to be HIV-infected, mothers are encouraged to breastfeed exclusively for the first 6 months of life and, after the introduction of complementary foods, should continue to breastfeed up to 2 years of age, as per recommendations for the general population.

Although the rate of acquisition of HIV infection among infants has decreased significantly in the United States, the rate of new HIV infections during adolescence and young adulthood continues to increase. HIV infection in adolescents occurs disproportionately among youth of minority race or ethnicity. Transmission of HIV to adolescents is attributable primarily to sexual exposure and secondarily to illicit intravenous drug use. It is estimated that, in 2011, males accounted for approximately 77% and 86% of adolescents 13 to 19 years of age and 20 to 24 years of age, respectively, diagnosed with HIV infection. Young men who have sex with men are particularly at high risk of acquiring HIV infection, and the rates of HIV infection in young men who have sex with men continue to increase. In the United States and 6 dependent areas in 2011, an estimated 77% and 91% of diagnoses of HIV infections among all adolescents and young adults 13 to 24 years of age and among male adolescent and young adults 13 to 24 years of age, respectively, were attributed to male-to-male sexual contact. In contrast, 92% of diagnoses of HIV infection in 2011 among young adolescent and adult women

13 to 24 years of age were attributed to heterosexual contact. In 2010, there were an estimated 39,035 adolescents and young adults living with a diagnosis of HIV infection in the United States and 6 dependent areas; 63% were black (African American), 19% Hispanic/Latino, and 15% non-Hispanic white. Rates of HIV infection among adolescents are particularly high in the Southeastern and Northeastern United States. Most HIV-infected adolescents and young adults are asymptomatic and, without testing, remain unaware of their infection. Youth 13 to 24 years of age represent 26% of new HIV infections annually, and 60% are unaware they are infected.

Incubation Period

Approximately 12 to 18 months of age for untreated children (mother-to-child transmission). However, some HIV-infected infants become ill in the first few months of life, whereas others remain relatively asymptomatic for more than 5 years and, rarely, until early adolescence. Following HIV acquisition in adolescents and adults, primary seroconversion syndrome can occur 7 to 14 days following viral acquisition and can last for 5 to 7 days.

Diagnostic Tests

Laboratory diagnosis of HIV-1 infection during infancy is based on detection of the virus or viral nucleic acid (see Table 69.2). Because neonates born to HIV-infected mothers acquire maternal antibodies passively, antibody assays are not informative for diagnosis of infection in children younger than 24 months unless assay results are negative. In children 24 months and older, HIV antibody assays can be used for diagnosis. Historically, 18 months was considered the age at which a positive antibody assay could accurately distinguish between presence of maternal and infant antibodies. However, using medical record data for a cohort of HIV-uninfected infants born from 2000 to 2007, it was demonstrated that clearance of maternal HIV antibodies occurred later than previously reported. Despite a median age of seroreversion of 13.9 months, 14% of children remained seropositive after 18 months, 4.3% after 21 months, and 1.2% after 24 months.

In the United States, the preferred test for diagnosis of HIV infection in neonates is the HIV DNA polymerase chain reaction (PCR) assay. The DNA PCR assay can detect 1 to 10 DNA copies of proviral DNA in peripheral blood mononuclear cells. Approximately 30% to 40% of HIV-infected neonates will have a positive HIV DNA PCR assay result in samples obtained before 48 hours of age. A positive result by 48 hours of age suggests in utero transmission. Approximately 93% of infected neonates have detectable HIV DNA by 2 weeks of age, and approximately 95% of HIV-infected neonates have a positive HIV DNA PCR assay result by 1 month of age. A single HIV DNA PCR assay has a sensitivity of 95% and a specificity of 97% for samples collected from infected children 1 to 36 months of age.

HIV isolation by culture is less sensitive, less available, and more expensive than the DNA PCR assay. Definitive results may take up to 28 days. This test is no longer recommended for routine diagnosis.

Detection of the p24 antigen (including immune complex dissociated) is less sensitive than the HIV DNA PCR assay or culture. False-positive test results occur in samples obtained from neonates younger than 1 month. This test generally should not be used, although newer assays have been reported to have sensitivities similar to HIV DNA PCR assays.

Plasma HIV RNA assays have also been used to diagnose HIV infection. However, a false-negative test result may occur in neonates receiving ART as prophylaxis. Although use of ART can reduce plasma viral loads to undetectable levels, results of DNA PCR assay, which detects cell-associated integrated HIV DNA, remain positive even among individuals with undetectable plasma viral loads.

In the absence of therapy, plasma viral loads among neonates who acquired HIV infection through mother-to-child transmission increase rapidly to very high levels (typically from several hundred thousand to more than 1 million copies/mL) after birth, decreasing only slowly to a "set point" by approximately 2 years of age. This is in contrast to infection in adults, in whom viral load generally does not reach the high levels that are seen in newly infected neonates and for whom the set point occurs approximately 6 months after acquisition of infection. An HIV RNA assay result with only low-level viral copy number in an HIV-exposed neonate may indicate a false-positive result, reinforcing the importance of repeating any positive assay result to confirm the diagnosis of HIV infection in infancy. Like HIV DNA PCR assays, the sensitivity of HIV RNA assays for diagnosing infections in the first week of life is low (25%–40%) because transmission usually occurs around the time of delivery. RNA assays provide quantitative results as a predictor of disease progression rather than for routine diagnosis of HIV infection in neonates. RNA assays are also useful in monitoring changes in viral load during the course of ART.

Diagnostic testing with HIV DNA or RNA assays is recommended at 14 to 21 days of age and, if results are negative, again at 1 to 2 months of age and at 4 to 6 months of age. An infant is considered infected if 2 samples from 2 different time points test positive by DNA or RNA PCR assay.

Viral diagnostic testing in the first 2 days of life is recommended by some experts to allow for early identification of neonates with presumed in utero infection. If testing is performed shortly after birth, umbilical cord blood should not be used because of possible contamination with maternal blood. Obtaining the sample as early as 14 days of age may facilitate decisions about initiating ART. HIV-infected neonates should be transitioned from neonatal antiretroviral prophylaxis to cART treatment. In nonbreastfed children younger than 18 months with negative HIV virologic test results, **presumptive** exclusion of HIV infection is based on

- Two negative HIV DNA or RNA virologic test results, from separate specimens, each obtained at 2 weeks or older and one obtained at 4 weeks or older; **OR**
- One negative HIV DNA or RNA virologic test result from a specimen obtained at 8 weeks or older; **OR**
- One negative HIV antibody test result obtained at 6 months or older; **AND**
- No other laboratory or clinical evidence of HIV infection (ie, no subsequent positive results from virologic tests if tests were performed and no AIDS-defining condition for which there is no other underlying condition of immunosuppression)

In nonbreastfed children younger than 18 months with negative HIV virologic test results, **definitive** exclusion of HIV is based on

- At least 2 negative HIV DNA or RNA virologic test results, from separate specimens, obtained at 1 month or older and obtained at 4 months or older; **OR**
- At least 2 negative HIV antibody test results from separate specimens obtained at 6 months or older; **AND**
- No other laboratory or clinical evidence of HIV infection (ie, no subsequent positive results from virologic tests if tests were performed and no AIDS-defining condition for which there is no other underlying condition of immunosuppression).

In children with 2 negative HIV DNA PCR test results, many clinicians will confirm the absence of antibody (ie, loss of passively acquired natural antibody) to HIV on testing at 12 through 24 months of age (seroreversion). In addition, some clinicians have a slightly more stringent requirement that the 2 separate antibody-negative blood samples obtained after 6 months of age be drawn at least 1 month apart for a child to be considered HIV uninfected.

Immunoassays (IAs) are used widely as the initial test for serum HIV antibody or for p24 antigen and HIV antibody. These tests are highly sensitive and specific. Repeated IA testing of initially reactive specimens is common practice and is followed by additional testing to establish the diagnosis of HIV. A positive HIV antibody test result (reactive IA followed by positive Western blot or HIV-1/HIV-2 antibody differentiation assay) in a child 18 months or older almost always indicates infection, although passively acquired maternal antibody can, rarely, persist beyond 18 months of age. HIV antibody tests can be performed on samples of blood or oral fluid; antigen/antibody tests can be performed only on serum or plasma. Rapid tests for HIV antibodies have been approved for use in the United States; these tests are used widely throughout the world, particularly to screen mothers of undocumented serostatus in maternity settings. As with laboratory IAs, additional testing is required after a reactive rapid test. Results from rapid tests are available within 20 minutes; however, IA results and follow-up testing might take 2 days or longer.

Neonates who acquire HIV infection through mother-to-child transmission commonly have high viral set points with progressive cellular immune dysfunction and immunosuppression resulting from a decrease in the total number of circulating $CD4^+$ T lymphocytes. Sometimes, T-lymphocyte counts do not decrease until late in the course of infection. Changes in cell populations frequently result in a decrease in the normal $CD4^+$ to $CD8^+$ T-lymphocyte ratio of 1.0 or greater. This nonspecific finding, although characteristic of HIV-1 infection, also occurs with other acute viral infections, including infections caused by CMV and Epstein-Barr virus, and tuberculosis. The risk of OIs correlates with the $CD4^+$ T-lymphocyte percentage and count. The normal values for peripheral $CD4^+$ T-lymphocyte counts are age related.

- **Adolescents and HIV testing.** Routine screening should be offered to all adolescents at least once by 16 through 18 years of age. Use of any licensed HIV antibody test is appropriate. For any positive test result, referral to an HIV specialist is appropriate to confirm diagnosis and initiate management. Adolescents with behaviors that increase risk of HIV acquisition (eg, multiple sex partners, illicit drug use, men who have sex with men) should be tested annually.
- **Consent for diagnostic testing.** The CDC recommends that diagnostic HIV testing and opt-out HIV screening should be part of routine clinical care in all health care settings for patients 13 through 64 years of age, thus preserving the patient's option to decline HIV testing and allowing a provider-patient relationship conducive to optimal clinical and preventive care. Patients or people responsible for the patient's care should be notified orally that testing is planned, advised of the indication for testing and the implications of positive and negative test results, and offered an opportunity to ask questions and to decline testing. With such notification, the patient's general consent for medical care is considered sufficient for diagnostic HIV testing. Although parental involvement in an adolescent's health care may be desirable, it is not typically required when the adolescent consents to HIV testing. However, laws on consent and confidentiality for HIV care differ among states. Public health statutes and legal precedents allow for evaluation and treatment of minors for sexually transmitted infections without parental knowledge or consent, but not every state has explicitly defined HIV infection as a condition for which testing or treatment may proceed without parental consent. Health care professionals should endeavor to respect an adolescent's request for privacy. HIV screening should be discussed with all adolescents and encouraged for adolescents who are sexually active. Providing information about HIV infection, diagnostic testing, transmission including secondary transmission, and implications of infection is an essential component of the anticipatory guidance provided to all adolescents as part of primary care. Access to clinical care, preventive counseling, and support services is essential for people with positive HIV test results.

Treatment

Because HIV treatment options and recommendations change with time and vary with occurrence of antiretroviral drug resistance and adverse event profile, consultation with an expert in pediatric HIV infection is recommended in the care of HIV-infected infants, children, and adolescents. Current treatment recommendations for HIV-infected children are available online (**http://aidsinfo.nih.gov**). Whenever possible, enrollment of HIV-infected children in clinical trials should be encouraged.

Combination antiretroviral therapy is indicated for most HIV-infected children. The principal objectives of therapy are to suppress viral replication maximally, to restore and preserve immune function, to reduce HIV-associated morbidity and mortality, to minimize drug toxicity, to maintain normal growth and development, and to improve quality of life. Initiation of cART depends on the age of the child and on a combination of virologic, immunologic, and clinical criteria. Data indicate that very early initiation of therapy reduces morbidity and mortality compared with starting treatment at onset of clinical symptoms or immune suppression. Effective administration of early therapy will maintain the viral load at low or undetectable concentrations and will reduce viral mutation and evolution.

Initiation of cART is recommended as follows:

1. HIV-infected infants 12 months or younger **should** receive cART irrespective of clinical symptoms, immune status, or viral load.
2. Children from 1 to 3 years of age **should** receive cART if they (a) have AIDS or significant HIV-related symptoms (CDC clinical categories C and B [except for the following category B condition: single episode of serious bacterial infection]), regardless of $CD4^+$ T-lymphocyte counts or plasma viral load values; (b) have a $CD4^+$ T-lymphocyte percentage below 25% or $CD4^+$ T-lymphocyte count below 1,000 cells/mm^3, regardless of symptoms or viral load; or (c) are asymptomatic or mildly symptomatic (CDC clinical category A or N or the following category B condition: single episode of serious bacterial infection) **and** have a $CD4^+$ T-lymphocyte percentage of 25% or greater **and** a viral load of 100,000 copies/mL or greater.
3. Children 3 to 5 years of age **should** receive cART if they (a) have AIDS or significant HIV-related symptoms (CDC clinical categories C and B [except for the following category B condition: single episode of serious bacterial infection]); (b) have a $CD4^+$ T-lymphocyte count at or below 750 cells/mm^3 or $CD4^+$ T-lymphocyte percentage below 25%; or (c) are asymptomatic or mildly symptomatic (CDC clinical category A or N or the following category B condition: single episode of serious bacterial infection) **and** have a $CD4^+$ T-lymphocyte count greater than 750 cells/mm^3 and a viral load of 100,000 copies/mL or greater.
4. Children 5 years and older **should** receive cART if they (a) have AIDS or significant HIV-related symptoms (CDC clinical categories C and B [except for the following B condition: single episode of serious bacterial infection]) or (b) have a $CD4^+$ T-lymphocyte count below 500 cells/mm^3.

Starting cART should be considered for HIV-infected children from 1 to 3 years of age who are asymptomatic or have mild symptoms (clinical category N or A, or the following clinical category B condition: single episode of serious bacterial infection) **and** have a $CD4^+$ T-lymphocyte percentage of 25% or greater **and** a viral load below 100,000 copies/mL. Initiation of cART should also be considered for HIV-infected children 5 years and older who are asymptomatic or have mild symptoms (clinical category N or A, or the following clinical category B condition: single episode of serious bacterial infection) **and** have a $CD4^+$ T-lymphocyte count above 500 cells/mm^3 **and** a viral load below 100,000 copies/mL. The child and the child's primary caregiver must be able to adhere to the prescribed regimen.

Initiation of treatment of adolescents generally follows guidelines for adults, for whom initiation of treatment is strongly recommended if an AIDS-defining illness is present or if the $CD4^+$ T-lymphocyte count is below 500 cells/mm^3, or regardless of $CD4^+$ T-lymphocyte count in patients with HIV-associated nephropathy or with hepatitis B virus infection when treatment of hepatitis B virus is recommended. Combination antiretroviral therapy should be considered for patients with $CD4^+$ T-lymphocyte counts above 500 cells/mm. In general, cART with at least 3 active drugs is recommended for all HIV-infected individuals requiring ART. Drug regimens most often include 2 nucleoside reverse transcriptase inhibitors plus a protease inhibitor or a non-nucleoside reverse transcriptase inhibitor (**http://aidsinfo.nih.gov**). Antiretroviral resistance testing (viral genotyping) is recommended before starting treatment. Suppression of virus to undetectable levels is the desired goal. A change in ART should be considered if there is evidence of disease progression (virologic, immunologic, or clinical), toxicity of or intolerance to drugs, initial presence or development of drug resistance, or availability of data suggesting the possibility of a superior regimen.

Intravenous immunoglobulin therapy has been used in combination with cART for HIV-infected children with hypogammaglobulinemia (IgG <400 mg/dL [4.0 g/L]) and can be considered for HIV-infected children who have recurrent, serious bacterial infections, such as bacteremia, meningitis, or pneumonia. Trimethoprim-sulfamethoxazole prophylaxis may provide comparable protection. Typically, neither form of prophylaxis is necessary for patients receiving effective cART.

Early diagnosis, prophylaxis, and aggressive treatment of OIs may prolong survival. This is particularly true for PCP, which accounts for approximately one-third of pediatric AIDS diagnoses overall and may occur early in the first year of life. Prophylaxis is not recommended for neonates who meet criteria for presumptive or definitive HIV-uninfected status. Thus, for neonates with negative HIV diagnostic test results at 2 and 4 weeks of age, PCP prophylaxis would not need to be initiated. Because mortality rates are high, PCP chemoprophylaxis should be given to all HIV-exposed infants with indeterminate HIV infection status starting at 4 to 6 weeks of age but can be stopped if the infant subsequently meets criteria for presumptive or definitive absence of HIV infection. All infants with HIV infection should receive PCP prophylaxis through 1 year of age regardless of immune status. The need for PCP prophylaxis for HIV-infected children 1 year and older is determined by the degree of immunosuppression from $CD4^+$ T-lymphocyte percentage and count.

Guidelines for prevention and treatment of OIs in children, adolescents, and adults provide indications for administration of drugs for infection with *M avium* complex, CMV, *T gondii*, and other organisms. Successful suppression of HIV replication in the blood to undetectable levels by cART has resulted in relatively normal $CD4^+$ and $CD8^+$ T-lymphocyte counts, leading to a dramatic decrease in the occurrence of most OIs. Limited data on the safety of discontinuing prophylaxis in HIV-infected children receiving cART are available; however, prophylaxis should not be discontinued in HIV-infected infants younger than 1 year irrespective of the viral or immunologic response. For older children, many experts consider discontinuing PCP prophylaxis on the basis of $CD4^+$ T-lymphocyte count for those who have received at least 6 months of effective cART as follows: for children 1 through 5 years of age, $CD4^+$ T-lymphocyte percentage of at least 15% or $CD4^+$ T-lymphocyte absolute count of at least 500 cells/µL for more than 3 consecutive months; and for children 6 years or older, $CD4^+$ T-lymphocyte percentage of at least 15% or the $CD4^+$ T-lymphocyte absolute count of at least 200 cells/µL for more than 3 consecutive months. Subsequently, the $CD4^+$ T-lymphocyte absolute count or percentage should be reevaluated at least every 3 months. Prophylaxis should be reinstituted if the original criteria for prophylaxis are reached again.

- **Immunization recommendations.** All recommended childhood immunizations should be given to HIV-exposed infants. If HIV infection is confirmed, guidelines for the HIV-infected child should be followed. Children with HIV infection should be immunized as soon as is age appropriate with inactivated vaccines. Inactivated influenza vaccine should be given annually according to the most current recommendations. Additionally, live-virus vaccines (measles-mumps-rubella [MMR] and varicella) can be given to asymptomatic HIV-infected children and adolescents without severe immunosuppression (ie, $CD4^+$ T-lymphocyte percentage >15% for at least 6 months in children 1 through 5 years of age and $CD4^+$ T-lymphocyte percentage >15% and a $CD4^+$ T-lymphocyte count >200 lymphocytes/mm^3 for a 6-month period in those 6 years and older). Severely immunocompromised HIV-infected infants, children, adolescents, and young adults should not receive measles virus–containing vaccine because vaccine-related pneumonia has been reported. The quadrivalent MMR-varicella vaccine should not be administered to any HIV-infected infants, regardless of degree of immunosuppression, because of lack of safety data in this population. Rotavirus vaccine can be given to HIV-exposed and HIV-infected infants irrespective of $CD4^+$ T-lymphocyte percentage or count. HIV-infected children should receive a dose of 23-valent polysaccharide pneumococcal vaccine after 24 months of age, with a minimal interval of 8 weeks since the last conjugate pneumococcal vaccine. Although HIV infection is not an indication for pneumococcal vaccine, people at increased risk of meningococcal disease and who are 2 years or older should receive a 2-dose primary series of the quadrivalent meningococcal vaccine at least 8 weeks apart. HIV-infected adolescents 11 through 18 years of age should receive all inactivated vaccines recommended for this age group, including the 3-dose series of human papillomavirus vaccine. The suggested schedule for administration of these vaccines is provided in the "Recommended Immunization Schedule for Persons Aged 0 Through 18 Years" (**http://redbook.solutions.aap.org/SS/Immunization_Schedules.aspx**).

- **Children who are HIV uninfected residing in the household of an HIV-infected person.** Members of households in which an adult or child has HIV infection can receive MMR vaccine because these vaccine viruses are not transmitted person to person. To decrease the risk of transmission of influenza to patients with symptomatic HIV infection, all household members 6 months or older should receive yearly influenza immunization. Immunization with varicella vaccine of siblings and susceptible adult caregivers of patients with HIV infection is encouraged to prevent acquisition of wild-type varicella-zoster virus infection, which can cause severe disease in immunocompromised hosts. Transmission of varicella vaccine virus from an immunocompetent host to a household contact is very uncommon.

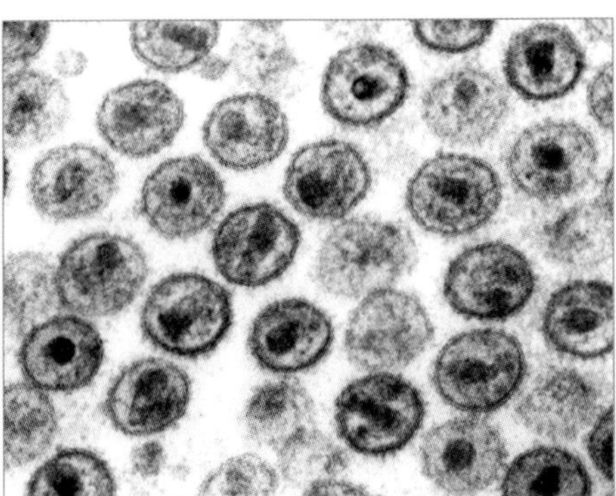

Image 69.1
HIV type 1. Transmission electron micrograph. Cone-shaped cores are sectioned in various orientations. Viral genomic RNA is located in the electron-dense wide end of core. Courtesy of Centers for Disease Control and Prevention/ Dr Edwin P. Ewing Jr.

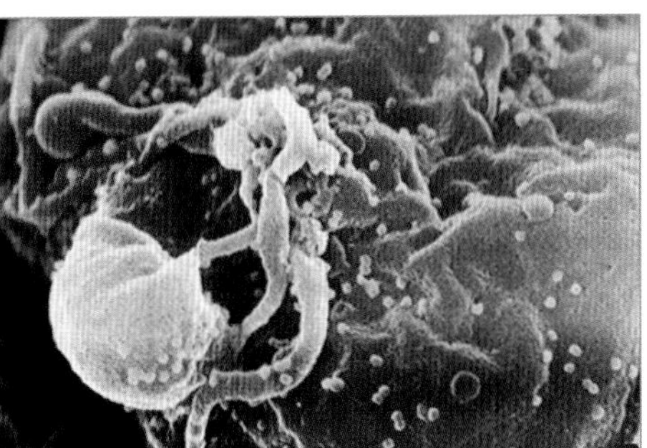

Image 69.2
Scanning electron micrograph of HIV type 1 budding from cultured lymphocyte. Courtesy of Centers for Disease Control and Prevention/ C. Goldsmith, P. Feorino, E. L. Palmer, W. R. McManus.

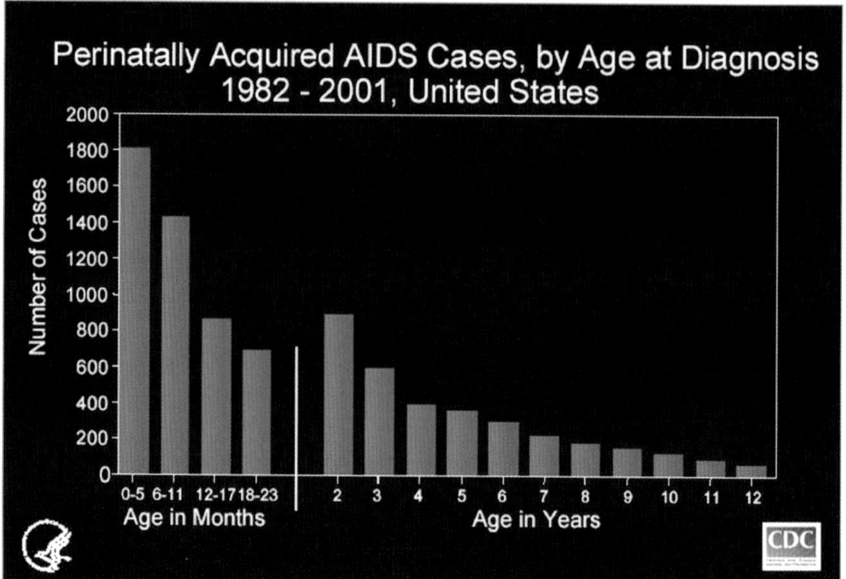

Image 69.3

Perinatally acquired AIDS cases, by age at diagnosis, 1982–2001, United States. Perinatally acquired AIDS was diagnosed for nearly 40% of infected infants within the first year of life and for 22% within the first 6 months. This distribution could change if more HIV-infected childbearing women become aware of their HIV status and seek medical care early in their infants' lives, when treatment could possibly prevent the progression from HIV infection to AIDS in their children. Courtesy of Centers for Disease Control and Prevention.

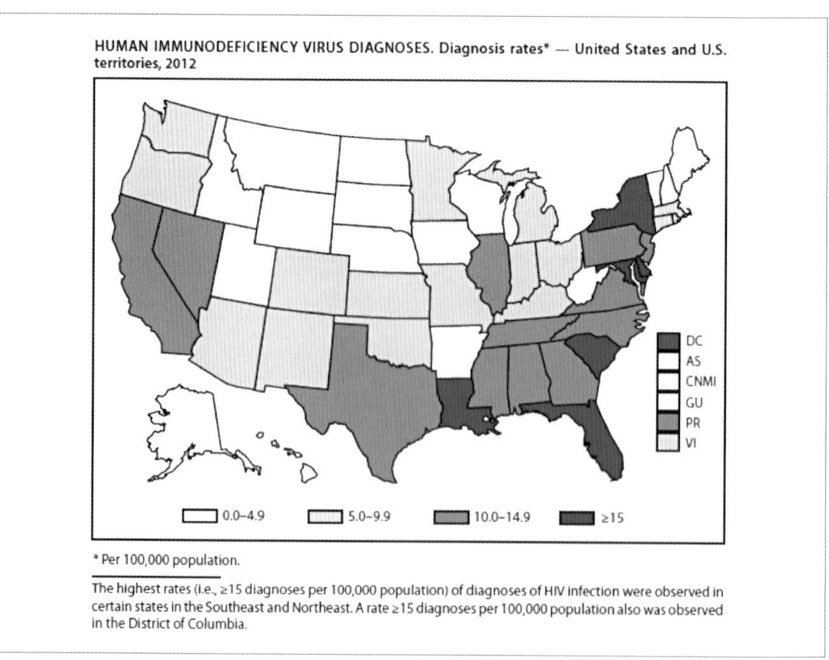

Image 69.4

Diagnosis rates—United States and US territories, 2012. Courtesy of *Morbidity and Mortality Weekly Report.*

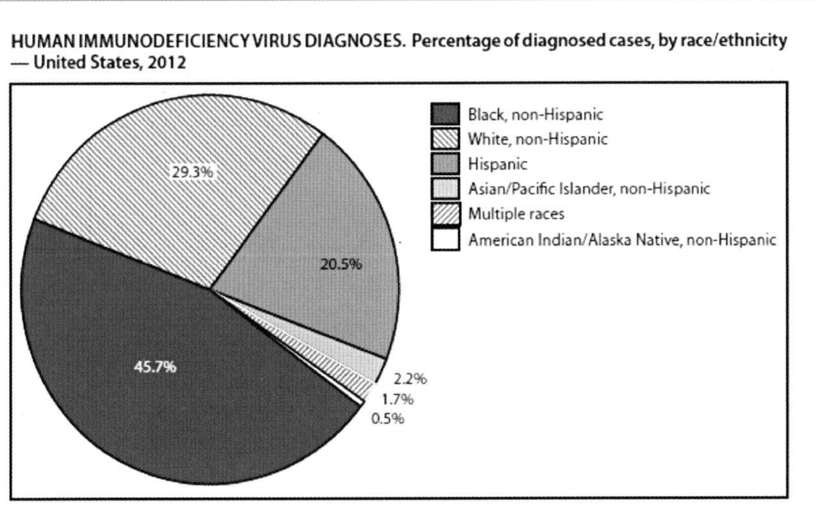

Image 69.5

Percentage of diagnosed cases, by race/ethnicity—United States, 2012. Courtesy of *Morbidity and Mortality Weekly Report.*

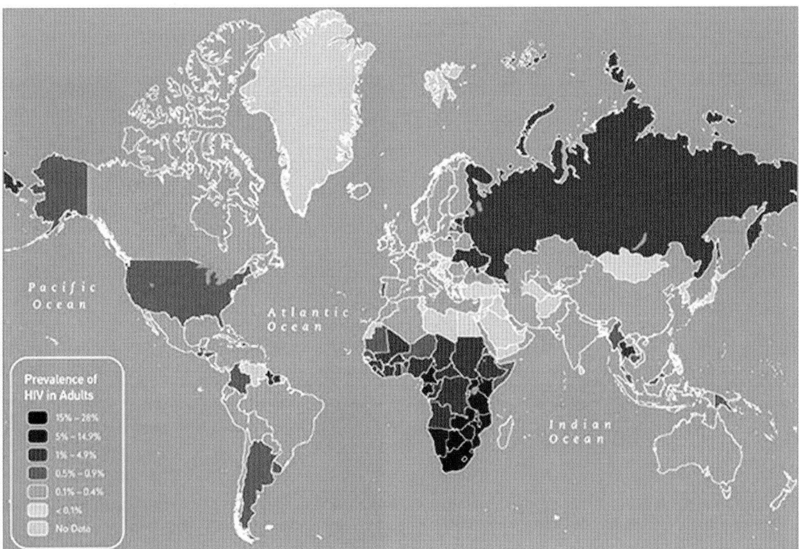

Image 69.6

HIV prevalence in adults, 2009. Centers for Disease Control and Prevention National Center for Emerging and Zoonotic Infectious Diseases (NCEZID) Division of Global Migration and Quarantine (DGMQ).

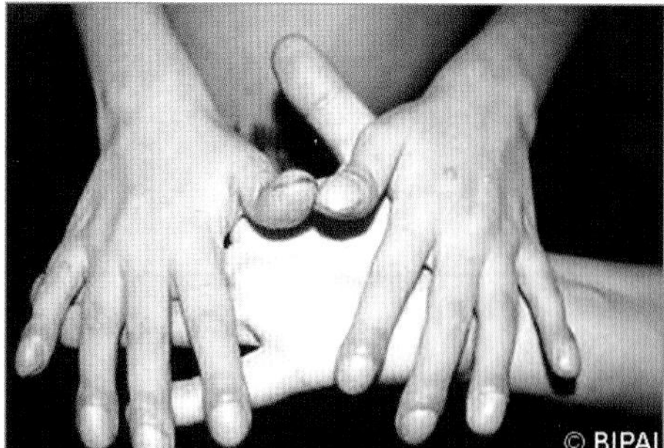

Image 69.7
Digital clubbing in a child with HIV infection and lymphoid interstitial pneumonitis/pulmonary lymphoid hyperplasia (LIP/PLH). Marked lymphadenopathy, hepatosplenomegaly, and salivary gland enlargement are also observed in many children with LIP/PLH. The clinical course of LIP/PLH is variable. Exacerbation of respiratory distress and hypoxemia can occur in association with intercurrent viral respiratory illnesses. Spontaneous clinical remission is sometimes observed. Copyright Baylor International Pediatric AIDS Initiative/Mark Kline, MD, FAAP.

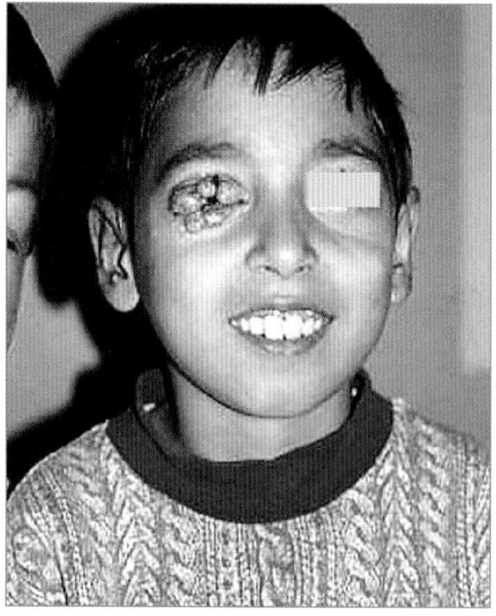

Image 69.9
Severe molluscum contagiosum in a boy with HIV infection. Some HIV-infected children develop molluscum contagiosum lesions that are unusually large or widespread. They are often seated more deeply in the epidermis. (See also **Molluscum Contagiosum.**) Copyright Baylor International Pediatric AIDS Initiative/Mark Kline, MD, FAAP.

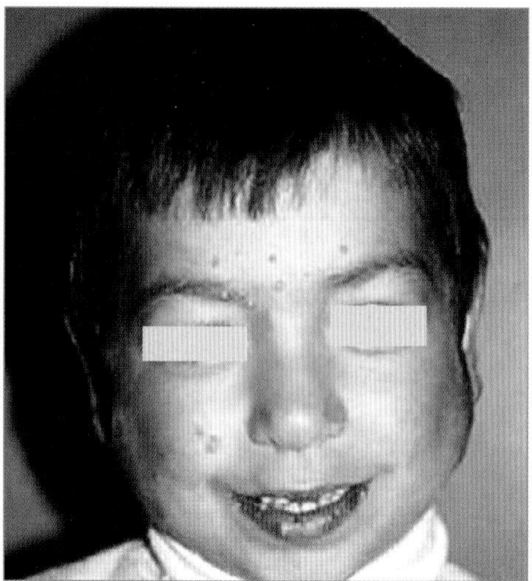

Image 69.8
Bilateral parotid gland enlargement in an HIV-infected male child with lymphoid interstitial pneumonitis/pulmonary lymphoid hyperplasia. Note the presence of multiple lesions of molluscum contagiosum, which are commonly seen in patients with HIV, particularly those with a low CD4 lymphocyte count. (See also **Molluscum Contagiosum.**) Copyright Baylor International Pediatric AIDS Initiative/Mark Kline, MD, FAAP.

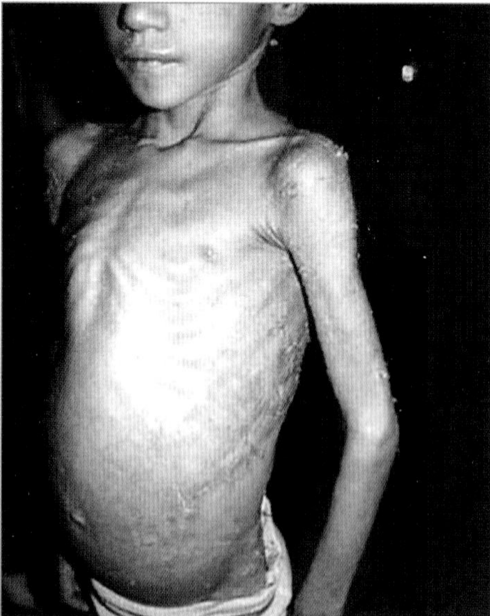

Image 69.10
Norwegian (crusted) scabies in a boy with HIV infection. Generalized scaling and hyperkeratotic, crusted plaques are present. (See also **Scabies.**) Copyright Baylor International Pediatric AIDS Initiative/Mark Kline, MD, FAAP.

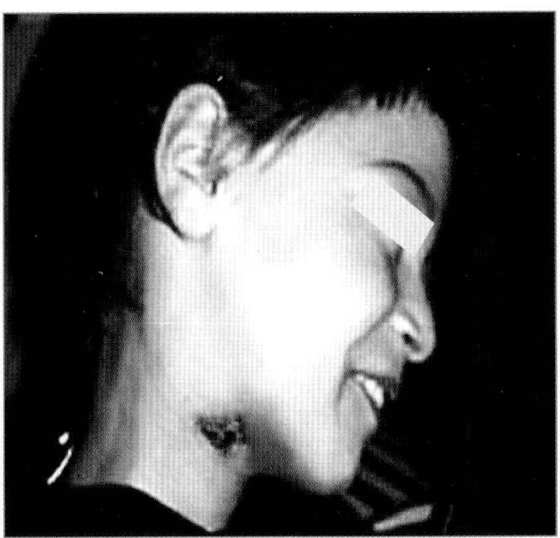

Image 69.11
An 8-year-old boy with HIV and tuberculous lymphadenitis (scrofula). Copious amounts of pus spontaneously drained from this lesion. In an immunocompromised child, other causes of lymphadenitis include infections with gram-positive bacteria, atypical mycobacterium, and *Bartonella henselae* (cat-scratch disease); malignant neoplasms such as lymphoma; masses such as branchial cleft cysts or cystic hygromas masquerading as lymph nodes; and adenitis due to HIV itself. (See also **Diseases Caused by Nontuberculous Mycobacteria.**) Copyright Baylor International Pediatric AIDS Initiative/Mark Kline, MD, FAAP.

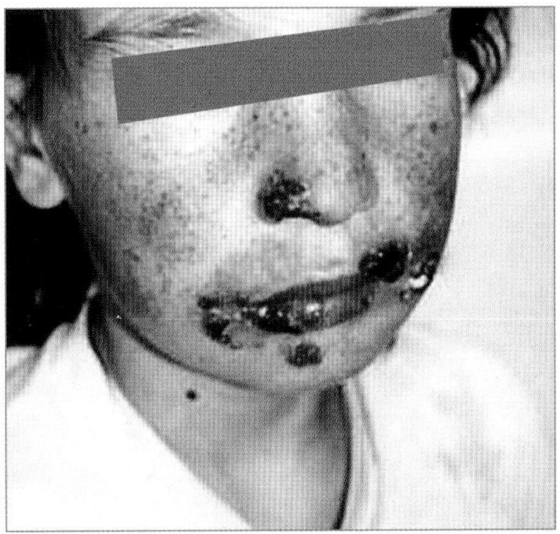

Image 69.12
Herpes simplex infection in a girl with HIV infection. Chronic or progressive herpetic skin lesions are observed occasionally in HIV-infected children, although, unlike varicella-zoster virus infections in these patients, herpes simplex infections much less commonly cause disseminated disease. (See also **Herpes Simplex.**) Copyright Baylor International Pediatric AIDS Initiative/Mark Kline, MD, FAAP.

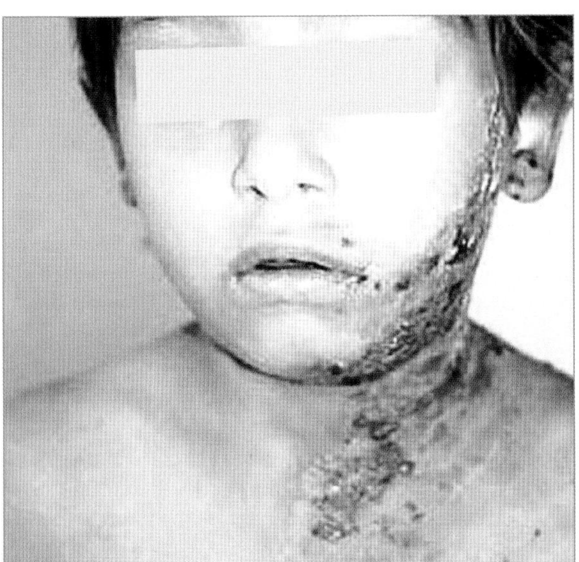

Image 69.13
Herpes zoster (shingles) in a boy with HIV infection. Such cases can be complicated by chronicity or dissemination. (See also **Varicella-Zoster Virus Infections.**) Copyright Baylor International Pediatric AIDS Initiative/Mark Kline, MD, FAAP.

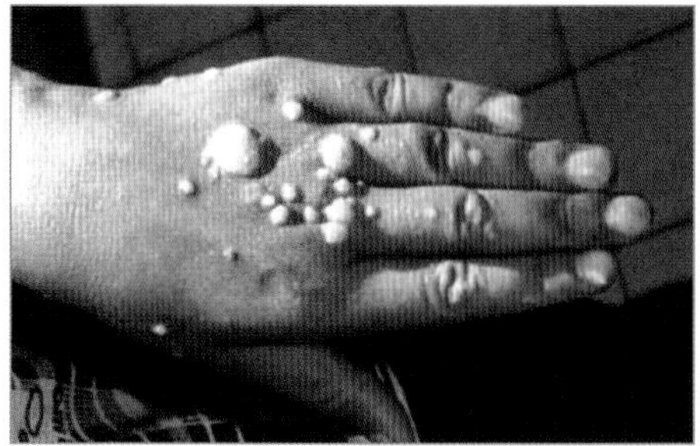

Image 69.14
Severe cutaneous warts (human papillomavirus infection) in a boy with HIV infection. Copyright Baylor International Pediatric AIDS Initiative/Mark Kline, MD, FAAP.

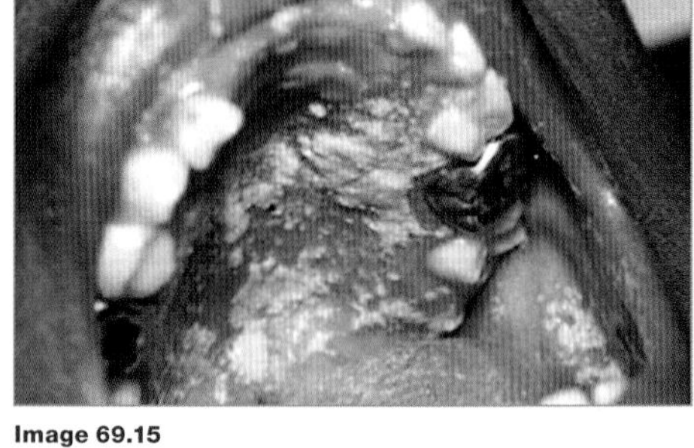

Image 69.15
Pseudomembranous candidiasis in a person with HIV infection. (See also **Candidiasis.**) Copyright Baylor International Pediatric AIDS Initiative/Mark Kline, MD, FAAP.

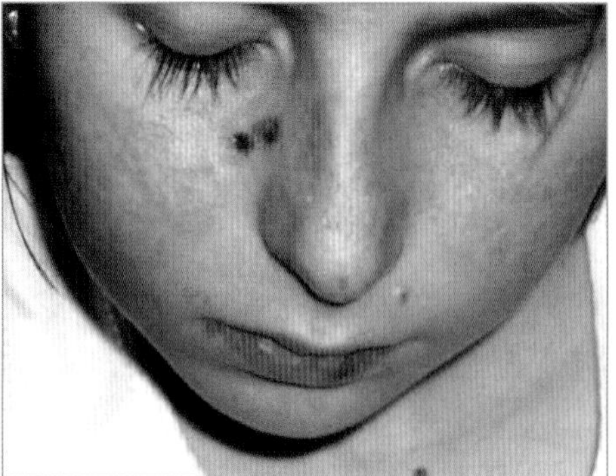

Image 69.16
A 9-year-old girl with HIV infection and cutaneous *Cryptococcus neoformans* infection. Skin lesions can be single or multiple and may appear as small papules, pustules, nodules, or ulcers with a base of granulation tissue. (See also ***Cryptococcus neoformans* and *Cryptococcus gattii* Infections.**) Copyright Baylor International Pediatric AIDS Initiative/Mark Kline, MD, FAAP.

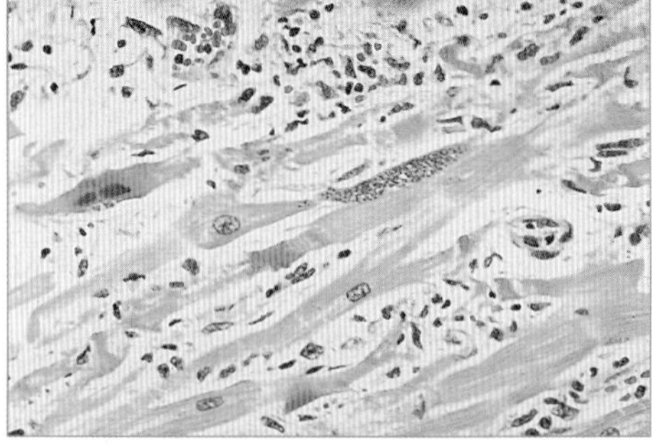

Image 69.17
Histopathology of toxoplasmosis of heart in fatal case of AIDS. Courtesy of Centers for Disease Control and Prevention/Dr Edwin P. Ewing Jr.

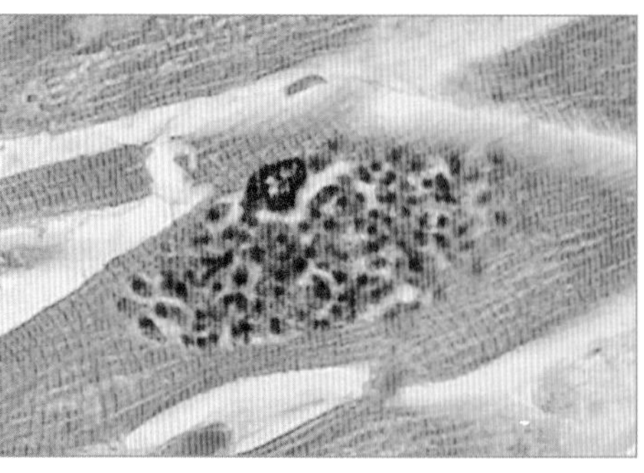

Image 69.18
Toxoplasmosis of the heart in a patient with AIDS. Courtesy of Centers for Disease Control and Prevention/Dr Edwin P. Ewing Jr.

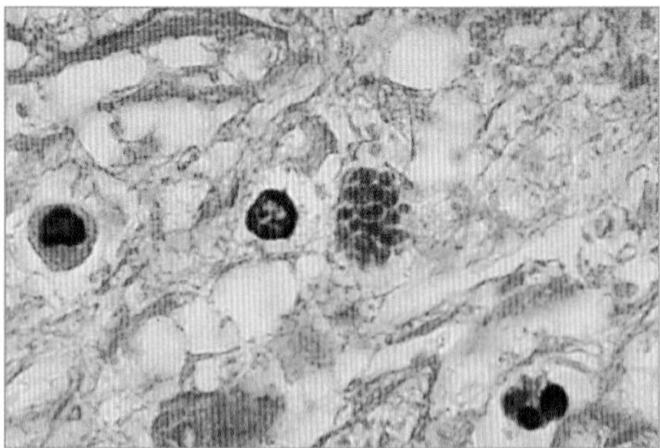

Image 69.19
Histopathology of toxoplasmosis of the brain in fatal case of AIDS. Courtesy of Centers for Disease Control and Prevention/Dr Edwin P. Ewing Jr.

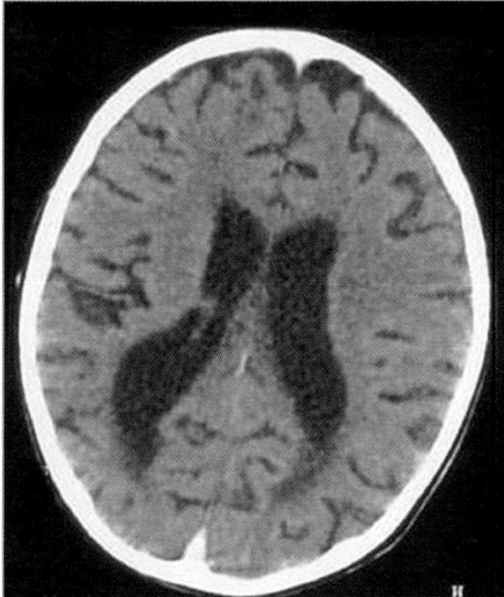

Image 69.20
Computed tomography scan of the brain of an 8-year-old boy with HIV infection and generalized brain atrophy. Cerebral atrophy is commonly observed among children with HIV-associated encephalopathy, but it may also be observed among children who are normal neurologically and developmentally. Copyright Baylor International Pediatric AIDS Initiative/Mark Kline, MD, FAAP.

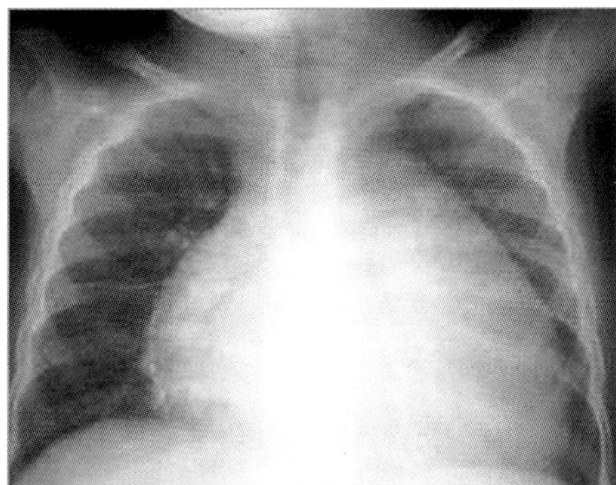

Image 69.22
Chest radiograph showing cardiomegaly in a 5-year-old girl with HIV infection, cardiomyopathy, and congestive heart failure. Many HIV-infected children with congestive heart failure respond well to medical management. Copyright Baylor International Pediatric AIDS Initiative/Mark Kline, MD, FAAP.

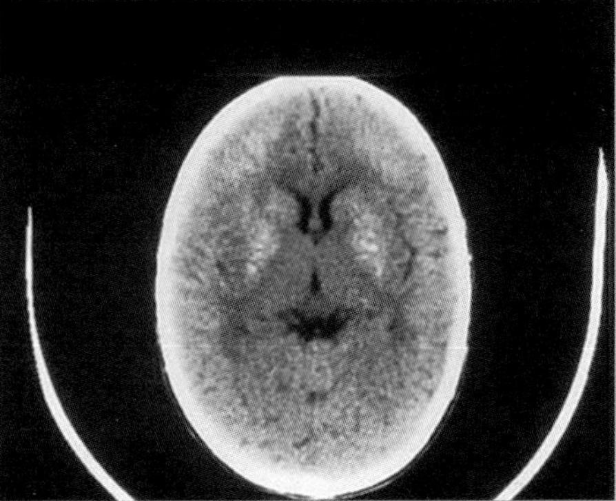

Image 69.21
Computed tomography scan of the brain of a 9-month-old girl with HIV infection and bilateral calcifications of the basal ganglia. This finding in an infant or young child strongly suggests HIV infection. Copyright Baylor International Pediatric AIDS Initiative/Mark Kline, MD, FAAP.

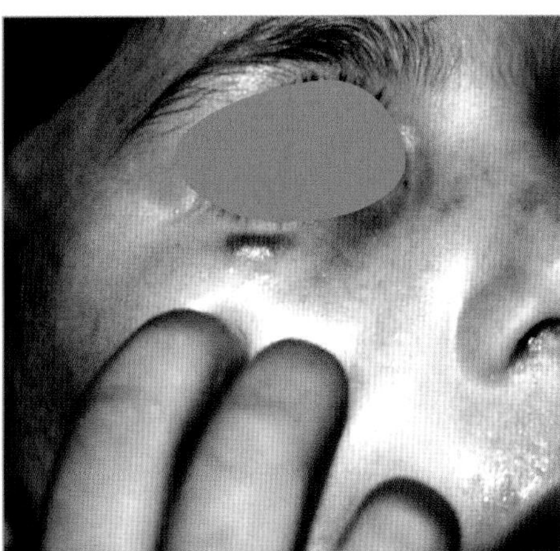

Image 69.23
A 7-year-old girl with HIV infection and a Kaposi sarcoma lesion. This tumor is rarely diagnosed among US children, with the occasional exceptions of children of Haitian descent with vertical HIV infection or older adolescents. Kaposi sarcoma is observed more commonly among HIV-infected children in some other geographic locales, including parts of Africa (eg, Zambia, Uganda) and Romania. Kaposi sarcoma has been linked to infection with a novel herpesvirus, now known as human herpesvirus 8 or Kaposi sarcoma–associated virus. Copyright Baylor International Pediatric AIDS Initiative/Mark Kline, MD, FAAP.

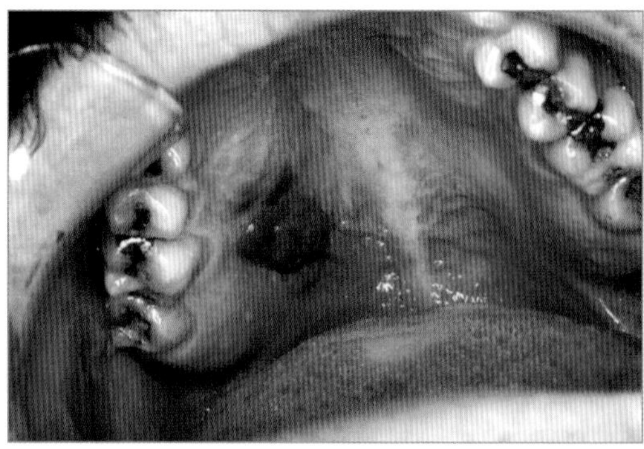

Image 69.24

This HIV patient presented with intraoral Kaposi sarcoma of the hard palate secondary to his AIDS infection. Approximately 7.5% to 10% of AIDS patients display signs of oral Kaposi sarcoma, which can range in appearance from small asymptomatic growths that are flat purple-red in color to larger nodular growths. Courtesy of Centers for Disease Control and Prevention/Sol Silverman Jr, DDS, University of California, San Francisco.

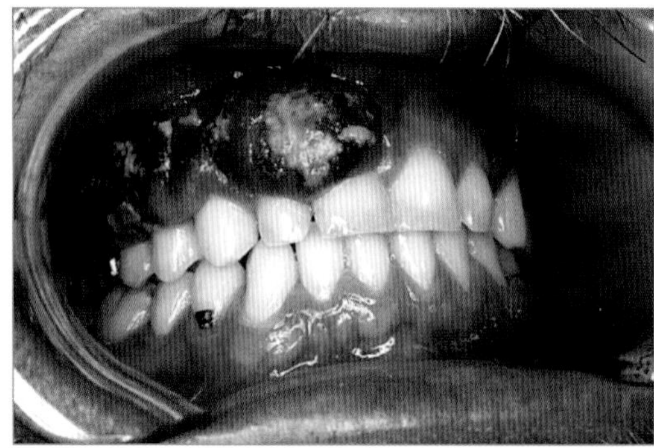

Image 69.25

This HIV-positive patient presented with an intraoral Kaposi sarcoma lesion with an overlying candidiasis infection. This AIDS patient exhibited a $CD4^{+}$ T-cell count less than 200 and a high viral load. Initially, the Kaposi sarcoma lesions are flattened and red, but as they age, they become raised and darker, tending to a purple coloration. Courtesy of Centers for Disease Control and Prevention/Sol Silverman Jr, DDS, University of California, San Francisco.

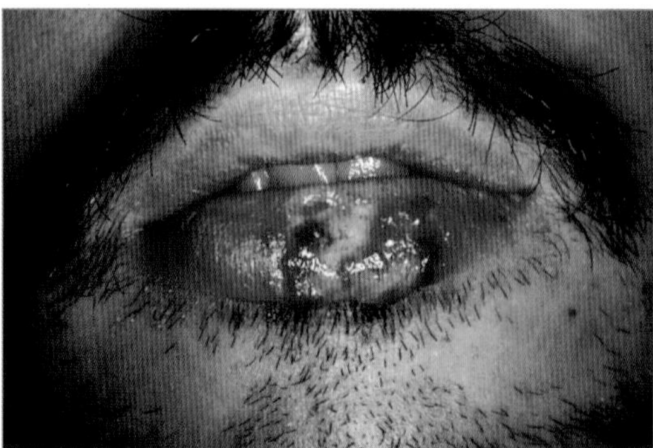

Image 69.26

This HIV-positive patient was exhibiting a chronic mucocutaneous herpes lesion for 1 month in duration. Courtesy of Centers for Disease Control and Prevention/Sol Silverman Jr, DDS, University of California, San Francisco.

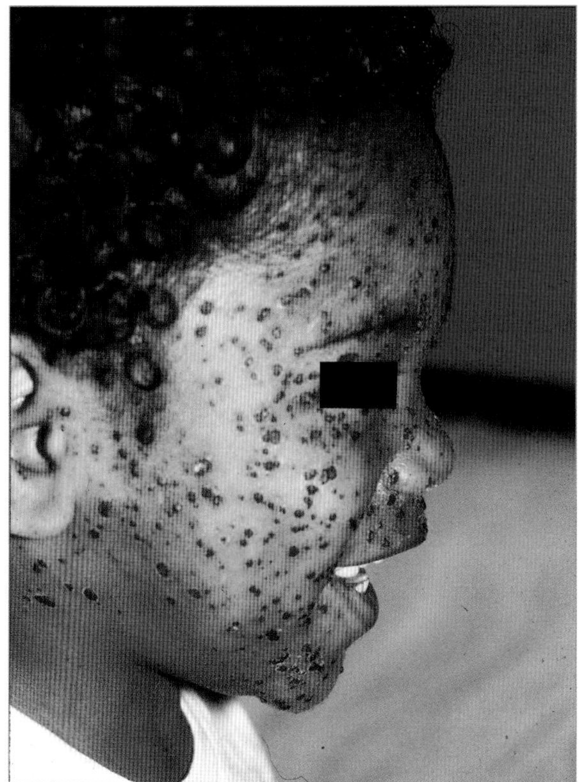

Image 69.27
A 5-year-old African American boy with HIV syndrome with varicella. Courtesy of Larry Frenkel, MD.

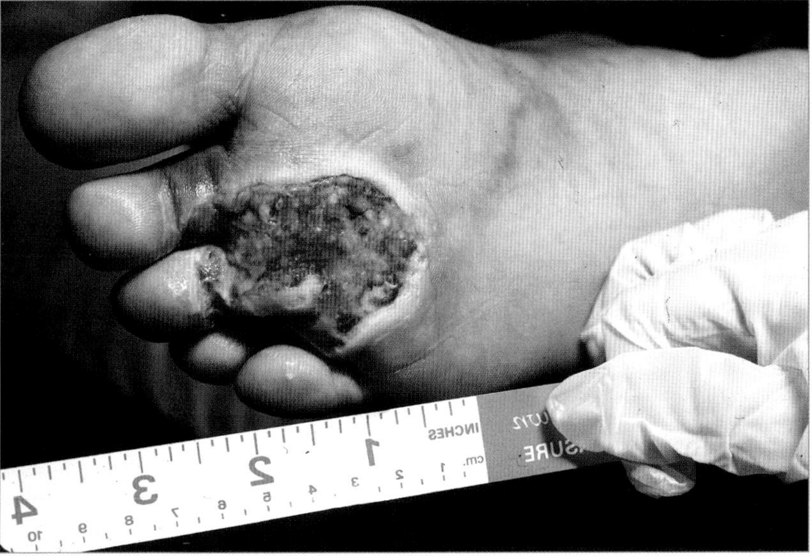

Image 69.28
A 17-year-old Hispanic male with HIV syndrome with an ulcerative lesion on the plantar surface of the left foot of several months' duration. A viral culture was positive for human herpesvirus, which led to the diagnosis of HIV. Courtesy of Larry Frenkel, MD.

70

Influenza

Clinical Manifestations

Influenza typically begins with sudden onset of fever, often accompanied by chills or rigors, headache, malaise, diffuse myalgia, and nonproductive cough. Subsequently, respiratory tract signs, including sore throat, nasal congestion, rhinitis, and cough, become more prominent. Conjunctival injection, abdominal pain, nausea, vomiting, and diarrhea are less commonly associated with influenza illness. In some children, influenza can appear as an upper respiratory tract infection or as a febrile illness with few respiratory tract symptoms. Influenza is an important cause of otitis media. Acute myositis characterized by calf tenderness and refusal to walk has been described. In infants, influenza can produce a sepsislike picture and can occasionally cause croup, bronchiolitis, or pneumonia. Although the large majority of children with influenza recover fully after 3 to 7 days, previously healthy children can have severe symptoms and complications. In the 2013–2014 influenza season, 43% of children hospitalized with influenza had no known underlying conditions. Neurologic complications associated with influenza range from febrile seizures to severe encephalopathy and encephalitis with status epilepticus, with resulting neurologic sequelae or death. Reye syndrome, which is now a very rare condition, has been associated with influenza infection and the use of aspirin therapy during the illness. Children with influenza or suspected influenza should not be given aspirin. Death from influenza-associated myocarditis has been reported. Invasive secondary infections or coinfections with group A streptococcus, *Staphylococcus aureus* (including methicillin-resistant *S aureus*), *Streptococcus pneumoniae*, or other bacterial pathogens can result in severe disease and death.

Etiology

Influenza viruses are orthomyxoviruses of 3 genera or types (A, B, and C). Epidemic disease is caused by influenza virus types A and B, and influenza A and B virus antigens are included in influenza vaccines. Type C influenza viruses cause sporadic, mild influenza-like illness in children and antigens are not included in influenza vaccines. The virus type or subtype may have an effect on the number of hospitalizations and deaths that season. For example, seasons with influenza A (H3N2) as the predominant circulating strain have had 2.7-times higher average mortality rates than other seasons. The 2009 influenza A (H1N1) pandemic combined exceptional pediatric virulence and lack of immunity, which resulted in nearly 4 times as many pediatric deaths as usually recorded.

Influenza A viruses are subclassified into subtypes by 2 surface antigens, hemagglutinin (HA) and neuraminidase (NA). Examples of these include H1N1 and H3N2 viruses. Specific antibodies to these various antigens, especially to HA, are important determinants of immunity. Minor antigenic variation within the same influenza B type or influenza A subtypes is called **antigenic drift.** Antigenic drift occurs continuously and results in new strains of influenza A and B viruses, leading to seasonal epidemics. On the basis of ongoing global surveillance data, there have only been 5 times since 1986 that the vaccine strains in the influenza vaccine have not changed from the previous season. Antigenic shifts are major changes in influenza A viruses that result in new subtypes that contain a new HA alone or with a new NA. Antigenic shift only occurs with influenza A viruses and can lead a to pandemic if the new strain can infect humans and be transmitted efficiently from person to person in a sustained manner in the setting of little or no preexisting immunity.

From April 2009 to August 2010, the World Health Organization declared such a pandemic caused by influenza A (H1N1) virus. There now have been 4 influenza pandemics caused by antigenic shift in the 20th and 21st centuries. The 2009 pandemic was associated with 2 waves of substantial activity in the United States, occurring in the spring and fall of 2009 and extending well into winter 2010. During this time, more than 99% of virus isolates characterized were the 2009 pandemic influenza A (H1N1) virus. As with previous antigenic shifts, the 2009 pandemic influenza A (H1N1) viral strain has replaced the previously circulating seasonal influenza A (H1N1) strain.

Humans of all ages are occasionally infected with influenza A viruses of swine or avian origin. Human infections with swine viruses have manifested as typical influenza-like illness, and confirmation of infection caused by an influenza virus of swine origin has been discovered retrospectively during routine typing of human influenza isolates. For example, influenza A (H3N2v) viruses with the matrix (M) gene from the 2009 H1N1 pandemic virus were first detected in people in 2011 and were responsible for a multistate outbreak in summer 2012. Most cases were associated with exposure to swine at agricultural fairs, and no sustained human-to-human transmission was observed. Similarly, human infections with avian influenza viruses are uncommon but may result in a spectrum of disease, including mild respiratory symptoms and conjunctivitis to severe lower respiratory tract disease, acute respiratory distress syndrome, and death. Most notable among avian influenza viruses are A (H5N1) and A (H7N9), both of which have been associated with severe disease and high case-fatality rates. Influenza A (H5N1) viruses emerged as human infections in 1997 and have since caused human disease in Asia, Africa, Europe, and the Middle East, areas where these viruses are present in domestic or wild birds. Influenza A (H7N9) infections were first detected in 2013 and have been associated with sporadic disease in China.

Epidemiology

Influenza is spread from person to person, primarily by respiratory tract droplets created by coughing or sneezing. Contact with respiratory tract droplet–contaminated surfaces followed by autoinoculation is another mode of transmission. During community outbreaks of influenza, the highest incidence occurs among school-aged children. Secondary spread to adults and other children within a family is common. Incidence and disease severity depend, in part, on immunity developed as a result of previous experience (by natural disease) or recent influenza immunization with the circulating strain or a related strain. Influenza A viruses, including 2 subtypes (H1N1 and H3N2), and influenza B viruses circulate worldwide, but the prevalence of each can vary among communities and within a single community over the course of an influenza season. Antigenic drift in the circulating strain(s) is associated with seasonal epidemics. In temperate climates, seasonal epidemics usually occur during winter months. Peak influenza activity in the United States can occur anytime from November to May but most commonly occurs between January and March. Community outbreaks can last 4 to 8 weeks or longer. Circulation of 2 or 3 influenza virus strains in a community may be associated with a prolonged influenza season of 3 months or more and bimodal peaks in activity. Influenza is highly contagious, especially among semi-enclosed, institutionalized populations and other ongoing, closed-group gatherings, such as school and preschool or child care classrooms. Patients may be infectious 24 hours before onset of symptoms. Viral shedding in nasal secretions usually peaks during the first 3 days of illness and ceases within 7 days but can be prolonged in young children and immunodeficient patients for 10 days or even longer. Viral shedding is correlated directly with degree of fever.

Incidence of influenza in healthy children is generally 10% to 40% each year, but illness rates as low as 3% have also been reported, depending on the circulating strain. Tens of thousands of children visit clinics and emergency departments because of influenza illness each season. Influenza and its complications have been reported to result in a 10% to 30% increase in the number of courses of antimicrobial agents prescribed to children during the influenza season. Although bacterial coinfections with a variety of pathogens, including methicillin-resistant *S aureus,* have been reported, medical care encounters for children with influenza are an important cause of inappropriate antimicrobial use.

Hospitalization rates among children younger than 2 years are similar to hospitalization rates among people 65 years and older. Rates vary among studies (190–480 per 100,000 population) because of differences in methodology and severity of influenza seasons. However, children younger than 24 months are consistently at a substantially higher risk of hospitalization than older children. Antecedent influenza infection is sometimes associated with development of pneumococcal or staphylococcal pneumonia in children. Methicillin-resistant staphylococcal community-acquired pneumonia, with a rapid clinical progression and a high fatality rate, has been reported in previously healthy children and adults with concomitant influenza infection. Rates of hospitalization and morbidity attributable to complications, such as bronchitis and pneumonia, are even greater in children with high-risk conditions, including asthma, diabetes mellitus, hemodynamically significant cardiac disease, immunosuppression, and neurologic and neurodevelopmental disorders. Influenza virus infection in neonates has also been associated with considerable morbidity, including a sepsislike syndrome, apnea, and lower respiratory tract disease.

Fatal outcomes, including sudden death, have been reported in chronically ill and previously healthy children. Since influenza-related pediatric deaths became nationally notifiable in 2004, the number of deaths among children reported annually in nonpandemic seasons has ranged from 46 (2005–2006 season) to 171 (2012–2013 season); during the 2009–2010 season, the number of pediatric deaths in the United States was 288. During the entire influenza A (H1N1) pandemic period lasting from April 2009 to August 2010, a total of 344 laboratory-confirmed, influenza-associated pediatric deaths were reported. Influenza A and B viruses have been associated with deaths in children, most of which have occurred in children younger than 5 years. Almost half of children who die do not have a high-risk condition as defined by the Advisory Committee on Immunization Practices. All influenza-associated pediatric deaths are nationally notifiable and should be reported to the Centers for Disease Control and Prevention through state health departments.

Incubation Period

Usually 1 to 4 days, with a mean of 2 days.

Influenza Pandemics

A pandemic is defined by emergence and global spread of a new influenza A virus subtype to which the population has little or no immunity and that spreads rapidly from person to person. Pandemics, therefore, can lead to substantially increased morbidity and mortality rates compared with seasonal influenza. During the 20th century, there were 3 influenza pandemics, in 1918 (H1N1), 1957 (H2N2), and 1968 (H3N2). The pandemic in 1918 killed at least 20 million people in the United States and perhaps as many as 50 million people worldwide. The 2009 influenza A (H1N1) pandemic was the first in the 21st century, lasting from April 2009 to August 2010; there were 18,449 deaths among laboratory-confirmed influenza cases. However, this is believed to represent only a fraction of the true number of deaths. On the basis of a modeling study from the Centers for Disease Control and Prevention, it is estimated the 2009 influenza A (H1N1) pandemic was associated with between 151,700 and 575,400 deaths worldwide. Public health authorities have developed plans for pandemic preparedness and response to a pandemic in the United States. Pediatricians should be familiar with national, state, and institutional pandemic plans, including recommendations for vaccine and antiviral drug use, health care surge capacity, and personal protective strategies that can be communicated to patients and families. Up-to-date information on pandemic influenza can be found at **www.flu.gov.**

Diagnostic Tests

Specimens for viral culture, reverse transcriptase-polymerase chain reaction (RT-PCR), rapid influenza molecular assays, or rapid diagnostic tests should be obtained, if possible, during the first 72 hours of illness because the quantity of virus shed decreases rapidly as illness progresses beyond that point. Specimens of nasopharyngeal secretions obtained by swab, aspirate, or wash should be placed in appropriate transport media for culture. After inoculation into eggs or cell culture, influenza virus can usually be isolated within 2 to 6 days. Rapid diagnostic tests for identification of influenza A and B antigens in respiratory tract specimens are available commercially, although their reported sensitivity (44%–97%) and specificity (76%–100%) compared with viral culture, RT-PCR, and rapid influenza molecular assays are variable and differ by test and specimen type. Additionally, many rapid diagnostic antigen tests cannot distinguish between influenza subtypes, a feature that can be critical during seasons with strains that differ in antiviral susceptibility or relative virulence. Results of rapid diagnostic tests should be interpreted in the context of clinical findings and local community influenza activity. Careful clinical judgment must be exercised because the prevalence of circulating influenza viruses influences the positive and negative predictive values of these influenza screening tests. False-positive results are more likely to occur during periods of low influenza activity; false-negative results are more likely to occur during periods of peak influenza activity. Decisions on treatment and infection control can be made on the basis of positive rapid diagnostic test results. Positive results are helpful because they may reduce additional testing to identify the cause of the child's influenza-like illness. Treatment should not be withheld in high-risk patients awaiting RT-PCR test results. Serologic diagnosis can be established retrospectively by a 4-fold or greater increase in antibody titer in serum specimens obtained during the acute and convalescent stages of illness, as determined by hemagglutination inhibition testing, complement fixation testing, neutralization testing, or enzyme immunoassay. However, serologic testing is rarely useful in patient management because 2 serum samples collected 10 to 14 days apart are required. Rapid influenza molecular assays are becoming more widely available. Reverse transcriptase-polymerase chain reaction, viral culture tests, and rapid influenza molecular assays offer potential for high sensitivity as well as specificity and are recommended as the tests of choice.

Treatment

In the United States, 2 classes of antiviral medications are currently approved for treatment or prophylaxis of influenza infections: neuraminidase inhibitors (oseltamivir and zanamivir) and adamantanes (amantadine and rimantadine). Guidance for use of these 4 antiviral agents is summarized in Table 70.1. Oseltamivir, an oral drug, remains the antiviral drug of choice that can be given to children as young as 2 weeks. Given preliminary pharmacokinetic data and limited safety data, oseltamivir can be used to treat influenza in term and preterm newborns from birth because benefits of therapy are likely to outweigh possible risks of treatment. Zanamivir, an inhaled drug, is an acceptable alternative but is more difficult to administer, especially to young children.

Widespread resistance to adamantanes has been documented among H3N2 and H1N1 influenza viruses since 2005 (influenza B

Table 70.1
Antiviral Drugs for Influenza[a]

Drug (Trade Name)	Virus	Administration	Treatment Indications	Chemoprophylaxis Indications	Adverse Effects
Oseltamivir (Tamiflu)	A and B	Oral	Birth or older[b]	3 mo or older	Nausea, vomiting
Zanamivir (Relenza)	A and B	Inhalation	7 y or older	5 y or older	Bronchospasm
Amantadine[c] (Symmetrel)	A	Oral	1 y or older	1 y or older	Central nervous system, anxiety, gastrointestinal
Rimantadine[c] (Flumadine)	A	Oral	13 y or older	1 y or older	Central nervous system, anxiety, gastrointestinal

[a] For current recommendations about treatment and chemoprophylaxis of influenza, including specific dosing information, see **www.cdc.gov/flu/professionals/antivirals/index.htm** or **www.aapredbook.org/flu**.

[b] Approved by the US Food and Drug Administration for children as young as 2 weeks. Given preliminary pharmacokinetic data and limited safety data, oseltamivir can be used to treat influenza in term and preterm newborns from birth because benefits of therapy are likely to outweigh possible risks of treatment.

[c] High levels of resistance to amantadine and rimantadine persist, and these drugs should not be used unless resistance patterns change significantly. Antiviral susceptibilities of viral strains are reported weekly at **www.cdc.gov/flu/weekly/fluactivitysurv.htm.**

viruses intrinsically are not susceptible to adamantanes). Since January 2006, neuraminidase inhibitors (oseltamivir, zanamivir) have been the only recommended influenza antiviral drugs against influenza viruses. Resistance to oseltamivir has been documented to be around 1%, at most, for any of the tested influenza viral samples during the past few years. Each year, options for treatment or chemoprophylaxis of influenza in the United States will depend on influenza strain resistance patterns.

Therapy for influenza virus infection should be offered to any hospitalized child who has severe, complicated, or progressive respiratory illness that may be influenza related, regardless of influenza-immunization status or whether onset of illness has been greater than 48 hours before admission. Outpatient therapy should be offered for influenza infection of any severity in children at high risk of complications of influenza infection, such as children younger than 2 years. Treatment may be considered for any otherwise healthy child with influenza infection for whom a decrease in duration of clinical symptoms is believed to be warranted by his or her pediatrician. Antiviral treatment should also be considered for symptomatic siblings of infants younger than 6 months or with underlying medical conditions that predispose them to complications of influenza. Children with severe influenza should be evaluated carefully for possible coinfection with bacterial pathogens (eg, *S aureus*) that might require antimicrobial therapy. Clinicians who want to have influenza isolates tested for susceptibility should contact their state health department.

The duration of treatment is 5 days for the neuraminidase inhibitors.

The most common adverse effects of oseltamivir are nausea and vomiting. Zanamivir use has been associated with bronchospasm in some people and is not recommended for use in patients with underlying airway disease.

Control of fever with acetaminophen or another appropriate nonsalicylate-containing antipyretic agent may be important in young children because fever and other symptoms of influenza could exacerbate underlying chronic conditions. Children and adolescents with influenza should not receive aspirin or any salicylate-containing products because of the potential risk of developing Reye syndrome.

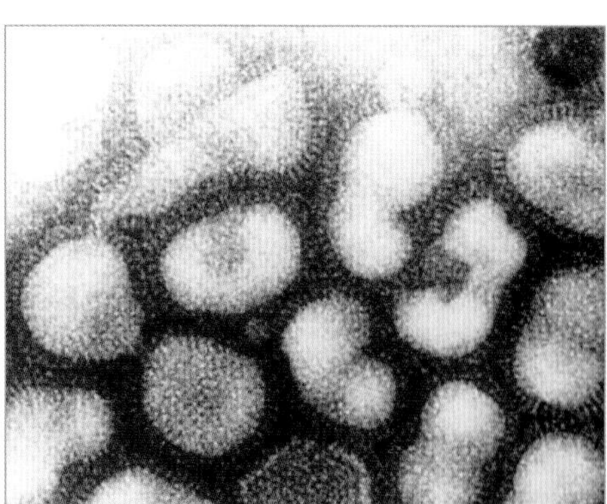

Image 70.1
Transmission electron micrograph of influenza A virus, late passage. Courtesy of Centers for Disease Control and Prevention/Dr Erskine Palmer.

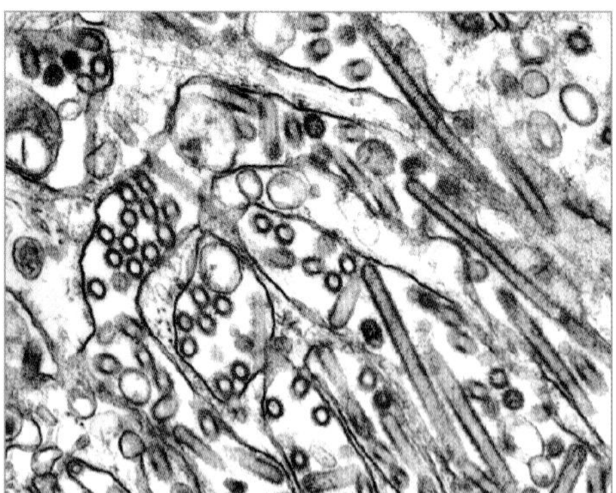

Image 70.2
Colorized transmission electron micrograph of avian influenza A (H5N1) viruses (seen in gold) grown in Madin-Darby canine kidney epithelial cells (seen in green). Avian influenza A viruses do not usually infect humans; however, several instances of human infections and outbreaks have been reported since 1997. When such infections occur, public health authorities monitor these situations closely. Courtesy of Centers for Disease Control and Prevention/Courtesy of Cynthia Goldsmith; Jacqueline Katz; Sherif R. Zaki.

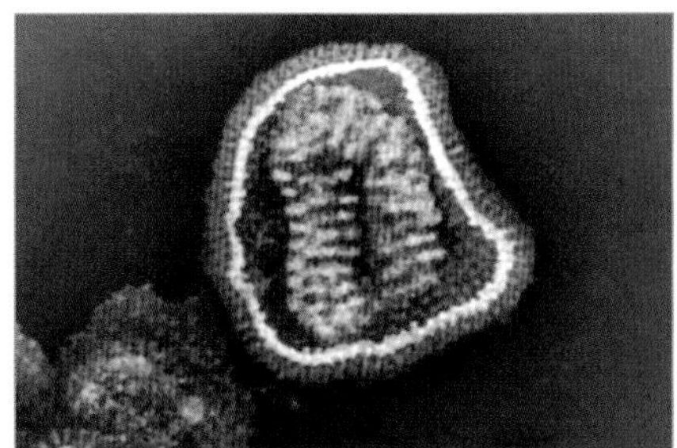

Image 70.3
This negative-stained transmission electron micrograph depicts the ultrastructural details of an influenza virus particle, or virion. Courtesy of Centers for Disease Control and Prevention/Erskine L. Palmer, MD/M. L. Martin, MD.

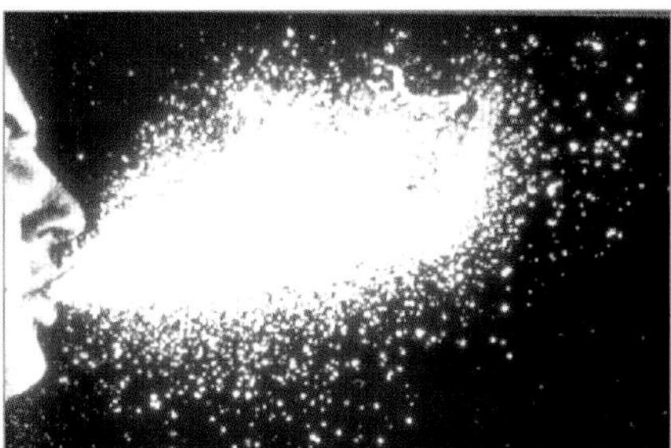

Image 70.4
Influenza, like many viral infections, is spread by droplet transmission or direct contact with items recently contaminated by infected nasopharyngeal secretions. Courtesy of Centers for Disease Control and Prevention.

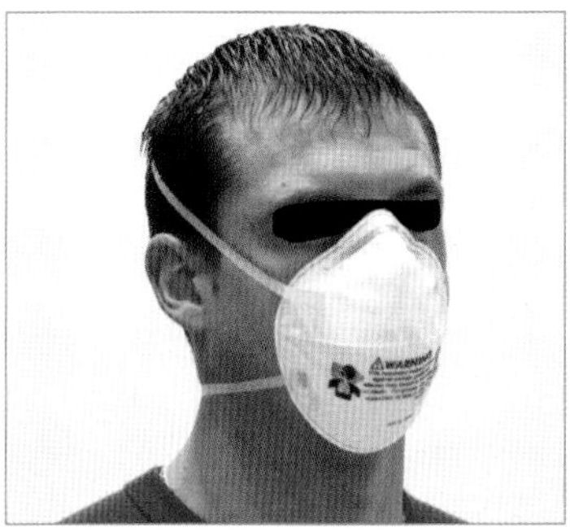

Image 70.5
Properly donned disposable N95 filtering facepiece respirator. To be properly donned, the respirator must be correctly oriented on the face and held in position with both straps. The straps must be correctly placed, with the upper strap high on the head and the lower strap below the ears. For persons with long hair, the lower strap should be placed under (not over) the hair. The nose clip must be tightened to avoid gaps between the respirator and the skin. Facial hair should be removed before donning. Appropriate respirator donning could be important in the event of an influenza epidemic. Courtesy of Centers for Disease Control and Prevention/*Emerging Infectious Diseases* and Kristin J. Cummings.

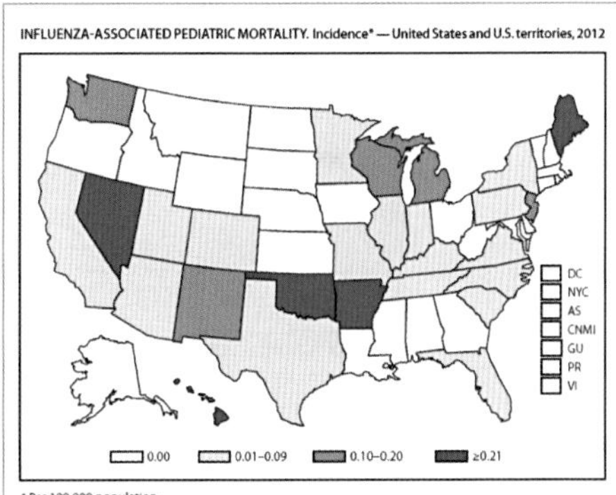

Image 70.6
Influenza-associated pediatric mortality. Incidence—United States and US territories, 2012. Courtesy of *Morbidity and Mortality Weekly Report.*

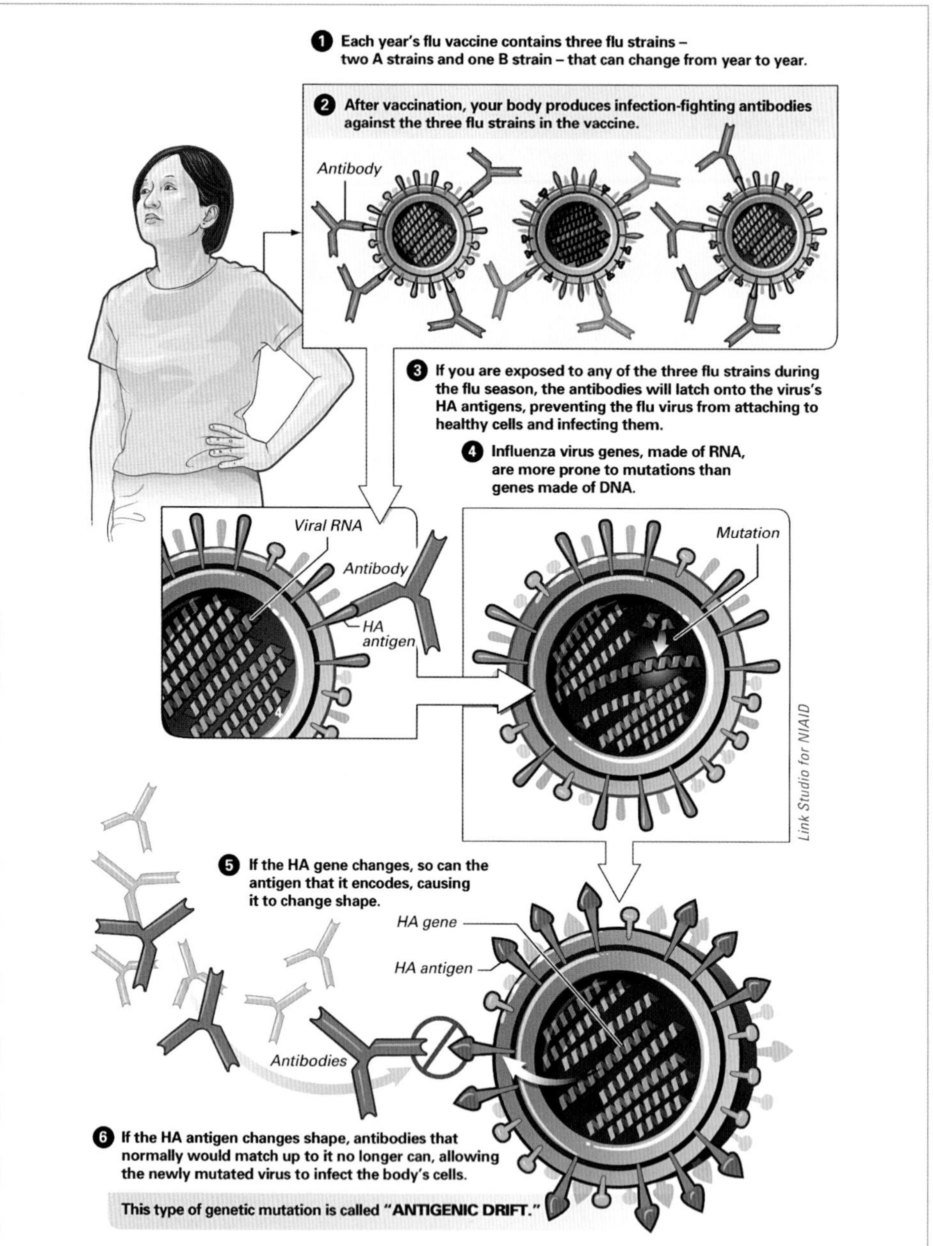

Image 70.7

Antigenic drift. Each year's flu vaccine contains 3 flu strains—2 A strains and 1 B strain—that can change from year to year. After vaccination, the body produces infection-fighting antibodies against the 3 flu strains in the vaccine. If a vaccinated individual is exposed to any of the 3 flu strains during the flu season, the antibodies will latch onto the virus hemagglutinin (HA) antigens, preventing the flu virus from attaching to healthy cells and infecting them. Influenza virus genes, made of RNA, are more prone to mutations than genes made of DNA. If the HA gene changes, so can the antigen that it encodes, causing it to change shape. If the HA antigen changes shape, antibodies that normally would match up to it no longer can, allowing the newly mutated virus to infect the body's cells. This type of genetic mutation is called antigenic drift. Courtesy of National Institute of Allergy and Infectious Diseases.

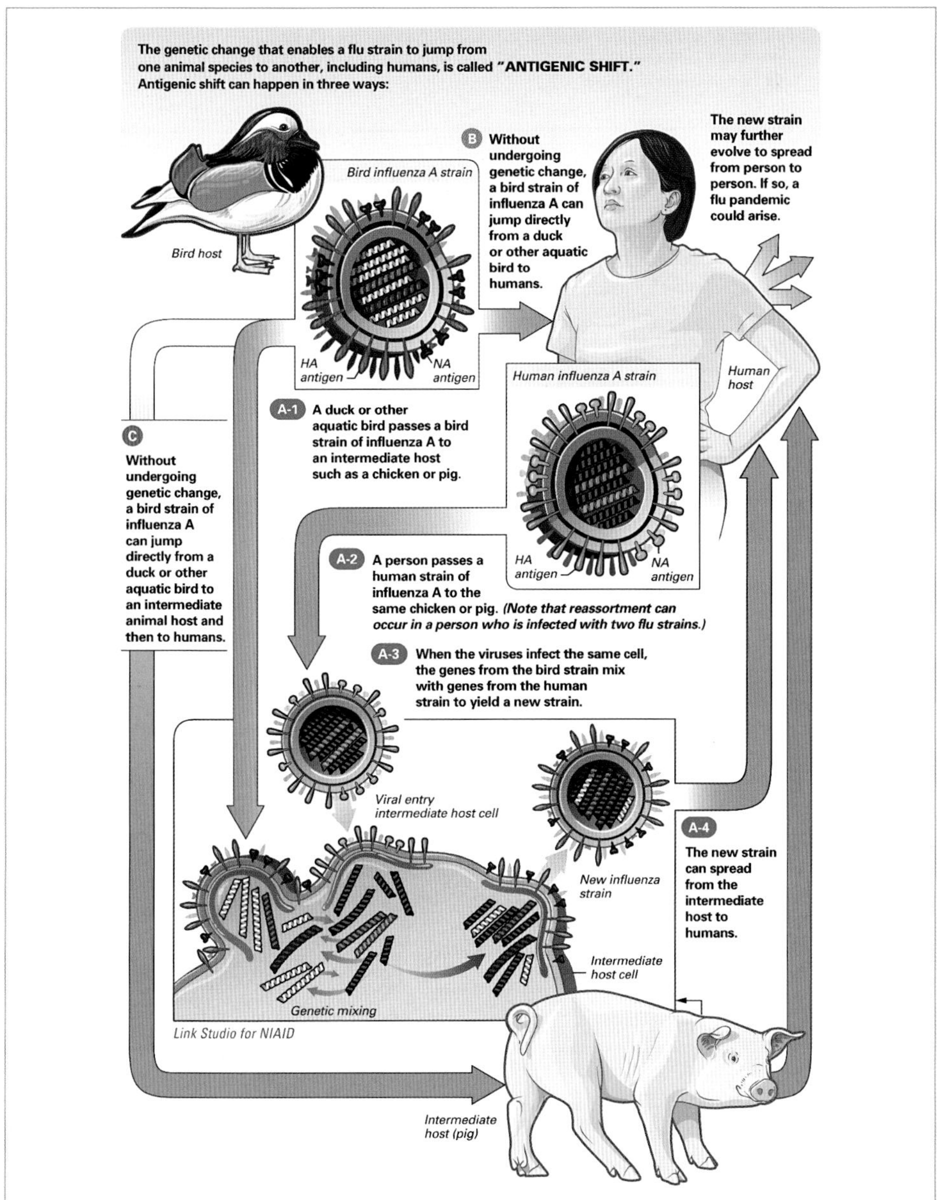

Image 70.8

Antigenic shift. The genetic change that enables a flu strain to jump from one animal species to another, including humans, is called antigenic shift. Antigenic shift can happen in 3 ways. **Antigenic shift 1:** A duck or other aquatic bird passes a bird strain of influenza A to an intermediate host, such as a chicken or pig. A person passes a human strain of influenza A to the same chicken or pig. When the viruses infect the same cell, genes from the bird strain mix with genes from the human strain to yield a new strain. The new strain can spread from the intermediate host to humans. **Antigenic shift 2:** Without undergoing genetic change, a bird strain of influenza A can jump directly from a duck or other aquatic bird to humans. **Antigenic shift 3:** Without undergoing genetic change, a bird strain of influenza A can jump directly from a duck or other aquatic bird to an intermediate animal host and then to humans. The new strain may further evolve to spread from person to person. If so, an influenza pandemic could arise. Courtesy of National Institute of Allergy and Infectious Diseases.

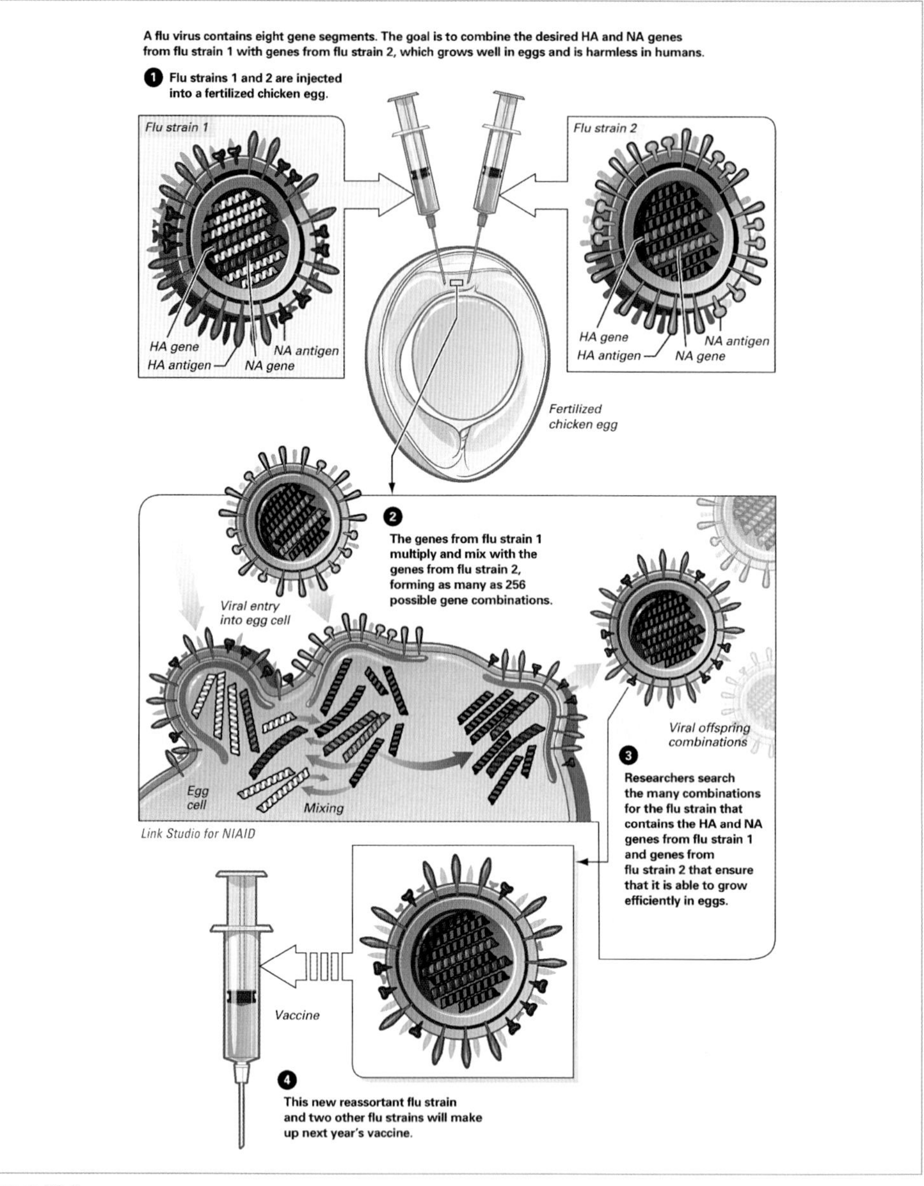

Image 70.9

Recombination. An influenza virus contains 8 gene segments. One of the gene segments codes for the surface antigen hemagglutinin (HA), and another codes for the surface antigen neuraminidase (NA). Each year, researchers predict which flu strains will be most prevalent and select 3—2 influenza A strains and 1 influenza B strain—to be included in that year's vaccine. The goal of recombination is to combine the desired HA and NA antigens from the target strain (flu strain 1) with genes from a harmless strain that grows well in an egg (flu strain 2). The illustration details the following steps in creating the vaccine: Flu strains 1 and 2 are injected into a fertilized chicken egg. The genes from flu strain 1 multiply and mix with the genes from flu strain 2, forming as many as 256 possible gene combinations. Researchers search the many combinations for the flu strain that contains the HA and NA genes from flu strain 1 and remaining genes from flu strain 2 that ensures it is able to grow efficiently in eggs. This new recombined flu strain and 2 other flu strains will make up next year's vaccine. Courtesy of National Institute of Allergy and Infectious Diseases.

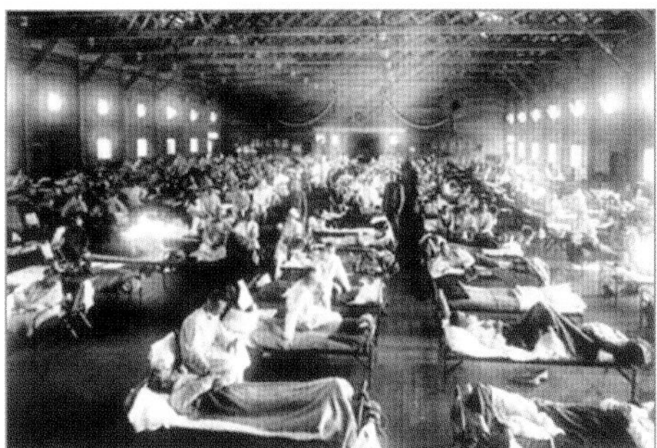

Image 70.10
Emergency hospital during 1918 influenza epidemic, Camp Funston, KS. Source: National Museum of Health and Medicine, Armed Forces Institute of Pathology, Washington, DC, Image NCP 1603. Courtesy of Immunization Action Coalition.

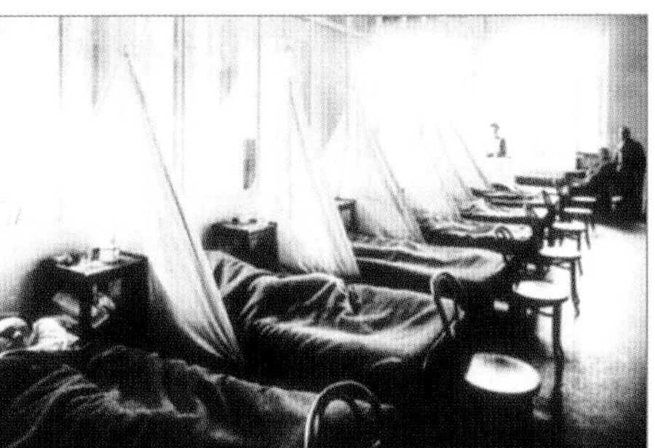

Image 70.11
US Army Camp Hospital No. 45, Aix-Les-Bains, France, influenza ward 1, 1918. Source: National Museum of Health and Medicine, Armed Forces Institute of Pathology, Washington, DC, Image Reeve 14682. Courtesy of Immunization Action Coalition.

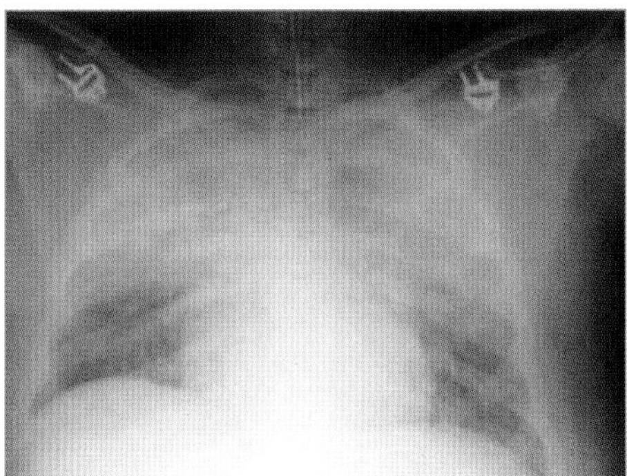

Image 70.12
Influenza pneumonia in a 12-year-old boy with respiratory failure. Courtesy of Benjamin Estrada, MD.

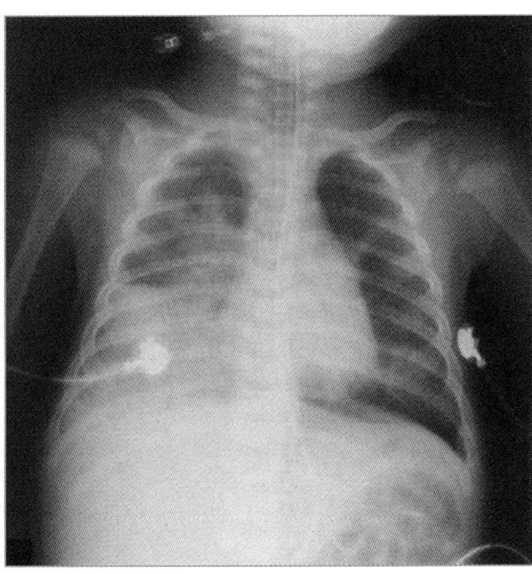

Image 70.13
Influenza A with *Staphylococcus aureus* pneumonia with empyema in a preschool-aged child. Courtesy of Benjamin Estrada, MD.

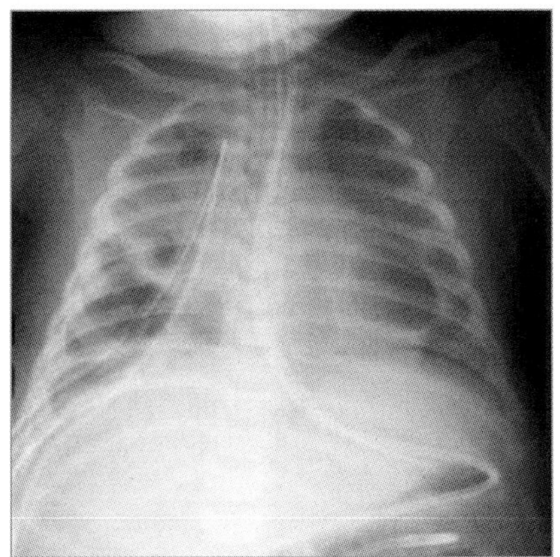

Image 70.14
Influenza A with *Staphylococcus aureus* superinfection in a 6-year-old. Note the presence of bilateral pneumatoceles. Courtesy of Benjamin Estrada, MD.

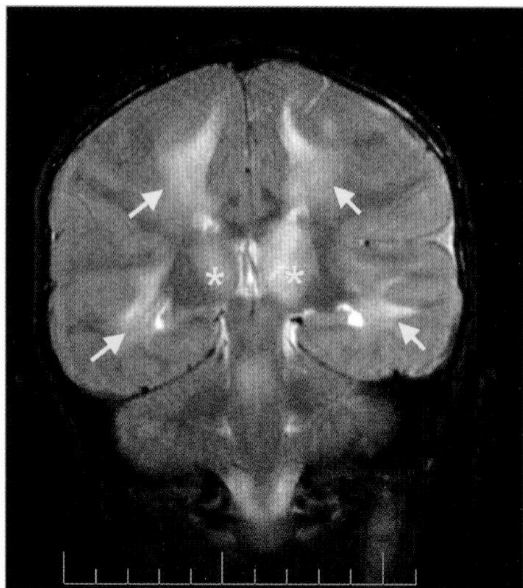

Image 70.15
Coronal T2-weighted magnetic resonance image of a 5-year-old with influenza-associated encephalopathy demonstrating bilateral confluent signal hyperintensity in the white matter (arrows) and thalami (asterisks). Courtesy of James Sejvar, MD.

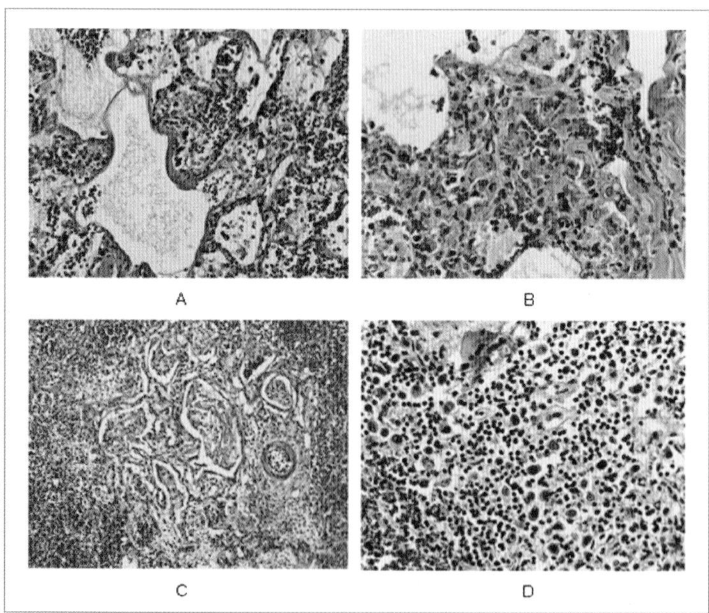

Image 70.16
Pathologic findings from a patient with confirmed influenza A (H5N1) infection (hematoxylin-eosin stain, magnification x40). A, Hyaline membrane formation lining the alveolar spaces of the lung and vascular congestion with a few infiltrating lymphocytes in the interstitial areas. Reactive fibroblasts are also present. B, An area of lung with proliferating reactive fibroblasts within the interstitial areas. Few lymphocytes are seen, and no viral intranuclear inclusions are visible. C, Fibrinous exudates filling the alveolar spaces, with organizing formation and few hyaline membranes. The surrounding alveolar spaces contain hemorrhage. D, A section of spleen showing numerous atypical lymphoid cells scattered around the white pulp. No viral intranuclear inclusions are seen. Courtesy of Centers for Disease Control and Prevention.

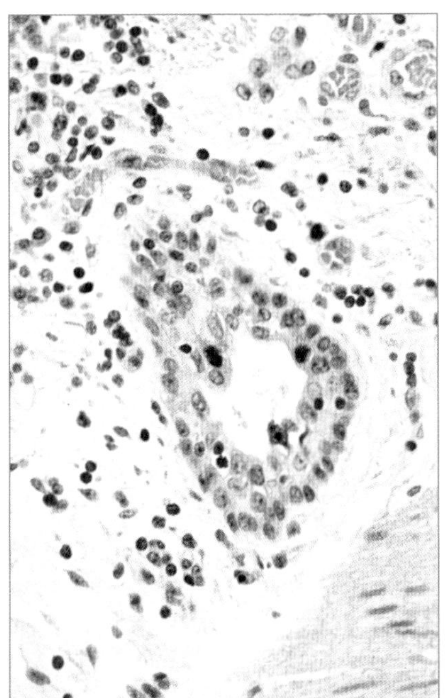

Image 70.17
Influenza viral antigens in bronchial epithelial lining cells as seen by immunohistochemistry. Courtesy of Centers for Disease Control and Prevention.

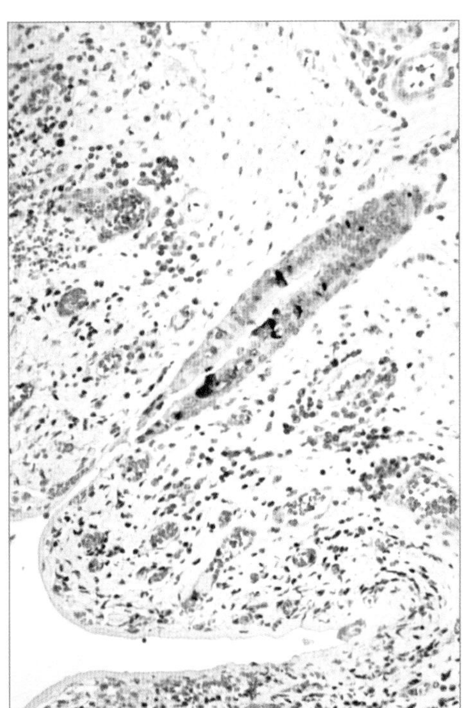

Image 70.18
Immunostaining for influenza B viral antigens. Note intracellular viral antigens in these areas. Courtesy of Centers for Disease Control and Prevention.

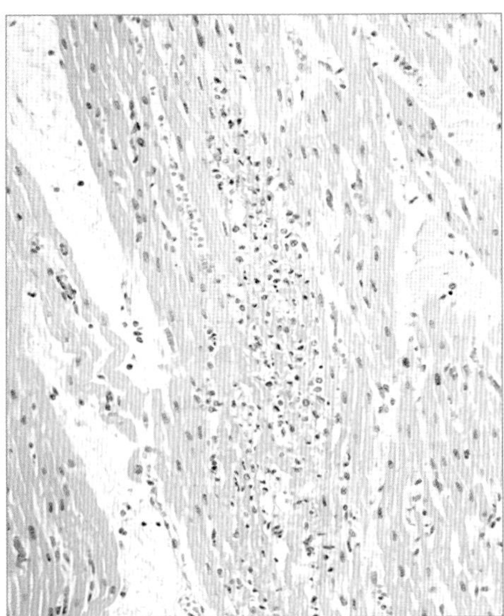

Image 70.19
Focal myocarditis seen in the patient in Image 70.18 with influenza B infection. Note myocardial necrosis associated with areas of mostly mononuclear inflammation. Courtesy of Centers for Disease Control and Prevention.

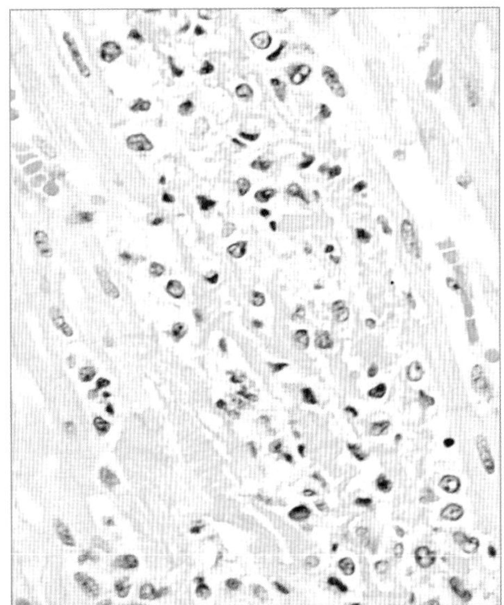

Image 70.20
This is Image 70.19 of influenza B myocarditis at a higher magnification. Courtesy of Centers for Disease Control and Prevention.

71

Isosporiasis (now designated as Cystoisosporiasis)

Clinical Manifestations

Watery diarrhea is the most common symptom of cystoisosporiasis and can be profuse and protracted, even in immunocompetent people. Manifestations are similar to those caused by other enteric protozoa (eg, *Cryptosporidium*, *Cyclospora* species) and can include abdominal pain, cramping, anorexia, nausea, vomiting, weight loss, and low-grade fever. Eosinophilia can also occur. The proportion of infected people who are asymptomatic is unknown. Severity of infection ranges from self-limiting in immunocompetent hosts to debilitating and life threatening in immunocompromised patients, particularly people infected with HIV. Infections of the biliary tract and reactive arthritis have also been reported.

Etiology

Cystoisospora (formerly *Isospora*) *belli* is a coccidian protozoan; oocysts (rather than cysts) are passed in stools.

Epidemiology

Infection occurs predominantly in tropical and subtropical regions of the world and can cause traveler's diarrhea. Infection results from ingestion of sporulated oocysts in contaminated food or water. Humans are the only known host for *C belli* and shed noninfective oocysts in feces. These oocysts must mature (sporulate) outside the host in the environment to become infective. Under favorable conditions, sporulation can be completed in 1 to 2 days and, perhaps, more quickly in some settings. Oocysts probably are resistant to most disinfectants and can remain viable for prolonged periods in a cool, moist environment.

Incubation Period

Uncertain, but ranges from 7 to 12 days in reported cases associated with accidental laboratory exposures.

Diagnostic Tests

Identification of oocysts in feces or in duodenal aspirates or finding developmental stages of the parasite in biopsy specimens (eg, of the small intestine) is diagnostic. Oocysts in stool are elongate and ellipsoidal (length, 25–30 µm). Oocysts can be shed in low numbers, even by people with profuse diarrhea. This constraint underscores the utility of repeated stool examinations, sensitive recovery methods (eg, concentration methods), and detection methods that highlight the organism (eg, oocysts stain bright red with modified acid-fast techniques and autofluoresce when viewed by ultraviolet fluorescent microscopy).

Treatment

Trimethoprim-sulfamethoxazole, typically for 7 to 10 days, is the drug of choice. Patients who are immunocompromised may need higher doses and a longer duration of therapy. Pyrimethamine (plus leucovorin, to prevent myelosuppression) is an alternative treatment for people who cannot tolerate trimethoprim-sulfamethoxazole. Ciprofloxacin is less effective than trimethoprim-sulfamethoxazole. In adolescents and adults, maintenance therapy is recommended to prevent recurrent disease for people infected with HIV.

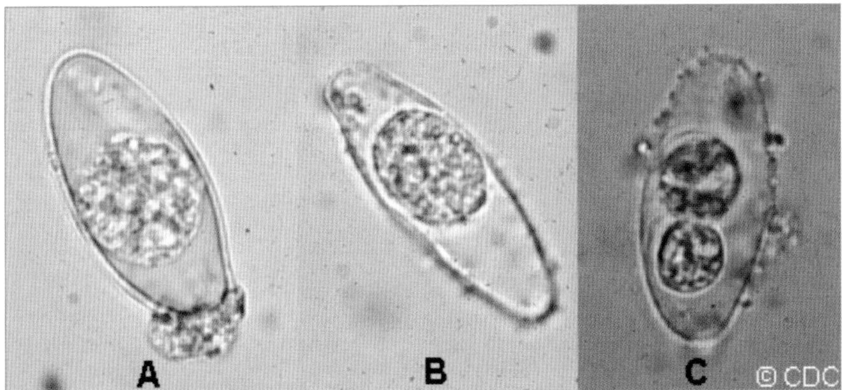

Image 71.1

Oocysts of *Cystoisospora* (formerly *Isospora*) *belli* (iodine stain). The oocysts are large (25–30 µm) and have a typical ellipsoidal shape. When excreted, they are immature and contain 1 sporoblast (A, B). The oocyst matures after excretion; the single sporoblast divides into 2 sporoblasts (C), which develop cyst walls, becoming sporocysts, which eventually contain 4 sporozoites each. Courtesy of Centers for Disease Control and Prevention.

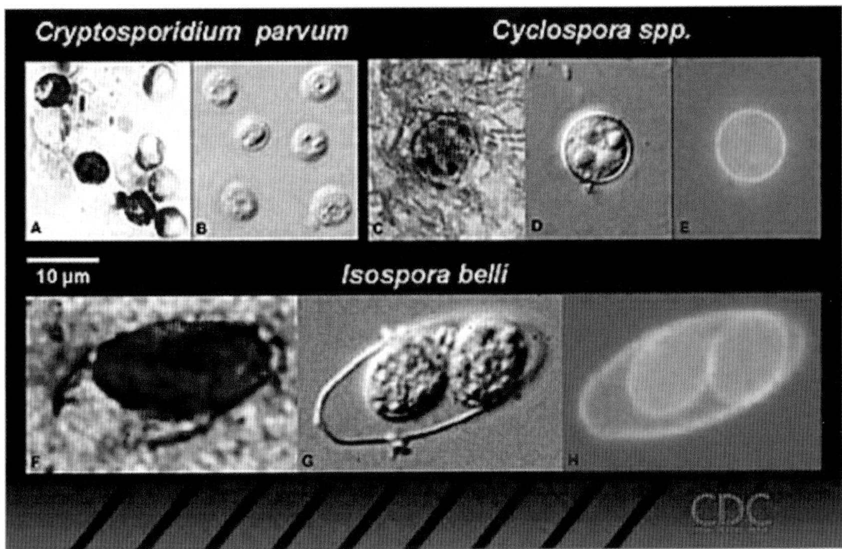

Image 71.2

Oocysts of *Cystoisospora* (formerly *Isospora*) *belli* can also be stained with acid-fast stain and visualized by epifluorescence on wet mounts, as illustrated. Three coccidian parasites that most commonly infect humans, seen in acid-fast stained smears (A, C, F), bright-field differential interference contrast (B, D, G), and epifluorescence (E, H, C; *Cryptosporidium parvum* oocysts do not autofluoresce). Courtesy of Centers for Disease Control and Prevention.

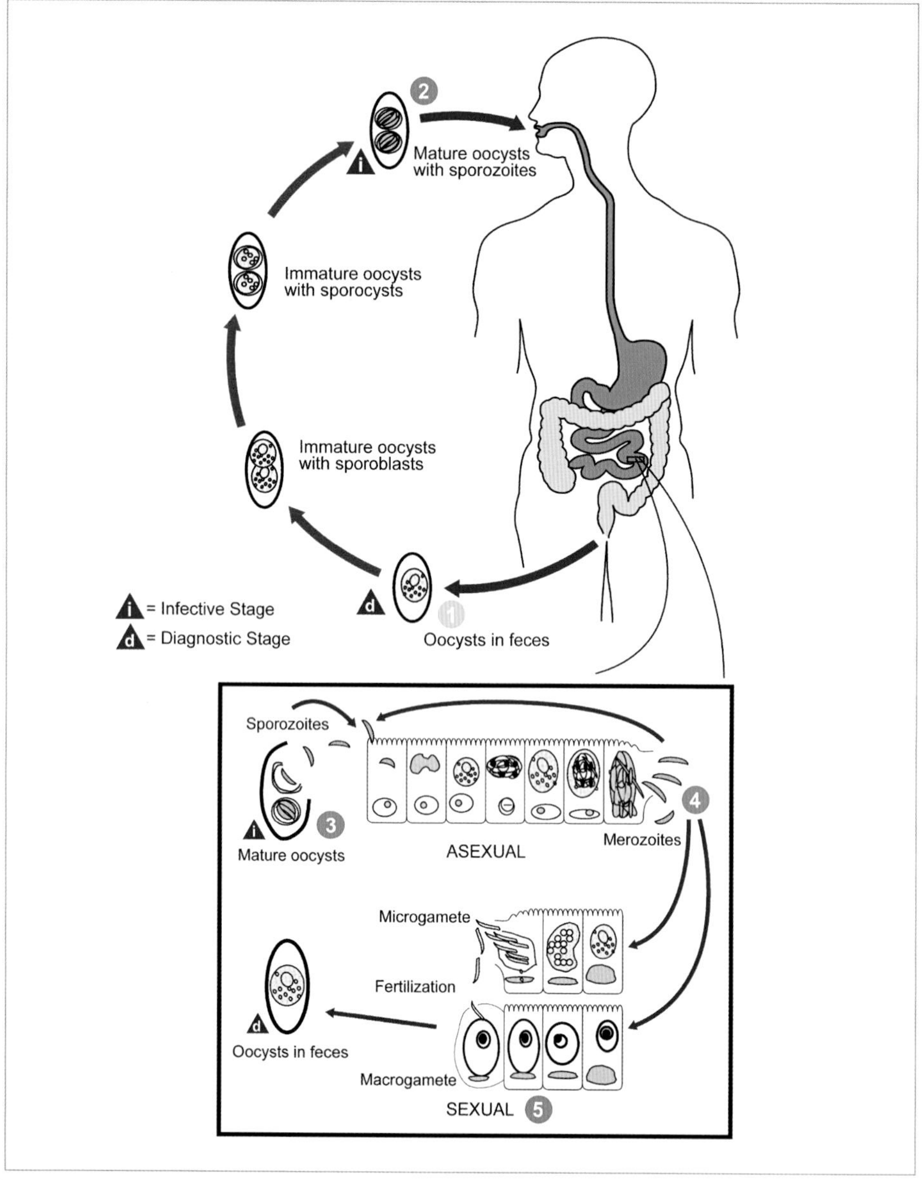

Image 71.3
At time of excretion, the immature oocyst usually contains 1 sporoblast (more rarely, 2) (1). In further maturation after excretion, the sporoblast divides into 2 (the oocyst now contains 2 sporoblasts); the sporoblasts secrete a cyst wall, thus becoming sporocysts; and the sporocysts divide twice to produce 4 sporozoites each (2). Infection occurs by ingestion of sporocyst-containing oocysts. The sporocysts excyst in the small intestine and release their sporozoites, which invade the epithelial cells and initiate schizogony (3). On rupture of the schizonts, the merozoites are released, invade new epithelial cells, and continue the cycle of asexual multiplication (4). Trophozoites develop into schizonts that contain multiple merozoites. After a minimum of 1 week, the sexual stage begins with the development of male and female gametocytes (5). Fertilization results in the development of oocysts that are excreted in the stool (1). *Cystoisospora* (formerly *Isospora*) *belli* infects humans and animals. Courtesy of Centers for Disease Control and Prevention/Alexander J. da Silva, PhD/ Melanie Moser.

72

Kawasaki Disease

Clinical Manifestations

Kawasaki disease (also called mucocutaneous lymph node syndrome) is a self-limited vasculitis characterized by fever and mucocutaneous signs that is recognized across the globe. If untreated, approximately 20% of children will develop coronary artery abnormalities, including aneurysms. The illness is characterized by fever and the following clinical features: bilateral bulbar conjunctival injection with limbic sparing and without exudate; erythematous mouth and pharynx, strawberry tongue, and red, cracked lips; a polymorphous, generalized, erythematous rash that can be morbilliform, maculopapular, or scarlatiniform or can resemble erythema multiforme; changes in the peripheral extremities consisting of induration of the hands and feet with erythematous palms and soles, often with later periungual desquamation; and acute, nonsuppurative, usually unilateral, cervical lymphadenopathy with at least 1 node 1.5 cm in diameter. Kawasaki disease diagnosis may be delayed in patients who come to attention because of fever and unilateral cervical lymphadenitis, which, mistakenly, is thought to be bacterial lymphadenitis; a distinguishing feature in Kawasaki disease is that lymphadenitis is unlikely to be necrotizing or suppurative by imaging studies. For diagnosis of classic Kawasaki disease, patients should have fever for at least 5 days (or fever until the date of treatment if given before the fifth day of illness) and at least 4 of the 5 previously listed features without alternative explanation for the findings. Presence of a concurrent or preceding viral upper respiratory infection does not exclude the diagnosis of Kawasaki disease. The epidemiologic case definition also allows diagnosis of incomplete Kawasaki disease when a patient has fewer than 4 principal clinical criteria in the presence of fever and coronary artery abnormalities. Irritability, abdominal pain, diarrhea, and vomiting are common associated symptoms. Other findings include urethritis with sterile pyuria (70% of cases), mild anterior uveitis (80%), mild elevation of hepatic transaminase levels (50%), arthritis or arthralgia (10%–20%), meningismus with cerebrospinal fluid pleocytosis (40%), pericardial effusion of at least 1 mm (<5%), gallbladder hydrops (<10%), and myocarditis manifested by congestive heart failure (<5%). A persistent resting tachycardia and the presence of an S_3 gallop are often appreciated. Fine desquamation in the groin area can occur in the acute phase of disease (Fink sign). Inflammation or ulceration may be observed at the inoculation scar of previous bacille Calmette-Guérin immunization. Rarely, Kawasaki disease can present with what appears to be "septic shock" with need for intensive care; these children often have significant thrombocytopenia at admission. Group A streptococcal or *Staphylococcus aureus* toxic shock syndrome should be excluded in such cases.

The diagnosis of incomplete Kawasaki disease should be considered in patients with fever for 5 days or longer plus the presence of 2 or more of the characteristic features with supportive laboratory data (eg, erythrocyte sedimentation rate ≥40 mm/h; C-reactive protein [CRP] concentration ≥3 mg/dL). If patients have purulent conjunctivitis, exudative pharyngitis, or splenomegaly, they are highly unlikely to have Kawasaki disease. The proportion of children with Kawasaki disease with incomplete manifestations is higher among infants younger than 12 months. Infants with Kawasaki disease have a higher risk of developing coronary artery aneurysms than do older children, making diagnosis and timely treatment especially important in this age group. Laboratory findings in incomplete cases are similar to findings in classic cases. Although laboratory findings in Kawasaki disease are nonspecific, they may prove useful in increasing or decreasing the likelihood of incomplete Kawasaki disease. Kawasaki disease should also be considered in any infant younger than 6 months with prolonged fever and no other explanation for the fever and in infants with shocklike syndrome in whom an inciting infection is not confirmed. If coronary artery aneurysm, ectasia, or dilation is evident, a presumptive diagnosis of Kawasaki disease should be made. A normal early echocardiographic study is typical and does not exclude the diagnosis but may be useful in evaluation of patients with suspected incomplete Kawasaki disease. In one study, 80% of patients with Kawasaki disease who ultimately developed coronary artery disease had abnormalities on their admission echocardiogram. Most of these patients were evaluated before day 10 of fever. The American Heart Association algorithm (Image 72.1) summarizes the approach for diagnosis and treatment of suspected incomplete Kawasaki disease.

The average duration of fever in untreated Kawasaki disease is 10 days; however, fever can last 2 weeks or longer. After fever resolves, patients can remain anorectic or irritable with decreased energy for 2 to 3 weeks. During this phase, desquamation of fingers and toes and fine desquamation of other areas can occur. Recurrent disease develops in approximately 2% of patients months to years later.

Coronary artery abnormalities are serious sequelae of Kawasaki disease and may occur in 20% of untreated children. Increased risk of developing coronary artery abnormalities is associated with male gender; age younger than 12 months or older than 8 years; fever for more than 10 days; high baseline relative neutrophil and band count (>80%); white blood cell count >15,000/mm^3; low hemoglobin concentration (<10 g/dL); hypoalbuminemia, hyponatremia, or thrombocytopenia at presentation; fever persisting or occurring after intravenous immunoglobulin (IVIG) administration; and persistence of elevated CRP concentration for more than 30 days or recurrent CRP elevations. Aneurysms of the coronary arteries have been demonstrated by echocardiography as early as 4 to 7 days after onset of illness but more typically occur between 1 and 4 weeks after onset of illness; onset later than 6 weeks is extremely uncommon. Giant coronary artery aneurysms (internal diameter ≥8 mm) are highly predictive of long-term complications. Aneurysms occurring in other medium-sized arteries (eg, iliac, femoral, renal, and axillary vessels) are uncommon and generally do not occur in the absence of significant coronary abnormalities. In addition to coronary artery disease, carditis can involve the pericardium, myocardium, or endocardium, and mitral or aortic regurgitation or both can develop. Carditis generally resolves when fever resolves.

In children with mild coronary artery dilation or ectasia, coronary artery dimensions often return to baseline within 6 to 8 weeks after onset of disease. Approximately 50% of coronary aneurysms (but only a small proportion of giant aneurysms) regress to normal luminal size within 1 to 2 years, although this process can be accompanied by development of coronary stenosis.

The current case-fatality rate for Kawasaki disease in the United States and Japan is less than 0.2%. The principal cause of death is myocardial infarction resulting from coronary artery occlusion attributable to thrombosis or progressive stenosis. Rarely, a large coronary artery aneurysm may rupture during the acute phase. The relative risk of mortality is highest within 6 weeks of onset of acute symptoms of Kawasaki disease, but myocardial infarction and sudden death can occur months to years after the acute episode. There is no current evidence that the vasculitis of Kawasaki disease predisposes to premature atherosclerotic coronary artery disease, although this seems plausible.

Etiology

The etiology is unknown. Epidemiologic and clinical features strongly suggest an infectious cause or trigger. Studies also suggest genetic susceptibility.

Epidemiology

Peak age of occurrence in the United States is between 18 and 24 months. Fifty percent of patients are younger than 2 years, and 80% are younger than 5 years; children older than 8 years less commonly develop the disease, but rare cases may occur even in adults. In children younger than 6 months, the diagnosis is often delayed because the symptom complex of Kawasaki disease is incomplete and individual features can be subtle. The prevalence of coronary artery abnormalities is higher when diagnosis and treatment are delayed beyond the 10th day of illness. The male to female ratio is approximately 1.5:1. In the United States, 4,000 to 5,500 cases are estimated to occur annually; the incidence is highest in children of Asian ancestry. More cases, including clusters, occur during winter and spring. No evidence indicates person-to-person or common-source spread, although the incidence is somewhat higher in siblings of children with the disease.

Incubation Period

Unknown.

Diagnostic Tests

No specific diagnostic test is available. The diagnosis is established by fulfillment of the clinical criteria after consideration of other possible illnesses, such as staphylococcal or streptococcal toxin-mediated disease; drug reactions (eg, Stevens-Johnson syndrome); viral infections, such as measles, adenovirus, Epstein-Barr virus, parvovirus B19, or enterovirus; rickettsial exanthems; leptospirosis; systemic-onset juvenile idiopathic arthritis; and reactive arthritis. The identification of a respiratory virus by molecular testing does not necessarily exclude the diagnosis of Kawasaki disease in infants and children who otherwise meet diagnostic criteria. Erythrocyte sedimentation rate and platelet count are usually normal within 6 to 8 weeks; CRP concentration returns to normal much sooner.

Treatment

Management during the acute phase is directed at decreasing inflammation of the myocardium and coronary artery wall and providing supportive care. Therapy should be initiated as soon as the diagnosis is established or strongly suspected. Once the acute phase has subsided, therapy is directed at prevention of coronary artery thrombosis. Specific recommendations for therapy include single, high-dose IVIG and high-dose aspirin therapy. Despite prompt treatment with IVIG and aspirin, approximately 4% of patients develop coronary artery aneurysms if treatment is initiated before the onset of coronary artery abnormalities. Many patients have fever in the 24 hours after completing the IVIG infusion. Persistent or recrudescent fever present 36 or more hours after the end of the IVIG infusion is used to define IVIG-resistant cases. Up to 15% of Kawasaki patients are resistant to IVIG therapy. In these situations, the diagnosis of Kawasaki disease should be reevaluated. If Kawasaki disease is still considered to be most likely, retreatment with IVIG and continued high-dose aspirin therapy is generally given.

Measles- and varicella-containing vaccines should be deferred for 11 months after receipt of high-dose IVIG for treatment of Kawasaki disease because of possible interference with the immune response. The schedule for administration of inactivated childhood vaccines should not be interrupted.

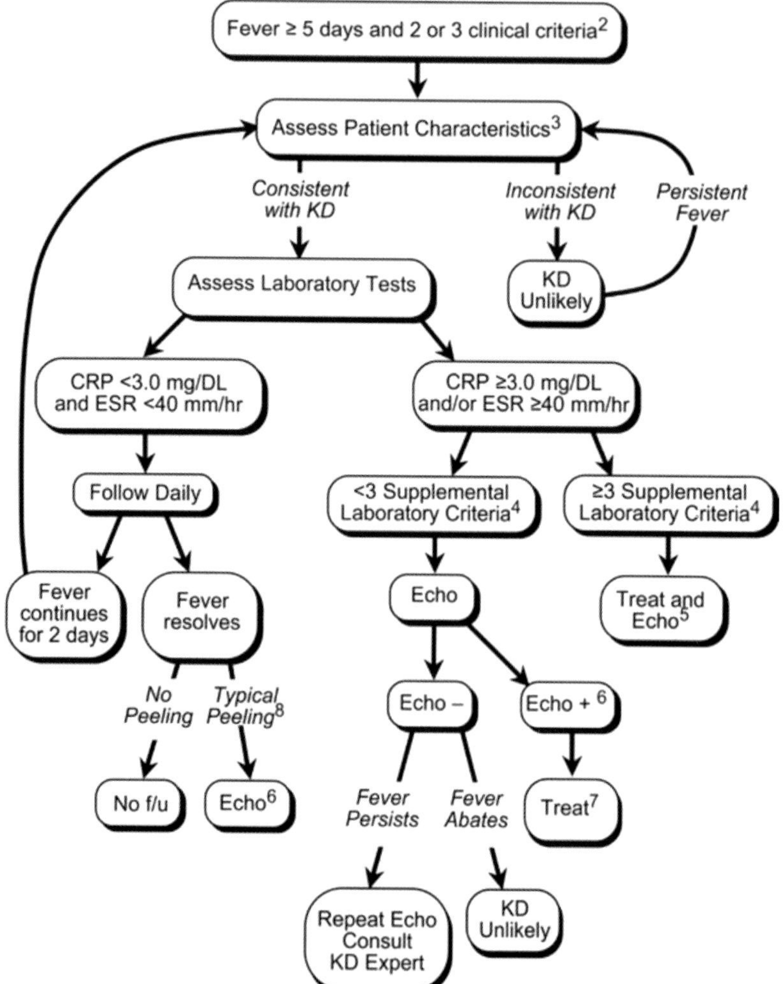

Evaluation of suspected incomplete Kawasaki disease. (1) In the absence of gold standard for diagnosis, this algorithm cannot be evidence based but rather represents the informed opinion of the expert committee. Consultation with an expert should be sought anytime assistance is needed. (2) Infants ≤6 months old on day ≥7 of fever without other explanation should undergo laboratory testing and, if evidence of systemic inflammation is found, an echocardiogram, even if the infants have no clinical criteria. (3) Patient characteristics suggesting Kawasaki disease are provided in text. Characteristics suggesting disease other than Kawasaki disease include exudative conjunctivitis, exudative pharyngitis, discrete intraoral lesions, bullous or vesicular rash, or generalized adenopathy. Consider alternative diagnoses. (4) Supplemental laboratory criteria include albumin ≤3.0 g/dL, anemia for age, elevation of alanine aminotransferase, platelets after 7 d ≥450 000/mm^3, white blood cell count ≥15 000/mm^3, and urine ≥10 white blood cells/high-power field. (5) Can treat before performing echocardiogram. (6) Echocardiogram is considered positive for purposes of this algorithm if any of 3 conditions are met: z score of LAD or RCA ≥2.5, coronary arteries meet Japanese Ministry of Health criteria for aneurysms, or ≥3 other suggestive features exist, including perivascular brightness, lack of tapering, decreased LV function, mitral regurgitation, pericardial effusion, or z scores in LAD or RCA of 2–2.5. (7) If the echocardiogram is positive, treatment should be given to children within 10 d of fever onset and those beyond day 10 with clinical and laboratory signs (CRP, ESR) of ongoing inflammation. (8) Typical peeling begins under nail bed of fingers and then toes.

Reprinted from Newburger JW, Takahashi M, Gerber MA, et al. Diagnosis, treatment, and long-term management of Kawasaki disease: a statement for health professionals from the Committee on Rheumatic Fever, Endocarditis, and Kawasaki Disease, Council on Cardiovascular Disease in the Young, American Heart Association. *Pediatrics.* 2004;114(6):1708–1733.

Image 72.1

Evaluation of suspected incomplete Kawasaki disease.

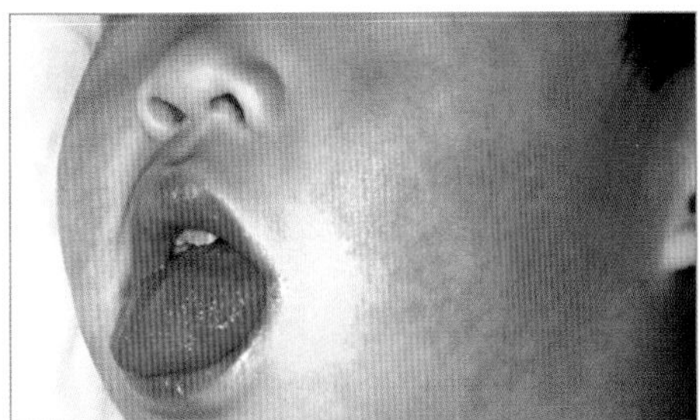

Image 72.2
A child with Kawasaki disease with striking facial rash and erythema of the oral mucous membrane.

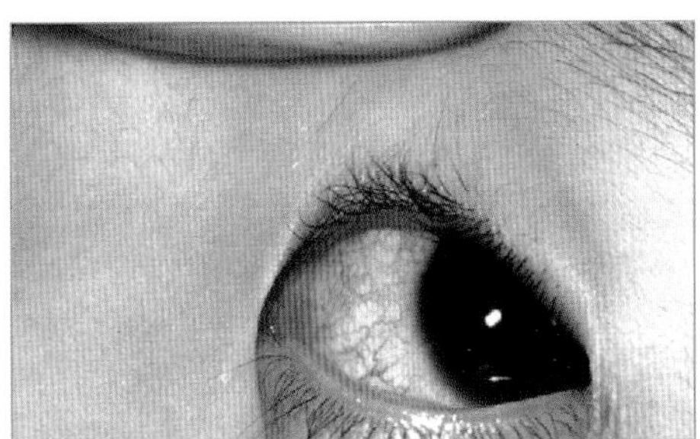

Image 72.3
A child with Kawasaki disease with conjunctivitis. Note the absence of conjunctival discharge.

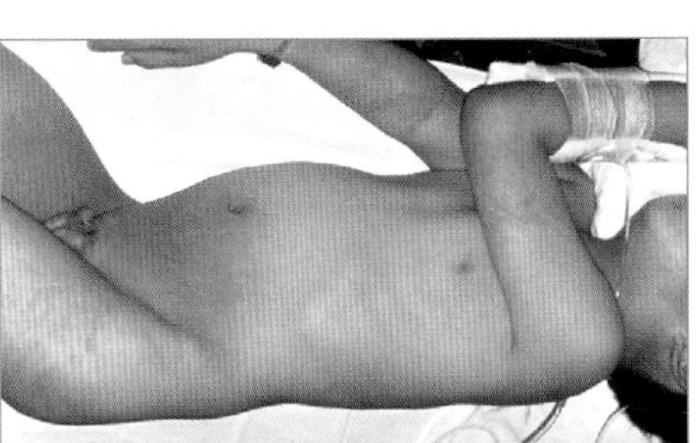

Image 72.4
Characteristic distribution of erythroderma of Kawasaki disease. The rash is accentuated in the perineal area in approximately two-thirds of patients.

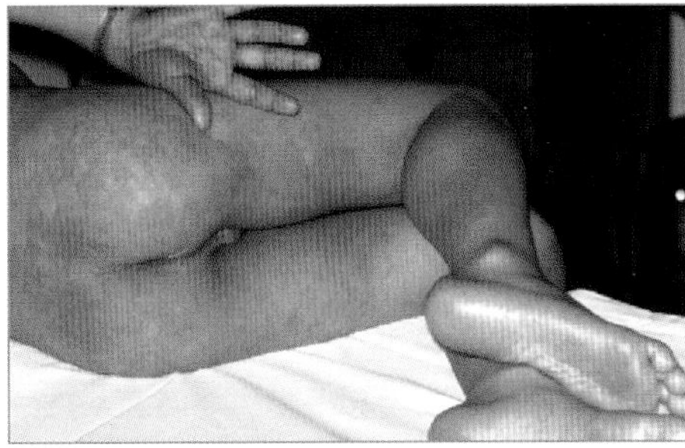

Image 72.5
Generalized erythema and early perianal and palmar desquamation. This is the same patient as in Image 72.4.

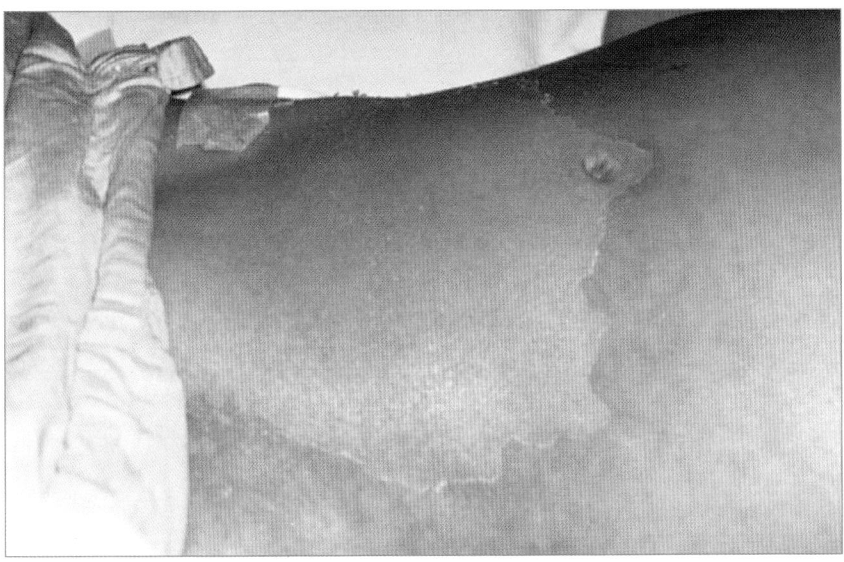

Image 72.6
Characteristic desquamation of the skin over the abdomen in a patient with Kawasaki disease. This is the same patient as in images 72.4 and 72.5.

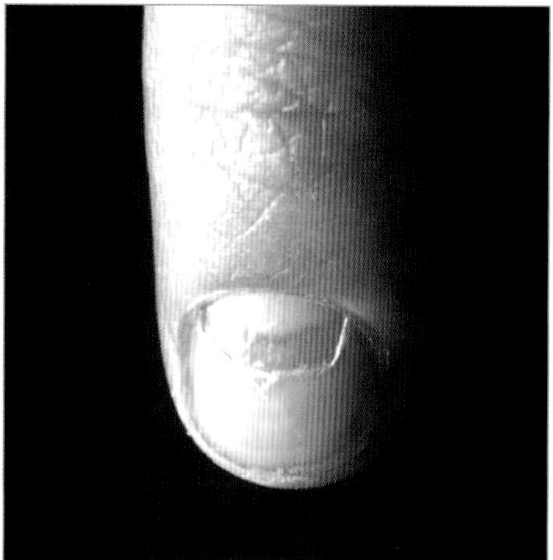

Image 72.7
Periungual desquamation of a patient with Kawasaki disease. This is the same patient as in images 72.4, 72.5, and 72.6.

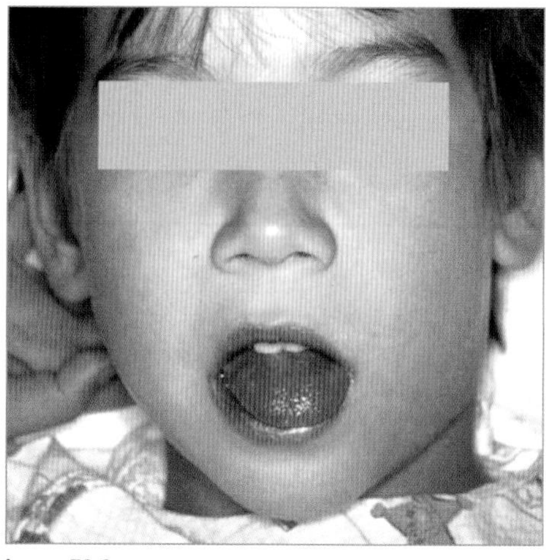

Image 72.8
Characteristic cutaneous and mucous membrane changes of Kawasaki disease. Courtesy of Neal Halsey, MD.

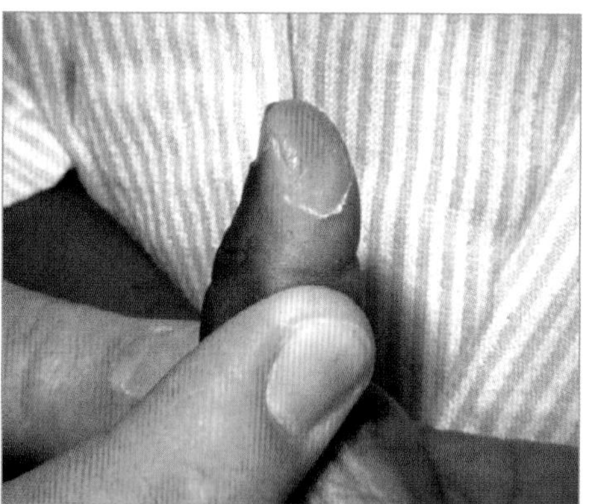

Image 72.9
Distal desquamation of Kawasaki disease. Courtesy of Neal Halsey, MD.

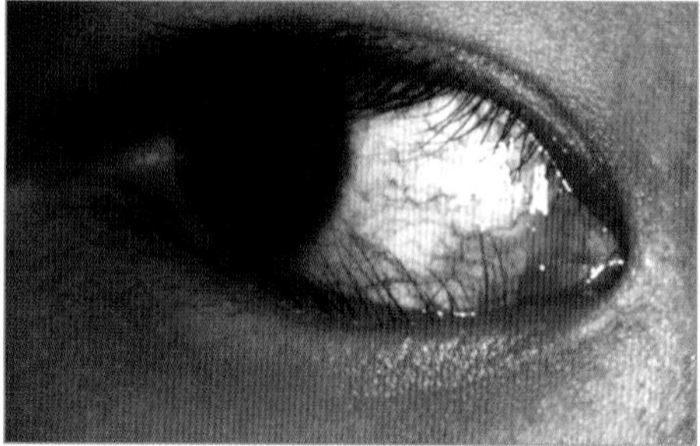

Image 72.10
Bulbar conjunctivitis in a patient with Kawasaki disease. Exudation is generally absent.

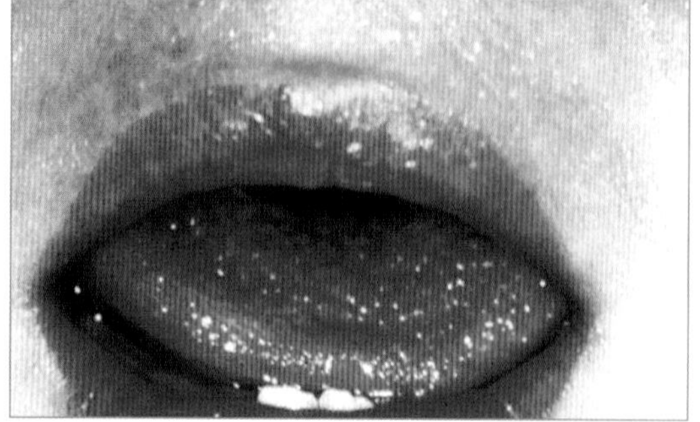

Image 72.11
Erythematous lips and injection of the oropharyngeal membranes in a patient with Kawasaki disease. Scarlet fever, toxic shock syndrome, staphylococcal scalded skin syndrome, and measles may be confused with this disease.

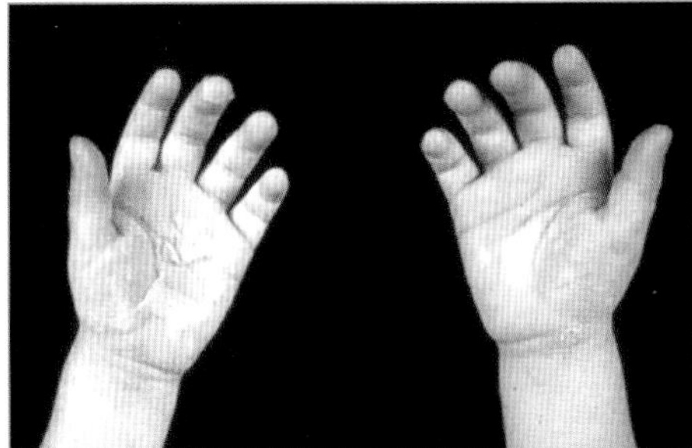

Image 72.12
A child with the characteristic desquamation of the hands in a later stage of Kawasaki disease. Copyright Charles Prober.

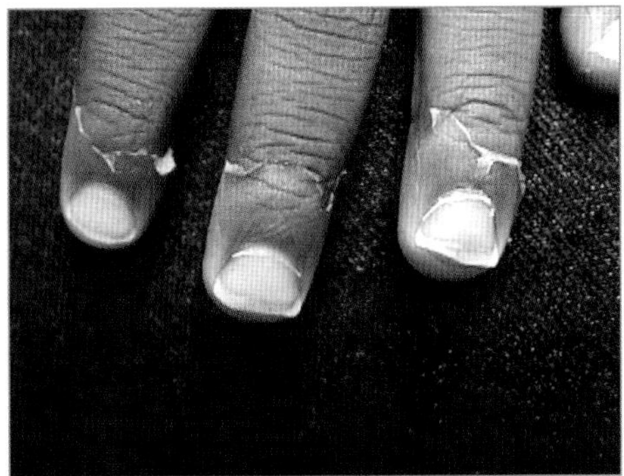

Image 72.13
Desquamation of the skin of the distal fingers following Kawasaki disease in a 4-year-old boy. Copyright Michael Rajnik, MD, FAAP.

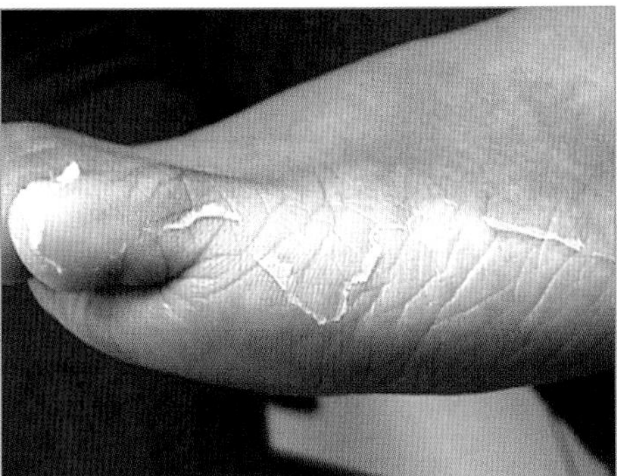

Image 72.14
Desquamation of the skin of the toes following Kawasaki disease. This is the same patient as in Image 72.13. Copyright Michael Rajnik, MD, FAAP.

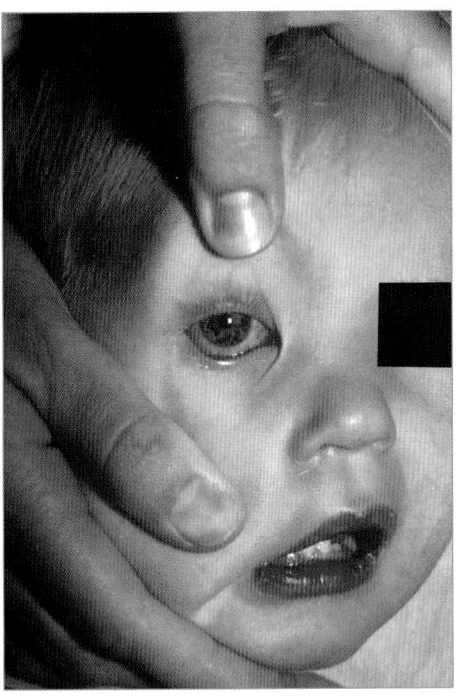

Image 72.15
This white 1-year-old presented with fever, generalized erythroderma, and conjunctivitis compatible with Kawasaki disease. Courtesy of George Nankervis, MD.

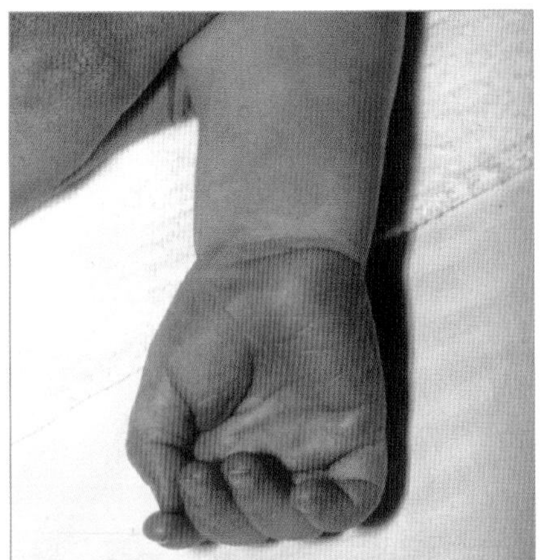

Image 72.16
Erythroderma of the palm of the hand of the child in Image 72.15 with Kawasaki disease. Courtesy of George Nankervis, MD.

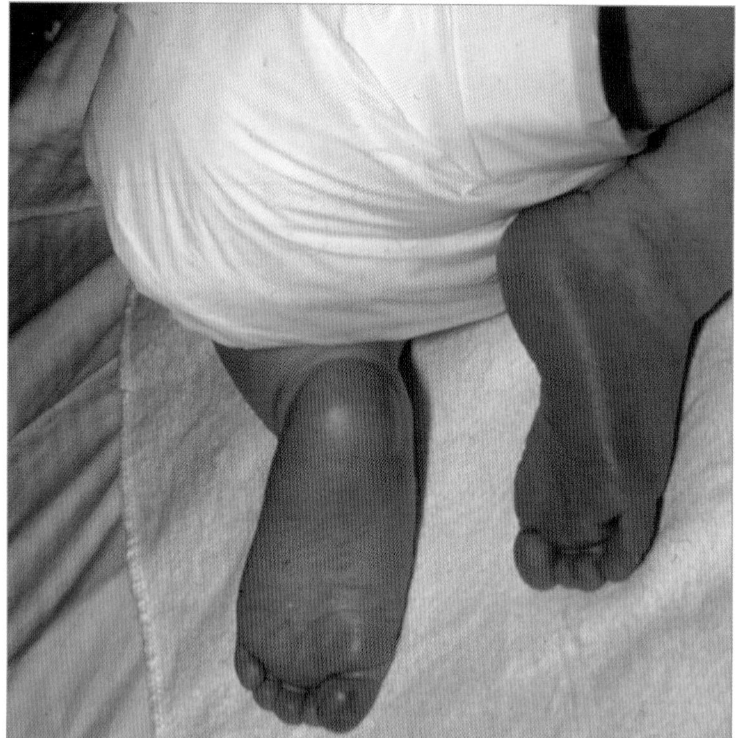

Image 72.17
Erythroderma of the plantar foot surface of the child in images 72.15 and 72.16 with Kawasaki disease. Courtesy of George Nankervis, MD.

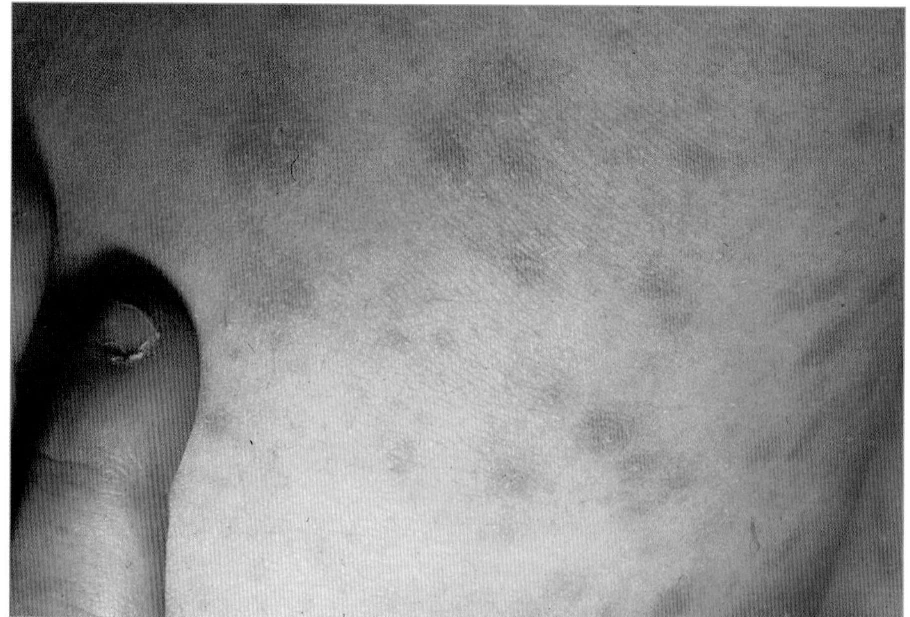

Image 72.18
A 7-year-old white girl with Kawasaki disease. Right arm. Courtesy of Larry Frenkel, MD.

73

Kingella kingae Infections

Clinical Manifestations

The most common infections attributable to *Kingella kingae* are pyogenic arthritis, osteomyelitis, and bacteremia. The vast majority of *K kingae* infections affect children, predominantly between 6 and 48 months of age, with most cases occurring in those younger than 2 years. *K kingae* is the most common cause of skeletal infections in children younger than 3 years in some geographic locations. *K kingae* pyogenic arthritis is generally monoarticular and most commonly involves the knee, hip, or ankle. *K kingae* osteomyelitis most often involves the femur or tibia and also has an unusual predilection for small bones, including the small bones of the foot. The clinical manifestations of *K kingae* pyogenic arthritis and osteomyelitis are similar to manifestations of skeletal infection due to other bacterial pathogens in immunocompetent children, although a subacute course may be more common. A Brodie abscess of bone attributable to *K kingae* is uncommon. Bacteremia can occur in previously healthy children and in children with preexisting chronic medical problems. Children with *K kingae* bacteremia present with fever and frequently have concurrent findings of respiratory or gastrointestinal tract disease. Other infections caused by *K kingae* include diskitis, endocarditis (*K kingae* belongs to the HACEK group of organisms), meningitis, and pneumonia.

Etiology

K kingae is a gram-negative organism that belongs to the Neisseriaceae family. It is a fastidious, facultative anaerobic, β-hemolytic small bacillus that appears as pairs or short chains with tapered ends and often resists decolorization, sometimes resulting in misidentification as a gram-positive organism.

Epidemiology

The usual habitat of *K kingae* is the posterior pharynx. The organism more frequently colonizes young children than adults and can be transmitted among children in child care centers, occasionally causing clusters of cases. Infection may be associated with preceding or concomitant stomatitis or upper respiratory tract infection.

Incubation Period

Variable.

Diagnostic Tests

K kingae can be isolated from blood, synovial fluid, bone, cerebrospinal fluid, respiratory tract secretions, and other sites of infection. Organisms grow better in aerobic conditions with supplemental carbon dioxide. In patients with *K kingae* pyogenic arthritis or osteomyelitis, blood cultures are often negative. *K kingae* is difficult to isolate on routine solid media, and synovial fluid and bone aspirates from patients with suspected *K kingae* infection should be inoculated into Bactec, BacT/Alert, or similar blood culture systems and held for at least 7 days to maximize recovery. Conventional and real-time polymerase chain reaction methods have improved detection of *K kingae*.

Treatment

K kingae is almost always highly susceptible to penicillins and cephalosporins, although β-lactamase production has been reported in rare isolates. Nearly all isolates are also susceptible to aminoglycosides, macrolides, trimethoprim-sulfamethoxazole, tetracyclines, and fluoroquinolones. Virtually all isolates are resistant to glycopeptide antibiotics (vancomycin and teicoplanin). Most cases of *K kingae* infection are treated with penicillin or ampicillin-sulbactam or a second- or third-generation cephalosporin.

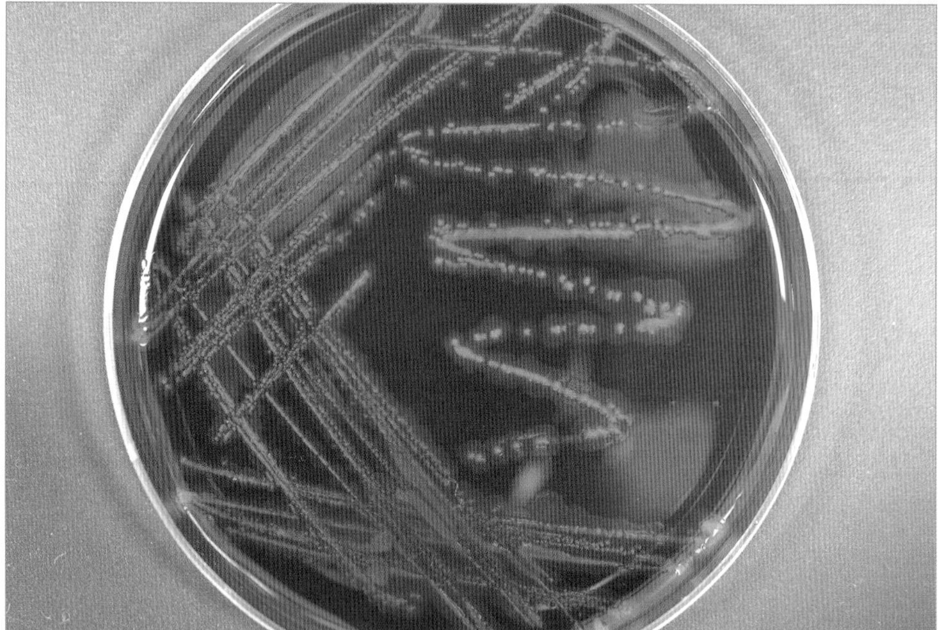

Image 73.1
Kingella kingae on blood agar. Smooth, gray colonies may pit the agar and are surrounded by a small but distinct zone of β-hemolysis on blood agar. Courtesy of Julia Rosebush, DO; Robert Jerris, PhD; and Theresa Stanley, M(ASCP).

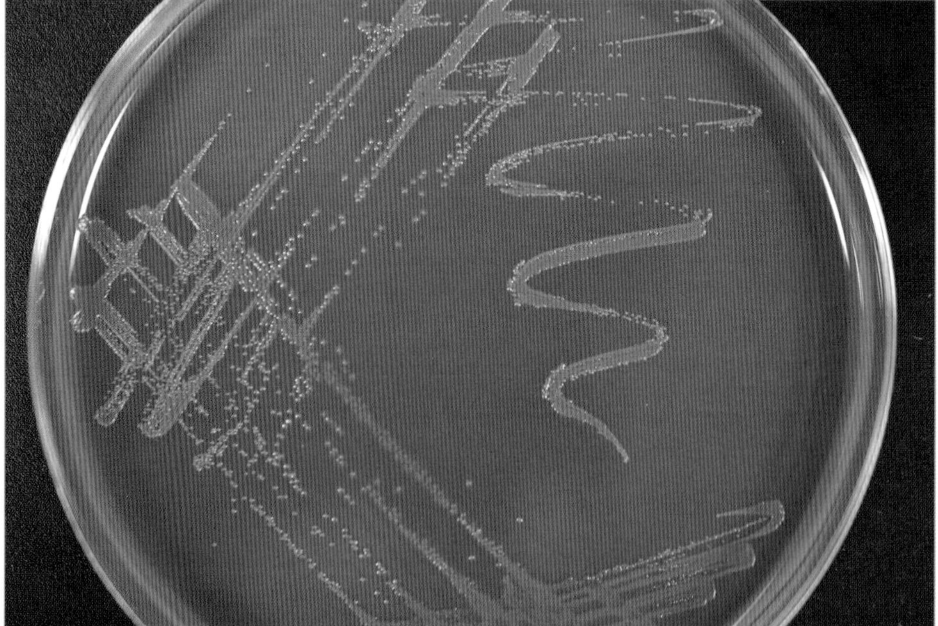

Image 73.2
Kingella kingae on chocolate agar. Colonies appear after 2 to 4 days of incubation on blood and chocolate agar. This species demonstrates β-hemolysis on blood agar. Courtesy of Julia Rosebush, DO; Robert Jerris, PhD; and Theresa Stanley, M(ASCP).

74

Legionella pneumophila Infections

Clinical Manifestations

Legionellosis is associated with 2 clinically and epidemiologically distinct illnesses: legionnaires' disease and Pontiac fever. **Legionnaires' disease** varies in severity from mild to severe pneumonia characterized by fever, cough, and progressive respiratory distress. Legionnaires' disease can be associated with chills, myalgia, and gastrointestinal tract, central nervous system, and renal manifestations. Respiratory failure and death can occur. **Pontiac fever** is a milder febrile illness without pneumonia that occurs in epidemics and is characterized by an abrupt onset and a self-limited, influenza-like illness.

Etiology

Legionella species are fastidious aerobic bacilli that stain gram negative after recovery on buffered charcoal yeast extract media. At least 20 different species have been implicated in human disease, but the most common species causing infections in the United States is *Legionella pneumophila,* with most isolates belonging to serogroup 1. Multiplication of *Legionella* organisms in water sources occurs optimally in temperatures between 25°C and 45°C (77°F and 113°F).

Epidemiology

Legionnaires' disease is acquired through inhalation of aerosolized water contaminated with *L pneumophila*. Person-to-person transmission has not been demonstrated. More than 80% of cases are sporadic; the sources of infection can be related to exposure to *L pneumophila*–contaminated water in the home, workplace, or hospitals or other medical facilities or to aerosol-producing devices in public places. Outbreaks have been ascribed to common-source exposure to contaminated cooling towers, evaporative condensers, potable water systems, whirlpool spas, humidifiers, and respiratory therapy equipment. Outbreaks have occurred in hospitals, hotels, and other large buildings, as well as on cruise ships. Health care–associated infections can occur and are often related to contamination of the hot water supply. In patients who develop pneumonia during or after their hospitalization, legionnaires' disease should be considered in the differential diagnosis. Legionnaires' disease occurs most commonly in people who are elderly, are immunocompromised, or have underlying lung disease. Infection in children is rare and is usually asymptomatic or mild and unrecognized. Severe disease has occurred in children with malignant neoplasms, severe combined immunodeficiency, chronic granulomatous disease, organ transplantation, end-stage renal disease, underlying pulmonary disease, and immunosuppression; in children receiving systemic corticosteroids; and as a health care–associated infection in newborns.

Incubation Period

For legionnaires' disease, 2 to 10 days; for Pontiac fever, 1 to 2 days.

Diagnostic Tests

Recovery of *Legionella* from respiratory tract secretions, lung tissue, pleural fluid, or other normally sterile fluid specimens using buffered charcoal yeast extract media provides definitive evidence of infection, but the sensitivity of culture is laboratory dependent. When a patient is suspected of having legionnaires' disease, culture of a respiratory specimen should be conducted in addition to urine antigen testing. Detection of *Legionella* antigen in urine by commercially available immunoassays is highly specific. Such tests are sensitive for *L pneumophila* serogroup 1. The bacterium can be demonstrated in specimens by direct immunofluorescent assay, but this test is less sensitive and the specificity is technician dependent and lower than culture or urine immunoassay. Genus-specific polymerase chain reaction–based assays have been developed that detect *Legionella* DNA in respiratory secretions as well as in blood and urine of some patients with pneumonia. For serologic diagnosis, a 4-fold increase in titer of antibodies to *L pneumophila* serogroup 1, measured by indirect immunofluorescent antibody assay, confirms a recent infection. Convalescent serum samples should be obtained 3 to 4 weeks after onset of symptoms; however, a titer increase can be delayed for 8 to 12 weeks. The positive predictive value of a single titer of 1:256 or greater is low and does not provide definitive evidence of infection. Antibodies to several gram-negative organisms, including *Pseudomonas* species, *Bacteroides fragilis,* and *Campylobacter jejuni,* can cause false-positive immunofluorescent antibody test results.

Treatment

Azithromycin is the drug of choice. Once the condition of a patient is improving, oral therapy can be substituted. Levofloxacin (or another fluoroquinolone) is the drug of choice for immunocompromised adults. Doxycycline and trimethoprim-sulfamethoxazole are alternative drugs. Duration of therapy is 5 to 10 days for azithromycin and 14 to 21 days for other drugs. Longer courses of therapy are recommended for patients who are immunocompromised or who have severe disease.

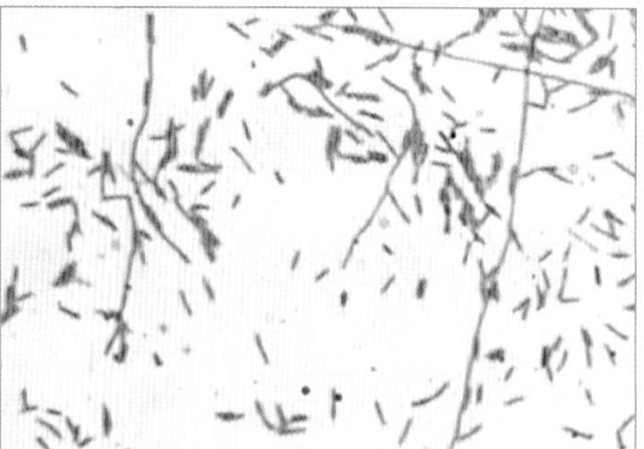

Image 74.1
This Gram-stained micrograph reveals chains and solitary gram-negative *Legionella pneumophila* bacteria found within a sample taken from a victim of the 1976 legionnaires' disease outbreak in Philadelphia, PA. Legionnaires' disease is the more severe form of legionellosis and is characterized by pneumonia, commencing 2 to 10 days after exposure. Pontiac fever is an acute-onset, flu-like, nonpneumonic illness, occurring within 1 to 2 days of exposure. Courtesy of Centers for Disease Control and Prevention.

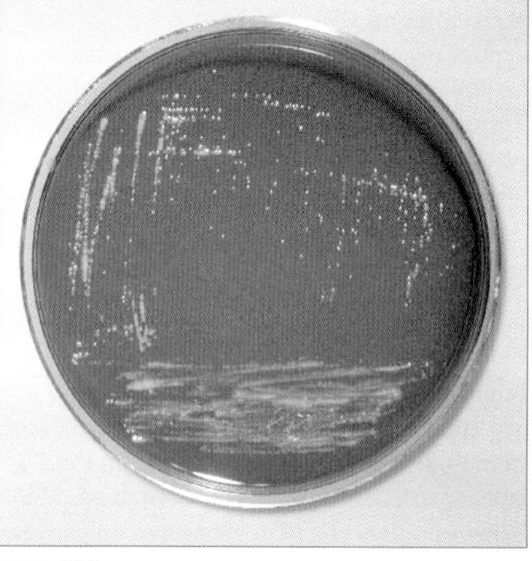

Image 74.2
Charcoal-yeast extract agar plate culture of *Legionella pneumophila*. Courtesy of Centers for Disease Control and Prevention/Dr Jim Feeley.

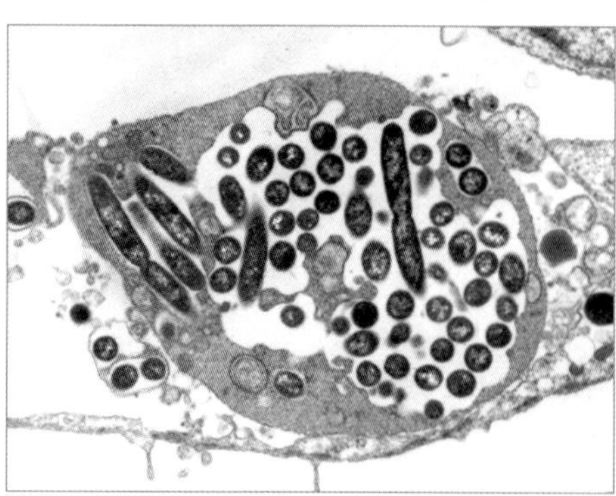

Image 74.3
Legionella pneumophila multiplying inside a cultured human lung fibroblast. Courtesy of Centers for Disease Control and Prevention/ Dr Edwin P. Ewing Jr.

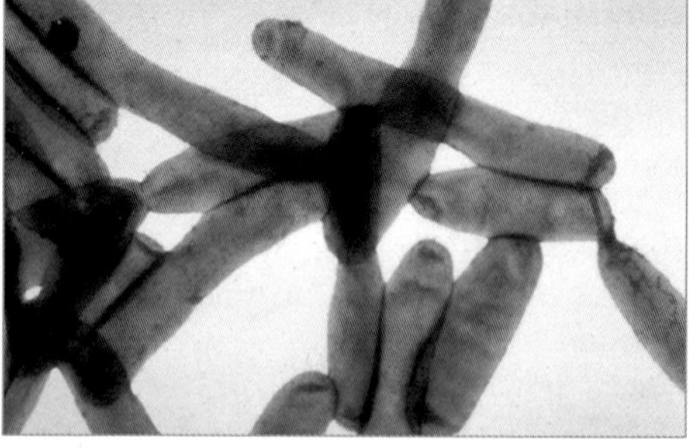

Image 74.4
Transmission electron micrograph of *Legionella pneumophila*. Courtesy of Centers for Disease Control and Prevention/Dr Francis Chandler.

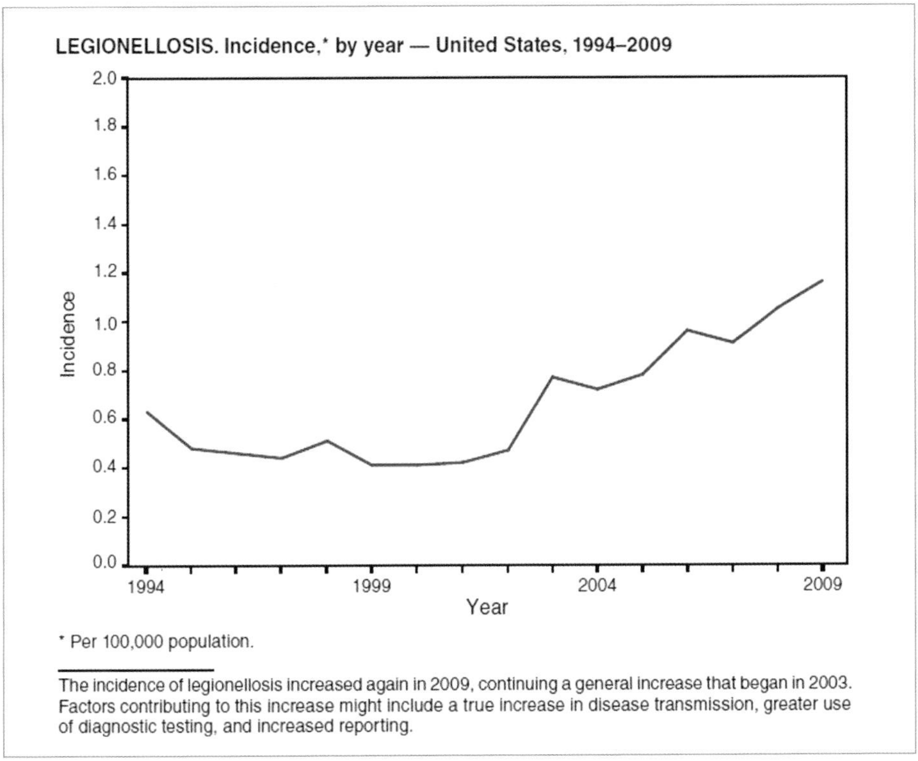

Image 74.5
Legionellosis. Incidence, by year—United States, 1997–2012. Courtesy of *Morbidity and Mortality Weekly Report.*

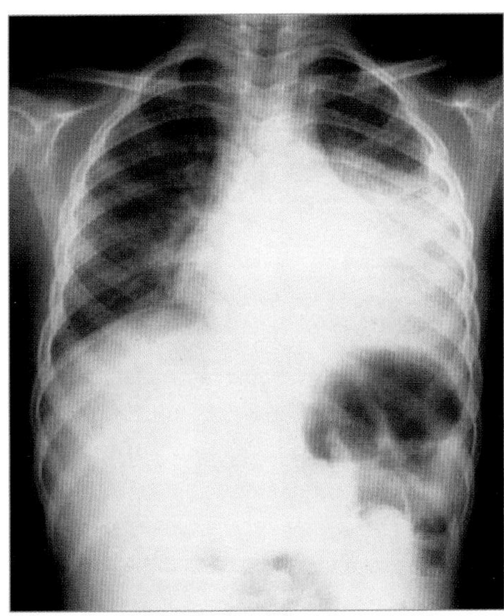

Image 74.6
An adult with pneumonia due to *Legionella pneumophila*. *Legionella* infections are rare in otherwise healthy children. Although nosocomial infections and hospital outbreaks are reported, this infection is not transmitted from person to person.

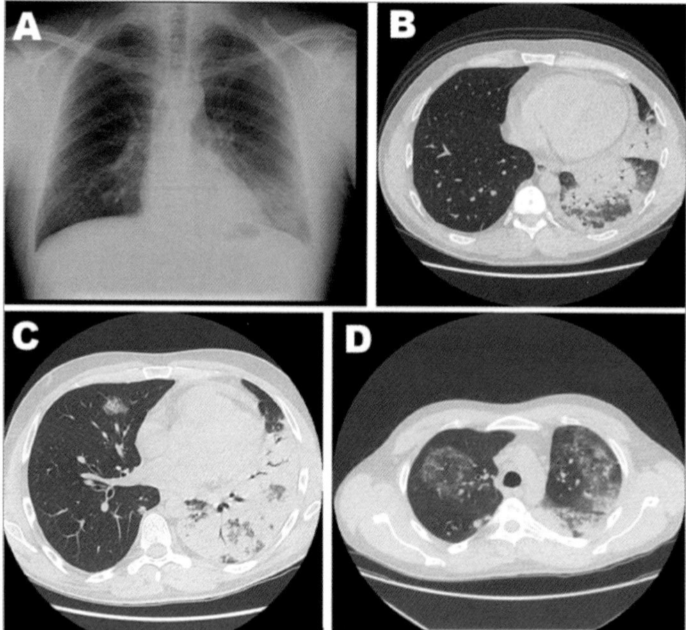

Image 74.7
Imaging studies of a 42-year-old man with severe pneumonia caused by *Legionella pneumophila* serogroup 11, showing lobar consolidation of the left lower lung lobe, with an air-bronchogram within the homogeneous airspace consolidation. Consensual mild pleural effusion was documented by a chest radiograph (A) and high-resolution computed tomography (B). A week after hospital admission, repeat high-resolution computed tomography of the chest showed extensive and homogeneous consolidation of left upper and lower lobes, accompanied by bilateral ground-glass opacities (C and D). Courtesy of *Emerging Infectious Diseases.*

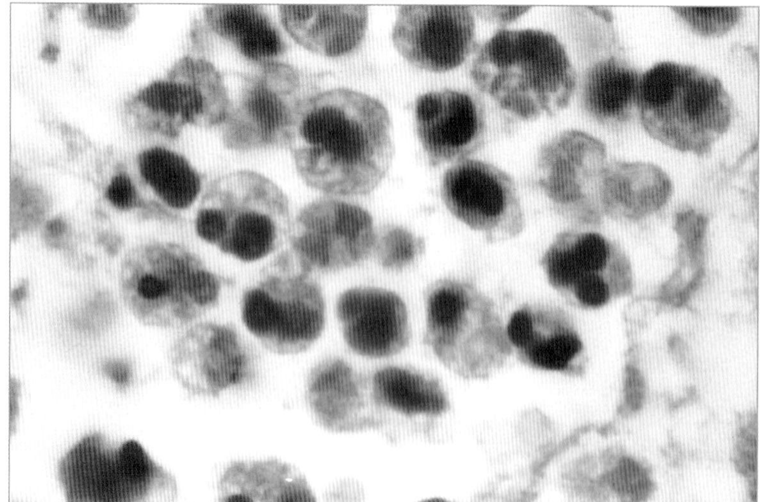

Image 74.8
This hematoxylin-eosin–stained micrograph of lung tissue biopsied from a patient with legionnaires' diseases revealed the presence of an intra-alveolar exudate consisting of macrophages and polymorphonuclear leucocytes. The *Legionella pneumophila* bacteria are not stained in this preparation (magnification x500). Courtesy of Centers for Disease Control and Prevention.

75

Leishmaniasis

Clinical Manifestations

The 3 main clinical syndromes are as follows:

- **Cutaneous leishmaniasis.** After inoculation by the bite of an infected female *Phlebotomus* species sand fly (approximately 2–3 mm long), parasites proliferate locally in mononuclear phagocytes, leading to an erythematous papule, which, typically, slowly enlarges to become a nodule and then an ulcerative lesion with raised, indurated borders. Ulcerative lesions can become dry and crusted or can develop a moist granulating base with an overlying exudate. Lesions can, however, persist as nodules or papules and can be single or multiple. Lesions are commonly on exposed areas of the body (eg, face, extremities) and may be accompanied by satellite lesions, sporotrichoid-like nodules, and regional adenopathy. Clinical manifestations of Old World and New World (American) cutaneous leishmaniasis are similar. Spontaneous resolution of lesions can take weeks to years—depending, in part, on the *Leishmania* species/strain—and usually results in a flat, atrophic scar.
- **Mucosal leishmaniasis (espundia)** traditionally refers to a metastatic sequela of New World cutaneous infection, which results from dissemination of the parasite from the skin to the naso-oropharyngeal mucosa; this form of leishmaniasis is typically caused by species in the *Viannia* subgenus. Mucosal disease usually becomes evident months to years after original cutaneous lesions heal; however, mucosal and cutaneous lesions can be noted simultaneously, as some affected people have subclinical cutaneous infection. Granulomatous inflammation may cause hypertrophy of the nose and lips. Untreated mucosal leishmaniasis can progress to cause ulcerative destruction (eg, perforation of the nasal septum) and facial disfigurement.
- **Visceral leishmaniasis (kala-azar).** After cutaneous inoculation by an infected sand fly, the parasite spreads throughout the reticuloendothelial system (eg, spleen, liver, bone marrow). The stereotypical clinical manifestations include fever, weight loss, pancytopenia, hypoalbuminemia, and hypergammaglobulinemia. Peripheral lymphadenopathy is quite common in East Africa (eg, South Sudan). Some patients in South Asia (the Indian subcontinent) develop grayish discoloration of their skin; this manifestation gave rise to the Hindi term kala-azar ("black sickness"). Untreated, advanced cases of visceral leishmaniasis are almost always fatal, directly from the disease or from complications such as secondary bacterial infections or hemorrhage. At the other end of the spectrum, visceral infection can be asymptomatic or oligosymptomatic. Latent visceral infection can activate years to decades postexposure in people who become immunocompromised (eg, because of coinfection with HIV; posttransplantation immunosuppression) or who receive immunomodulatory therapy (eg, with an antitumor necrosis factor-α agent) because of other medical conditions.

Etiology

In the human host, *Leishmania* species are obligate intracellular parasites of mononuclear phagocytes. To date, approximately 20 *Leishmania* species (in the *Leishmania* and *Viannia* subgenera) are known to infect humans. Cutaneous leishmaniasis is typically caused by Old World species *Leishmania tropica, Leishmania major,* and *Leishmania aethiopica* and by New World species *Leishmania mexicana, Leishmania amazonensis, Leishmania* (*Viannia*) *braziliensis, Leishmania* (*V*) *panamensis, Leishmania* (*V*) *guyanensis,* and *Leishmania* (*V*) *peruviana.* Mucosal leishmaniasis is typically caused by species in the *Viannia* subgenus (especially *L* [*V*] *braziliensis* but also *L* [*V*] *panamensis* and, sometimes, *L* [*V*] *guyanensis*). Most cases of visceral leishmaniasis are caused by *Leishmania donovani* or *Leishmania infantum* (*Leishmania chagasi* is synonymous). *L donovani* and *L infantum* can also cause cutaneous leishmaniasis; however, people with typical cutaneous leishmaniasis caused by these organisms rarely develop visceral leishmaniasis.

Epidemiology

In most settings, leishmaniasis is a zoonosis, with mammalian reservoir hosts, such as rodents or dogs. However, some transmission cycles are anthroponotic; infected humans are the primary or only reservoir hosts of *L donovani* in South Asia (potentially also in East Africa) and of *L tropica*. Congenital and parenteral transmission have also been reported.

Overall, leishmaniasis is endemic in more than 90 countries in the tropics, subtropics, and southern Europe. Visceral leishmaniasis (an estimated 0.2–0.4 million new cases annually) is found in focal areas of more than 60 countries: in the Old World, in parts of Asia (particularly South, Southwest, and Central Asia), Africa (particularly East Africa), the Middle East, and southern Europe; in the New World, particularly in Brazil, with scattered foci elsewhere. Most (>90%) of the world's cases of visceral leishmaniasis occur in South Asia (India, Bangladesh, and Nepal), East Africa (Sudan, South Sudan, and Ethiopia), and Brazil. Cutaneous leishmaniasis is more common (an estimated total of 0.7–1.2 million new cases annually) and more widespread than visceral leishmaniasis. Cutaneous leishmaniasis is found in focal areas of more than 90 countries: in the Old World, in parts of the Middle East, Asia (particularly Southwest and Central Asia), Africa (particularly North and East Africa, with some cases elsewhere), and southern Europe; in the New World, in parts of Mexico, Central America, and South America (not in Chile or Uruguay). Occasional cases of cutaneous leishmaniasis have been acquired in Texas and Oklahoma. The geographic distribution of leishmaniasis cases identified in the United States reflects immigration and travel patterns (eg, the locations of popular tourist destinations in Latin America and of various military activities).

Incubation Period

Ranges from weeks to years. In **cutaneous** leishmaniasis, skin lesions typically appear within several weeks; in **visceral**, from 2 to 6 months.

Diagnostic Tests

Definitive diagnosis is made by detecting the parasite in infected tissue by light-microscopic examination of stained slides (eg, of aspirates, touch preparations, histologic sections), by in vitro culture, or by molecular methods. In cutaneous and mucosal disease, tissue can be obtained by a 3-mm punch biopsy, lesion scrapings, or needle aspiration of the raised nonnecrotic edge of the lesion. In visceral leishmaniasis, although the sensitivity is highest for splenic aspiration (approximately 95%), the procedure can be associated with life-threatening hemorrhage; bone marrow aspiration is safer. Other potential sources of specimens include liver, lymph node, and, in some patients (eg, those coinfected with HIV), whole blood or buffy coat. Identification of the *Leishmania* species may affect prognosis and influence treatment decisions. The Centers for Disease Control and Prevention (CDC) (**www.cdc.gov/parasites/leishmaniasis**) can assist in all aspects of diagnostic testing. Serologic testing is not usually helpful in cases of cutaneous leishmaniasis but can provide supportive evidence for the diagnosis of visceral or mucosal leishmaniasis, particularly if the patient is immunocompetent.

Treatment

Systemic antileishmanial treatment is always indicated for patients with visceral or mucosal leishmaniasis, but not all patients with cutaneous leishmaniasis need to be treated. Consultation with infectious disease or tropical medicine specialists or with staff of the CDC Division of Parasitic Diseases and Malaria is recommended (telephone: 404/718-4745; e-mail: **parasites@cdc.gov**; CDC Emergency Operations Center [after business hours and on weekends]: 770/488-7100). The relative merits of various treatment approaches or regimens for an individual patient should be considered, taking into account that the therapeutic response may vary not only for different *Leishmania* species but also for the same species in different geographic regions. In addition, special considerations apply in the United States for the availability of particular medications. For example, the pentavalent antimonial compound sodium stibogluconate is not commercially available but can be obtained through the CDC Drug Service (404/639-3670), under an investigational new drug protocol. Liposomal amphotericin B, which is administered by intravenous infusion, is recommended for treatment of visceral leishmaniasis. The oral agent, miltefosine, is approved for treatment of cutaneous and mucosal as well as visceral leishmaniasis but is limited to infection caused by particular *Leishmania* species and for patients 12 years and older who are not pregnant or breastfeeding.

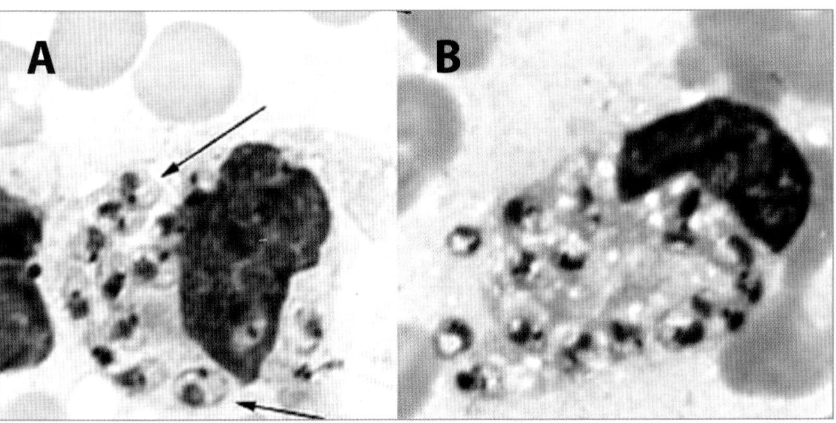

Image 75.1
Leishmania tropica amastigotes from a skin touch preparation. A, Still intact macrophage is practically filled with amastigotes, several of which have a clearly visible nucleus and a kinetoplast (arrows). B, Amastigotes are being freed from a rupturing macrophage. The patient has a history of travel to Egypt, Africa, and the Middle East. Culture in Novy-MacNeal-Nicolle medium followed by isoenzyme analysis identified the species as *L tropica* minor. Courtesy of Centers for Disease Control and Prevention.

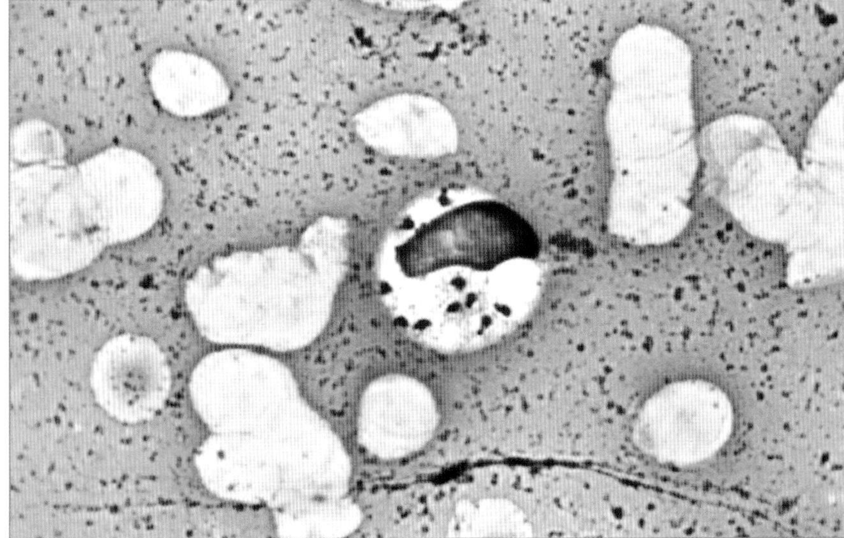

Image 75.2
Leishmania donovani in bone marrow cell. Smear. Courtesy of Centers for Disease Control and Prevention/L. L. Moore Jr, MD.

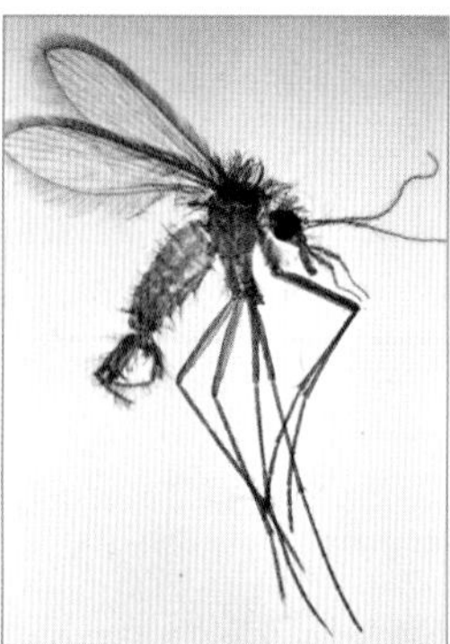

Image 75.3

This image depicts a mounted male *Phlebotomus* species fly, which, due to its resemblance, may be mistaken for a mosquito. *Phlebotomus* species sand flies are bloodsucking insects that are very small and sometimes act as the vectors for various diseases, such as leishmaniasis and bartonellosis (also known as Carrión disease). Courtesy of Centers for Disease Control and Prevention/Donated by the World Health Organization.

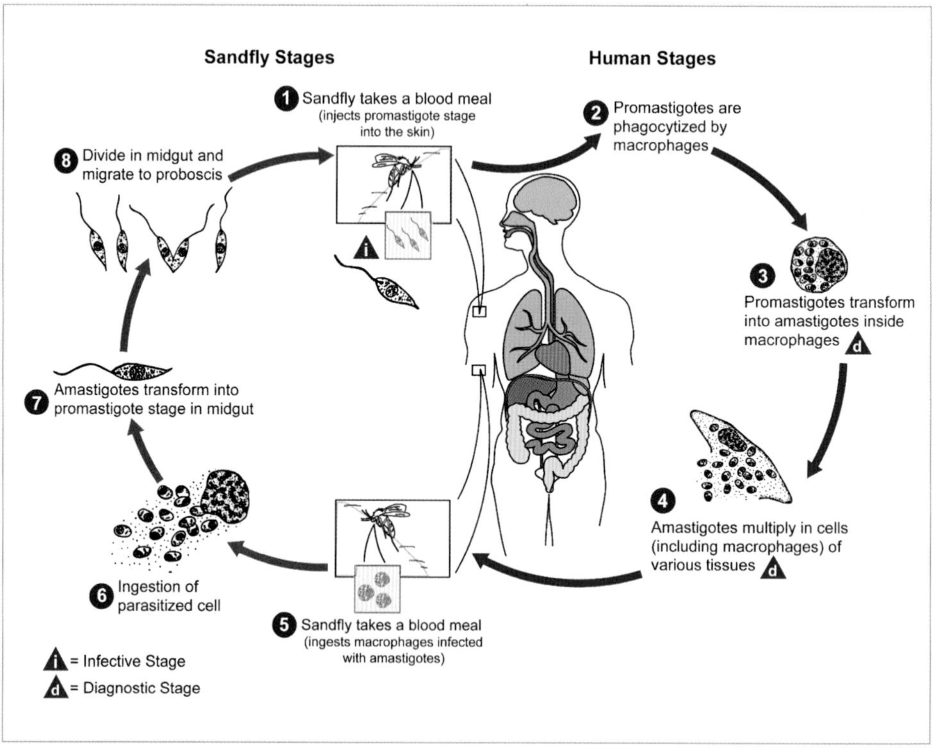

Sandfly Stages

Human Stages

1 Sandfly takes a blood meal (injects promastigote stage into the skin)

2 Promastigotes are phagocytized by macrophages

3 Promastigotes transform into amastigotes inside macrophages d

4 Amastigotes multiply in cells (including macrophages) of various tissues d

5 Sandfly takes a blood meal (ingests macrophages infected with amastigotes)

6 Ingestion of parasitized cell

7 Amastigotes transform into promastigote stage in midgut

8 Divide in midgut and migrate to proboscis

i = Infective Stage

d = Diagnostic Stage

Image 75.4

Leishmaniasis is transmitted by the bite of female *Phlebotomus* species sand flies. The sand flies inject the infective stage, promastigotes, during blood meals (1). Promastigotes that reach the puncture wound are phagocytized by macrophages (2) and transform into amastigotes (3). Amastigotes multiply in infected cells and affect different tissues, depending, in part, on the *Leishmania* species (4). This originates the clinical manifestations of leishmaniasis. Sand flies become infected during blood meals on an infected host when they ingest macrophages infected with amastigotes (5, 6). In the sand fly's midgut, the parasites differentiate into promastigotes (7), which multiply and migrate to the proboscis (8). Courtesy of Centers for Disease Control and Prevention/Alexander J. da Silva, PhD/Blaine Mathison.

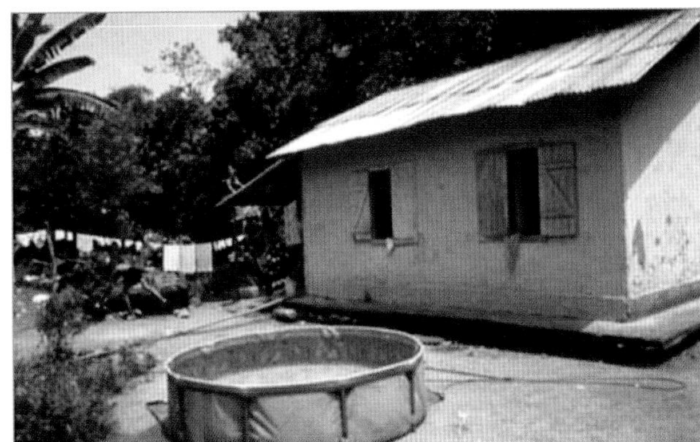

Image 75.5
Homes built in newly cleared forest areas (here, outside Rio de Janeiro) expose settlers to the sand flies that transmit leishmaniasis. Courtesy of World Health Organization.

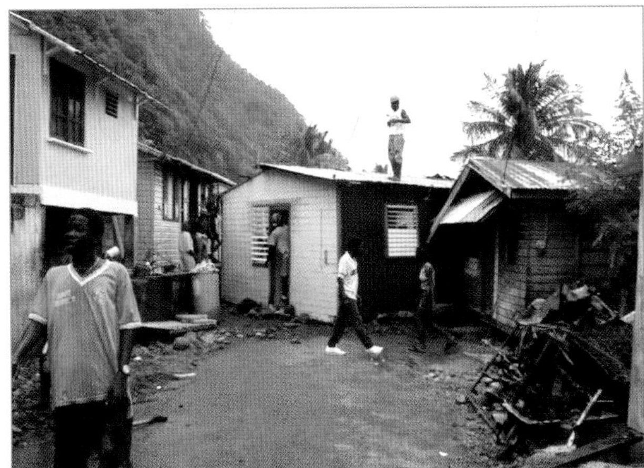

Image 75.6
A shantytown, another environment where *Leishmania* infection proliferates due to inadequate housing and lack of sanitation. Courtesy of World Health Organization.

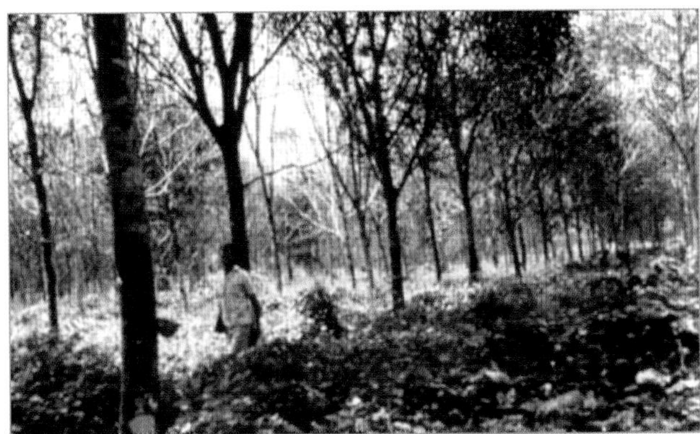

Image 75.7
Natural uncut forests are transmission sites for leishmaniasis. People who collect rubber or clear such areas for agriculture are prone to infection. Courtesy of World Health Organization/TDR/Lainson/Wellcome Trust.

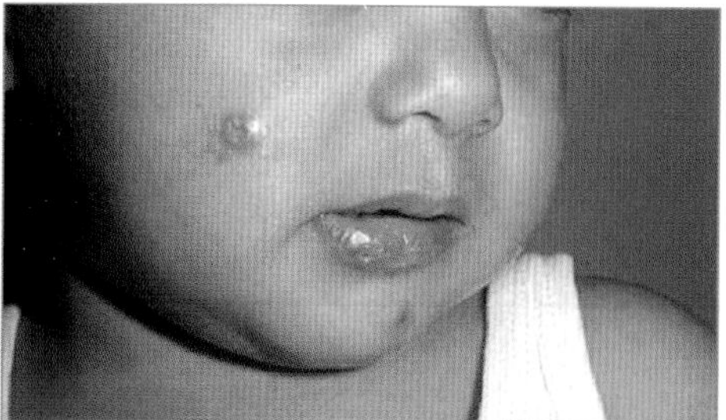

Image 75.8
Cutaneous leishmaniasis, as in this boy from India, seldom disseminates in immunocompetent persons. Multiple organisms can usually be found on biopsy of the border of a lesion.

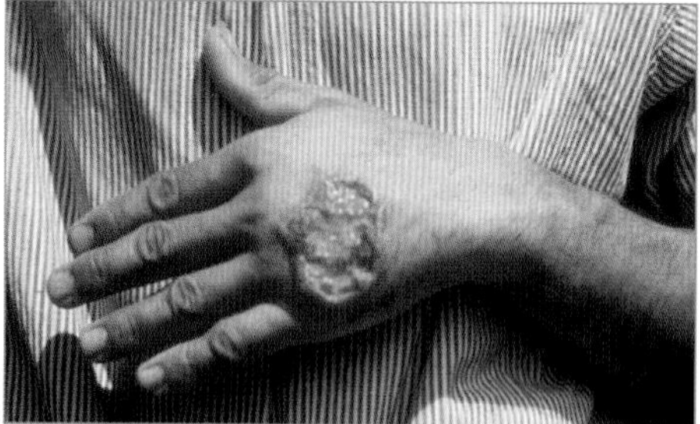

Image 75.10
Skin ulcer due to leishmaniasis, hand of Central American adult. Courtesy of Centers for Disease Control and Prevention/Dr D.S. Martin.

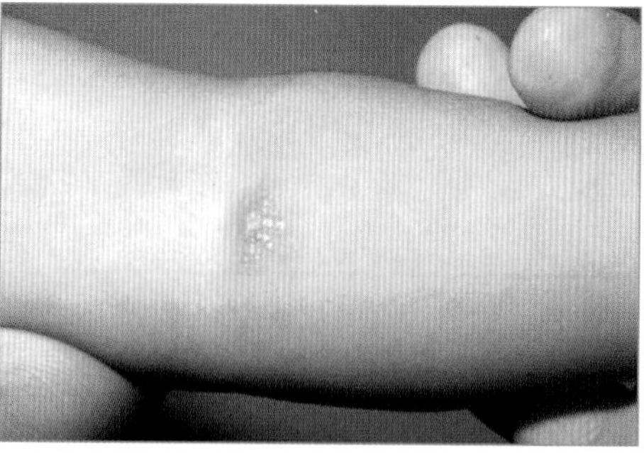

Image 75.9
Cutaneous leishmaniasis. Infected sand fly inoculation site with satellite lesions. The organism may be demonstrated by punch biopsy of the margin of a cutaneous lesion. This is the same child as in Image 75.9.

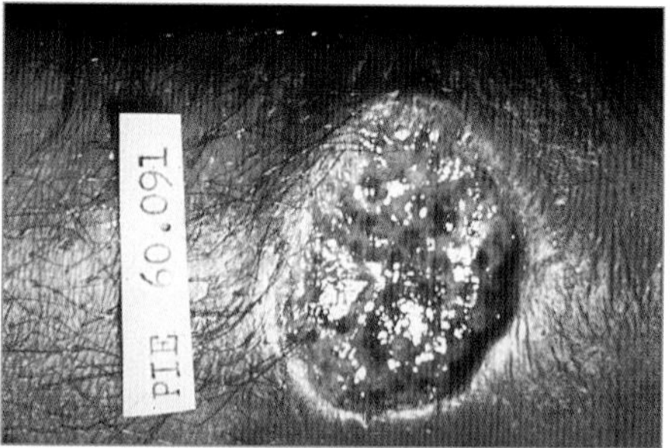

Image 75.11
Crater lesion of leishmaniasis, skin. Courtesy of Centers for Disease Control and Prevention.

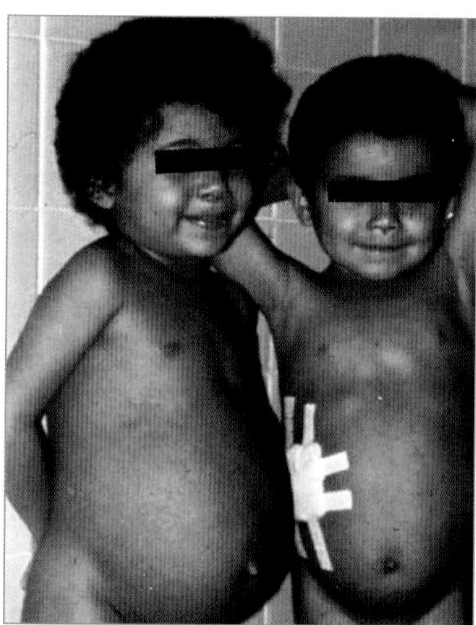

Image 75.12
Two young boys suffering visceral leishmaniasis, with distended abdomens due to hepatosplenomegaly. Courtesy of World Health Organization/TDR/Lainson/Wellcome Trust.

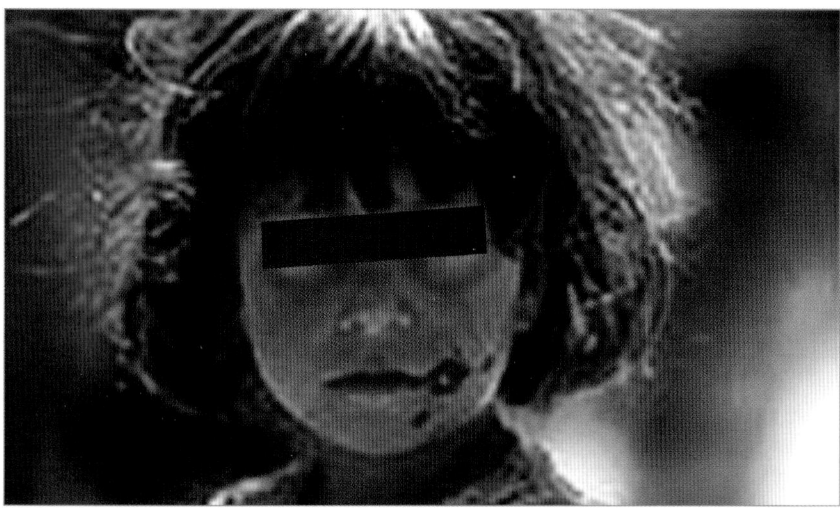

Image 75.13
A young girl with cutaneous leishmaniasis. Courtesy of World Health Organization.

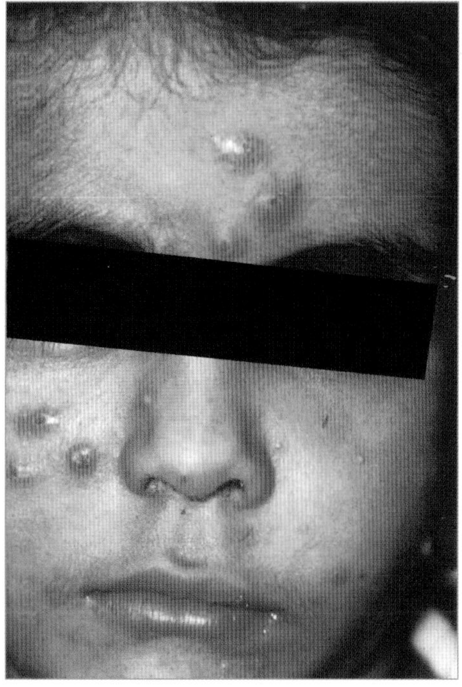

Image 75.14
A young girl with cutaneous leishmaniasis with multiple cutaneous lesions. Courtesy of World Health Organization.

76

Leprosy

Clinical Manifestations

Leprosy (Hansen disease) is a curable infection involving skin, peripheral nerves, mucosa of the upper respiratory tract, and testes. The clinical forms of leprosy reflect the cellular immune response to *Mycobacterium leprae* and, in turn, the number, size, structure, and bacillary content of the lesions. The organism has unique tropism for peripheral nerves, and all forms of leprosy exhibit nerve involvement. Leprosy lesions usually do not itch or hurt. They lack sensation to heat, touch, and pain but otherwise may be difficult to distinguish from other common maladies. There can be madarosis (loss of eyelashes or eyebrows) and ocular problems. However, the stereotypical presentations of leonine facies with nasal deformity or clawed hands with loss of digits are manifestations of late-stage untreated disease that are seldom seen today. Although the nerve injury caused by leprosy is irreversible, early diagnosis and drug therapy can prevent sequelae.

Leprosy manifests over a broad clinical and histopathologic spectrum. In the United States, the Ridley-Jopling scale is used to classify patients according to the histopathologic features of their lesions and organization of the underlying granuloma. The scale includes tuberculoid, borderline tuberculoid, borderline, borderline lepromatous, and lepromatous. A simplified scheme introduced by the World Health Organization for circumstances in which pathologic examination and diagnosis are unavailable is based purely on clinical skin examination. Under this scheme, leprosy is classified by the number of skin patches seen on skin examination, classifying disease as paucibacillary (1–5 lesions, usually tuberculoid or borderline tuberculoid) or multibacillary (>5 lesions, usually borderline, borderline lepromatous, or lepromatous). Patients in the tuberculoid spectrum have active cell-mediated immunity with low antibody responses to *M leprae* and few well-defined lesions containing few bacilli. Lepromatous spectrum cases have high antibody responses with little cell-mediated immunity to *M leprae* and several somewhat-diffuse lesions usually containing numerous bacilli.

Serious consequences of leprosy occur from immune reactions and nerve involvement with resulting anesthesia, which can lead to repeated unrecognized trauma, ulcerations, fractures, and even bone resorption. Injuries can have a significant effect on life quality. Leprosy is a leading cause of permanent physical disability among communicable diseases worldwide. Eye involvement can occur, and patients should be examined by an ophthalmologist. A diagnosis of leprosy should be considered in any patient with hypoesthetic or anesthetic skin rash or skin patches, especially those that do not respond to ordinary therapies, and among those with a history of residence in areas with endemic leprosy or contact with armadillos.

- **Leprosy reactions.** Acute clinical exacerbations reflect abrupt changes in the immunologic balance. They are especially common during initial years of treatment but can occur in the absence of therapy. Two major types of leprosy reactions (LRs) are seen: type 1 (reversal reaction, LR-1) is predominantly observed in borderline tuberculoid and borderline lepromatous leprosy and is the result of a sudden increase in effective cell-mediated immunity. Acute tenderness and swelling at the site of cutaneous and neural lesions with development of new lesions are major manifestations. Ulcerations can occur, but polymorphonuclear leukocytes are absent from the LR-1 lesion. Fever and systemic toxicity are uncommon. Type 2 (erythema nodosum leprosum, LR-2) occurs in borderline and lepromatous forms as a systemic inflammatory response. Tender, red dermal papules or nodules resembling erythema nodosum, along with high fever, migrating polyarthralgia, painful swelling of lymph nodes and spleen, iridocyclitis, and, rarely, nephritis, can occur.

Etiology

Leprosy is caused by *M leprae,* an obligate intracellular bacterium that can have variable staining by Gram stain. It is best visualized using the Fite method. *M leprae* is the only bacterium known to infect peripheral nerves.

Epidemiology

Leprosy is considered a neglected tropical disease and is most prevalent in tropical and subtropical zones. It is not highly infectious. Fewer than 5% of people appear to be genetically susceptible to the infection. Accordingly, spouses of leprosy patients are not likely to develop leprosy, but biological parents, children, and siblings who are household contacts of untreated patients with leprosy are at increased risk.

Transmission is thought to be through long-term close contact with an infected individual, and it likely occurs through respiratory shedding of infectious droplets by untreated cases or individuals incubating subclinical infections. The 9-banded armadillo (*Dasypus novemcinctus*) and 6-banded armadillo (*Euphractus sexcinctus*) are the only known nonhuman reservoirs of *M leprae;* zoonotic transmission is reported in the southern United States. Like many other chronic infectious diseases, onset of leprosy is increasingly associated with use of anti-inflammatory autoimmune therapies and immunologic senescence among elderly patients.

There are approximately 6,500 people with leprosy living in the United States, with 3,300 under active medical management. During 1994–2011, there were 2,323 new cases of leprosy. Over this period, a decline in the rate of new diagnoses from 0.52 (1994–1996) to 0.43 (2009–2011) per million was observed. The rate among foreign-born people decreased from 3.66 to 2.29, whereas the rate among US-born people was 0.16 in both 1994–1996 and 2009–2011. The majority of leprosy cases reported in the United States occurred among residents of Texas, California, and Hawaii or among immigrants or those who lived or worked in leprosy-endemic countries. More than 65% of the world's leprosy patients reside in South and Southeast Asia— primarily India. Other areas of high endemicity include Angola, Brazil, Central African Republic, Democratic Republic of Congo, Madagascar, Mozambique, the Republic of the Marshall Islands, South Sudan, the Federated States of Micronesia, and the United Republic of Tanzania.

Incubation Period

Usually 3 to 5 years (range, 1–20 years).

Diagnostic Tests

Histopathologic examination of skin biopsy by an experienced pathologist is the best method of establishing the diagnosis and is the basis for classification of leprosy. These specimens can be sent to the National Hansen's Disease (Leprosy) Program (NHDP) [800/642-2477; **www.hrsa.gov/hansensdisease**] in formalin or embedded in paraffin. Acid-fast bacilli may be found in slit smears or biopsy specimens of skin lesions of patients with lepromatous forms but are rarely visualized from patients with tuberculoid and indeterminate forms of disease. A polymerase chain reaction assay for *M leprae* is available to assist diagnosis after consultation with the NHDP and can be performed on the basis of clinical suspicion.

Treatment

Leprosy is curable. The primary goal of therapy is prevention of permanent nerve damage, which can be accomplished by early diagnosis and treatment. Combination antimicrobial multidrug therapy can be obtained free of charge from the NHDP in the United States and from the World Health Organization in other countries. Certain criteria must be met for physicians wishing to obtain the antimicrobial therapy from the NHDP (**www.hrsa.gov/hansensdisease/diagnosis/recommendedtreatment.html**).

It is important to treat *M leprae* infections with more than 1 antimicrobial agent to minimize development of antimicrobial-resistant organisms. Adults are treated with dapsone, rifampin, and clofazimine. Resistance to all 3 drugs has been documented but is rare. The infectivity of leprosy patients ceases within a few days of initiating standard multidrug therapy.

- **Multibacillary leprosy (6 patches or more).** Dapsone **and** rifampin **and** clofazimine for 24 months are recommended. Clarithromycin can be used in place of clofazimine for children. Clofazimine is not available commercially; in the United States, it is available only as an investigational drug for treatment of leprosy and is obtained through the NHDP.
- **Paucibacillary leprosy (1–5 patches).** Dapsone **and** rifampin for 12 months are recommended. Before beginning antimicrobial therapy, patients should be tested for glucose-6-phosphate dehydrogenase deficiency, have baseline complete blood cell counts and liver function test results documented, and be evaluated for any evidence of tuberculosis infection, especially if the patient is infected with HIV. Skin darkening typically resolves within several months of completing therapy.

Leprosy reactions should be treated aggressively to prevent peripheral nerve damage. Treatment with prednisone can be initiated. All patients with leprosy should be educated about signs and symptoms of neuritis and cautioned to report signs and symptoms of neuritis immediately so corticosteroid therapy can be instituted. Patients should receive counseling because of the social and psychological effects of this disease.

Relapse of disease after completing multidrug therapy is rare (0.01%–0.14%); the presentation of new skin patches is usually attributable to a late type 1 reaction. When it does occur, relapse is usually attributable to reactivation of drug-susceptible organisms. People with relapses of disease require another course of multidrug therapy. Therapy for patients with leprosy should be undertaken in consultation with an expert in leprosy.

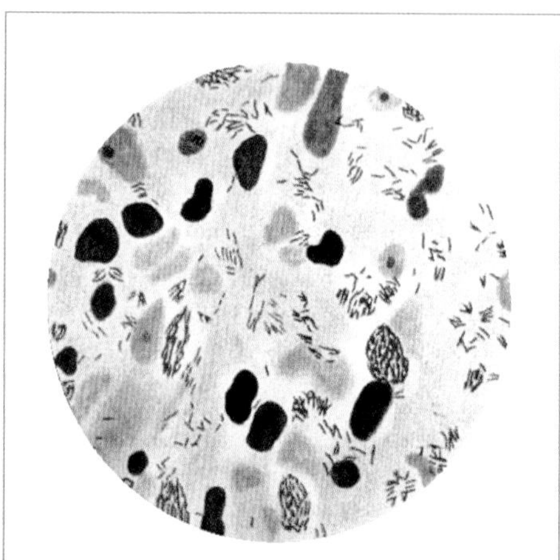

Image 76.1
A photomicrograph of *Mycobacterium leprae* taken from a leprous skin lesion. *M leprae* is the cause of leprosy, or Hansen disease. A slow-multiplying bacterium, it mainly affects the skin, nerves, and mucous membranes. In 1999, the world incidence level was estimated to be 640,000; in 2000, 738,284 cases were identified. In 2007, 101 new cases of leprosy were reported in the United States. Courtesy of Centers for Disease Control and Prevention.

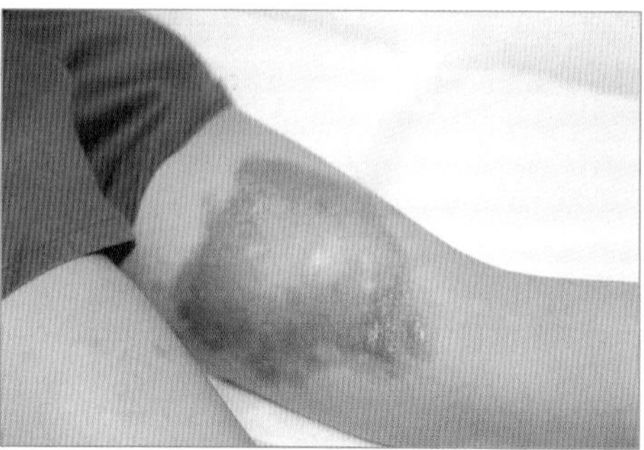

Image 76.2
Hansen disease. A young Vietnamese boy who spent 2 years in a refugee camp in the Philippines presented with the nodular violaceous skin lesion shown. The results of a biopsy of the lesion showed acid-fast organisms surrounding blood vessels. A diagnosis of lepromatous leprosy was made and the child was treated with a multidrug regimen. Copyright Barbara Jantausch, MD, FAAP.

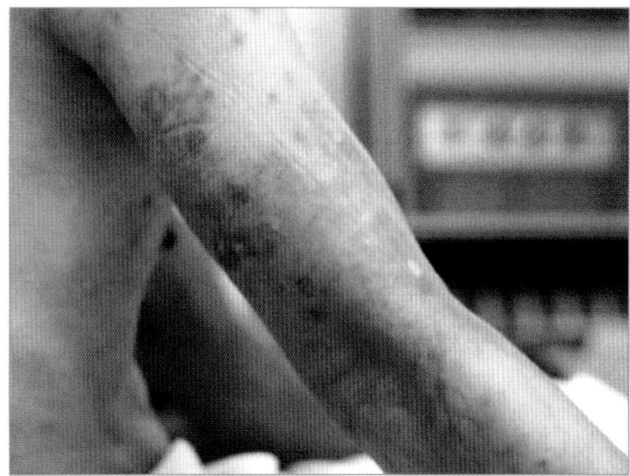

Image 76.3
Erythema nodosum leprosum in a 29-year-old Asian man. Copyright Gary Williams.

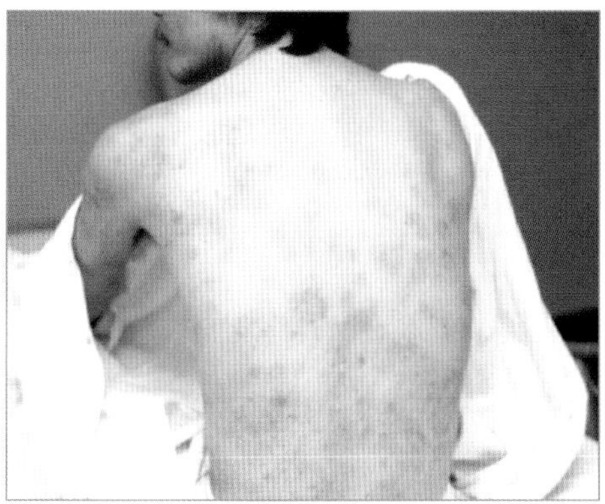

Image 76.4
Erythema nodosum leprosum in the same patient as in Image 76.3. Copyright Gary Williams.

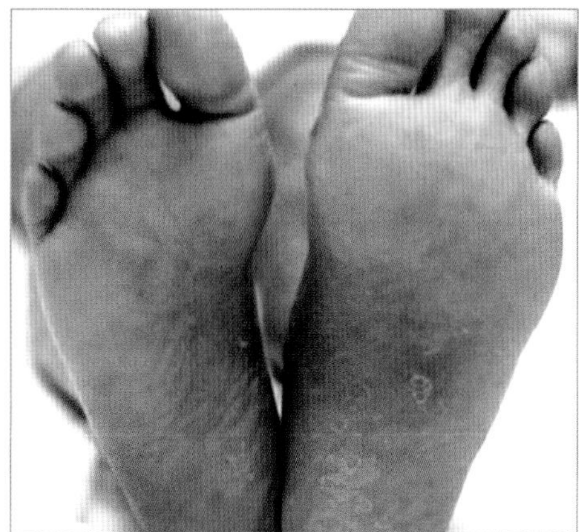

Image 76.5
Erythema nodosum leprosum in the same patient as in images 76.3 and 76.4. Copyright Gary Williams.

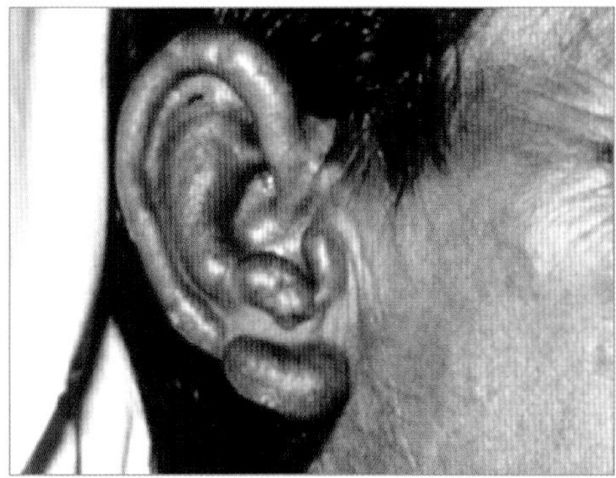

Image 76.6
Lepromatous leprosy in an Asian man. Newly diagnosed cases are considered contagious until treatment is established and should be reported to local and state public health departments. Courtesy of Hugh Moffet, MD.

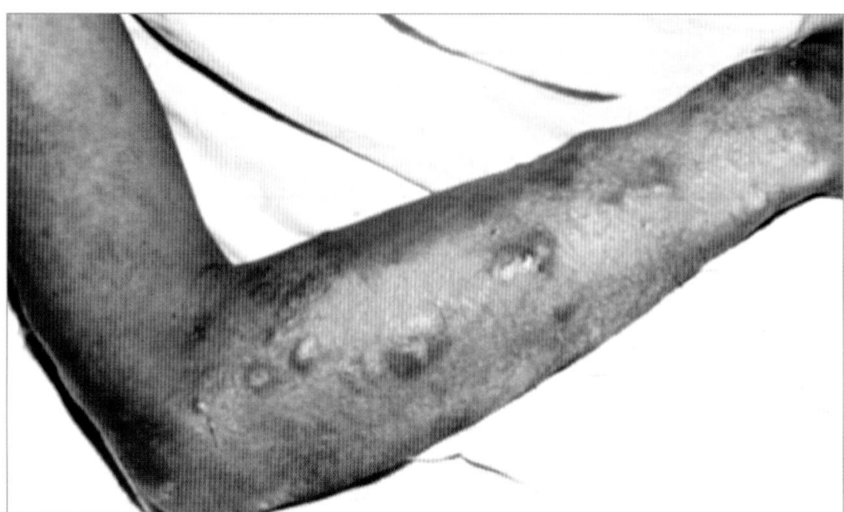

Image 76.7
An adult male with lepromatous leprosy. Courtesy of Hugh Moffet, MD.

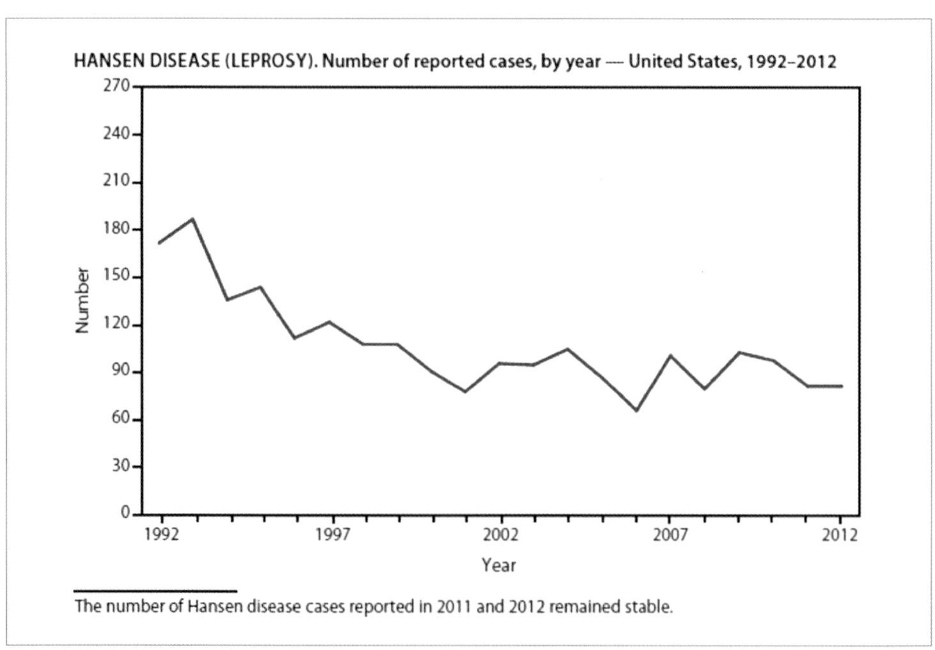

Image 76.8
Number of reported cases, by year—United States, 1992–2012. Courtesy of *Morbidity and Mortality Weekly Report.*

77

Leptospirosis

Clinical Manifestations

Leptospirosis is an acute febrile disease with varied manifestations. The severity of disease ranges from asymptomatic or subclinical to self-limited systemic illness (approximately 90% of patients) to life-threatening illness with jaundice, renal failure (oliguric or nonoliguric), myocarditis, hemorrhage (particularly pulmonary), and refractory shock. Clinical presentation may be monophasic or biphasic. Classically described biphasic leptospirosis has an acute septicemia phase, usually lasting 1 week, when *Leptospira* organisms are present in blood, followed by a second immune-mediated phase that does not respond to antibiotic therapy. Regardless of its severity, the acute phase is characterized by nonspecific symptoms, including fever, chills, headache, nausea, and vomiting, occasionally accompanied by rash or conjunctival suffusion. Distinct clinical findings include notable conjunctival suffusion without purulent discharge (30%–99% of cases) and myalgia of the calf and lumbar regions (40%–100% of cases). Findings commonly associated with the immune-mediated phase include fever, aseptic meningitis, and uveitis; between 5% and 10% of *Leptospira*-infected patients are estimated to experience severe illness. Severe manifestations include any combination of jaundice and renal dysfunction (Weil syndrome), pulmonary hemorrhage, cardiac arrhythmias, and circulatory collapse. The estimated case-fatality rate from severe illness is 5% to 15%, although it can increase to greater than 50% in patients with pulmonary hemorrhage. Asymptomatic or subclinical infection with seroconversion is frequent, especially in settings of endemic infection.

Etiology

Leptospirosis is caused by pathogenic spirochetes of the genus *Leptospira*. Leptospires are classified by species and subdivided into more than 250 antigenically defined serovars and grouped into serogroups on the basis of antigenic relatedness.

Epidemiology

Leptospirosis is among the most globally important zoonoses, affecting people in resource-rich and resource-limited countries in urban and rural contexts. It has been estimated that approximately 868,000 people annually worldwide are currently infected (range, 327,000–1,520,000), with approximately 49,200 (range, 19,000–88,900) deaths occurring each year. The reservoirs for *Leptospira* species include a range of wild and domestic animals, primarily rats, dogs, and livestock (eg, cattle, pigs), that can shed organisms asymptomatically for years. *Leptospira* organisms excreted in animal urine can remain viable in moist soil or water for weeks to months in warm climates. Humans usually become infected via entry of leptospires through contact of mucosal surfaces (especially conjunctivae) or abraded skin with contaminated environmental sources. Unusually, infection may be acquired through direct contact with infected animals or their tissues, infective urine or fluids from carrier animals, or urine-contaminated soil or water. Epidemic exposure is associated with seasonal flooding and natural disasters, including hurricanes and monsoons. Populations in tropical regions of high endemicity likely encounter *Leptospira* organisms commonly during routine activities of daily living. People who are predisposed by occupation include abattoir and sewer workers, miners, veterinarians, farmers, and military personnel. Recreational exposures and clusters of disease have been associated with adventure travel; sporting events, including triathlons; and wading, swimming, or boating in contaminated water, particularly during flooding or following heavy rainfall. Being submerged in or swallowing water during these activities is a common historical finding. Person-to-person transmission does not occur.

Incubation Period

5 to 14 days; range, 2 to 30 days.

Diagnostic Tests

Leptospira organisms can be isolated from blood or cerebrospinal fluid during the early septicemic phase (first 7–10 days) of illness and from urine specimens 14 days or more after illness onset. Specialized culture media are required but are not routinely available in most laboratories. *Leptospira* organisms can be grown on *Leptospira* semisolid medium (ie, Ellinghausen-McCullough-Johnson-Harris) from blood culture bottles used in automated systems within 1 week of inoculation. However, isolation of the organism may be difficult, requiring incubation for up to 16 weeks, and the sensitivity of culture for diagnosis is low. For these reasons, serum specimens should always be obtained to facilitate diagnosis. Antibodies can develop as early as 5 to 7 days after onset of illness and can be measured by commercially available immunoassays. However, these assays have variable sensitivity according to regional differences of the various *Leptospira* species and increases in antibody titer may not be detected until more than 10 days after onset, especially if antimicrobial therapy is initiated early. Antibody increases can be transient, delayed, or absent in some patients. Microscopic agglutination, the gold standard serologic test, is performed only in reference laboratories and requires seroconversion demonstrated between acute and convalescent specimens obtained at least 10 days apart. Immunohistochemical and immunofluorescent techniques can detect leptospiral antigens in infected tissues. Polymerase chain reaction assays for detection of *Leptospira* DNA in blood and urine have been developed but are only available in research laboratories.

Treatment

Intravenous penicillin is the drug of choice for patients with severe infection requiring hospitalization; penicillin has been shown to be effective in shortening duration of fever as late as 7 days into the course of illness. Penicillin G decreases the duration of systemic symptoms and persistence of associated laboratory abnormalities and may prevent development of leptospiruria. As with other spirochetal infections, a Jarisch-Herxheimer reaction (an acute febrile reaction accompanied by headache, myalgia, and an aggravated clinical picture lasting less than 24 hours) can develop after initiation of penicillin therapy. Parenteral cefotaxime, ceftriaxone, and doxycycline have been demonstrated in randomized clinical trials to be equal in efficacy to penicillin G for treatment of severe leptospirosis. Severe cases also require appropriate supportive care, including fluid and electrolyte replacement. Patients with oliguric renal insufficiency and pulmonary hemorrhage syndrome require prompt dialysis and mechanical ventilation, respectively, to improve clinical outcome. For patients with mild disease, oral doxycycline has been shown to shorten the course of illness and decrease occurrence of leptospiruria; ampicillin or amoxicillin can also be used to treat mild disease. Azithromycin has been demonstrated in a clinical trial to be as effective as doxycycline and can be used as an alternative in patients for whom doxycycline is contraindicated (eg, pregnant women).

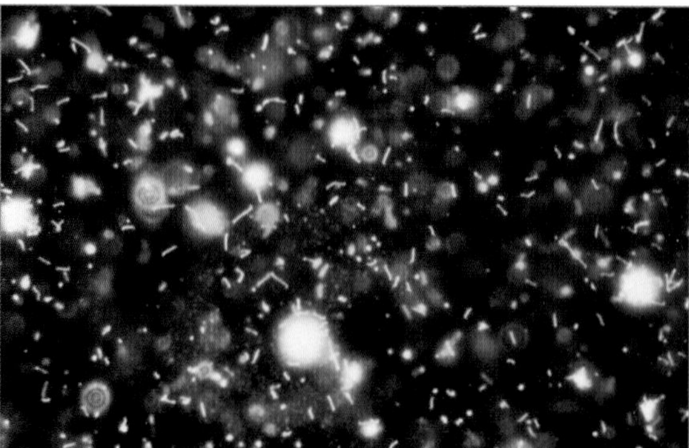

Image 77.1
Photomicrograph of leptospiral microscopic agglutination test with live antigen (darkfield microscopy technique). Leptospirosis is a common global zoonotic disease of humans and several warm-blooded animals, especially in subtropic regions of the world, caused by the spirochete bacteria *Leptospira*. Courtesy of Centers for Disease Control and Prevention/Mrs M. Gatton.

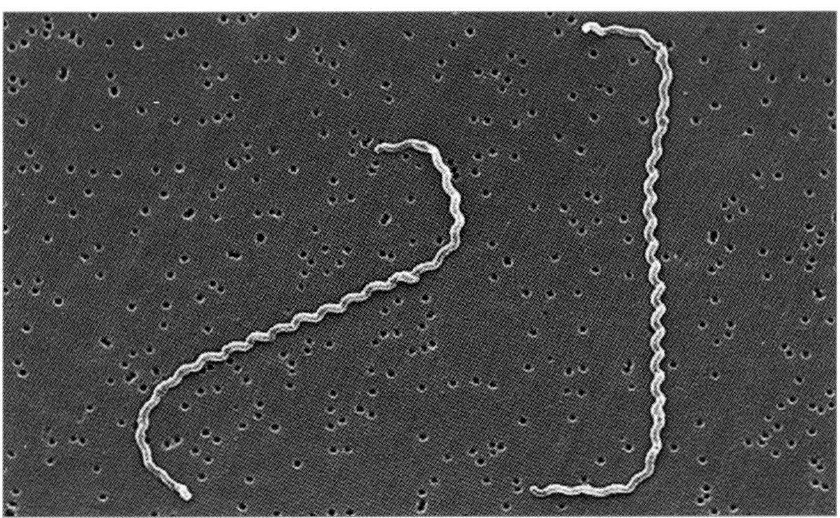

Image 77.2
Scanning electron micrograph of *Leptospira interrogans* strain RGA. Courtesy of Centers for Disease Control and Prevention National Center for Infectious Disease/Rob Weyant/Janice Haney Carr.

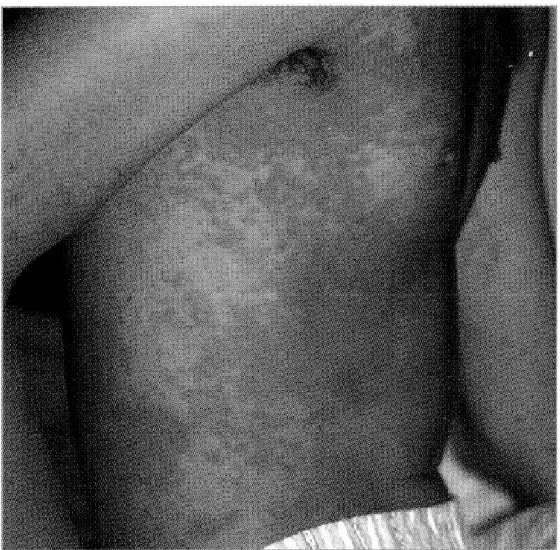

Image 77.3
Leptospirosis rash in an adolescent male that shows the generalized vasculitis caused by this infection.

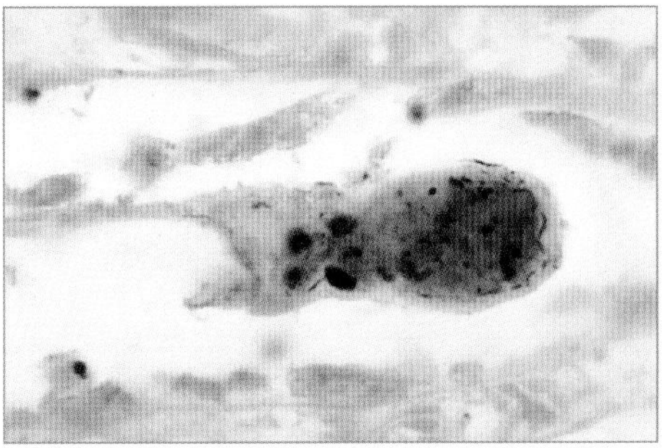

Image 77.4
Photomicrograph of kidney tissue, using a silver staining technique, revealing the presence of *Leptospira* bacteria. Courtesy of Centers for Disease Control and Prevention/Martin Hicklin, MD.

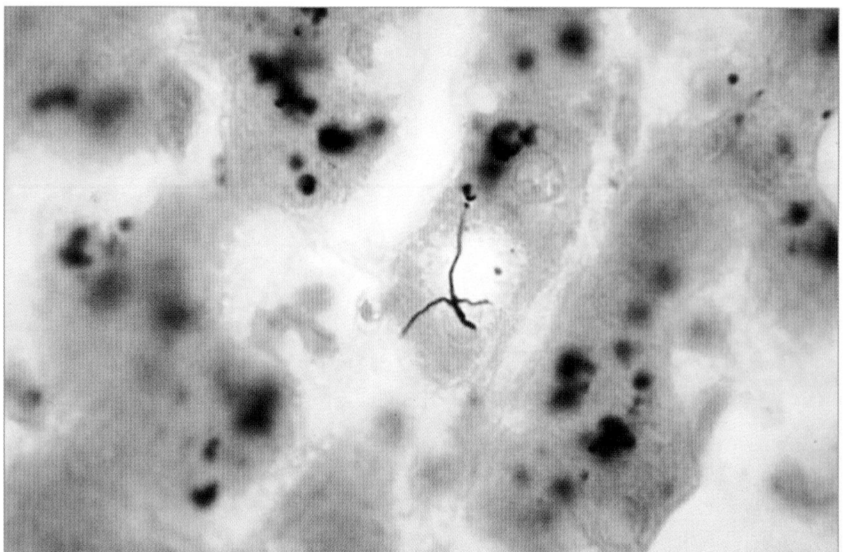

Image 77.5

Photomicrograph of liver tissue revealing the presence of *Leptospira* bacteria. Humans become infected by swallowing water contaminated by infected animals or through skin contact, especially with mucosal surfaces, such as the eyes or nose, or with broken skin. The disease is not known to be spread from person to person. Courtesy of Centers for Disease Control and Prevention/Martin Hicklin, MD.

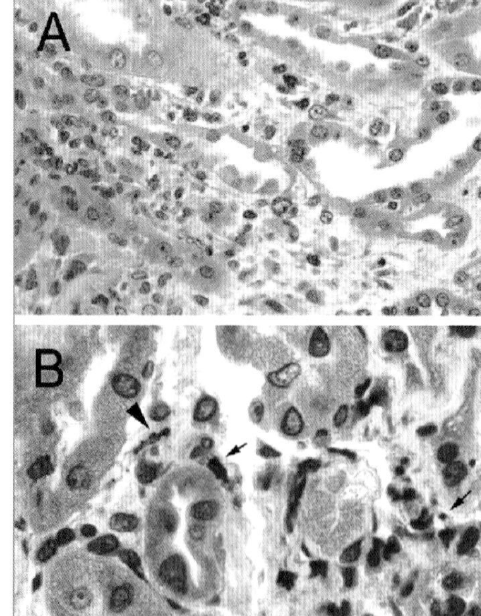

Image 77.6

A, Renal biopsy shows inflammatory cell infiltrate in the interstitium and focal denudation of tubular epithelial cells (hematoxylin-eosin, original magnification x100). B, Immunostaining of fragmented leptospire (arrowhead) and granular form of bacterial antigens (arrows) (original magnification x158). Meites E, Jay MT, Deresinski S, et al. Reemerging leptospirosis, California. *Emerg Infect Dis.* 2004; 10(3):406–412.

78

Listeria monocytogenes Infections

(Listeriosis)

Clinical Manifestations

Listeriosis is a relatively uncommon but severe invasive infection caused by *Listeria monocytogenes.* Transmission predominantly is foodborne, and illness occurs most frequently among pregnant women and their fetuses or newborns, older adults, and people with impaired cell-mediated immunity resulting from underlying illness or treatment (eg, organ transplant, hematologic malignancy, immunosuppression resulting from therapy with corticosteroid or antitumor necrosis factor agents, AIDS). Pregnancy-associated infections can result in spontaneous abortion, fetal death, preterm delivery, and neonatal illness or death. In pregnant women, infections can be asymptomatic or associated with a nonspecific febrile illness with myalgia, back pain, and, occasionally, gastrointestinal tract symptoms. Fetal infection results from transplacental transmission following maternal bacteremia. Approximately 65% of pregnant women with *Listeria* infection experience a prodromal illness before the diagnosis of listeriosis in their newborn. Amnionitis during labor, brown staining of amniotic fluid, or asymptomatic perinatal infection can occur. Neonates can present with early-onset and late-onset syndromes similar to those of group B streptococcal disease. Preterm birth, pneumonia, and septicemia are common in early-onset disease (within the first week of life), with fatality rates of 14% to 56%. An erythematous rash with small, pale papules characterized histologically by granulomas, termed "granulomatosis infantisepticum," can occur in severe newborn infection. Late-onset infections occur at 8 to 30 days of life following term deliveries and usually result in meningitis with fatality rates of approximately 25%. Late-onset infection may result from acquisition of the organism during passage through the birth canal or, rarely, from environmental sources.

Clinical features characteristic of invasive listeriosis outside pregnancy or the neonatal period are bacteremia and meningitis with or without parenchymal brain involvement and, less commonly, brain abscess or endocarditis. *L monocytogenes* can also cause rhombencephalitis (brainstem encephalitis) in otherwise healthy adolescents and young adults. Outbreaks of febrile gastroenteritis caused by food contaminated with a large inoculum of *L monocytogenes* have been reported; this illness typically lasts 2 to 3 days. The prevalence of stool carriage of *L monocytogenes* among healthy, asymptomatic adults is estimated to be 1% to 5%.

Etiology

L monocytogenes is a facultatively anaerobic, nonspore-forming, nonbranching, motile, gram-positive rod that multiplies intracellularly. The organism grows readily on blood agar and produces incomplete hemolysis. *L monocytogenes* serotypes 1/2a, 4b, and 1/2b cause most human cases of invasive listeriosis. Unlike most bacteria, *L monocytogenes* grows well at refrigerator temperatures (4°C–10°C [39°F–50°F]).

Epidemiology

L monocytogenes causes approximately 1,600 cases of invasive disease and 260 deaths annually in the United States. This saprophytic organism is distributed widely in the environment and is an important cause of illness in ruminants. Foodborne transmission causes outbreaks and sporadic infections in humans. Commonly incriminated foods include deli-style, ready-to-eat meats, particularly poultry, and unpasteurized milk and soft cheeses, including Mexican-style cheese. The US incidence of listeriosis decreased substantially during the 1990s, when US regulatory agencies began enforcing rigorous screening guidelines for *L monocytogenes* in processed foods. The last large outbreak in the United States occurred in 2011, resulting in 143 hospitalizations, and was linked to contaminated cantaloupe.

Incubation Period

For pregnancy-associated cases, 2 to 4 weeks; for nonpregnancy-associated cases, 1 to 14 days; for febrile gastroenteritis, 24 hours.

Diagnostic Tests

L monocytogenes can be recovered readily on blood agar from cultures of blood, cerebrospinal fluid (CSF), meconium, placental or fetal tissue specimens, amniotic fluid, and other infected tissue specimens, including joint, pleural, or peritoneal fluid. Gram stain of meconium, placental tissue, biopsy specimens of the rash of early-onset infection, or CSF from an infected patient may demonstrate the organism. The organisms can be gram-variable and resemble diphtheroids, cocci, or diplococci. Laboratory misidentification is not uncommon, and the isolation of a "diphtheroid" from blood or CSF should always alert one to the possibility that the organism is *L monocytogenes*.

Treatment

No controlled trials have established the drug(s) of choice or duration of therapy for *Listeria* infection. Combination therapy using intravenous ampicillin and an aminoglycoside, usually gentamicin, is recommended for severe infections, including meningitis, encephalitis, endocarditis, and infections in neonates and immunocompromised patients. Use of an alternative to an aminoglycoside that is active intracellularly (eg, trimethoprim-sulfamethoxazole, a quinolone, linezolid, rifampin) is supported by clinical reports in adults. In the penicillin-allergic patient, trimethoprim-sulfamethoxazole or a quinolone has been used successfully as monotherapy for *Listeria* central nervous system infections. Cephalosporins are not active against *L monocytogenes*. For bacteremia without associated central nervous system infection, 14 days of treatment is sufficient. For *L monocytogenes* meningitis, most experts recommend 21 days of treatment. Longer courses are necessary for patients with endocarditis or parenchymal brain infection (cerebritis, rhombencephalitis, brain abscess).

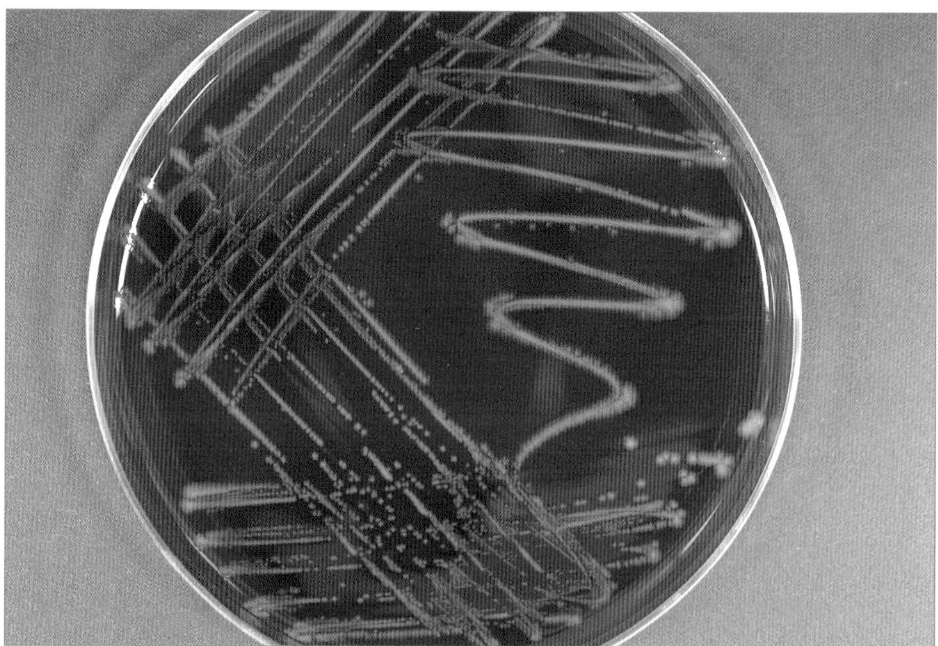

Image 78.1
Listeria monocytogenes on blood agar. Courtesy of Julia Rosebush, DO; Robert Jerris, PhD; and Theresa Stanley, M(ASCP).

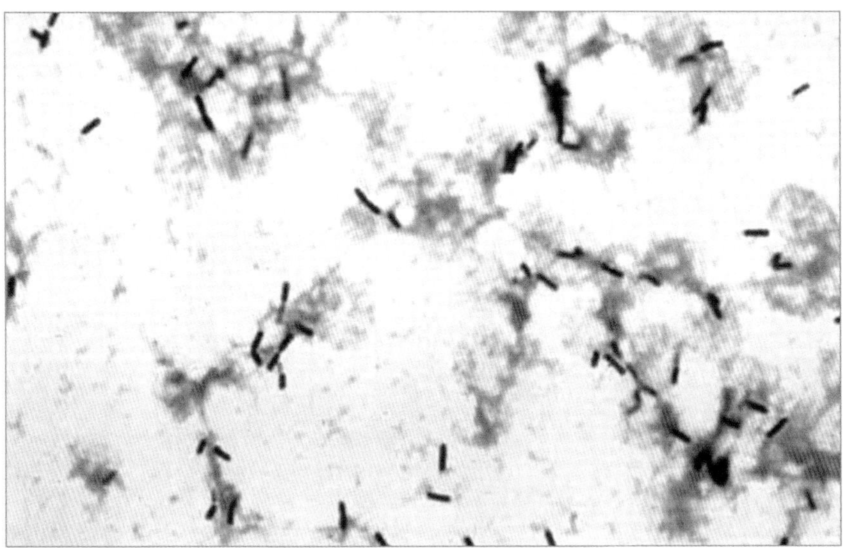

Image 78.2
Cerebrospinal fluid showing characteristic gram-positive rods (Gram stain). Listeriosis is a severe but relatively uncommon infection. Listeriosis occurs most frequently among pregnant women and their fetuses or newborns, people of advanced age, or immunocompromised people. Copyright Martha Lepow, MD.

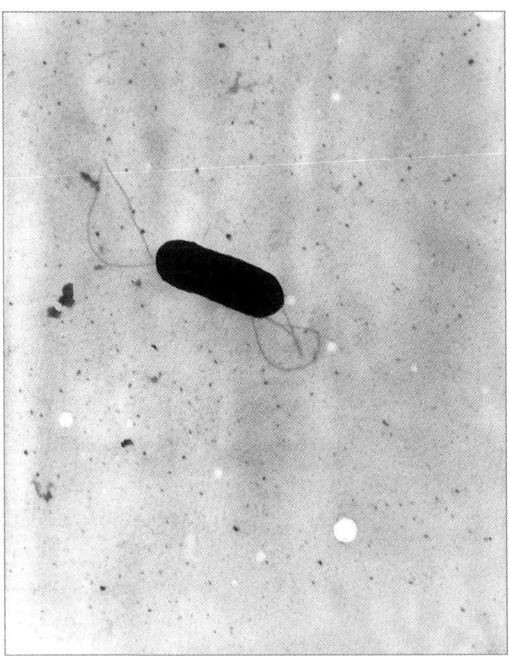

Image 78.3
Electron micrograph of a flagellated *Listeria monocytogenes* bacterium (magnification x41,250). Courtesy of Centers for Disease Control and Prevention/Dr Balasubr Swaminathan; Peggy Hayes.

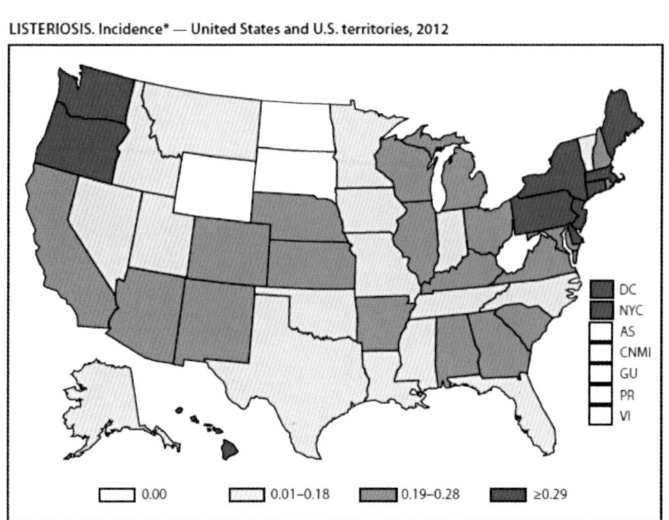

Image 78.4
Listeriosis. Incidence—United States and US territories, 2012. Courtesy of *Morbidity and Mortality Weekly Report.*

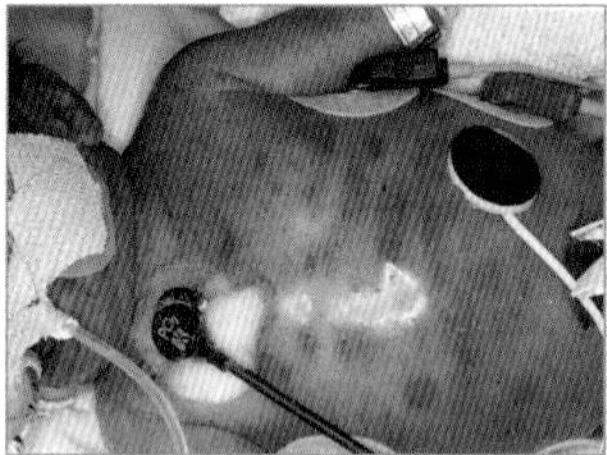

Image 78.5
Skin lesions present at birth in a neonate with congenital pneumonia. *Listeria monocytogenes* was isolated from blood and skin lesion cultures.

79

Lyme Disease

(Lyme Borreliosis, *Borrelia burgdorferi* Infection)

Clinical Manifestations

Clinical manifestations of Lyme disease are divided into 3 stages: early localized, early disseminated, and late disease. Early localized disease is characterized by a distinctive lesion, erythema migrans, at the site of a recent tick bite. Erythema migrans is, by far, the most common manifestation of Lyme disease in children. Erythema migrans begins as a red macule or papule that usually expands over days to weeks to form a large, annular, erythematous lesion that typically increases in size to 5 cm or more in diameter, sometimes with partial central clearing. The lesion is usually but not always painless, and it is not pruritic. Localized erythema migrans can vary greatly in size and shape and can be confused with cellulitis; lesions may have a purplish discoloration or central vesicular or necrotic areas. A classic bull's-eye appearance with concentric rings appears in a minority of cases. Factors that distinguish erythema migrans from local allergic reaction to a tick bite include larger size (>5 cm), gradual expansion, lack of pruritus, and slower onset. Constitutional symptoms, such as malaise, headache, mild neck stiffness, myalgia, and arthralgia, often accompany the rash of early localized disease. Fever can be present but is not universal and is generally mild.

In early disseminated disease, multiple erythema migrans lesions may appear several weeks after an infective tick bite and consist of secondary annular, erythematous lesions similar to, but usually smaller than, the primary lesion. Other manifestations of early disseminated illness (which may occur with or without rash) are palsies of the cranial nerves (especially cranial nerve VII), lymphocytic meningitis, and polyradiculitis. Ophthalmic conditions (eg, conjunctivitis, optic neuritis, keratitis, uveitis) can occur, usually in concert with other neurologic manifestations. Systemic symptoms, such as low-grade fever, arthralgia, myalgia, headache, and fatigue, are also common during the early disseminated stage. Lymphocytic meningitis can occur and often is associated with cranial neuropathy or papilledema; patients with lymphocytic meningitis typically have a more subacute onset, lower temperature, and fewer white blood cells in cerebrospinal fluid (CSF) than those with viral meningitis. Carditis, which usually manifests as various degrees of heart block, can occur in children but is relatively less common. Occasionally, people with early Lyme disease have concurrent human granulocytic anaplasmosis or babesiosis, which are transmitted by the same tick. Coinfection can present as more severe disease than Lyme monoinfection, and the presence of a high fever with Lyme disease or inadequate response to treatment should raise suspicion of concurrent anaplasmosis or babesiosis. Certain laboratory abnormalities, such as leukopenia, thrombocytopenia, anemia, or abnormal hepatic transaminase concentrations, should raise concern for coinfection.

Late disease occurs in patients who are not treated at an earlier stage of illness and most commonly manifests as Lyme arthritis in children, which is characterized by inflammatory arthritis that is usually pauciarticular and affects large joints, particularly knees. Although arthralgias can be present at any stage of Lyme disease, Lyme arthritis has objective evidence of joint swelling. Arthritis can occur without a history of earlier stages of illness (including erythema migrans). Compared with pyogenic arthritis, Lyme arthritis tends to manifest with joint swelling or effusion out of proportion to pain or disability and with lower peripheral blood neutrophilia and erythrocyte sedimentation rate. Polyneuropathy, encephalopathy, and encephalitis are extremely rare manifestations of late disease. Children who are treated with antimicrobial agents in the early stage of disease almost never develop late disease.

Lyme disease does not cause a congenital infection syndrome. No evidence suggests Lyme disease can be transmitted via human milk.

Some patients with demonstrated Lyme disease have persistent subjective symptoms, such as fatigue and arthralgia, after appropriate treatment, a condition known as posttreatment Lyme disease syndrome. Although the cause is unknown, ongoing infection with *Borrelia burgdorferi* has not been demonstrated, and long-term antibiotics have not been shown to be beneficial. Patients with posttreatment Lyme disease syndrome usually respond to symptomatic treatment and recover gradually.

"Chronic Lyme disease" is a nonspecific term that lacks a clinical definition. It is used by a small minority of clinicians and patient advocates to refer to patients with chronic, unexplained syndromes usually characterized by pain and fatigue. Alternative diagnoses may be responsible for symptoms and should be considered. In none of these situations is there credible evidence that persistent infection with *B burgdorferi* is demonstrable.

Etiology

In the United States, Lyme disease is caused by the spirochete *B burgdorferi* sensu stricto. In Eurasia, *B burgdorferi, Borrelia afzelii,* and *Borrelia garinii* cause borreliosis.

Epidemiology

Lyme disease primarily occurs in 2 distinct geographic regions of the United States. More than 90% of cases occur in New England and in the eastern Mid-Atlantic States, as far south as Virginia. The disease also occurs, but with lower frequency, in the upper Midwest, especially Wisconsin and Minnesota. Transmission also occurs at a low level on the West Coast, especially northern California. The occurrence of cases in the United States correlates with the distribution and frequency of infected tick vectors—*Ixodes scapularis* in the east and Midwest and *Ixodes pacificus* in the west. In Southern states, *I scapularis* ticks are rare compared with the northeast. Ticks that are present in Southern states do not commonly feed on competent reservoir mammals and are less likely to bite humans because of different questing habits. Reported cases from states without known enzootic risks may have been acquired in states with endemic infection or may be misdiagnoses resulting from false-positive serologic test results or results that are misinterpreted as positive.

Most cases of early Lyme disease occur between April and October; more than 50% of cases occur during June and July. People of all ages can be affected, but incidence in the United States is highest among children 5 through 9 years of age and adults 55 through 59 years of age.

A lesion similar to erythema migrans known as "southern tick-associated rash illness" or STARI has been reported in south central and southeastern states without endemic *B burgdorferi* infection. The etiology and appropriate treatment of this condition remain unknown. Southern tick-associated rash illness results from the bite of the lone star tick, *Amblyomma americanum*, which is abundant in southern states and is biologically incapable of transmitting *B burgdorferi*. Patients with STARI may present with constitutional symptoms in addition to erythema migrans; however, STARI has not been associated with any of the disseminated complications of Lyme disease.

Clinical manifestations of Lyme disease in eastern Canada, Europe, states of the former Soviet Union, China, and Japan vary somewhat from manifestations seen in the United States. In particular, European Lyme disease may cause borrelial lymphocytoma and acrodermatitis chronica atrophicans and is more likely to produce neurologic disease, whereas arthritis is uncommon. These differences are attributable to the different genospecies of *Borrelia* responsible for European Lyme disease. The primary tick vector in Europe is *Ixodes ricinus*, and the primary tick vector in Asia is *Ixodes persulcatus*.

Incubation Period

From tick bite to appearance of single or multiple erythema migrans lesions is 1 to 32 days (median 11 days). Late manifestations can occur months after the tick bite.

Diagnostic Tests

The diagnosis of Lyme disease rests first and foremost on the recognition of a consistent clinical illness in people who have had plausible geographic exposure. Early localized

Lyme disease is diagnosed clinically on recognition of an erythema migrans lesion. Although erythema migrans is not strictly pathognomonic for Lyme disease, it is highly distinctive and characteristic. If a patient has a small lesion (<5-cm diameter) that resembles erythema migrans, the patient can be followed over several days to see if the lesion expands to greater than 5 cm; this will improve the specificity of a clinical diagnosis. In areas endemic for Lyme disease during the warm months of the year, it is expected that the vast majority of erythema migrans is attributable to *B burgdorferi* infection, and early initiation of treatment is appropriate.

Diagnostic testing is based on serology; during early infection, the sensitivity is low and serologic testing is not recommended because only approximately one-third of patients with solitary erythema migrans lesions are seropositive. Furthermore, immunoglobulin (Ig) M–based Lyme disease serologic testing carries a substantial risk of false-positive results. Patients who have multiple lesions of erythema migrans are also diagnosed clinically, although the likelihood of seropositivity is higher. Diagnosis of disseminated Lyme disease requires a typical clinical illness, plausible geographic exposure, and a positive serologic test result.

The standard testing method for Lyme disease is a 2-tier serologic assay. The initial test is a quantitative screening for antibodies to a whole-cell sonicate or C6 antigen of *B burgdorferi*. This test is performed using an enzyme-linked immunosorbent assay (ELISA) or immunofluorescent antibody (IFA) test. It should be noted that clinical laboratories vary somewhat in their description of this test. It may be described as "Lyme ELISA," "Lyme antibody screen," "total Lyme antibody," or "Lyme IgG/IgM." Many commercial laboratories offer enzyme immunoassay (EIA) or IFA tests with reflex to Western immunoblot if the first-tier assay result is positive. This is the most foolproof way of ordering the appropriate 2-tier test for Lyme disease.

The initial EIA or IFA test result may be reported as a titer, but the role of the numerical titer is solely to categorize the result as negative, equivocal, or positive. If the first-tier ELISA result is negative, the patient is considered seronegative and no further testing is indicated. If the result is equivocal or positive, a second-tier test is required. Although sensitive, the first-tier test is not specific and has a rate of false-positive results that may exceed 5% in clinically compatible cases and far higher in clinically nonsuggestive cases. This is partly because the test is not well standardized and because there are antigenic components of *B burgdorferi* that are not specific to this species. In particular, other spirochetal infections, normal spirochetes from our oral flora, other acute infections, and certain autoimmune diseases may be cross-reactive. The EIA or IFA test is the important, helpful first-tier test but is too nonspecific to determine, in itself, a patient's serologic status.

Serum specimens that yield positive or equivocal EIA results should then be tested by the second-tier standardized Western immunoblot. This assay tests for the presence of antibodies to specific *B burgdorferi* antigens. Three IgM antibodies (to the 23/24, 39, and 41 kDa polypeptides) and 10 IgG antibodies (to the 18, 23/24, 28, 30, 39, 41, 45, 60, 66, and 93 kDa polypeptides) are tested. The presence of at least 2 IgM bands or 5 IgG bands is considered a positive immunoblot result. Laboratory reporting practices can produce some confusion when physicians are interpreting results. It is common for clinical laboratories to report the titers of all 13 bands and describe them as positive or negative; laboratories often print positive bands in bold, which frequently results in misinterpretation of the overall result as positive despite the fact that 4 or fewer IgG bands are present. The presence of 4 or fewer IgG bands is too nonspecific to meet criteria for positivity. It is imperative the physician review the interpretive criteria for the test overall rather than risk overinterpretation of what may be a negative test result.

The IgM assay is only useful for patients in the first 30 days after symptom onset. The IgM immunoblot should be disregarded (or, if possible, not ordered to begin with) in patients who have had symptoms for longer than

4 to 6 weeks because false-positive IgM assay results are common, and most untreated patients with disseminated Lyme disease will have a positive IgG result by week 6 of illness. Immunoblot testing should not be performed if the EIA result is negative or without a prior EIA; the specificity of immunoblot testing diminishes if this test is performed alone. The EIA and Western blot should not be thought of as "screening" and "confirmatory," respectively. They are interdependent parts of an overall testing method.

A licensed, commercially available serologic test (C6) that detects antibody to a peptide of the immunodominant conserved region of the variable surface antigen (VlsE) of *B burgdorferi* appears to have improved sensitivity for patients with early Lyme disease and Lyme disease acquired in Europe. However, when used alone, its specificity is lower than that of standard 2-tier testing. In the future, the C6 EIA may replace immunoblotting in the 2-tier method.

Polymerase chain reaction testing (using a laboratory with excellent quality-control procedures) has been used to detect *B burgdorferi* DNA in joint fluid. This test, however, is not necessary for the diagnosis of Lyme arthritis, a late disseminated manifestation in which patients are almost invariably seropositive. For patients with persistent arthritis after a standard course of therapy, polymerase chain reaction testing of synovial fluid or tissue may help discriminate ongoing infection from antibiotic-refractory arthritis. Polymerase chain reaction testing can also detect *B burgdorferi* in skin biopsy specimens of erythema migrans lesions, although this invasive procedure is not recommended for routine clinical practice. Polymerase chain reaction has poor sensitivity for CSF and blood specimens.

Suspected central nervous system Lyme disease can be confirmed by demonstration of intrathecal production of antibodies against *B burgdorferi,* which is indicated by CSF/serum IgG optical density ratio greater than 1.3 in specimens collected simultaneously. Cerebrospinal fluid antibody tests, however, can be falsely positive in a variety of other central nervous system inflammatory processes; in particular, the presence of CSF antibodies to *B burgdorferi* cannot confirm a diagnosis of Lyme disease if a different diagnosis is more plausible.

The widespread practice of ordering serologic tests for patients with nonspecific symptoms, such as fatigue or arthralgia, or testing for Lyme disease because of parental or patient pressure, is strongly discouraged. Almost all positive serologic test results in these patients are false-positive results. In areas with endemic infection, previous subclinical infection with seroconversion may occur, and the patient's symptoms may be merely coincidental. Patients with active Lyme disease almost always have objective signs of infection (eg, erythema migrans, facial nerve palsy, arthritis). Nonspecific symptoms commonly accompany these specific signs but almost never are the only evidence of Lyme disease.

Some patients who are treated with antimicrobial agents for early Lyme disease never develop detectable antibodies against *B burgdorferi;* they are cured and are not at risk of late disease. Development of antibodies in patients treated for early Lyme disease does not indicate lack of cure or presence of persistent infection. Ongoing infection without development of antibodies ("seronegative Lyme") has not been demonstrated. Most patients with early disseminated disease and virtually all patients with late disease have antibodies against *B burgdorferi.* Once such antibodies develop, they persist for many years. Consequently, tests for antibodies should not be repeated or used to assess the success of treatment.

Treatment

Consensus practice guidelines for assessment, treatment, and prevention of Lyme disease have been published by the Infectious Diseases Society of America and recommendations for children are summarized in Table 79.1. Antimicrobial therapy for nonspecific symptoms or for asymptomatic seropositivity is discouraged. Doxycycline is the drug of choice for treatment of early Lyme disease in children

Table 79.1
Recommended Treatment of Lyme Disease in Children

Disease Category	Drug(s) and Dose[a]
Early localized disease[a]	
8 y or older	Doxycycline, 4 mg/kg per day, orally, divided into 2 doses (maximum 200 mg/d) for 14 days[b]
Younger than 8 y or unable to tolerate doxycycline[b]	Amoxicillin, 50 mg/kg per day, orally, divided into 3 doses (maximum 1.5 g/d) for 14 days **OR** Cefuroxime, 30 mg/kg per day in 2 divided doses (maximum 1,000 mg/d or 1 g/d) for 14 days
Early disseminated and late disease	
Multiple erythema migrans	Same oral regimen as for early localized disease, for 14 days
Isolated facial palsy	Same oral regimen as for early localized disease, for 14 days (range 14–21 days)[c,d]
Arthritis	Same oral regimen as for early localized disease, for 28 days
Recurrent arthritis	Same oral regimen as for first-episode arthritis, for 28 days **OR** Preferred parenteral regimen: Ceftriaxone sodium, 50–75 mg/kg, IV, once a day (maximum 2 g/d) for 14 days (range 14–28 days) Alternative parenteral regimen: Penicillin, 200,000–400,000 U/kg per day, IV, given in divided doses every 4 hours (maximum 18–24 million U/d) for 14 days (range 14–28 days) **OR** Cefotaxime 150–200 mg/kg per day, IV, divided into 3 or 4 doses (maximum 6 g/d) for 14 days (range 14–28 days)
Antibiotic-refractory/ persistent arthritis[e]	Symptomatic therapy
Atrioventricular heart block or carditis	Oral regimen as for early disease if asymptomatic[f] or not hospitalized, for 14 days (range 14–21 days) **OR** Parenteral regimen initially for hospitalized patients, dosing as for recurrent arthritis, for 14 days (range 14–21 days); oral therapy can be substituted to complete the 14–21 day course.
Meningitis	Ceftriaxone[g] or alternatives of cefotaxime or penicillin[g]: dosing as for recurrent arthritis, for 14 days (range 10–21 days) **OR** Doxycycline, 4–8 mg/kg per day, orally, divided into 2 doses (maximum 100–200 mg) for 14 days (range 14-21 days)[b]
Encephalitis or other late neurologic disease[h]	Ceftriaxone[g] or alternatives of cefotaxime or penicillin[g]: dosing as for recurrent arthritis, for 14 days (range 14–28 days)

Abbreviation: IV, intravenously.

[a] For patients who are allergic to penicillin, alternatives are cefuroxime, azithromycin, and erythromycin.

[b] Tetracycline-based antimicrobial agents, including doxycycline, may cause permanent tooth discoloration for children younger than 8 years if used for repeated treatment courses. However, doxycycline binds less readily to calcium compared with older tetracyclines, and in some studies, doxycycline was not associated with visible teeth staining in younger children (see Tetracyclines).

[c] Corticosteroids should not be given.

[d] Treatment has no effect on the resolution of facial nerve palsy; its purpose is to prevent late disease.

[e] Arthritis is not considered persistent unless objective evidence of synovitis exists at least 2 months after completion of a course of parenteral therapy or of two 28-day courses of oral therapy. Some experts administer a second course of an oral agent before using an IV-administered antimicrobial agent.

[f] Symptoms for heart block or carditis include syncope, dyspnea, or chest pain.

[g] For treatment of meningitis or encephalitis with ceftriaxone, cefotaxime, or penicillin, drug should be administered IV.

[h] Other late neurologic manifestations include peripheral neuropathy or encephalopathy.

8 years and older and, unlike amoxicillin, also treats patients with anaplasmosis. For children younger than 8 years, amoxicillin is recommended. For patients who are allergic to penicillin, the alternative drug is cefuroxime. Erythromycin and azithromycin are less effective. Early Lyme disease should be treated orally for 14 days.

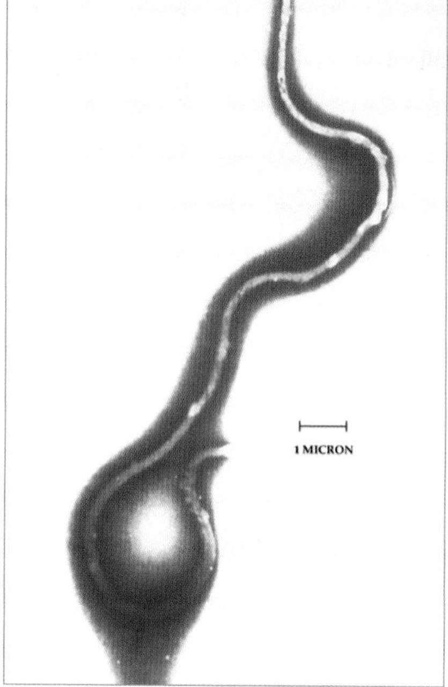

Image 79.1
Photomicrograph of *Borrelia burgdorferi*, the bacteria that cause Lyme disease. This is a spiral-shaped bacteria that is frequently carried by deer ticks of the genus *Ixodes*. When the deer tick bites a human being, the bacteria are transmitted to the human bloodstream. Courtesy of Centers for Disease Control and Prevention.

Patients with Lyme disease and simultaneously infected with *Babesia microti* (babesiosis), *Anaplasma phagocytophilum* (human granulocytic anaplasmosis), or both should be treated for each infection.

Isolation of the Hospitalized Patient

Standard precautions are recommended.

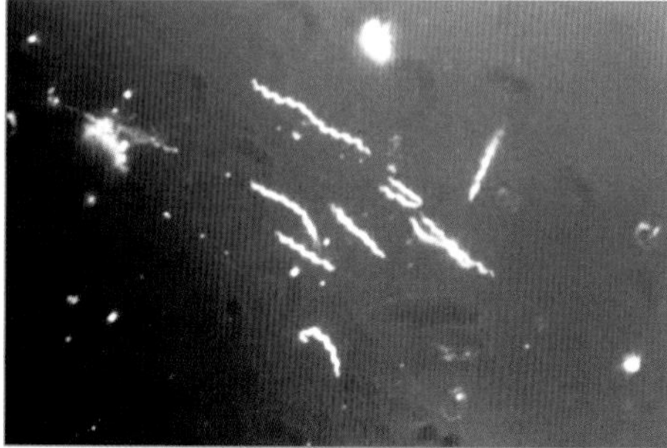

Image 79.2
Using darkfield microscopy technique, this photomicrograph reveals the presence of spirochetes, or corkscrew-shaped bacteria known as *Borrelia burgdorferi*, which is the pathogen responsible for causing Lyme disease (magnification x400). *B burgdorferi* are helical-shaped bacteria and are about 10 to 25 µm long. These bacteria are transmitted to humans by the bite of an infected deer tick. Courtesy of Centers for Disease Control and Prevention.

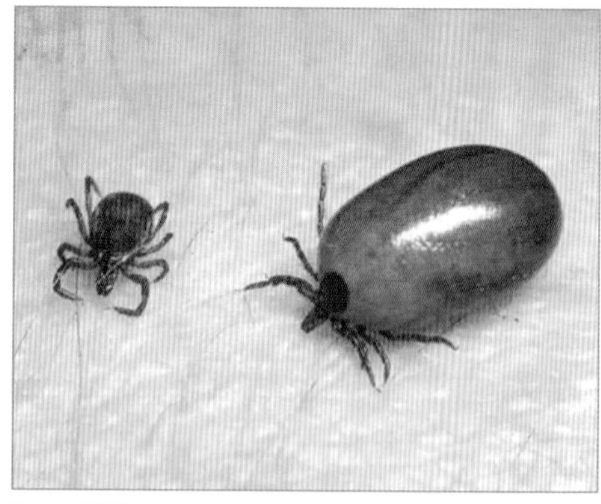

Image 79.3
Two deer ticks of the *Ixodes* genus that transmit *Borrelia burgdorferi* to humans. The engorged tick on the right demonstrates increased size from a blood meal. Both are magnified for this photograph.

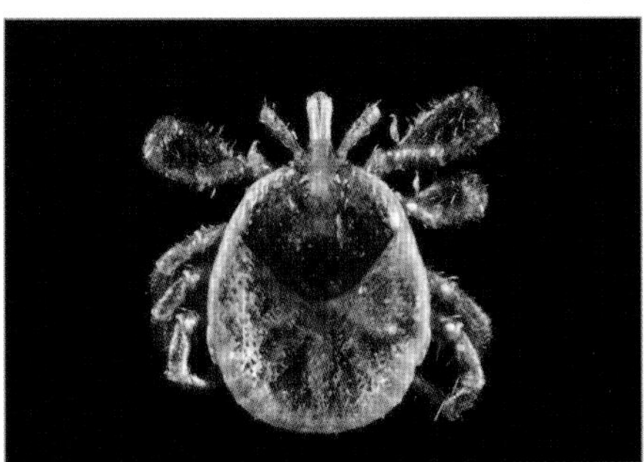

Image 79.4
This photograph depicts a dorsal view of an immature, or nymphal, lone star tick, *Amblyomma americanum.* Nymphal ticks are much smaller than adult ticks, and people might not notice a nymph until it has been feeding for a few days. Nymphs are, therefore, more likely than adult ticks to transmit diseases to people. Courtesy of Centers for Disease Control and Prevention/ Amanda Loftis, MD; William Nicholson, MD; Will Reeves, MD; Chris Paddock, MD.

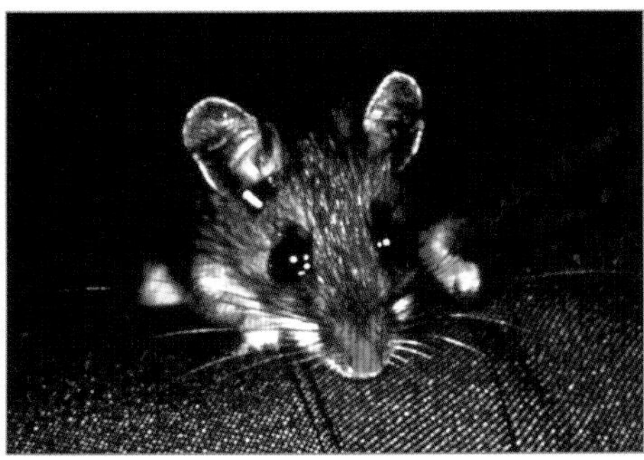

Image 79.6
This photograph depicts a white-footed mouse, *Peromyscus leucopus*, which is a wild rodent reservoir host of ticks, which are known to carry *Borrelia burgdorferi*, the bacteria responsible for Lyme disease. During their larval stage, *Ixodidae,* or hard ticks, feed on small mammals, particularly the white-footed mouse, which serves as the primary reservoir for *B burgdorferi.* Courtesy of Centers for Disease Control and Prevention.

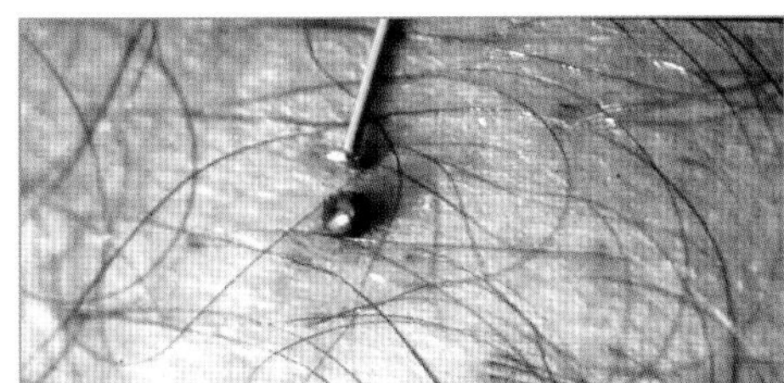

Image 79.5
Despite engorgement, the deer tick is still small and its size approximates the head of a small nail. The ticks that transmit *Rickettsia rickettsii*, usually the dog or lone star ticks, are larger, particularly when engorged.

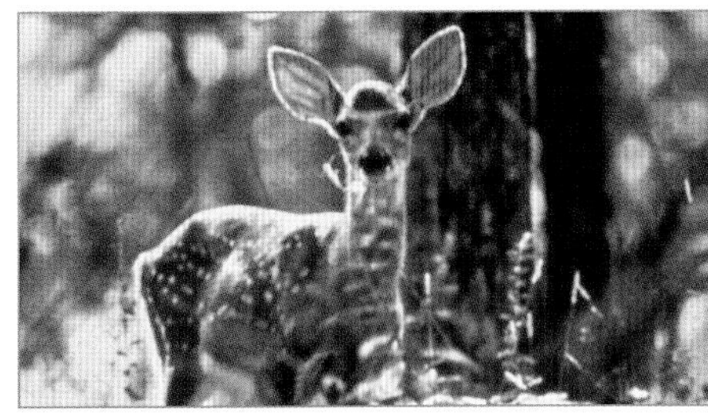

Image 79.7
This photograph of a white-tailed deer, *Odocoileus virginianus*, was taken during a Lyme disease field investigation in 1993. White-tailed deer are investigated during outbreaks of Lyme disease because they serve as hosts to the ticks which carry *Borrelia burgdorferi*, the bacteria responsible for Lyme disease. Courtesy of Centers for Disease Control and Prevention.

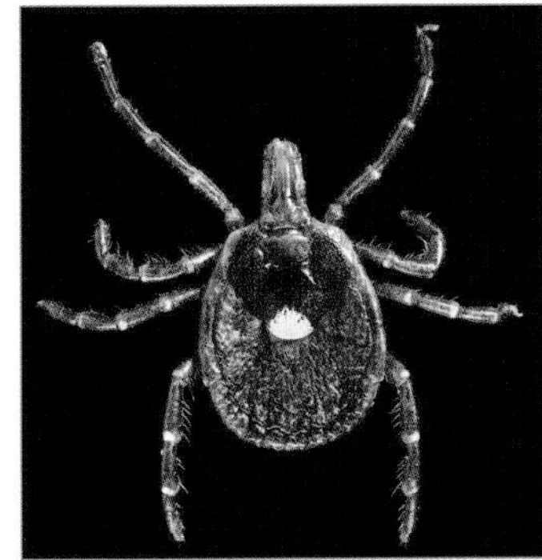

Image 79.8
This photograph depicts a dorsal view of a female lone star tick, *Amblyomma americanum.* Note the characteristic lone star marking located centrally on its dorsal surface, at the distal tip of its scutum. Courtesy of Centers for Disease Control and Prevention/Amanda Loftis, MD; William Nicholson, MD; Will Reeves, MD; Chris Paddock, MD/James Gathany.

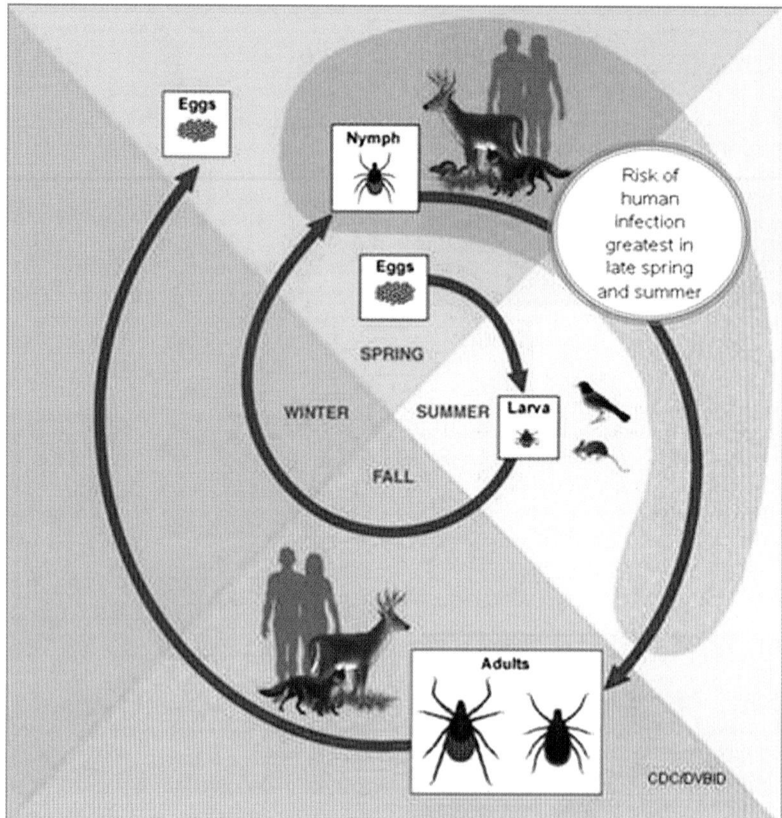

Image 79.9

Life cycle of black-legged ticks, which live for 2 years and have 3 feeding stages: larvae, nymph, and adult. Tick eggs are laid in the spring and hatch as larvae in the summer. Larvae feed on mice, birds, and other small animals in the summer and early fall. When a young tick feeds on an infected animal, the tick takes bacteria into its body along with the blood meal, and it remains infected for the rest of its life. After this initial feeding, the larvae become inactive as they grow into nymphs. The following spring, nymphs seek blood meals to fuel their growth into adults. When the tick feeds again, it can transmit the bacterium to its new host. Usually, the new host is another small rodent, but, sometimes, the new host is a human. Most cases of human illness occur in the late spring and summer when the tiny nymphs are most active and human outdoor activity is greatest. Adult ticks feed on large animals and, sometimes, on humans. In the spring, adult female ticks lay their eggs on the ground, completing the life cycle. Although adult ticks often feed on deer, these animals do not become infected. Deer are, nevertheless, important in transporting ticks and maintaining tick populations. Courtesy of Centers for Disease Control and Prevention.

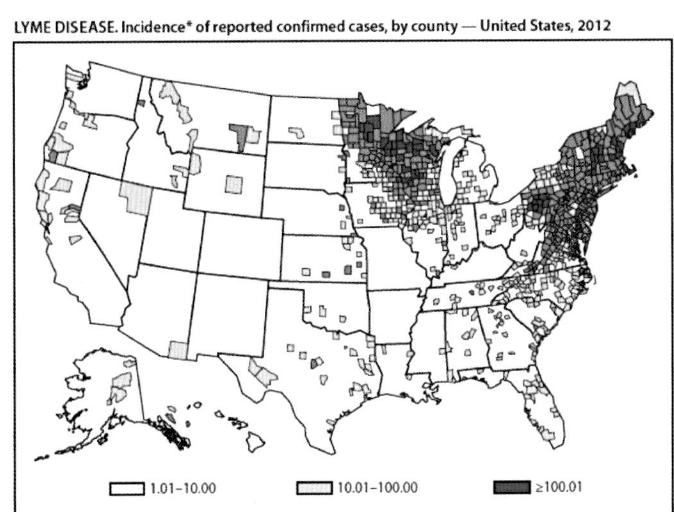

* Per 100,000 population.

Approximately 95% of confirmed Lyme disease cases were reported from states in the Northeast, mid-Atlantic, and upper Midwest. A rash that can be confused with early Lyme disease sometimes occurs following bites of the lone star tick (*Amblyomma americanum*). These ticks, which do not transmit the Lyme disease bacterium, are common human-biting ticks in the southern and southeastern United States.

Image 79.10
Incidence of reported confirmed cases, by county—United States, 2012. Courtesy of *Morbidity and Mortality Weekly Report.*

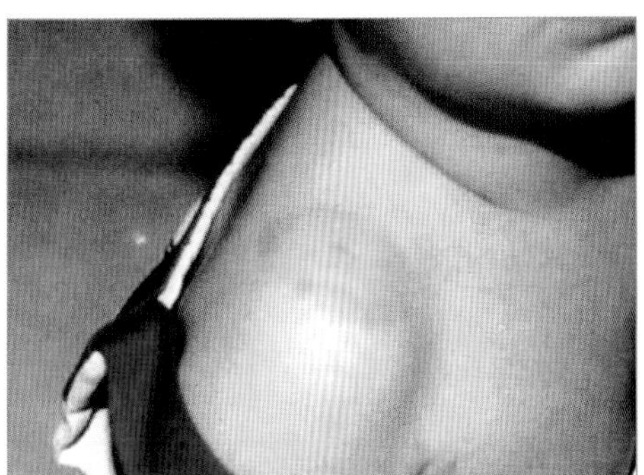

Image 79.11
Lyme disease. The rash of erythema migrans in a 4-year-old boy with infection due to *Borrelia burgdorferi*. Copyright Richard Jacobs.

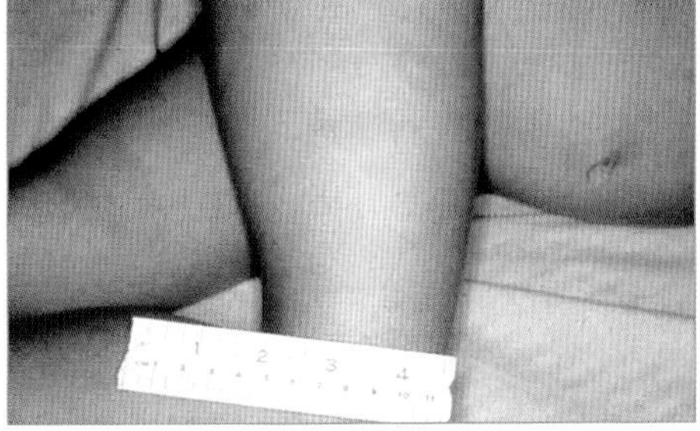

Image 79.12
Erythema migrans lesion at the site of a tick bite characteristic of early localized Lyme disease. It is annular with central clearing (ie, a target lesion), but in other cases, the initial lesion can be uniformly erythematous and occasionally have a vesicular or necrotic center, as illustrated in Image 79.17. Systemic symptoms, such as fever, myalgia, headache, or malaise, can occur at this stage of infection.

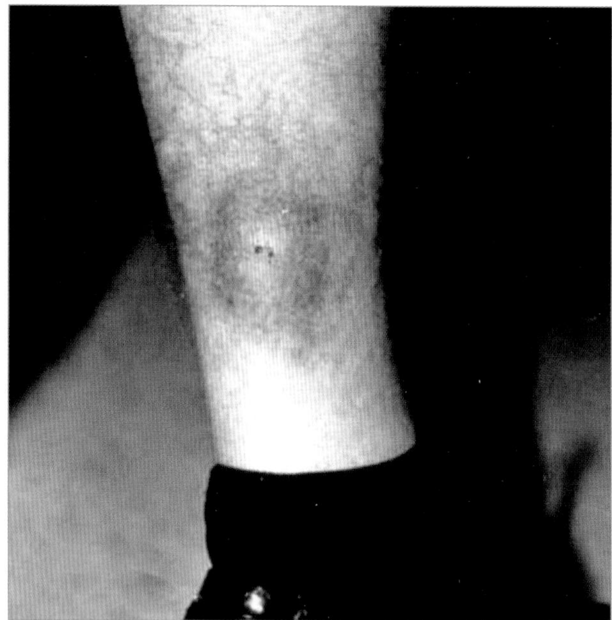

Image 79.13
The rash at the site of a tick bite on the lower leg is indicative of the variation in the initial rash of Lyme disease. Central clearing is incomplete, and a central necrotic area is apparent at the presumed site of the tick bite.

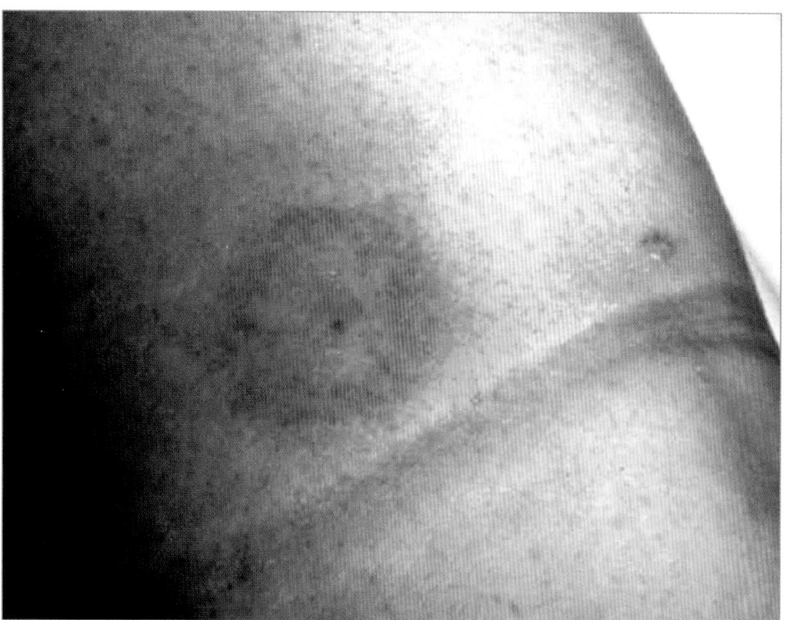

Image 79.14
The rash on the lower leg is similar to that in Image 79.17, but it does not have a necrotic center.

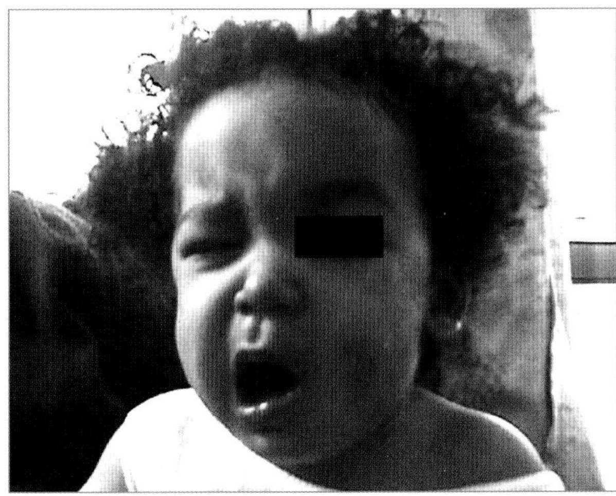

Image 79.15
A 15-month-old girl with left facial nerve palsy complicating Lyme disease. Copyright Michael Rajnik, MD, FAAP.

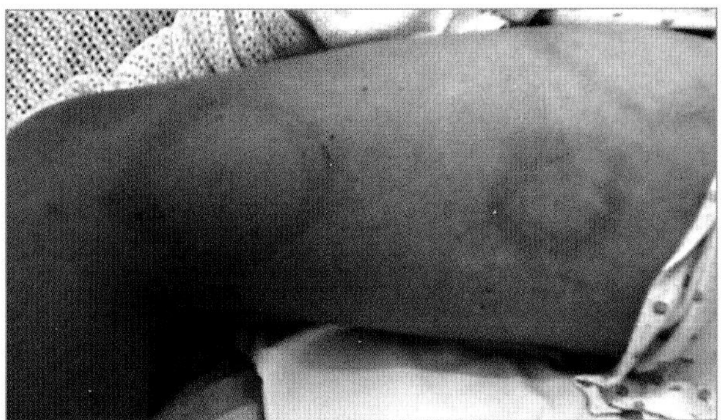

Image 79.16
Erythema migrans lesions in a 12-year-old boy who contracted Lyme disease in Maryland. Copyright Michael Rajnik, MD, FAAP.

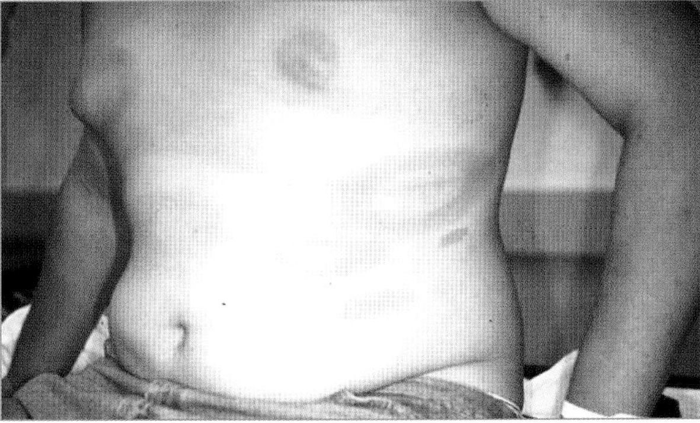

Image 79.17
A 14-year-old boy with multiple annular skin lesions and worsening headache associated with photophobia. Results from a lumbar puncture revealed a cerebrospinal fluid pleocytosis and aseptic meningitis. The characteristic erythema migrans skin lesions helped to determine the diagnosis of Lyme disease. The patient was treated with intravenous ceftriaxone. Copyright Barbara Jantausch, MD, FAAP.

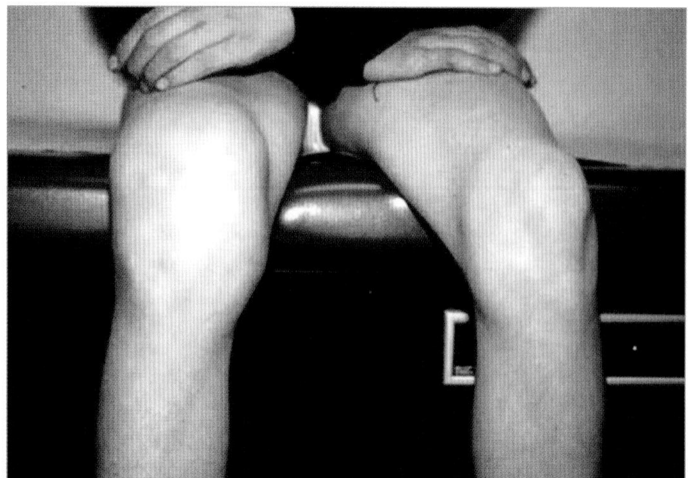

Image 79.18
Borrelia burgdorferi synovitis with marked swelling and only mild tenderness. Arthritis usually occurs within 1 to 2 months following the appearance of erythema migrans, and the knees are the most commonly affected joints.

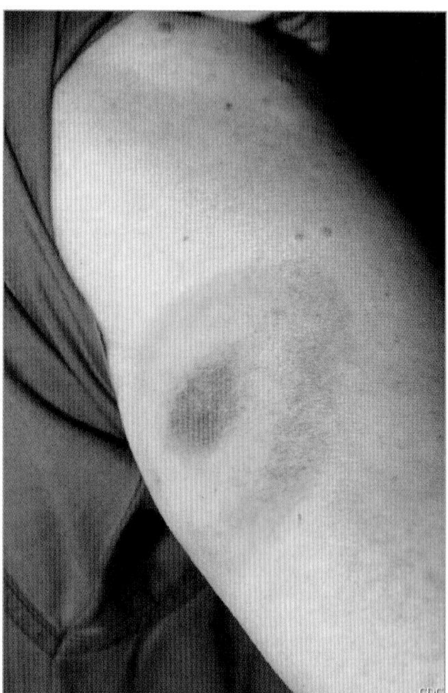

Image 79.19
This photograph depicts the pathognomonic erythematous rash in the pattern of a bull's-eye, which developed at the site of a tick bite on this Maryland woman's posterior right upper arm. Courtesy of Centers for Disease Control and Prevention/James Gathany.

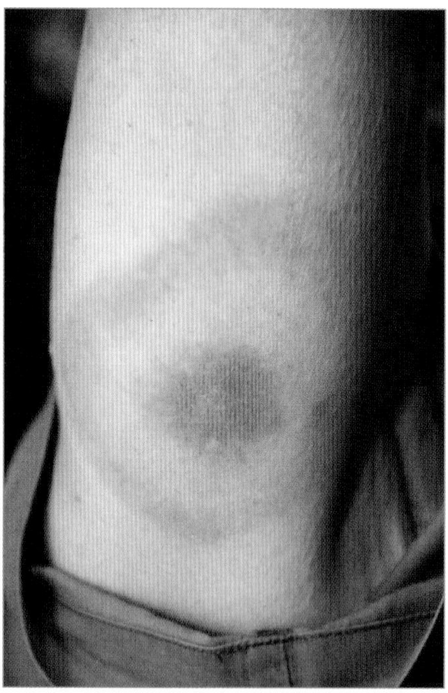

Image 79.20
This photograph depicts the pathognomonic erythematous rash (erythema migrans) in the pattern of a bull's-eye, which developed at the site of a tick bite on this Maryland woman's posterior right upper arm. The expanding rash reflects migration of the spirochetes after introduction of the organism during the tick bite. Courtesy of Centers for Disease Control and Prevention/James Gathany.

80

Lymphatic Filariasis

(Bancroftian, Malayan, and Timorian)

Clinical Manifestations

Lymphatic filariasis is caused by infection with the filarial parasites, *Wuchereria bancrofti*, *Brugia malayi*, or *Brugia timori*. Adult worms cause lymphatic dilatation and dysfunction, result in abnormal lymph flow, and, eventually, may lead to lymphedema in the legs, scrotal area (for *W bancrofti* only), and arms. Recurrent secondary bacterial infections hasten progression of lymphedema to the more severe form known as elephantiasis. Although the infection occurs commonly in young children living in lymphatic filariasis–endemic areas, chronic manifestations of infection, such as hydrocele and lymphedema, occur infrequently in people younger than 20 years. Most filarial infections remain clinically asymptomatic but still commonly cause subclinical lymphatic dilatation and dysfunction. Lymphadenopathy, most frequently of the inguinal, crural, and axillary lymph nodes, is the most common clinical sign of lymphatic filariasis in children. When the adult worm dies, there is an acute inflammatory response that progresses distally (retrograde) along the affected lymphatic vessel, usually in the limbs. Accompanying systemic symptoms, such as headache or fever, are generally mild. In postpubertal males, adult *W bancrofti* organisms are most commonly found in the intrascrotal lymphatic vessels; thus, inflammation around dead or dying adult worms can present as funiculitis (inflammation of the spermatic cord), epididymitis, or orchitis. A tender granulomatous nodule may be palpable at the site of dying or dead adult worms. Chyluria can occur as a manifestation of bancroftian filariasis. Tropical pulmonary eosinophilia, characterized by cough, fever, marked eosinophilia, and high serum immunoglobulin E concentrations, is a rare manifestation of lymphatic filariasis.

Etiology

Filariasis is caused by 3 filarial nematodes: *W bancrofti*, *B malayi*, and *B timori*.

Epidemiology

The parasite is transmitted by the bite of infected species of various genera of mosquitoes, including *Culex*, *Aedes*, *Anopheles*, and *Mansonia*. *W bancrofti*, the most prevalent cause of lymphatic filariasis, is found in Haiti, the Dominican Republic, Guyana, northeast Brazil, sub-Saharan and North Africa, and Asia, extending from India through the Indonesian archipelago to the western Pacific islands. Humans are the only definitive host for the parasite. *B malayi* is found mostly in Southeast Asia and parts of India. *B timori* is restricted to certain islands at the eastern end of the Indonesian archipelago. Live adult worms release microfilariae into the bloodstream. Adult worms live for an average of 5 to 8 years, and reinfection is common. Microfilariae that can infect mosquitoes may remain in the patient's blood for decades; individual microfilaria have a life span up to 1.5 years. The adult worm is not transmissible from person to person or by blood transfusion, but microfilariae may be transmitted by transfusion.

Incubation Period

From acquisition to the appearance of microfilariae in blood, 3 to 12 months, depending on the species of parasite.

Diagnostic Tests

Microfilariae can generally be detected microscopically on blood smears obtained at night (10:00 pm–4:00 am), although variations in the periodicity of microfilaremia have been described depending on the parasite strain and geographic location. Adult worms or microfilariae can be identified in tissue specimens obtained at biopsy. Serologic enzyme immunoassays are available, but interpretation of results is affected by cross-reactions of filarial antibodies with antibodies against other helminths. Assays for circulating parasite antigen of *W bancrofti* are available commercially but are not cleared by the US Food and Drug Administration. Ultrasonography can be used to visualize adult worms. Patients with lymphedema may no longer have microfilariae or filarial antibody present.

Treatment

The main goal of treatment of an infected person is to kill the adult worm. Diethylcarbamazine citrate, which is microfilaricidal and active against the adult worm, is the drug of choice for lymphatic filariasis. Ivermectin is effective against the microfilariae of *W bancrofti* but has no effect on the adult parasite. Albendazole has demonstrated macrofilaricidal activity. In some studies, combination therapy with single-dose diethylcarbamazine citrate–albendazole or ivermectin-albendazole has been shown to be more effective than any one drug alone in suppressing microfilaremia and is the basis for the World Health Organization Global Programme to Eliminate Lymphatic Filariasis. Doxycycline (up to 6 weeks), a drug that targets the *Wolbachia* (intracellular rickettsial-like bacteria) endosymbiont, has been shown to be macrofilaricidal as well. Tetracycline-based antimicrobial agents, including doxycycline, may cause permanent tooth discoloration for children younger than 8 years if used for repeated treatment courses. For early forms of lymphedema, antifilarial chemotherapy has been shown to have limited efficacy for reversing or stabilizing the lymphedema. Doxycycline, in limited studies, has been shown to decrease the severity of lymphedema. Complex decongestive physiotherapy may be effective for treating lymphedema and requires strict attention to hygiene in the affected anatomic areas. Chyluria originating in the bladder responds to fulguration; chyluria originating in the kidney usually cannot be corrected. Prompt identification and treatment of bacterial superinfections, particularly streptococcal and staphylococcal infections, and careful treatment of intertriginous and ungual fungal infections are important aspects of therapy for lymphedema.

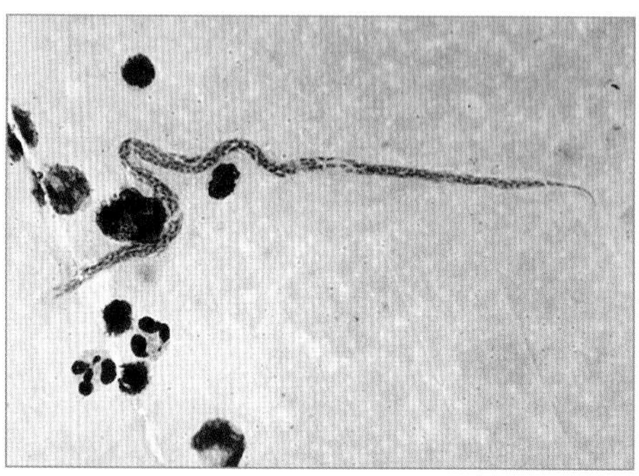

Image 80.1
Mansonella ozzardi, infectious agent of filariasis. Courtesy of Centers for Disease Control and Prevention/Dr Lee Moore.

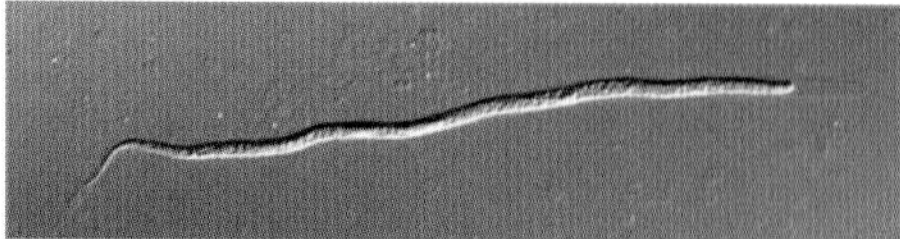

Image 80.3
Microfilaria of *Brugia malayi* collected by the Knott (centrifugation) concentration technique, in 2% formalin wet preparation. Note the erythrocyte ghosts (for size comparison) and the clearly visible sheath that extends beyond the anterior and posterior ends of the microfilaria. (There are 4 sheathed species: *Wuchereria bancrofti, Brugia malayi, Brugia timori,* and *Loa loa.*) Courtesy of Centers for Disease Control and Prevention.

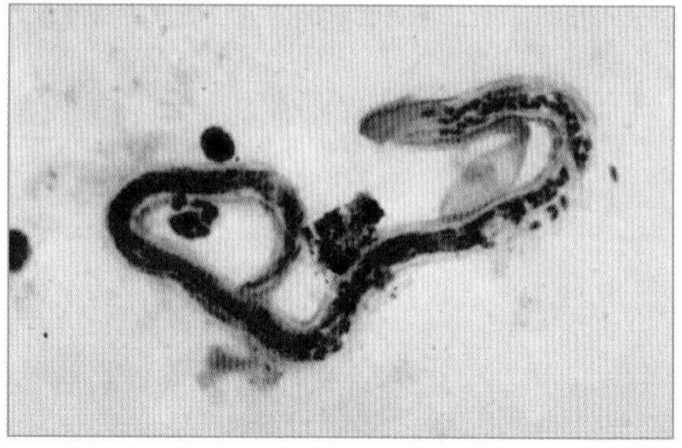

Image 80.2
This photomicrograph shows the inner body and cephalic space of a *Brugia malayi* microfilaria in a thick blood smear. *B malayi,* a nematode that can inhabit the lymphatics and subcutaneous tissues in humans, is one of the causative agents for lymphatic filariasis. The vectors for this parasite are mosquito species from the genera *Mansonia* and *Aedes.* Courtesy of Centers for Disease Control and Prevention/Mae Melvin, MD.

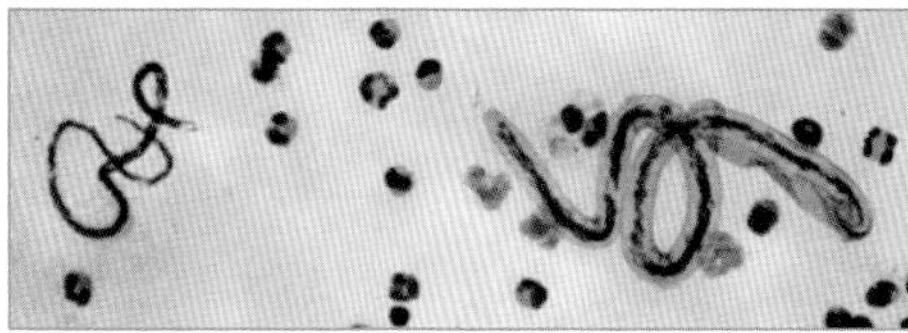

Image 80.4
Microfilariae of *Loa loa* (right) and *Mansonella perstans* (left) in a patient in Cameroon (thick blood smear; hematoxylin stain). *L loa* is sheathed, with a relatively dense nuclear column; its tail tapers and is frequently coiled, and nuclei extend to the end of the tail. *M perstans* is smaller, has no sheath, and has a blunt tail with nuclei extending to the end of the tail. Courtesy of Centers for Disease Control and Prevention.

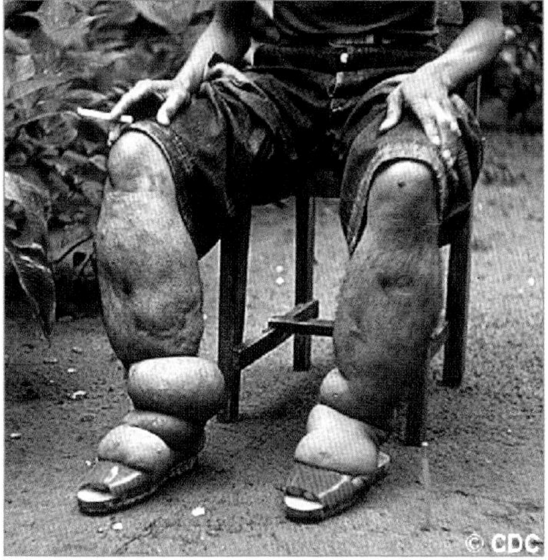

Image 80.6
Elephantiasis of both legs due to filariasis. Luzon, Philippines. Courtesy of Centers for Disease Control and Prevention.

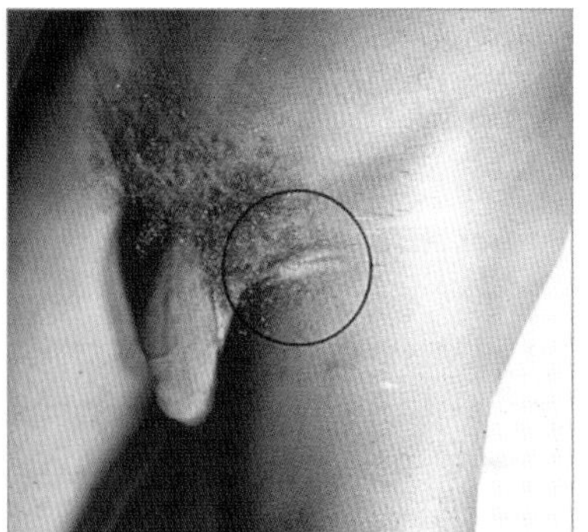

Image 80.8
Inguinal lymph nodes enlarged due to filariasis. Courtesy of Centers for Disease Control and Prevention.

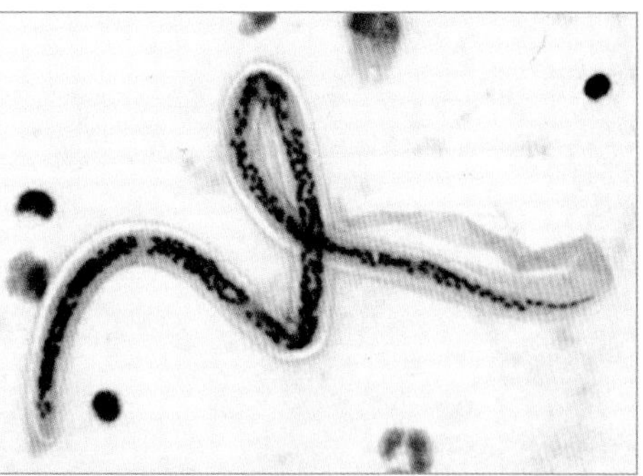

Image 80.5
Microfilaria of *Wuchereria bancrofti* from a patient in Haiti (thick blood smear; hematoxylin stain). The microfilaria is sheathed, its body is gently curved, and the tail is tapered to a point. The nuclear column (ie, the cells that constitute the body of the microfilaria) is loosely packed; the cells can be visualized individually and do not extend to the tip of the tail. The sheath is slightly stained by hematoxylin. Courtesy of Centers for Disease Control and Prevention.

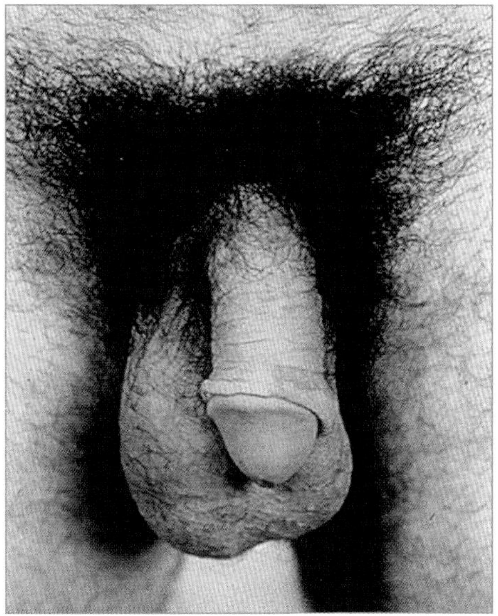

Image 80.7
Scrotal lymphangitis due to filariasis. Courtesy of Centers for Disease Control and Prevention.

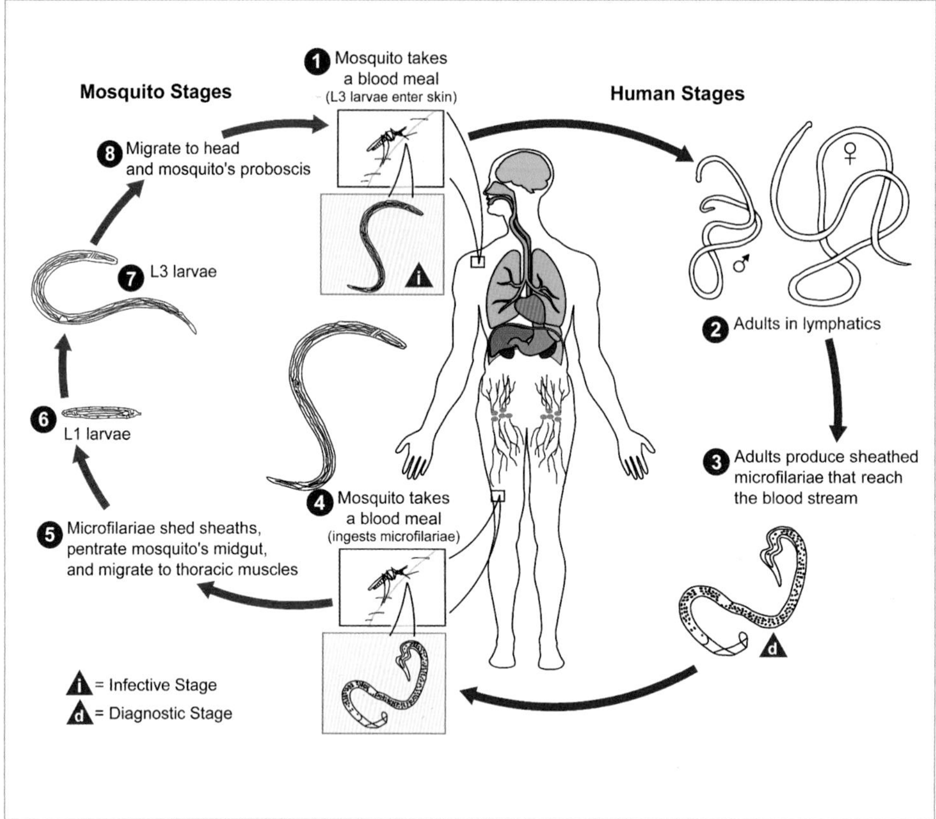

Image 80.9

The typical vector for *Brugia malayi* filariasis are mosquito species from the genera *Mansonia* and *Aedes.* During a blood meal, an infected mosquito introduces third-stage filarial larvae onto the skin of the human host, where they penetrate into the bite wound (1). They develop into adults that commonly reside in the lymphatics (2). The adult worms resemble those of *Wuchereria bancrofti* but are smaller. Female worms measure 43 to 55 mm in length by 130 to 170 µm in width, and males measure 13 to 23 mm in length by 70 to 80 µm in width. Adults produce microfilariae, measuring 177 to 230 µm in length and 5 to 7 µm in width, that are sheathed and have nocturnal periodicity. The microfilariae migrate into lymph and enter the bloodstream, reaching the peripheral blood (3). A mosquito ingests the microfilariae during a blood meal (4). After ingestion, the microfilariae lose their sheaths and work their way through the wall of the proventriculus and cardiac portion of the midgut to reach the thoracic muscles (5). There, the microfilariae develop into first-stage larvae (6) and, subsequently, into third-stage larvae (7). The third-stage larvae migrate through the hemocoel to the mosquito's proboscis (8) and can infect another human when the mosquito takes a blood meal (1). Courtesy of Centers for Disease Control and Prevention.

81

Lymphocytic Choriomeningitis

Clinical Manifestations

Child and adult infections are asymptomatic in approximately one-third of cases. Symptomatic infection can result in a mild to severe illness that includes fever, malaise, myalgia, retro-orbital headache, photophobia, anorexia, and nausea. Initial symptoms can last up to 1 week. A biphasic febrile course is common; after a few days without symptoms, the second phase can occur in up to half of symptomatic patients, consisting of neurologic manifestations that vary from aseptic meningitis to severe encephalitis. Transmission of lymphocytic choriomeningitis (LCM) virus through organ transplantation can result in fatal disseminated infection with multiple organ failure. In the past, LCM virus caused up to 10% to 15% of all cases of aseptic meningitis, and it was a common cause of aseptic meningitis during winter months. Arthralgia or arthritis, respiratory tract symptoms, orchitis, and leukopenia develop occasionally. Recovery without sequelae is the usual outcome. Lymphocytic choriomeningitis virus infection should be suspected in presence of aseptic meningitis or encephalitis during the fall/winter season; febrile illness, followed by brief remission, followed by onset of neurologic illness; and cerebrospinal fluid (CSF) findings of lymphocytosis and hypoglycorrhachia.

Infection during pregnancy has been associated with spontaneous abortion. Congenital infection can cause severe abnormalities, including hydrocephalus, chorioretinitis, intracranial calcifications, microcephaly, and mental retardation. Congenital LCM etiology should be considered when TORCH (**t**oxoplasma, **o**ther [syphilis], **r**ubella, **c**ytomegalovirus, **h**erpes simplex) infections are suspected. Patients with immune abnormalities may experience severe or fatal illness, as observed in patients receiving organs from LCM virus–infected donors.

Etiology

Lymphocytic choriomeningitis virus is a single-stranded RNA virus that belongs to the family Arenaviridae.

Epidemiology

Lymphocytic choriomeningitis is a chronic infection of common house mice, which are often infected asymptomatically and chronically shed virus in urine and other excretions. Congenital murine infection is common and results in a normal-appearing litter with chronic viremia and particularly high virus excretion. In addition, pet hamsters, laboratory mice, guinea pigs, and colonized golden hamsters can have chronic infection and can be sources of human infection. Humans are infected by aerosol or by ingestion of dust or food contaminated with the virus from the urine, feces, blood, or nasopharyngeal secretions of infected rodents. The disease is observed more frequently in young adults. Human-to-human transmission has occurred during pregnancy from infected mothers to their fetuses and through solid organ transplantation from an undiagnosed, acutely LCM virus–infected organ donor. Several such clusters of cases have been described following transplantation, and index case was traced to a pet hamster purchased by the donor. A number of laboratory-acquired LCM virus infections have occurred through infected laboratory animals and contaminated tissue-culture stocks.

Incubation Period

Usually 6 to 13 days; occasionally 3 weeks.

Diagnostic Tests

In patients with central nervous system disease, mononuclear pleocytosis, often exceeding 1,000 cells/µL, is present in CSF. Hypoglycorrhachia can occur. Lymphocytic choriomeningitis virus can usually be isolated from CSF obtained during the acute phase of illness and, in severe disseminated infections, also from blood, urine, and nasopharyngeal secretion specimens. Reverse transcriptase-polymerase chain reaction assays can be used on CSF. Serum specimens from the acute and convalescent phases of illness can be tested for increases in antibody titers by enzyme immunoassays. Demonstration of virus-specific immunoglobulin M antibodies in serum or CSF specimens is useful. In congenital infections, diagnosis is usually suspected at the sequela phase, and diagnosis is usually made by serologic testing. In immunosuppressed patients, the seroconversion can take several weeks. Diagnosis can be made retrospectively by immunohistochemical assay of fixed tissues obtained from necropsy.

Treatment

Supportive.

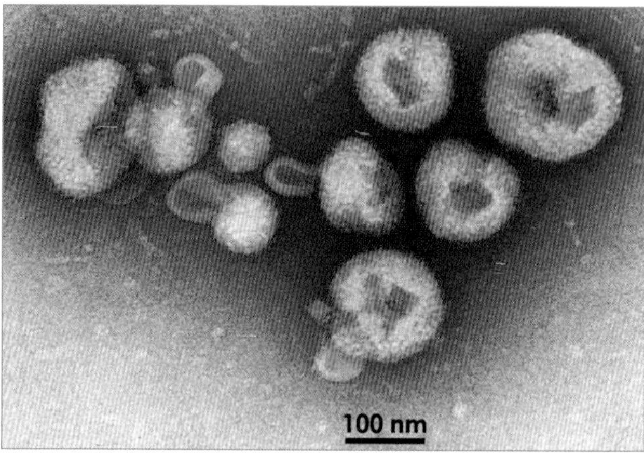

Image 81.1
This transmission electron micrograph depicted 8 virions (viral particles) of a newly discovered virus, which was determined to be a member of the genus *Arenavirus*. A cause of fatal hemorrhagic fever, it was confirmed that this virus was responsible for causing illness in 5 South Africans, 4 of whom died having succumbed to its devastating effects. Ultrastructurally, these round *Arenavirus* virions displayed the characteristic "sandy" or granular capsid (ie, outer skin), an appearance from which the Latin name, arena, was derived. Other members of the genus *Arenavirus* include the West African Lassa virus, lymphocytic choriomeningitis, and Bolivian hemorrhagic fever, also known as Machupo virus, all of which are spread to humans through their inhalation of airborne particulates originating from rodent excrement, which can occur during the simple act of sweeping a floor. Courtesy of Centers for Disease Control and Prevention/Charles Humphrey.

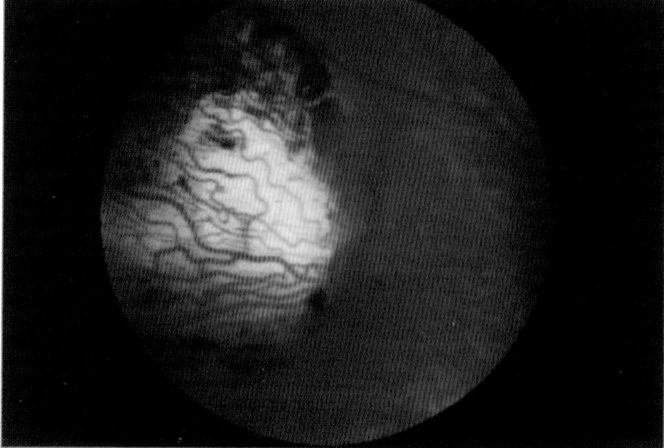

Image 81.2
Fundus photograph of a 9-month-old girl with congenital lymphocytic choriomeningitis virus infection. Extensive chorioretinal scarring is visible. Hydrocephalus and periventricular calcification were visible on computed tomography scan and magnetic resonance imaging. Copyright Leslie L. Barton, MD, FAAP.

82

Malaria

Clinical Manifestations

The classic symptoms of malaria are high fever with chills, rigor, sweats, and headache, which may be paroxysmal. If appropriate treatment is not administered, fever and paroxysms may occur in a cyclic pattern. Depending on the infecting species, fever classically appears every other (*Plasmodium falciparum*, *Plasmodium vivax*, and *Plasmodium ovale*) or every third day (*Plasmodium malariae*), although, in general practice, this pattern is infrequently observed, especially in children. Other manifestations as the clinical disease progresses can include nausea, vomiting, diarrhea, cough, tachypnea, arthralgia, myalgia, and abdominal and back pain. Anemia and thrombocytopenia, along with pallor and jaundice caused by hemolysis, are common in severe illness. Hepatosplenomegaly may be present. More severe disease may occur in people without immunity acquired as a result of previous infections, young children, and people who are pregnant or immunocompromised.

Infection with *P falciparum*, 1 of the 5 *Plasmodium* species that infect humans, is potentially fatal and most commonly manifests as a febrile nonspecific illness without localizing signs. Severe disease (most commonly caused by *P falciparum*, although, recently, also caused by *P vivax* from India, Southeast Asia, and South America) can manifest as one of the following clinical syndromes, each of which are medical emergencies, and can be fatal:

- **Cerebral malaria,** characterized by unarousable coma, can manifest with a range of neurologic signs and symptoms, including generalized seizures, signs of increased intracranial pressure (confusion and progression to stupor, coma), and death.
- **Hypoglycemia,** which can present with metabolic acidosis and hypotension associated with hyperparasitemia or result from quinine or quinidine-induced hyperinsulinemia.
- **Renal failure** caused by acute tubular necrosis (rare in children younger than 8 years).
- **Respiratory failure,** without pulmonary edema.
- **Metabolic acidosis,** usually attributed to lactic acidosis, hypovolemia, liver dysfunction, and impaired renal function.
- **Severe anemia** attributable to high parasitemia and hemolysis, sequestration of infected erythrocytes to capillaries, and hemolysis of infected erythrocytes associated with hypersplenism.
- **Vascular collapse and shock** associated with hypothermia and adrenal insufficiency. People with asplenia who become infected may be at increased risk of more severe illness and death.

Syndromes primarily associated with *P vivax* and *P ovale* infection are as follows:

- **Anemia** attributable to acute parasitemia
- **Hypersplenism** with danger of late splenic rupture
- **Relapse of infection,** for as long as 3 to 5 years after the primary infection, attributable to latent hepatic stages (hypnozoites)

Syndromes associated with *P malariae* infection include

- **Chronic asymptomatic parasitemia** for as long as decades after the primary infection
- **Nephrotic syndrome** resulting from deposition of immune complexes in the kidney

Plasmodium knowlesi is a nonhuman primate malaria parasite that can also infect humans. *P knowlesi* malaria has been commonly misdiagnosed as the more benign *P malariae* malaria. Disease can be characterized by very rapid replication of the parasite and hyperparasitemia resulting in severe disease. Severe disease in patients with *P knowlesi* infection should be treated aggressively because hepatorenal failure and death have been documented.

Congenital malaria resulting from perinatal transmission occurs infrequently. Most congenital cases have been caused by *P vivax* and *P falciparum; P malariae* and *P ovale* account for fewer than 20% of such cases. Manifestations can resemble those of neonatal sepsis, including fever and nonspecific symptoms of poor appetite, irritability, and lethargy.

Etiology

The genus *Plasmodium* includes species of intraerythrocytic parasites that infect a wide range of mammals, birds, and reptiles. The 5 species that infect humans are *P falciparum, P vivax, P ovale, P malariae,* and *P knowlesi.* Coinfection with multiple species is increasingly recognized as polymerase chain reaction technology is applied to the diagnosis of malaria.

Epidemiology

Malaria is endemic throughout the tropical areas of the world and is acquired from the bite of the female nocturnal-feeding *Anopheles* genus of mosquito. Half of the world's population lives in areas where transmission occurs. Worldwide, 216 million cases and 655,000 deaths were reported in 2010. Most deaths occur in young children. Infection by the malaria parasite poses substantial risks to pregnant women, especially primigravidae, and their fetuses and can result in spontaneous abortion and stillbirth. Malaria also contributes significantly to low birth weight in countries where *P falciparum* is endemic. The risk of malaria is highest, but variable, for travelers to sub-Saharan Africa, Papua New Guinea, the Solomon Islands, and Vanuatu; the risk is intermediate on the Indian subcontinent and is low in most of Southeast Asia and Latin America. The potential for malaria transmission is ongoing in areas where malaria was previously eliminated if infected people return and the mosquito vector is still present. These conditions have resulted in recent cases in travelers to areas such as Jamaica, the Dominican Republic, and the Bahamas. Transmission is possible in more temperate climates, including areas of the United States where anopheline mosquitoes are present. Nearly all of the approximately 1,500 annual reported cases in the United States result from infection acquired abroad. Rarely, mosquitoes in airplanes flying from areas with endemic malaria have been the source of cases in people working or residing near international airports. Local transmission also, rarely, occurs in the United States.

P vivax and *P falciparum* are the most common species worldwide. *P vivax* malaria is prevalent on the Indian subcontinent and in Central America. *P falciparum* malaria is prevalent in Africa, in Papua New Guinea, and on the island of Hispaniola (Haiti and the Dominican Republic). *P vivax* and *P falciparum* species are the most common malaria species in southern and Southeast Asia, Oceania, and South America. *P malariae,* although much less common, has a wide distribution. *P ovale* malaria occurs most often in West Africa but has been reported in other areas. Cases of human infections with *P knowlesi* reported, so far, have been from certain countries of Southeast Asia like Borneo, Malaysia, Philippines, Thailand, the Thai-Burmese border, Singapore, and Cambodia.

Relapses may occur in *P vivax* and *P ovale* malaria because of a persistent hepatic (hypnozoite) stage of infection. Recrudescence of *P falciparum* and *P malariae* infection occurs when a persistent low-concentration parasitemia causes recurrence of symptoms of the disease or when drug resistance prevents elimination of the parasite. In areas of Africa and Asia with hyperendemic infection, repeated infection in people with partial immunity results in a high prevalence of asymptomatic parasitemia.

The spread of chloroquine-resistant *P falciparum* strains throughout the world is of increasing concern. In addition, resistance to other antimalarial drugs is also occurring in many areas where the drugs are used widely. *P falciparum* resistance to sulfadoxine-pyrimethamine is common throughout Africa; mefloquine resistance has been documented in Burma (Myanmar), Laos, Thailand, Cambodia, China, and Vietnam; and emerging resistance to artemisinin has been observed at the Cambodia-Thailand border. Chloroquine-resistant *P vivax* has been reported in Indonesia, Papua New Guinea, the Solomon Islands, Myanmar, India, and Guyana. Malaria symptoms can develop as soon as 7 days after exposure in an area with endemic malaria to as late as several months after departure. More than 80% of cases diagnosed in the United States occur in people who have onset of symptoms after their return to the United States. Beginning in 2012, the Centers for Disease Control and Prevention has tested samples from US patients for molecular markers associated with antimalarial drug resistance. Of the 65 *P falciparum*–positive samples, genetic polymorphisms were associated with pyrimethamine drug resistance in 53 (82%), sulfadoxine resistance in 61 (94%), chloroquine resistance in 29 (45%), mefloquine resistance in 1 (2%), and atovaquone resistance in 2 (3%); none had genetic polymorphisms associated with artemisinin resistance.

Diagnostic Tests

Definitive diagnosis relies on identification of the parasite microscopically on stained blood films. Thick and thin blood films should be examined. The thick film allows for concentration of the blood to find parasites that may be present in small numbers, whereas the thin film is most useful for species identification and determination of the degree of parasitemia (the percentage of erythrocytes harboring parasites). If initial blood smear test results are negative for *Plasmodium* species but malaria remains a possibility, the smear test should be repeated every 12 to 24 hours during a 72-hour period.

Confirmation and identification of the species of malaria parasites on the blood smear is important in guiding therapy. Serologic testing is generally not helpful, except in epidemiologic surveys. Polymerase chain reaction assay is available in reference laboratories and many state health departments. An approved test for antigen detection is available in the United States; however, this product has poor sensitivity for detecting low-density *P vivax* infections. Positive and negative rapid diagnostic test results should be confirmed by microscopic examination because low-level parasitemia may not be detected, false-positive results occur, and mixed infections may not be detected accurately. Also, information about the sensitivity of rapid diagnostic tests for the 2 less common species of malaria, *P ovale* and *P malariae,* is limited.

Treatment

The choice of malaria chemotherapy is based on the infecting species, possible drug resistance, and severity of disease. Severe malaria is defined as any one or more of the following signs or symptoms: parasitemia greater than 5% of red blood cells, signs of central nervous system or other end-organ involvement, shock, acidosis, thrombocytopenia, or hypoglycemia. Patients with severe malaria require intensive care and parenteral treatment with intravenous quinidine until the parasite density decreases to less than 1% and they are able to tolerate oral therapy. Concurrent treatment with tetracycline, doxycycline, or clindamycin should begin orally or intravenously if oral treatment is not tolerated. Exchange transfusion for severe disease is not efficacious.

For patients with severe malaria in the United States who do not tolerate or cannot easily access quinidine, intravenous artesunate has become available through a Centers for Disease Control and Prevention investigational new drug protocol. For patients with *P falciparum* malaria, sequential blood smears to determine percentage of erythrocytes harboring parasites can be useful in monitoring treatment.

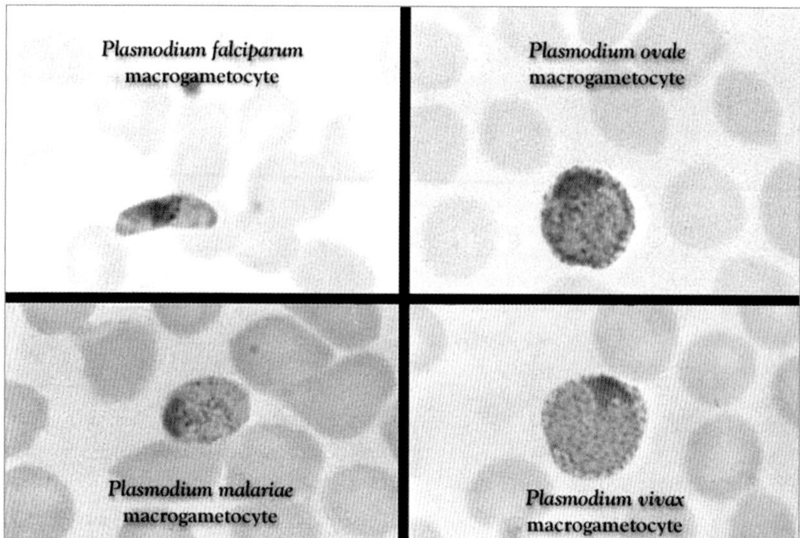

Image 82.1

This Giemsa-stained slide reveals a *Plasmodium falciparum, Plasmodium ovale, Plasmodium malariae,* and *Plasmodium vivax* gametocyte. The male (microgametocytes) and female (macrogametocytes) are ingested by an *Anopheles* mosquito during its blood meal. Known as the sporogonic cycle, while in the mosquito's stomach, the microgametes penetrate the macrogametes, generating zygotes. Courtesy of Centers for Disease Control and Prevention/Steven Glenn, Laboratory & Consultation Division.

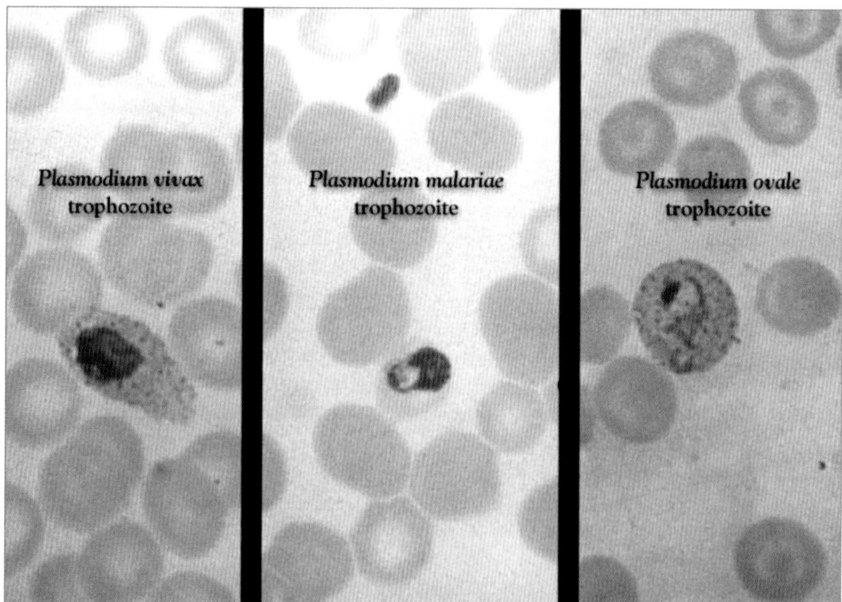

Image 82.2

This thin-film Giemsa-stained micrograph reveals growing *Plasmodium vivax, Plasmodium malariae,* and *Plasmodium ovale* trophozoites. As the parasite increases in size, the ring morphology of the early trophozoite disappears and becomes what is referred to as a mature trophozoite, which undergoes further transformation, maturing into a schizont. Courtesy of Centers for Disease Control and Prevention/Steven Glenn, Laboratory & Consultation Division.

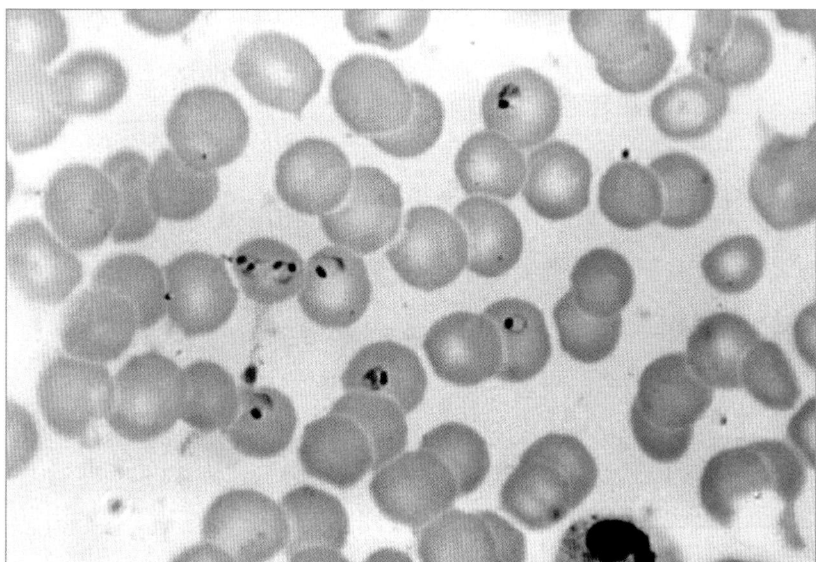

Image 82.3
This thin-film Giemsa-stained micrograph reveals a ringform *Plasmodium falciparum* trophozoite. As *P falciparum* trophozoites mature, they tend to retain their ringlike shape and, sometimes, trace amounts of yellow pigment can be seen within the cytoplasm. In this case, the presence of debris can make microscopic diagnosis more difficult. Courtesy of Centers for Disease Control and Prevention/ Steven Glenn, Laboratory & Consultation Division.

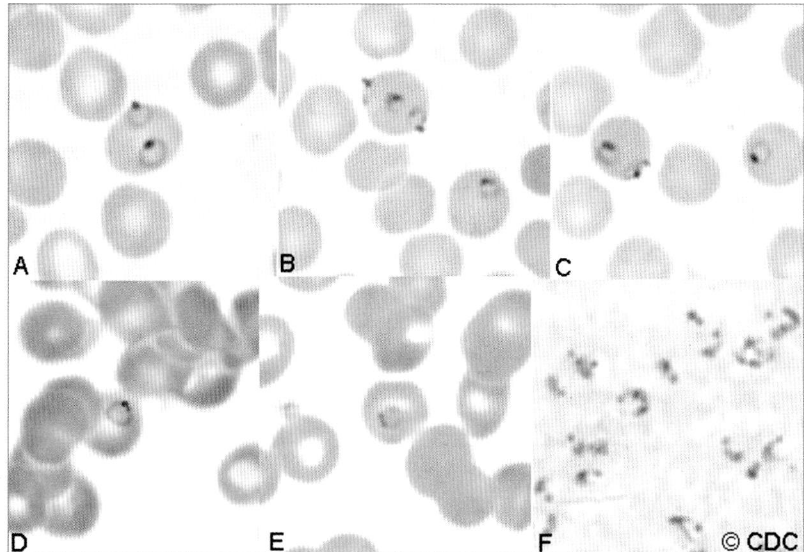

Image 82.4
Plasmodium falciparum ring-stage smears from patients. *P falciparum* rings have delicate cytoplasm and 1 or 2 small chromatin dots. Red blood cells (RBCs) that are infected are not enlarged; multiple infection of RBCs is more common in *P falciparum* than in other species. Occasional appliqué forms (rings appearing on the periphery of the RBC) can be present. A–C, Multiple infected RBCs with appliqué forms in thin blood smears. D, Signet ring form. E, Double chromatin dot. F, A thick blood smear showing many ringforms of *P falciparum.* Courtesy of Centers for Disease Control and Prevention.

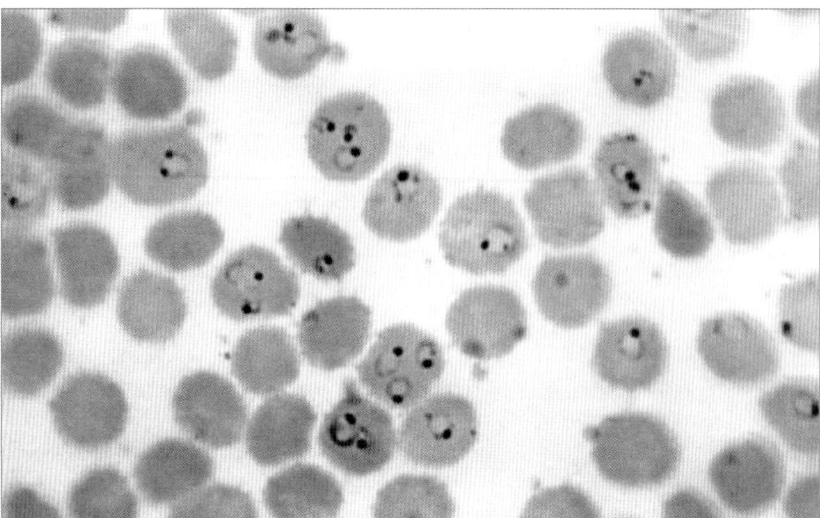

Image 82.5
This thin-film Giemsa-stained micrograph depicts a number of ringform *Plasmodium falciparum* trophozoites. During the parasite's development, the trophozoite represents an asexual, erythrocytic stage in which the organism loses its ring appearance and begins to accumulate pigment, which is yellow to black in coloration. Courtesy of Centers for Disease Control and Prevention/Steven Glenn, Laboratory & Consultation Division.

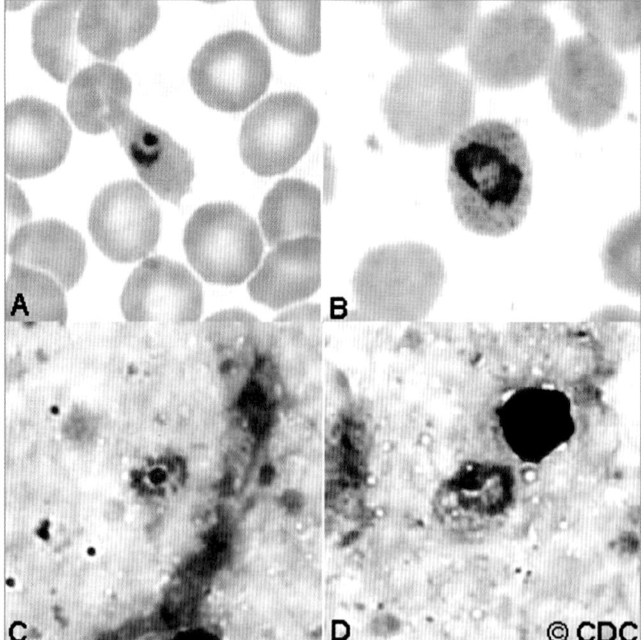

Image 82.6
Plasmodium ovale ring-stage parasites (smears from patients). *P ovale* rings have sturdy cytoplasm and large chromatin dots. Red blood cells (RBCs) are normal to slightly enlarged (x1.25), may be round to oval, and are sometimes fimbriated. Schüffner dots are visible under optimal conditions. A–B, *P ovale* rings in thin blood smears. A, Fimbriation of the infected RBC. B, Schüffner dots. C–D, Rings of *P ovale* in thick blood smears. Courtesy of Centers for Disease Control and Prevention.

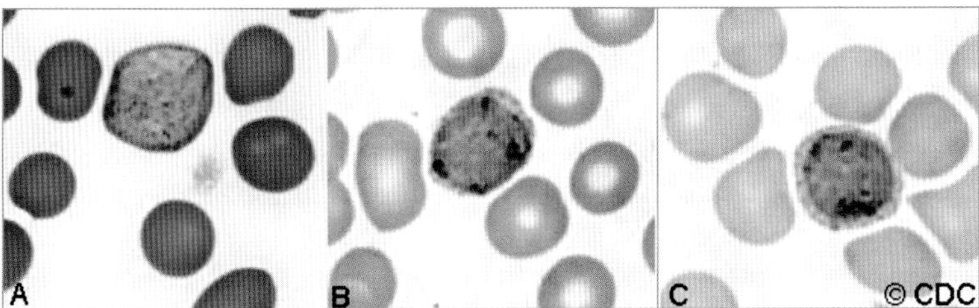

Image 82.7
Plasmodium vivax gametocytes (smears from patients). *P vivax* gametocytes are round to oval with scattered brown pigment and may almost fill the red blood cell. Red blood cells are enlarged 1.5 to 2 times and may be distorted. Under optimal conditions, Schüffner dots may appear more fine than those seen in *Plasmodium ovale*. Courtesy of Centers for Disease Control and Prevention.

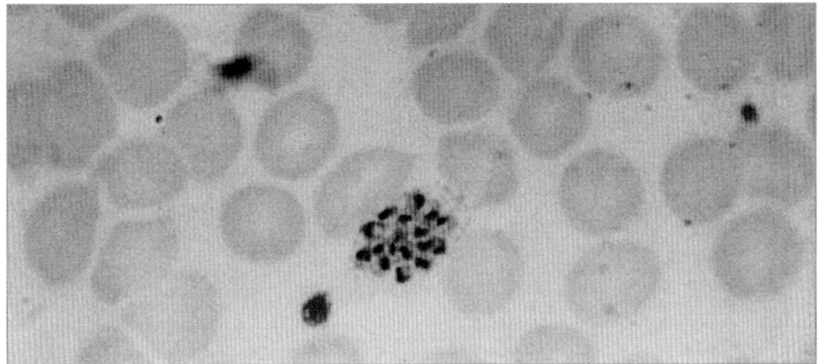

Image 82.8
This thin-film Giemsa-stained micrograph depicts a mature *Plasmodium vivax* schizont containing 16 merozoites. Note the similarities seen in this platelet artifact to characteristics displayed by a late-staged malarial schizont containing a number of merozoites. Maturing schizonts will eventually rupture and release their cache of merozoites into the blood. Courtesy of Centers for Disease Control and Prevention/Steven Glenn, Laboratory Training & Consultation Division.

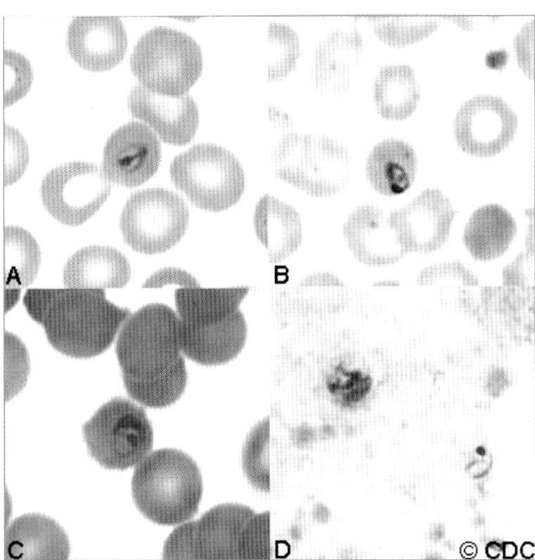

Image 82.9
Plasmodium malariae ring-stage parasites (smears from patients). *P malariae* rings have sturdy cytoplasm and a large chromatin dot. The red blood cells are normal to smaller than normal (x0.075) in size. A–C, Ringforms in thin blood smears. D, A thick blood smear showing 2 rings (lower right) and a gametocyte. Courtesy of Centers for Disease Control and Prevention.

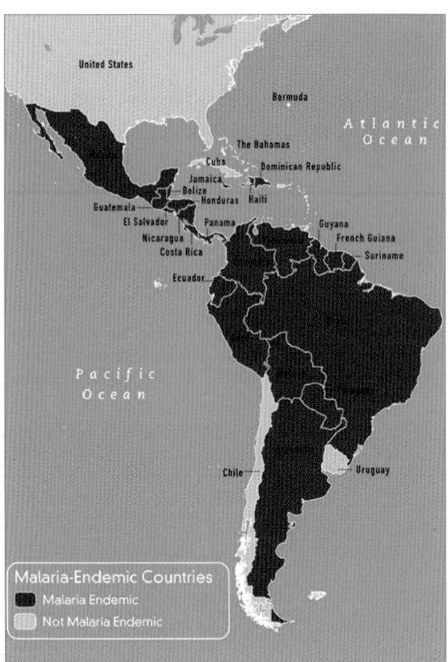

Image 82.10
Malaria-endemic countries in the western hemisphere. Centers for Disease Control and Prevention.

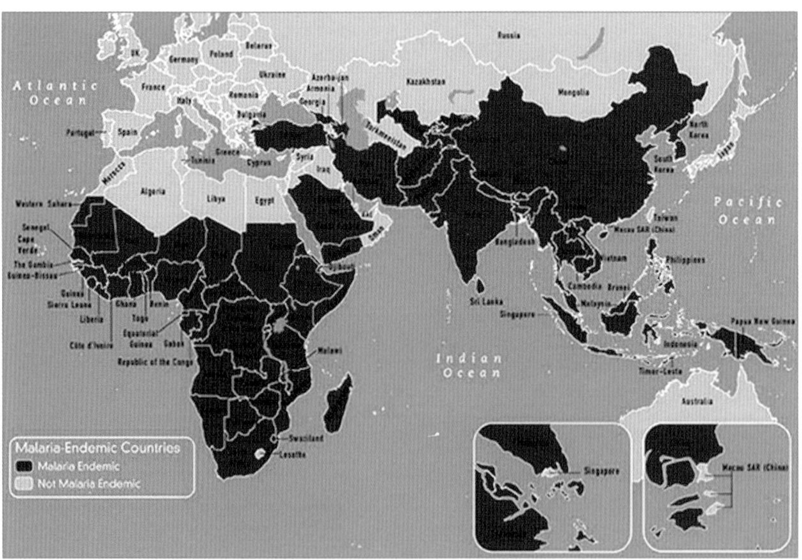

Image 82.11
Malaria-endemic countries in the eastern hemisphere. Centers for Disease Control and Prevention National Center for Emerging and Zoonotic Infectious Diseases (NCEZID) Division of Global Migration and Quarantine (DGMQ).

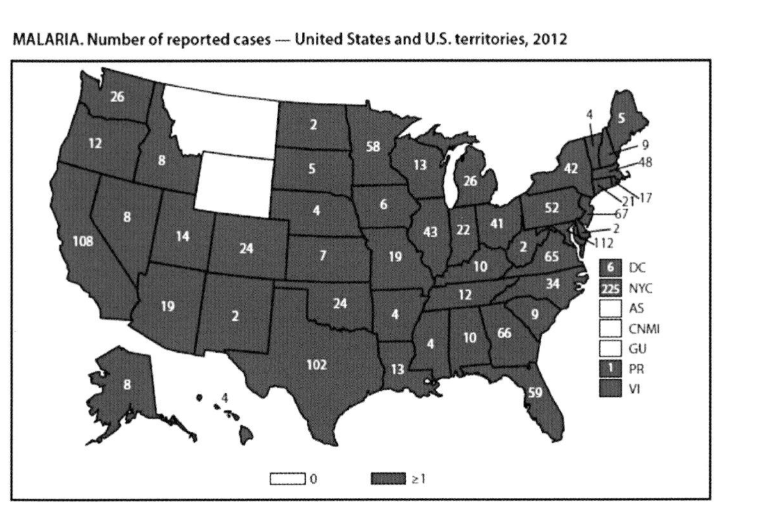

Image 82.12

Number of reported cases—United States and US territories, 2012. Courtesy of *Morbidity and Mortality Weekly Report.*

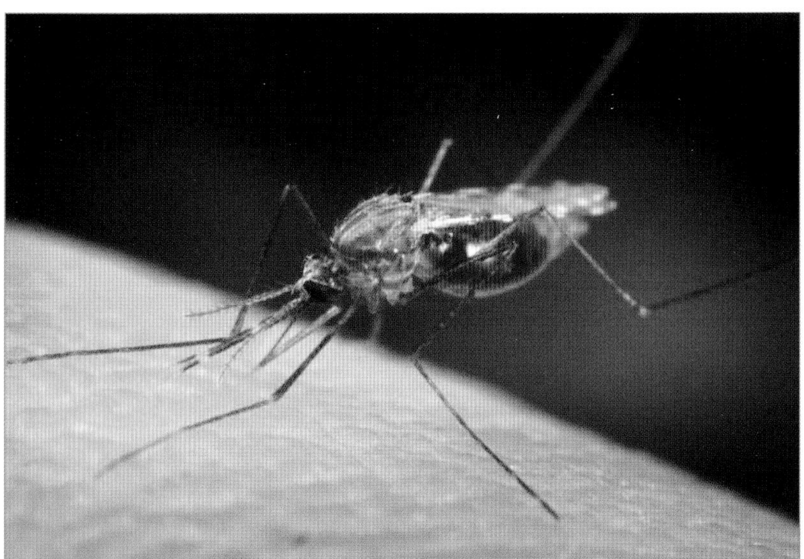

Image 82.13

This photograph depicts an *Anopheles funestus* mosquito partaking in a blood meal from its human host. Note the blood passing through the proboscis, which has penetrated the skin and entered a miniscule cutaneous blood vessel. The *A funestus* mosquito, which, along with *A gambiae*, is 1 of the 2 most important malaria vectors in Africa, where more than 80% of the world's malarial disease and deaths occurs. Courtesy of Centers for Disease Control and Prevention/James Gathany.

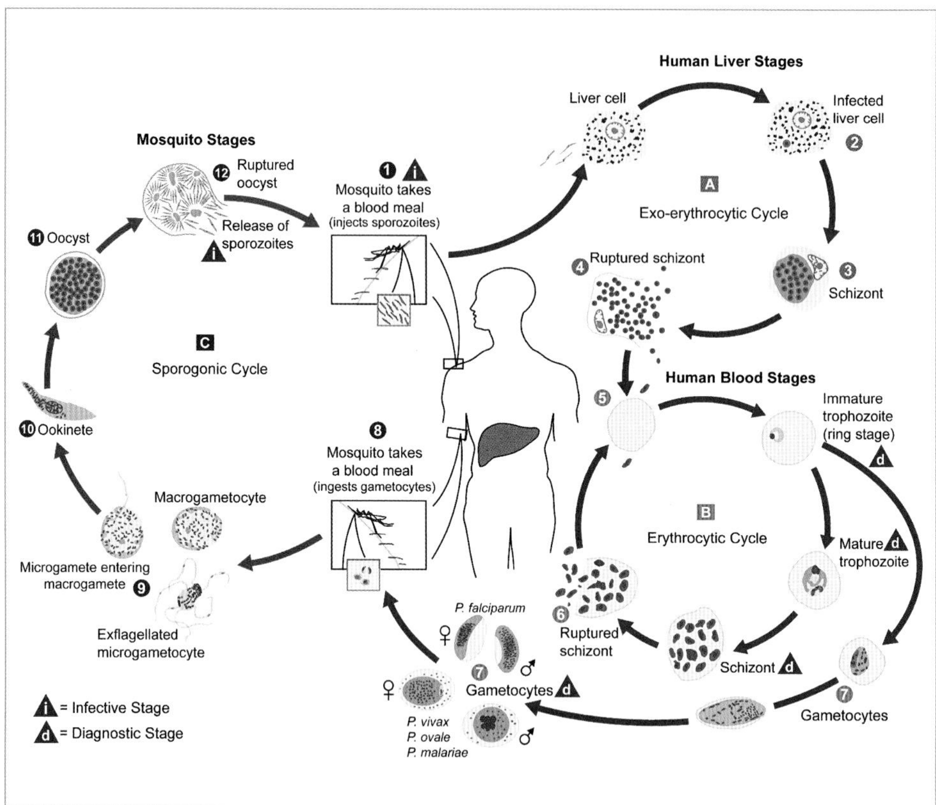

Image 82.14

The malaria parasite life cycle involves 2 hosts. During a blood meal, a malaria-infected female *Anopheles* species mosquito inoculates sporozoites into the human host (1). Sporozoites infect liver cells (2) and mature into schizonts (3), which rupture and release merozoites (4). (Of note, in *Plasmodium vivax* and *Plasmodium ovale,* a dormant stage [hypnozoites] can persist in the liver and cause relapses by invading the bloodstream weeks, or even years, later.) After this initial replication in the liver (exoerythrocytic schizogony) (A), the parasites undergo asexual multiplication in the erythrocytes (erythrocytic schizogony) (B). Merozoites infect red blood cells (5). The ring-stage trophozoites mature into schizonts, which rupture, releasing merozoites (6). Some parasites differentiate into sexual erythrocytic stages (gametocytes) (7). Blood stage parasites are responsible for the clinical manifestations of the disease. The gametocytes, male (microgametocytes) and female (macrogametocytes), are ingested by an *Anopheles* species mosquito during a blood meal (8). The parasite multiplication in the mosquito is known as the sporogonic cycle (C). While in the mosquito's stomach, the microgametes penetrate the macrogametes, generating zygotes (9). The zygotes, in turn, become motile and elongated (ookinetes) (10) and invade the midgut wall of the mosquito, where they develop into oocysts (11). The oocysts grow, rupture, and release sporozoites (12), which make their way to the mosquito's salivary glands. Inoculation of the sporozoites into a new human host perpetuates the malaria life cycle (1). Courtesy of Centers for Disease Control and Prevention/DPDx/Alexander J. da Silva, PhD, Melanie Moser.

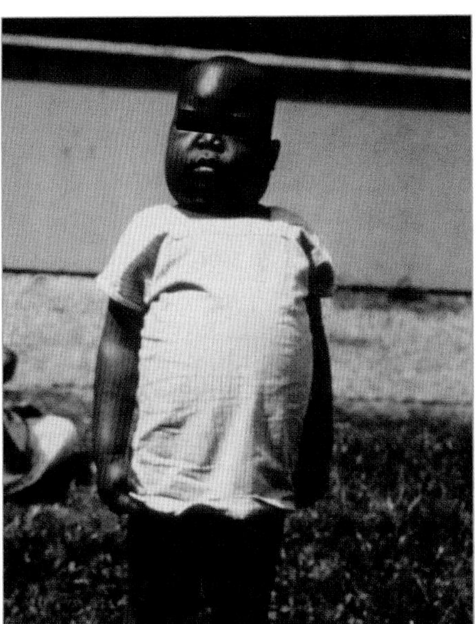

Image 82.15
The edema exhibited by this African child was brought on by nephrosis associated with malaria. Infection with one type of malaria, *Plasmodium falciparum*, if not promptly treated, may cause kidney failure. Swelling of the abdomen, eyes, feet, and hands are some of the symptoms of nephrosis brought on by the damaged kidneys. Courtesy of Centers for Disease Control and Prevention/Dr Myron Schultz.

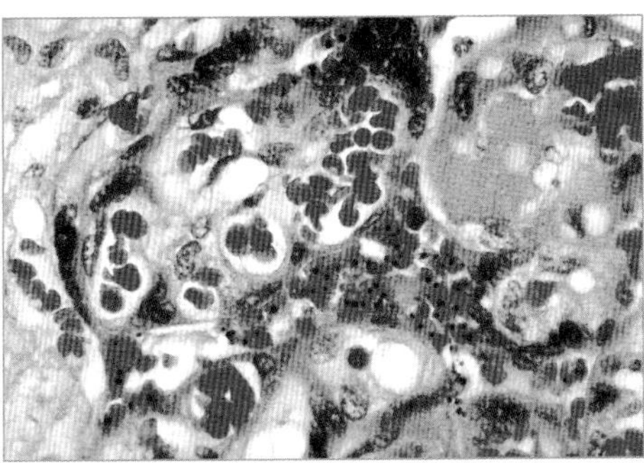

Image 82.18
A photomicrograph of placental tissue revealing the presence of the malarial parasite *Plasmodium falciparum*. Maternal or placental malaria predisposes the newborn to a low birth weight, premature delivery, and increased mortality, and the mother to maternal anemia. Courtesy of Centers for Disease Control and Prevention/ Edwin P. Ewing Jr, MD.

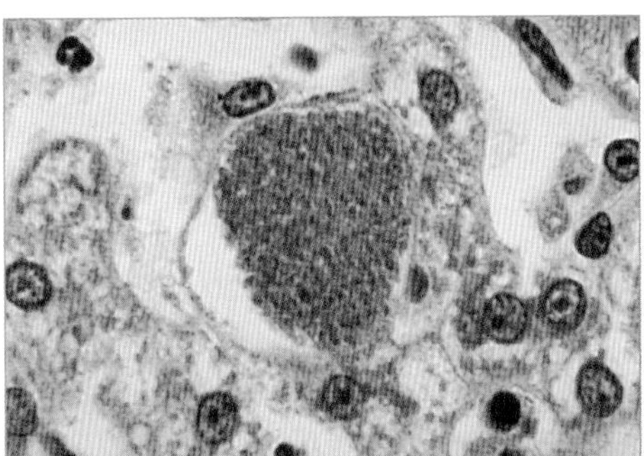

Image 82.16
Histopathology of malaria exoerythrocytic forms in liver. Courtesy of Centers for Disease Control and Prevention/Dr Mae Melvin.

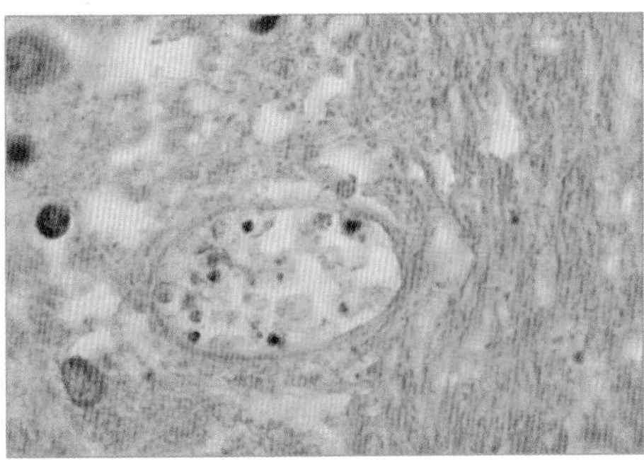

Image 82.17
Histopathology of malaria of brain. Mature schizonts. Courtesy of Centers for Disease Control and Prevention/Dr Martin D. Hicklin.

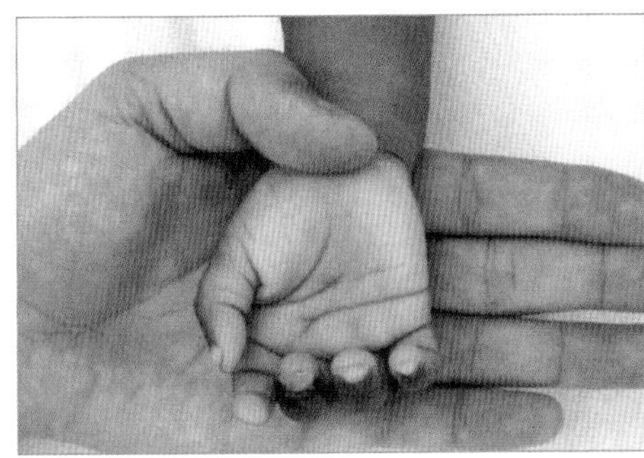

Image 82.19
Severe *Plasmodium vivax* malaria, Brazilian Amazon. Hand of a 2-year-old (patient no. 1) with severe anemia (hemoglobin level 3.6 g/dL) and showing intense pallor, compared with the hand of a healthy physician. Courtesy of *Emerging Infectious Diseases*.

83

Measles

Clinical Manifestations

Measles is an acute viral disease characterized by fever, cough, coryza, and conjunctivitis, followed by a maculopapular rash beginning on the face and spreading cephalocaudally and centrifugally. During the prodromal period, a pathognomonic enanthema (Koplik spots) may be present. Complications include otitis media, bronchopneumonia, laryngotracheobronchitis (croup), and diarrhea and occur commonly in young children and immunocompromised hosts. Acute encephalitis often results in permanent brain damage and occurs in approximately 1 of every 1,000 cases. In the postmeasles-elimination era, death, predominantly resulting from respiratory and neurologic complications, has occurred in 1 to 3 of every 1,000 cases in the United States. Case-fatality rates are increased in children younger than 5 years and immunocompromised children. Sometimes, the characteristic rash does not develop in immunocompromised patients.

Subacute sclerosing panencephalitis (SSPE) is a rare degenerative central nervous system disease characterized by behavioral and intellectual deterioration and seizures that occur 7 to 11 years after wild-type measles (incidence, 4 to 11 per 100,000 measles cases). Widespread measles immunization has led to the virtual disappearance of SSPE in the United States.

Etiology

Measles virus is an enveloped RNA virus with one serotype, classified as a member of the genus *Morbillivirus* in the Paramyxoviridae family.

Epidemiology

The only natural host of measles virus is humans. Measles is transmitted by direct contact with infectious droplets or, less commonly, by airborne spread. Measles is one of the most highly communicable of all infectious diseases. In temperate areas, the peak incidence of infection usually occurs during late winter and spring. In the prevaccine era, most cases of measles in the United States occurred in preschool- and young school-aged children, and few people remained susceptible by 20 years of age. The childhood and adolescent immunization program in the United States has resulted in a greater than 99% decrease in the reported incidence of measles and interruption of endemic disease transmission since measles vaccine was first licensed in 1963.

From 1989 to 1991, the incidence of measles in the United States increased because of low immunization rates in preschool-aged children, especially in urban areas. Following improved coverage in preschool-aged children and implementation of a routine second dose of measles-mumps-rubella vaccine for children, the incidence of measles declined to extremely low levels (<1 case per 1 million population). In 2000, an independent panel of internationally recognized experts unanimously agreed that measles was no longer endemic in the United States. From 2001 through 2012, a median of 60 measles cases were reported annually (range, 37–220). In 2008, 2011, and 2013, the numbers of reported cases were 140, 220, and 189, respectively; these larger numbers of cases were attributable to an increase in the number of importations or spread from importations. The number of measles outbreaks (≥3 cases linked in time and space) that occurred ranged from 2 to 16 per year. In the first half of 2014, 514 measles cases from 16 outbreaks were reported in 20 states. Forty-eight separate importations occurred; 81% were in unvaccinated people, 12% of those infected had an unknown vaccination status (78% of those were adults), and 7% of those infected were vaccinated (including 5% with 2 or more doses). Among the unvaccinated people who became infected, 87% cited personal belief exemptions for not being immunized, 3% were unvaccinated travelers 6 months to 2 years of age, and 5% were too young to be vaccinated. This is the largest number of measles cases in the United States since 1994.

Vaccine failure occurs in as many as 5% of people who have received a single dose of vaccine at 12 months or older. Although waning immunity after immunization may be a factor in some cases, most cases of measles in previously immunized children seem to occur in people in whom response to the vaccine was inadequate (ie, primary vaccine failures). This was the main reason a 2-dose vaccine schedule was routinely recommended for children and high-risk adults.

Patients are contagious from 4 days before the rash to 4 days after appearance of the rash. Immunocompromised patients who may have prolonged excretion of the virus in respiratory tract secretions can be contagious for the duration of the illness. Patients with SSPE are not contagious.

Incubation Period

8 to 12 days from exposure to onset; in family studies, average interval between rash in the index case is 14 days (range, 7–21 days).

Diagnostic Tests

Measles virus infection can be diagnosed by a positive serologic test result for measles immunoglobulin (Ig) M antibody, a significant increase in measles IgG antibody concentration in paired acute and convalescent serum specimens (at least 10 days apart) by any standard serologic assay, or isolation of measles virus or identification of measles RNA (by reverse transcriptase-polymerase chain reaction assay) from clinical specimens, such as throat or nasopharyngeal secretions. The simplest method of establishing the diagnosis of measles is testing for IgM antibody on a single serum specimen obtained during the first encounter with a person suspected of having disease; if the result is positive, it is a good measure for a presumptive case. The sensitivity of measles IgM assays varies by timing of specimen collection, immunization status of the case, and the assay. IgM capture assays often have positive results on the day of rash onset. However, up to 20% of assays for IgM may be negative in the first 72 hours after rash onset. IgM is detectable for at least 1 month after rash onset in unimmunized people but might be absent or present only transiently in people immunized with 1 or 2 vaccine doses. In populations with high vaccine coverage, such as the United States, it is recommended that diagnostic testing for measles include serologic and virologic testing. People with febrile rash illness who are seronegative for measles IgM should be tested for rubella using the same specimens. Genotyping of viral isolates allows determination of patterns of importation and transmission, and genome sequencing can be used to differentiate between wild-type and vaccine virus infection in those who have been immunized recently. All cases of suspected measles should be immediately reported to the local or state health department.

Treatment

No specific antiviral therapy is available. Vitamin A treatment of children with measles in developing countries has been associated with decreased morbidity and mortality rates. Low serum concentrations of vitamin A have also been found in children in the United States. All children with measles should receive vitamin A, regardless of their country of residence, once daily for 2 days.

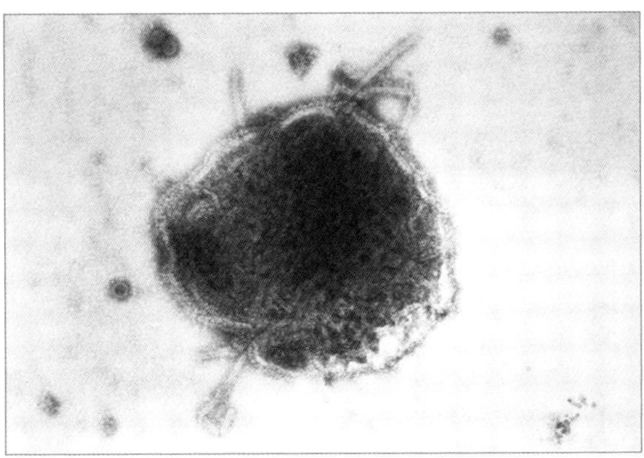

Image 83.1
This electron micrograph reveals a paramyxovirus measles virus and virions of the polyomavirus, simian virus 40. Courtesy of Centers for Disease Control and Prevention/Dr Erskine Palmer.

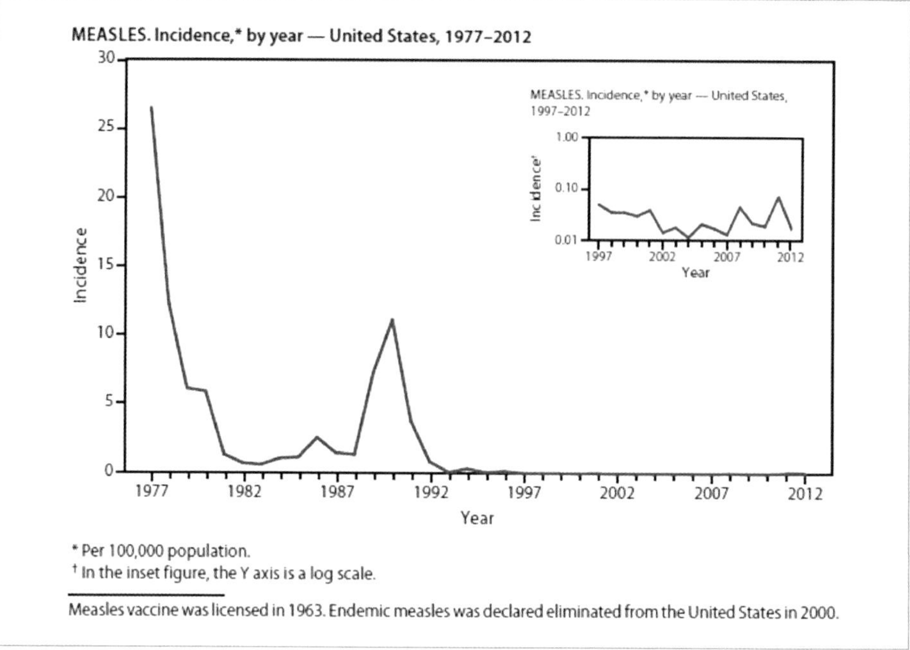

Image 83.2
Measles. Incidence, by year—United States, 1977–2012. Courtesy of *Morbidity and Mortality Weekly Report.*

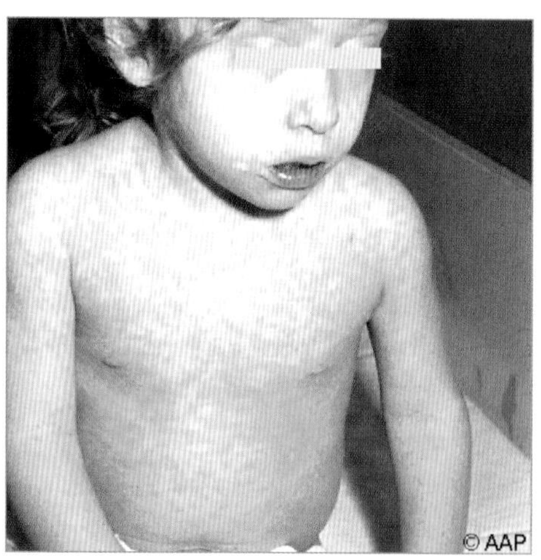

Image 83.3
Child with measles who exhibited an appearance of feeling miserable.

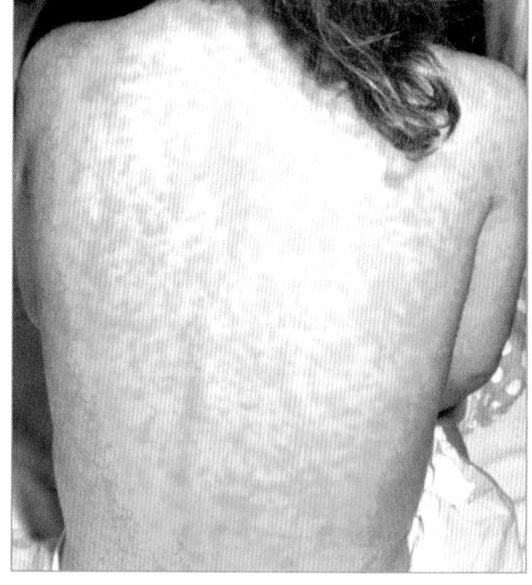

Image 83.4
Measles. This is the same patient as in Image 83.3.

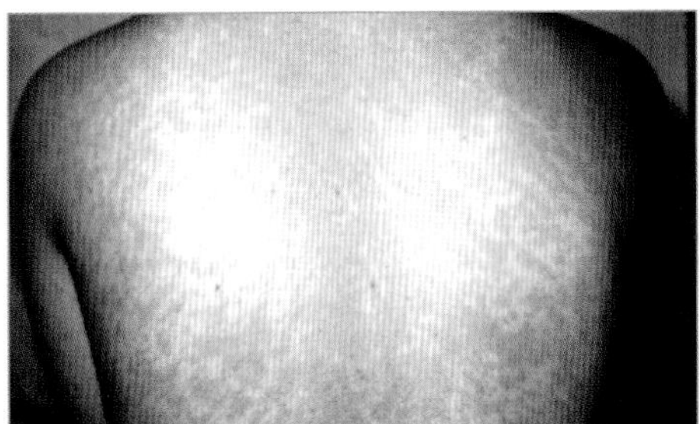

Image 83.5
Characteristic confluent measles rash over the back of this child.

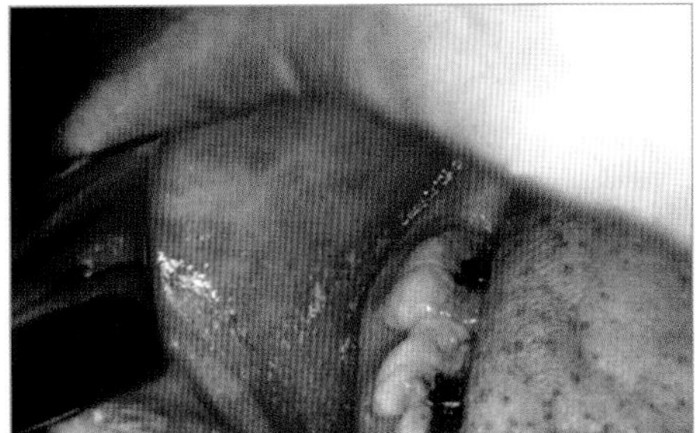

Image 83.6
Measles with Koplik spots.

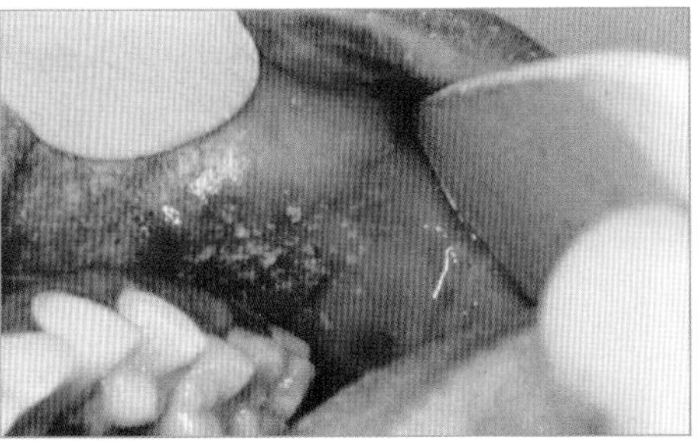

Image 83.7
Koplik spots of measles in a 7-year-old white boy. Courtesy of Larry Frenkel, MD.

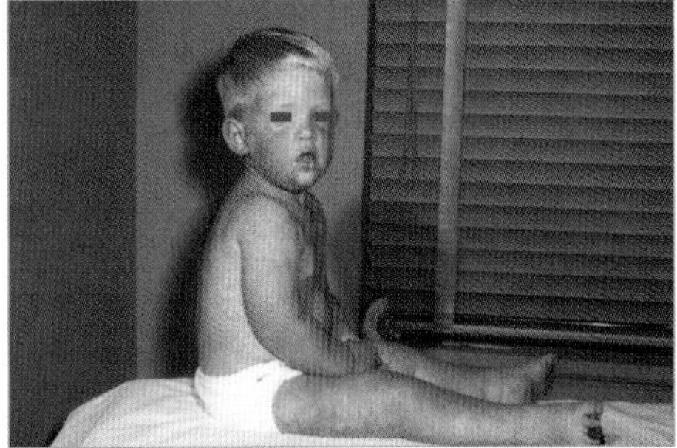

Image 83.8
This child with measles is displaying the characteristic red, blotchy pattern on his face and body during the third day of the rash. Courtesy of Centers for Disease Control and Prevention.

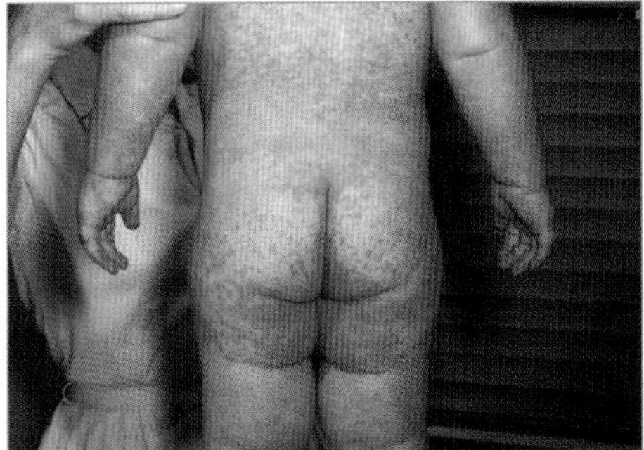

Image 83.9
This child with measles is showing the characteristic red, blotchy rash on his buttocks and back during the third day of the rash. Measles is an acute, highly communicable viral disease with prodromal fever, conjunctivitis, coryza, cough, and Koplik spots on the buccal mucosa. A red, blotchy rash appears around day 3 of the illness, first on the face and then becoming generalized. Courtesy of Centers for Disease Control and Prevention.

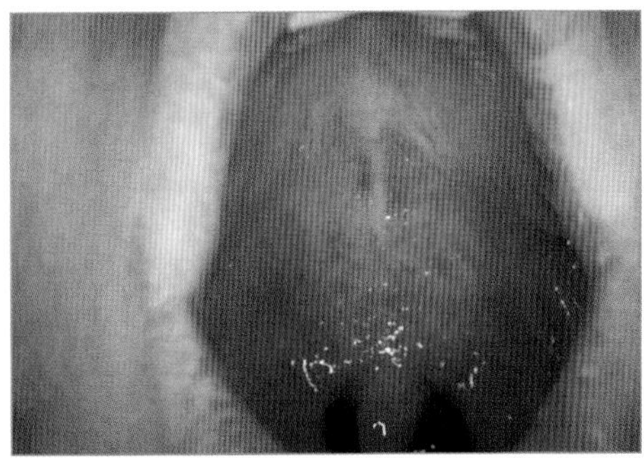

Image 83.10
This was a patient who presented with Koplik spots on the palate due to preeruptive measles on day 3 of the illness. Measles is an acute, highly communicable viral disease with fever, conjunctivitis, coryza, cough, and Koplik spots. Koplik spots are small, red, irregularly shaped spots with blue-white centers found on the mucosal surface of the oral cavity. Courtesy of Centers for Disease Control and Prevention/ Heinz F. Eichenwald, MD.

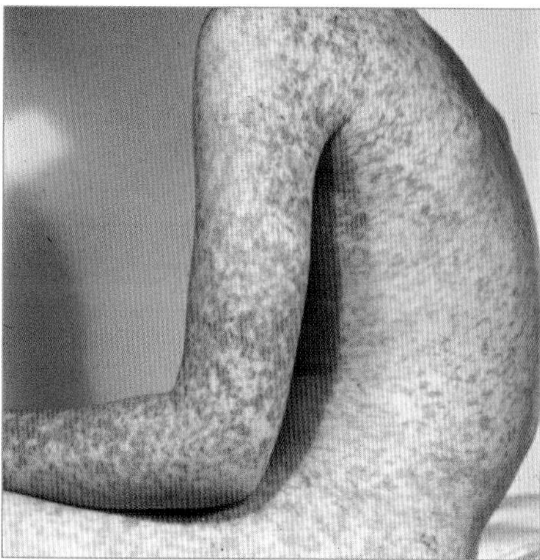

Image 83.11
Measles in a 7-year-old white boy. Courtesy of Paul Wehrle, MD.

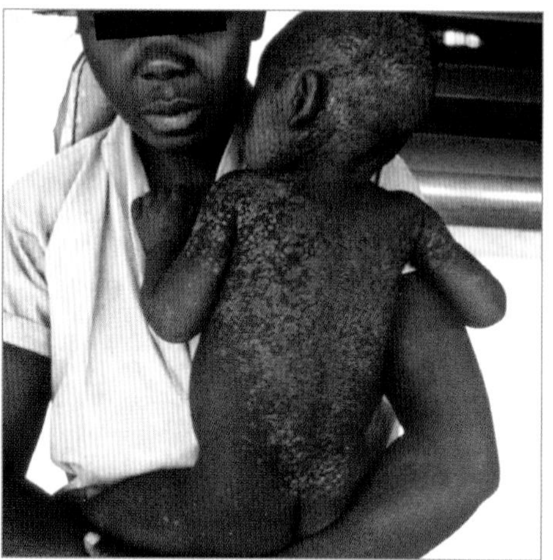

Image 83.13
This late 1960s photograph shows a Nigerian mother and her child, who was recovering from measles. Note the skin is sloughing on the child as he heals from his measles infection. This child was among many who were cared for in camps set up during the Centers for Disease Control and Prevention–led refugee relief effort during the Nigerian-Biafran war. Measles was a constant threat in these camps. Sloughing of the skin in recovering measles patients was often extensive and resembled that of a burn victim. Due to their weakened state, children like the one shown here needed nursing care to avoid subsequent infections. Courtesy of Centers for Disease Control and Prevention/Dr Lyle Conrad.

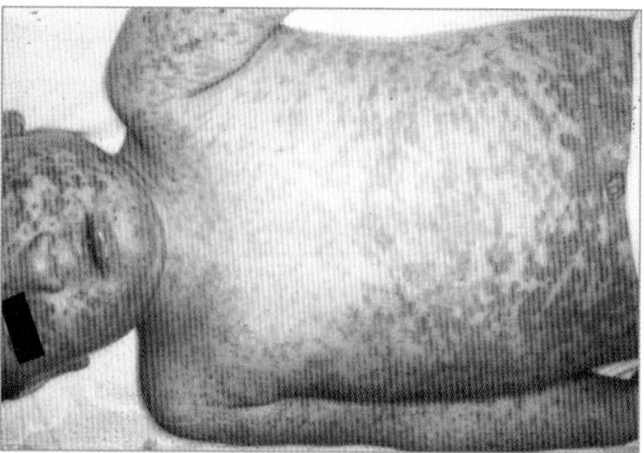

Image 83.12
The near-confluent exanthem of measles in a 2-year-old white boy. Courtesy of Paul Wehrle, MD.

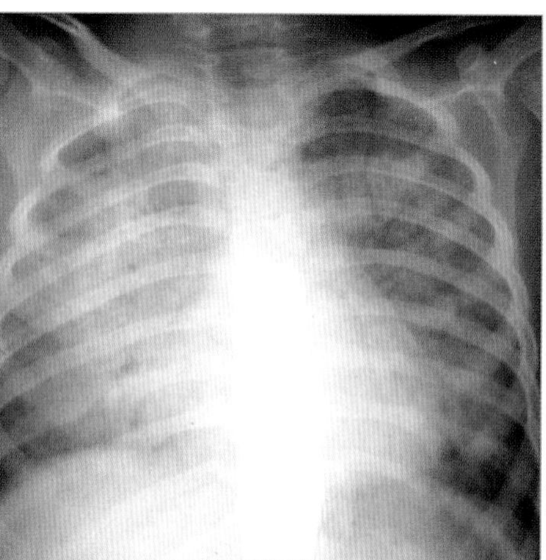

Image 83.14
Measles pneumonia in a 6-year-old with acute lymphoblastic leukemia. The child died of respiratory failure.

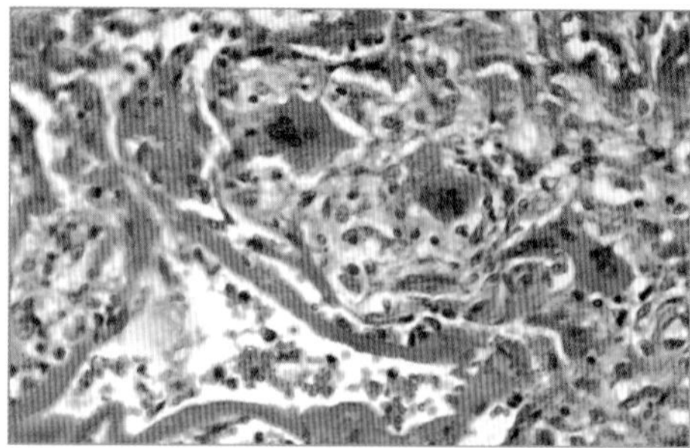

Image 83.15
Measles pneumonia with interstitial mononuclear cell infiltration, multinucleated giant cells, and hyaline membranes (hematoxylin-eosin stain, original magnification x250).

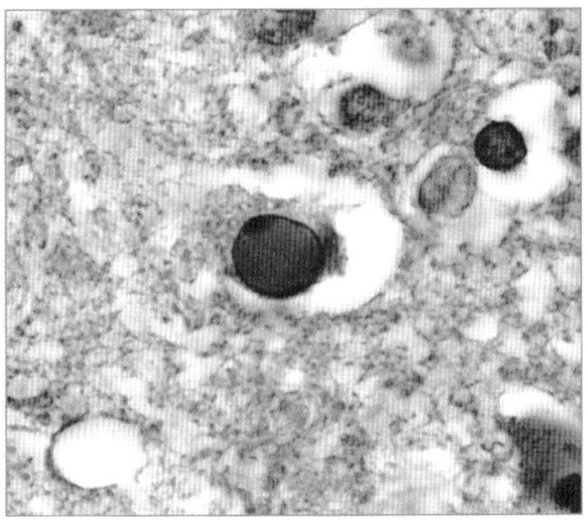

Image 83.16
Measles encephalitis in an immunosuppressed patient who underwent renal transplantation with viral intranuclear inclusion. Courtesy of Dimitris P. Agamanolis, MD.

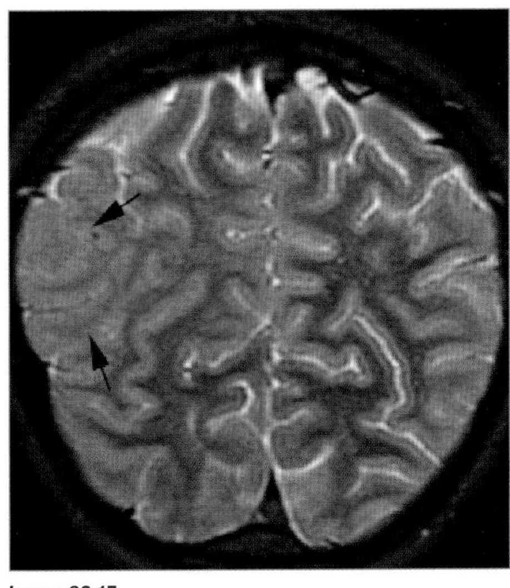

Image 83.17
This coronal T2-weighted magnetic resonance image shows swelling and hyperintensity of the right parietal occipital cortex (arrows) in a patient with measles encephalitis.

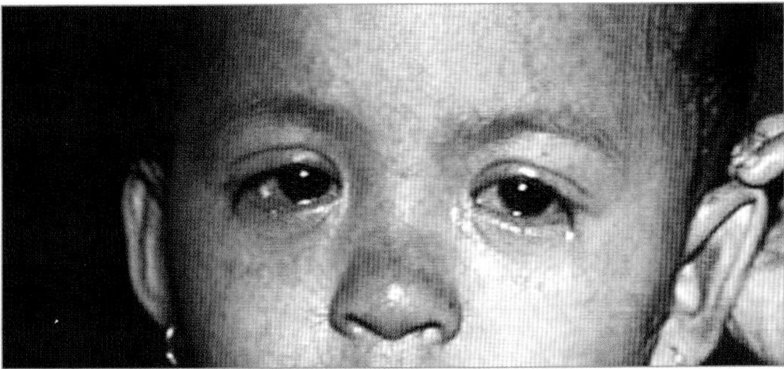

Image 83.18
A child with measles rash and conjunctivitis. Courtesy of Centers for Disease Control and Prevention.

84

Meningococcal Infections

Clinical Manifestations

Invasive infection usually results in meningitis (~50% of cases), bacteremia (~35%–40% of cases), or both. Bacteremic pneumonia is uncommon (~9% of cases). Onset can be insidious and nonspecific but is typically abrupt, with fever, chills, malaise, myalgia, limb pain, prostration, and a rash that can initially be macular, maculopapular, petechial, or purpuric (meningococcemia). The maculopapular and petechial rash is indistinguishable from the rash caused by some viral infections. Purpura can also occur in severe sepsis caused by other bacterial pathogens. In fulminant cases, purpura, limb ischemia, coagulopathy, pulmonary edema, shock, coma, and death can ensue within hours despite appropriate therapy. Signs and symptoms of meningococcal meningitis are indistinguishable from those associated with acute meningitis caused by other meningeal pathogens (eg, *Streptococcus pneumoniae*). In severe and fatal cases of meningococcal meningitis, raised intracranial pressure is a predominant presenting feature. The overall case-fatality rate for meningococcal disease is 10% to 15% and is somewhat higher in adolescents than infants. Death is more common in those with coma, hypotension, leukopenia, and thrombocytopenia and absence of meningitis. Less common manifestations of meningococcal infection include conjunctivitis, febrile occult bacteremia, septic arthritis, and chronic meningococcemia. Invasive infections can be complicated by arthritis, myocarditis, pericarditis, and endophthalmitis. A self-limiting postinfectious inflammatory syndrome occurs in fewer than 10% of cases 4 or more days after onset of meningococcal infection and most commonly presents as fever, arthritis, or vasculitis. Iritis, scleritis, conjunctivitis, pericarditis, and polyserositis are less common manifestations of postinfectious inflammatory syndrome.

Sequelae associated with meningococcal disease occur in 11% to 19% of survivors and include hearing loss, neurologic disability, digit or limb amputations, and skin scarring. In addition, some patients may also experience subtle long-term neurologic deficits, such as impaired school performance, behavioral problems, and attention-deficit/hyperactivity disorder.

Etiology

Neisseria meningitidis is a gram-negative diplococcus with at least 13 serogroups based on capsular type.

Epidemiology

Strains belonging to groups A, B, C, W, and Y are most commonly implicated in invasive disease worldwide. Serogroup A has been frequently associated with epidemics outside the United States, primarily in sub-Saharan Africa. A serogroup A meningococcal conjugate vaccine was introduced in the "meningitis belt" of sub-Saharan Africa in December 2010. This novel vaccine is highly effective and has the potential to end epidemic meningitis as a public health concern in sub-Saharan Africa. An increase in cases of serogroup W meningococcal disease has been associated with the hajj pilgrimage in Saudi Arabia. Since 2002, serogroup W meningococcal disease has been reported in sub-Saharan African countries during epidemic seasons. More recently, serogroup W outbreaks have occurred in South America. Prolonged outbreaks of serogroup B meningococcal disease have occurred in New Zealand, France, and Oregon. More recently, several clusters of serogroup B meningococcal disease have occurred on college campuses in the United States. Serogroup X causes a substantial number of cases of meningococcal disease in parts of Africa but is rare on other continents.

The incidence of meningococcal disease varies over time and by age and location. During the past 60 years, the annual incidence of meningococcal disease in the United States has varied from less than 0.3 to 1.5 cases per 100,000 population. Incidence cycles have occurred over multiple years. Since the early 2000s, annual incidence rates have decreased, and since 2005, only an estimated 800 to 1,000 US cases have been reported annually. The reasons for this decrease, which preceded introduction of meningococcal polysaccharide-protein conjugate vaccine into the immunization schedule, are not known but may be related to immunity of the population to circulating meningococcal strains and changes in behavioral risk factors (eg, smoking and exposure to secondhand smoke among adolescents and young adults).

Distribution of meningococcal serogroups in the United States has shifted in the past 2 decades. Serogroups B, C, and Y each account for approximately 30% of reported cases, but serogroup distribution varies by age, location, and time. Approximately three-quarters of cases among adolescents and young adults are caused by serogroups C, W, or Y and potentially are preventable with available vaccines. In infants and children younger than 5 years, 60% of cases are caused by serogroup B and, therefore, are not preventable with vaccines licensed in the United States for those ages.

Since introduction in the United States of *Haemophilus influenzae* type b and pneumococcal polysaccharide-protein conjugate vaccines for infants, *N meningitidis* has become the leading cause of bacterial meningitis in children and remains an important cause of septicemia. The peak incidence occurs in infants. Other peaks occur in adolescents and young adults 16 through 21 years of age and adults older than 65 years. Close contacts of patients with meningococcal disease are at increased risk of becoming infected. Patients with persistent complement component deficiencies (eg, C5–C9, properdin, factor H or factor D deficiencies) or anatomic or functional asplenia are at increased risk of invasive and recurrent meningococcal disease. Asymptomatic colonization of the upper respiratory tract provides the source from which the organism is spread. The highest rates of meningococcal colonization occur in older adolescents and young adults. Transmission occurs from person to person through droplets from the respiratory tract and requires close contact.

Outbreaks occur in communities and institutions, including child care centers, schools, colleges, and military recruit camps. However, most cases of meningococcal disease are sporadic, with fewer than 5% associated with outbreaks. The attack rate for household contacts is 500 to 800 times the rate for the general population. Serologic typing, multilocus sequence typing, multilocus enzyme electrophoresis, and pulsed-field gel electrophoresis of enzyme-restricted DNA fragments can be useful epidemiologic tools during a suspected outbreak to detect concordance among invasive strains.

Incubation Period

1 to 10 days (usually <4 days).

Diagnostic Tests

Cultures of blood and cerebrospinal fluid are indicated for patients with suspected invasive meningococcal disease. Culture of a petechial or purpuric lesion scraping, synovial fluid, and other, usually sterile body fluid specimens yield the organism in some patients. A Gram stain of a petechial or purpuric scraping, cerebrospinal fluid, and buffy coat smear of blood can be helpful. Because *N meningitidis* can be a component of the nasopharyngeal flora, isolation of *N meningitidis* from this site is not helpful diagnostically. A serogroup-specific polymerase chain reaction (PCR) test to detect *N meningitidis* from clinical specimens is used routinely in the United Kingdom and some European countries, where up to 56% of cases are confirmed by PCR testing alone. This test is particularly useful in patients who receive antimicrobial therapy before cultures are obtained. In the United States, PCR-based assays are available in some research and public health laboratories. A recently described multiplex PCR assay appears to have a sensitivity and specificity approaching 100% for detection of serogroups A, B, C, W, and Y.

Case definitions for invasive meningococcal disease are given in Box 84.1.

Treatment

The priority in management of meningococcal disease is treatment of shock in meningococcemia and of raised intracranial pressure in severe cases of meningitis. Empirical therapy for suspected meningococcal disease should include an extended-spectrum cephalosporin, such as cefotaxime or ceftriaxone. Once the microbiologic diagnosis is established, definitive treatment with penicillin G (300,000 U/kg/d), ampicillin, or an extended-spectrum cephalosporin is recommended. Ceftriaxone clears nasopharyngeal

Box 84.1
Surveillance Case Definitions for Invasive Meningococcal Disease

Confirmed Case

A clinically compatible case and isolation of *Neisseria meningitidis* from a usually sterile site; for example

- Blood
- Cerebrospinal fluid
- Synovial fluid
- Pleural fluid
- Pericardial fluid
- Isolation from skin scraping of petechial or purpuric lesions

Probable Case

A clinically compatible case with **either** a positive result of antigen test or immunohistochemistry of formalin-fixed tissue **or** a positive polymerase chain reaction test of blood or cerebrospinal fluid, without a positive sterile site culture.

Suspect

- A clinically compatible case and gram-negative diplococcic in any sterile fluid, such as cerebrospinal fluid, synovial fluid, or scraping from a petechial or purpuric lesion
- Clinical purpura fulminans without a positive culture

carriage effectively after one dose and allows outpatient management for completion of therapy when appropriate. For patients with a life-threatening penicillin allergy characterized by anaphylaxis, chloramphenicol is recommended, if available. If chloramphenicol is not available, meropenem can be used, although the rate of cross-reactivity in penicillin-allergic adults is 2% to 3%. For travelers from areas where penicillin resistance has been reported, cefotaxime, ceftriaxone, or chloramphenicol is recommended. In meningococcemia, early and rapid fluid resuscitation and early use of inotropic and ventilatory support may reduce mortality. The postinfectious inflammatory syndromes associated with meningococcal disease often respond to nonsteroidal anti-inflammatory drugs.

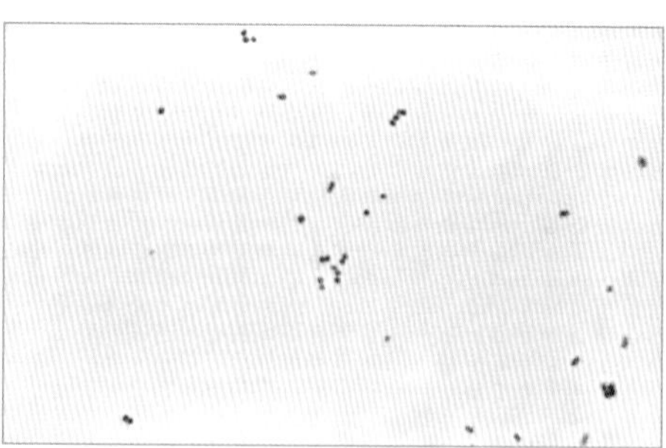

Image 84.1
This micrograph depicts the presence of aerobic gram-negative *Neisseria meningitidis* diplococcal bacteria (magnification x1,150). Meningococcal disease is an infection caused by a bacterium called *N meningitidis* or meningococcus. Courtesy of Centers for Disease Control and Prevention/Dr Brodsky.

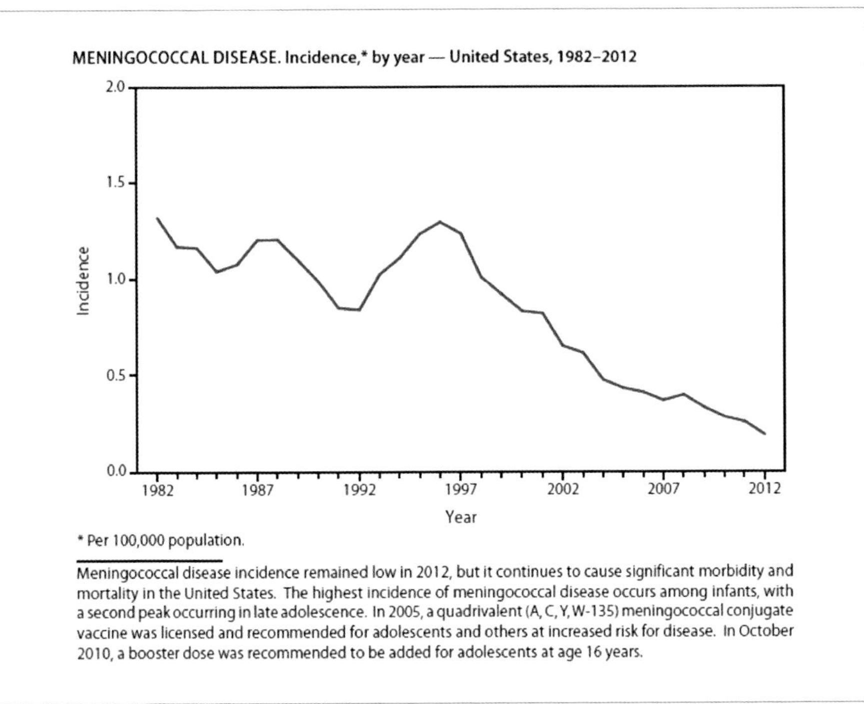

Image 84.2
Meningococcal disease. Incidence, by year—United States, 1982–2012. Courtesy of *Morbidity and Mortality Weekly Report.*

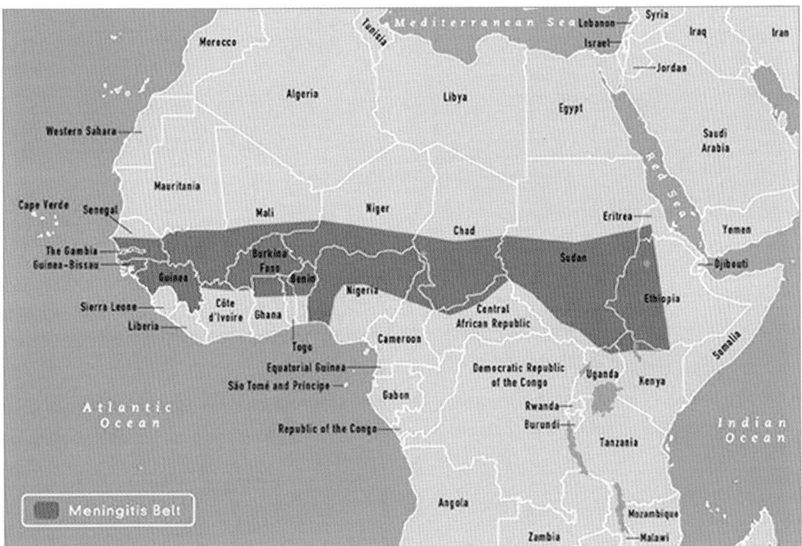

Image 84.3
Areas with frequent epidemics of meningococcal meningitis. Centers for Disease Control and Prevention National Center for Emerging and Zoonotic Infectious Diseases (NCEZID) Division of Global Migration and Quarantine (DGMQ).

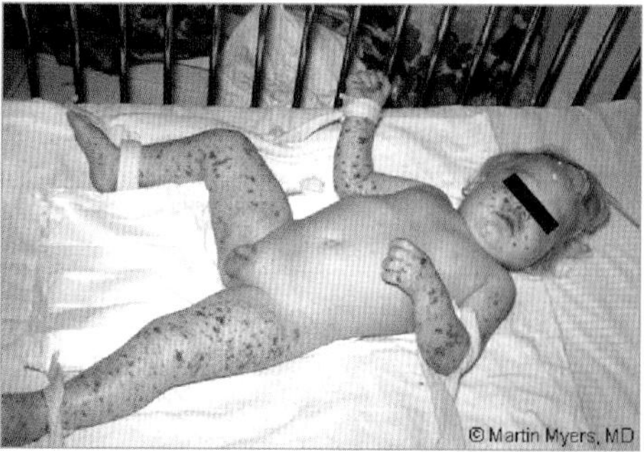

Image 84.4
Young boy with meningococcemia that demonstrates striking involvement of the extremities with sparing of the trunk. Copyright Martin G. Myers, MD.

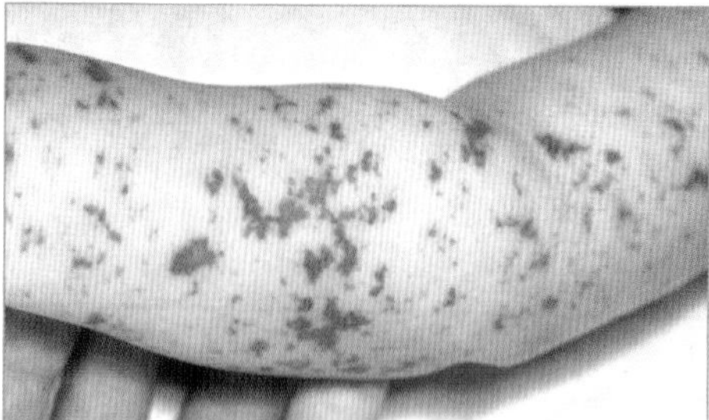

Image 84.5
The arm of the boy shown in Image 84.4, which demonstrates striking extremity involvement and characteristic angular lesions. Copyright Martin G. Myers, MD.

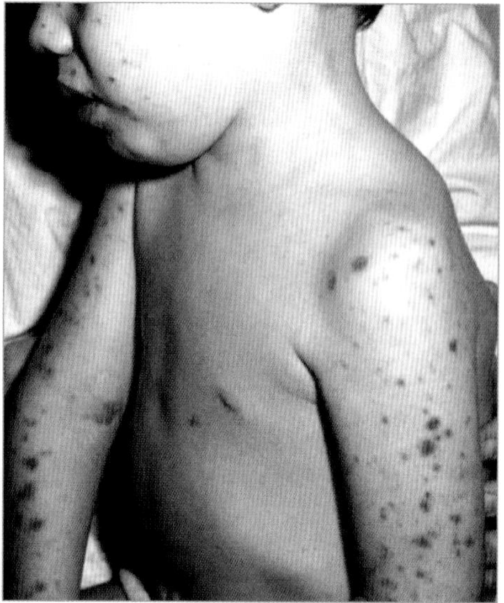

Image 84.6
Meningococcemia showing striking involvement of the extremities with relative sparing of the skin of the child's body surface.

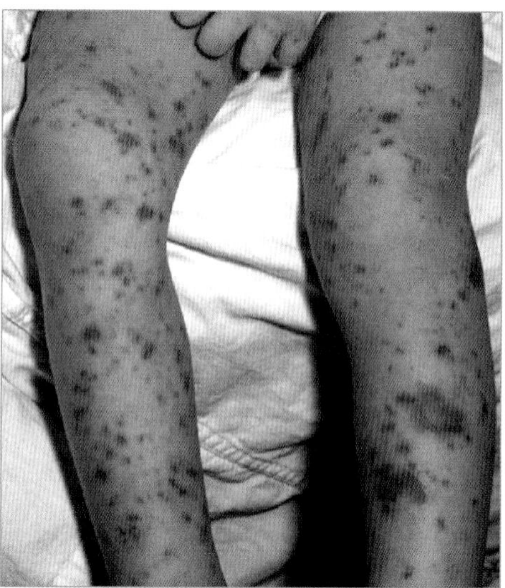

Image 84.7
Meningococcemia. This image shows the lower extremities of the patient in Image 84.6.

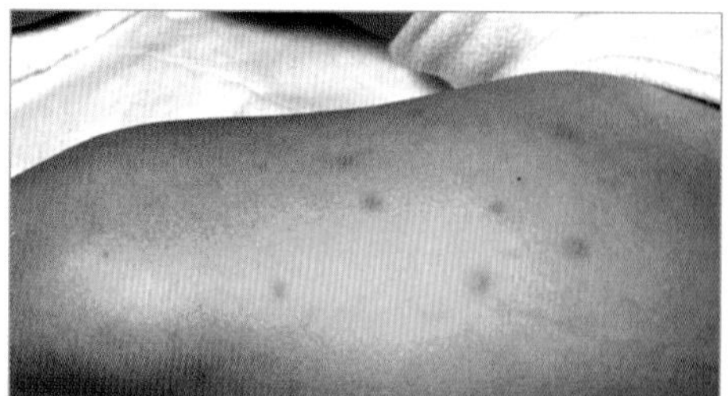

Image 84.8
Papular skin lesions of early meningococcemia.

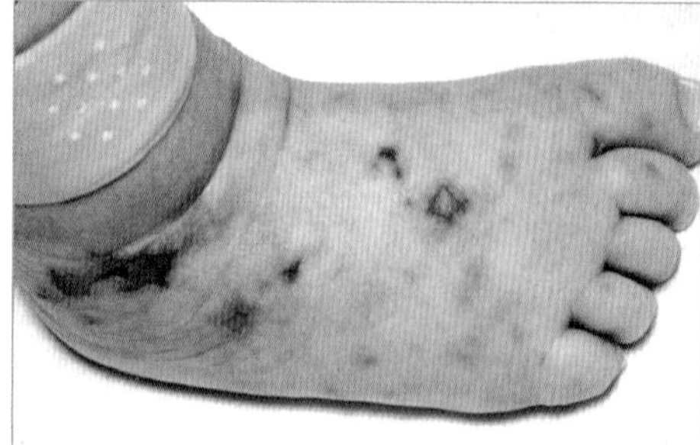

Image 84.9
Characteristic, angular, necrotic lesions on the foot of infant boy with meningococcemia (after 2 days of intravenous penicillin treatment).

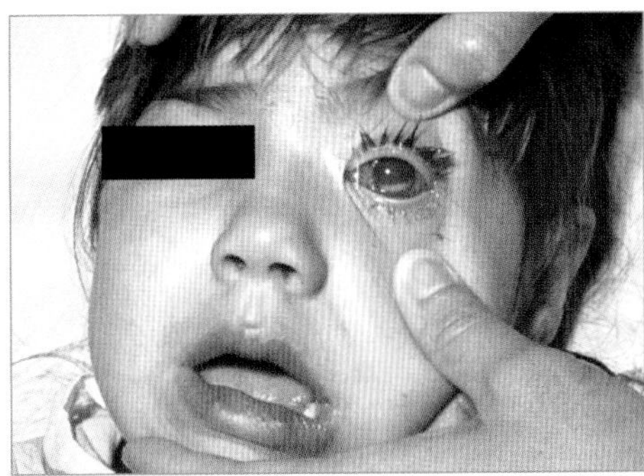

Image 84.10
Preschool-aged girl with meningococcal panophthalmitis. An infant sibling had meningococcal meningitis 1 week prior to the onset of this child's illness.

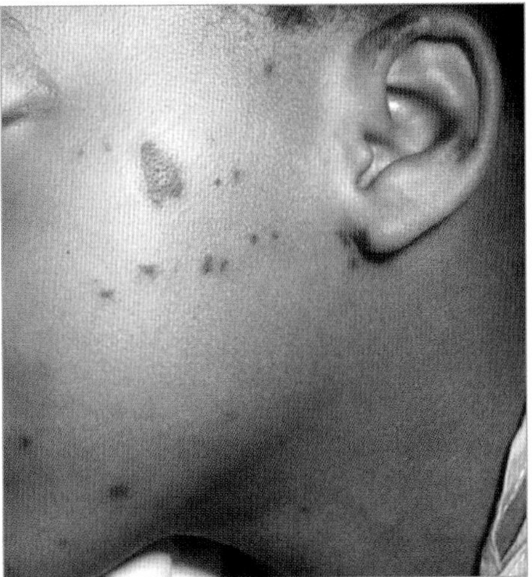

Image 84.12
Meningococcemia in an adolescent female with disseminated intravascular coagulation.

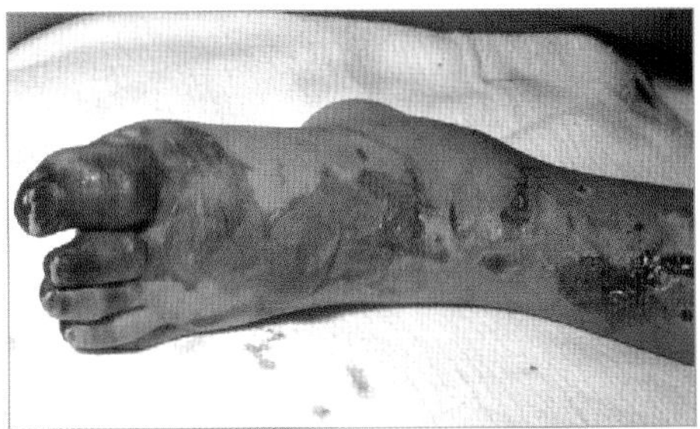

Image 84.14
Patient shown in images 84.12 and 84.13 with gangrene of the toes.

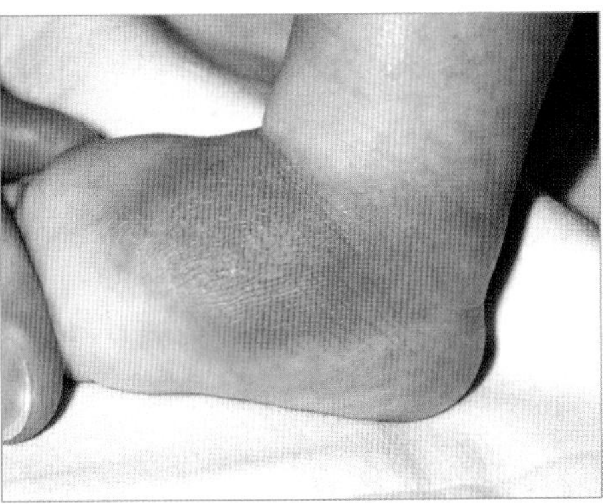

Image 84.11
This 6-month-old boy presented with fever and erythema and tenderness over the ankle. Blood culture and needle aspirate of the cellulitis grew *Neisseria meningitidis*. Courtesy of Neal Halsey, MD.

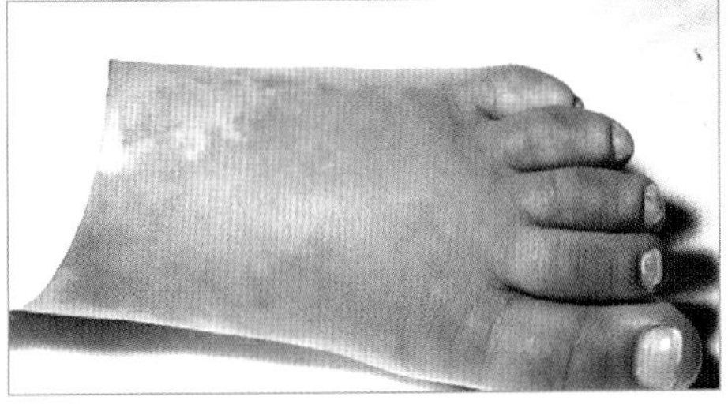

Image 84.13
Patient shown in Image 84.12 with marked purpura of the left foot.

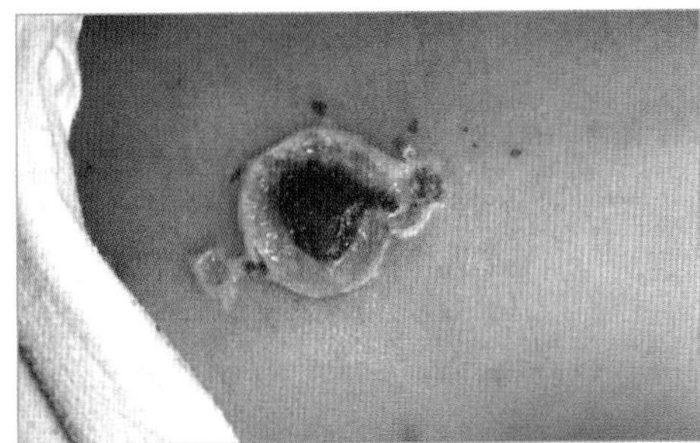

Image 84.15
Patient shown in images 84.12, 84.13, and 84.14 with cutaneous necrosis.

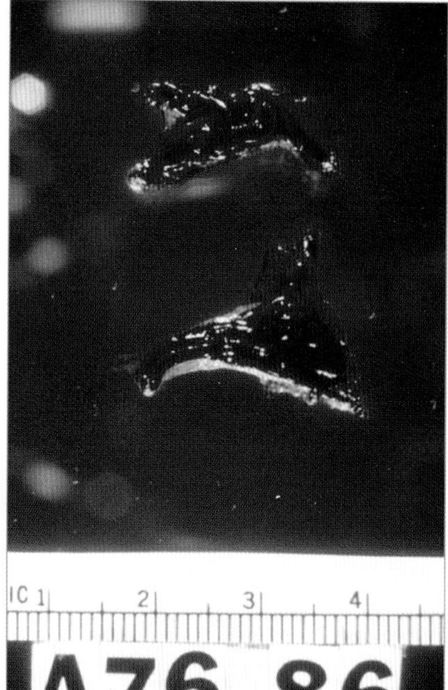

Image 84.16
Hemorrhagic adrenal glands from a 2-year-old who had the characteristic histopathology of Waterhouse-Friderichsen syndrome at autopsy. Courtesy of George Nankervis, MD.

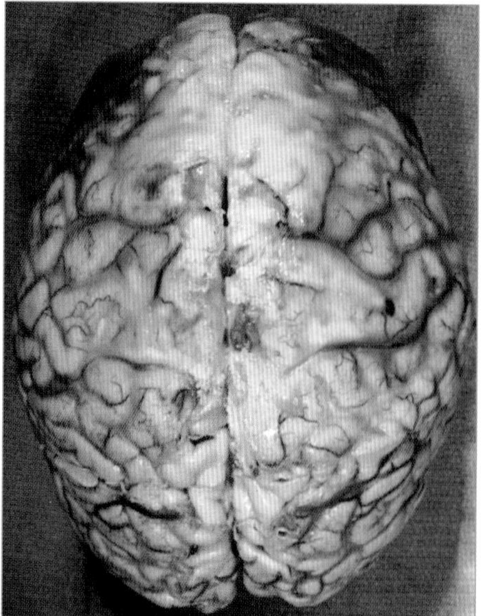

Image 84.18
Fatal meningococcal meningitis with purulent exudate in the subarachnoid space covering the cerebral convexities. Courtesy of Dimitris P. Agamanolis, MD.

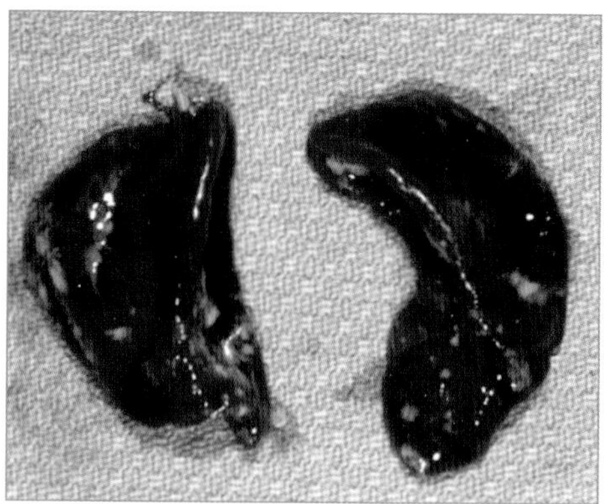

Image 84.17
Adrenal hemorrhage in a patient with gram-negative sepsis, a major complication of meningococcal disease with increased mortality. Courtesy of Dimitris P. Agamanolis, MD.

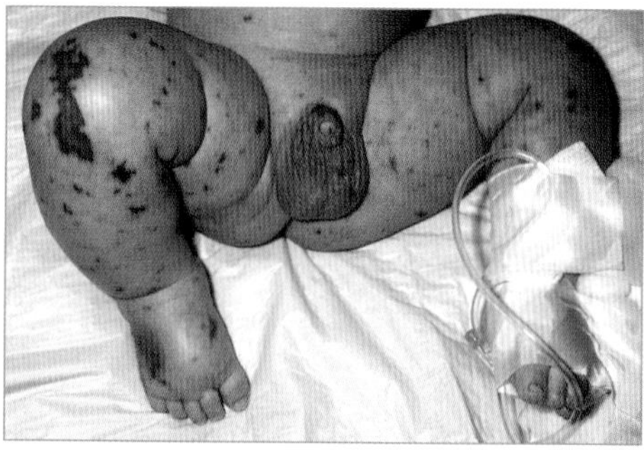

Image 84.19
Meningococcemia in an infant boy. Courtesy of Ed Fajardo, MD.

85

Human Metapneumovirus

Clinical Manifestations

Since its discovery in 2001, human metapneumovirus (hMPV) has been shown to cause acute respiratory tract illness in people of all ages. Human metapneumovirus is one of the leading causes of bronchiolitis in infants and also causes pneumonia, asthma exacerbations, croup, and upper respiratory tract infections with concomitant acute otitis media in children. Human metapneumovirus is also associated with acute exacerbations of chronic obstructive pulmonary disease and pneumonia in adults. Otherwise healthy young children infected with hMPV usually have mild or moderate symptoms, but some young children have severe disease requiring hospitalization. Human metapneumovirus infection in immunosuppressed people can result in severe disease, and fatalities have been reported in hematopoietic stem cell or lung transplant recipients. Preterm birth and underlying cardiopulmonary disease are likely risk factors, but degree of risk associated with these conditions is not fully defined. Recurrent infection occurs throughout life and, in previously healthy people, is usually mild or asymptomatic.

Etiology

Human metapneumovirus is a single-stranded, negative-sense RNA virus of the family Paramyxoviridae. Four major genotypes of virus have been identified with 2 major antigenic subgroups (designated A and B). These different subgroups cocirculate each year.

Epidemiology

Humans are the only source of infection. Transmission studies have not been reported, but spread is likely to occur by direct or close contact with contaminated secretions. Health care–associated infections have been reported. Human metapneumovirus infections usually occur annually during winter and early spring in temperate climates, coinciding or overlapping with the latter half of the respiratory syncytial virus (RSV) season. Sporadic infection may occur throughout the year. In otherwise healthy infants, the duration of viral shedding is 1 to 2 weeks. Prolonged shedding (months) has been reported in severely immunocompromised hosts.

Serologic studies suggest most children are infected at least once by 5 years of age. The population incidence of hospitalizations attributable to hMPV is generally thought to be lower than that attributable to RSV but comparable to that of influenza and parainfluenza virus 3 in children younger than 5 years. Large studies have shown that hMPV is detected in 6% to 7% of children with lower respiratory illnesses who are hospitalized or seen in the outpatient and emergency departments. Overall annual rates of hospitalization associated with hMPV infection are about 1 per 1,000 children younger than 5 years, 2 per 1,000 infants 6 to 11 months of age, and 3 per 1,000 infants younger than 6 months. Coinfection with RSV and other respiratory viruses can occur.

Incubation Period

An estimated 3 to 5 days.

Diagnostic Tests

Human metapneumovirus can be difficult to isolate in cell culture. Reverse transcriptase-polymerase chain reaction assays are the diagnostic method of choice for hMPV. Several reverse transcriptase-polymerase chain reaction assays for hMPV are available commercially. Immunofluorescence assays using monoclonal antibodies for hMPV antigen are also available, with reported sensitivities varying from 65% to 90%.

Treatment

Treatment is supportive and includes hydration and careful clinical assessment of respiratory status, including measurement of oxygen saturation, use of supplemental oxygen, and, if necessary, mechanical ventilation. Antimicrobial agents are not indicated in the treatment of infants hospitalized with uncomplicated hMPV bronchiolitis or pneumonia unless evidence exists for the presence of a concurrent bacterial infection.

86

Microsporidia Infections

(Microsporidiosis)

Clinical Manifestations

Patients with intestinal infection have watery, nonbloody diarrhea, generally without fever. Abdominal cramping can occur. Data suggest asymptomatic infection is more common than previously thought. Symptomatic intestinal infection is most common in immunocompromised people, especially in organ transplant recipients and people who are infected with HIV with low $CD4^+$ lymphocyte counts, in whom infection often results in chronic diarrhea. The clinical course can be complicated by malnutrition and progressive weight loss. Chronic infection in immunocompetent people is rare. Other clinical syndromes that can occur in HIV-infected and immunocompromised patients include keratoconjunctivitis, encephalitis, sinusitis, dermatitis, myositis, osteomyelitis, nephritis, hepatitis, cholangitis, peritonitis, prostatitis, urethritis, cystitis, disseminated disease, pulmonary disease, cardiac disease, and wasting syndrome.

Etiology

Microsporidia are obligate intracellular, spore-forming organisms classified as fungi. *Enterocytozoon bieneusi* and *Encephalitozoon intestinalis* are the most commonly reported pathogens in humans and are most often associated with chronic diarrhea in HIV-infected people. Multiple genera, including *Encephalitozoon, Enterocytozoon, Nosema, Pleistophora, Trachipleistophora, Anncaliia, Vittaforma,* and *Microsporida,* have been implicated in human infection, as have unclassified species.

Epidemiology

Most microsporidia infections are transmitted by oral ingestion of spores. Microsporidia spores are commonly found in surface water, and human strains have been identified in municipal water supplies and ground water. Several studies indicate waterborne transmission occurs. Person-to-person spread by the fecal-oral route also occurs. Spores have also been detected in other body fluids, but their role in transmission is unknown. Data suggest the possibility of zoonotic transmission.

Incubation Period

Unknown.

Diagnostic Tests

Infection with gastrointestinal *Microsporida* species can be documented by identification of organisms in biopsy specimens from the small intestine. *Microsporida* species spores can also be detected in formaldehyde solution–fixed stool specimens or duodenal aspirates stained with a chromotrope-based stain and examined by an experienced microscopist. Chemofluorescent agents like calcofluor, as well as Gram, acid-fast, periodic acid-Schiff, Warthin-Starry silver, and Giemsa stains, can also be used to detect organisms in tissue sections. Organisms are not often noticed because they are small (1–4 µm), stain poorly, and evoke minimal inflammatory response. Stool concentration techniques do not improve the ability to detect *E bieneusi* spores. Polymerase chain reaction assay can also be used for diagnosis. Identification for classification purposes and diagnostic confirmation of species requires transmission electron microscopy or molecular techniques.

Treatment

Restoration of immune function is critical for control of any microsporidia infection. For a limited number of patients, albendazole, fumagillin, metronidazole, atovaquone, and nitazoxanide have been reported to decrease diarrhea but without eradication of the organism. Albendazole is the drug of choice for infections caused by *E intestinalis* but is ineffective against *E bieneusi* and *Vittaforma corneae* infections, which may respond to fumagillin. However, fumagillin is associated with bone marrow toxicity, recurrence of diarrhea is common after therapy is discontinued, and the drug is not available in the United States. In patients infected with HIV, antiretroviral therapy, which is associated with improvement in the $CD4^+$ T-lymphocyte count, can modify the course of disease favorably and should be considered as a main part of the treatment plan. None of these therapies have been studied in children.

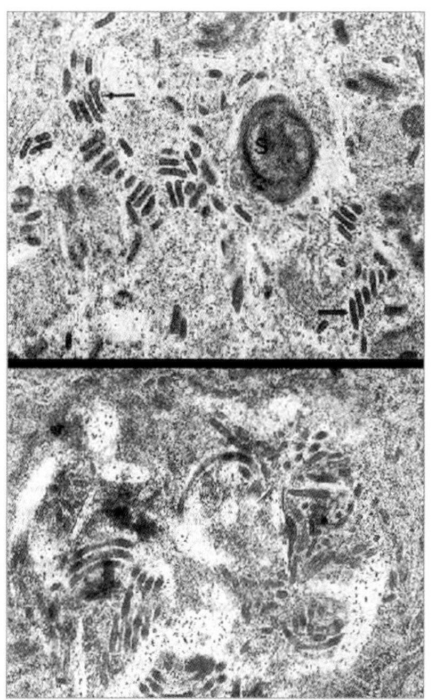

Image 86.1
Transmission electron micrographs showing developmental intracellular stages of microsporidia. Courtesy of Centers for Disease Control and Prevention.

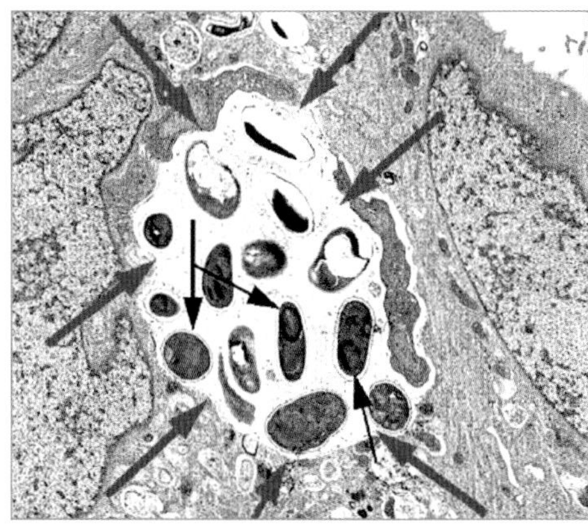

Image 86.2
Transmission electron micrograph showing developing forms of *Encephalitozoon intestinalis* inside a parasitophorous vacuole (red arrows) with mature spores (black arrows). Microsporidiosis, parasite. Courtesy of Centers for Disease Control and Prevention.

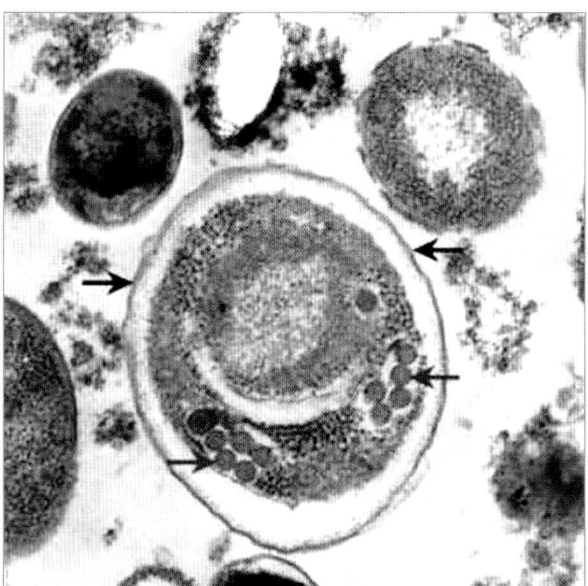

Image 86.3
Transmission electron micrograph of a mature microsporidia spore. Black arrows indicate the electron dense cell wall and red arrows, the coils of polar tubule. Although polymerase chain reaction can be used for diagnosis, serologic tests are unreliable. Courtesy of Centers for Disease Control and Prevention.

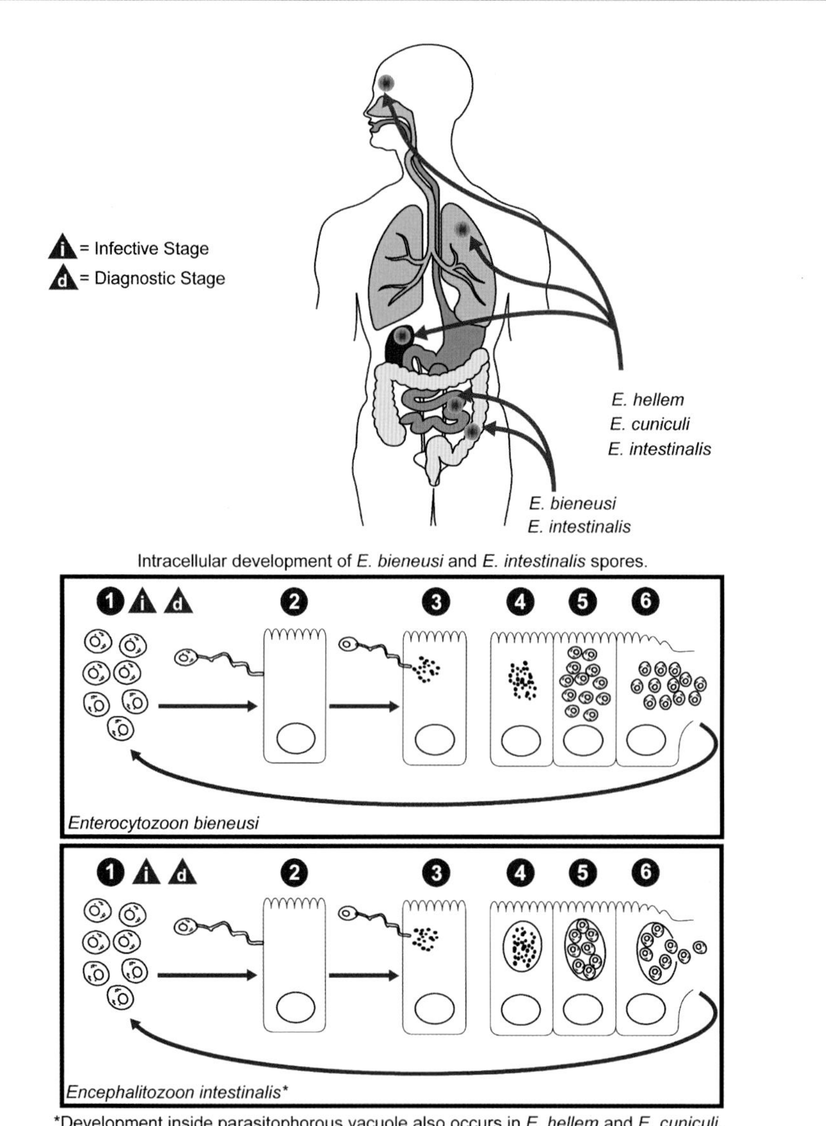

Image 86.4

The infective form of microsporidia is the resistant spore and it can survive for a long time in the environment (1). The spore extrudes its polar tubule and infects the host cell (2). The spore injects the infective sporoplasm into the eukaryotic host cell through the polar tubule (3). Inside the cell, the sporoplasm undergoes extensive multiplication by merogony (binary fission) (4) or schizogony (multiple fission). This development can occur in direct contact with the host cell cytoplasm (eg, *Enterocytozoon bieneusi*) or inside a vacuole termed parasitophorous vacuole (eg, *Enterocytozoon intestinalis*). Free in the cytoplasm or inside a parasitophorous vacuole, microsporidia develop by sporogony to mature spores (5). During sporogony, a thick wall is formed around the spore that provides resistance to adverse environmental conditions. When the spores increase in number and completely fill the host cell cytoplasm, the cell membrane is disrupted and releases the spores to the surroundings (6). These free mature spores can infect new cells, thus continuing the cycle. Courtesy of Centers for Disease Control and Prevention/Alexander J. da Silva, PhD/Melanie Moser.

87

Molluscum Contagiosum

Clinical Manifestations

Molluscum contagiosum is a benign viral infection of the skin with no systemic manifestations. It is usually characterized by 1 to 20 discrete, 2- to 5-mm–diameter, flesh-colored to translucent, dome-shaped papules, some with central umbilication. Lesions commonly occur on the trunk, face, and extremities but are rarely generalized. Molluscum contagiosum is a self-limited epidermal infection that usually resolves spontaneously in 6 to 12 months but may take as long as 4 years to disappear completely. An eczematous reaction encircles lesions in approximately 10% of patients. People with eczema, immunocompromising conditions, and HIV infection tend to have more widespread and prolonged eruptions.

Etiology

The cause is a poxvirus, which is the sole member of the genus *Molluscipoxvirus*.

Epidemiology

Humans are the only known source of the virus, which is spread by direct contact, including sexual contact, or by fomites. Vertical transmission has been suggested in case reports of neonatal molluscum contagiosum infection. Lesions can be disseminated by autoinoculation. Infectivity is generally low, but occasional outbreaks have been reported, including outbreaks in child care centers. The period of communicability is unknown.

Incubation Period

2 to 7 weeks, but can be as long as 6 months.

Diagnostic Tests

The diagnosis can usually be made clinically from the characteristic appearance of the lesions. Wright or Giemsa staining of cells expressed from the central core of a lesion reveals characteristic intracytoplasmic inclusions. Electron microscopic examination of these cells identifies typical poxvirus particles. Adolescents and young adults with genital molluscum contagiosum should be tested for sexually transmitted infections.

Treatment

There is no consensus on management of molluscum contagiosum in children and adolescents. Genital lesions should be treated to prevent spread to sexual contacts. Treatment of nongenital lesions is mainly for cosmetic reasons. Lesions in healthy people are typically self-limited, and treatment may not be necessary. However, therapy may be warranted to alleviate discomfort, including itching; reduce autoinoculation; limit transmission of the virus to close contacts; reduce cosmetic concerns; and prevent secondary infection. Physical destruction of the lesions is the most rapid and effective means of curing molluscum contagiosum. Modalities available include curettage, cryotherapy with liquid nitrogen, electrodesiccation, and chemical agents designed to initiate a local inflammatory response (eg, podophyllin, tretinoin, cantharidin, 25%–50% trichloroacetic acid, liquefied phenol, silver nitrate, tincture of iodine, potassium hydroxide). Cidofovir is a cytosine nucleotide analogue with in vitro activity against molluscum contagiosum; cidofovir should be reserved for extreme cases because of potential carcinogenicity and known toxicities. Solitary genital lesions in children are usually not acquired by sexual transmission but rather other modes of direct contact with the virus, including autoinoculation.

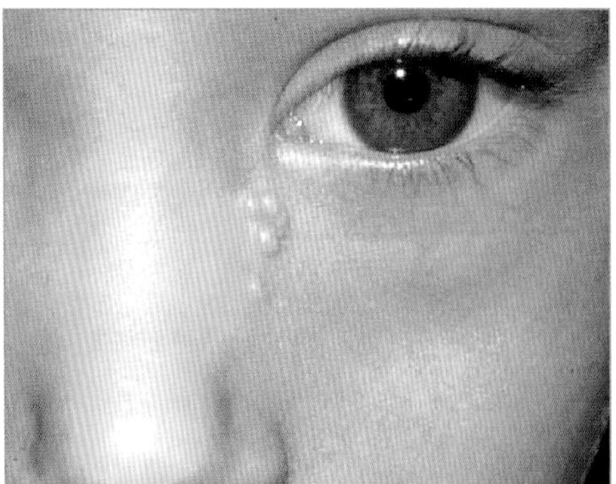

Image 87.1
Molluscum contagiosum lesions adjacent to nasal bridge. Copyright Edgar K. Marcuse, MD.

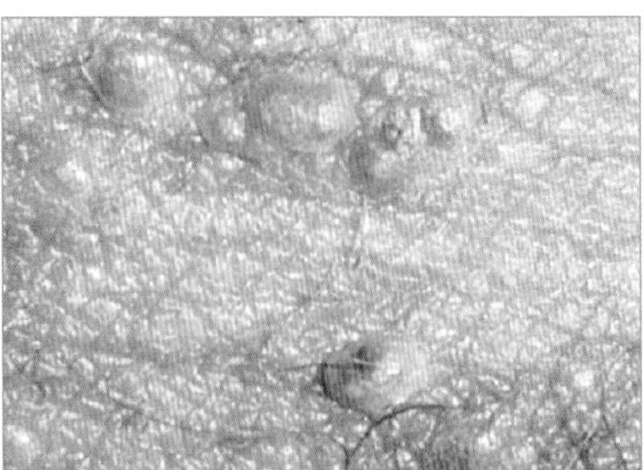

Image 87.2
A central dimple or umbilication is the hallmark of molluscum contagiosum. The lesions of molluscum contagiosum vary in size from 1 to 6 mm and, unlike venereal warts, are smooth and pearly and have an umbilicated center.

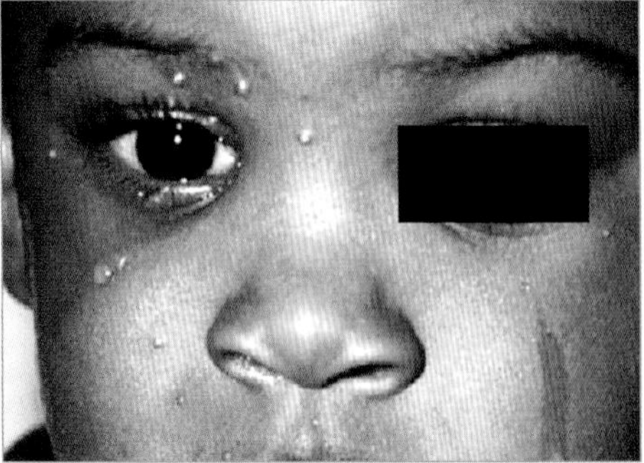

Image 87.3
Molluscum contagiosum is characterized by one or more translucent or white papules. Intracytoplasmic inclusions may be seen with Wright or Giemsa staining of material expressed from the core of a lesion.

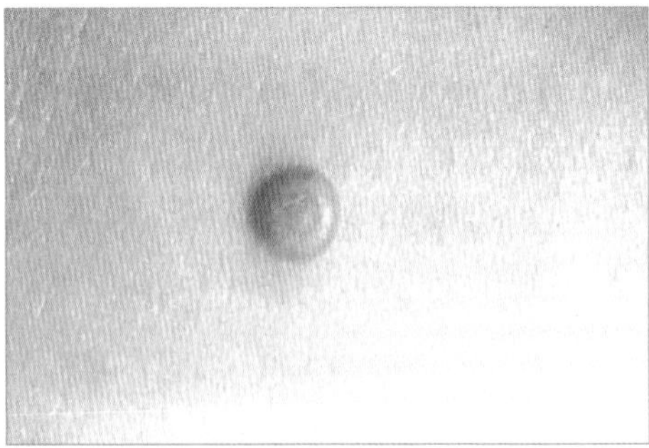

Image 87.4
A molluscum contagiosum lesion with characteristic umbilication.

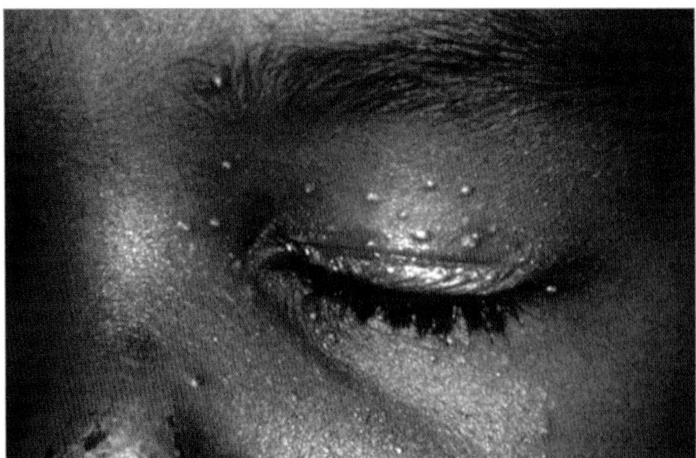

Image 87.5
Pearly papules on the forehead and eyelid in a child with molluscum contagiosum lesions, which commonly occur on the face.

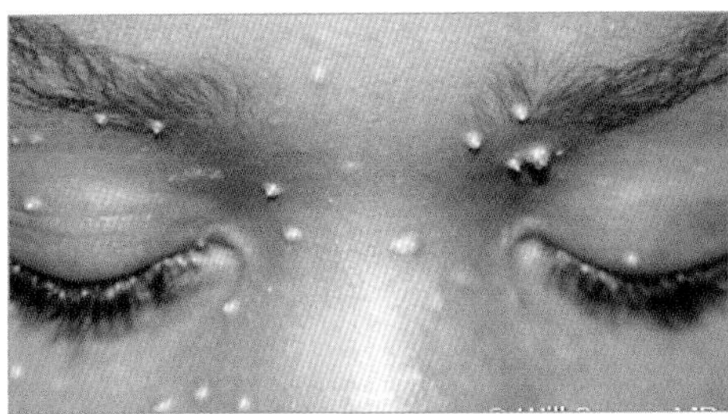

Image 87.6
This 10-year-old girl has had multiple small bumps on the face for the past month. These started as a solitary papule on her eyebrow but spread over several weeks. They have developed a small pointed core and are an embarrassment to the child. School pictures are pending. The family demands treatment. There is a family history of keloids. The family was counseled on the limited treatment options due to the potential for permanent scarring and keloid formation. Consultation with a dermatologist was arranged at the parents' request. Courtesy of Will Sorey, MD.

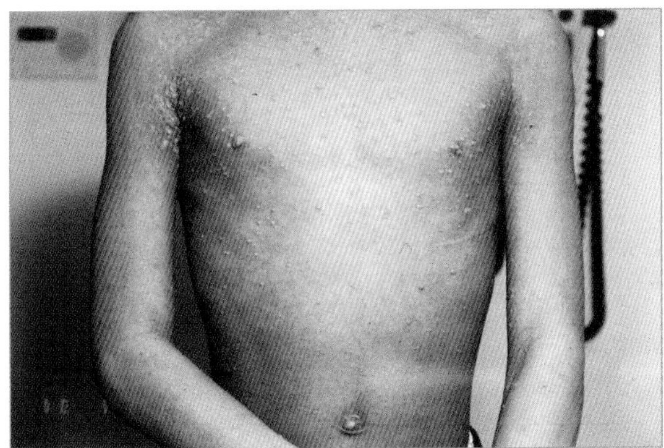

Image 87.7
A 15-year-old boy with HIV with numerous and widespread molluscum contagiosum lesions. Courtesy of Larry Frenkel, MD.

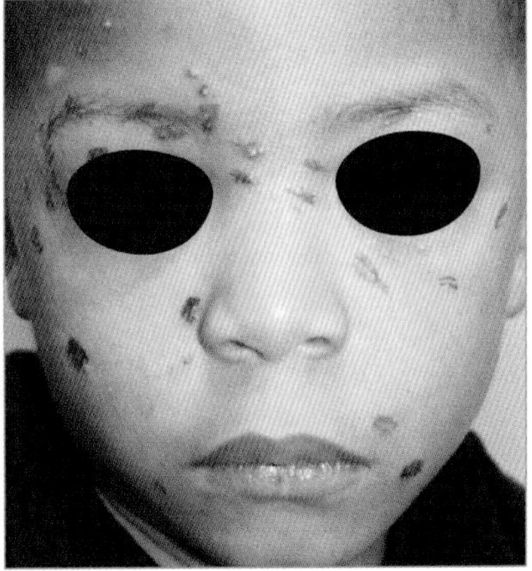

Image 87.8
This healthy 5-year-old boy with widespread molluscum was started on home treatment with a topical liquid salicylic acid preparation. He developed itchy crusted erosions around the treated lesions. Topical therapy was discontinued and a topical antibiotic ointment was prescribed with rapid clearing of the irritant dermatitis. Courtesy of H. Cody Meissner, MD, FAAP.

88

Mumps

Clinical Manifestations

Mumps is a systemic disease characterized by swelling of one or more of the salivary glands, usually the parotid glands. Approximately one-third of infections do not cause clinically apparent salivary gland swelling and can be asymptomatic (subclinical) or manifest primarily as respiratory tract infection. More than 50% of people with mumps have cerebrospinal fluid pleocytosis, but fewer than 10% have symptoms of viral meningitis. Orchitis is a commonly reported complication after puberty, although sterility rarely results. Rare complications include arthritis, thyroiditis, mastitis, glomerulonephritis, myocarditis, endocardial fibroelastosis, thrombocytopenia, cerebellar ataxia, transverse myelitis, encephalitis, pancreatitis, oophoritis, and permanent hearing impairment. Infection in adults is more likely to result in complications. Whether first trimester maternal mumps causes spontaneous abortion or intrauterine fetal death is uncertain, and this does not result in congenital malformation.

Etiology

Mumps is an RNA virus in the Paramyxoviridae family. Other infectious causes of parotitis include Epstein-Barr virus, cytomegalovirus, parainfluenza virus, influenza A virus, enteroviruses, lymphocytic choriomeningitis virus, HIV, nontuberculous mycobacteria, and gram-positive and, less often, gram-negative bacteria.

Epidemiology

Mumps occurs worldwide, and humans are the only known natural hosts. The virus is spread by contact with infectious respiratory tract secretions and saliva. Mumps virus is the only known cause of epidemic parotitis. Historically, the peak incidence of mumps was between January and May and among children younger than 10 years. Mumps vaccine was recommended for routine childhood immunization in 1977. After implementation of the one-dose mumps vaccine recommendation, the incidence of mumps in the United States declined from 50 to 251 per 100,000 in the prevaccine era to 2 per 100,000 in 1988. After implementation of the 2-dose measles-mumps-rubella vaccine recommendation in 1989, mumps further declined to extremely low levels, with an incidence of 0.1 per 100,000 by 1999. From 2000 to 2005, seasonality was no longer evident, and there were fewer than 300 reported cases per year (incidence of 0.1 per 100,000), representing a greater than 99% reduction in disease incidence. In early 2006, a large-scale mumps outbreak occurred in the Midwestern United States, with 6,584 reported cases (incidence of 2.2 per 100,000). Most of the cases occurred among people 18 through 24 years of age, many of whom were college students who had received 2 doses of mumps vaccine. Another outbreak in 2009–2010 affected more than 3,500 people, mainly students in grades 6 through 12 who were members of traditional observant religious communities in New York and New Jersey and who had received 2 doses of measles-mumps-rubella vaccine. Two doses of the mumps vaccine are approximately 88% effective in preventing disease. The period of maximum communicability begins several days before parotitis onset. The recommended isolation period is for 5 days after onset of parotid swelling.

Incubation Period

16 to 18 days, but occasionally 12 to 25 days after exposure.

Diagnostic Tests

Despite the outbreaks in 2006 and 2009–2010, mumps remains an uncommon infection in the United States, and parotitis has other etiologies, including other infectious agents. People with parotitis without other apparent cause should undergo diagnostic testing to confirm mumps virus as the cause or to diagnose other etiologies. Mumps can be confirmed by detection of mumps virus nucleic acid via reverse transcriptase-polymerase chain reaction assay in specimens from buccal swabs (Stensen duct exudates), throat washings, saliva, or spinal fluid; by detection of mumps-specific immunoglobulin (Ig) M antibody; or by a significant increase between acute and convalescent titers in serum mumps IgG antibody titer determined by standard quantitative or semiquantitative serologic assay.

Confirming the diagnosis of mumps in highly immunized populations is challenging because the IgM response may be absent or short lived; acute IgG titers might already be high, so no significant increase can be detected between acute and convalescent specimens. Emphasis should be placed on obtaining clinical specimens within 1 to 3 days after onset of parotitis. In immunized people, a negative IgM result does not rule out mumps.

Treatment

There is no antiviral therapy, so therapy is supportive.

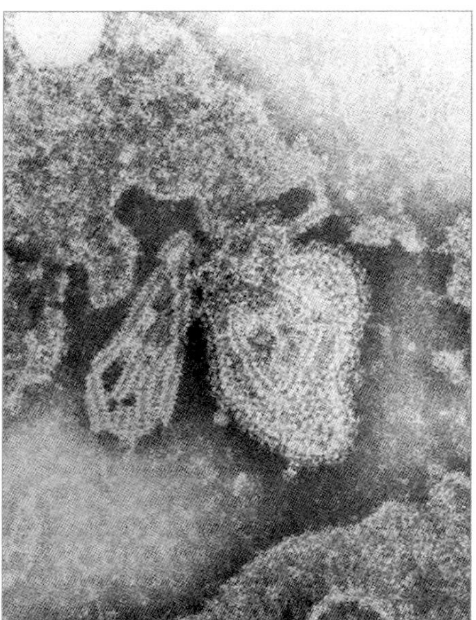

Image 88.1
Electron micrograph of the mumps virus. The mumps virus is a member of the Paramyxoviridae family and is enveloped by a helical ribonucleic-protein capsid, which has a Herring-body–like appearance. Courtesy of Centers for Disease Control and Prevention/Dr F. A. Murphy.

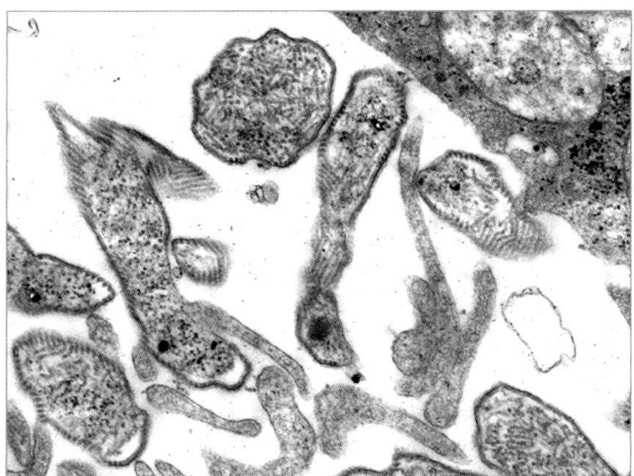

Image 88.2
Thin-section electron micrograph of mumps virus. Filamentous nucleocapsids can be seen within viral particles and juxtaposed along the viral envelope. Courtesy of Centers for Disease Control and Prevention/Courtesy of A. Harrison and F. A. Murphy.

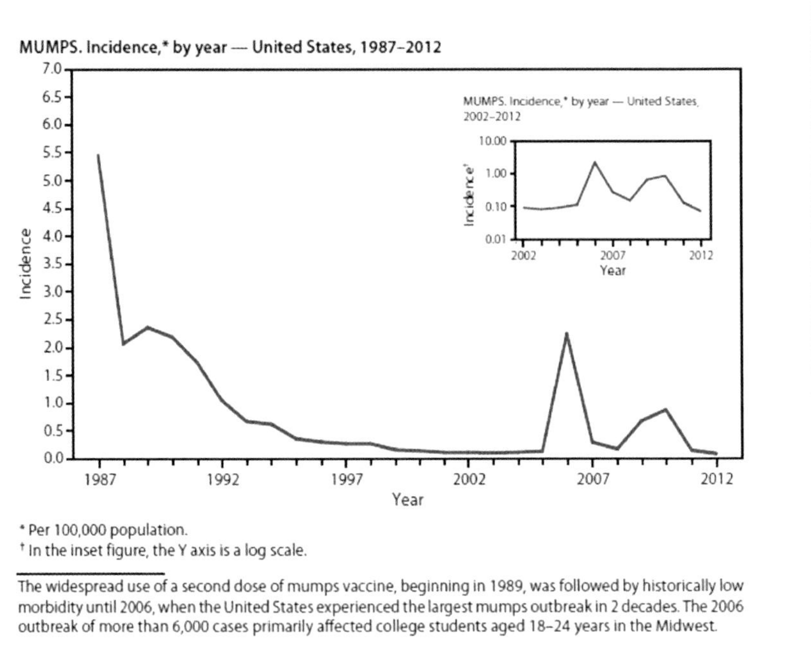

Image 88.3
Mumps. Incidence, by year—United States, 1987–2012. Courtesy of *Morbidity and Mortality Weekly Report.*

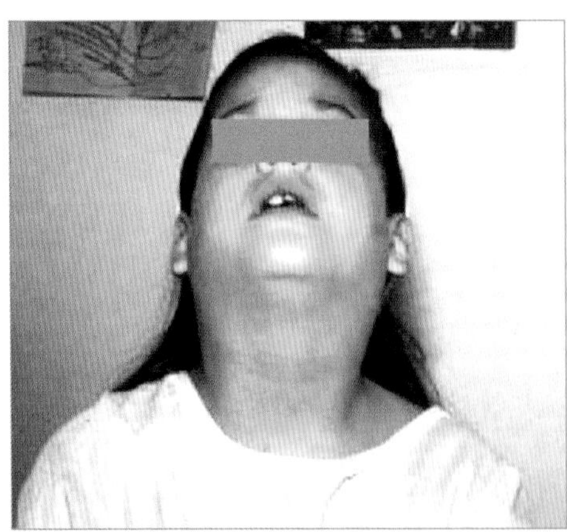

Image 88.4
Mumps with parotid and submandibular involvement bilaterally. The differential diagnosis for acute infectious parotitis includes cytomegalovirus, parainfluenza viruses, lymphocytic choriomeningitis, coxsackieviruses and other enteroviruses, HIV, nontuberculous mycobacterium, and certain bacteria. Copyright Martha Lepow.

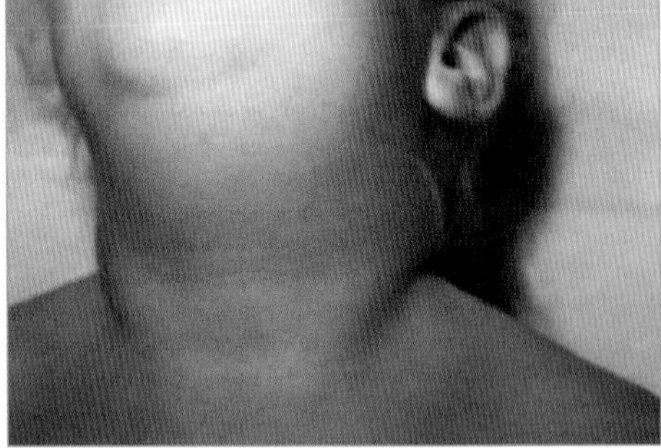

Image 88.5
This is a photograph of a patient with bilateral swelling in the submaxillary regions due to mumps. Prior to vaccine licensure in 1967, 100,000 to 200,000 mumps cases are estimated to have occurred in the United States each year. Courtesy of Centers for Disease Control and Prevention/Dr Heinz F. Eichenwald.

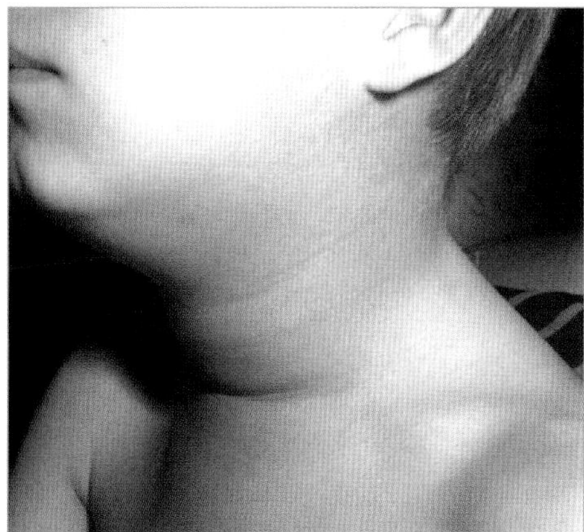

Image 88.6
Mumps parotitis with cervical and presternal edema and erythema that resolved spontaneously.

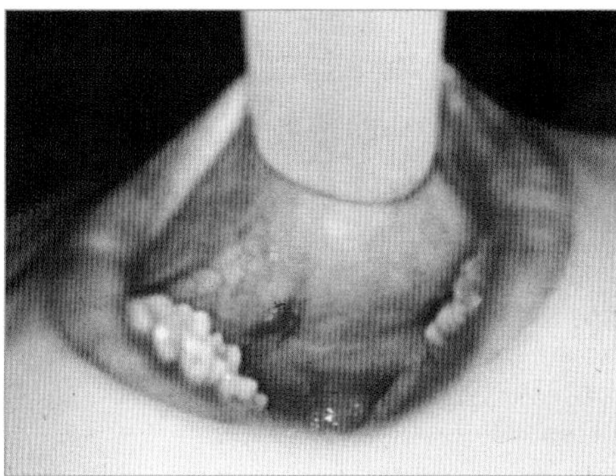

Image 88.7
Swelling and erythema of the Stensen duct in a 10-year-old white boy with mumps parotitis. Courtesy of Paul Wehrle, MD.

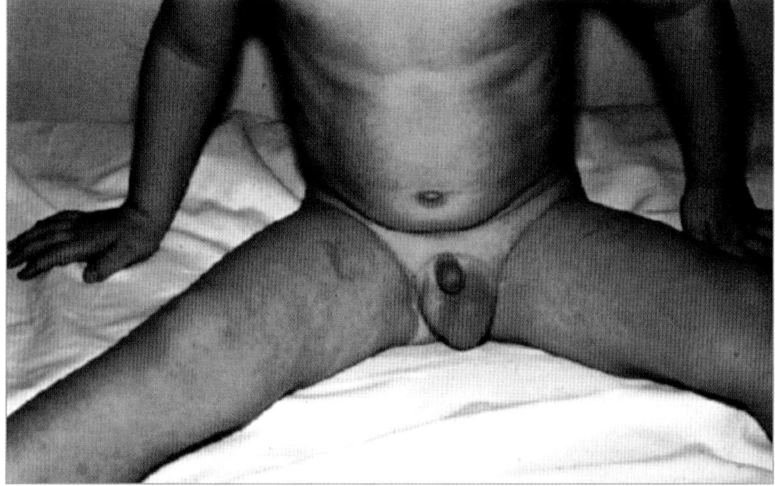

Image 88.8
Mumps orchitis in a 6-year-old boy. This complication is unusual in prepubertal boys. The highest risk for orchitis is in males between 15 and 29 years of age.

89

Mycoplasma pneumoniae and Other *Mycoplasma* Species Infections

Clinical Manifestations

Mycoplasma pneumoniae is a frequent cause of upper and lower respiratory tract infections in children, including pharyngitis, acute bronchitis, and pneumonia. Acute otitis media is uncommon. Bullous myringitis, once considered pathognomonic for mycoplasma, is now known to occur with other pathogens as well. Coryza, sinusitis, and croup are rare. Symptoms are variable and include cough, malaise, fever, and, occasionally, headache. Acute bronchitis and upper respiratory tract illness caused by *M pneumoniae* are generally mild and self-limited. Approximately 10% of infected school-aged children will develop pneumonia with cough and widespread rales on physical examination within days after onset of constitutional symptoms. Cough is often initially nonproductive but later can become productive. Cough can persist for 3 to 4 weeks and can be accompanied by wheezing. Approximately 10% of children with *M pneumoniae* infection will exhibit a rash, which is most often maculopapular. Radiographic abnormalities are variable. Bilateral diffuse infiltrates or focal abnormalities, such as consolidation, effusion, or hilar adenopathy, can occur.

Unusual manifestations include nervous system disease (eg, aseptic meningitis, encephalitis, acute disseminated encephalomyelitis, cerebellar ataxia, transverse myelitis, peripheral neuropathy), as well as myocarditis, pericarditis, arthritis, erythema nodosum, polymorphous mucocutaneous eruptions (including classic and atypical Stevens-Johnson syndrome), hemolytic anemia, thrombocytopenic purpura, and hemophagocytic syndromes. In patients with sickle cell disease, Down syndrome, immunodeficiencies, and chronic cardiorespiratory disease, severe pneumonia with pleural effusion can develop. Acute chest syndrome and pneumonia have been associated with *M pneumoniae* in patients with sickle cell disease. Infection has also been associated with exacerbations of asthma.

Several other *Mycoplasma* species colonize mucosal surfaces of humans and can produce disease in children. *Mycoplasma hominis* infection has been reported in neonates (especially at scalp electrode monitor site) and children (immunocompetent and immunocompromised). Intra-abdominal abscesses, septic arthritis, endocarditis, pneumonia, meningoencephalitis, brain abscess, and surgical wound infections have all been reported.

Etiology

Mycoplasmas, including *M pneumoniae,* are pleomorphic bacteria that lack a cell wall. Mycoplasmas cannot be detected using light microscopy.

Epidemiology

Mycoplasmas are ubiquitous in animals and plants, but *M pneumoniae* causes disease only in humans. *M pneumoniae* is transmissible by respiratory droplets during close contact with a symptomatic person. Outbreaks have been described in hospitals, military bases, colleges, and summer camps. Occasionally, *M pneumoniae* causes ventilator-associated pneumonia. *M pneumoniae* is a leading cause of pneumonia in school-aged children and young adults but is an infrequent cause of community-acquired pneumonia in preschool-aged children. In the United States, an estimated 2 million infections are caused by *M pneumoniae* each year; approximately 20% of hospitalized community-acquired pneumonia cases may be caused by *M pneumoniae.* Infections occur throughout the world, in any season, and in all geographic settings. In family studies, approximately 30% of household contacts develop pneumonia. Asymptomatic carriage after infection may occur for weeks to months. Immunity after infection is not long lasting.

Incubation Period

2 to 3 weeks (range, 1 to 4 weeks).

Diagnostic Tests

M pneumoniae can be grown in special enriched broth followed by passage to SP4 agar media or on commercially available mixed liquid broth/agar slant media, but most clinical facilities lack the capacity to perform this culture. Serologic tests using immunofluorescence and enzyme immunoassays that detect *M pneumoniae*–specific immunoglobulin (Ig) M and IgG antibodies are available commercially. IgM antibodies are not generally detectable within the first 7 days after onset of symptoms. IgM antibody titer peaks at approximately 3 to 6 weeks and persists for 2 to 3 months after infection. Although the presence of IgM antibodies may indicate recent *M pneumoniae* infection, false-positive test results occur and may not indicate current infection. Serologic diagnosis is best made by demonstrating a 4-fold or greater increase in antibody titer between acute and convalescent serum specimens. Measurement of serum cold hemagglutinin titer has limited value.

Polymerase chain reaction (PCR) tests for *M pneumoniae* are available commercially and are increasingly replacing other tests because PCR tests performed on respiratory tract specimens (nasal wash, nasopharyngeal swab, pharyngeal swab) have sensitivity and specificity between 80% and 100%, yield positive results earlier in the course of illness than serologic tests, and are rapid. Identification of *M pneumoniae* by PCR or culture in a patient with compatible clinical manifestations suggests causation; attributing a nonclassic clinical disorder to *Mycoplasma* is problematic, however, because *M pneumoniae* can colonize the respiratory tract for several weeks after acute infection, even after appropriate antimicrobial therapy. Polymerase chain reaction assay of body fluids for *M hominis* is available at reference laboratories.

Treatment

Evidence of benefit of antimicrobial therapy for nonhospitalized children with lower respiratory tract disease attributable to *M pneumoniae* is limited. Some data suggest benefit of appropriate antimicrobial therapy in hospitalized children. Antimicrobial therapy is not recommended for preschool-aged children with community-acquired pneumonia because viral pathogens are responsible for the great majority of cases. There is no evidence that treatment of other possible manifestations of *M pneumoniae* infection (eg, upper respiratory tract infection, extrapulmonary infection) with antimicrobial agents alters the course of illness. Macrolides, including azithromycin, clarithromycin, and erythromycin, are the preferred antimicrobial agents for treatment of pneumonia in school-aged children who have moderate to severe infection and those with underlying conditions, such as sickle cell disease. Fluoroquinolones and doxycycline are also effective in adolescents. Macrolide-resistant strains are increasingly common.

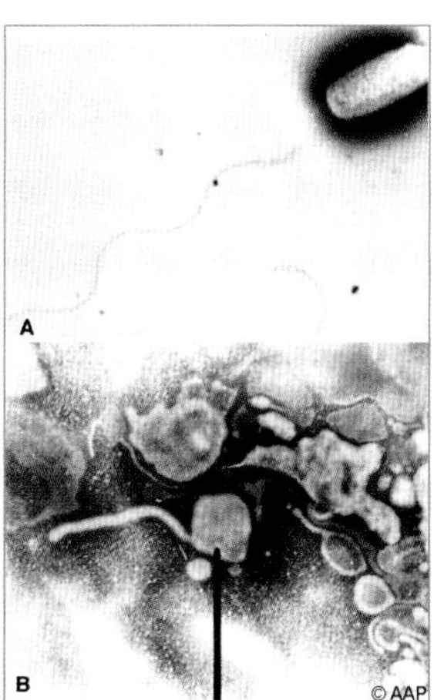

Image 89.1

A, Typical structure of a common gram-negative bacterium (*Pseudomonas aeruginosa*) and its flagellum, as seen on electron microscopy. B, Pleomorphic structure of *Mycoplasma pneumoniae*, as seen on electron microscopy. The bacterium is indicated by the black pointer. Mycoplasmas, including *M pneumoniae*, lack a cell wall.

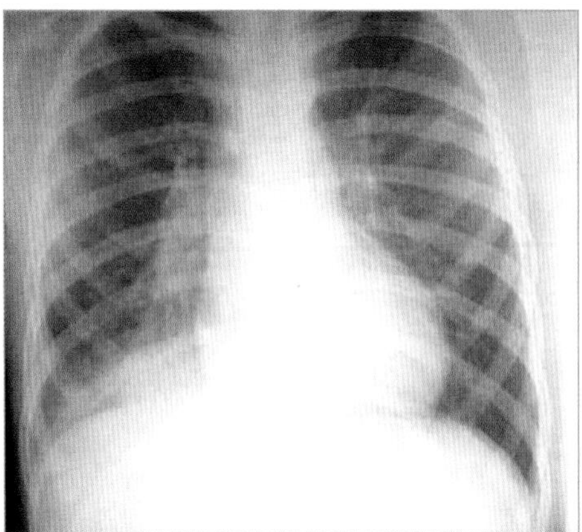

Image 89.2
A preadolescent boy with bilateral perihilar infiltration and right lower lobe pneumonia and pleural effusion due to *Mycoplasma pneumoniae*. Courtesy of Edgar O. Ledbetter, MD, FAAP.

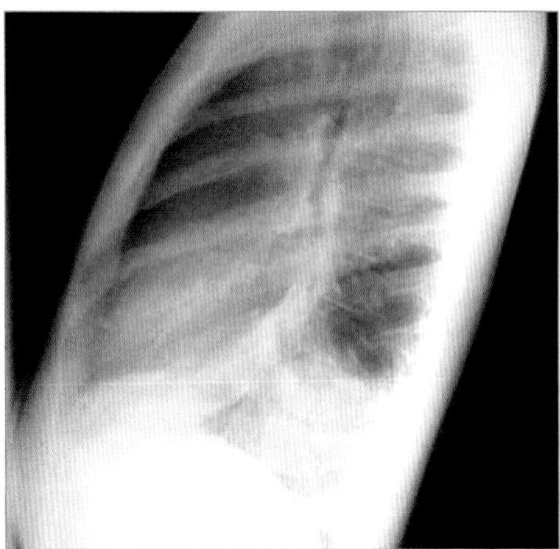

Image 89.3
Right lateral radiograph of the patient in Image 89.2 with pneumonia and pleural effusion. Pleural effusions associated with *Mycoplasma pneumoniae* infections generally resolve spontaneously without drainage. Courtesy of Edgar O. Ledbetter, MD, FAAP.

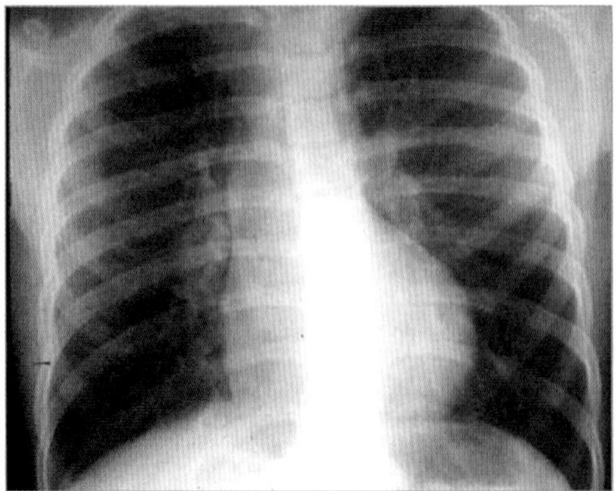

Image 89.4
Preadolescent boy with bilateral perihilar infiltrates caused by *Mycoplasma pneumoniae*.

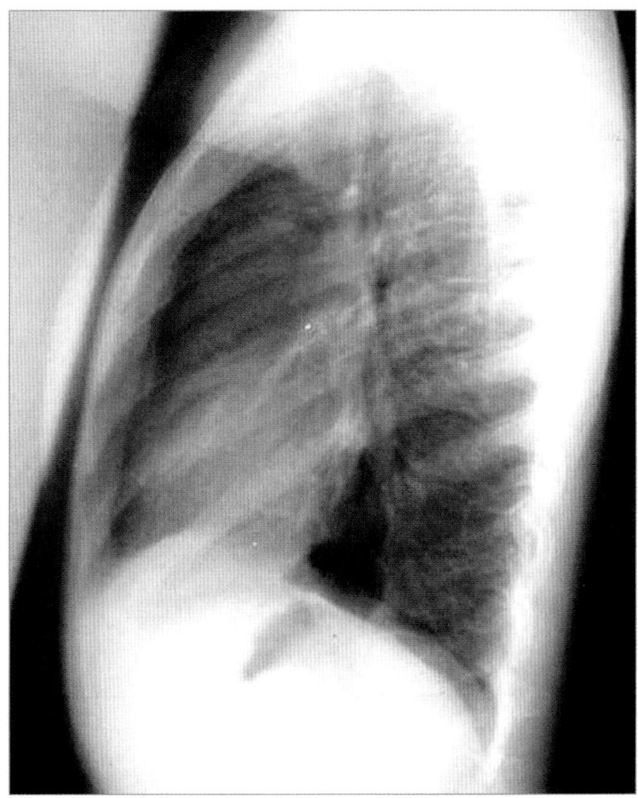

Image 89.5
Lateral radiograph of the patient in Image 89.4 with pneumonia caused by *Mycoplasma pneumoniae.*

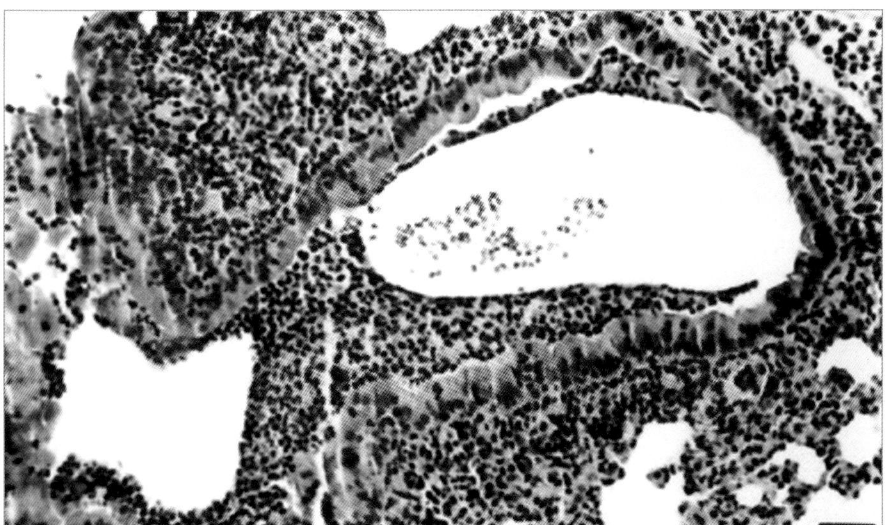

Image 89.6
Histopathologic study of *Mycoplasma pneumoniae*–infected lung tissue. The respiratory bronchiole is surrounded by an inflammatory mononuclear cell response. The intraluminal site is approximately 30% occluded by mucus and white blood cells. *M pneumoniae* is a common cause of pneumonia and tracheobronchitis in school-aged children and adolescents.

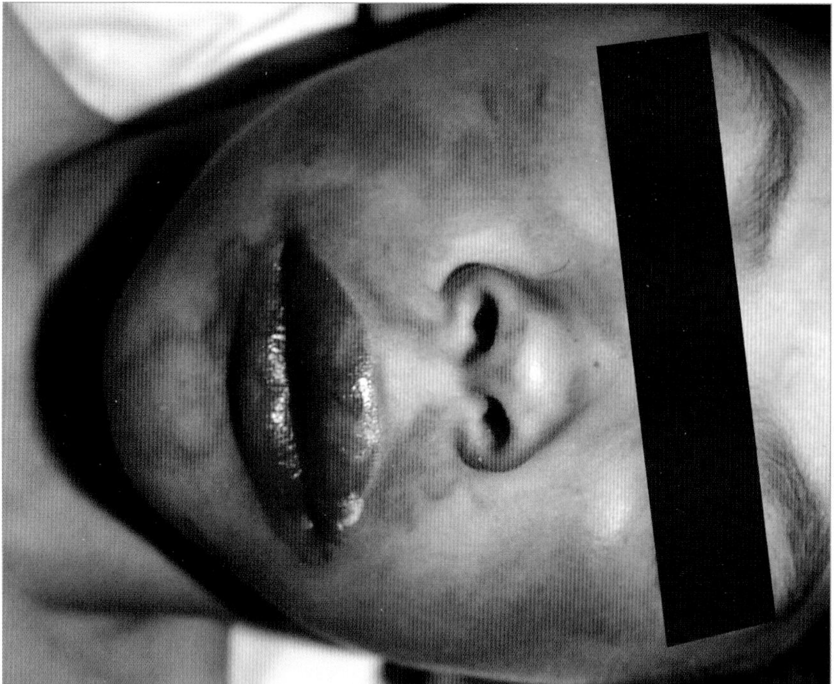

Image 89.7
Erythema multiforme associated with mycoplasma infection. This 10-year-old boy presented with fever and macular lesions on the face, chest, arms, and back, as well as facial swelling. He had a 4-day period of increasing cough and low-grade fever prior to the onset of the skin lesions and facial swelling. Chest radiograph revealed mild increased infiltrates in the right lung. Cold agglutinins were markedly elevated and he had a greater than 4-fold rise in complement fixation antibody to *Mycoplasma pneumoniae*. Courtesy of Neal Halsey, MD.

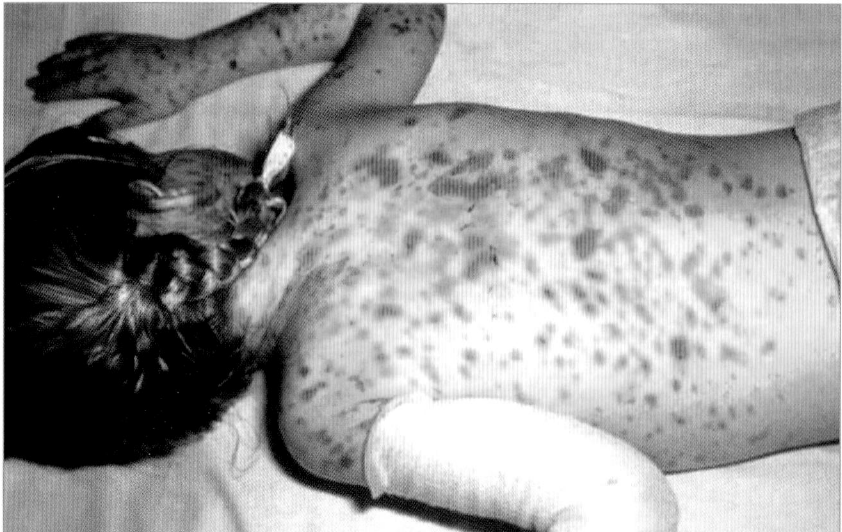

Image 89.8
Erythema multiforme rash (Stevens-Johnson syndrome) associated with *Mycoplasma pneumoniae* infection in a preadolescent girl. Copyright Charles Prober, MD.

90

Nocardiosis

Clinical Manifestations

Immunocompetent children typically develop cutaneous or lymphocutaneous disease with pustular or ulcerative lesions that remain localized after soil contamination of a skin injury. Invasive disease occurs most commonly in people with chronic granulomatous disease, organ transplantation, HIV infection, or disease requiring long-term systemic corticosteroid therapy. Infection has occurred in adults receiving tumor necrosis factor inhibitors, especially infliximab. In immunocompromised children, infection characteristically begins in the lungs, and illness can be acute, subacute, or chronic. Pulmonary disease commonly manifests as rounded nodular infiltrates that can undergo cavitation. Hematogenous spread may occur from the lungs to the brain (single or multiple abscesses), in skin (pustules, pyoderma, abscesses, mycetoma), or, occasionally, in other organs. Some experts recommend neuroimaging in patients with pulmonary disease attributable to the frequency of concurrent central nervous system disease, which can initially be asymptomatic. *Nocardia* organisms can be recovered from patients with cystic fibrosis, but their role as a lung pathogen in these patients is not clear.

Etiology

Nocardia species are gram-positive, filamentous bacteria that belong to a group informally known as the aerobic actinomycetes. Other members of this group include *Actinomadura madurae,* one of several species that are the causative agent of actinomycetoma; *Rhodococcus equi;* and *Gordonia bronchialis.* In the United States, the most prevalent species isolated from human sources are from the *Nocardia asteroides* complex (*Nocardia nova, Nocardia farcinica, Nocardia cyriacigeorgica,* and *Nocardia abscessus*). Primary cutaneous infection is most often associated with *Nocardia brasiliensis.* Other, less common pathogenic species include *Nocardia brevicatena, Nocardia otitidiscaviarum, Nocardia pseudobrasiliensis, Nocardia transvalensis* complex, and *Nocardia veterana.*

Epidemiology

Nocardia species are ubiquitous environmental saprophytes, living in soil, organic matter, and water. Infections caused by *Nocardia* species are typically the result of environmental exposure through inhalation of soil or dust particles or through traumatic inoculation with a soil-contaminated object. Person-to-person and animal-to-human transmission does not occur.

Incubation Period

Unknown.

Diagnostic Tests

Isolation of *Nocardia* species from body fluid, abscess material, or tissue provides a definitive diagnosis. Isolation of *Nocardia* species can require extended incubation periods because of their slow growth. Recovery of *Nocardia* species from tissue can be improved if the laboratory is requested to observe cultures for 3 to 4 weeks in an appropriate liquid medium. Stained smears of sputum, body fluids, or pus demonstrating beaded, branching rods that stain weakly gram positive and partially acid fast by the modified Kinyoun method suggest the diagnosis. Brown-Brenn tissue Gram-stain method and Grocott-Gomori methenamine silver stains are recommended to demonstrate microorganisms in tissue specimens. Serologic tests for *Nocardia* species are not useful.

Treatment

Trimethoprim-sulfamethoxazole or a sulfonamide alone (eg, sulfisoxazole, sulfamethoxazole) has been the drug of choice for mild infections. Sulfonamides that are less urine soluble, such as sulfadiazine, should be avoided. For immunocompromised patients and patients with severe disease, disseminated disease, or central nervous system involvement, combination therapy for the first 4 to 12 weeks is recommended. Suggested combinations include trimethoprim-sulfamethoxazole plus amikacin, meropenem or imipenem, or ceftriaxone. Immunocompetent patients with primary lymphocutaneous disease usually respond after 6 to 12 weeks of therapy. Drainage of abscesses is beneficial. Immunocompromised patients and patients with serious disease should be treated for 6 to 12 months and for at least 3 months after apparent cure because of the propensity for relapse. Patients with AIDS may need even longer therapy, and suppressive therapy should be considered for life.

If infection does not respond to trimethoprim-sulfamethoxazole, other agents, such as clarithromycin (*N nova*), amoxicillin-clavulanate (*N brasiliensis* and *N abscessus*), imipenem, or meropenem, may be beneficial. A case series including a small number of patients demonstrated that linezolid may be effective for treatment of some invasive infections.

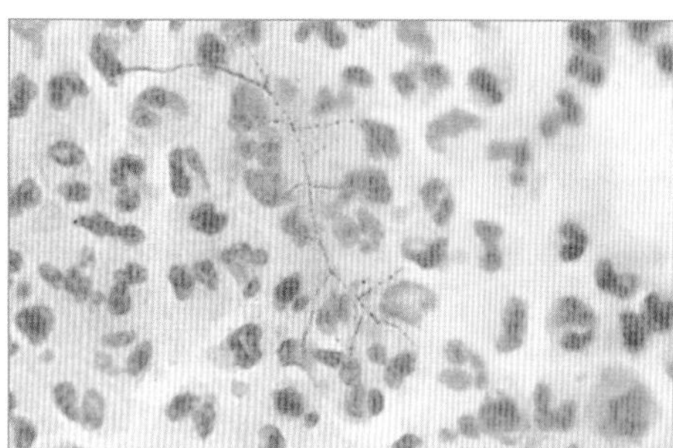

Image 90.1
Nocardia asteroides (Gram stain). Courtesy of Edgar O. Ledbetter, MD, FAAP.

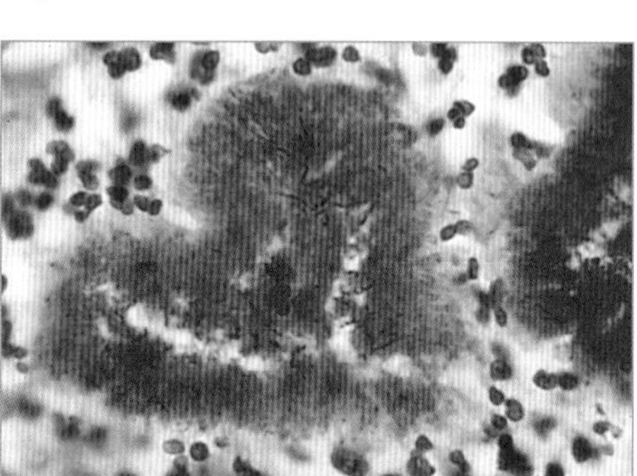

Image 90.3
Note the presence of the gram-positive acid-fast *Nocardia brasiliensis* bacteria using a modified Fite-Faraco stain. Courtesy of Centers for Disease Control and Prevention/Dr Lucille Georg.

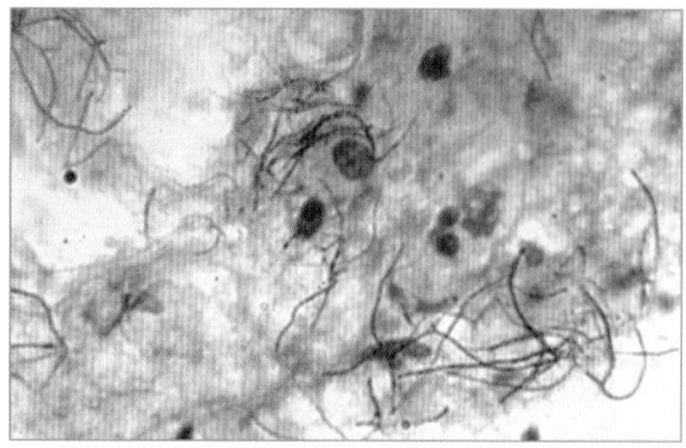

Image 90.5
Nocardia asteroides colony (tissue acid-fast stain).

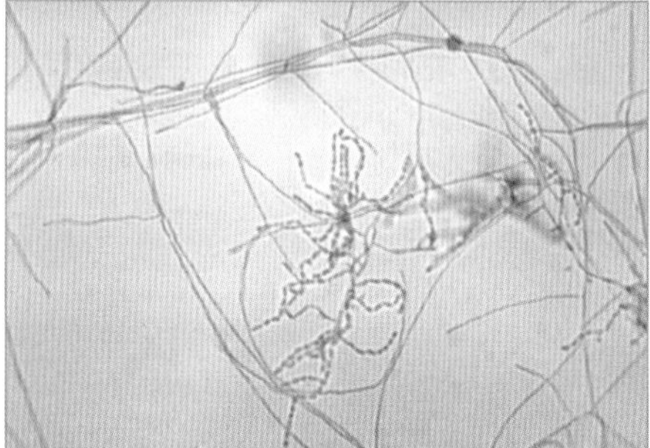

Image 90.2
This gram-positive aerobic *Nocardia asteroides* slide culture reveals chains of aerial mycelia. The filamentous structure of these bacteria tend toward a branching pattern terminating in a rod or coccoid-shaped morphologic appearance. Courtesy of Centers for Disease Control and Prevention/Lucille K. Georg, MD.

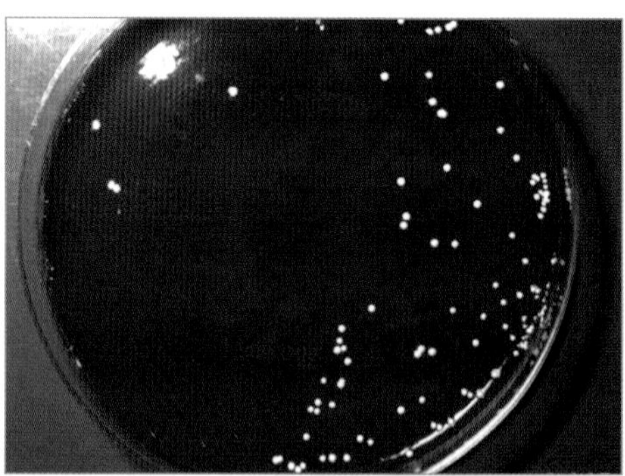

Image 90.4
Nocardia asteroides colonies (white, chalklike colonies on blood agar plate).

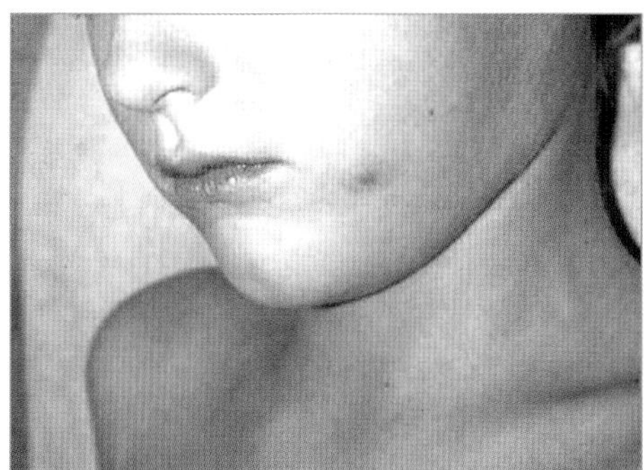

Image 90.6
Cutaneous *Nocardia asteroides* lesion in a 10-year-old boy with no evidence of disseminated disease. Courtesy of Edgar O. Ledbetter, MD, FAAP.

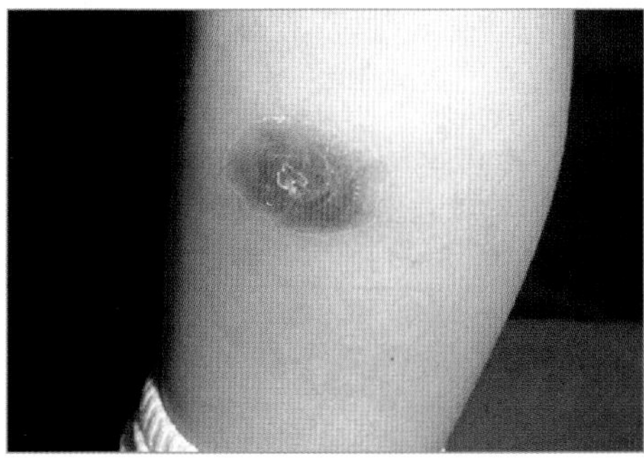

Image 90.8
Cutaneous nocardiosis of lower leg of immunocompetent preschool-aged girl.

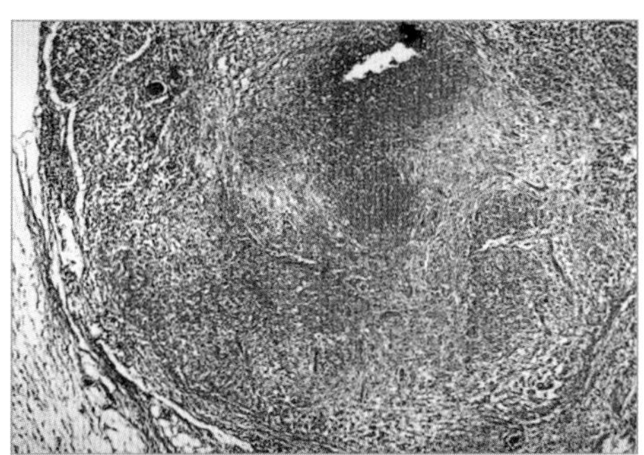

Image 90.10
This photomicrograph depicts the histopathologic changes due to nocardiosis of a mesenteric lymph node. Courtesy of Centers for Disease Control and Prevention/Dr Martin Hicklin.

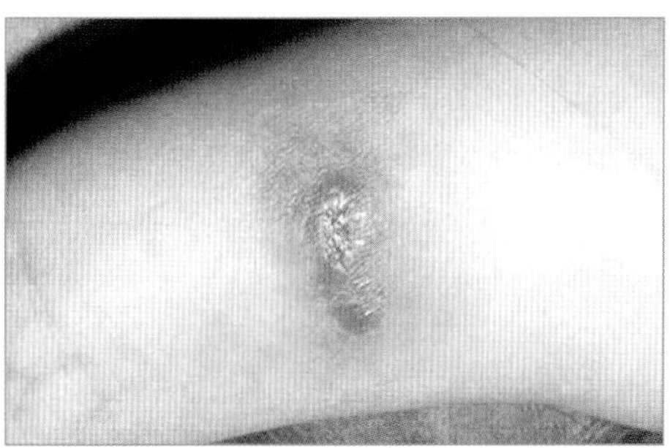

Image 90.7
Cutaneous nocardiosis of forearm in an immunocompetent preschool-aged boy.

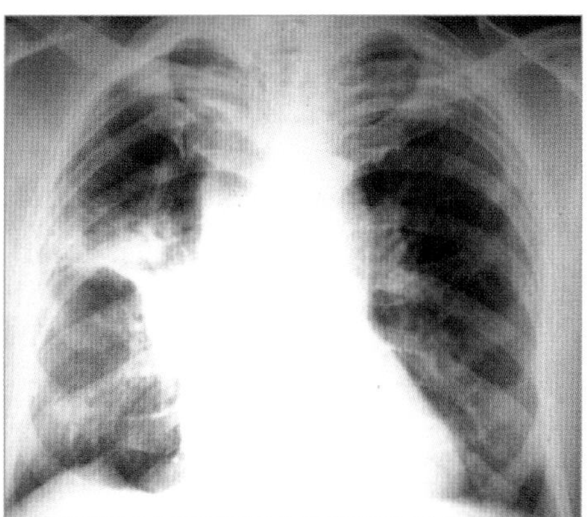

Image 90.9
Nocardia pneumonia, bilateral, in an immuno-compromised child. Invasive nocardiosis is unusual in immunocompetent children.

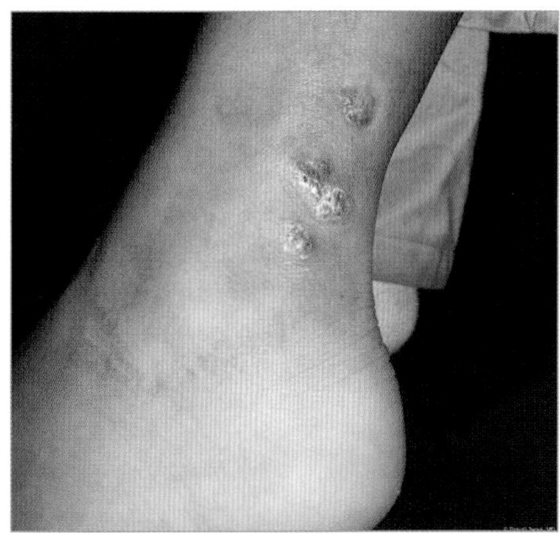

Image 90.11
Hispanic school-aged child with chronic rash on the lower left ankle. Histopathology confirmed *Nocardia brasiliensis*. Courtesy of Preeti Jaggi, MD.

91

Norovirus and Other Human Calicivirus Infections

Clinical Manifestations

Abrupt onset of vomiting accompanied by watery diarrhea, abdominal cramps, and nausea are characteristic of norovirus gastroenteritis. Acute diarrhea without vomiting can also occur. Symptoms last from 24 to 60 hours, but longer courses of illness can occur, particularly among young children. Systemic manifestations, including fever, myalgia, malaise, anorexia, and headache, may accompany gastrointestinal tract symptoms. Since introduction of rotavirus vaccines, noroviruses have become the leading cause of gastroenteritis in the United States.

Etiology

Noroviruses are 27- to 40-nm, RNA viruses of the family Caliciviridae. This family has at least 5 genera (*Lagovirus*, *Nebovirus*, *Vesivirus*, *Sapovirus*, and *Norovirus*), with noroviruses and *Sapovirus* species often referred to as human caliciviruses. Noroviruses are currently divided into 6 genogroups (1–6), of which 3 (1, 2, and 4) can cause human illness.

Epidemiology

Noroviruses are a major cause of sporadic cases and outbreaks of gastroenteritis. Norovirus causes an estimated 1 in 15 US residents to become ill each year, with 56,000 to 71,000 hospitalizations and 570 to 800 deaths. Noroviruses have become the predominant agent of pediatric viral gastroenteritis in the United States. *Sapovirus* infections are reported among children with sporadic acute diarrhea, although, increasingly, *Sapovirus* species have been recognized as a cause of outbreaks. Asymptomatic norovirus excretion is common in children. Outbreaks tend to occur in closed populations (eg, long-term care facilities, schools, cruise ships). Transmission is person to person via fecal-oral or vomitus-oral routes, through contaminated food or water, or by contaminated environmental surfaces. Norovirus is recognized as the most common cause of foodborne illness and foodborne disease outbreaks in the United States. Common-source outbreaks have been described after ingestion of ice, shellfish, and a variety of ready-to-eat foods, including salads, berries, and bakery products, usually contaminated by infected food handlers. Norovirus has been detected in raw or unpasteurized milk or milk products. Viral excretion may start before onset of symptoms, peaks several days after exposure, and can persist for 3 weeks or more. Prolonged excretion has been reported in immunocompromised hosts. Infection occurs year-round but is more common during winter.

Incubation Period

12 to 48 hours.

Diagnostic Tests

A multiplex nucleic acid–based assay for the detection of gastrointestinal pathogens, which includes norovirus, is approved by the US Food and Drug Administration, although it may not be widely available. An enzyme immunoassay kit is also approved for preliminary identification of norovirus. Most state and local public health laboratories use real-time reverse transcriptase-polymerase chain reaction assay for detection of norovirus RNA in stool.

Treatment

Supportive therapy includes oral or intravenous rehydration solutions to replace and maintain fluid and electrolyte balance.

92

Onchocerciasis

(River Blindness, Filariasis)

Clinical Manifestations

The disease involves skin, subcutaneous tissues, lymphatic vessels, and eyes. Subcutaneous, nontender nodules that can be up to several centimeters in diameter containing male and female worms develop 6 to 12 months after initial infection. In patients in Africa, nodules tend to be found on the lower torso, pelvis, and lower extremities, whereas in patients in Central and South America, the nodules are more often located on the upper body (head and trunk) but can occur on the extremities. After the worms mature, fertilized females produce microfilariae that migrate to the dermis and may cause a papular dermatitis. Pruritus is often highly intense, resulting in patient-inflicted excoriations over the affected areas. After a period of years, skin can become lichenified and hypopigmented or hyperpigmented. Microfilariae may invade ocular structures, leading to inflammation of the cornea, iris, ciliary body, retina, choroid, and optic nerve. Loss of visual acuity and blindness can result if the disease is untreated.

Etiology

Onchocerca volvulus is a filarial nematode.

Epidemiology

O volvulus has no significant animal reservoir. Microfilariae in human skin infect *Simulium* species flies (blackflies) when they take a blood meal and then, in 10 to 14 days, develop into infectious larvae that are transmitted with subsequent bites. Blackflies breed in fast-flowing streams and rivers (hence, the colloquial name for the disease, river blindness). The disease occurs primarily in equatorial Africa, but small foci are found in southern Mexico, Guatemala, northern South America, and Yemen. Prevalence is greatest among people who live near vector breeding sites. The infection is not transmissible by person-to-person contact or blood transfusion.

Incubation Period

12 to 18 months from larval inoculation to microfilariae in the skin, but can be as long as 3 years.

Diagnostic Tests

Direct examination of a 1- to 2-mg shaving or biopsy specimen of the epidermis and upper dermis (usually taken from the posterior iliac crest area) can reveal microfilariae. Microfilariae are not found in blood. Adult worms may be demonstrated in excised nodules that have been sectioned and stained. A slit lamp examination of an involved eye may reveal motile microfilariae in the anterior chamber or "snowflake" corneal lesions. Eosinophilia is common. Specific serologic tests and polymerase chain reaction techniques for detection of microfilariae in skin are only available in research laboratories.

Treatment

Ivermectin, a microfilaricidal agent, is the drug of choice for treatment of onchocerciasis. Treatment decreases dermatitis and the risk of developing severe ocular disease but does not kill the adult worms (which can live for more than a decade) and, thus, is not curative. One single oral dose of ivermectin should be given every 6 to 12 months until asymptomatic. Adverse reactions to treatment are caused by death of microfilariae and can include rash, edema, fever, myalgia, and, rarely, asthma exacerbation and hypotension. Such reactions are more common in people with higher skin loads of microfilaria and decrease with repeated treatment in the absence of reexposure. Precautions to ivermectin treatment include pregnancy, central nervous system disorders, and high levels of circulating *Loa loa* microfilaremia. Treatment of patients with high levels of circulating *L loa* microfilaremia with ivermectin can sometimes result in fatal encephalopathy. The American Academy of Pediatrics notes that ivermectin is usually compatible with breastfeeding. A 6-week course of doxycycline can be used to kill adult worms through depletion of the endosymbiotic rickettsia-like bacteria, which appear to be required for survival of *O volvulus*. This approach may be used as adjunctive therapy for children 8 years or older and nonpregnant adults. Doxycycline treatment should be initiated several days after treatment with ivermectin.

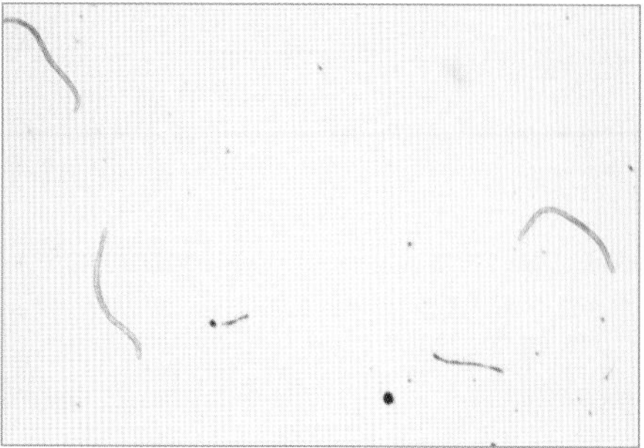

Image 92.1
This is a glycerin mount photomicrograph of the microfilarial pathogen *Onchocerca volvulus* in its larval form. Courtesy of Centers for Disease Control and Prevention/Ladene Newton.

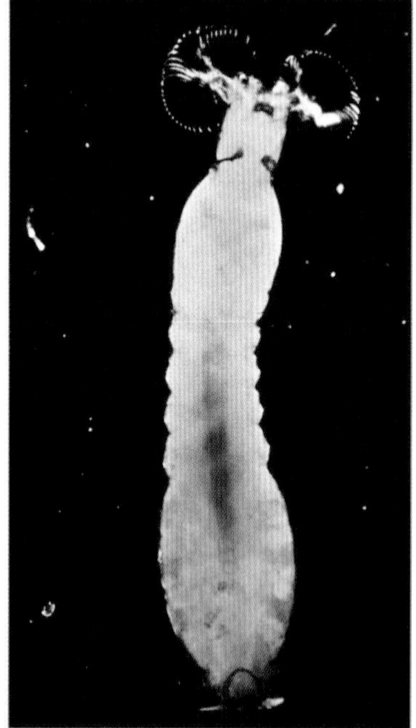

Image 92.3
As an adult, this *Simulium* species larva, or blackfly, is a vector of the disease onchocerciasis, or river blindness. The blackfly larva is usually a filter-feeder, feeding on nutrients extracted from passing currents. Prior to entering the pupal stage, a *Simulium* species larva passes through 6 larval stages and then encases itself in a silken, submerged cocoon. Courtesy of Centers for Disease Control and Prevention/Dr Martin Hicklin.

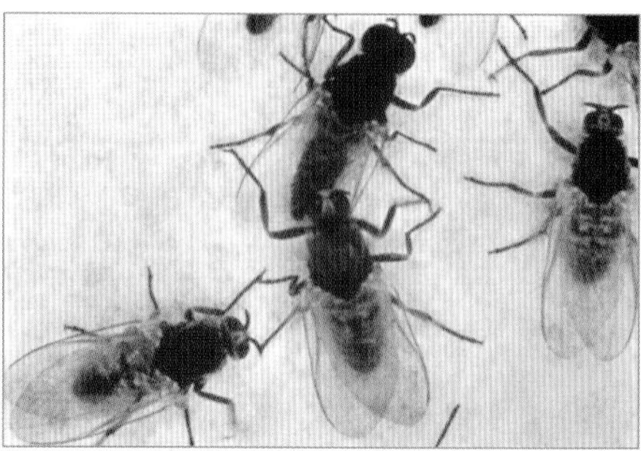

Image 92.2
These are *Simulium* species of flies, or blackflies, a vector of the disease onchocerciasis, or river blindness. Courtesy of World Health Organization.

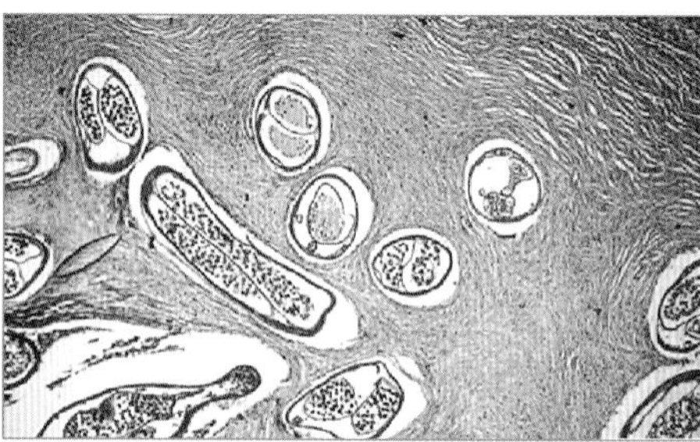

Image 92.4
Histopathologic features of *Onchocerca* nodule in onchocerciasis. Courtesy of Centers for Disease Control and Prevention/Dr Mae Melvin.

93

Human Papillomaviruses

Clinical Manifestations

Human papillomaviruses (HPVs) are a large family of viruses. Most HPV infections are not apparent. However, HPVs can cause benign epithelial proliferation (warts) of the skin and mucous membranes and are associated with cancers. Human papillomaviruses can be grouped into cutaneous and genital (mucosal) types. The cutaneous types cause nongenital warts, including common skin warts, plantar warts, flat warts, threadlike (filiform) warts, and epidermodysplasia verruciformis. Some mucosal types (low risk) are associated with warts or papillomas of mucous membranes, including the upper respiratory tract, anogenital, oral, nasal, and conjunctival areas. Other mucosal types (high risk) are associated with cancers and precancers, including cervical, anogenital, and oropharyngeal cancers.

Common **skin warts** are dome-shaped with conical projections that give the surface a rough appearance. They are usually painless and multiple, commonly occurring on the hands and around or under the nails. When small dermal vessels become thrombosed, black dots appear in the warts.

Plantar warts on the foot are often larger than warts at other sites and may not project through much of the skin surface. They can be painful when walking and are characterized by marked hyperkeratosis, sometimes with black dots.

Flat warts ("juvenile warts") are commonly found on the face and extremities of children and adolescents. They are usually small, multiple, and flat topped; seldom exhibit papillomatosis; and, rarely, cause pain. Filiform warts occur on the face and neck. Cutaneous warts are benign.

Anogenital warts, also called **condylomata acuminata,** are skin-colored warts with a papular, flat, or cauliflowerlike surface that range in size from a few millimeters to several centimeters; these warts often occur in groups. In males, these warts may be found on the penis, scrotum, or anal or perianal area. In females, these lesions can occur on the vulva, anal or perianal area, and, less commonly, in the vagina or on the cervix. Warts usually are painless, although they can cause itching, burning, local pain, or bleeding.

Anogenital **low-grade squamous intraepithelial lesions** can result from persistent infection with low-risk and high-risk HPV types, whereas **high-grade squamous intraepithelial lesions** result from persistent infection with high-risk HPV types. High-grade squamous intraepithelial lesions are considered precancers. In the cervix, these lesions are detected through routine screening with cytologic testing (Papanicolaou [Pap] test); tissue biopsy is required to make the diagnosis. In the past, cervical lesions have been called dysplasias (mild, moderate, severe) or cervical intraepithelial neoplasia (CIN grades 1, 2, or 3, with only grades 2 or 3 being considered cancer precursors). Endocervical glandular precancer, **adenocarcinoma in situ,** also may result from high-risk HPV types. **Invasive cancers** associated with HPV include cervical, vaginal, vulvar, penile, anal, and oropharyngeal.

Juvenile recurrent respiratory papillomatosis is a rare condition characterized by recurring papillomas in the larynx or other areas of the upper respiratory tract. This condition is most commonly diagnosed in children aged 2 to 5 years and manifests as voice change (eg, hoarseness), stridor, or abnormal cry. Respiratory papillomas can cause respiratory tract obstruction in young children. Adult onset has also been described.

Epidermodysplasia verruciformis is a rare, inherited disorder believed to be a consequence of a deficiency of cell-mediated immunity resulting in an abnormal susceptibility to certain HPV types and manifesting as chronic cutaneous HPV infection and frequent development of skin cancer. Lesions may resemble flat warts but are often similar to tinea versicolor, covering the torso and upper extremities. Most appear during the first decade of life, but malignant transformation, which occurs in 30% to 60% of affected people, is usually delayed until adulthood.

Etiology

Human papillomaviruses are DNA viruses of the Papillomaviridae family, which can be grouped into cutaneous and mucosal types. In children, the most common lesions from cutaneous HPVs are hand and foot warts. Mucosal HPVs infect the genital tract and other mucosal surfaces and are grouped into low-risk and high-risk types based on their association with cancers. Low-risk types 6 and 11 are associated with about 90% of condylomata acuminata, recurrent respiratory papillomatosis, and conjunctival papillomas. High-risk types (16, 18, 31, 33, 35, 39, 45, 51, 52, 56, 58, 59, 68, 69, 73, and 82) can cause low-grade cervical cell abnormalities, high-grade cervical cell abnormalities that are precursors to cancer, and anogenital cancers. High-risk HPV types are detected in 99% of cervical cancers. Type 16 is the cause of approximately 50% of cervical cancers worldwide, and types 16 and 18 together account for approximately 70% of cervical cancers. Type 16 is also the cause of most HPV-related oropharyngeal cancers.

Epidemiology

Human papillomavirus types involved in common hand and foot warts are quite different from mucosal types. Nongenital hand and foot warts commonly occur among school-aged children; the prevalence rate is as high as 50%. These can be acquired through casual contact and facilitated through minor skin trauma. Autoinoculation can result in spread of lesions. The intense and often widespread appearance of cutaneous warts in patients with compromised cellular immunity suggests that alterations in T-lymphocyte immunity impair clearance.

Genital HPV infections are transmitted primarily by skin-to-skin contact, usually through sexual intercourse; other genital contact has been associated with transmission. In US females, the highest prevalence of infection is in 20- to 24-year-olds. Most infections are subclinical and clear within 2 years. Persistent infection with high-risk types of HPV is associated with development of cervical cancer, resulting in approximately 12,000 new US cases and 4,000 deaths annually. Cervical cancer is a rare outcome of infection that generally requires decades of persistent infection. Human papillomavirus is also the cause of most vulvar, vaginal, penile, and anal cancers, as well as a significant percentage of oropharyngeal cancers. Nearly 27,000 US cases of HPV-related cancers are diagnosed annually. The risk of development of cancer precursor lesions is greater in people with HIV infection and cellular immune deficiencies.

Rarely, infection is transmitted to a neonate through the birth canal during delivery or from nongenital sites. Respiratory papillomatosis is believed to be acquired by aspiration of infectious maternal secretions intrapartum. When anogenital warts are identified in a child who is beyond infancy but is prepubertal, sexual abuse must be considered.

Incubation Period

Estimated range, 3 months to several years. Human papillomavirus acquired intrapartum by neonates may never cause clinical disease or become apparent over several years.

Diagnostic Tests

Most cutaneous and anogenital warts are diagnosed clinically. Respiratory papillomatosis is diagnosed using endoscopy and biopsy. Cytologic screening (Pap test) and, sometimes, HPV testing of cervical specimens will identify women requiring follow-up with colposcopy and biopsy. Vulvar, vaginal, penile, and anal lesions may be identified using visual inspection; in some cases, cytologic screening (Pap test) is used and suspicious lesions are biopsied. For all anogenital lesions, diagnosis is made on the basis of histologic findings.

Although cytologic and histologic changes can be suggestive of HPV, these findings are not diagnostic of HPV. Detection of HPV infection is based on detection of viral nucleic acid (DNA or RNA) or capsid protein. Clinical tests for high-risk HPV may be used in combination with Pap testing for cervical cancer screening in women 30 years or older and for triage of equivocal Pap test abnormalities (atypical squamous cells of undetermined significance) in women 21 years or older. These HPV tests are not recommended for use in adolescents or men.

Treatment

Treatment of HPV infection is directed toward eliminating lesions. Treatment of anogenital warts may differ from treatment of cutaneous nongenital warts. Regression of nongenital and genital warts occurs in approximately 30% of cases within 6 months. Most methods of treatment of cutaneous warts use chemical or physical destruction of the infected epithelium, including cryotherapy with liquid nitrogen, laser or surgical removal of warts, application of salicylic acid products, or application of topical immune-modulating agents. Daily treatment with tretinoin has been useful for widespread flat warts in children. Care must be taken to avoid a deleterious cosmetic result with therapy.

Treatments for genital warts are characterized as patient applied or provider administered. No one treatment is superior to another. Interventions include ablation or excisional treatments, antiproliferative methods, and immune-modulating therapy. Many agents used for treatment have not been tested for safety and efficacy in children, and some are contraindicated in pregnancy. Although most forms of therapy are successful for initial removal of warts, treatment may not eradicate HPV infection from the surrounding tissue. Recurrences are common and may be attributable to reactivation rather than reinfection.

Cancer precursor lesions that are identified in the cervix (ie, high-grade squamous intraepithelial lesions, adenocarcinoma in situ) and elsewhere in the genital tract require excision or destruction. Overtreatment of cervical lesions can cause substantial economic, emotional, and reproductive adverse effects, including higher risk of preterm birth. Management of invasive cervical and other anogenital and oropharyngeal cancers requires a specialist and should be conducted according to existing guidance.

Respiratory papillomatosis is difficult to treat and is best managed by an experienced otolaryngologist. Local recurrence is common, and repeated surgical procedures for removal are often necessary. Extension or dissemination of respiratory papillomas from the larynx into the trachea, bronchi, or lung parenchyma is rare but can result in increased morbidity and mortality; carcinoma can occur rarely. Intralesional interferon, indole-3-carbinole, photodynamic therapy, intralesional mumps vaccine, and intralesional cidofovir have been used as investigational treatments, but the efficacy of these therapies is uncertain. Oral warts can be removed through cryotherapy, electrocautery, or surgical excision.

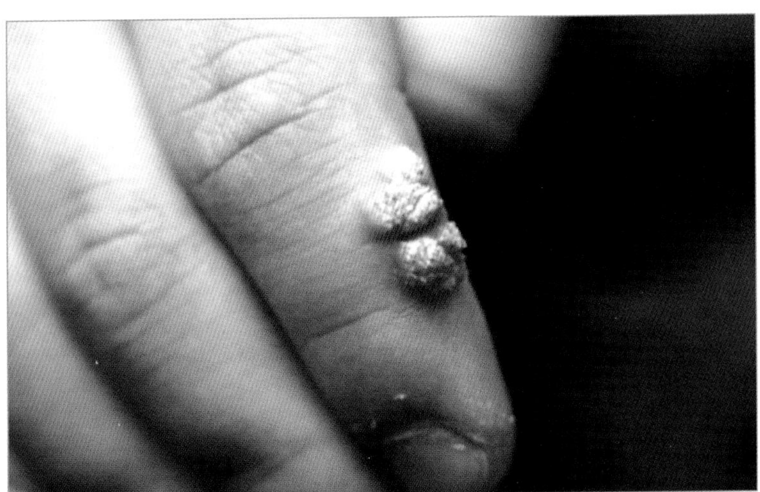

Image 93.1
Digitate human papillomavirus wart with fingerlike projections on a child's index finger. Copyright Gary Williams.

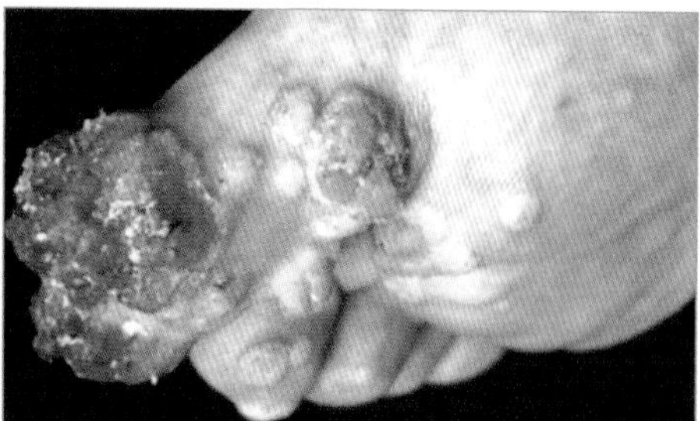

Image 93.2
Human papillomavirus warts on the foot of an immunocompromised 14-year-old boy. Copyright Gary Williams.

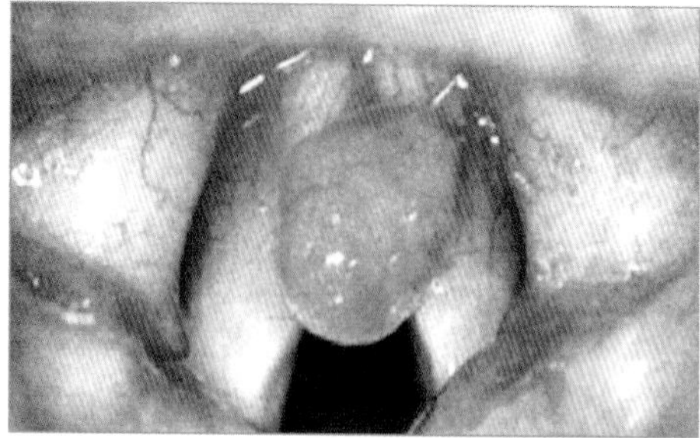

Image 93.3
Laryngeal papillomas may cause hoarseness. Although rare, they can occur in infants of mothers infected with human papillomavirus.

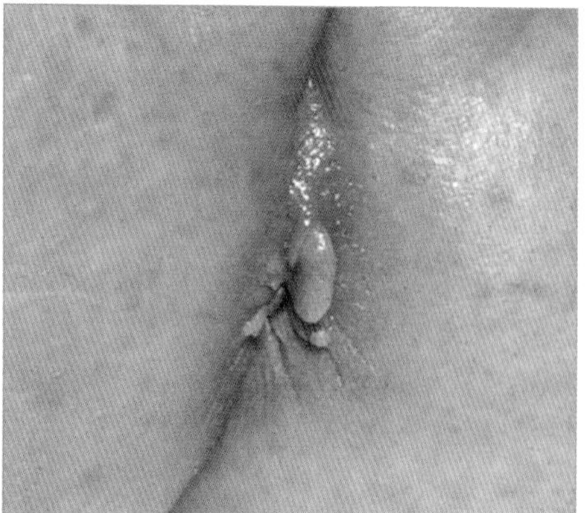

Image 93.4
A 13-month-old girl with condyloma acuminata around the anus from sexual abuse (sodomy). Copyright Martin G. Myers, MD.

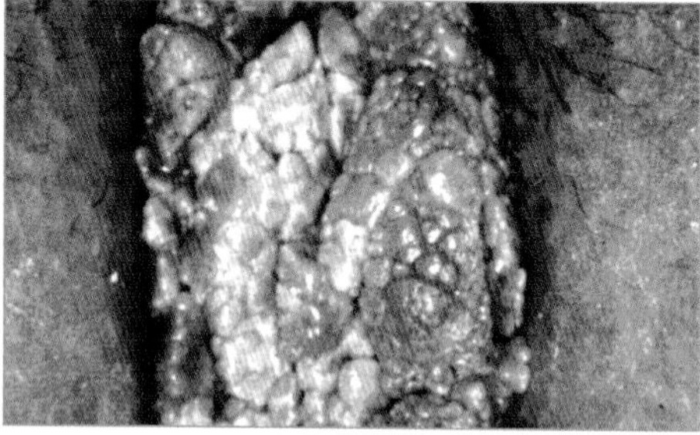

Image 93.5
Massive condyloma acuminata (genital warts) in a 10-year-old girl who had been sexually abused. These genital warts are commonly caused by human papillomavirus, especially types 6 and 11.

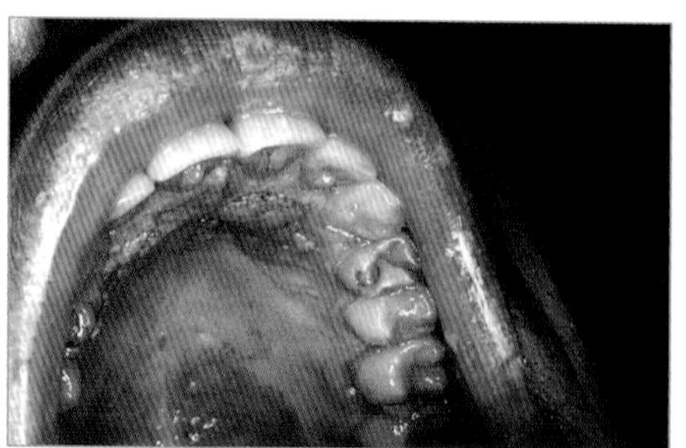

Image 93.6
This HIV-positive patient was exhibiting signs of a secondary condyloma acuminata infection (ie, venereal warts). This intraoral eruption of condyloma acuminata was caused by human papillomavirus (HPV). Although oral HPV is a rare occurrence, HIV reduces the body's immune response and, therefore, such secondary infections can manifest themselves. Courtesy of Centers for Disease Control and Prevention/Sol Silverman Jr, DDS.

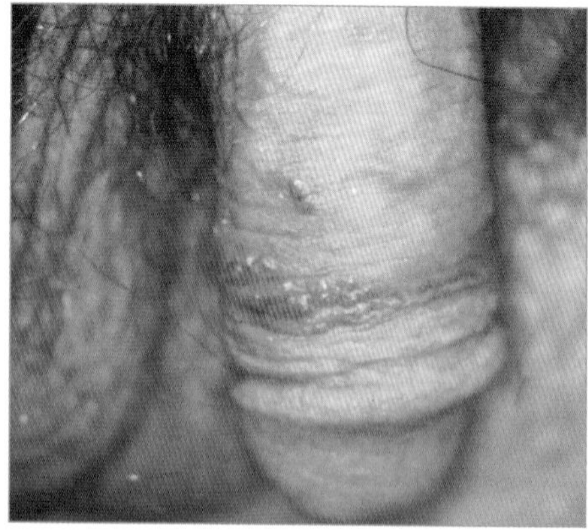

Image 93.7
This patient with condylomata acuminata presented with soft, wartlike growths on the penis (12 hours postpodophyllin application). Condylomata acuminata refers to an epidermal manifestation caused by epidermotropic human papillomavirus. The most commonly affected areas are the penis, vulva, vagina, cervix, perineum, and perianal area. Courtesy of Centers for Disease Control and Prevention/Susan Lindsley.

94

Paracoccidioidomycosis

(South American Blastomycosis)

Clinical Manifestations

Disease occurs primarily in adults, in whom the site of initial infection is the lungs. Disease is infrequent in children, in whom approximately 5% to 10% of all cases occur. Clinical patterns can include subclinical infection or progressive disease that can be acute-subacute (juvenile type) or chronic (adult type). In both forms, constitutional symptoms, such as fever, malaise, anorexia, and weight loss, are common. In the juvenile form, the initial pulmonary infection is usually asymptomatic, and manifestations are related to dissemination of infection to the reticuloendothelial system, resulting in enlarged lymph nodes and involvement of liver, spleen, and bone marrow. Skin lesions are observed regularly and are typically located on the face, neck, and trunk. Involvement of bones, joints, and mucous membranes is less common. Enlarged lymph nodes occasionally coalesce and form abscesses or fistulas. The chronic form of the illness can be localized to the lungs or can disseminate. Oral mucosal lesions are observed in 50%. Skin involvement is common but occurs in a smaller proportion than in patients with the acute-subacute form. Infection can be latent for years before causing illness.

Etiology

Paracoccidioides brasiliensis is a thermally dimorphic fungus with yeast and mycelia phases.

Epidemiology

The infection occurs in Latin America, from Mexico to Argentina. The natural reservoir is unknown, although soil is suspected. The mode of transmission is unknown, but transmission most likely occurs via inhalation of contaminated soil or dust; person-to-person transmission does not occur.

Incubation Period

Highly variable; range, 1 month to many years.

Diagnostic Tests

Round, multiple-budding cells with a distinguishing pilot's wheel appearance can be seen in preparations of sputum, bronchoalveolar lavage specimens, scrapings from ulcers, and material from lesions or in tissue biopsy specimens. Several procedures, including wet or KOH wet preparations, or histologic staining are adequate for visualization of fungal elements. The mycelia form of *P brasiliensis* can be cultured on most enriched media. Its appearance is not distinctive. A number of serologic tests are available; quantitative immunodiffusion is the preferred test. The antibody titer by immunodiffusion usually is 1:32 or greater in acute infection.

Treatment

Amphotericin B is preferred by many experts for initial treatment of severe paracoccidioidomycosis. An alternative is intravenous trimethoprim-sulfamethoxazole. Children treated initially by the intravenous route can transition to orally administered therapy after clinical improvement has been observed, usually after 3 to 6 weeks.

Oral therapy with itraconazole is the treatment of choice for less severe or localized infection and to complete treatment when amphotericin B is used initially. Prolonged therapy for 6 to 12 months is necessary to minimize the relapse rate. Children with severe disease can require a longer course. Voriconazole is as well tolerated and as effective as itraconazole in adults, but data for its use in children with paracoccidioidomycosis are not available. Trimethoprim-sulfamethoxazole orally is an alternative, but treatment must be continued for 2 years or longer to lessen the risk of relapse, which occurs in 10% to 15% of optimally treated patients.

Serial serologic testing by quantitative immunodiffusion is useful for monitoring the response to therapy. The expected response is a progressive decline in titers after 1 to 3 months of treatment with stabilization at a low titer.

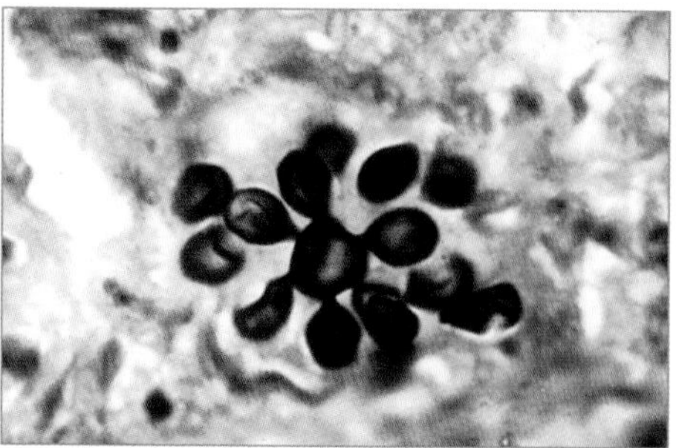

Image 94.1
Histopathologic features of paracoccidioidomycosis. Budding cell of *Paracoccidioides brasiliensis* (methenamine silver stain). Courtesy of Centers for Disease Control and Prevention.

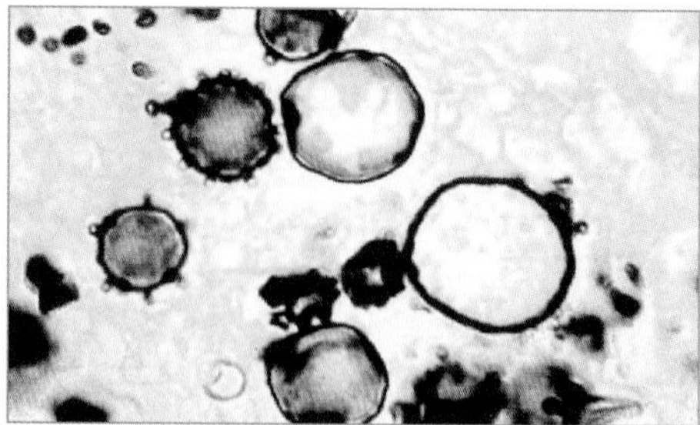

Image 94.2
Histopathologic features of paracoccidioidomycosis, liver. Minute buds on several cells of *Paracoccidioides brasiliensis* (methenamine silver stain). Courtesy of Centers for Disease Control and Prevention/Dr Lucille K. Georg.

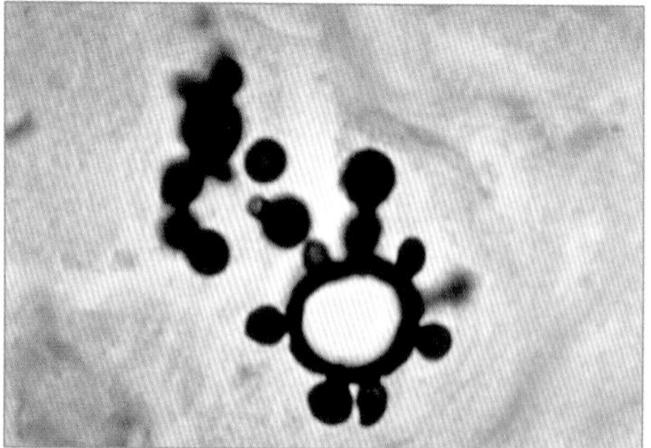

Image 94.3
Histopathology of paracoccidioidomycosis. Budding cells of *Paracoccidioides brasiliensis* (methenamine silver stain). Courtesy of Centers for Disease Control and Prevention/Dr Lucille K. Georg.

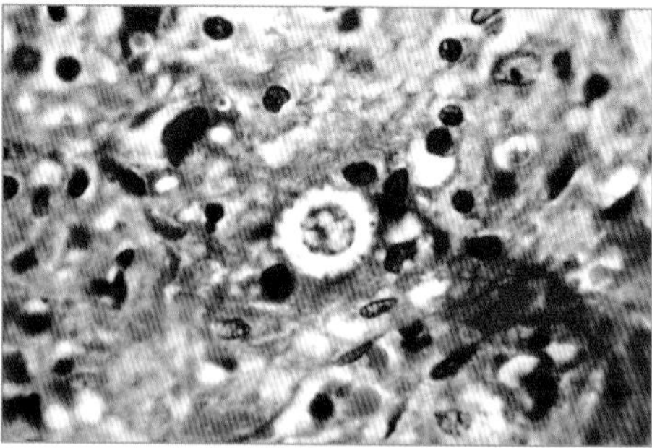

Image 94.4
This micrograph depicts the histopathologic changes associated with paracoccidioidomycosis due to *Paracoccidioides brasiliensis.* This is the only etiological agent for the disease paracoccidioidomycosis. The *P brasiliensis* fungus is geographically restricted to areas of South and Central America. A cell of *P brasiliensis* is centrally located. Courtesy of Centers for Disease Control and Prevention/Dr Lucille K. Georg.

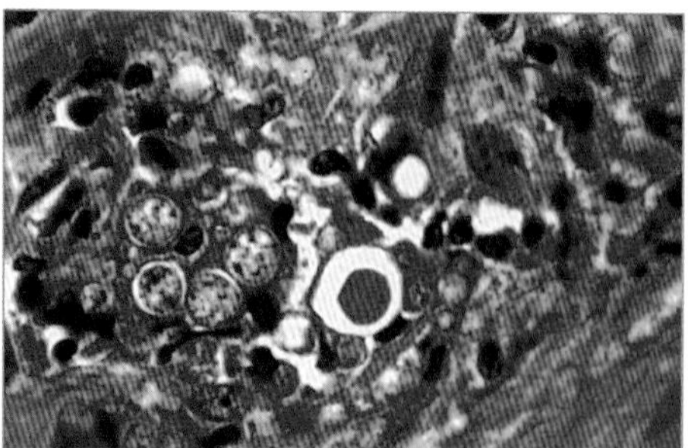

Image 94.5
Histopathologic features of paracoccidioidomycosis from skin sample. Cells of *Paracoccidioides brasiliensis* are visible. Courtesy of Centers for Disease Control and Prevention/Dr Lucille K. Georg.

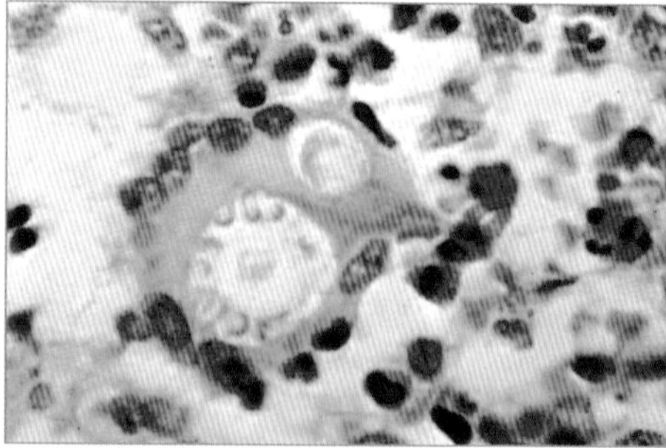

Image 94.6
Histopathologic features of paracoccidioidomycosis, skin. Budding cell of *Paracoccidioides brasiliensis* within multinucleated giant cell. Courtesy of Centers for Disease Control and Prevention/Dr Lucille K. Georg.

95

Paragonimiasis

Clinical Manifestations

There are 2 major forms of paragonimiasis: disease attributable to *Paragonimus westermani, Paragonimus heterotrema, Paragonimus africanus, Paragonimus uterobilateralis,* and *Paragonimus kellicotti* causing primary pulmonary disease with or without extrapulmonary manifestations, and disease attributable to other species of *Paragonimus,* most notably *Paragonimus skrjabini,* for which humans are accidental hosts and manifestations generally are extrapulmonary, resulting in a larva migrans syndrome similar to that caused by *Toxocara canis.* The former disease is especially likely to have an insidious onset and a chronic course. Pulmonary disease is associated with chronic cough and dyspnea, but most infections are probably inapparent or result in mild symptoms. Heavy infestations cause paroxysms of coughing, which often produce blood-tinged sputum that is brown because of the presence of *Paragonimus* species eggs. Hemoptysis can be severe. Pleural effusion, pneumothorax, bronchiectasis, and pulmonary fibrosis with clubbing can develop. Extrapulmonary manifestations also may involve liver, spleen, abdominal cavity, intestinal wall, intra-abdominal lymph nodes, skin, and central nervous system, with meningoencephalitis, seizures, and space-occupying tumors attributable to invasion of the brain by adult flukes, usually occurring within a year of pulmonary infection. Symptoms tend to subside after approximately 5 years but can persist for as many as 20 years.

Extrapulmonary paragonimiasis is associated with migratory allergic subcutaneous nodules containing juvenile worms. Pleural effusion is common, as is invasion of the brain.

Etiology

In Asia, classical paragonimiasis is caused by adult flukes and eggs of *P westermani* and *P heterotrema.* In Africa, the adult flukes and eggs of *P africanus* and *P uterobilateralis* produce the disease, whereas in North America, the endemic species is *P kellicotti.* In North America, disease has also been caused by *P westermani,* present in imported crab. The adult flukes of *P westermani* are up to 12 mm long and 7 mm wide and occur throughout Asia. A triploid parthenogenetic form of *P westermani,* which is larger, produces more eggs, and elicits greater disease, has been described in Japan, Korea, Taiwan, and parts of eastern China. *P heterotrema* occurs in Southeast Asia and adjacent parts of China.

Extrapulmonary paragonimiasis (ie, visceral larva migrans) is caused by larval stages of *P skrjabini* and *Paragonimus miyazakii.* The worms rarely mature in infected human tissues. *P skrjabini* occurs in China, whereas *P miyazakii* occurs in Japan. *Paragonimus mexicanus* and *Paragonimus ecuadoriensis* occur in Mexico, Costa Rica, Ecuador, and Peru. *P kellicotti,* a lung fluke of mink and opossums in the United States, can also cause infection in humans.

Epidemiology

Transmission occurs when raw or undercooked freshwater crabs or crayfish containing larvae (metacercariae) are ingested. Numerous cases have been associated with ingestion of uncooked crawfish during river raft trips in the Midwestern United States. The metacercariae excyst in the small intestine and penetrate the abdominal cavity, where they remain for a few days before migrating to the lungs. *P westermani* and *P heterotrema* mature within the lungs over 6 to 10 weeks, when they begin egg production. Eggs escape from pulmonary capsules into the bronchi and exit from the human host in sputum or feces. Eggs hatch in freshwater within 3 weeks, giving rise to miracidia. Miracidia penetrate freshwater snails and emerge several weeks later as cercariae, which encyst within the muscles and viscera of freshwater crustaceans before maturing into infective metacercariae. A less common mode of transmission that may also occur is human infection through the ingestion of raw pork, usually from wild pigs, containing the juvenile stages of *Paragonimus* species (described as occurring in Japan).

Humans are accidental ("dead-end") hosts for *P skrjabini* and *P miyazakii* in visceral larva migrans. These flukes cannot mature in humans and, hence, do not produce eggs.

Paragonimus species also infect a variety of other mammals, such as canids, mustelids, felids, and rodents, which serve as animal reservoir hosts.

Incubation Period

Variable; egg production begins by approximately 8 weeks after ingestion of *P westermani* metacercariae.

Diagnostic Tests

Microscopic examination of stool, sputum, pleural effusion, cerebrospinal fluid, and other tissue specimens may reveal eggs. A Western blot serologic antibody test based on *P westermani* antigen, available at the Centers for Disease Control and Prevention, is sensitive and specific; antibody concentrations detected by immunoblot decrease slowly after the infection is cured by treatment. Charcot-Leyden crystals and eosinophils in sputum are useful diagnostic elements. Chest radiographs can appear normal or resemble radiographs from patients with tuberculosis. Misdiagnosis is likely unless paragonimiasis is suspected.

Treatment

Praziquantel in a 2-day course is the treatment of choice and is associated with high cure rates as demonstrated by disappearance of egg production and radiographic lesions in the lungs. The drug is also effective for some extrapulmonary manifestations. An alternative drug for patients unable to take praziquantel is triclabendazole; it is not commercially available but may be obtained from the Centers for Disease Control and Prevention under an investigational drug protocol. For patients with central nervous system paragonimiasis, a short course of steroids may be beneficial in addition to the praziquantel.

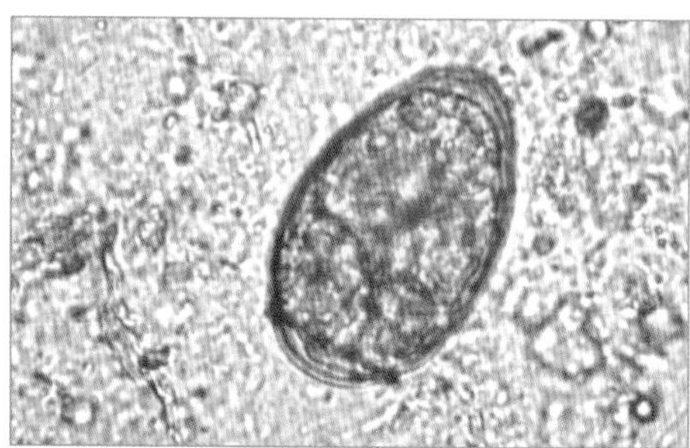

Image 95.1
Paragonimus westermani ova in stool preparation (original magnification x400).

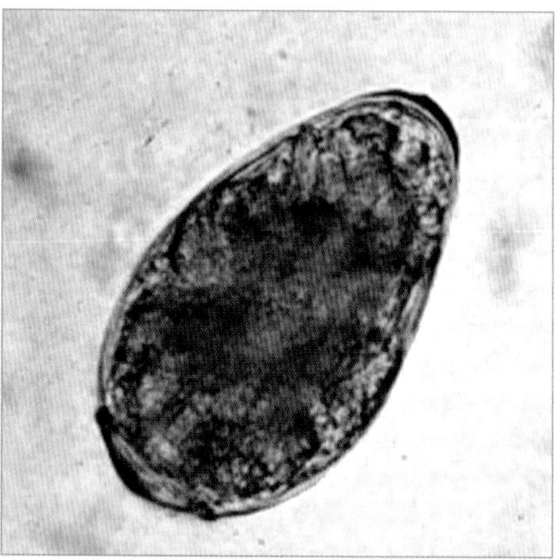

Image 95.2
Ovum of *Paragonimus westermani*. The average ovum size is 85 by 53 µm (range, 68–118 µm by 39–67 µm). They are yellow-brown and ovoid or elongate, with a thick shell, and often asymmetric, with one end slightly flattened. At the large end, the operculum is clearly visible. The opposite (abopercular) end is thickened. The ova of *P westermani* are excreted unembryonated and may be found in the stool or sputum. Courtesy of Centers for Disease Control and Prevention.

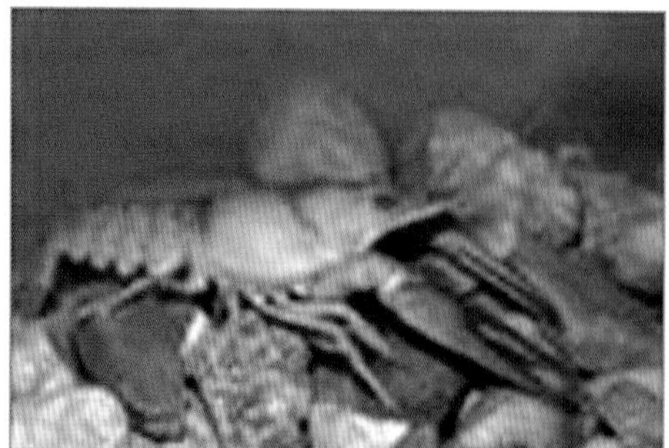

Image 95.3
Eating raw or undercooked crabs or crayfish can result in human paragonimiasis, a parasitic disease caused by *Paragonimus westermani* and *Paragonimus heterotrema*. Courtesy of Centers for Disease Control and Prevention.

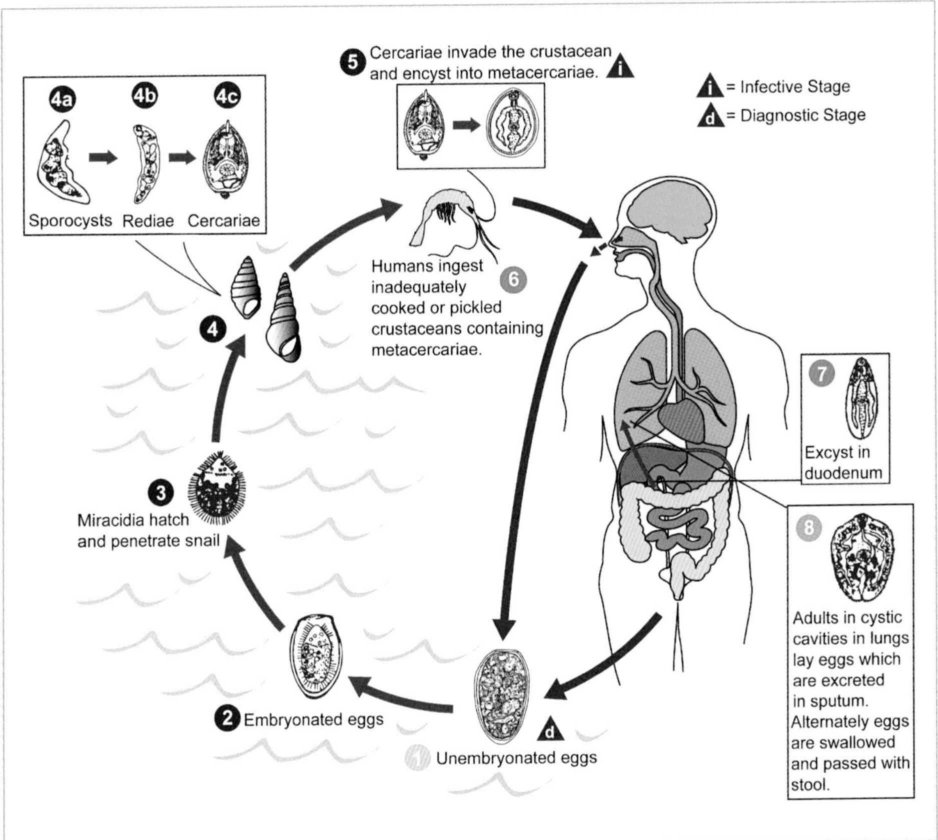

Image 95.4

Life cycle of *Paragonimus westermani*. The eggs are excreted unembryonated in the sputum or, alternately, they are swallowed and passed with stool (1). In the external environment, the eggs become embryonated (2), and miracidia hatch and seek the first intermediate host, a snail, and penetrate its soft tissues (3). Miracidia go through several developmental stages inside the snail (4): sporocysts (4a), rediae (4b), with the latter giving rise to many cercariae (4c), which emerge from the snail. The cercariae invade the second intermediate host, a crustacean such as a crab or crayfish, where they encyst and become metacercariae. This is the infective stage for the mammalian host (5). Human infection with *P westermani* occurs by eating inadequately cooked or pickled crab or crayfish that harbor metacercariae of the parasite (6). The metacercariae excyst in the duodenum (7), penetrate through the intestinal wall into the peritoneal cavity, then through the abdominal wall and diaphragm into the lungs, where they become encapsulated and develop into adults (8) (7.5–12 mm by 4–6 mm). The worms can also reach other organs and tissues, such as the brain and striated muscles, respectively. However, when this takes place, completion of the life cycles is not achieved because the eggs laid cannot exit these sites. Time from infection to oviposition is 65 to 90 days. Infections may persist for 20 years in humans. Animals such as pigs, dogs, and a variety of feline species can also harbor *P westermani*. Courtesy of Centers for Disease Control and Prevention/Alexander J. da Silva, PhD/Melanie Moser.

96

Parainfluenza Viral Infections

Clinical Manifestations

Parainfluenza viruses (PIVs) are the major cause of laryngotracheobronchitis (croup) but also upper respiratory tract infection, bronchiolitis, and pneumonia. Parainfluenza virus 1 (PIV1) and, to a lesser extent, 2 (PIV2) are the most common pathogens associated with croup. Parainfluenza virus 3 (PIV3) is most commonly associated with bronchiolitis and pneumonia in infants and young children. Infections with parainfluenza virus 4 (PIV4) are less well characterized, but studies using sensitive molecular assays suggest they may be more common than previously appreciated. Rarely, PIVs have been isolated from patients with parotitis, aseptic meningitis, encephalitis, or Guillain-Barré syndrome. Parainfluenza virus infections can exacerbate symptoms of chronic lung disease and asthma in children and adults. In children with immunodeficiency and recipients of hematopoietic stem cell transplants, PIVs can cause refractory infections with persistent shedding, severe pneumonia with viral dissemination, and even fatal disease, most commonly caused by PIV3. Parainfluenza virus infections do not confer complete protective immunity; reinfections can occur with all serotypes and at any age, but reinfections usually cause a mild illness limited to the upper respiratory tract.

Etiology

Parainfluenza viruses are enveloped, single-stranded, negative-sense RNA viruses classified in the family Paramyxoviridae. Four antigenically distinct types—1, 2, 3, and 4 (with 2 subtypes, 4A and 4B)—that infect humans have been identified.

Epidemiology

Parainfluenza viruses are transmitted from person to person by direct contact and exposure to contaminated nasopharyngeal secretions through respiratory tract droplets and fomites. Parainfluenza virus infections can be sporadic or associated with outbreaks of acute respiratory tract disease. Seasonal patterns of infection are distinct, predictable, and cyclic in temperate regions. Different serotypes have distinct epidemiologic patterns. Parainfluenza virus 1 tends to produce outbreaks of respiratory tract illness, usually croup, in the autumn of every other year. Parainfluenza virus 2 can also cause outbreaks of respiratory tract illness in the autumn, often in conjunction with PIV1 outbreaks, but PIV2 outbreaks tend to be less severe, irregular, and less common. Parainfluenza virus 3 is endemic and usually is prominent during spring and summer in temperate climates but often continues into autumn, especially in years when autumn outbreaks of PIV1 or PIV2 are absent. Infections with PIV4 are recognized less commonly and can be associated with illnesses ranging from mild to severe.

The age of primary infection varies with serotype. Primary infection with all types usually occurs by 5 years of age. Infection with PIV3 occurs more often in infants and is a prominent cause of bronchiolitis and pneumonia in this age group. By 12 months of age, 50% of infants have acquired PIV3 infection. Infections between 1 and 5 years of age more commonly are associated with PIV1 and, to a lesser extent, PIV2. Age at acquisition of PIV4 infection is not well defined. Rates of PIV-associated hospitalizations for children vary depending on clinical syndrome, PIV type, and patient age.

Immunocompetent children with primary PIV infection can shed virus for up to 1 week before onset of clinical symptoms and for 1 to 3 weeks after symptoms have disappeared, depending on serotype. Severe lower respiratory tract disease with prolonged shedding of the virus can develop in immunodeficient people. In these patients, infection may spread beyond the respiratory tract to the liver and lymph nodes.

Incubation Period

2 to 6 days.

Diagnostic Tests

Parainfluenza viruses may be isolated from nasopharyngeal secretions, usually within 4 to 7 days of culture inoculation or earlier by use of centrifugation of the specimen onto a monolayer of susceptible cells (shell vial assay). Highly sensitive reverse transcriptase-polymerase chain reaction assays are also available commercially for detection and differentiation of PIVs. Rapid antigen identification techniques, including immunofluorescence assays, can be used to detect the viruses in nasopharyngeal secretions, but sensitivities of the tests vary. Serologic diagnosis, made retrospectively by a significant increase in antibody titer between serum specimens obtained during acute infection and convalescence, is less useful.

Treatment

Specific antiviral therapy is not available. Most infections are self-limited and require no treatment. Monitoring for hypoxia and hypercapnia in more severely affected children with lower respiratory tract disease is useful. For laryngotracheobronchitis, racemic epinephrine aerosol is commonly given to severely affected hospitalized patients with croup. Parenteral, oral, and nebulized corticosteroids have been demonstrated to lessen the severity and duration of symptoms and hospitalization in patients with moderate to severe laryngotracheobronchitis. Oral steroids are also effective for outpatients with less severe croup. Management is otherwise supportive.

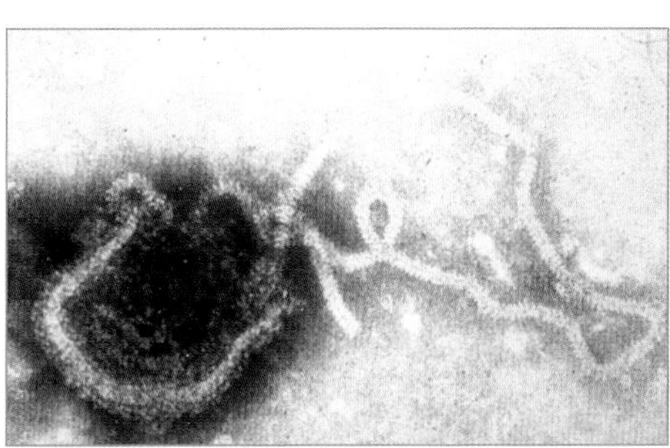

Image 96.1
Electron micrograph of parainfluenza virus. Copyright Charles Prober.

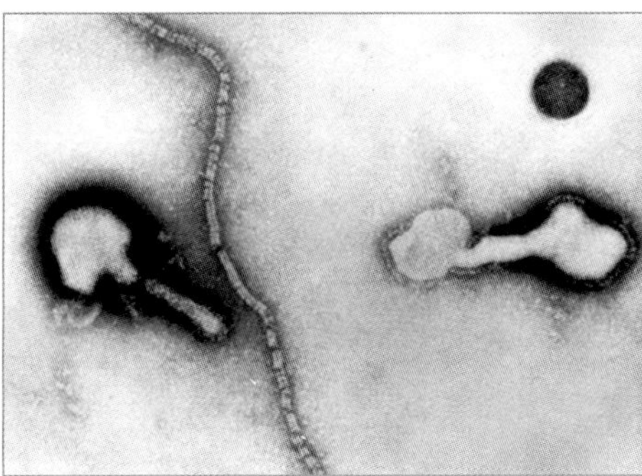

Image 96.2
Transmission electron micrograph of parainfluenza virus showing 2 intact particles and a free filamentous nucleocapsid. Courtesy of Centers for Disease Control and Prevention/Dr Erskine Palmer.

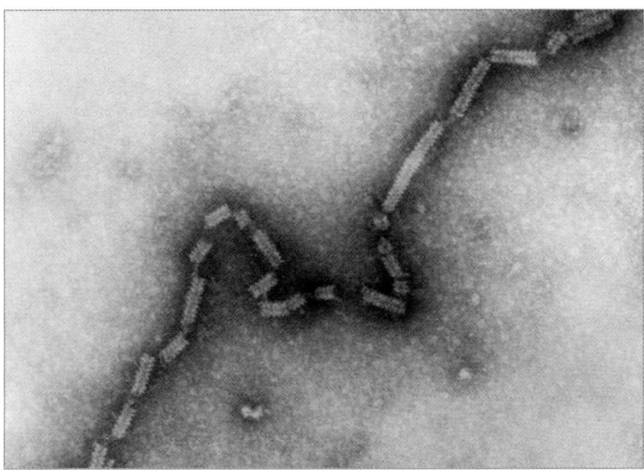

Image 96.3
This electron micrograph depicts the paramyxovirus 4A nucleocapsid with its herringbone-shaped RNA core. Courtesy of Centers for Disease Control and Prevention/Dr Fred Murphy.

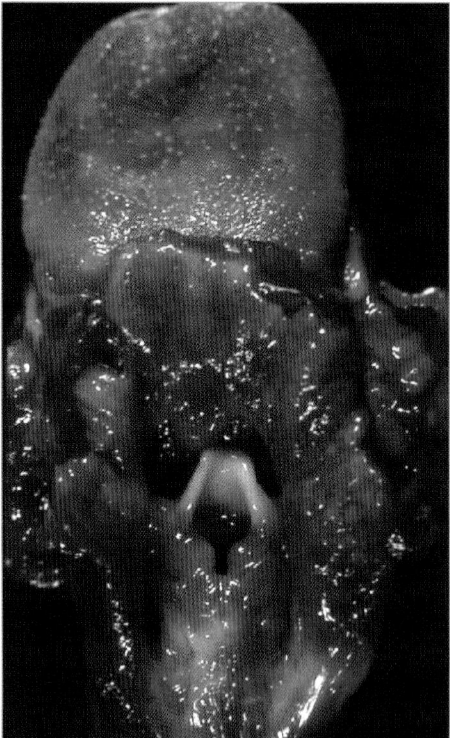

Image 96.4
Fatal croup. Edema, congestion, and inflammation of larynx and pharynx. Courtesy of Dimitris P. Agamanolis, MD.

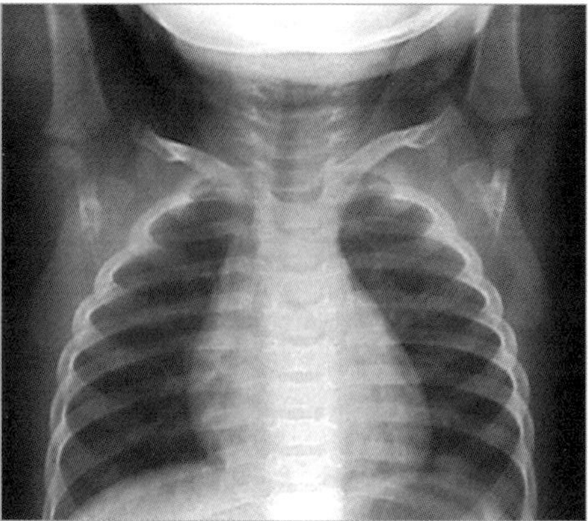

Image 96.5
Parainfluenza laryngotracheitis in a 2-year-old boy. Courtesy of Benjamin Estrada, MD.

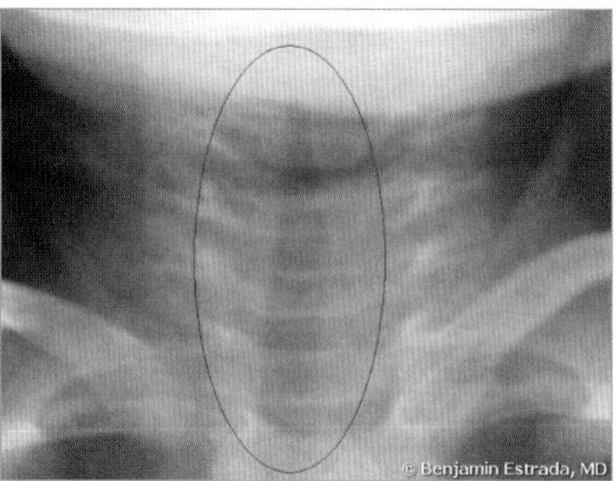

Image 96.6
Parainfluenza laryngotracheitis with the steeple sign in a 2-year-old. Courtesy of Benjamin Estrada, MD.

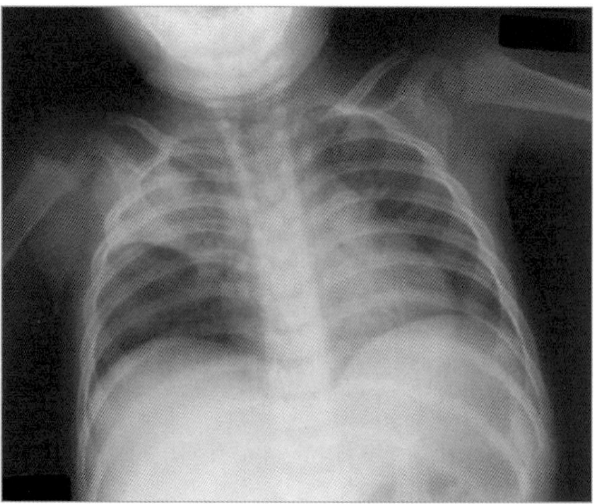

Image 96.7
Parainfluenza pneumonia in a 2-year-old boy. Courtesy of Benjamin Estrada, MD.

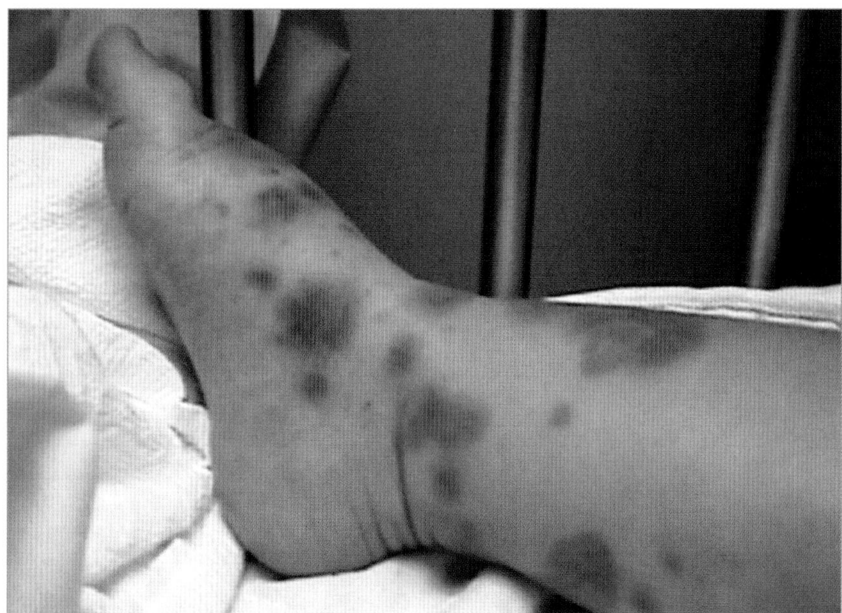

Image 96.8
Erythema multiforme minor in a 2-year-old boy with parainfluenza. Courtesy of Larry Frenkel, MD.

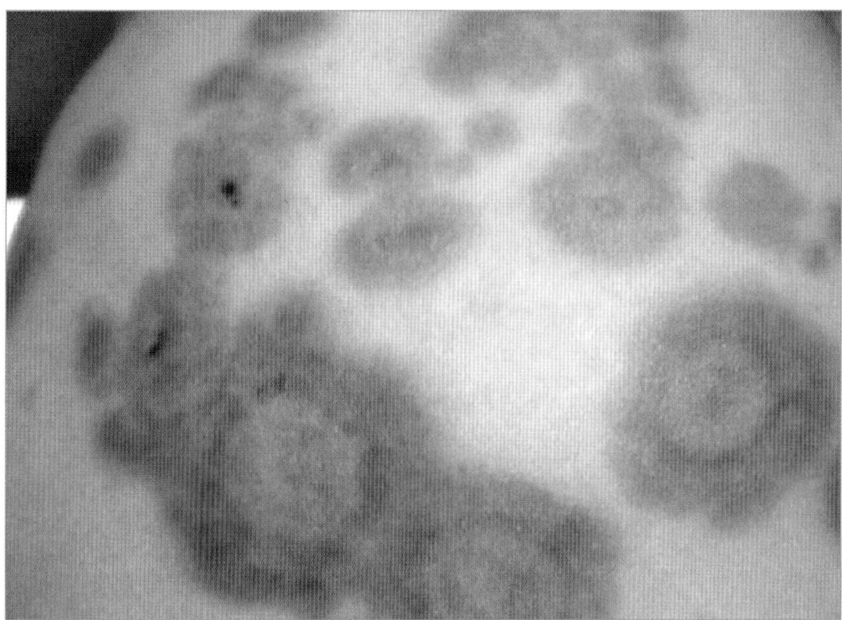

Image 96.9
Erythema multiforme minor in a 2-year-old boy with parainfluenza. Courtesy of Larry Frenkel, MD.

97

Parasitic Diseases

Many parasitic diseases have traditionally been considered exotic and, therefore, frequently are not included in differential diagnoses of patients in the United States, Canada, and Europe. Nevertheless, a number of these organisms are endemic in industrialized countries, and, overall, parasites are among the most common causes of morbidity and mortality in various and diverse geographic locations worldwide. Outside the tropics and subtropics, parasitic diseases are particularly common among tourists returning to their own countries, immigrants from areas with highly endemic infection, and people who are immunocompromised. Some of these infections disproportionately affect impoverished populations, such as black and Hispanic people living in the United States and aboriginal people living in Alaska and the Canadian Arctic. Physicians and clinical laboratory personnel need to be aware of where these infections can be acquired, their clinical presentations, and methods of diagnosis and should advise people how to prevent infection (Table 97.1).

Consultation and assistance in diagnosis and management of parasitic diseases are available from the Centers for Disease Control and Prevention, state health departments, and university departments or divisions of geographic medicine, tropical medicine, pediatric infectious diseases, global health, and public health. Important human parasitic infections are discussed in individual chapters; the diseases are arranged alphabetically. The recommendation for drugs is found in the disease-specific chapters.

Table 97.1
Parasitic Diseases Not Covered Elsewhere

Disease/Agent	Where Infection May Be Acquired	Definitive Host	Intermediate Host	Modes of Human Infection	Directly Communicable (Person to Person)	Diagnostic Laboratory Tests in Humans	Causative Form of Parasite	Manifestations in Humans
Angiostrongylus cantonensis (neurotropic disease)	Widespread in the tropics, particularly Pacific Islands, Southeast Asia, Central and South America, the Caribbean, and the United States	Rats	Snails and slugs	Eating improperly cooked infected mollusks or food contaminated by mollusk secretions containing larvae; prawns, fish, and land crabs that have ingested infected mollusks also may be infectious.	No	Eosinophils in CSF; rarely, identification of larvae in CSF or at autopsy; serologic test	Larval worms	Eosinophilia, meningo-encephalitis
Angiostrongylus costaricensis (gastrointestinal tract disease)	Central and South America	Rodents	Snails and slugs	Eating improperly/poorly cooked infected mollusks or food contaminated by mollusk secretions containing larvae	No	Gel diffusion; identification of larvae and eggs in tissue	Larval worms	Abdominal pain, eosinophilia
Anisakiasis	Cosmopolitan, most common where eating raw fish is practiced	Marine mammal	Certain salt-water fish, squid, and octopus	Eating uncooked or inadequately treated infected marine fish	No	Identification of recovered larvae in granulomas or vomitus	Larval worms	Acute gastrointestinal tract disease
Opisthorchis (*Clonorchis*) *sinensis, Opisthorchis viverrini, Opisthorchis felineus* (flukes)	East Asia, Eastern Europe, Russian Federation	Humans, cats, dogs, other mammals	Certain fresh-water snails	Eating uncooked infected freshwater fish	No	Eggs in stool or duodenal fluid	Larvae and mature flukes	Abdominal pain; hepatobiliary disease Cholangio-carcinoma

Table 97.1
Parasitic Diseases Not Covered Elsewhere (*continued*)

Disease/Agent	Where Infection May Be Acquired	Definitive Host	Intermediate Host	Modes of Human Infection	Directly Communicable (Person to Person)	Diagnostic Laboratory Tests in Humans	Causative Form of Parasite	Manifestations in Humans
Dracunculiasis (*Dracunculus medinensis*) (guinea worm)	Foci in Africa Global eradication nearly achieved	Humans	Crustacea (copepods)	Drinking water infested with infected copepods	No	Identification of emerging or adult worm in subcutaneous tissues	Adult female worm	Emerging roundworm; inflammatory response; systemic and local blister or ulcer in skin
Fasciolopsiasis (*Fasciolopsis buski*)	East Asia	Humans, pigs, dogs	Certain freshwater snails, plants	Eating uncooked infected plants	No	Eggs or worm in feces or duodenal fluid	Larvae and mature worms	Diarrhea, constipation, vomiting, anorexia, edema of face and legs, ascites
Intestinal capillariasis (*Capillaria philippinensis*)	Philippines, Thailand	Humans, fish-eating birds	Fish	Ingestion of uncooked infected fish	Uncertain	Eggs and parasite in feces	Larvae and mature worms	Protein-losing enteropathy, diarrhea, malabsorption, ascites, emaciation

Abbreviation: CSF, cerebrospinal fluid.

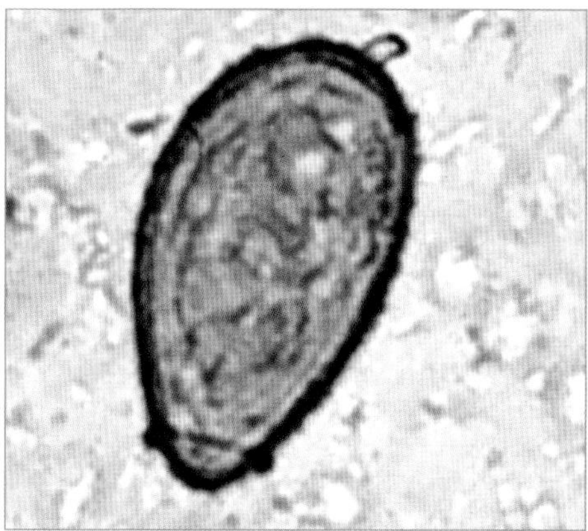

Image 97.1
Opisthorchis (formerly *Clonorchis*) *sinensis* (Chinese liver fluke) egg. These are small, operculated eggs, 27 to 35 µm by 11 to 20 µm. The operculum, at the smaller end of the egg, is convex and rests on a visible "shoulder." At the opposite (larger, abopercular) end, a small knob or hooklike protrusion is often visible (as is the case here). The miracidium is visible inside the egg. (Also referred to as opisthorchiasis.) Courtesy of Centers for Disease Control and Prevention/Dr Mae Melvin.

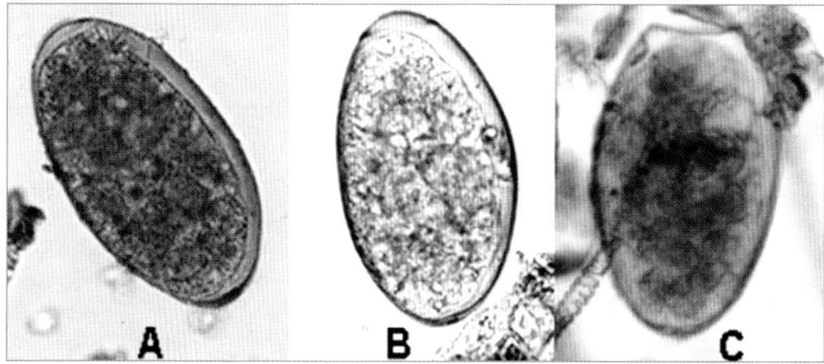

Image 97.2
Fasciola hepatica eggs (wet mounts with iodine). The eggs are ellipsoidal. They have a small, barely distinct operculum (A, B, upper end of the eggs). The operculum can be opened (egg C), for example, when a slight pressure is applied to the coverslip. The eggs have a thin shell that is slightly thicker at the abopercular end. They are passed unembryonated. The size ranges from 120 to 150 µm by 63 to 90 µm. Fascioliasis is caused by the sheep liver fluke infecting the liver and biliary system. Courtesy of Centers for Disease Control and Prevention.

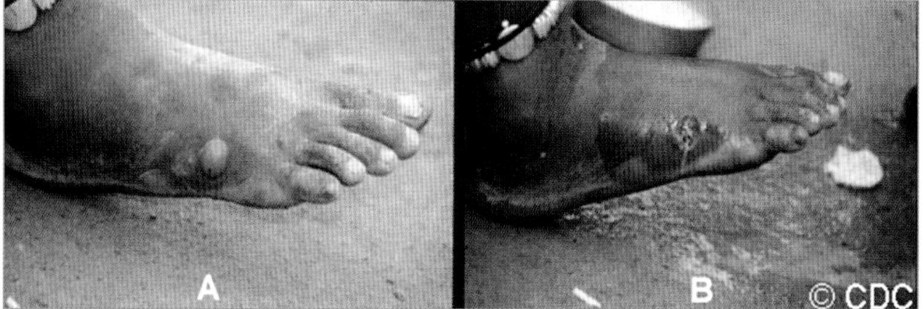

Image 97.3
Dracunculiasis. The female *Dracunculus medinensis* (guinea worm) induces a painful blister (A); after rupture of the blister, the worm emerges as a whitish filament (B) in the center of a painful ulcer, which is often secondarily infected. Courtesy of Centers for Disease Control and Prevention.

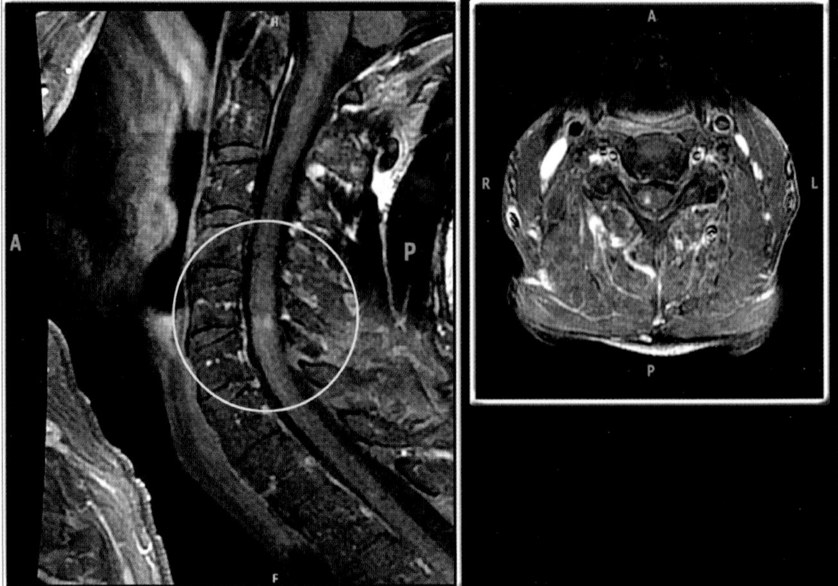

Image 97.4
Saggital and axial T2-weighted magnetic resonance images of a focal lesion of the cervical spine in an 18-year-old patient with spinal cord involvement of infection with *Gnathostoma spinigerum,* a nematode found throughout Asia that can be acquired by humans through consumption of undercooked shellfish or meat. Courtesy of James Sejvar, MD.

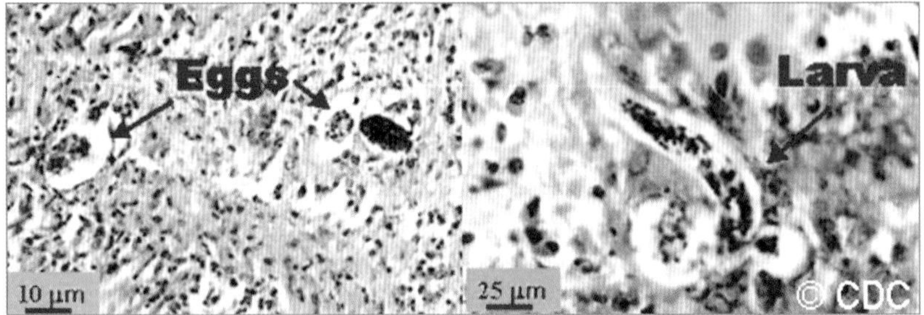

Image 97.5
Eggs and larva of *Angiostrongylus costaricensis*. In humans, eggs and larvae are not normally excreted but remain sequestered in tissues. Eggs and larvae (occasionally adult worms) of *A costaricensis* can be identified in biopsy or surgical specimens of intestinal tissue. The larvae need to be distinguished from larvae of *Strongyloides stercoralis;* however, the presence of granulomas containing thin-shelled eggs or larvae serve to distinguish *A costaricensis* infections. The larval infection can cause mesenteric arteritis and abdominal pain, occurring primarily in people in Central and South America. Courtesy of Centers for Disease Control and Prevention.

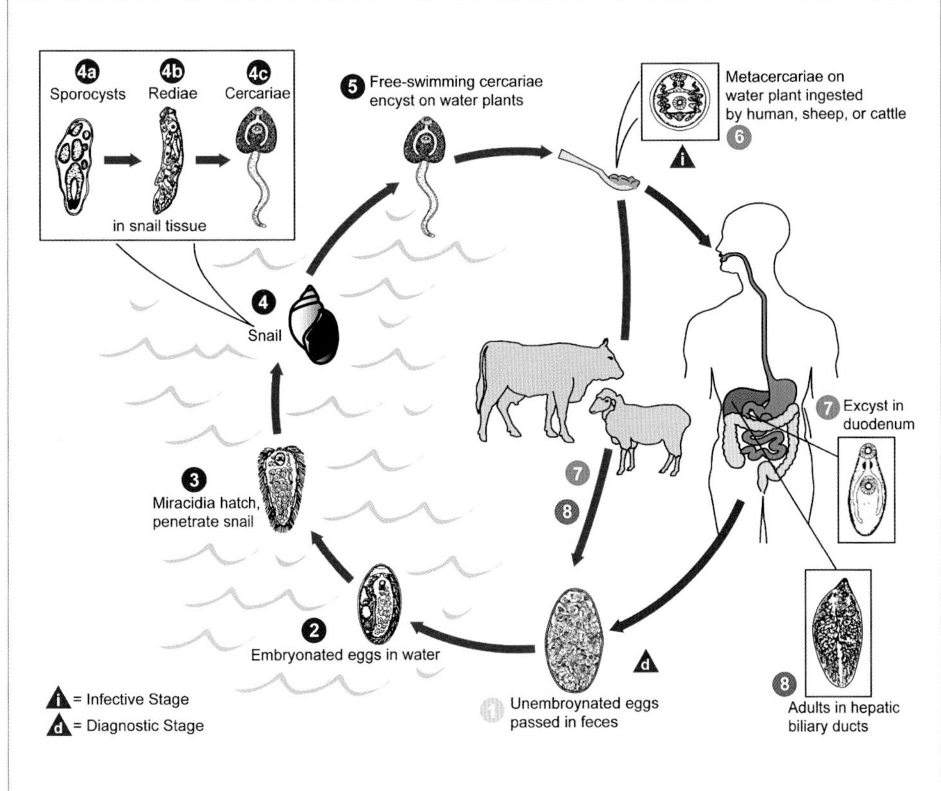

Image 97.6

Fasciola hepatica (life cycle). Immature eggs are discharged in the biliary ducts and in the stool (1). Eggs become embryonated in water (2) and release miracidia (3), which invade a suitable snail intermediate host (4), including many species of the genus *Lymnaea.* In the snail, the parasites undergo several developmental stages (sporocysts [4a], rediae [4b], and cercariae [4c]). The cercariae are released from the snail (5) and encyst as metacercariae on aquatic vegetation or other surfaces. Mammals acquire the infection by eating vegetation containing metacercariae. Humans can become infected by ingesting metacercariae-containing freshwater plants, especially watercress (6). After ingestion, the metacercariae excyst in the duodenum (7) and migrate through the intestinal wall, the peritoneal cavity, and the liver parenchyma into the biliary ducts, where they develop into adults (8). In humans, maturation from metacercariae into adult flukes takes approximately 3 to 4 months. The adult flukes (*F hepatica,* up to 30 by 13 mm; *Fasciola gigantica,* up to 75 mm) reside in the large biliary ducts of the mammalian host. *F hepatica* infect various animal species, mostly herbivores. Courtesy of Centers for Disease Control and Prevention.

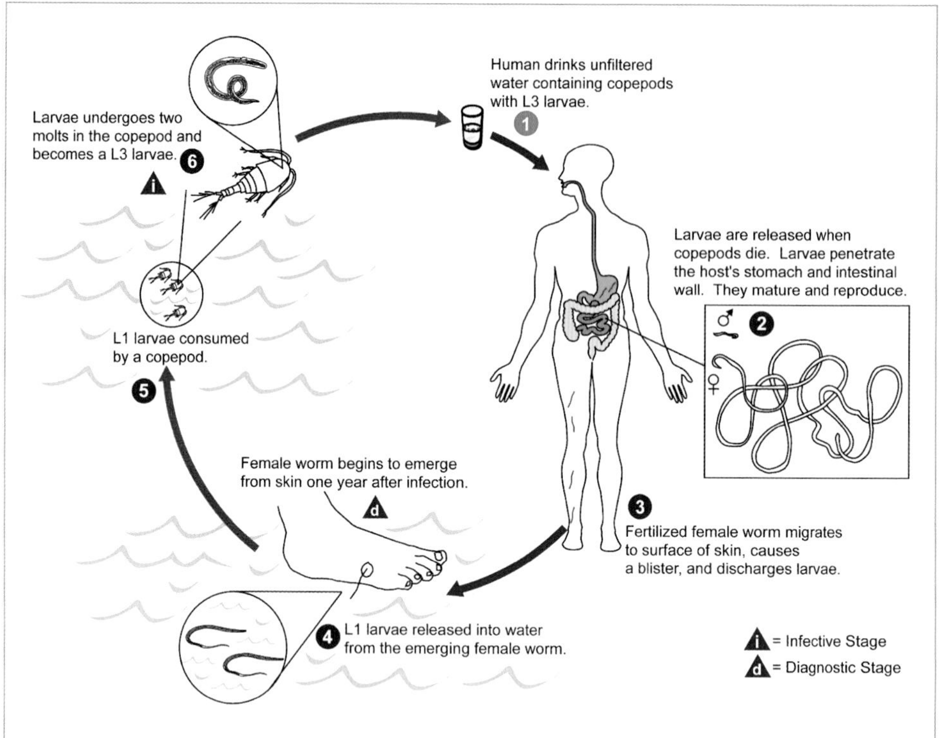

Image 97.7

Dracunculus medinensis. Humans become infected by drinking unfiltered water containing copepods (small crustaceans) that are infected with larvae of *D medinensis* (1). Following ingestion, the copepods die and release the larvae, which penetrate the host stomach and intestinal wall and enter the abdominal cavity and retroperitoneal space (2). After maturation into adults and copulation, the male worms die and the females (length, 70–120 cm) migrate in the subcutaneous tissues toward the skin surface (3). Approximately 1 year after infection, the female worm induces a blister on the skin, generally on the distal lower extremity, which ruptures. When this lesion comes into contact with water, a contact that the patient seeks to relieve the local discomfort, the female worm emerges and releases larvae (4). The larvae are ingested by a copepod (5) and after 2 weeks (and 2 molts) have developed into infective larvae (6). Ingestion of the copepods closes the cycle. Courtesy of Centers for Disease Control and Prevention/Alexander J. da Silva, PhD/Melanie Moser.

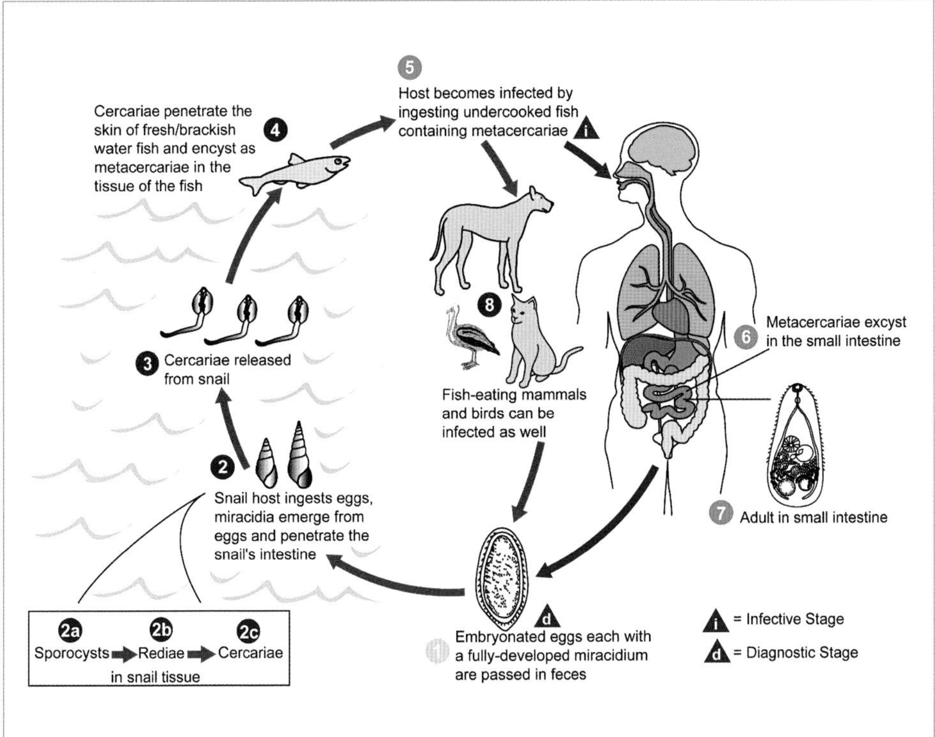

Image 97.8

Heterophyes heterophyes. Adults release embryonated eggs each with a fully developed miracidium, and eggs are passed in the host's feces (1). After ingestion by a suitable snail (first intermediate host), the eggs hatch and release miracidia, which penetrate the snail's intestine (2). Genera *Cerithidia* and *Pironella* are important snail hosts in Asia and the Middle East, respectively. The miracidia undergo several developmental stages in the snail (sporocysts [2a], rediae [2b], and cercariae [2c]). Many cercariae are produced from each redia. The cercariae are released from the snail (3) and encyst as metacercariae in the tissues of a suitable freshwater or brackish water fish (second intermediate host) (4). The definitive host becomes infected by ingesting undercooked or salted fish containing metacercariae (5). After ingestion, the metacercariae excyst, attach to the mucosa of the small intestine (6), and mature into adults (measuring 1.0–1.7 mm by 0.3–0.4 mm) (7). In addition to humans, various fish-eating mammals (eg, cats, dogs) and birds can be infected by *H heterophyes* (8). Geographic distribution: Egypt, the Middle East, and Far East. Courtesy of Centers for Disease Control and Prevention/Alexander J. da Silva, PhD/Melanie Moser.

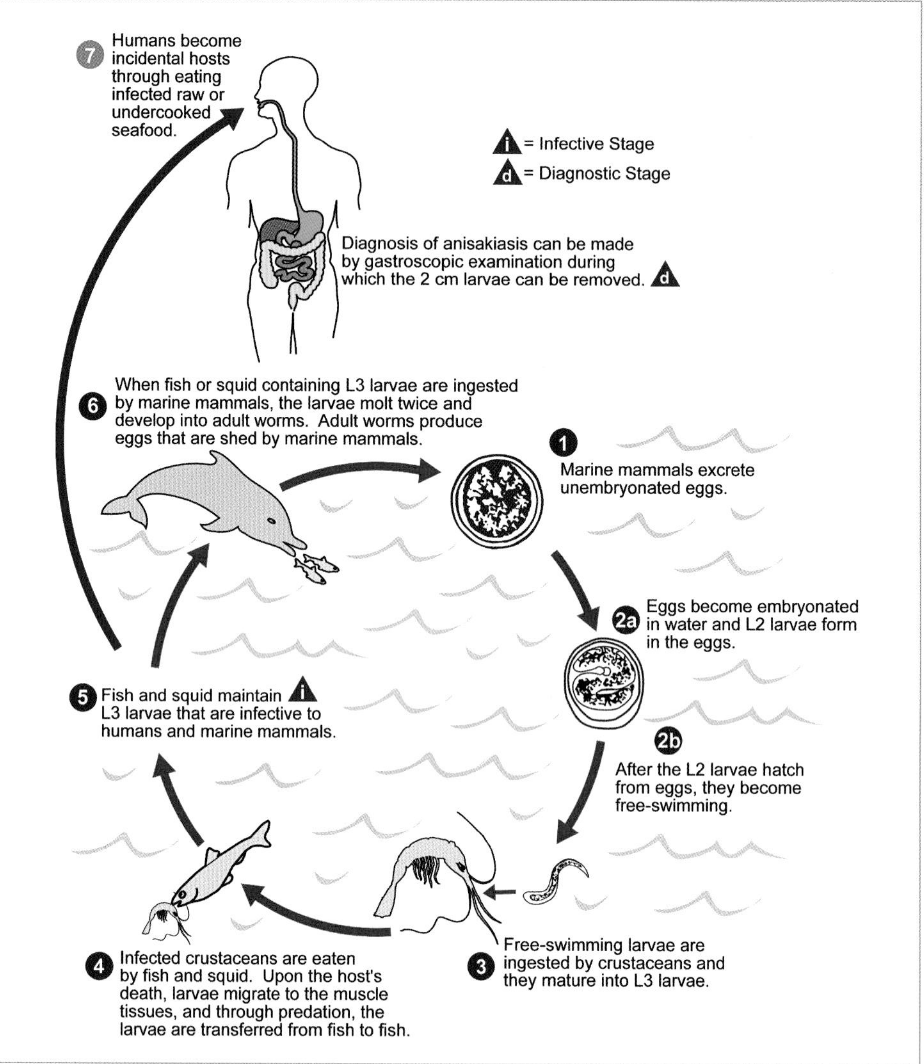

Image 97.9

Anisakiasis is caused by the accidental ingestion of larvae of the nematodes (roundworms) *Anisakis* simplex or *Pseudoterranova decipiens*. Adult stages of *Anisakis* simplex or *P decipiens* reside in the stomach of marine mammals, where they are embedded in the mucosa, in clusters. Unembryonated eggs produced by adult females are passed in the feces of marine mammals (1). The eggs become embryonated in water, and first-stage larvae are formed in the eggs. The larvae molt, becoming second-stage larvae (2a), and, after the larvae hatch from the eggs, they become free-swimming (2b). Larvae released from the eggs are ingested by crustaceans (3). The ingested larvae develop into third-stage larvae that are infective to fish and squid (4). The larvae migrate from the intestine to the tissues in the peritoneal cavity and grow up to 3 cm in length. On the host's death, larvae migrate to the muscle tissues and, through predation, are transferred from fish to fish. Fish and squid maintain third-stage larvae that are infective to humans and marine mammals (5). When fish or squid containing third-stage larvae are ingested by marine mammals, the larvae molt twice and develop into adult worms. The adult females produce eggs that are shed by marine mammals (6). Humans become infected by eating raw or undercooked infected marine fish (7). After ingestion, the *Anisakis* larvae penetrate the gastric and intestinal mucosa, causing the symptoms of anisakiasis. Courtesy of Centers for Disease Control and Prevention/Alexander J. da Silva, PhD/Melanie Moser.

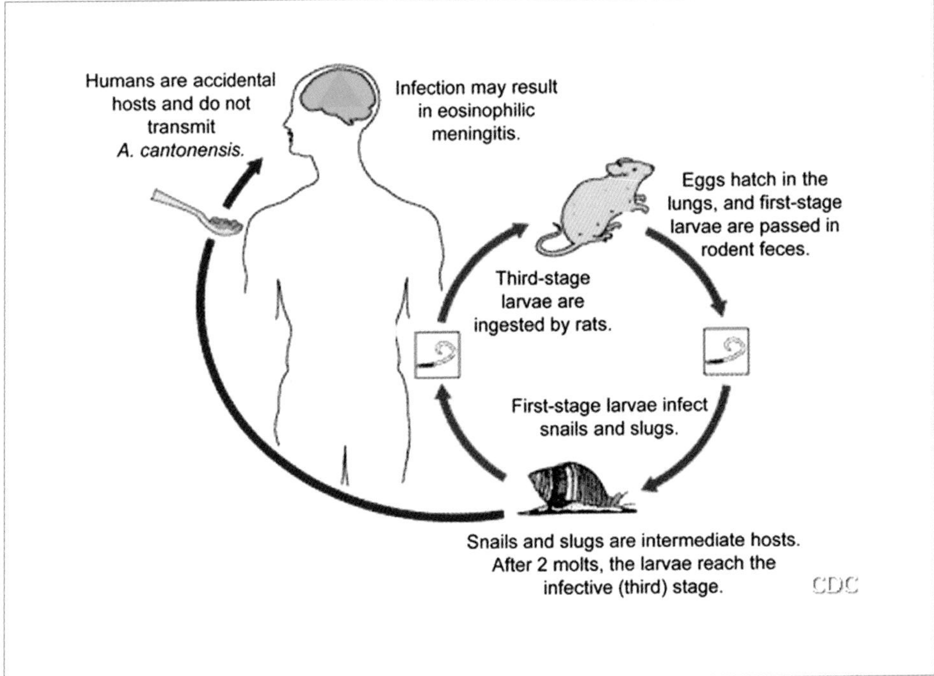

Image 97.10
Life cycle of *Angiostrongylus cantonensis*. Courtesy of Centers for Disease Control and Prevention/ *Emerging Infectious Diseases.*

98

Parvovirus B19

(Erythema Infectiosum, Fifth Disease)

Clinical Manifestations

Infection with human parvovirus B19 is recognized most often as erythema infectiosum (EI), or fifth disease, which is characterized by a distinctive rash that may be preceded by mild systemic symptoms, including fever in 15% to 30% of patients. The facial rash can be intensely red with a "slapped cheek" appearance that often is accompanied by circumoral pallor. A symmetric, macular, lacelike, and, often, pruritic rash also occurs on the trunk, moving peripherally to involve the arms, buttocks, and thighs. The rash can fluctuate in intensity and recur with environmental changes, such as temperature and exposure to sunlight, for weeks to months. A brief, mild, nonspecific illness consisting of fever, malaise, myalgia, and headache often precedes the characteristic exanthema by approximately 7 to 10 days. Arthralgia and arthritis occur in fewer than 10% of infected children but commonly among adults, especially women. Knees are involved most often in children, but symmetric polyarthropathy of knees, fingers, and other joints can occur in adults.

Human parvovirus B19 can also cause asymptomatic infections. Other manifestations (Table 98.1) include a mild respiratory tract illness with no rash, a rash atypical for EI that may be rubelliform or petechial, papular-purpuric gloves-and-socks syndrome (painful and pruritic papules, petechiae, and purpura of hands and feet, often with fever and an enanthem), polyarthropathy syndrome (arthralgia and arthritis in adults in the absence of other manifestations of EI), chronic erythroid hypoplasia with severe anemia in immunodeficient patients, and transient aplastic crisis lasting 7 to 10 days in patients with hemolytic anemias (eg, sickle cell disease, autoimmune hemolytic anemia). For children with other conditions associated with low hemoglobin concentrations, including hemorrhage, severe anemia, and thalassemia, parvovirus B19 infection will not result in aplastic crisis but might result in prolongation of recovery from the anemia resulting from these conditions. Patients with transient aplastic crisis may have a prodromal illness with fever, malaise, and myalgia, but rash is usually absent. Human parvovirus B19 infection sometimes has been associated with decreases in numbers of platelets, lymphocytes, and neutrophils.

Human parvovirus B19 infection occurring during pregnancy can cause fetal hydrops, intrauterine growth restriction, isolated pleural and pericardial effusions, and death, but the virus does not cause congenital anomalies. The risk of fetal death is between 2% and 6% when infection occurs during pregnancy. The greatest risk appears to occur during the first half of pregnancy.

Etiology

Human parvovirus B19 is a small, nonenveloped, single-stranded DNA virus in the family Parvoviridae, genus *Erythrovirus*. There are 3 distinct genotypes. Parvovirus B19 replicates in human erythrocyte precursors. Human parvovirus B19–associated red blood cell aplasia is related to caspase-mediated apoptosis of erythrocyte precursors.

Table 98.1
Clinical Manifestations of Human Parvovirus B19 Infection

Conditions	Usual Hosts
Erythema infectiosum (fifth disease)	Immunocompetent children
Polyarthropathy syndrome	Immunocompetent adults (more common in women)
Chronic anemia/pure red cell aplasia	Immunocompromised hosts
Transient aplastic crisis	People with hemolytic anemia (ie, sickle cell anemia)
Hydrops fetalis/congenital anemia	Fetus (first 20 weeks of pregnancy)
Petechial, papular-purpuric gloves-and-socks syndrome	Immunocompetent adults

Epidemiology

Parvovirus B19 is distributed worldwide and is a common cause of infection in humans, who are the only known hosts. Modes of transmission include contact with respiratory tract secretions, percutaneous exposure to blood or blood products, and vertical transmission from mother to fetus. Human parvovirus B19 infections are ubiquitous, and cases of EI can occur sporadically or in outbreaks in elementary or junior high schools during late winter and early spring. Secondary spread among susceptible household members is common, with infection occurring in approximately 50% of susceptible contacts in some studies. The transmission rate in schools is lower, but infection can be an occupational risk for school and child care personnel, with approximately 20% of susceptible contacts becoming infected. In young children, antibody seroprevalence is generally 5% to 10%. In most communities, approximately 50% of young adults and, often, more than 90% of elderly people are seropositive. The annual seroconversion rate in women of childbearing age has been reported to be approximately 1.5%. Timing of the presence of high-titer parvovirus B19 DNA in serum and respiratory tract secretions indicates that people with EI are infectious before and after rash onset or joint symptoms. In contrast, patients with aplastic crises are contagious from before the onset of symptoms for at least a week after onset. Symptoms of papular-purpuric gloves-and-socks syndrome can occur in association with viremia and before development of antibody response, and affected patients should be considered infectious.

Incubation Period

Usually 4 to 14 days, but can be as long as 21 days.

Diagnostic Tests

Parvovirus B19 cannot be propagated in standard cell culture. In the immunocompetent host, detection of serum parvovirus B19–specific immunoglobulin (Ig) M antibodies is the preferred diagnostic test for parvovirus B19–associated rash illness. A positive IgM test result indicates infection probably occurred within the previous 2 to 3 months. On the basis of immunoassay results, IgM antibodies can be detected in 90% or more of patients at the time of the EI rash and by the third day of illness in patients with transient aplastic crisis. Serum IgG antibodies appear by approximately day 2 of EI and persist for life. These assays are available through commercial laboratories; however, their sensitivity and specificity can vary, particularly for IgM. The optimal method for detecting transient aplastic crisis or chronic infection in the immunocompromised patient is demonstration of high titer of viral DNA by polymerase chain reaction (PCR) assays. Because parvovirus B19 DNA can be detected at low levels by PCR assay in serum for months and even years after the acute viremic phase, detection does not necessarily indicate acute infection. Low levels of parvovirus B19 DNA can also be detected by PCR in tissues (skin, heart, liver, bone marrow), independent of active disease.

Treatment

For most patients, only supportive care is indicated. Patients with aplastic crisis may require transfusion. For treatment of chronic infection in immunodeficient patients, intravenous immunoglobulin therapy is often effective and should be considered. Some cases of parvovirus B19 infection concurrent with hydrops fetalis have been treated successfully with intrauterine blood transfusions of the fetus.

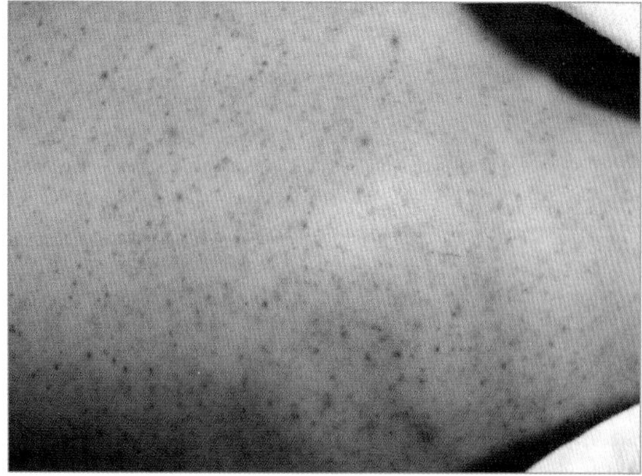

Image 98.1
Parvovirus B19 infection with a generalized rash in a 9-year-old boy. Courtesy of Benjamin Estrada, MD.

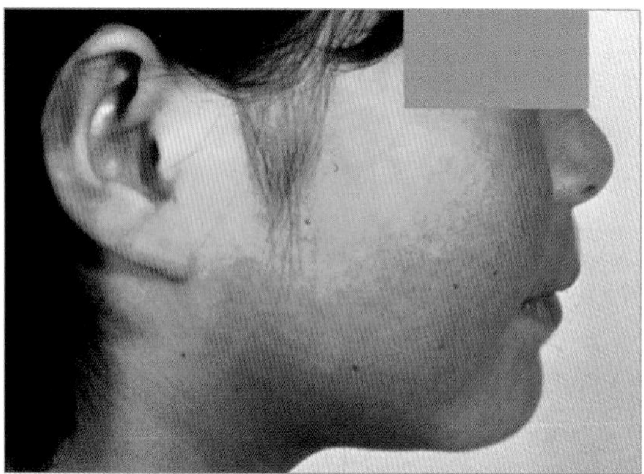

Image 98.2
Parvovirus B19 infection (erythema infectiosum, fifth disease) with typical facial erythema, commonly referred to as the "slapped cheek" sign.

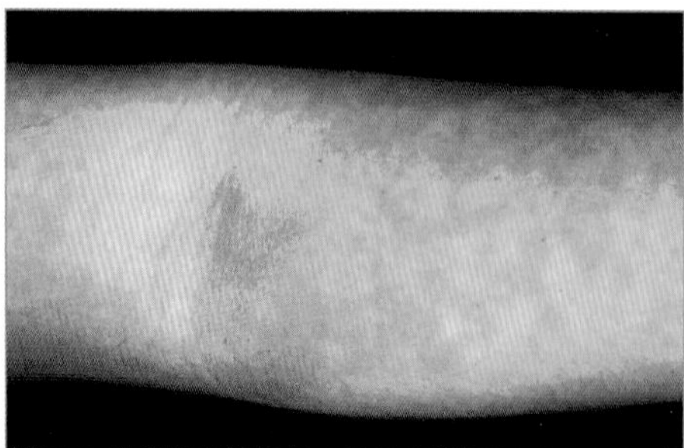

Image 98.3
Parvovirus B19 infection. Characteristic lacelike pattern on the back of the leg. This is the same patient as in Image 98.2.

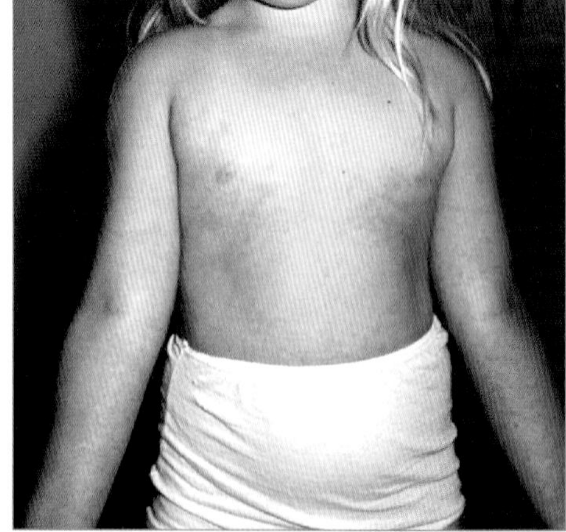

Image 98.4
Parvovirus B19 infection (erythema infectiosum, fifth disease) in a 5-year-old girl.

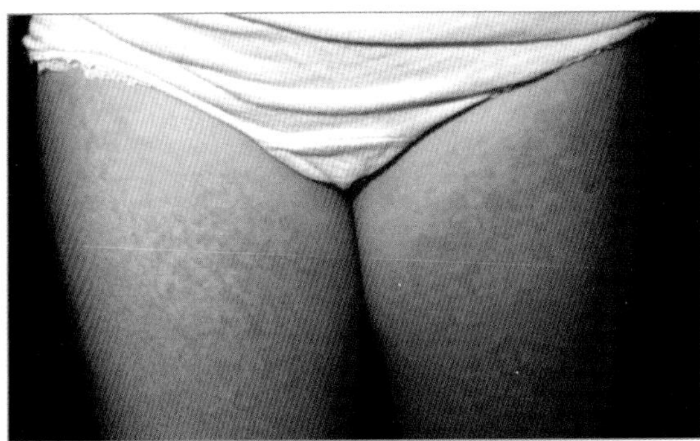

Image 98.5
Parvovirus B19 infection (erythema infectiosum, fifth disease). This is the same child as in Image 98.4.

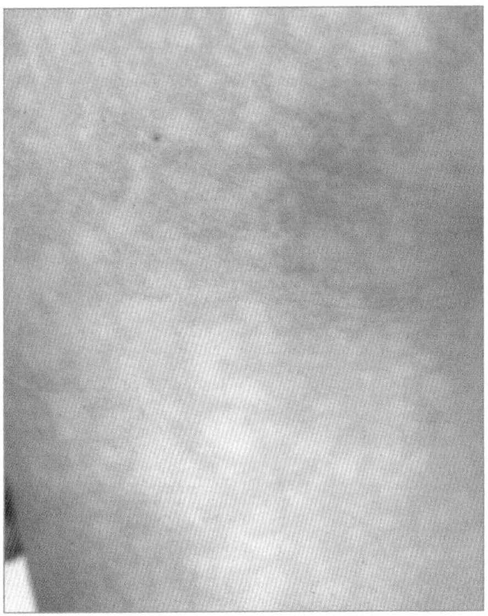

Image 98.6
Close-up view of the lacelike pattern of fifth disease in a 6-year-old girl. Courtesy of George Nankervis, MD.

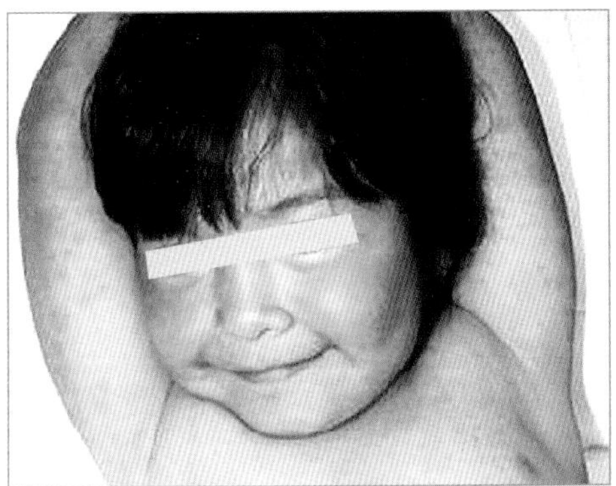

Image 98.7
Characteristic "slapped cheek" appearance of the face in a child who has fifth disease. The characteristic rash is also present on the arms.

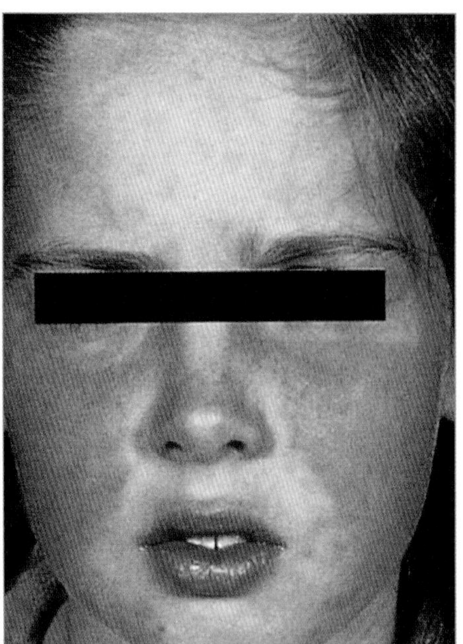

Image 98.8
An 8-year-old white girl with the facial erythema of erythema infectiosum. Courtesy of Larry Frenkel, MD.

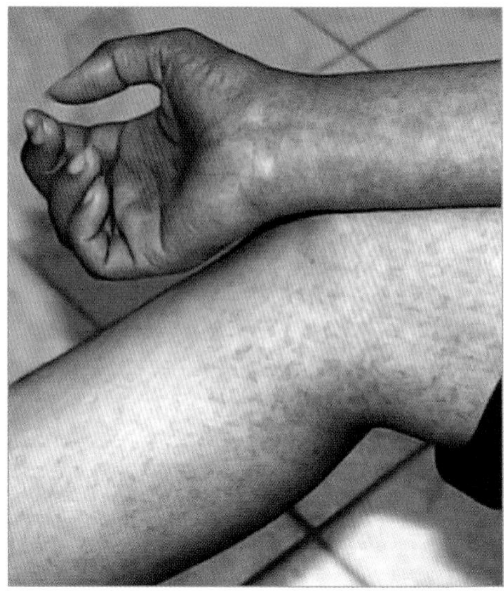

Image 98.9
Stocking glove purpura. This 18-year-old girl awoke one morning with asymptomatic symmetric purpura of the hands and feet, which spread to involve the proximal extremities. The exanthem faded over 7 to 10 days. Although an enanthem is not usually reported with parvovirus infection, she also developed some erythema of the buccal mucosa and white plaques on a red base on the dorsum of the tongue. Courtesy of H. Cody Meissner, MD, FAAP.

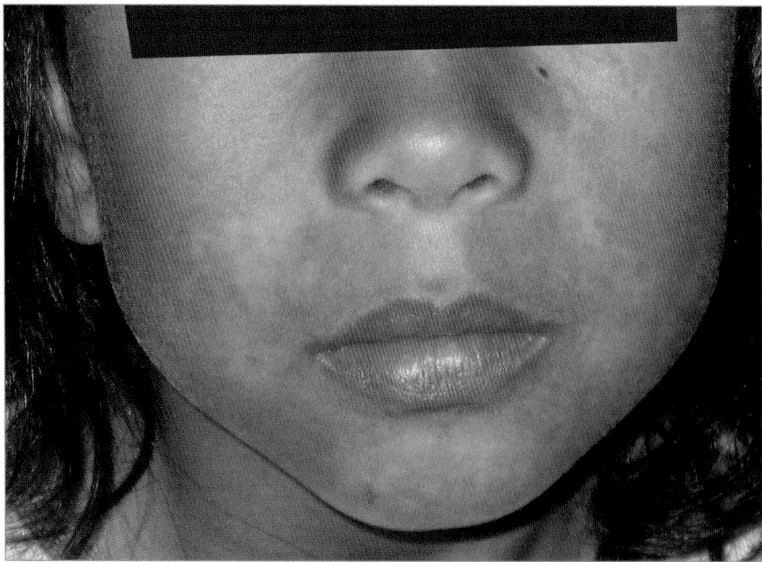

Image 98.10
This healthy 6-year-old girl developed an asymptomatic symmetric red papular eruption on her face, extremities, and trunk, which became confluent on her face 1 week earlier. Courtesy of H. Cody Meissner, MD, FAAP.

99

Pasteurella Infections

Clinical Manifestations

The most common manifestation in children is cellulitis at the site of a bite or scratch of a cat, dog, or other animal. Cellulitis typically develops within 24 hours of the injury and includes swelling, erythema, tenderness, and serous or sanguinopurulent discharge at the site. Regional lymphadenopathy, chills, and fever can occur. Local complications, such as abscesses and tenosynovitis, are frequent, but septic arthritis and osteomyelitis are also reported. Less common manifestations of infection include septicemia, meningitis, endocarditis, respiratory tract infections (eg, pneumonia, pulmonary abscesses, pleural empyema), appendicitis, hepatic abscess, peritonitis, and ocular infections (eg, corneal ulcers, endophthalmitis). People with liver disease, solid organ transplant, or underlying host defense abnormalities are predisposed to bacteremia with *Pasteurella multocida*.

Etiology

Members of the genus *Pasteurella* are nonmotile, facultatively anaerobic, mostly catalase and oxidase positive, gram-negative coccobacilli that are primarily respiratory tract pathogens in animals. The most common human pathogen is *P multocida* subsp *multocida* (causing >50% of infections).

Epidemiology

Pasteurella species are found in the oral flora of 70% to 90% of cats, 25% to 50% of dogs, and many other animals. Transmission can occur from the bite or scratch or licking of a previous wound by a cat or dog or, less commonly, from another animal. Rarely, respiratory tract spread occurs from animals to humans; in a significant proportion of cases, no animal exposure can be identified. Although rare, human-to-human transmission has been documented vertically from mother to neonate, horizontally from colonized humans, and by contaminated blood products.

Incubation Period

Usually less than 24 hours.

Diagnostic Tests

The isolation of *Pasteurella* species from skin lesion drainage or other sites of infection (eg, blood, joint fluid, cerebrospinal fluid, sputum, pleural fluid, suppurative lymph nodes) is diagnostic. *Pasteurella* species are somewhat fastidious but may be cultured on several media generally used in clinical laboratories, including sheep blood and chocolate agars. Although they resemble several other organisms morphologically, laboratory identification to the genus level is generally not difficult.

Treatment

The drug of choice is penicillin. Other oral agents that are usually effective include ampicillin, amoxicillin, cefuroxime, cefixime, cefpodoxime, doxycycline, and fluoroquinolones. *Pasteurella* species are usually resistant to vancomycin, clindamycin, and erythromycin. For patients who are allergic to β-lactam agents, azithromycin or trimethoprim-sulfamethoxazole are alternative choices. For suspected polymicrobial infected bites, oral amoxicillin-clavulanate or, for severe infection, intravenous ampicillin-sulbactam or piperacillin-tazobactam can be given. The duration of therapy is usually 7 to 10 days for local infections and 10 to 14 days for more severe infections. Antimicrobial therapy should be continued for 4 to 6 weeks for bone and joint infections. Wound drainage or debridement may be necessary.

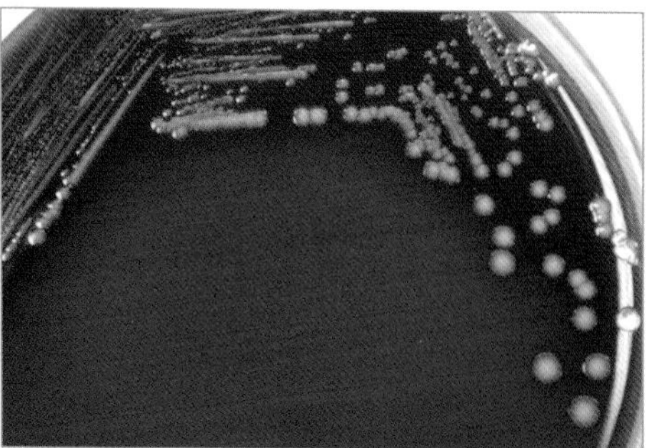

Image 99.1
This photograph depicts the colonial morphology displayed by gram-negative *Yersinia pestis* bacteria, which was grown on a medium of sheep blood agar for a 72-hour period at a temperature of 37°C (98.6°F). Courtesy of Centers for Disease Control and Prevention/Todd Parker, MD, and Audra Marsh.

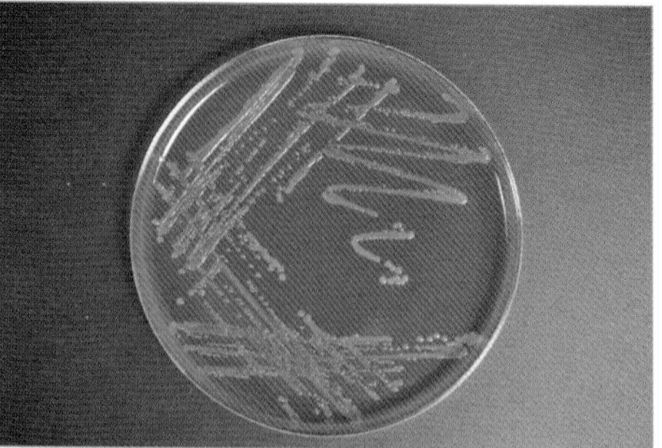

Image 99.2
Pasteurella multocida on chocolate agar. Colonies are small, gray, smooth, and nonhemolytic. Courtesy of Julia Rosebush, DO; Robert Jerris, PhD; and Theresa Stanley, M(ASCP).

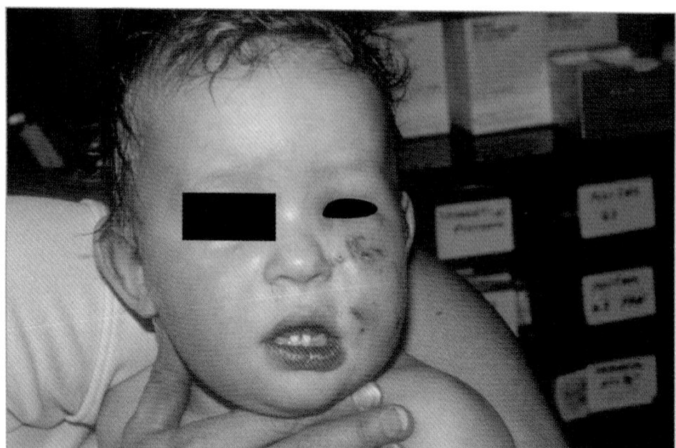

Image 99.3
Pasteurella multocida cellulitis secondary to multiple cat bites about the face of a 1-year-old. Courtesy of George Nankervis, MD.

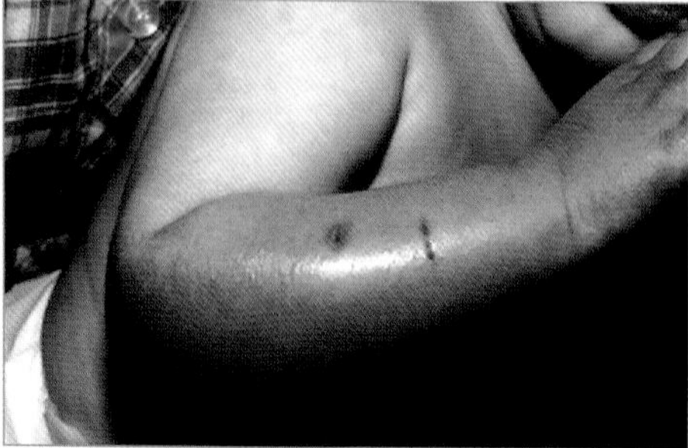

Image 99.4
Right forearm of 1-year-old boy bitten by a stray cat. The child developed fever, redness, and swelling 10 hours after the bite. He was taking amoxicillin for otitis media at the time of the bite. The child responded to treatment with intravenous cefuroxime, although the fever persisted for 36 hours. *Pasturella multocida* was cultured from purulent material obtained from the wound the day after admission. Courtesy of Larry I. Corman, MD.

100

Pediculosis Capitis

(Head Lice)

Clinical Manifestations

Itching is the most common symptom of head lice infestation, but many children are asymptomatic. Adult lice or eggs (nits) are found on the hair and are most readily apparent behind the ears and near the nape of the neck. Excoriations and crusting caused by secondary bacterial infection may occur and are often associated with regional lymphadenopathy. Head lice usually deposit their eggs on a hair shaft 4 mm or less from the scalp. Because hair grows at a rate of approximately 1 cm per month, the duration of infestation can be estimated by the distance of the nit from the scalp.

Etiology

Pediculus humanus capitis is the head louse. Nymphs and adult lice feed on human blood.

Epidemiology

In the United States, head lice infestation is most common in children attending child care and elementary school. Head lice infestation is not a sign of poor hygiene or influenced by hair length. All socioeconomic groups are affected. In the United States, infestations are less common in black children than in children of other races and ethnicities. Head lice are not a health hazard because they are not responsible for spread of any disease. Head lice are only able to crawl; therefore, transmission occurs mainly by direct head-to-head contact with hair of infested people. Transmission by contact with personal belongings, such as combs, hairbrushes, and hats, is uncommon. Away from the scalp, head lice survive fewer than 2 days at room temperature, and their eggs generally become nonviable within a week and cannot hatch at a lower ambient temperature than that near the scalp.

Incubation Period

From the laying of eggs to hatching of first nymph, 8 to 9 days, varying from 7 to 12 days, but shorter in hot climates. Lice mature to the adult stage 9 to 12 days later. Adult females then may lay eggs (nits), but only if the female has mated.

Diagnostic Tests

Identification of eggs (nits), nymphs, and lice with the naked eye is possible; diagnosis can be confirmed by using a hand lens, dermatoscope (epiluminescence microscope), or traditional microscope. Nymphal and adult lice shun light, move rapidly, and conceal themselves. Wetting the hair with water, oil, or a conditioner and using a fine-tooth comb may improve ability to diagnose infestation and shorten examination time. It is important to differentiate nits from dandruff, benign hair casts (a layer of follicular cells that may slide easily off the hair shaft), plugs of desquamated cells, external hair debris, and fungal infections of the hair. Because nits remain affixed to the hair firmly, even if dead or hatched, the mere presence of nits is not a sign of an active infestation.

Treatment

A number of effective pediculicidal agents are available to treat head lice infestation (Table 100.1). Safety is a major concern with pediculicides because the infestation itself

Table 100.1
Topical Pediculicides for the Treatment of Head Lice

Product	Availability	Cost Estimate[a]
Permethrin 1% lotion (Nix)	Over the counter	$
Pyrethrins + piperonyl butoxide (Rid)	Over the counter	$
Malathion 0.5% (Ovide)	Prescription	$$$$
Benzyl alcohol 5% (Ulesfia)	Prescription	$$–$$$$[b]
Spinosad 0.9% suspension (Natroba)	Prescription	$$$$
Ivermectin 0.5% lotion (Sklice)	Prescription	$$$$

[a] $, <$25; $$, $26–$99; $$$, $100–$199; $$$$, $200–$299.

[b] Cost varies by length of hair, which affects number of units of product required.

presents minimal risk to the host. Pediculicides should be used only as directed and with care. Instructions on proper use of any product should be explained carefully. Therapy can be started with over-the-counter 1% permethrin or with a pyrethrin combined with piperonyl butoxide product; both have good safety profiles. However, resistance to these compounds has been documented in the United States. For treatment failures not attributable to improper use of an over-the-counter pediculicide, malathion, benzyl alcohol lotion, spinosad suspension, or ivermectin lotion should be used. When lice are resistant to all topical agents, oral ivermectin may be used. Drugs that have residual activity may kill nymphs as they emerge from eggs. Pediculicides that are not sufficiently ovicidal usually require more than one application. Ideally, retreatment should occur after the eggs that are present at initial treatment have hatched but before any new eggs have been produced.

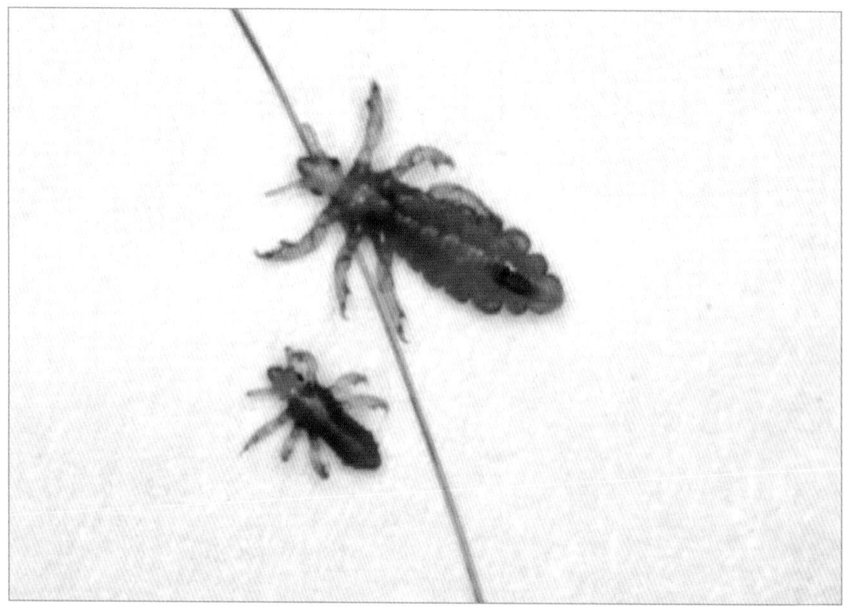

Image 100.1
Head louse, baby louse, and hair. Copyright Gary Williams, MD.

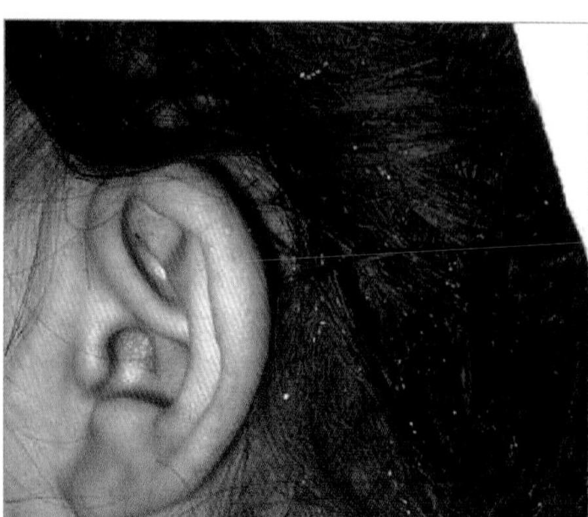

Image 100.2
Nits on the hair shafts. Copyright Edward K. Marcuse, MD.

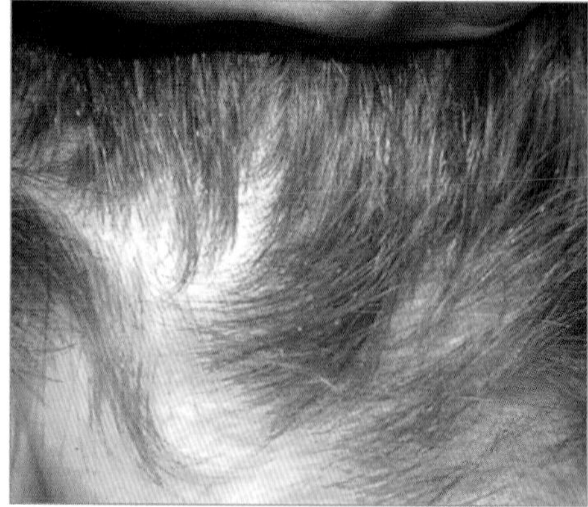

Image 100.3
Nits on the hair shaft. Copyright Edgar K. Marcuse, MD.

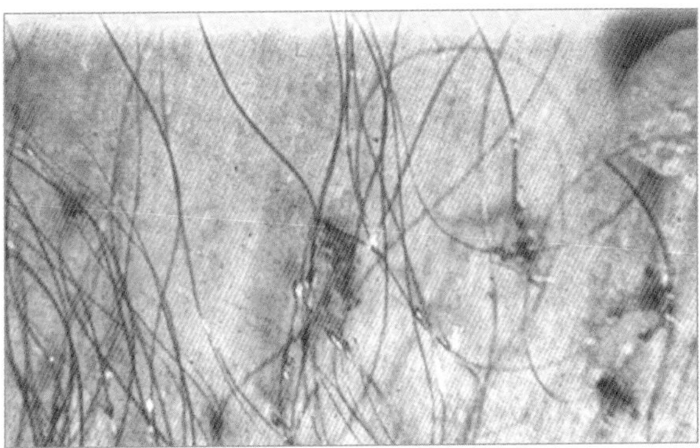

Image 100.4
Pediculosis (head lice) with nits and excoriations of the scalp. Courtesy of Centers for Disease Control and Prevention.

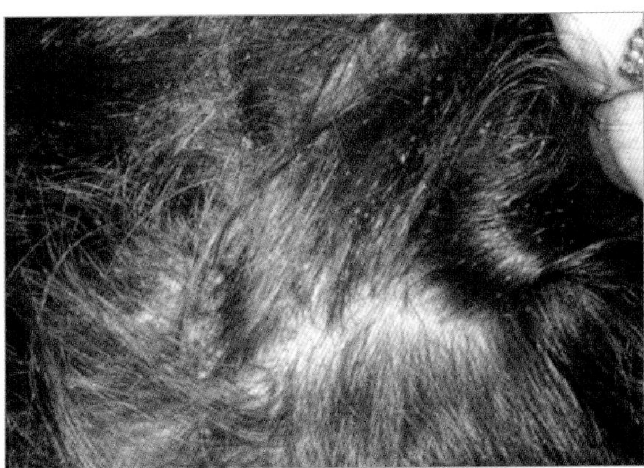

Image 100.5
An 8-year-old girl with an earache. This child complained of otalgia. During the course of otoscopic evaluation, she was noted to have a very large number of nits in her hair as well as active lice. On questioning, she stated she has had itching of the scalp. She was treated with topical permethrin with temporary resolution. Reinfestation occurred after sharing a riding helmet with a cousin. Courtesy of Will Sorey, MD.

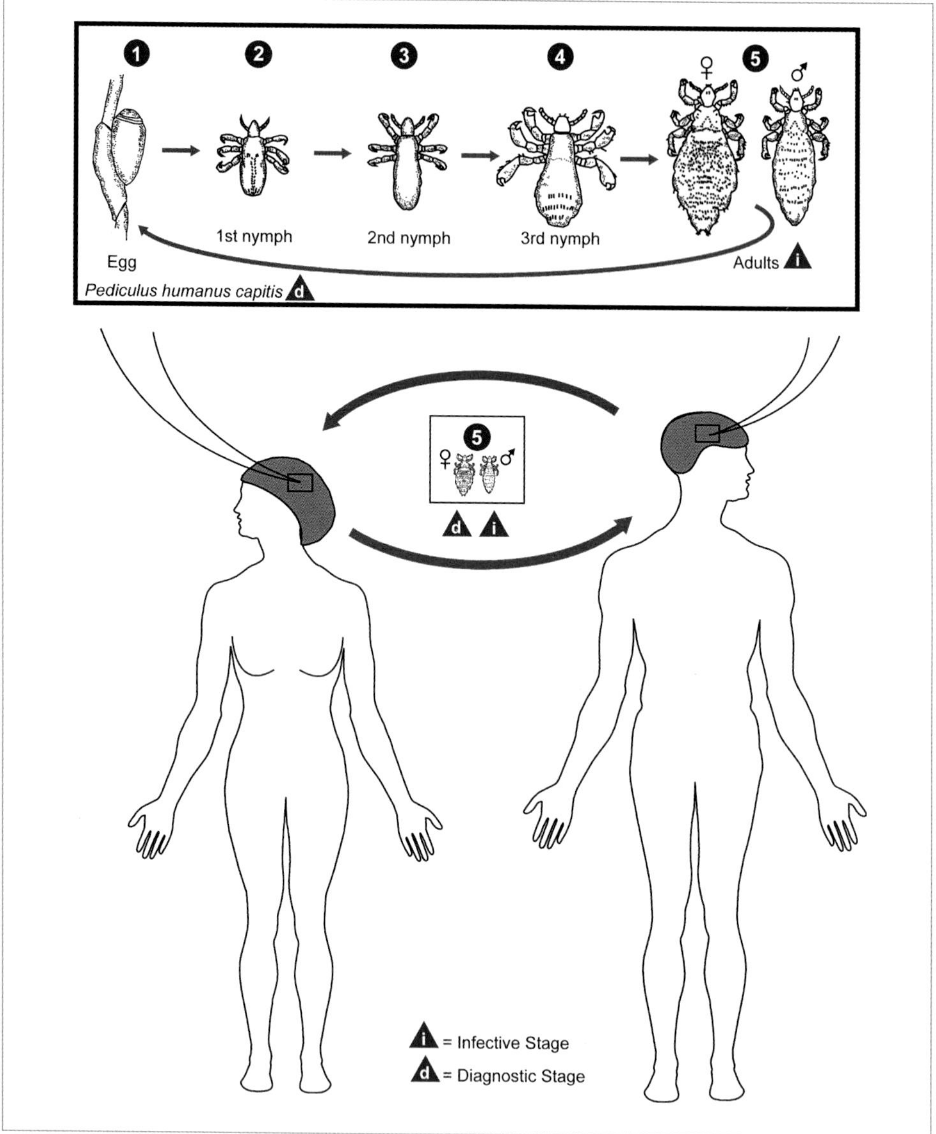

Image 100.6

The life cycle of the head louse has 3 stages: egg, nymph, and adult. **Eggs:** Nits are head lice eggs. They are hard to see and are often confused for dandruff or hair spray droplets. Nits are laid by the adult female and are cemented at the base of the hair shaft nearest the scalp (1). They are 0.8 by 0.3 mm, oval, and, usually, yellow to white. Nits take about 1 week to hatch (range, 6–9 days). Viable eggs are usually located within 6 mm of the scalp. **Nymphs:** The egg hatches to release a nymph (2). The nit shell then becomes a more visible dull yellow and remains attached to the hair shaft. The nymph looks like an adult head louse but is about the size of a pin head. Nymphs mature after 3 molts (3, 4) and become adults about 7 days after hatching. **Adults:** The adult louse is about the size of a sesame seed, has 6 legs (each with claws), and is tan to grayish-white (5). In persons with dark hair, the adult louse will appear darker. Females are usually larger than males and can lay up to 8 nits per day. Adult lice can live up to 30 days on a person's head. To live, adult lice need to feed on blood several times daily. Without blood meals, the louse will die within 1 to 2 days off the host. Courtesy of Centers for Disease Control and Prevention/Alexander J. da Silva, PhD/Melanie Moser.

101

Pediculosis Corporis

(Body Lice)

Clinical Manifestations

Intense itching, particularly at night, is common with body lice infestations. Bites manifest as small erythematous macules, papules, and excoriations primarily on the trunk. In heavily bitten areas, typically around the midsection, the skin can become thickened and discolored. Secondary bacterial infection of the skin (pyoderma) caused by scratching is common.

Etiology

Pediculus humanus humanus (or *corporis*) is the body louse. Nymphs and adult lice feed on human blood.

Epidemiology

Body lice are generally restricted to people living in crowded conditions without access to regular bathing or changes of clothing (eg, refugees, victims of war or natural disasters, homeless people). Under these conditions, body lice can spread rapidly through direct contact or contact with contaminated clothing or bedding. Body lice live in clothes or bedding, lay their eggs on or near the seams of clothing, and move to the skin to feed. Body lice cannot survive away from a blood source for longer than approximately 5 to 7 days at room temperature. In contrast with head lice, body lice are well-recognized vectors of disease (eg, epidemic typhus, trench fever, epidemic relapsing fever, bacillary angiomatosis).

Incubation Period

From laying eggs to hatching of first nymph, 1 to 2 weeks. Lice mature and are capable of reproducing 9 to 19 days after hatching.

Diagnostic Tests

Identification of eggs, nymphs, and lice with the naked eye is possible; diagnosis can be confirmed by using a hand lens, dermatoscope (epiluminescence microscope), or a traditional microscope. Adult and nymphal body lice are seldom seen on the body because they are generally sequestered in clothing.

Treatment

Treatment consists of improving hygiene and regular changes of clean clothes and bedding. Infested materials can be decontaminated by washing in hot water (at least 53.5°C [128.3°F]), by machine drying at hot temperatures, by dry cleaning, or by pressing with a hot iron. Temperatures exceeding 53.5°C (128.3°F) for 5 minutes are lethal to lice and eggs. Pediculicides are not usually necessary if materials are laundered at least weekly. Some people with much body hair may require full-body treatment with a pediculicide because lice and eggs may adhere to body hair.

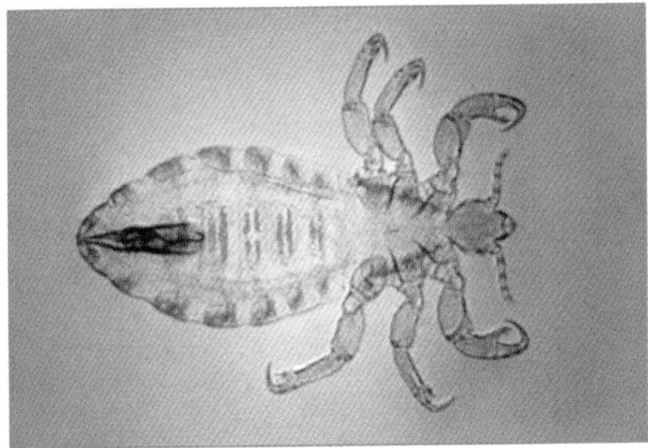

Image 101.1
This body louse, *Pediculus humanus humanus,* was photographed during a 1972 study of migrant labor camp disease vectors. Body lice, family Pediculidae, are parasitic insects that live on the body and in the clothing or bedding of infested humans. Infestation is common and is found worldwide. Itching and rash are common with lice infestation. Courtesy of Centers for Disease Control and Prevention.

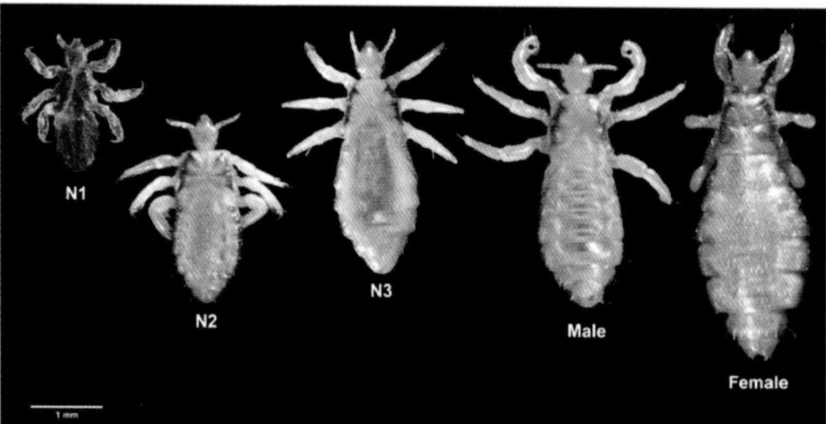

Image 101.2
This 2006 image depicted 5 body lice, *Pediculus humanus humanus,* which, from left to right, include 3 nymphal-staged lice, beginning with a stage N1, then N2, and, thirdly, an N3-staged nymph, followed by an adult male louse and, finally, an adult female louse. Courtesy of Centers for Disease Control and Prevention/Joseph Strycharz, PhD; Kyong Sup Yoon, PhD; Frank Collins, PhD.

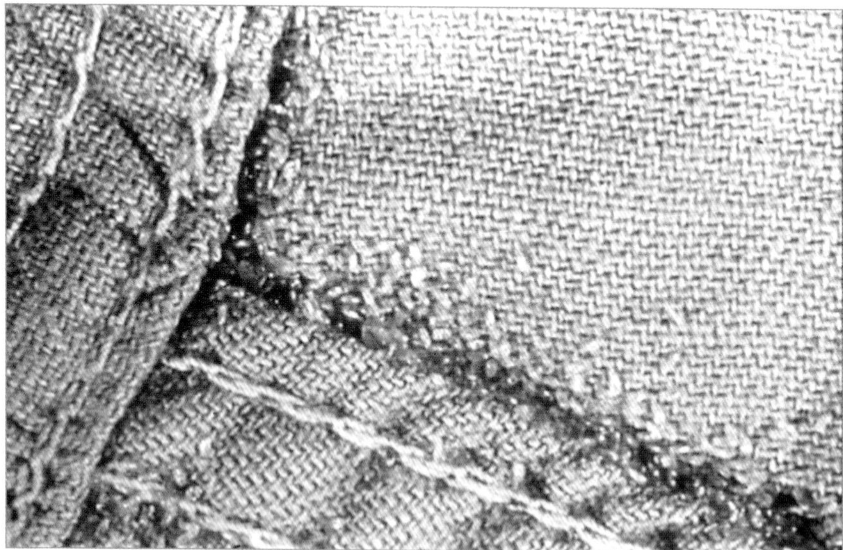

Image 101.3
This is a piece of clothing, the seams of which contained lice eggs from the body louse *Pediculus humanus humanus.* The most important factor in the control of body lice infestation is the ability to change and wash clothing. Courtesy of Centers for Disease Control and Prevention/Reed & Carnrick Pharmaceuticals.

102

Pediculosis Pubis

(Pubic Lice, Crab Lice)

Clinical Manifestations

Pruritus of the anogenital area is a common symptom in pubic lice infestations ("crabs" or "phthiriasis"). The parasite is found most frequently in the pubic region, but infestation can involve the eyelashes, eyebrows, beard, axilla, perianal area, and, rarely, scalp. A characteristic sign of heavy pubic lice infestation is the presence of bluish or slate-colored macules (maculae ceruleae) on the chest, abdomen, or thighs.

Etiology

Phthirus pubis is the pubic or crab louse. Nymphs and adult lice feed on human blood.

Epidemiology

Pubic lice infestations are more prevalent in adults and are usually transmitted through sexual contact. Transmission by contaminated items, such as towels, is uncommon. Pubic lice on the eyelashes or eyebrows of children may be evidence of sexual abuse, although other modes of transmission are possible. Infested people should be examined for other sexually transmitted infections. Adult pubic lice can survive away from a host for up to 36 hours, and their eggs can remain viable for up to 10 days under suitable environmental conditions.

Incubation Period

From the laying of eggs to the hatching of first nymph, 6 to 10 days. Adult lice become capable of reproducing approximately 2 to 3 weeks after hatching.

Diagnostic Tests

Identification of eggs (nits), nymphs, and lice with the naked eye is possible; the diagnosis can be confirmed by using a hand lens, microscope, or dermatoscope.

Treatment

All areas of the body with coarse hair should be examined for evidence of pubic lice infestation. Lice and their eggs can be removed manually, or the hairs can be shaved to eliminate infestation immediately. Caution should be used when inspecting, removing, or treating lice on or near the eyelashes. Pediculicides used to treat other kinds of louse infestations are effective for treatment of pubic lice. Retreatment is recommended as for head lice. For treatment of pubic lice infestation of eyelashes, an ophthalmic-grade petrolatum ointment is applied to the eyelashes 2 to 4 times daily for 8 to 10 days.

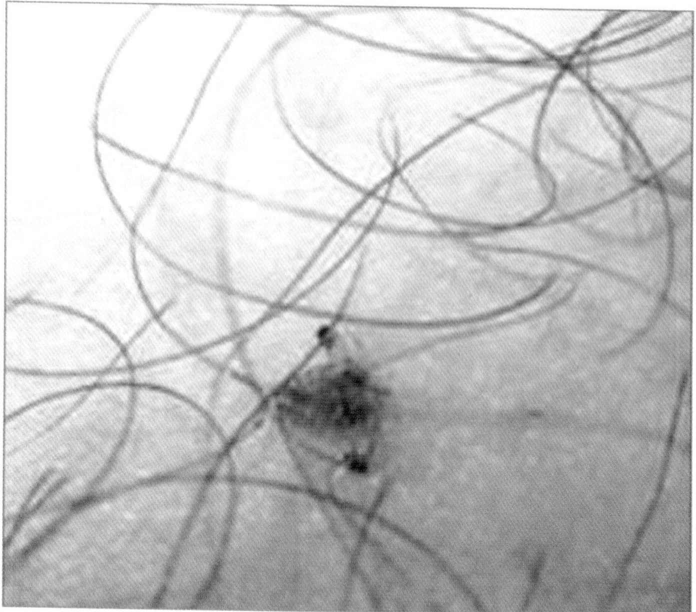

Image 102.1
Pediculosis, the infestation of humans by lice, has been documented for millennia. Three species of lice infest humans: *Pediculus humanus humanus,* the body louse; *Pediculus humanus capitis,* the head louse; and *Pthirus pubis,* the pubic or crab louse. The hallmark of louse infestation is pruritus at the site of bites. Lice are more active at night, frequently disrupting the sleep of the host, which is the derivation of the term "feeling lousy." Adult pubic lice can survive without a blood meal for 36 hours. Unlike head lice, which may travel up to 23 cm per minute, pubic lice are sluggish, traveling a maximum of 10 cm per day. Viable eggs on pubic hairs may hatch up to 10 days later. Pubic louse infestation is localized most frequently to the pubic and perianal regions but may spread to the mustache, beard, axillae, eyelashes, or scalp hair. Infestation is usually acquired through sexual contact, and the finding of pubic lice in children (often limited to the eyelashes) should raise concern for possible sexual abuse. Courtesy of H. Cody Meissner, MD, FAAP.

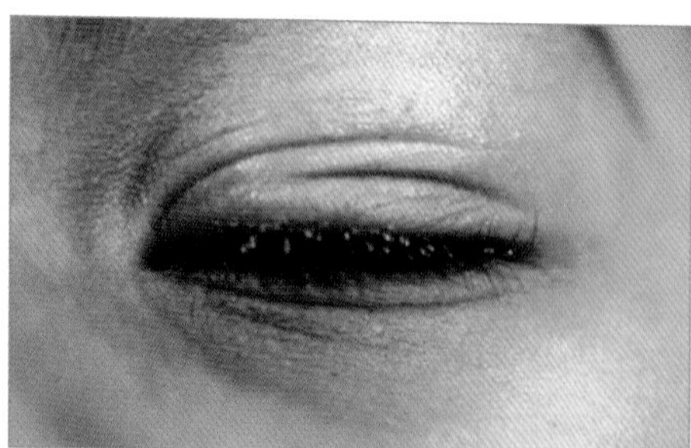

Image 102.2
Pubic lice *(Phthirus pubis)* in the eyelashes of a 3-year-old boy. The diagnosis can be confirmed by the use of a hand lens or microscope. Copyright Gary Williams.

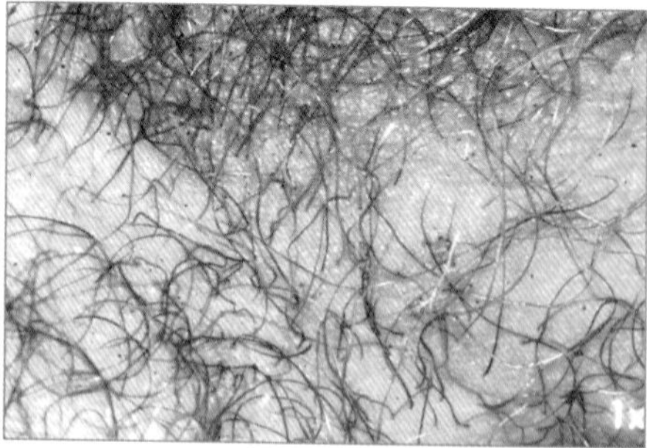

Image 102.3
This photograph reveals the presence of pubic or crab lice, *Pthirus pubis,* with reddish-brown feces. Pubic lice are generally found in the genital area on pubic hair but may occasionally be found on other coarse body hair, such as leg hair, armpit hair, mustache, beard, eyebrows, and eyelashes. Courtesy of Centers for Disease Control and Prevention/Reed & Carnrick Pharmaceuticals.

103

Pertussis (Whooping Cough)

Clinical Manifestations

Pertussis begins with mild upper respiratory tract symptoms similar to the common cold (catarrhal stage) and progresses to cough and then usually to paroxysms of cough (paroxysmal stage), characterized by inspiratory whoop and commonly followed by vomiting. Fever is absent or minimal. Symptoms wane gradually over weeks to months (convalescent stage). Cough illness in immunized children and adults can range from typical to mild and unrecognized. The duration of classic pertussis is 6 to 10 weeks. Approximately half of adolescents with pertussis cough for 10 weeks or longer. Complications among adolescents and adults include syncope, weight loss, sleep disturbance, incontinence, rib fractures, and pneumonia; among adults, complications increase with age. Pertussis is most severe when it occurs during the first 6 months of life, particularly in preterm and unimmunized or underimmunized infants. Disease in infants younger than 6 months can be atypical with a short catarrhal stage, followed by gagging, gasping, bradycardia, or apnea (67%) as prominent early manifestations; absence of whoop; and prolonged convalescence. Sudden unexpected death can be caused by pertussis. Complications among infants include pneumonia (23%) and pulmonary hypertension, as well as complications related to severe coughing spells, such as subdural or conjunctival bleeding and hernia, and severe coughing spells leading to hypoxia and complications such as seizures (2%), encephalopathy (<0.5%), apnea, and death. More than two-thirds of infants with pertussis are hospitalized. Case-fatality rates are approximately 1% in infants younger than 2 months and less than 0.5% in infants 2 through 11 months of age.

Etiology

Pertussis is caused by a fastidious, gram-negative, pleomorphic bacillus, *Bordetella pertussis*. Other causes of sporadic prolonged cough illness include *Bordetella parapertussis*, *Mycoplasma pneumoniae*, *Chlamydia trachomatis*, *Chlamydophila pneumoniae*, *Bordetella bronchiseptica* (the cause of kennel cough), *Bordetella holmesii*, and certain respiratory tract viruses, particularly adenoviruses and respiratory syncytial viruses.

Epidemiology

Humans are the only known hosts of *B pertussis*. Transmission occurs by close contact with cases via aerosolized droplets. Cases occur year-round, typically with a late summer-autumn peak. Neither infection nor immunization provides lifelong immunity. Lack of natural booster events and waning immunity since the most recent immunization, particularly when acellular pertussis vaccine is used for the entire immunization series, are responsible for increased cases reported in school-aged children, adolescents, and adults. Additionally, waning maternal immunity and reduced transplacental antibody in mothers who have not received tetanus, diphtheria, acellular pertussis vaccine during pregnancy contribute to an increase in pertussis in very young infants. More than 41,000 cases of pertussis were reported in the United States in 2012, the highest in people older than 50 years. Up to 80% of previously immunized household contacts of symptomatic cases are infected with pertussis. Symptoms in these contacts vary from asymptomatic infection to classic pertussis. Older siblings (including adolescents) and adults with mild or unrecognized atypical disease are important sources of pertussis for infants and young children. Infected people are most contagious during the catarrhal stage through the third week after onset of paroxysms. Factors affecting the length of communicability include age, immunization status or previous infection, and appropriate antimicrobial therapy.

Incubation Period

7 to 10 days; range, 5 to 21 days.

Diagnostic Tests

Culture is considered the gold standard for laboratory diagnosis of pertussis. Although culture is 100% specific, it is not optimally sensitive because *B pertussis* is a fastidious organism. Culture requires collection of an appropriate nasopharyngeal specimen, obtained by aspiration or with Dacron (polyethylene terephthalate) or calcium alginate swabs. Specimens must be placed into special transport media immediately and not allowed to dry while being transported promptly to the laboratory. Culture results can be negative if taken from a previously immunized person, if antimicrobial therapy has been started, if more than 2 weeks has elapsed since cough onset, or if the specimen is not handled appropriately.

Polymerase chain reaction (PCR) assay is now the most commonly used laboratory method for detection of *B pertussis* because of its improved sensitivity and more rapid turnaround time. The PCR test requires collection of an adequate nasopharyngeal specimen. Calcium alginate swabs are inhibitory to PCR and should not be used for PCR tests. The PCR test has optimal sensitivity during the first 3 weeks of cough, is unlikely to be useful if antimicrobial therapy has been given for more than 5 days, and lacks sensitivity in previously immunized people. Unacceptably high rates of false-positive results are reported from some laboratories, and pseudo-outbreaks linked to contaminated specimens have also been reported. The Centers for Disease Control and Prevention has released a best practices document to guide pertussis PCR assays (**www.cdc.gov/pertussis/clinical/diagnostic-testing/diagnosis-pcr-bestpractices.html**) as well as a video demonstrating optimal specimen collection. Multiple DNA target sequences are required to distinguish between *Bordetella* species. Direct fluorescent antibody testing is no longer recommended.

Commercial serologic tests for pertussis infection can be helpful for diagnosis, especially later in illness and in adolescents and adults. In the absence of recent immunization, an elevated serum immunoglobulin (Ig) G antibody to pertussis toxin (PT) after 2 weeks of onset of cough is suggestive of recent *B pertussis* infection. An increasing titer, a single IgG anti-PT value of approximately 100 IU/mL or greater, or a decreasing titer, if obtained later in the illness, are considered diagnostic.

An increased white blood cell count attributable to absolute lymphocytosis is suggestive of pertussis in infants and young children but is often absent in adolescents and adults with pertussis. A markedly elevated white blood cell count is associated with a poor prognosis in young infants.

Treatment

Antimicrobial agents administered during the catarrhal stage may ameliorate the disease. Clinicians should begin antimicrobial therapy prior to test results if the clinical history is strongly suggestive of pertussis or the patient is at high risk of severe or complicated disease (eg, young infants). After the cough is established, antimicrobial agents have no discernible effect on the course of illness but are recommended to limit spread of organisms to others. A 5-day course of azithromycin is appropriate for treatment. Azithromycin should be used with caution in people with long QT syndrome and proarrhythmic conditions. Resistance of *B pertussis* to macrolide antimicrobial agents has been reported, but rarely. Penicillins and first- and second-generation cephalosporins are not effective against *B pertussis*.

Antimicrobial agents used for infants younger than 6 months require special consideration. An association between orally administered erythromycin and azithromycin with infantile hypertrophic pyloric stenosis has been reported in neonates younger than 1 month. Azithromycin is the drug of choice for treatment or prophylaxis of pertussis in neonates younger than 1 month in whom the risk of developing severe pertussis and life-threatening complications outweighs the potential risk of infantile hypertrophic pyloric stenosis.

Trimethoprim-sulfamethoxazole is an alternative for patients older than 2 months who cannot tolerate macrolides or who are infected with a macrolide-resistant strain, but studies evaluating trimethoprim-sulfamethoxazole as treatment for pertussis are limited.

Young infants are at increased risk of respiratory failure, secondary bacterial pneumonia, and cardiopulmonary failure and death from severe pulmonary hypertension. Hospitalized young infants with pertussis should be managed in a setting where these complications can be recognized and managed urgently.

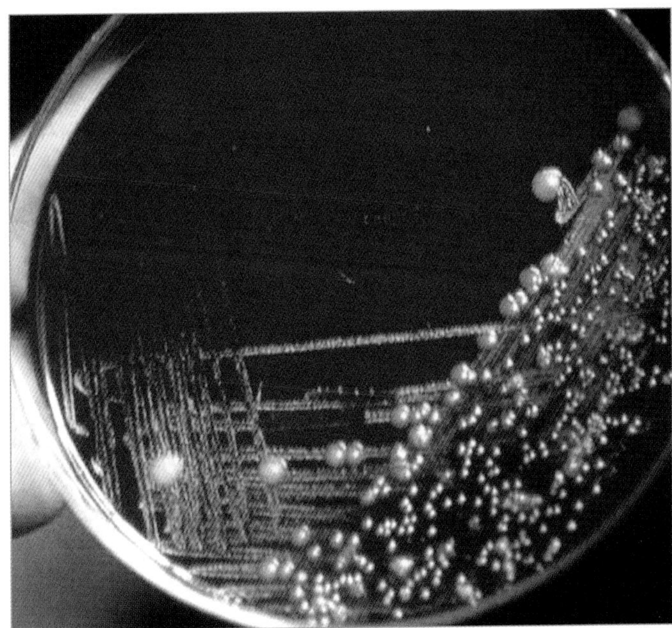

Image 103.1
Colonies of *Bordetella pertussis* growing on Bordet-Gengou agar. Courtesy of Edgar O. Ledbetter, MD, FAAP.

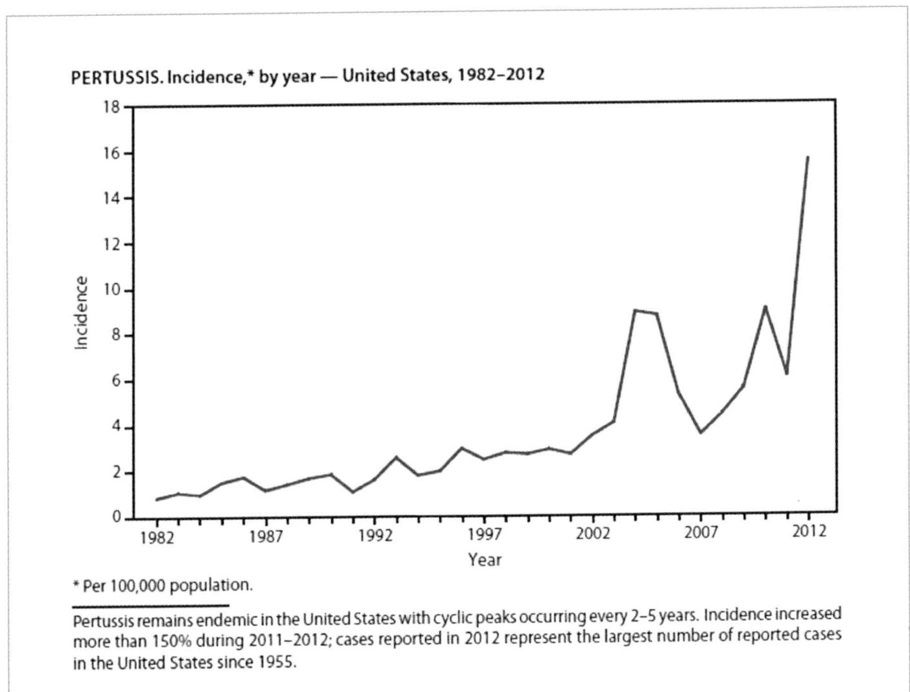

Image 103.2
Pertussis. Incidence, by year—United States, 1982–2012. Courtesy of *Morbidity and Mortality Weekly Report.*

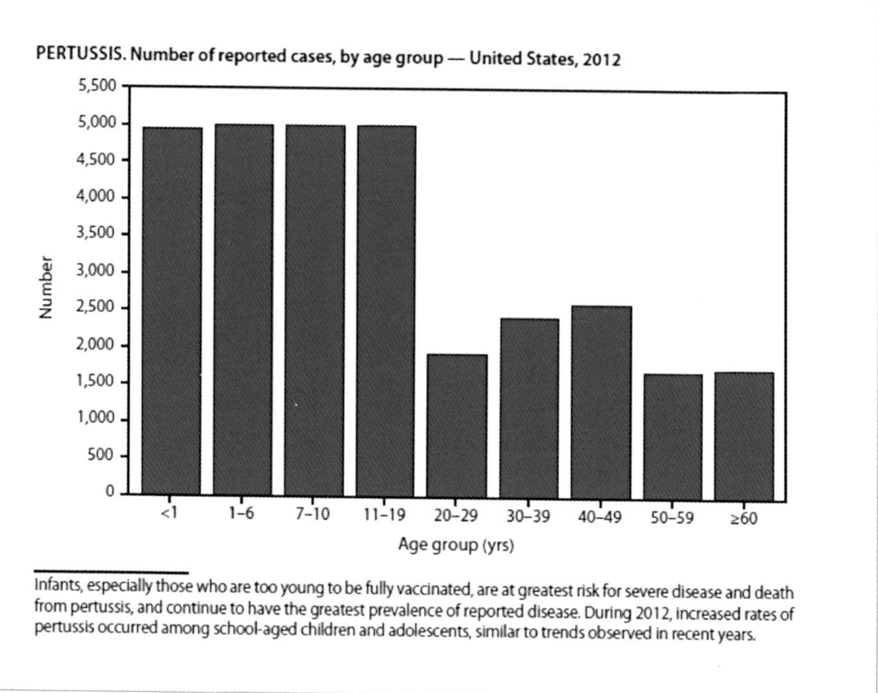

Image 103.3

Pertussis. Number of reported cases, by age group—United States, 2012. Courtesy of *Morbidity and Mortality Weekly Report.*

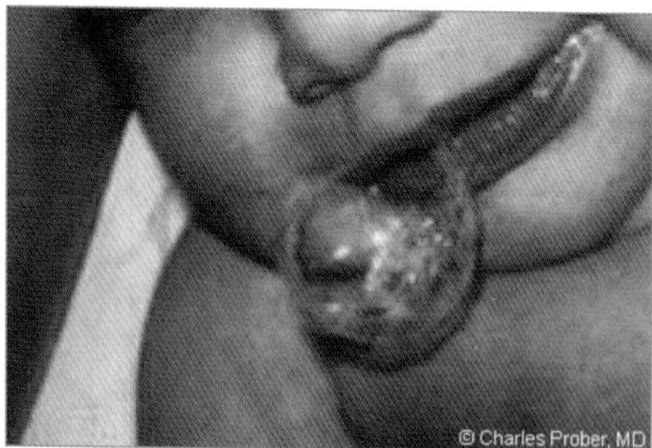

Image 103.4

Thick bronchopulmonary secretions of pertussis in an infant. Copyright Charles Prober, MD.

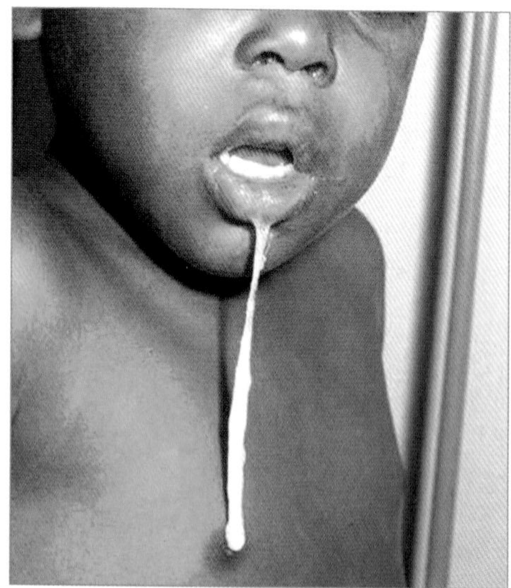

Image 103.5

A preschool-aged boy with pertussis. Thick respiratory secretions were produced by a paroxysmal coughing spell. Courtesy of Edgar O. Ledbetter, MD, FAAP.

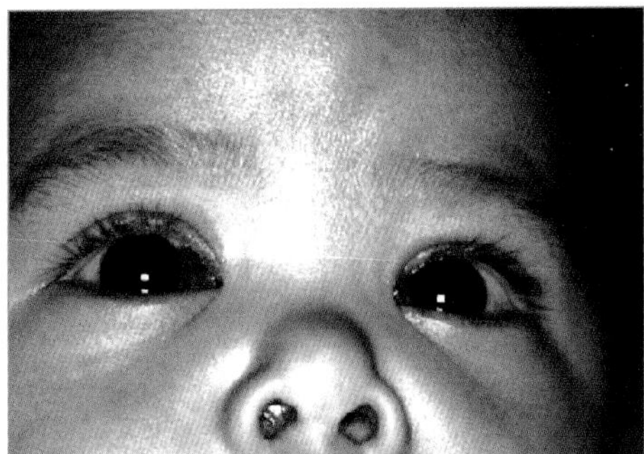

Image 103.6
Bilateral subconjunctival hemorrhages and thick nasal mucus in an infant with pertussis.

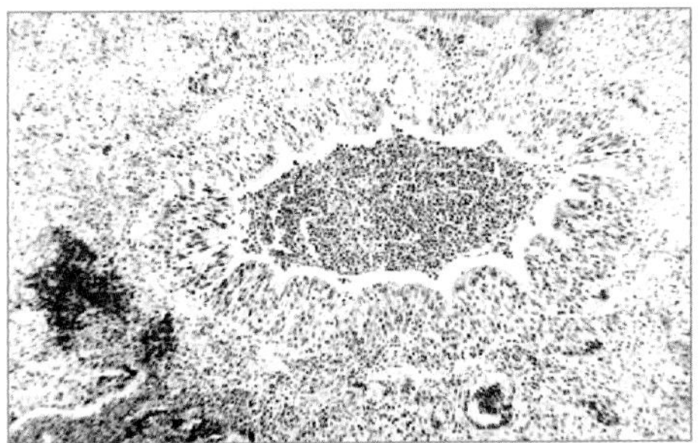

Image 103.8
Bronchiolar plugging in the neonate in Image 103.7 who died of pertussis pneumonia. Neonates, infants, and children often acquire pertussis from an infected adult or sibling contact.

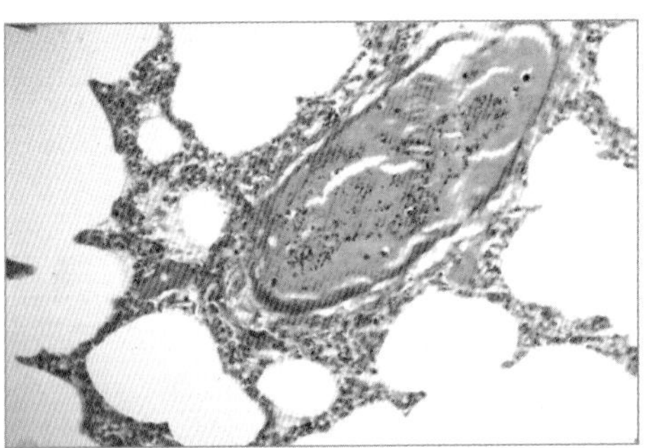

Image 103.10
Plugging and alveolar dilatation of pertussis pneumonia in an infant who died. Courtesy of Edgar O. Ledbetter, MD, FAAP.

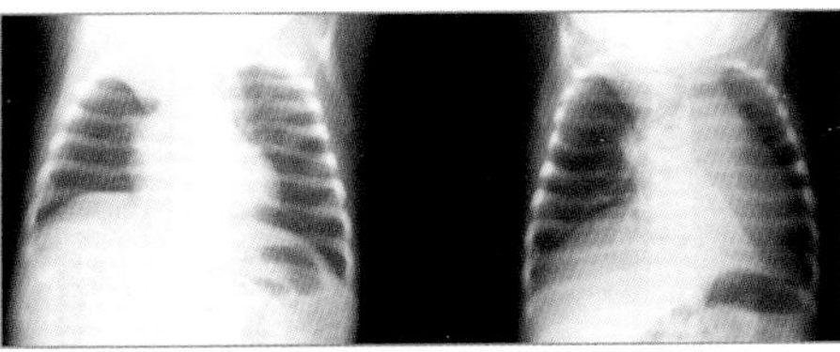

Image 103.7
A 4-week-old with pertussis pneumonia with pulmonary air trapping and progressive atelectasis confirmed at autopsy. The neonate acquired the infection from the mother shortly after birth. Segmented and lobar atelectasis are not uncommon complications of pertussis.

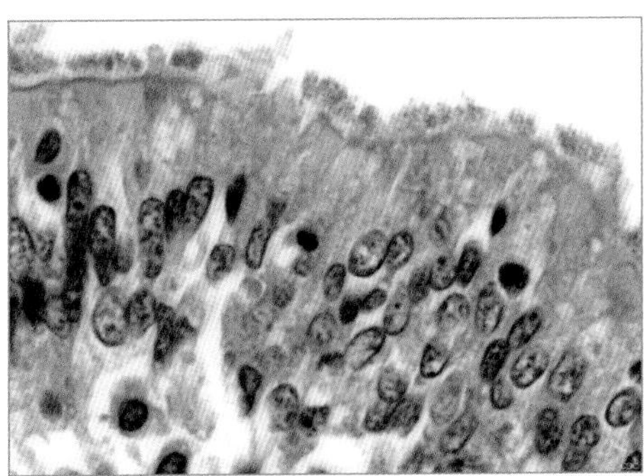

Image 103.9
Bordetella pertussis bacteria enmeshed in the cilia of respiratory epithelial cells lining a bronchiole in an infant with fatal pertussis (hematoxylin-eosin stain, original magnification x100). Courtesy of Christopher Paddock, MD.

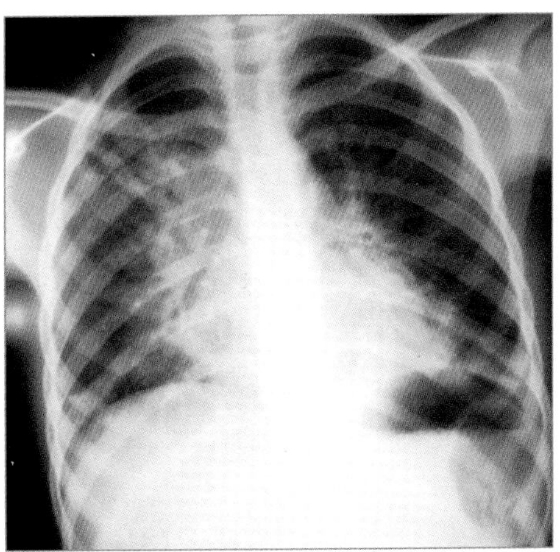

Image 103.11
Pertussis pneumonia in a 7-year-old who was exhausted from persistent coughing. Obliteration of cardiac borders on the chest radiograph is a common radiographic change of pertussis pneumonia.

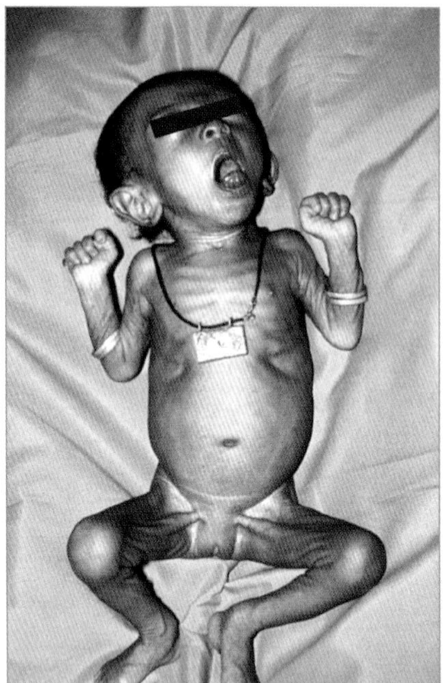

Image 103.12
This image depicts a malnourished female infant who presented to a clinic suffering from what was diagnosed as pertussis. Pertussis is a highly communicable, vaccine-preventable disease caused by *Bordetella pertussis,* a gram-negative coccobacillus, that lasts for many weeks and typically afflicts children with severe coughing, whooping, and posttussive vomiting. Courtesy of Centers for Disease Control and Prevention.

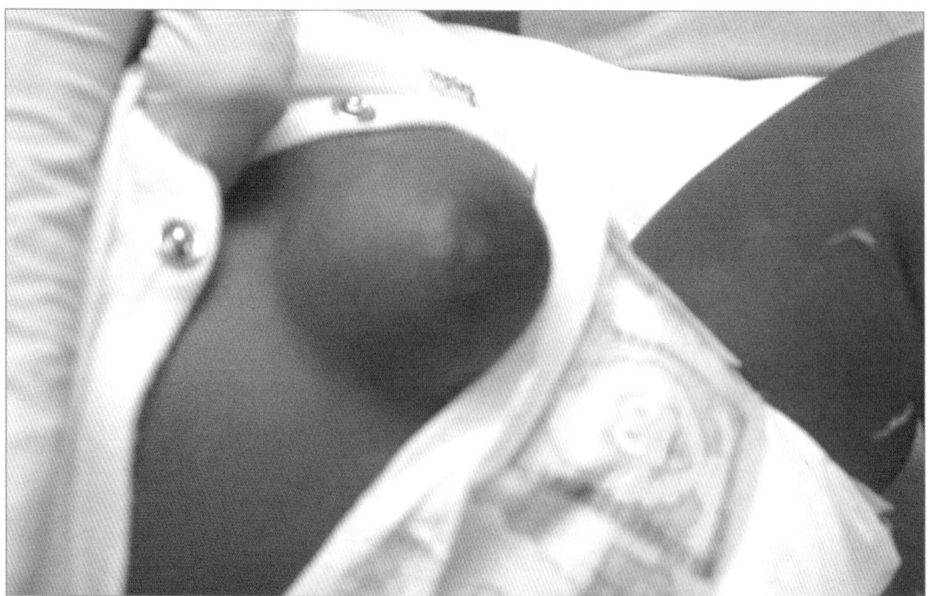

Image 103.13
Umbilical hernia more prominent as a result of persistent pertussis cough in a 4-month-old boy. Courtesy of Benjamin Estrada, MD.

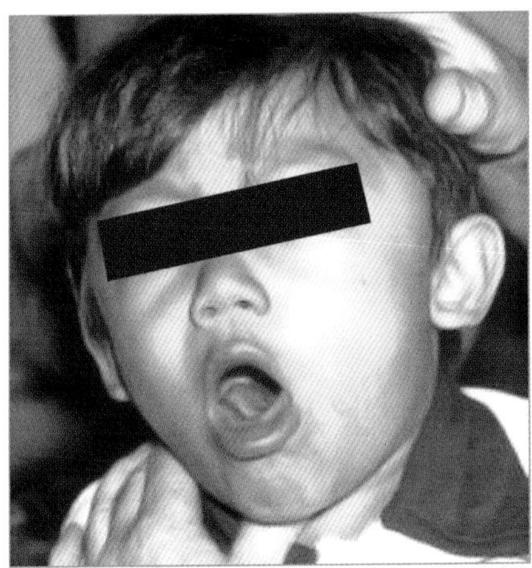

Image 103.14
This child has pertussis (whooping cough). He has severe coughing spasms, which are often followed by a whooping sound. It is difficult for him to stop coughing and catch his breath. Courtesy of Centers for Disease Control and Prevention.

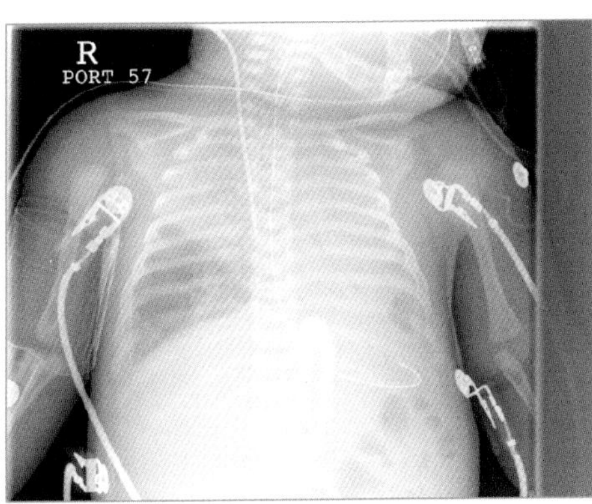

Image 103.15
Pertussis pneumonia in a 2-month-old 2 days after hospital admission. His mother had been coughing since shortly after delivery. Courtesy of Carol J. Baker, MD, FAAP.

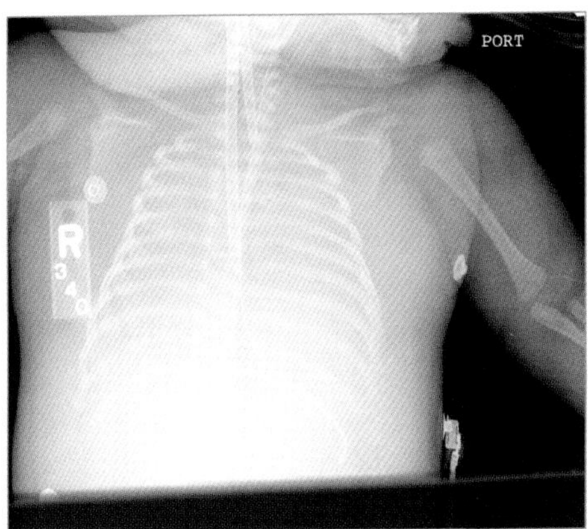

Image 103.16
The infant in Image 103.15 required mechanical ventilation because of respiratory failure. Courtesy of Carol J. Baker, MD, FAAP.

104

Pinworm Infection

(*Enterobius vermicularis*)

Clinical Manifestations

Although some people are asymptomatic, pinworm infection (enterobiasis) can cause pruritus ani and, rarely, pruritus vulvae. Bacterial superinfections can result from scratching and excoriation of an area. Although pinworms have been found in the lumen of the appendix and, in some cases, these intraluminal parasites have been associated with acute appendicitis, pinworms have also been observed in histologically normal appendixes. Many clinical findings, such as grinding of teeth at night, weight loss, and enuresis, have been attributed to pinworm infections, but proof of a causal relationship has not been established. Urethritis, vaginitis, salpingitis, or pelvic peritonitis may occur from aberrant migration of an adult worm from the perineum.

Etiology

Enterobius vermicularis is a nematode or roundworm.

Epidemiology

Enterobiasis occurs worldwide and commonly clusters within families. Prevalence rates are higher in preschool- and school-aged children, in primary caregivers of infected children, and in institutionalized people; up to 50% of these populations may be infected.

Egg transmission occurs by the fecal-oral route directly or indirectly via contaminated hands or fomites such as shared toys, bedding, clothing, toilet seats, and baths. Female pinworms usually die after depositing up to 10,000 fertilized eggs within 24 hours on the perianal skin. Reinfection occurs by autoinfection, from pinworms crawling into the rectum after hatching, or by infection following ingestion of eggs from another person. A person remains infectious as long as female nematodes are discharging eggs on perianal skin. Eggs usually remain infective in an indoor environment for 2 to 3 weeks. Humans are the only known natural hosts; dogs and cats do not harbor *E vermicularis*.

Incubation Period

From ingestion of an egg until an adult gravid female migrates to the perianal region, 1 to 2 months or longer.

Diagnostic Tests

Diagnosis is made when adult worms are visualized in the perianal region, which is best examined 2 to 3 hours after the child is asleep. No egg shedding occurs inside the intestinal lumen; thus, very few ova are present in stool, so examination of stool specimens for ova and parasites is not recommended. Alternatively, diagnosis is made by touching the perianal skin with transparent (not translucent) adhesive tape to collect any eggs that may be present; the tape is then applied to a glass slide and examined under a low-power microscopic lens. Specimens should be obtained on 3 consecutive mornings when the child first awakens. Eosinophilia is unusual and should not be attributed to pinworm infection.

Treatment

Because pinworms are largely innocuous, the risk versus benefit of treatments should be weighed. Drugs of choice for treatment are pyrantel pamoate and albendazole, which are given in a single dose and repeated in 2 weeks because none of these drugs are completely effective against the egg or developing larvae stages. Pyrantel pamoate is available without prescription. Reinfection with pinworms occurs easily; prevention should be discussed when treatment is given. Infected people should bathe in the morning; bathing removes a large proportion of eggs. Frequently changing the infected child's underclothes, bedclothes, and bedsheets may decrease the egg contamination of the local environment and risk of reinfection. Specific personal hygiene measures (eg, exercising hand hygiene before eating or preparing food, keeping fingernails short, avoiding scratching of the perianal region, avoiding nail biting) may decrease risk of autoinfection and continued transmission. All household members should be treated as a group in situations in which multiple or repeated symptomatic infections occur. Vaginitis is self-limited and does not require separate treatment.

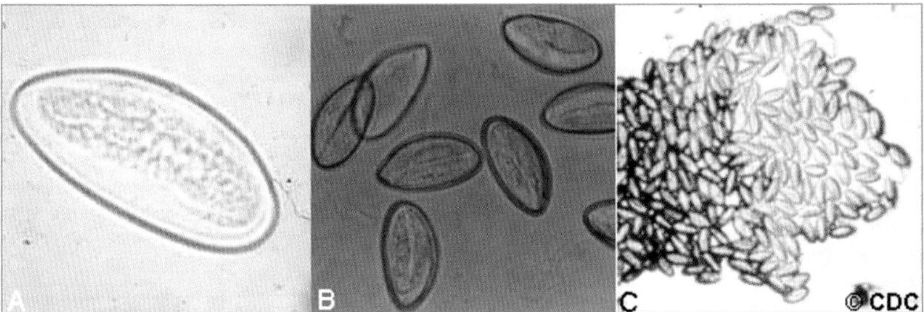

Image 104.1
A, B, Enterobius egg(s). C, Enterobius eggs on cellulose tape preparation. Courtesy of Centers for Disease Control and Prevention.

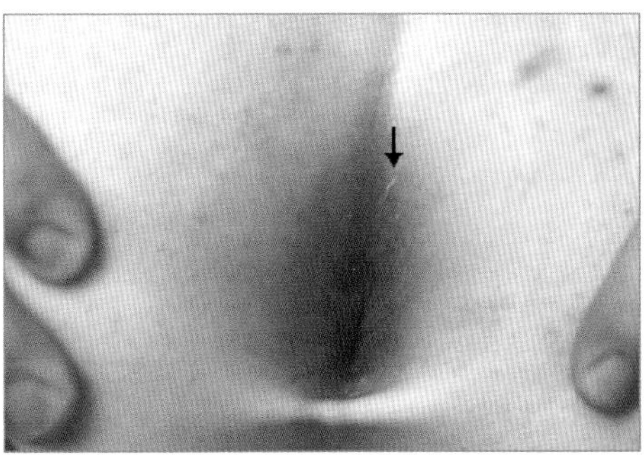

Image 104.2
Adult pinworm (*Enterobius vermicularis*) in the perianal area of a 14-year-old boy. Perianal inspection 2 to 3 hours after the child goes to sleep may reveal pinworms that have migrated outside of the intestinal tract. Copyright Gary Williams.

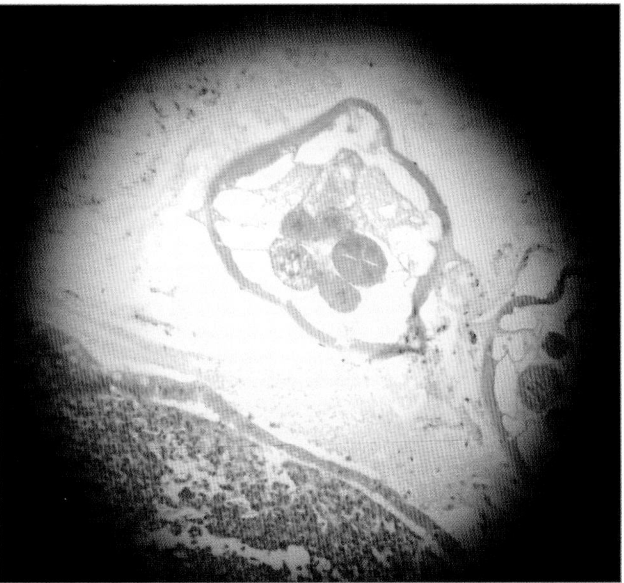

Image 104.3
Enterobius vermicularis in the lumen of the appendix of a 10-year-old. Pinworms can be found in the lumen of the appendix, but most evidence indicates they do not cause acute appendicitis. Courtesy of Benjamin Estrada, MD.

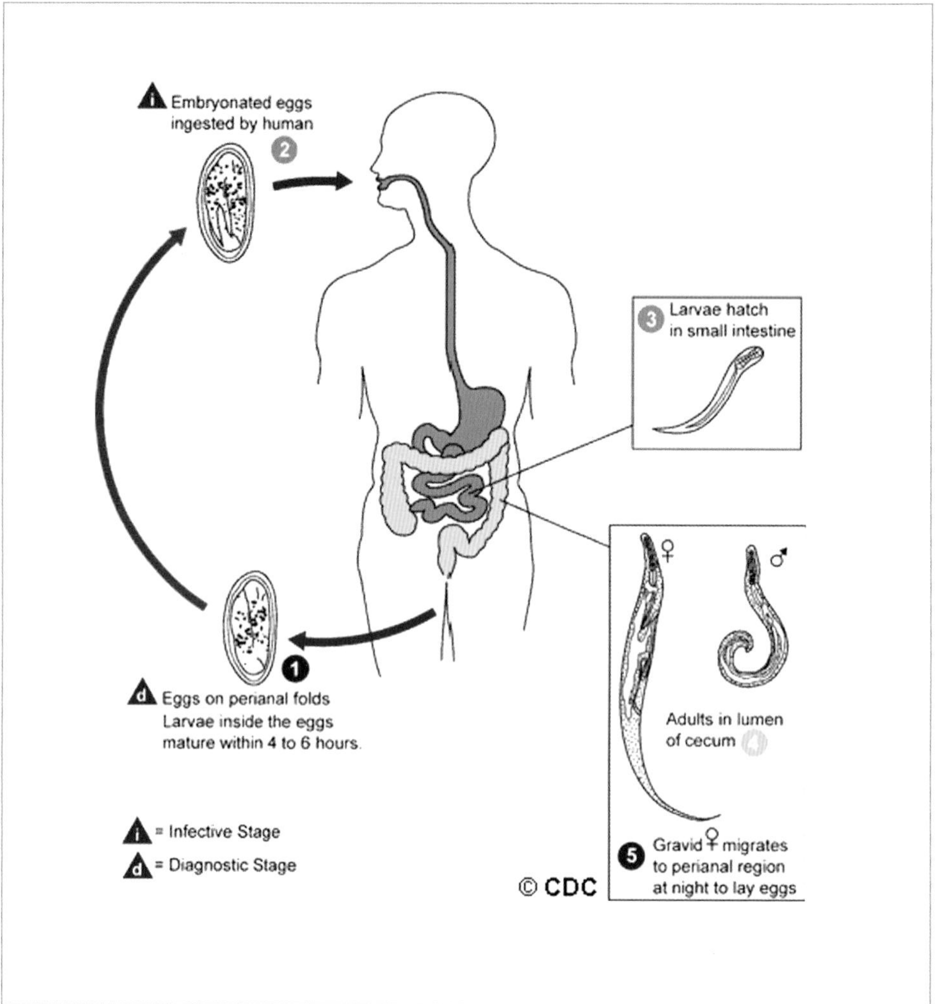

Image 104.4

Eggs are deposited on perianal folds (1). Self-infection occurs by transferring infective eggs to the mouth with hands that have scratched the perianal area (2). Person-to-person transmission can also occur through handling of contaminated clothes or bed linens. Enterobiasis may also be acquired through surfaces in the environment that are contaminated with pinworm eggs (eg, curtains, carpeting). Some small number of eggs may become airborne and inhaled. These could be swallowed and follow the same development as ingested eggs. Following ingestion of infective eggs, the larvae hatch in the small intestine (3) and the adults establish themselves in the colon (4). The time interval from ingestion of infective eggs to oviposition by the adult females is about 1 month. The life span of the adults is about 2 months. Gravid females migrate nocturnally outside the anus and oviposit while crawling on the skin of the perianal area (5). The larvae contained inside the eggs develop (the eggs become infective) in 4 to 6 hours under optimal conditions (1). Retroinfection, or the migration of newly hatched larvae from the anal skin back into the rectum, may occur, but the frequency with which this happens is unknown. Courtesy of Centers for Disease Control and Prevention.

105

Pityriasis Versicolor

(Tinea Versicolor)

Clinical Manifestations

Pityriasis versicolor (formerly tinea versicolor) is a common and benign superficial infection of the skin. It classically occurs in adolescence and involves the upper trunk and neck. Infants and children are more likely to exhibit facial involvement. The condition can occur at any age and may involve other areas, including the scalp, genital area, and thighs. Symmetric involvement with ovoid discrete or coalescent lesions of varying size is typical; these macules or patches vary in color, even in the same person. White, pink, tan, or brown coloration is often surmounted by faint dusty scales. Common conditions confused with this disorder include pityriasis alba, vitiligo, seborrheic dermatitis, pityriasis rosea, progressive macular hypopigmentation, pityriasis lichenoides, and secondary syphilis.

Etiology

The cause of pityriasis versicolor is *Malassezia* species, a group of lipid-dependent yeasts that exist on healthy skin in yeast phase and cause clinical lesions only when substantial growth of hyphae occurs. Lesions fail to tan during the summer and are relatively darker during the winter, hence the term versicolor.

Epidemiology

Pityriasis versicolor can occur in any climate or age group but tends to favor adolescents and young adults, particularly in tropical climates. Moisture, heat, and the presence of lipids from the sebaceous glands seem to encourage hyphal overgrowth. These organisms can also cause systemic infections in neonates, particularly those receiving total parenteral nutrition with lipids, and folliculitis, particularly in immunocompromised individuals.

Incubation Period

Unknown.

Diagnostic Tests

The presence of symmetrically distributed, faintly scaling macules and patches of varying color concentrated on the upper back and chest is diagnostic. The "evoked scale" sign consists of stretching or scraping involved skin, which elicits a visible layer of thin scale. Involved areas fluoresce yellow-green under Wood lamp evaluation. Potassium hydroxide wet mount preparation of scraped scales reveals the classic "spaghetti and meatballs" short hyphae and clusters of yeast forms. Because this yeast is a common inhabitant of the skin, culture from the surface is nondiagnostic. Growth requires media enriched with sterile olive oil or another long-chain fatty acid.

Treatment

Multiple topical and systemic agents are efficacious, and recommendations vary substantially. The most cost-effective treatments are selenium sulfide shampoo/lotion and clotrimazole cream for 2 to 3 weeks. Effective topical agents include ketoconazole, bifonazole, miconazole, econazole, oxiconazole, clotrimazole, terbinafine, and ciclopirox, as well as zinc pyrithione shampoo. Systemic therapies, including fluconazole and ketoconazole, are easy to use and are effective. Single doses do not appear to be as efficacious as multiple doses over several days or weeks. Although oral agents are easier to use, they are not necessarily more effective and have possible serious side effects. For uncomplicated cases, most experts recommend initiating therapy with topical agents; selenium sulfide shampoo used for 3 to 7 days for 5 to 10 minutes and then showered off; or a topical azole applied twice daily for 2 to 3 weeks. Systemic therapy is reserved for resistant infection or extensive involvement. Repigmentation may not occur for several months after treatment.

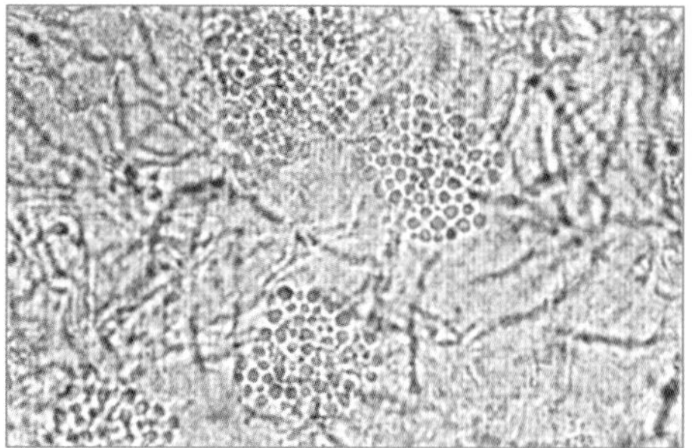

Image 105.1
The spores and pseudohyphae of *Malassezia furfur* (a yeast that can cause pityriasis versicolor) resemble spaghetti and meatballs on a potassium hydroxide slide.

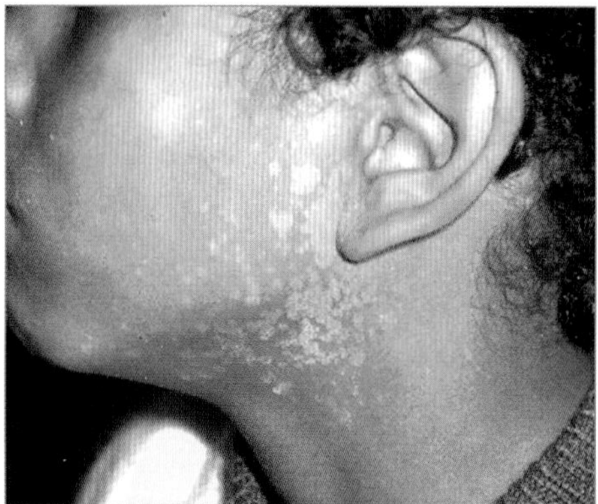

Image 105.3
Pityriasis versicolor. Courtesy of Edgar K. Marcuse, MD.

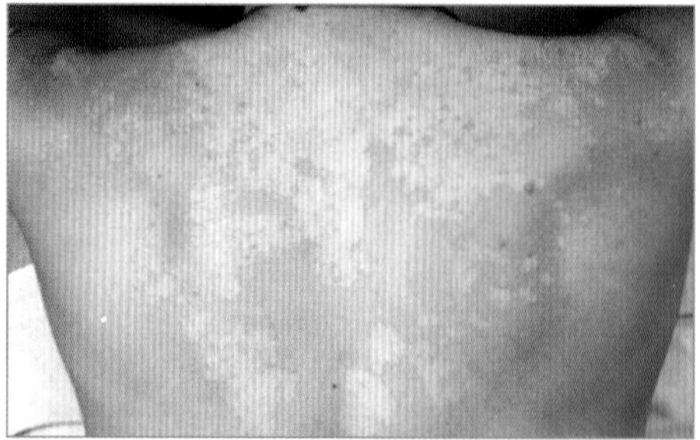

Image 105.5
Pityriasis versicolor in a 16-year-old boy. Courtesy of Gary Williams, MD/Dr Lucille K. Georg.

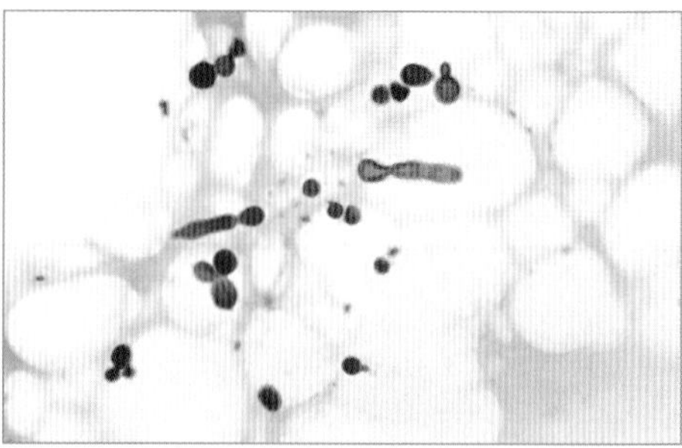

Image 105.2
Note the yeastlike fungal cells and short hyphae of *Malassezia furfur* in skin scale from a patient with pityriasis versicolor. Usually, *M furfur* grows sparsely without causing a rash. In some individuals, it grows more actively for reasons unknown, resulting in pale brown, flaky patches on the trunk, neck, or arms, a condition called pityriasis versicolor (formerly called tinea versicolor). Courtesy of Centers for Disease Control and Prevention/Dr Lucille K. Georg.

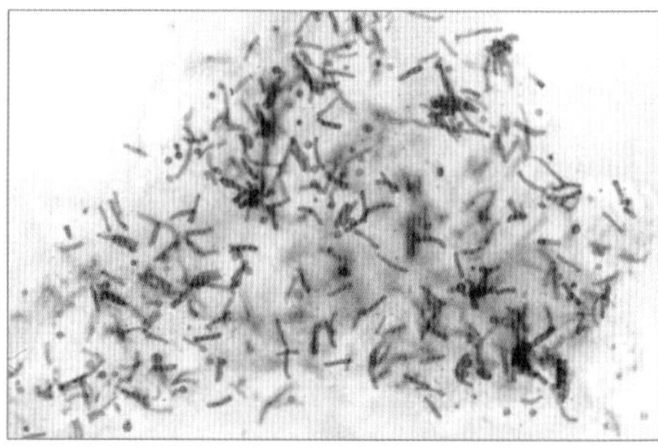

Image 105.4
This photomicrograph of a skin scale reveals the presence of the fungus *Malassezia furfur.* Usually, *M furfur* grows sparsely without causing a rash. In some individuals, it grows more actively for reasons unknown, resulting in pale brown, flaky patches on the trunk, neck, or arms, a condition called pityriasis versicolor (formerly called tinea versicolor). Courtesy of Centers for Disease Control and Prevention.

106

Plague

Clinical Manifestations

Naturally acquired plague most commonly manifests in the **bubonic form,** with acute onset of fever and painful swollen regional lymph nodes (buboes). Buboes most commonly develop in the inguinal region but also occur in axillary or cervical areas. Less commonly, plague manifests in the **septicemic form** (ie, hypotension, acute respiratory distress, purpuric skin lesions, intravascular coagulopathy, organ failure) or as **pneumonic plague** (ie, cough, fever, dyspnea, and hemoptysis) and, rarely, as **meningeal, pharyngeal, ocular,** or **gastrointestinal plague.** Abrupt onset of fever, chills, headache, and malaise are characteristic in all cases. Occasionally, patients have symptoms of mild lymphadenitis or prominent gastrointestinal tract symptoms, which may obscure the correct diagnosis. When left untreated, plague will often progress to overwhelming sepsis with renal failure, acute respiratory distress syndrome, instability, diffuse intravascular coagulation, necrosis of distal extremities, and death. Plague has been referred to as the black death.

Etiology

Plague is caused by *Yersinia pestis,* a pleomorphic, bipolar-staining, gram-negative coccobacillus.

Epidemiology

Plague is a zoonotic infection primarily maintained in rodents and their fleas. Humans are incidental hosts who typically develop bubonic or primary septicemic manifestations through the bite of infected rodent fleas or direct contact with tissues of infected animals. Secondary pneumonic plague arises from hematogenous seeding of the lungs with *Y pestis* in patients with untreated bubonic or septicemic plague. Primary pneumonic plague is acquired by inhalation of respiratory tract droplets from a human or animal with pneumonic plague. Only the pneumonic form has been shown to be transmitted from person to person, and the last known case of person-to-person transmission in the United States occurred in 1924. Rarely, humans can develop primary pneumonic plague following exposure to domestic cats with respiratory tract plague infections. Plague occurs worldwide with enzootic foci in parts of Asia, Africa, and the Americas. Most human plague cases are reported from rural, underdeveloped areas and mainly occur as isolated cases or in small, focal clusters. Since 2000, more than 95% of the approximately 22,000 cases reported to the World Health Organization have been from countries in sub-Saharan Africa. In the United States, plague is endemic in western states, with most (approximately 85%) of the 37 cases reported from 2006 through 2010 being from New Mexico, Colorado, Arizona, and California. Cases of peripatetic plague have been identified in states without endemic plague, such as Connecticut (2008) and New York (2002).

Incubation Period

2 to 8 days for bubonic plague; 1 to 6 days for primary pneumonic plague.

Diagnostic Tests

Y pestis has a bipolar (safety-pin) appearance when stained with Wright-Giemsa or Wayson stains. A positive fluorescent antibody test result for the presence of *Y pestis* in direct smears or cultures of blood, bubo aspirate, sputum, or another clinical specimen provides presumptive evidence of *Y pestis* infection. Diagnosis of plague is usually confirmed by culture of *Y pestis* from blood, bubo aspirate, sputum, or another clinical specimen. Automated blood culture identification systems can misidentify *Y pestis.* Many clinical laboratories provide preliminary identification of *Yersinia* species, with definitive identification performed at state or federal laboratory. Isolation of *Yersinia* species from an automated system should trigger additional evaluation to determine whether the clinical presentation is consistent with plague. A single positive serologic test result from passive hemagglutination assay or enzyme immunoassay in an unimmunized patient who has not previously had plague also provides presumptive evidence of infection. Seroconversion, defined as a 4-fold difference in antibody titer between 2 serum specimens obtained at least 2 weeks apart, also confirms the diagnosis of plague. Polymerase chain reaction assay and immunohistochemical staining for rapid diagnosis of *Y pestis* are available in some reference or public health laboratories.

Treatment

For children, gentamicin and streptomycin administered intramuscularly or intravenously appear to be equally effective. Tetracycline, doxycycline, chloramphenicol, and trimethoprim-sulfamethoxazole are alternative drugs. Trimethoprim-sulfamethoxazole should not be used as monotherapy to treat pneumonic or septicemic plague because of higher treatment failure rates. Fluoroquinolones have been shown to be highly effective in animal and in vitro studies, and levofloxacin has been approved for treatment of plague. The usual duration of antimicrobial treatment is 7 to 10 days or several days after fever has resolved. Fluoroquinolones, especially those with higher cerebrospinal fluid penetration (ie, levofloxacin), should be used for plague meningitis in the United States, but chloramphenicol is also effective. Drainage of abscessed buboes may be necessary; drainage material is infectious until effective antimicrobial therapy has been administered.

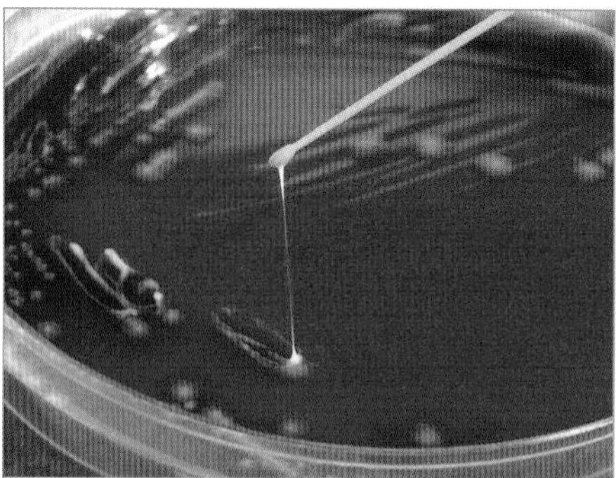

Image 106.1
This photograph depicts the colonial morphology displayed by gram-negative *Yersinia pestis* bacteria, which were grown on a medium of sheep blood agar for a 48-hour period at a temperature of 37°C (98.6°F). There is a tenacious nature of these colonies when touched by an inoculation loop, and they tend to form "stringy," sticky strands. Morphologic characteristics after 48 hours of *Y pestis* colonial growth include an average colonial diameter of 1.0 to 2.0 mm and an opaque coloration that ranges from gray-white to yellowish. If permitted to continue growing, *Y pestis* colonies take on what is referred to as a "fried egg" appearance, which becomes more prominent as the colonies age. Older colonies also display what is termed a "hammered copper" texture to their surfaces. Courtesy of Centers for Disease Control and Prevention/Pete Seidel.

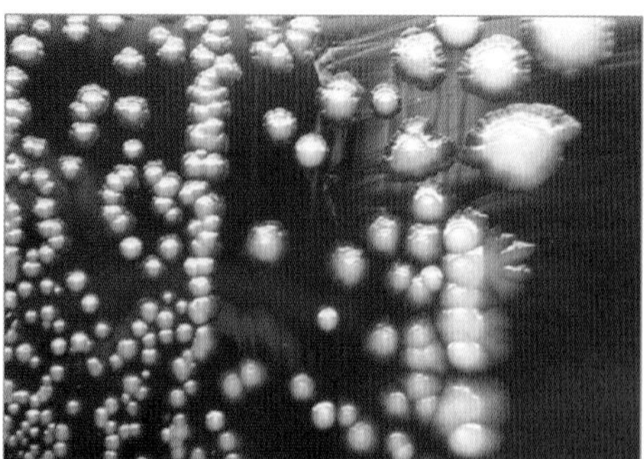

Image 106.2
Yersinia pestis on sheep blood agar, 72 hours. *Y pestis* grows well on most standard laboratory media, after 48 to 72 hours, gray-white to slightly yellow opaque raised, irregular "fried egg" morphology; alternatively, colonies may have a "hammered copper" shiny surface. Courtesy of Centers for Disease Control and Prevention/Courtesy of Larry Stauffer, Oregon State Public Health Laboratory.

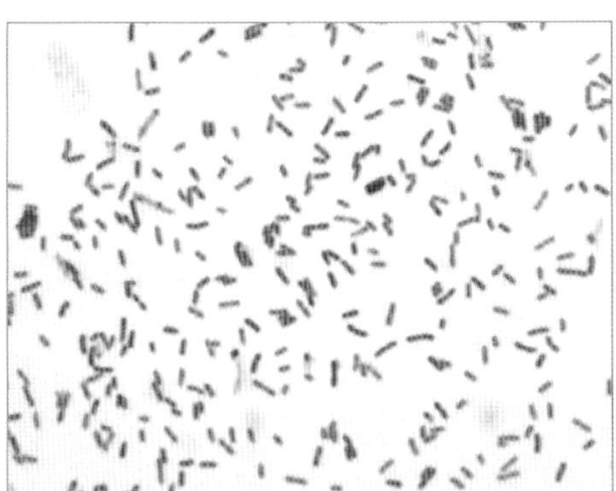

Image 106.3
Yersinia pestis is a small (0.5 x 1.0 µm) gram-negative bacillus (magnification x1,000). Bipolar staining occurs when using Wayson, Wright, Giemsa, or methylene blue stain and may occasionally be seen in Gram-stained preparations. Courtesy of Centers for Disease Control and Prevention/Courtesy of Larry Stauffer, Oregon State Public Health Laboratory.

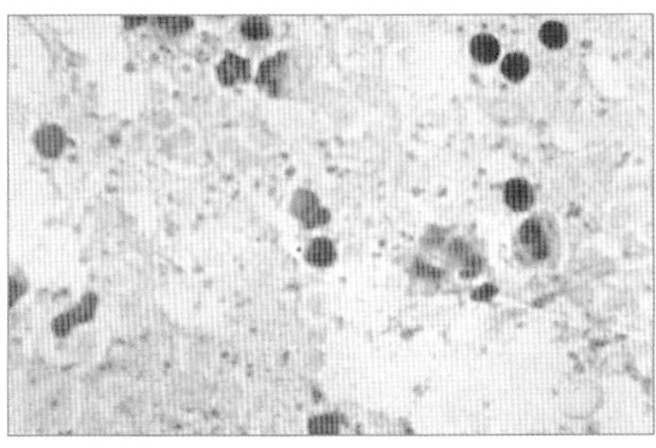

Image 106.5
Bubo aspirate (Gram stain) showing many gram-negative bacilli, *Yersinia pestis*.

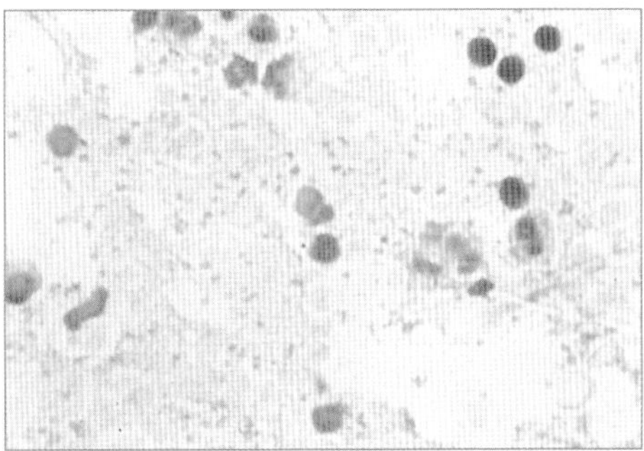

Image 106.4
Plague bubo aspirate. Courtesy of Gary Overturf, MD.

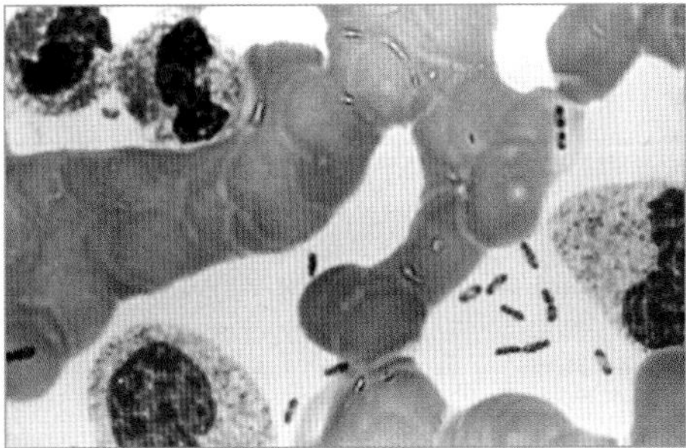

Image 106.6
Dark-stained bipolar ends of *Yersinia pestis* can clearly be seen in this Wright stain of blood from a plague victim. The actual cause of the disease is the plague bacillus, *Y pestis*. It is a nonmotile, nonspore-forming, gram-negative, nonlactose-fermenting, bipolar, ovoid, safety-pin–shaped bacterium. Courtesy of Centers for Disease Control and Prevention.

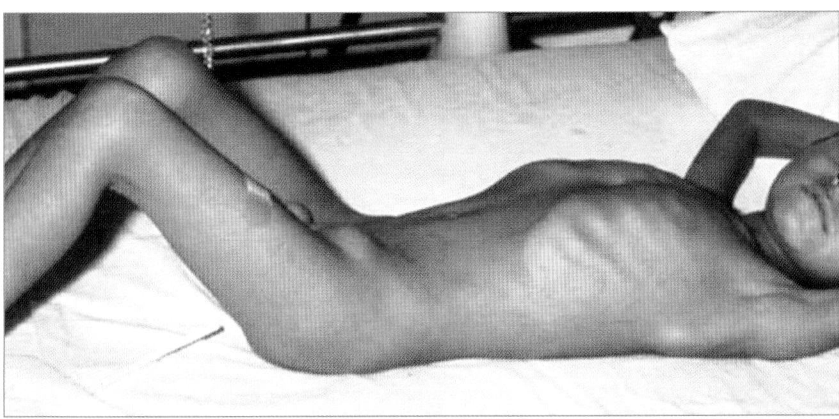

Image 106.7
Inguinal plague buboes in an 8-year-old boy. If left untreated, bubonic plague often becomes septicemic, with meningitis occurring in 6% of cases.

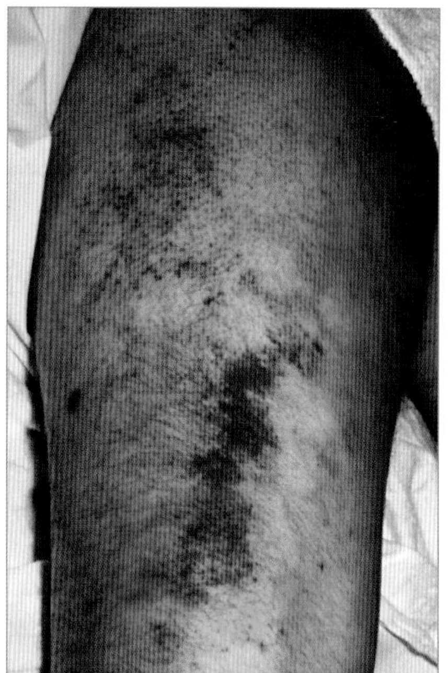

Image 106.8
This patient acquired a plague infection through abrasions on his upper right leg. Bubonic plague is transmitted through the bite of an infected flea or, as in this case, exposure to inoculated material through a break in the skin. Symptoms include swollen, tender lymph glands known as buboes. Courtesy of Centers for Disease Control and Prevention/Dr Jack Poland.

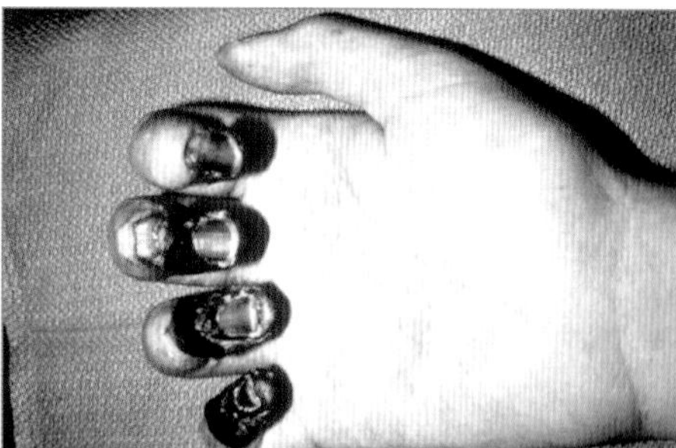

Image 106.10
Right hand of a plague patient displaying acral gangrene. Gangrene is one of the manifestations of plague and is the origin of the term black death given to plague throughout the ages. Disseminated intravascular coagulation is not uncommon in septicemic plague. Courtesy of Centers for Disease Control and Prevention.

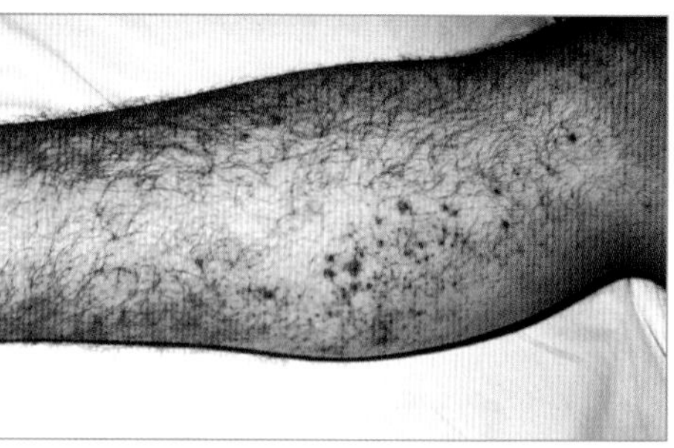

Image 106.9
Small hemorrhages on the skin of a plague victim. Capillary fragility is one of the manifestations of a plague infection, evident here on the leg of an infected patient. Courtesy of Centers for Disease Control and Prevention.

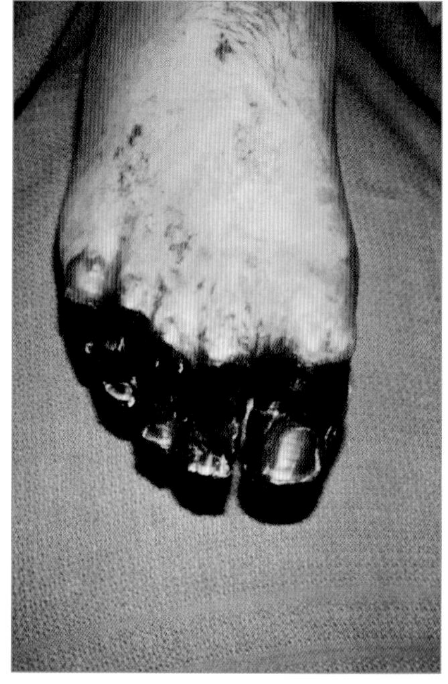

Image 106.11
This patient presented with symptoms of plague that included gangrene of the right foot causing necrosis of the toes. Courtesy of Centers for Disease Control and Prevention/William Archibald.

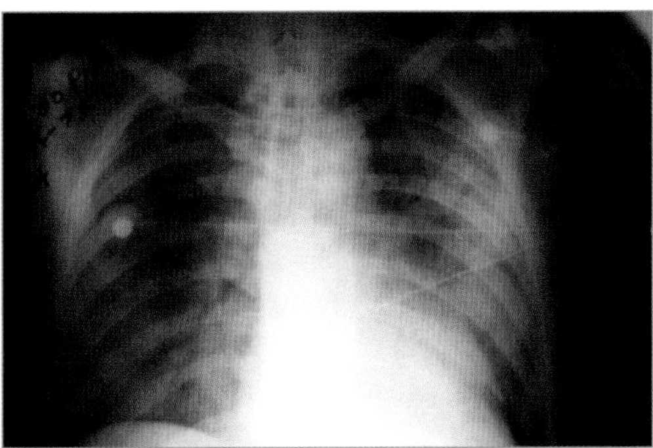

Image 106.12
This anteroposterior radiograph reveals a bilaterally progressive plague infection involving both lung fields. The first signs of plague are fever, headache, weakness, and rapidly developing pneumonia with shortness of breath, chest pain, cough, and, sometimes, bloody or watery sputum, eventually progressing for 2 to 4 days into respiratory failure and shock. Courtesy of Centers for Disease Control and Prevention/Dr Jack Poland.

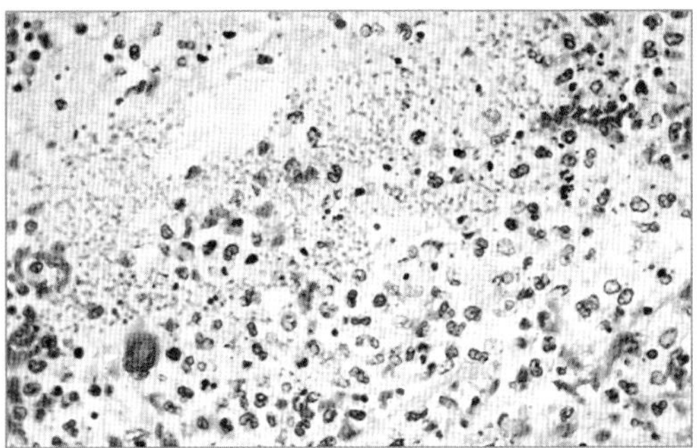

Image 106.13
Photomicrograph of lung tissue (Giemsa stain) from a patient with fatal human plague, revealing pneumonia and an abundance of *Yersinia pestis* organisms. Courtesy of Centers for Disease Control and Prevention.

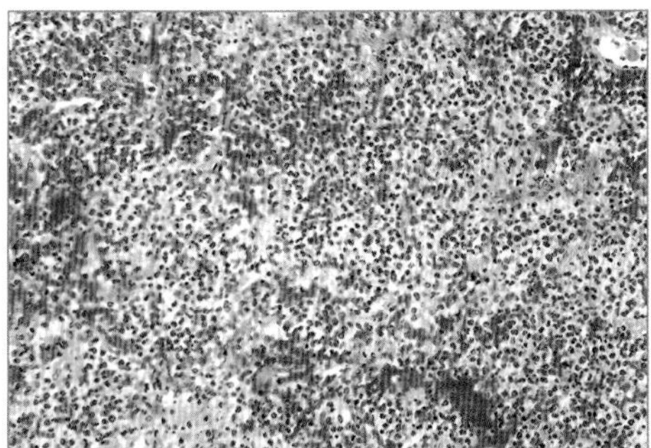

Image 106.14
Histopathology of lung in fatal human plague. Area of marked fibrinopurulent pneumonia. Courtesy of Centers for Disease Control and Prevention/Dr Marshall Fox.

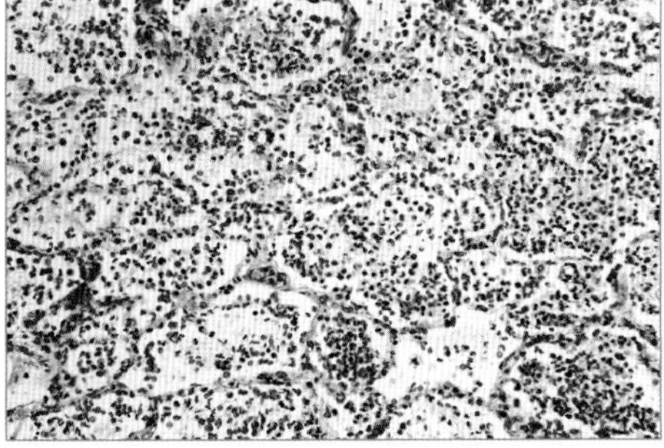

Image 106.15
This photomicrograph depicts the histopathologic changes in lung tissue in a case of fatal human plague pneumonia (hematoxylin-eosin stain, magnification x160). Note the presence of many polymorphonuclear leukocytes, capillary engorgement, and intra-alveolar debris, all indicative of an acute infection. Courtesy of Centers for Disease Control and Prevention/Dr Marshall Fox.

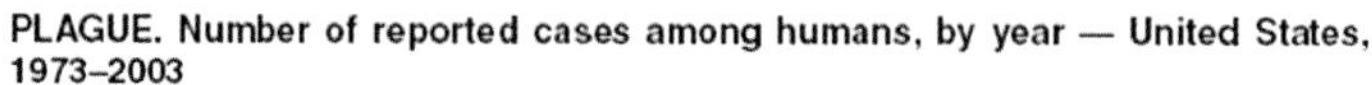

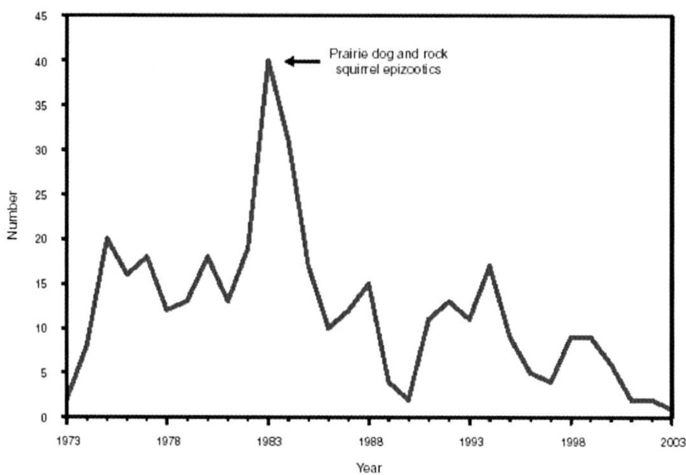

In 2003, a single case of plague was reported, bringing the 3-year total for 2001–2003 to five cases. This is the lowest sustained rate of naturally occurring plague in the United States in 40 years. The low number of cases was expected because of prolonged drought conditions in the Southwest during the past 5 years. Increased precipitation in the Southwest in 2004 might result in increased human cases in 2005.

Image 106.16
Plague. Number of reported cases among humans by year in the United States, 1973–2003. The World Health Organization reports 1,000 to 3,000 cases of plague each year globally. Courtesy of *Morbidity and Mortality Weekly Report.*

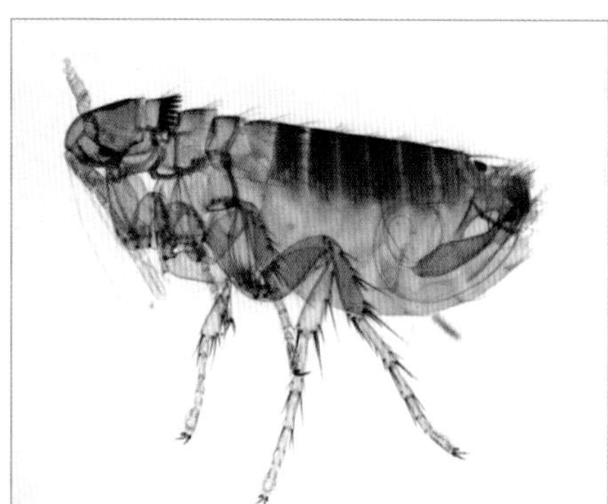

Image 106.17
This photograph depicts an adult male *Diamanus montana* flea, formerly known as *Oropsylla montana*. This flea is a common ectoparasite of the rock squirrel, *Citellus variegatus,* and, in the western United States, is an important vector for the bacterium *Yersinia pestis,* the pathogen responsible for causing plague. Courtesy of Centers for Disease Control and Prevention/ John Montenieri.

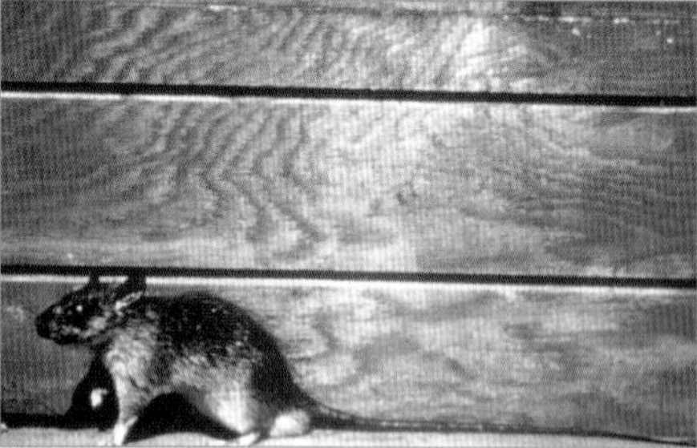

Image 106.18
This image shows the roof rat or black rat, *Rattus rattus,* a carrier of the plague bacterium, *Yersinia pestis*. The roof rat can be differentiated from the Norway (brown) rat by its smaller size; its body is generally 16 to 20 cm (6–8 inches) in length with a 19- to 25-cm (7- to 10-inch) tail. It is a climber and nests largely in buildings and trees. Courtesy of Centers for Disease Control and Prevention.

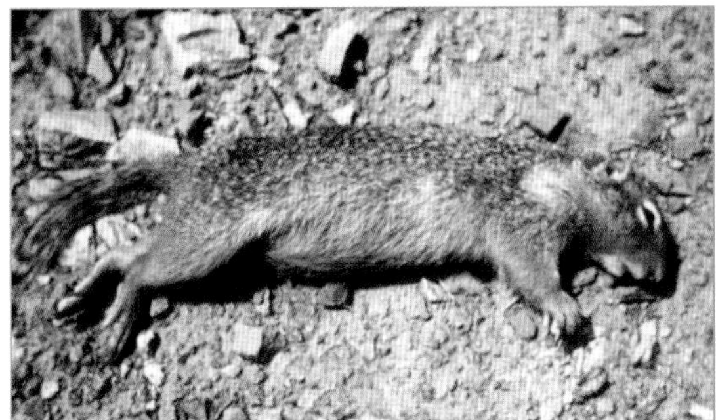

Image 106.19
This photograph shows a ground squirrel that died due to a plague infection, *Yersinia pestis*. Field rodents, such as western ground squirrels and prairie dogs, may be a threat when their burrows are beside labor camps and residential areas because they and their fleas are carriers of the plague bacteria. Courtesy of Centers for Disease Control and Prevention.

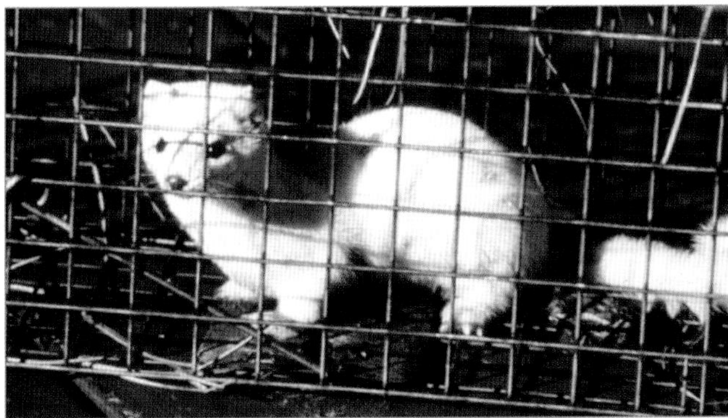

Image 106.20
The long-tailed weasel, *Mustela frenata,* here seen in its winter pelage, is a carrier of plague vectors. Long-tailed weasels have been identified as carriers of fleas inoculated with *Yersinia pestis,* the plague bacteria. This animal was found during a 1975 plague and Colorado tick fever study. Courtesy of Centers for Disease Control and Prevention.

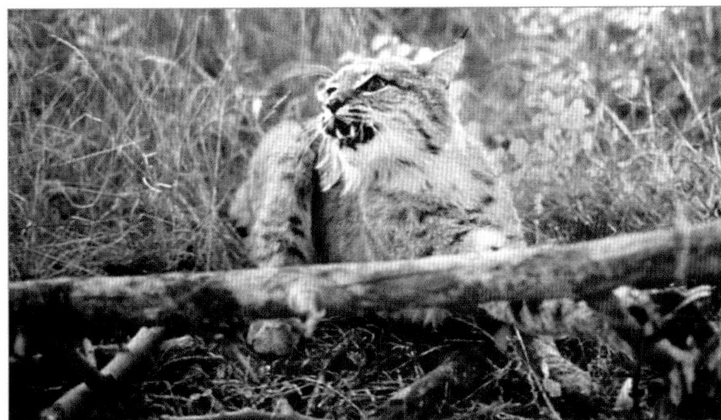

Image 106.21
The bobcat, *Felis rufus,* can be a source of plague infection for humans. People involved in trapping and skinning wild carnivores, especially bobcats, should be extremely cautious about exposure to *Yersinia pestis* vectors. Courtesy of Centers for Disease Control and Prevention.

107

Pneumococcal Infections

Clinical Manifestations

Streptococcus pneumoniae is a common cause of invasive bacterial infections in children, including febrile bacteremia. Pneumococci are also a common cause of acute otitis media (AOM), sinusitis, community-acquired pneumonia, pleural empyema, and conjunctivitis. As of 2008, *S pneumoniae* remained the most common cause of bacterial meningitis and subdural hygromas in infants and children from 2 months of age in the United States. Pneumococci occasionally cause mastoiditis, periorbital cellulitis, endocarditis, osteomyelitis, pericarditis, peritonitis, pyogenic arthritis, soft tissue infection, overwhelming septicemia in patients with splenic dysfunction, and neonatal septicemia. Hemolytic uremic syndrome can accompany complicated invasive disease (eg, pneumonia with pleural empyema).

Etiology

S pneumoniae organisms (pneumococci) are lancet-shaped, gram-positive, catalase-negative diplococci. More than 90 pneumococcal serotypes have been identified on the basis of unique polysaccharide capsules.

Epidemiology

Pneumococci are ubiquitous, with many people having transient colonization of the upper respiratory tract. In children, nasopharyngeal carriage rates range from 21% in industrialized countries to more than 90% in resource-limited countries. Transmission is from person to person by respiratory droplet contact. The period of communicability may be as long as the organism is present in respiratory tract secretions but is probably less than 24 hours after effective antimicrobial therapy is begun. Among young children who acquire a new pneumococcal serotype in the nasopharynx, illness (eg, otitis media) occurs in approximately 15%, usually within a few days of acquisition. Viral upper respiratory tract infections, including influenza, can predispose to pneumococcal infection and transmission. Pneumococcal infections are most prevalent during winter months. Incidence is highest in infants, young children, elderly people, and black, Alaska Native, and some American Indian populations. The incidence and severity of infections are increased in people with congenital or acquired humoral immunodeficiency, HIV infection, absent or deficient splenic function (eg, sickle cell disease, congenital or surgical asplenia), diabetes mellitus, chronic liver disease, chronic renal failure or nephrotic syndrome, or abnormal innate immune responses. Children with cochlear implants have high rates of pneumococcal meningitis, as do children with congenital or acquired cerebrospinal fluid (CSF) leaks. Other categories of children at presumed high risk or at moderate risk of developing invasive pneumococcal disease (IPD) are outlined in Table 107.1. Since introduction of pneumococcal conjugate vaccine (PCV7 [2000] and PCV13 [2010]), racial disparities have diminished; however, rates of IPD among some American Indian (Alaska Native and Apache) populations remain more than 5-fold higher than the rate among children in the general US population.

From 1998 to 2007, the incidence of vaccine-type invasive pneumococcal infections decreased by 99%, and the incidence of all IPD decreased by 76% in children younger than 5 years. In adults 65 years and older, IPD caused by PCV7 serotypes decreased 92% compared with baseline and all serotype invasive disease by 37%. The reduction in cases in these latter groups indicates the significant indirect benefits of PCV7 immunization by interruption of transmission of pneumococci from children to adults. Further reductions in disease in children of all ages, also associated with herd protection, have been demonstrated to date for at least 3 of the additional 6 serotypes in PCV13, including serotype 19A.

Incubation Period

Varies by type of infection but can be as short as 1 to 3 days.

Diagnostic Tests

Recovery of *S pneumoniae* from a normally sterile site (eg, blood, CSF, peritoneal fluid, middle ear fluid, joint fluid) or from a suppurative focus confirms the diagnosis. The finding

Table 107.1
Underlying Medical Conditions That Are Indications for Pneumococcal Immunization Among Children, by Risk Group[a]

Risk Group	Condition
Immunocompetent children	Chronic heart disease[b]
	Chronic lung disease[c]
	Diabetes mellitus
	Cerebrospinal fluid leaks
	Cochlear implant
Children with functional or anatomic asplenia	Sickle cell disease and other hemoglobinopathies Chronic or acquired asplenia, or splenic dysfunction
Children with immuno-compromising conditions	HIV infection
	Chronic renal failure and nephrotic syndrome
	Diseases associated with treatment with immunosuppressive drugs or radiation therapy, including malignant neoplasms, leukemias, lymphomas, and Hodgkin disease; or solid organ transplantation
	Congenital immunodeficiency[d]

[a] Centers for Disease Control and Prevention. Licensure of a 13-valent pneumococcal conjugate vaccine (PCV13) and recommendations for use among children. Advisory Committee on Immunization Practices (ACIP), 2010. *MMWR Morb Mortal Wkly Rep.* 2010;59(9):258–261.
[b] Particularly cyanotic congenital heart disease and cardiac failure.
[c] Including asthma if treated with prolonged high-dose oral corticosteroids.
[d] Include B-(humoral) or T-lymphocyte deficiency; complement deficiencies, particularly C1, C2, C3, and C4 deficiency; and phagocytic disorders (excluding chronic granulomatous disease).

of lancet-shaped gram-positive organisms and white blood cells in expectorated sputum or pleural exudate suggests pneumococcal pneumonia or pleural empyema in older children and adults. Recovery of pneumococci by culture of an upper respiratory tract swab specimen is of no diagnostic significance. Real-time polymerase chain reaction assay using *lyt*A is investigational but may be specific and significantly more sensitive than culture of pleural fluid, CSF, and blood, particularly in patients who have received recent antimicrobial therapy.

- **Susceptibility testing.** All *S pneumoniae* isolates from normally sterile body fluids (eg, CSF, blood, middle ear fluid, pleural fluid, joint fluid) should be tested for antimicrobial susceptibility to determine the minimum inhibitory concentration of penicillin, cefotaxime or ceftriaxone, and clindamycin. Cerebrospinal fluid isolates should also be tested for susceptibility to vancomycin and meropenem. **Nonsusceptible** includes **intermediate** and **resistant** isolates. Breakpoints vary depending on whether an isolate is from a nonmeningeal or meningeal site. Accordingly, current definitions by the Clinical and Laboratory Standards Institute for susceptibility and nonsusceptibility are provided in Table 107.2 for nonmeningeal and meningitis presentations. If the patient has a nonmeningeal infection caused by an isolate that is nonsusceptible to penicillin, cefotaxime, and ceftriaxone, susceptibility testing to other agents, such as clindamycin, erythromycin, trimethoprim-sulfamethoxazole, linezolid, meropenem, and vancomycin, should be performed.

Quantitative minimum inhibitory concentration testing using reliable methods, such as broth microdilution or antimicrobial gradient strips (E-test), should be performed on isolates from children with invasive infections. When quantitative testing methods are not available or for isolates from noninvasive infections, the qualitative screening test using a 1-mcg oxacillin disk on an agar plate reliably identifies all penicillin-**susceptible** pneumococci using meningitis breakpoints (ie, disk-zone diameter of ≥20 mm). Organisms with an oxacillin

Table 107.2
Clinical and Laboratory Standards Institute Definitions of In vitro Susceptibility and Nonsusceptibility of Nonmeningeal and Meningeal Pneumococcal Isolates

Drug and Isolate Location	Susceptible, mcg/mL	Nonsusceptible, mcg/mL	
		Intermediate	Resistant
Penicillin (oral)[a]	≤0.06	0.12–1.0	≥2.0
Penicillin (intravenous)[b]			
Nonmeningeal	≤2.0	4.0	≥8.0
Meningeal	≤0.06	None	≥0.12
Cefotaxime **OR** ceftriaxone			
Nonmeningeal	≤1.0	2.0	≥4.0
Meningeal	≤0.5	1.0	≥2.0

[a] Without meningitis.
[b] Treated with intravenous penicillin.

From Clinical and Laboratory Standards Institute. *Performance Standards for Antimicrobial Susceptibility Testing: 18th Informational Supplement.* CLSI Publication No. M100-S23. Wayne, PA: Clinical and Laboratory Standards Institute; 2013.

disk-zone size of less than 20 mm are potentially nonsusceptible for treatment of meningitis and require quantitative susceptibility testing. The oxacillin disk test is used as a screening test for resistance to β-lactam drugs (ie, penicillins and cephalosporins).

Treatment

S pneumoniae strains that are nonsusceptible to penicillin G, cefotaxime, ceftriaxone, and other antimicrobial agents using meningitis breakpoints have been identified throughout the United States and worldwide but are uncommon using nonmeningeal breakpoints. Recommendations for treatment of pneumococcal infections are as follows:

- **Bacterial meningitis possibly or proven to be caused by *S pneumoniae*.** Combination therapy with vancomycin and cefotaxime or ceftriaxone should be administered initially to all infants and children 1 month or older with definite or probable bacterial meningitis because of the possibility of *S pneumoniae* resistant to penicillin, cefotaxime, and ceftriaxone.

  For children with serious hypersensitivity reactions to β-lactam antimicrobial agents (ie, penicillins and cephalosporins), the combination of vancomycin and rifampin should be considered. Vancomycin should not be given alone because bactericidal concentrations in CSF are difficult to sustain, and clinical experience to support use of vancomycin as monotherapy is minimal. Rifampin also should not be given as monotherapy because resistance can develop during therapy. Meropenem alone can be given as an alternative drug.

  Once results of susceptibility testing are available, therapy should be modified. Vancomycin should be discontinued and penicillin or cefotaxime or ceftriaxone should be continued if the organism is susceptible; if the isolate is penicillin nonsusceptible, cefotaxime or ceftriaxone should be continued. If the organism is nonsusceptible to penicillin and cefotaxime or ceftriaxone, consultation with an infectious disease specialist should be considered.

- **Dexamethasone.** For infants and children 6 weeks and older, adjunctive therapy with dexamethasone may be considered after weighing the potential benefits and possible risks. If used, dexamethasone should be given before or concurrently with the first dose of antimicrobial agents.

- **Nonmeningeal invasive pneumococcal infections requiring hospitalization.** For nonmeningeal invasive infections in previously healthy children who are not critically ill, antimicrobial agents currently used to treat infections with *S pneumoniae* and other potential pathogens should be initiated at the usually recommended dosages. For critically ill infants and children with invasive infections potentially attributable to *S pneumoniae,* vancomycin, in addition to empirical antimicrobial therapy (ie, cefotaxime or ceftriaxone or others), can be considered. Such patients include those with presumed septic shock, severe pneumonia with empyema, or significant hypoxia or myopericardial involvement. If vancomycin is administered, it should be discontinued as soon as antimicrobial susceptibility test results demonstrate effective alternative agents.

If the organism has in vitro resistance to penicillin, cefotaxime, and ceftriaxone, therapy should be modified on the basis of clinical response, susceptibility to other antimicrobial agents, and results of follow-up cultures of blood and other infected body fluids. Consultation with an infectious disease specialist should be considered.

- **Nonmeningeal invasive pneumococcal infections in the immunocompromised host.** The preceding recommendations for management of possible pneumococcal infections requiring hospitalization also apply to immunocompromised children. Vancomycin should be discontinued as soon as antimicrobial susceptibility test results indicate effective alternative antimicrobial agents are available.
- **Acute otitis media.** According to clinical practice guidelines of the American Academy of Pediatrics and the American Academy of Family Physicians on AOM, high-dose amoxicillin is recommended, except in select cases in which the option of observation without antimicrobial therapy is warranted. Optimal duration of therapy is uncertain. For younger children and children with severe disease at any age, a 10-day course is recommended; for children 6 years and older with mild or moderate disease, a duration of 5 to 7 days is appropriate.

  Patients who fail to respond to initial management should be reassessed at 48 to 72 hours to confirm the diagnosis of AOM and exclude other causes of illness. If AOM is confirmed in the patient managed initially with observation, amoxicillin should be given. If the patient has failed initial antibacterial therapy, a change in antibacterial agent is indicated. Suitable alternative agents should be active against penicillin-nonsusceptible pneumococci as well as β-lactamase–producing *Haemophilus influenzae* and *Moraxella catarrhalis.* Such agents include high-dose oral amoxicillin-clavulanate; oral cefdinir, cefpodoxime, or cefuroxime; or intramuscular ceftriaxone in a 3-day course. Macrolide resistance among *S pneumoniae* is high, so clarithromycin and azithromycin are not generally considered appropriate alternatives for initial therapy.

  Myringotomy or tympanocentesis should be considered for children failing to respond to second-line therapy and for severe cases to obtain cultures to guide therapy. For multidrug-resistant strains of *S pneumoniae,* use of levofloxacin or other agents should be considered in consultation with an expert in infectious diseases.
- **Sinusitis.** Antimicrobial agents effective for treatment of AOM are also likely to be effective for acute sinusitis and are recommended.

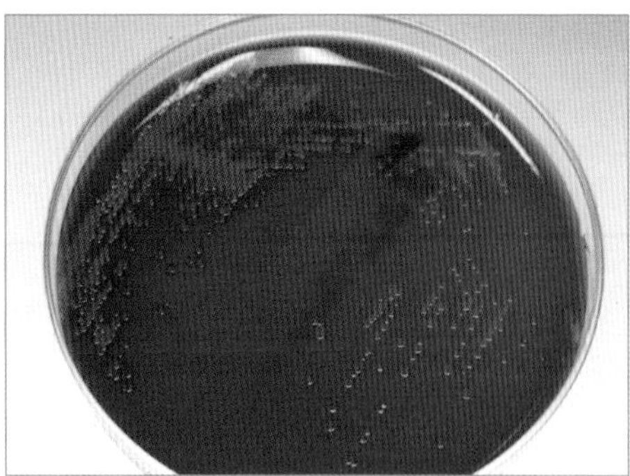

Image 107.1
Streptococcus pneumoniae, 24-hour sheep blood agar plate, with alpha hemolysis. Courtesy of Robert Jerris, MD.

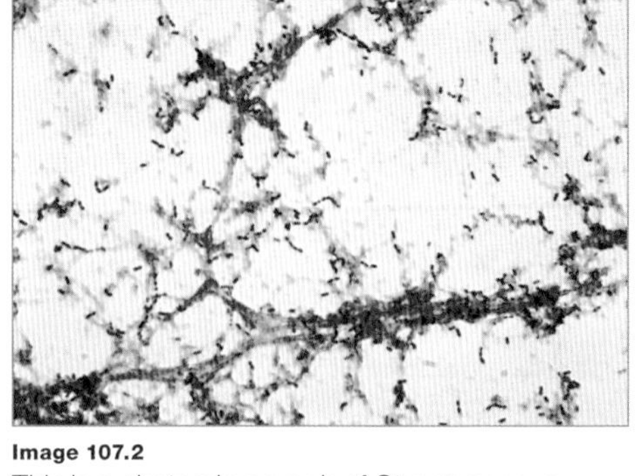

Image 107.2
This is a photomicrograph of *Streptococcus pneumoniae* grown from a blood culture (Gram stain). Courtesy of Centers for Disease Control and Prevention/Dr Mike Miller.

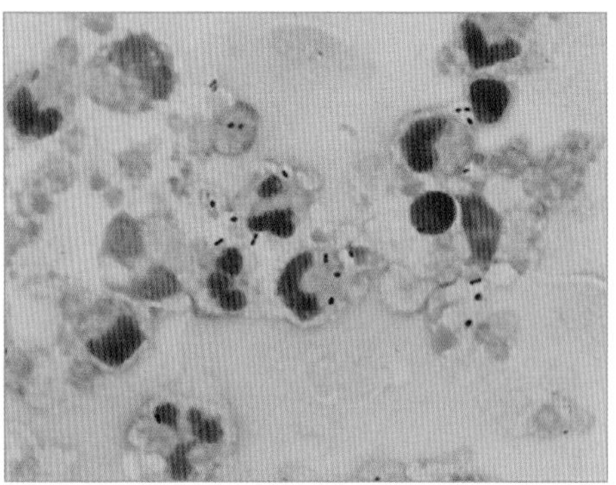

Image 107.3
Streptococcus pneumoniae (pneumococcus) in a Gram stain of cerebrospinal fluid. Courtesy of H. Cody Meissner, MD, FAAP.

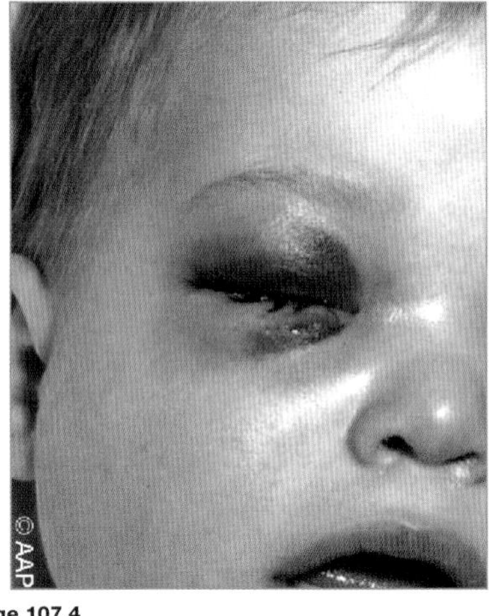

Image 107.4
Periorbital cellulitis with purulent exudate from which *Streptococcus pneumoniae* and *Haemophilus influenzae* type b were grown on culture. *S pneumoniae* was isolated on blood culture. The cerebrospinal fluid culture result was negative.

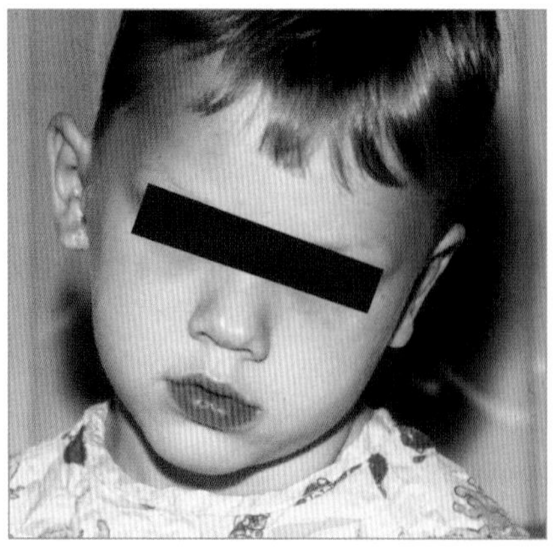

Image 107.5
A 3½-year-old boy with acute suppurative otitis media and mastoiditis due to *Streptococcus pneumoniae*. Note the protuberance of the right external ear secondary to mastoid swelling. Courtesy of George Nankervis, MD.

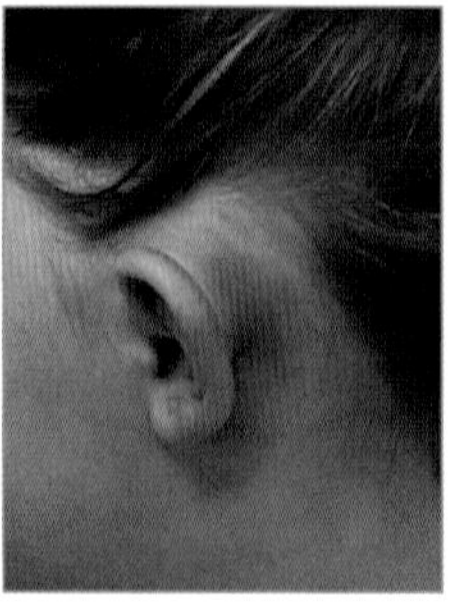

Image 107.6
Streptococcus pneumoniae mastoiditis in a 7-year-old girl. Courtesy of Benjamin Estrada, MD.

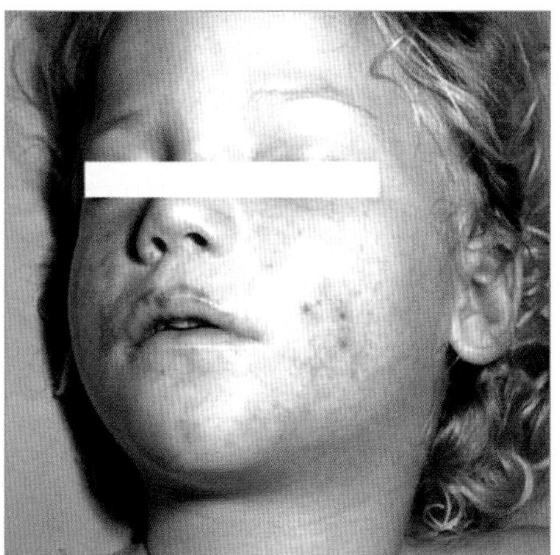

Image 107.7
Streptococcus pneumoniae sepsis with purpura fulminans in a child who had undergone splenectomy for refractory idiopathic thrombocytopenic purpura.

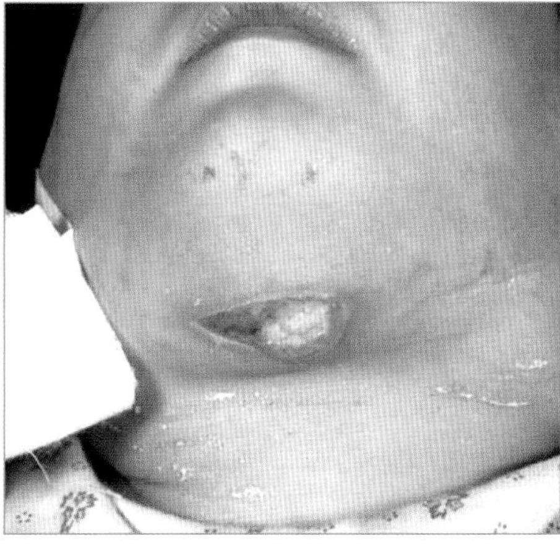

Image 107.8
Streptococcus pneumoniae submental abscess in a 5-year-old girl with dysgammaglobulinemia. There is an increased incidence of pneumococcal disease in immunocompromised children. Courtesy of Edgar O. Ledbetter, MD, FAAP.

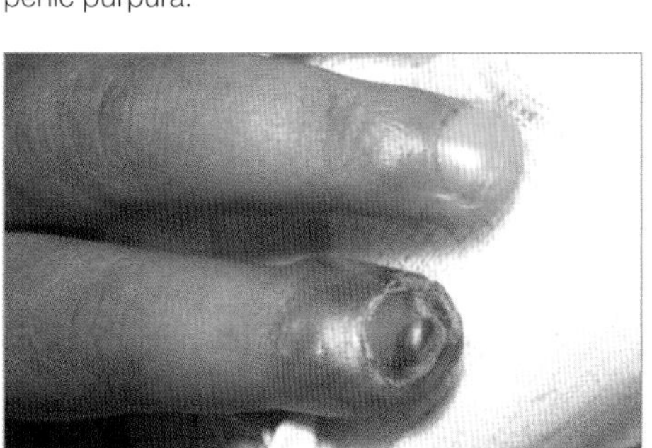

Image 107.9
Perionychial abscess caused by *Streptococcus pneumoniae* in a child with acute lymphoblastic leukemia.

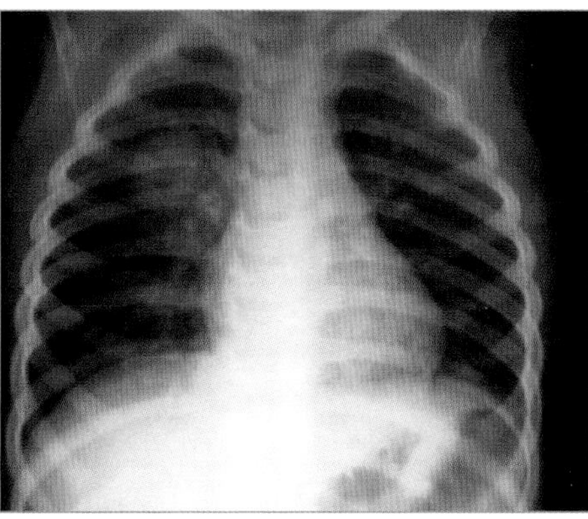

Image 107.10
Segmental (nodular) pneumonia due to *Streptococcus pneumoniae.*

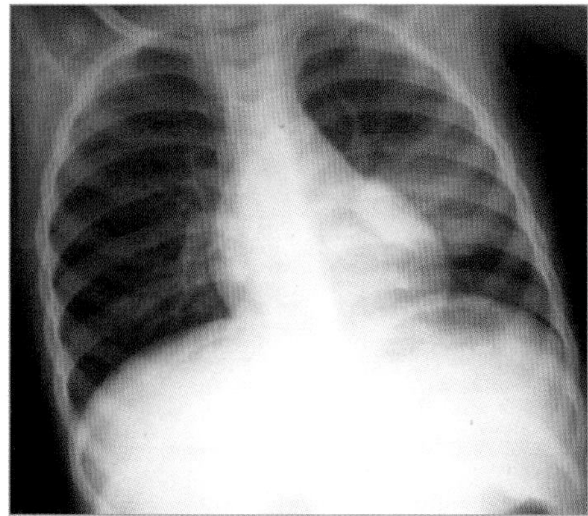

Image 107.11
Segmental (nodular) pneumonia due to *Streptococcus pneumoniae.*

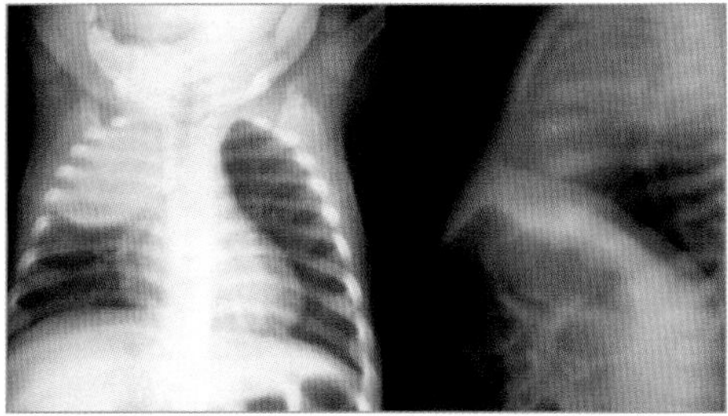

Image 107.12
Streptococcus pneumoniae pneumonia of the upper lobe of the right lung. The blood culture result was positive, and the infant had a prompt response to penicillin therapy.

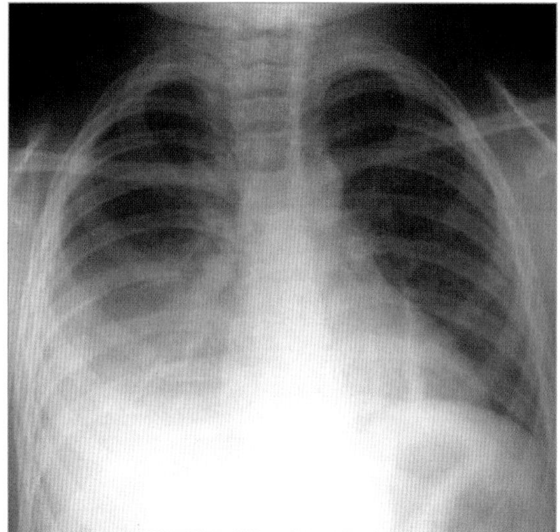

Image 107.13
Pneumococcal pneumonia with pleural effusion on the right. Courtesy of Edgar O. Ledbetter, MD, FAAP.

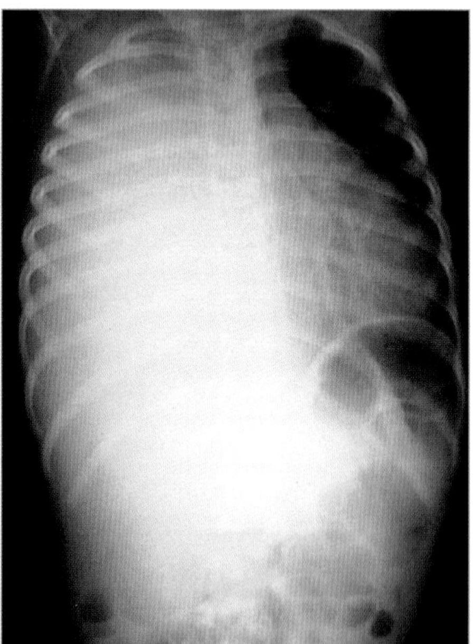

Image 107.14
Pneumococcal pneumonia with massive effusion pushing the mediastinal structures into the left area of the chest. A delayed clinical response to treatment was not surprising. Courtesy of Edgar O. Ledbetter, MD, FAAP.

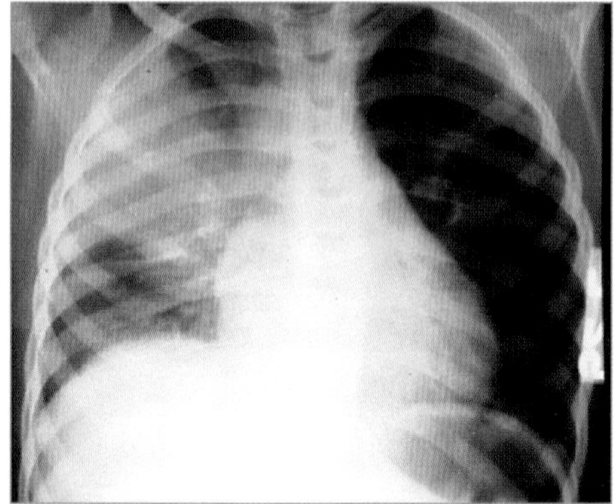

Image 107.15
Pneumonia with right subpleural empyema due to *Streptococcus pneumoniae* in a child with sickle cell disease.

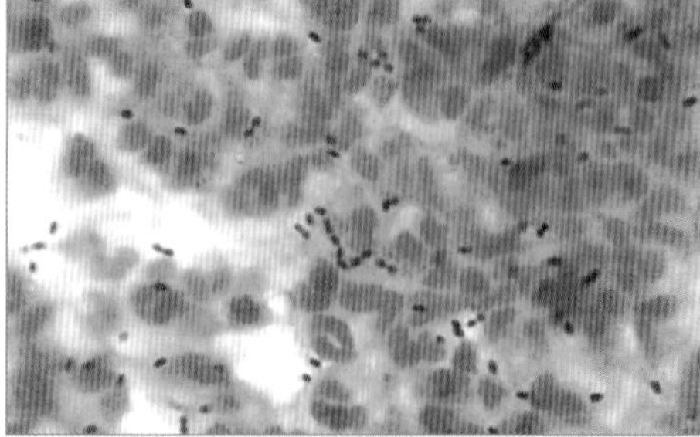

Image 107.16
Streptococcus pneumoniae in pleural exudate (Gram stain).

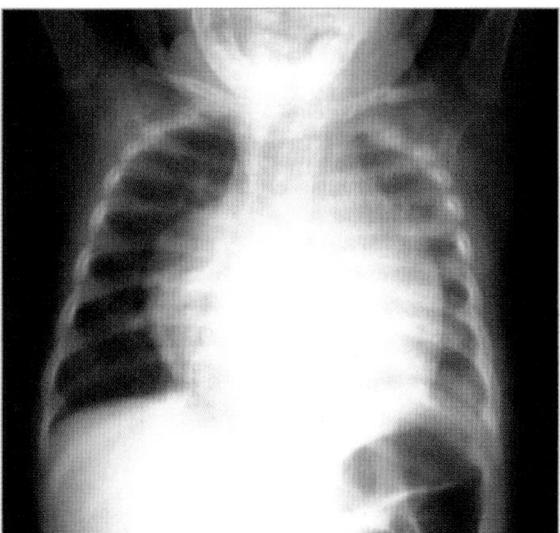

Image 107.17
Pneumonia and purulent pericarditis due to *Streptococcus pneumoniae* in a previously healthy infant. Despite clinical improvement with penicillin therapy and repeated needle aspiration of the pericardial space, the infant died of constrictive pericarditis.

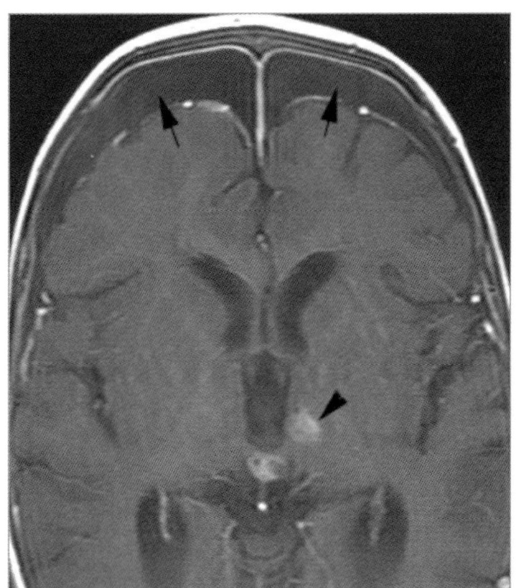

Image 107.19
An axial T1-weighted magnetic resonance image following contrast shows frontal subdural hygromas (arrows). Also note the enhancing left thalamic infarction secondary to penetrating artery spasm (arrowhead) in a patient with pneumococcal meningitis.

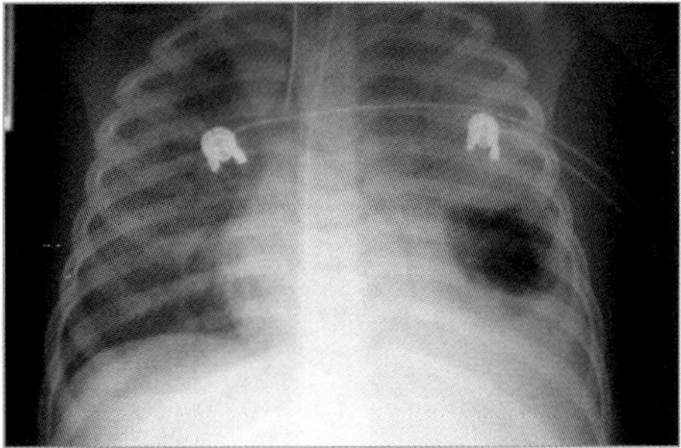

Image 107.18
Streptococcus pneumoniae pneumonia with pneumatocele formation in the left lung. Courtesy of Benjamin Estrada, MD.

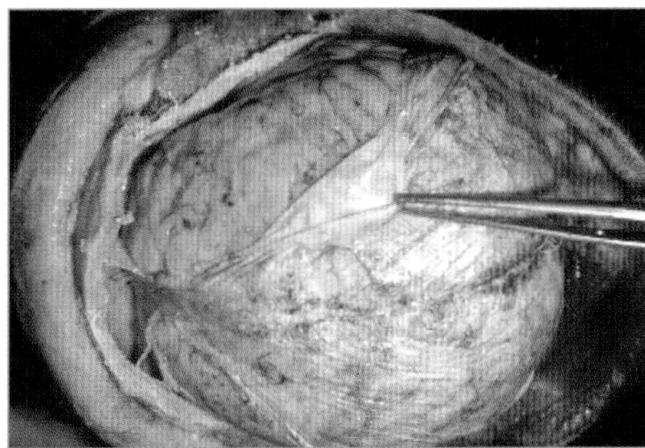

Image 107.20
Skull opened at autopsy revealing purulent inflammation of leptomeninges beneath reflected dura in a patient who died of pneumococcal meningitis. Courtesy of Centers for Disease Control and Prevention/Dr Edwin P. Ewing Jr.

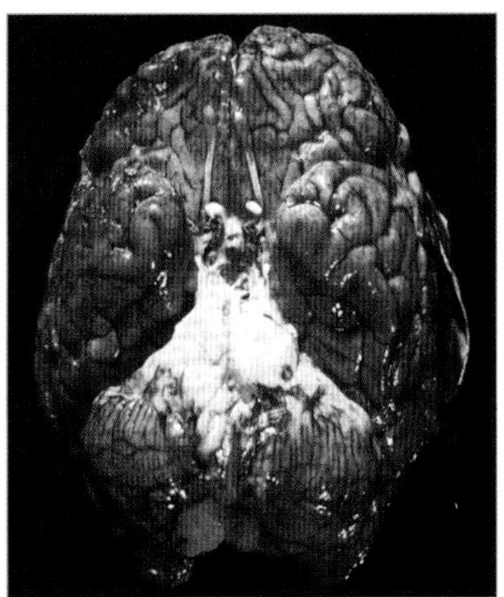

Image 107.21
A ventral view of the brain depicting purulent exudate from fatal *Streptococcus pneumoniae* meningitis. Courtesy of Centers for Disease Control and Prevention.

108

Pneumocystis jiroveci Infections

Clinical Manifestations

Symptomatic infection is extremely rare in healthy people. Disease in immunocompromised infants and children can produce a respiratory illness characterized by dyspnea, tachypnea, significant oxygen desaturation, nonproductive cough, and fever. The intensity of these signs and symptoms vary and, in some immunocompromised children and adults, the onset can be acute and fulminant. Chest radiographs often show bilateral diffuse interstitial or alveolar disease; rarely, lobar, miliary, cavitary, and nodular lesions or even no lesions are seen. Most children with *Pneumocystis* pneumonia (PCP) are significantly hypoxic. The mortality rate in immunocompromised patients ranges from 5% to 40% in treated patients and approaches 100% without therapy.

Etiology

Originally considered a protozoan, *Pneumocystis* is now classified as a fungus on the basis of DNA sequence analysis. Human *Pneumocystis* now is called *Pneumocystis jiroveci,* while *Pneumocystis carinii* is used for organisms infecting rats. *P carinii* f sp *hominis* or "human *P carinii*" are sometimes still used to refer to human *Pneumocystis. P jiroveci* is an atypical fungus, with several morphologic and biologic similarities to protozoa, including susceptibility to a number of antiprotozoal agents but resistance to most antifungal agents. In addition, the organism exists as 2 distinct morphologic forms: the 5- to 7-µm–diameter cysts, which contain up to 8 intracystic bodies, and the smaller, 1- to 5-µm–diameter trophozoite or trophic form.

Epidemiology

Pneumocystis species are ubiquitous in mammals worldwide, particularly rodents, and have a tropism for growth on respiratory tract epithelium. *Pneumocystis* isolates recovered from mice, rats, and ferrets differ genetically from each other and from human *P jiroveci*. Asymptomatic or mild human infection occurs early in life, with more than 85% of healthy children acquiring antibody by 20 months of age. In resource-limited countries and in times of famine, PCP can occur in epidemics, primarily affecting malnourished infants and children. Epidemics have also occurred among preterm neonates. In industrialized countries, PCP occurs almost entirely in immunocompromised people with deficient cell-mediated immunity, particularly people with HIV infection, recipients of immunosuppressive therapy after solid organ transplantation or treatment for malignant neoplasm, and children with congenital immunodeficiency syndromes. Although decreasing in frequency because of effective prophylaxis and antiretroviral therapy, PCP remains one of the most common serious opportunistic infections in infants and children with perinatally acquired HIV infection and adolescents with advanced immunosuppression. Although onset of disease can occur at any age, including rare instances during the first month of life, PCP most commonly occurs in HIV-infected children in the first year of life, with peak incidence at 3 through 6 months of age. The single most important factor in susceptibility to PCP is the status of cell-mediated immunity of the host, reflected by a marked decrease in $CD4^+$ T-lymphocyte count and percentage. The mode of transmission is unknown. Animal studies have demonstrated animal-to-animal transmission by the airborne route. Although reactivation of latent infection with immunosuppression has been proposed as an explanation for disease after the first 2 years of life, animal models of PCP do not support the existence of latency. Studies of patients with AIDS with more than one episode of PCP suggest reinfection rather than relapse. In patients with cancer, the disease can occur during remission or relapse. The period of communicability is unknown.

Incubation Period

Unknown, but possibly a median of 53 days from exposure to clinically apparent infection.

Diagnostic Tests

A definitive diagnosis of PCP is made by visualization of organisms (*Pneumocystis* cysts) in lung tissue or respiratory tract secretion specimens. The most sensitive and specific diagnostic procedures involve specimen collection from open lung biopsy and, in older children, transbronchial biopsy. However, bronchoscopy with bronchoalveolar lavage, induction of sputum in older children and adolescents, and intubation with deep endotracheal aspiration are less invasive, can be diagnostic, and are sensitive in patients who have a large number of *Pneumocystis* organisms. Methenamine silver, toluidine blue O, calcofluor white, and fluorescein-conjugated monoclonal antibody are the most useful stains for identifying the thick-walled cysts of *P jiroveci*. Extracystic trophozoite forms can also be identified with special stains. The sensitivity of all microscopy-based methods depends on the skill of the laboratory technician. Polymerase chain reaction assays for detecting *P jiroveci* infection have been shown to be highly sensitive and cost-effective even with noninvasive specimens, such as oral wash or expectorated sputum.

Treatment

The drug of choice is trimethoprim-sulfamethoxazole (TMP-SMX), usually administered intravenously. Oral therapy should be reserved for patients with mild disease who do not have malabsorption or diarrhea and for patients with a favorable clinical response to initial intravenous therapy. Duration of therapy is 14 to 21 days. The rate of adverse reactions to TMP-SMX (eg, rash, neutropenia, anemia, thrombocytopenia, renal toxicity, hepatitis, nausea, vomiting, diarrhea) is higher in HIV-infected children than in non–HIV-infected patients. It is not necessary to discontinue therapy for most mild adverse reactions. At least half of the patients with more severe reactions (excluding anaphylaxis) requiring interruption of therapy will subsequently tolerate TMP-SMX if rechallenged after the reaction resolves.

Intravenously administered pentamidine is an alternative drug for children and adults who cannot tolerate TMP-SMX or who have severe disease and have not responded to TMP-SMX after 5 to 7 days of therapy. Pentamidine is associated with a high incidence of adverse reactions, including pancreatitis, diabetes mellitus, renal toxicity, electrolyte abnormalities, hypoglycemia, hyperglycemia, hypotension, cardiac arrhythmias, fever, and neutropenia. Atovaquone is approved for oral treatment of mild to moderate PCP in adults who are intolerant of TMP-SMX. Experience with use of atovaquone in children is limited, although atovaquone-azithromycin appears to be as effective as TMP-SMX for preventing serious bacterial infections as well as PCP. Adverse reactions to atovaquone are limited to rash, nausea, and diarrhea.

Corticosteroids appear to be beneficial in treatment of HIV-infected adults with moderate to severe PCP (as defined by a Pao_2 of <70 mm Hg in room air or an arterial-alveolar gradient of >35 mm Hg). Studies have shown that use of corticosteroids can lead to reduced acute respiratory failure, decreased need for ventilation, and reduced mortality in children with PCP. Although no controlled studies of the use of corticosteroids in young children have been performed, most experts would recommend corticosteroids as part of therapy for children with moderate to severe PCP disease.

Coinfection with other organisms, such as cytomegalovirus or pneumococcus, has been reported in HIV-infected children. Children with dual infections can have more severe disease.

Chemoprophylaxis is highly effective in preventing PCP among some high-risk groups. Prophylaxis against a first episode of PCP is indicated for many patients with significant immunosuppression, including people with HIV infection and people with primary or acquired cell-mediated immunodeficiency.

Prophylaxis for PCP is recommended for children who have received hematopoietic stem cell transplants or solid organ transplants; children with hematologic malignancies (eg, leukemia, lymphoma) and some nonhematologic malignancies; children with severe cell-mediated immunodeficiency, including children who received adrenocorticotropic hormone for treatment of infantile spasm; and children who are otherwise immunosuppressed and who have had a previous episode of PCP. In general, for this diverse group of immunocompromised hosts, the risk of PCP increases with duration and intensity of chemotherapy, with other immunosuppressive therapies, and with coinfection with immunosuppressive viruses (eg, cytomegalovirus) and rates of PCP for similar patients in a given locale. Consequently, the recommended duration of PCP prophylaxis will vary depending on individual circumstances.

The recommended drug regimen for PCP prophylaxis for all immunocompromised patients is TMP-SMX, administered orally on 3 consecutive days each week. Alternatively, TMP-SMX can be administered daily, 7 days a week. For patients who cannot tolerate TMP-SMX, alternative choices include oral atovaquone or dapsone.

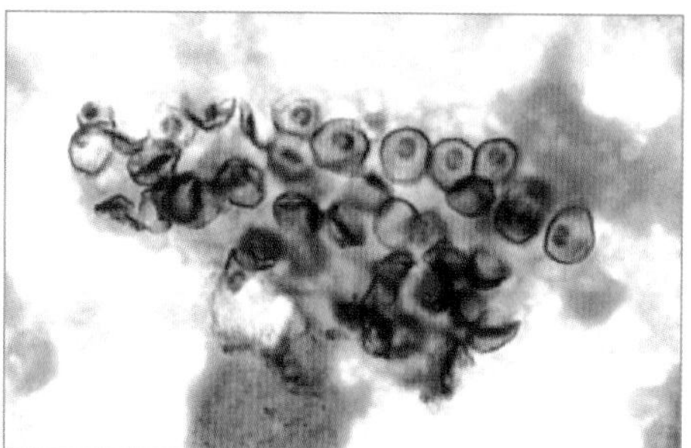

Image 108.1
Pneumocystis jiroveci organisms in tracheal aspirate (Gomori methenamine silver stain). Courtesy of Russell Byrnes.

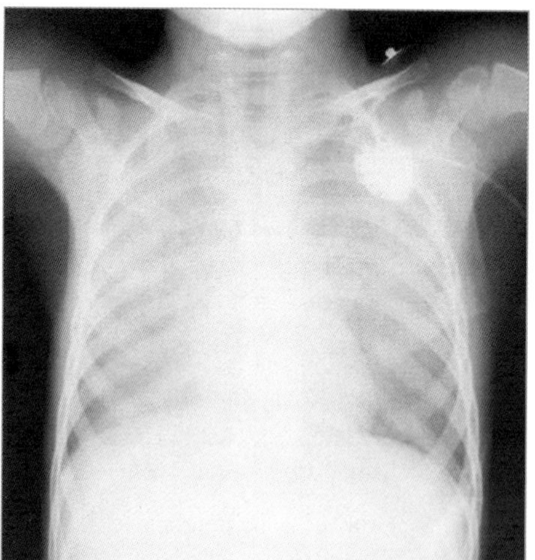

Image 108.3
An infant with bilateral *Pneumocystis jiroveci* pneumonia. Courtesy of Benjamin Estrada, MD.

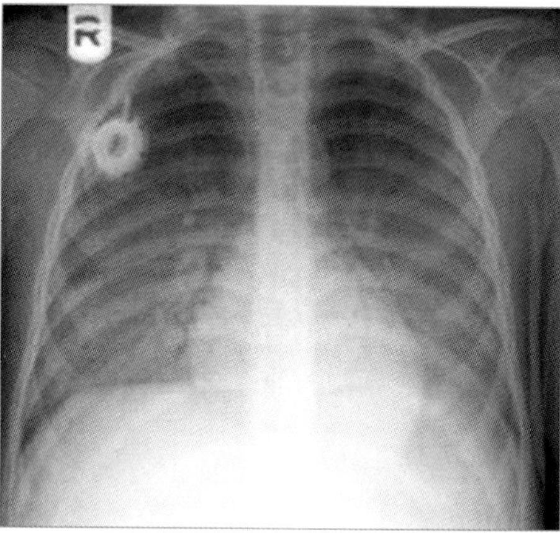

Image 108.2
Pneumocystis jiroveci pneumonia. This pathogen is an important cause of pulmonary infections in patients who are immunocompromised. Characteristic signs and symptoms include dyspnea at rest, tachypnea, nonproductive cough, fever, and hypoxia with an increased oxygen requirement. The intensity of the signs and symptoms can vary, and onset may be acute and fulminant. Chest radiographs frequently demonstrate diffuse bilateral interstitial or alveolar disease. This is a chest radiograph from a 5-year-old boy demonstrating bilateral perihilar infiltrates due to *P jiroveci*. Courtesy of Beverly P. Wood, MD, MSEd, PhD, FAAP.

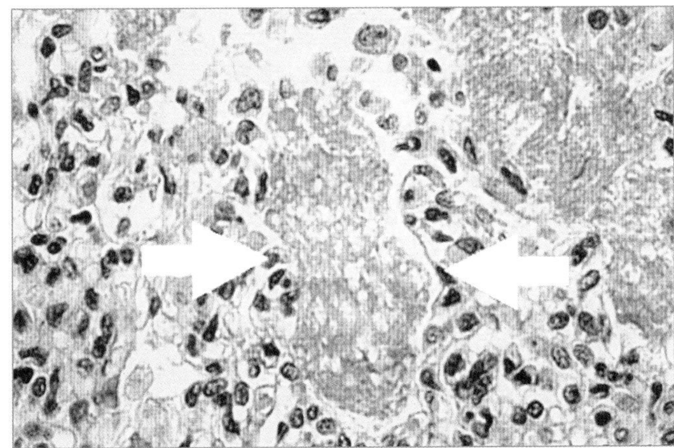

Image 108.4
Foamy intra-alveolar exudate in lung biopsy specimen from a patient with *Pneumocystis jiroveci* pneumonia (hematoxylin-eosin stain).

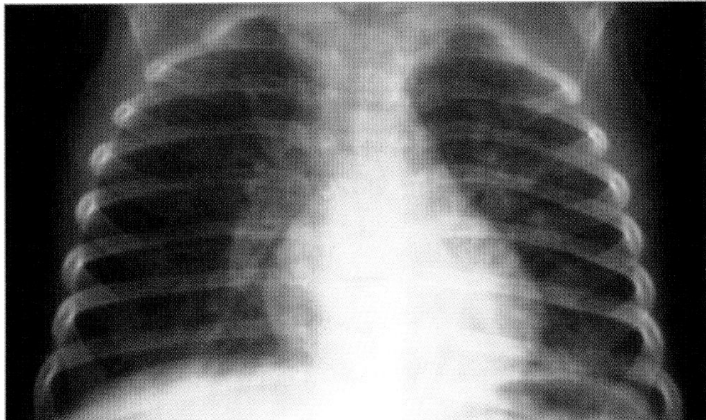

Image 108.5
Pneumocystis jiroveci pneumonia with hyperaeration in an infant with congenital agammaglobulinemia.

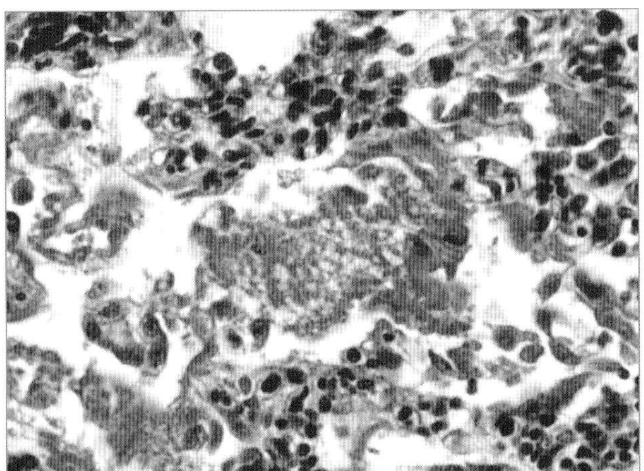

Image 108.6
Pneumocystis jiroveci in the lung. Frothy exudate in alveolar spaces. Courtesy of Dimitris P. Agamanolis, MD.

109

Poliovirus Infections

Clinical Manifestations

Approximately 72% of poliovirus infections in susceptible children are asymptomatic. Nonspecific illness with low-grade fever and sore throat (minor illness) occurs in 24% of people who become infected. Viral meningitis, sometimes with paresthesias, occurs in 1% to 5% of patients a few days after the minor illness has resolved. Rapid onset of asymmetric acute flaccid paralysis with areflexia of the involved limb occurs in fewer than 1% of infections; residual paralytic disease occurs in approximately two-thirds of people with acute motor neuron disease. The classical case of paralytic polio begins with a minor illness characterized by fever, sore throat, headache, nausea, constipation, or malaise for several days, followed by a symptom-free period of 1 to 3 days. Rapid onset of paralysis then follows, but paralysis can occur without this prodrome. Typically, paralysis is asymmetric and affects the proximal muscles more than the distal muscles. Cranial nerve involvement (bulbar poliomyelitis, often showing a tripod sign) and paralysis of respiratory tract muscles can occur. Sensation is usually intact. Findings in cerebrospinal fluid are characteristic of viral meningitis, with mild pleocytosis and lymphocytic predominance. Adults who contracted paralytic poliomyelitis during childhood can develop the noninfectious postpolio syndrome 15 to 40 years later. Postpolio syndrome is characterized by slow and irreversible exacerbation of weakness, most likely occurring in those muscle groups involved during the original infection. Muscle and joint pain are also common. The prevalence of postpolio syndrome is unclear, but the estimated range is 25% to 40%.

Etiology

Polioviruses are classified as members of the family Picornaviridae, genus *Enterovirus*, in the species enterovirus C, and include 3 serotypes (1, 2, and 3). Acute paralytic disease may be caused by naturally occurring (wild) polioviruses or by circulating vaccine-derived polioviruses as a result of sustained person-to-person circulation in the absence of adequate population immunity. In addition, rare cases of vaccine-associated paralytic poliomyelitis (VAPP) occur in recipients of oral poliovirus vaccine (OPV) or their close contacts. People with primary β-lymphocyte immunodeficiencies are at increased risk of VAPP and of chronic infection (immunodeficiency-associated vaccine-derived polioviruses). With recent progress in the World Health Organization Global Polio Eradication Initiative, more cases of paralytic disease are caused by vaccine-related viruses (VAPP and circulating vaccine-derived polioviruses) than by wild polioviruses.

Epidemiology

Humans are the only natural reservoir for poliovirus. Spread is by contact with feces and respiratory secretions. Infection is more common in infants and young children and occurs at an earlier age among children living in poor hygienic conditions. In temperate climates, poliovirus infections are most common during summer and autumn; in the tropics, the seasonal pattern is less pronounced.

The last reported case of poliomyelitis attributable to indigenously acquired, naturally occurring wild poliovirus in the United States occurred in 1979 during an outbreak among unimmunized people that resulted in 10 paralytic cases. The only identified imported case of paralytic poliomyelitis since 1986 occurred in 1993 in a child transported to the United States for medical care. Since 1986, all other cases acquired in the United States have been VAPP cases attributable to OPV. From 1980 to 1997, the average annual number of cases of VAPP reported in the United States was 8. Implementation of an all–inactivated poliovirus vaccine schedule in 2000 halted the occurrence of VAPP cases in the United States. In 2005, however, a healthy, unimmunized young adult from the United States acquired VAPP in Central America, most likely from an infant grandchild of the host family who had recently been immunized with OPV. In 2005, a type 1 vaccine-derived poliovirus was identified in the stool of an asymptomatic, unimmunized, immunodeficient child in Minnesota. Subsequently, poliovirus infections in 7 other unimmunized children (35% of all children tested) within the index patient's community were documented. None of the infected children had paralysis. Phylogenetic analysis suggested the vaccine-derived poliovirus circulated in the community for approximately 2 months before the infant's infection was detected and the initiating OPV dose had been given (likely in another country) before the index child's birth. In 2009, a woman with long-standing common-variable immunodeficiency was diagnosed with VAPP and died of polio-associated complications. Molecular characterization of the poliovirus isolate suggested the infection likely occurred approximately 12 years earlier, coinciding with OPV immunization of her child. Circulation of indigenous wild poliovirus strains ceased in the United States several decades ago, and the risk of contact with imported wild polioviruses has decreased in parallel with the success of the global eradication program. Of the 3 poliovirus serotypes, type 2 wild poliovirus appears to have been eradicated globally, with the last naturally occurring case detected in 1999 in India. No cases of type 3 wild poliovirus were detected during 2013, suggesting this type is also on the verge of eradication. Type 1 poliovirus now accounts for all polio cases attributable to wild poliovirus.

Communicability of poliovirus is greatest shortly before and after onset of clinical illness, when the virus is present in the throat and excreted in high concentrations in feces. Virus persists in the throat for approximately 1 to 2 weeks after onset of illness and is excreted in feces for 3 to 6 weeks. Patients are potentially contagious as long as fecal excretion persists. In recipients of OPV, virus also persists in the throat for 1 to 2 weeks and is excreted in feces for several weeks or, in rare cases, for more than 2 months. Immunocompromised patients with significant β-lymphocyte immune deficiencies have excreted immunodeficiency-associated vaccine-derived polioviruses for periods of more than 20 years.

Incubation Period

Nonparalytic poliomyelitis, 3 to 6 days; paralytic poliomyelitis, 7 to 21 days to paralysis (range, 3–35 days).

Diagnostic Tests

Poliovirus can be detected in specimens from the pharynx and feces, less commonly from urine, and, rarely, from cerebrospinal fluid by isolation in cell culture or reverse transcriptase-polymerase chain reaction. Two or more stool and throat swab specimens for enterovirus isolation or detection should be obtained at least 24 hours apart from patients with suspected paralytic poliomyelitis as early in the course of illness as possible (within 14 days of symptom onset). Fecal material is most likely to yield virus in cell culture. However, poliovirus may be excreted intermittently, and a single negative test result does not rule out infection.

Because OPV is no longer available in the United States, the chance of exposure to vaccine-type polioviruses is remote. If a poliovirus is isolated in the United States, the isolate should be reported immediately to the state health department and sent to the Centers for Disease Control and Prevention for further testing. The diagnostic test of choice for confirming poliovirus disease is viral culture of stool and throat swab specimens. Interpretation of acute and convalescent serologic test results can be difficult because of high levels of population immunity.

Treatment

Supportive.

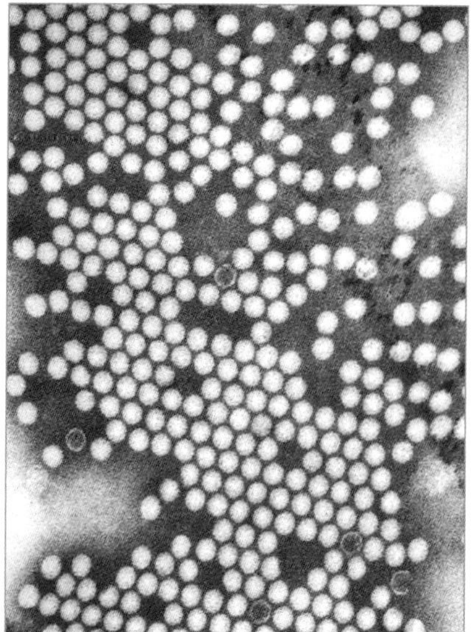

Image 109.1
Electron micrograph of the poliovirus. Poliovirus is a species of Enterovirus, which is a genus in the family of Picornaviridae and an RNA virus. Courtesy of Centers for Disease Control and Prevention/Fred Murphy, MD, and Sylvia Whitfield.

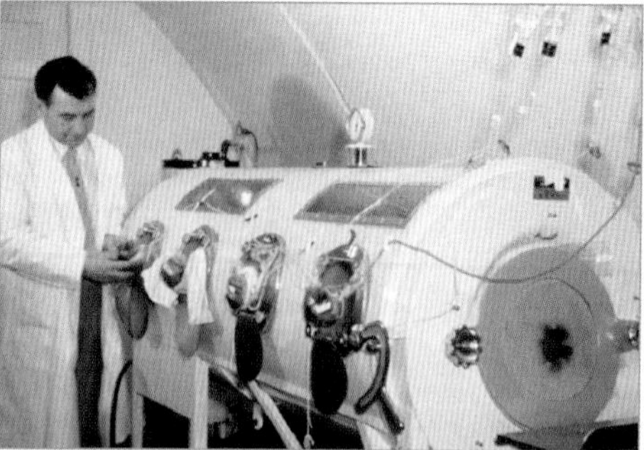

Image 109.2
A physician examines a tank respirator, also known as an iron lung, during a polio epidemic. The iron lung encased the thoracic cavity externally in an airtight chamber. The chamber was used to create a negative pressure around the thoracic cavity, thereby causing air to rush into the lungs to equalize intrapulmonary pressure. Courtesy of Centers for Disease Control and Prevention.

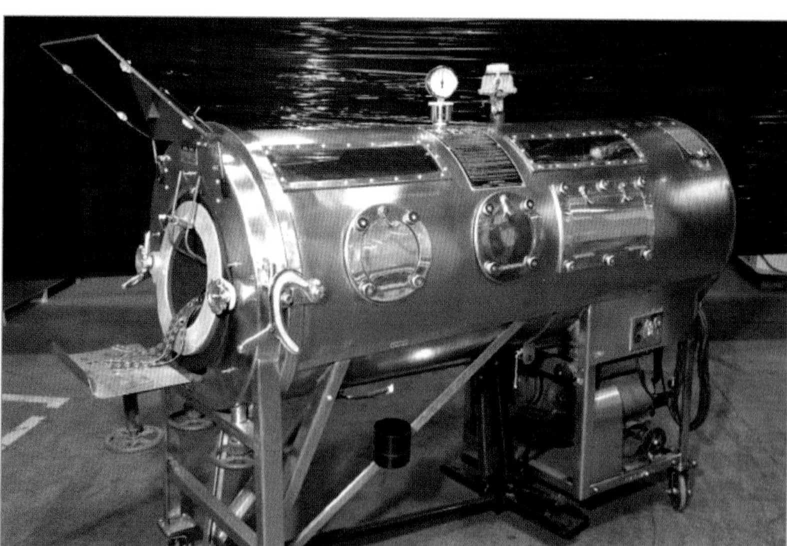

Image 109.3
Made of stainless steel and still in good working order, this Emerson Respirator, also known as an iron lung, was used by polio patients whose ability to breath was paralyzed due to this crippling viral disease. This iron lung was donated to the David J. Sencer Centers for Disease Control and Prevention Museum by the family of polio patient Barton Hebert of Covington, LA, who had used the device from the late 1950s until his death in 2003. Iron lungs encase the thoracic cavity externally in an airtight chamber. The chamber is used to create a negative pressure around the thoracic cavity, thereby causing air to rush into the lungs to equalize intrapulmonary pressure. Courtesy of Centers for Disease Control and Prevention/Jim Gathany.

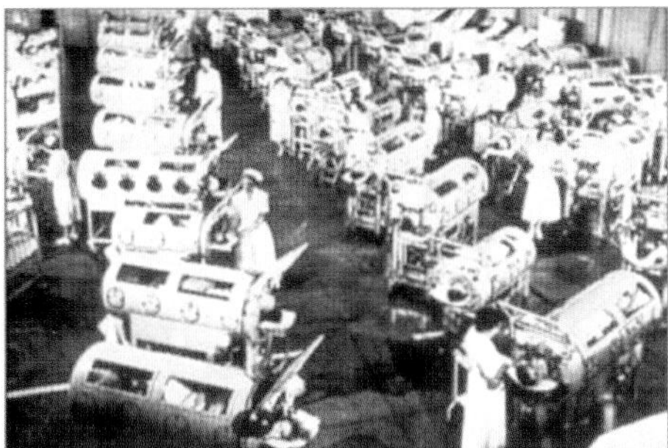

Image 109.4
This 1952 photo of a Los Angeles, CA, hospital respiratory ward shows polio patients in iron lungs—machines that were necessary to help them breathe. Courtesy of Centers for Disease Control and Prevention.

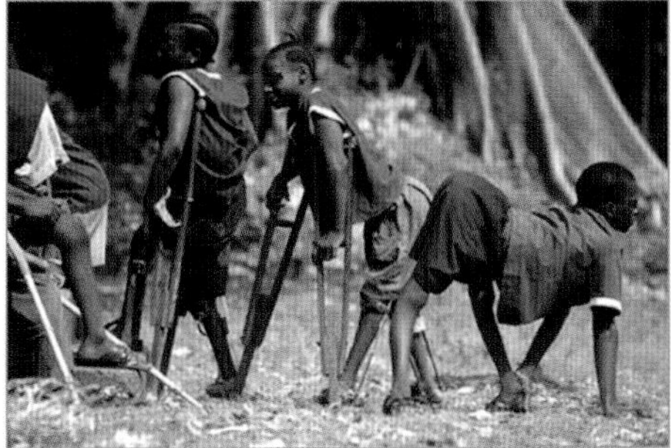

Image 109.6
Cheshire Home for Handicapped Children, Freetown, Sierra Leone. Courtesy of World Health Organization/Immunization Action Coalition.

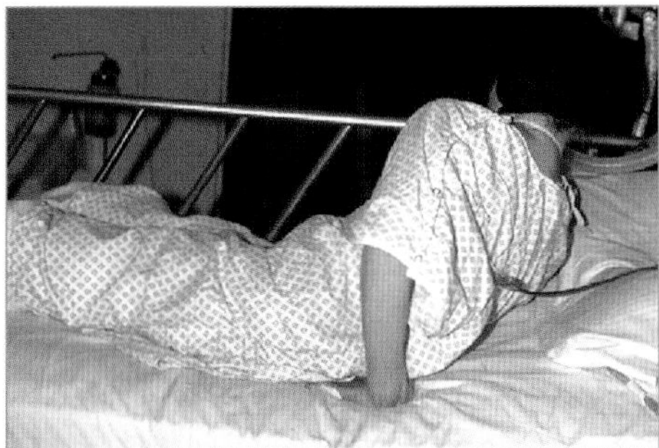

Image 109.8
A young girl with bulbar polio with tripod sign attempts to sit upright. Copyright Martin G. Myers, MD.

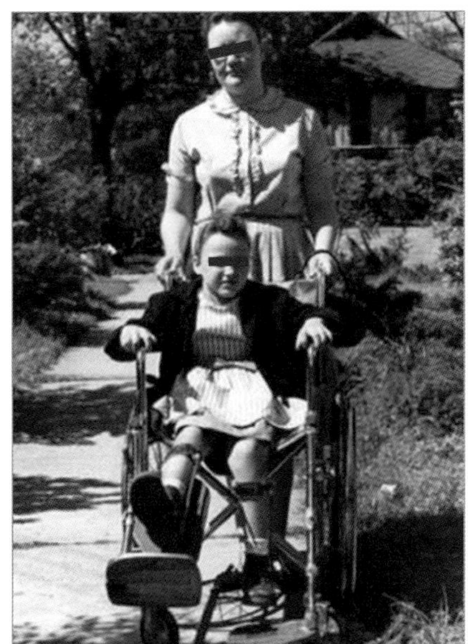

Image 109.5
Images like this were used to encourage polio vaccination. Courtesy of Centers for Disease Control and Prevention.

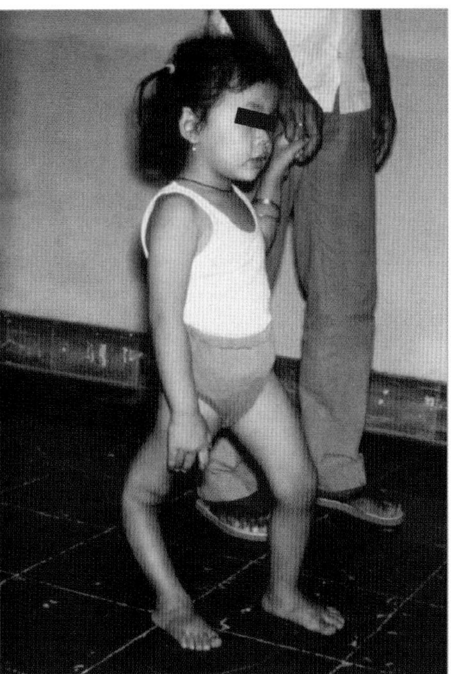

Image 109.7
This child is displaying a deformity of her right lower extremity caused by the poliovirus. Courtesy of Centers for Disease Control and Prevention.

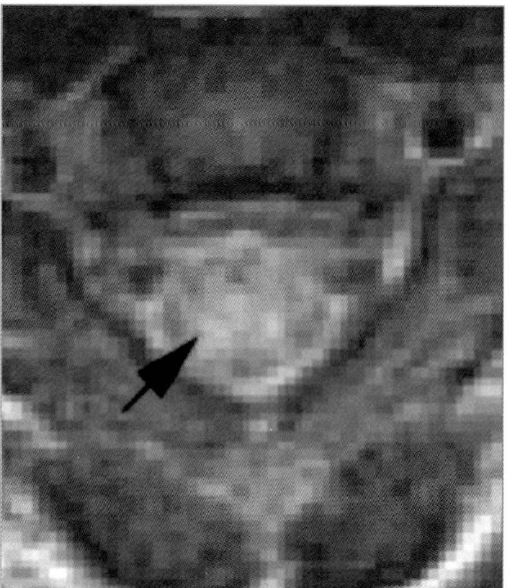

Image 109.9
Axial T2-weighted magnetic resonance image shows cervical spinal cord hyperintensity involving the central gray matter (arrow).

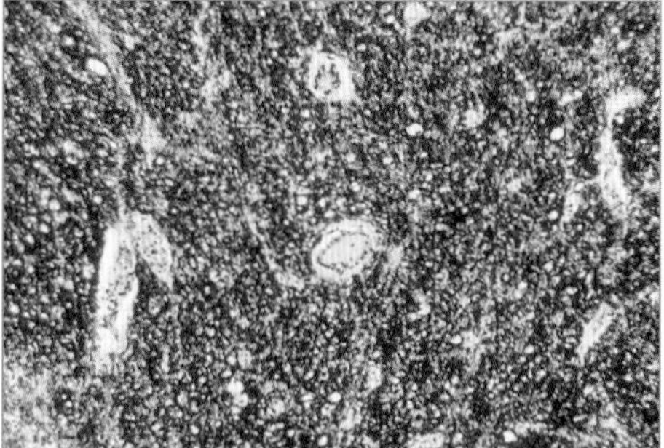

Image 109.10
A photomicrograph of the cervical spinal cord in the region of the anterior horn revealing polio type 3 degenerative changes. The poliovirus has an affinity for the anterior horn motor neurons of the cervical and lumbar regions of the spinal cord. Death of these cells causes muscle weakness of those muscles once innervated by the now-dead neurons. Courtesy of Centers for Disease Control and Prevention/Dr Karp, Emory University.

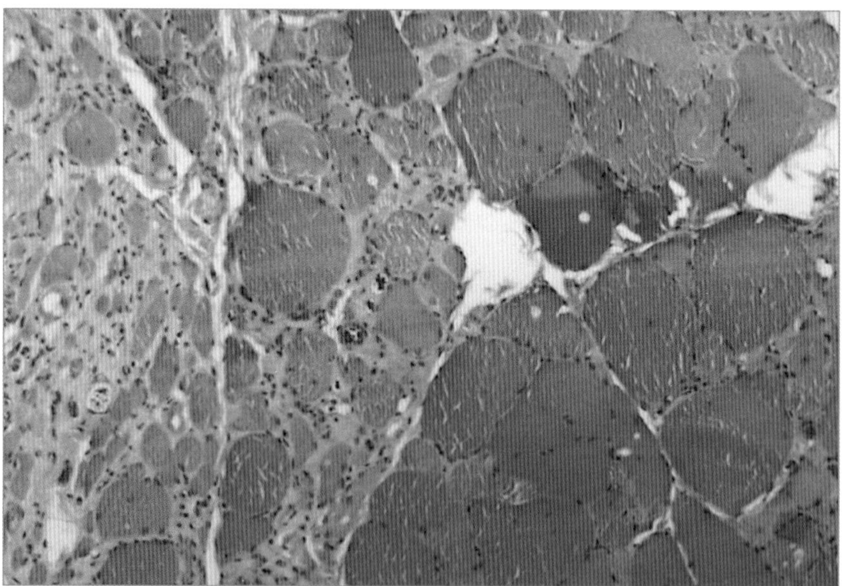

Image 109.11
A photomicrograph of skeletal muscle tissue revealing myotonic dystrophic changes as a result of polio type 3. When spinal neurons die, wallerian degeneration takes place, resulting in muscle weakness of those muscles once innervated by the now-dead neurons (denervated). The degree of paralysis is directly correlated to the number of deceased neurons. Courtesy of Centers for Disease Control and Prevention/Dr Karp, Emory University.

110

Prion Diseases: Transmissible Spongiform Encephalopathies

Clinical Manifestations

Transmissible spongiform encephalopathies (TSEs), or prion diseases, constitute a group of rare, rapidly progressive, universally fatal neurodegenerative diseases of humans and animals that are characterized by neuronal degeneration, spongiform change, gliosis, and accumulation of abnormal misfolded protease-resistant prion protein (PrP) (protease-resistant prion protein [PrP-res], variably called scrapie prion protein [PrP^{Sc}] or, as suggested by the World Health Organization, TSE-associated PrP [PrP^{TSE}]) that distributes diffusely throughout the brain or forms plaques of various morphology.

Human TSEs include several diseases: Creutzfeldt-Jakob disease (CJD), Gerstmann-Sträussler-Scheinker syndrome, fatal familial and sporadic fatal insomnia, kuru, and variant CJD (vCJD, presumably caused by the agent of bovine spongiform encephalopathy [BSE], commonly called "mad cow disease"). Classic CJD can be sporadic (~85% of cases), familial (~15% of cases), or iatrogenic (<1% of cases). Sporadic CJD is most commonly a disease of older adults (median age of death in the United States, 68 years) but also, rarely, has been described in adolescents older than 13 years and young adults. Iatrogenic CJD has been acquired through intramuscular injection of contaminated cadaveric pituitary hormones (growth hormone and human gonadotropin), dura mater allografts, corneal transplantation, and use of contaminated instrumentation at neurosurgery or during depth-electrode electroencephalographic (EEG) recording. In 1996, an outbreak of vCJD linked to exposure to tissues from BSE-infected cattle was reported in the United Kingdom. Since the end of 2003, 4 presumptive cases of transfusion-transmitted vCJD have been reported: 3 clinical cases, as well as 1 probable asymptomatic case in which PrP^{TSE} was detected in spleen and lymph nodes but not brain tissues. A fifth iatrogenic vCJD infection in a hemophiliac patient in the United Kingdom, also preclinical with a finding of PrP^{TSE} in spleen, was attributed to treatment with potentially vCJD-contaminated, UK-sourced fractionated plasma products. The best-known TSEs affecting animals include scrapie of sheep, BSE, and a chronic wasting disease of North American deer, elk, and moose. Except for vCJD, no other human TSE has been attributed to infection with an agent of animal origin.

Creutzfeldt-Jakob disease manifests as a rapidly progressive neurologic disease with escalating defects in memory, personality, and other higher cortical functions. At presentation, approximately one-third of patients have cerebellar dysfunction, including ataxia and dysarthria. Iatrogenic CJD can also manifest as dementia with cerebellar signs. Myoclonus develops in at least 80% of affected patients at some point in the course of disease. Death usually occurs in weeks to months (median, 4–5 months); approximately 10% to 15% of patients with sporadic CJD survive for more than 1 year.

Variant CJD is distinguished from classic CJD by younger age of onset, early "psychiatric" manifestations, and other features, such as painful sensory symptoms, delayed onset of overt neurologic signs, relative absence of diagnostic EEG changes, and a more prolonged duration of illness (median, 13–14 months). In vCJD, a high proportion of people exhibit high signal abnormalities on T2-weighted brain magnetic resonance imaging in the pulvinar region of the posterior thalamus (known as the pulvinar sign). In vCJD, the neuropathologic examination reveals numerous florid plaques (surrounded by vacuoles) and exceptionally striking accumulation of PrP^{TSE} in the brain. In addition, PrP^{TSE} is detectable in the tonsils and other lymphoid tissues of patients with vCJD.

Etiology

The infectious particle or prion responsible for human and animal prion diseases is believed to be a misfolded form of a normal ubiquitous PrP found on the surface of neurons and many other cells in humans and animals. The precise protein structure and mechanism of propagation is unknown. It is generally postulated that sporadic CJD arises from a spontaneous structural change into the pathogenic form of the normal cellular protease-sensitive host-encoded glycoprotein (PrP^{C} or PrP-sen). Prion propagation is postulated to occur by a "recruitment" reaction (the nature of which is under investigation), in which abnormal PrP^{TSE} serves as a template or lattice for the conversion of neighboring PrP^{C} molecules into misfolded protein with high potential to aggregate.

Epidemiology

Classic CJD is rare, occurring in the United States at a rate of approximately 1 case per 1 million people annually. The onset of disease peaks at ages 60 through 74 years. Case-control studies of sporadic CJD have not identified any consistent environmental risk factor. No statistically significant increase in cases of sporadic CJD has been observed in people previously treated with blood, blood components, or plasma derivatives. The incidence of sporadic CJD is not increased in patients with several diseases associated with frequent exposure to blood or blood products, suggesting that the risk of transfusion transmission of classic CJD, if any, is very low and appropriately regarded as theoretical. Creutzfeldt-Jakob disease has not been reported in neonates born to infected mothers. Familial or genetic form of TSEs, inherited as autosomal-dominant disorder, is associated with a variety of mutations of the PrP-encoding gene (*PRNP*) located on chromosome 20. Familial CJD onset of disease is approximately 10 years earlier than sporadic CJD.

As of June 2014, the total number of vCJD cases reported was 177 patients in the United Kingdom, 27 in France, 5 in Spain, 4 in Ireland, 4 in the United States, 3 in the Netherlands, 2 in Portugal, 2 in Italy, 2 in Canada, and 1 each in Taiwan, Japan, and Saudi Arabia. Two of the 4 patients in the United States, 2 of the 4 in Ireland, and 1 each of the patients in France and Canada are believed to have acquired vCJD during prolonged residence in the United Kingdom. The Centers for Disease Control and Prevention and Health Canada have concluded that one of the vCJD patients in the United States and in Canada probably were infected during their residencies as children in Saudi Arabia. Authorities suspect the Japanese patient was infected during a short visit of 24 days to the United Kingdom in 1990, 12 years before the onset of vCJD. Most patients with vCJD were younger than 30 years, and several were adolescents. All but 3 of the primary 174 United Kingdom patients with noniatrogenic vCJD died before 60 years of age; all but 14 patients died before 50 years of age; and 151 patients (87%) died before age 40 years. The median age at death of the 174 primary vCJD cases was 27 years. The ages at death of the 3 iatrogenic vCJD transfusion transmission cases were 32, 69, and 75 years. On the basis of animal inoculation studies, comparative PrP immunoblotting, and epidemiologic investigations, almost all cases of vCJD are believed to have resulted from exposure to tissues from cattle infected with BSE. As noted, 3 clinically symptomatic patients and 1 patient with no clinical signs of the disease are believed to have been infected with vCJD through transfusion of nonleukoreduced red blood cells, and 1 hemophiliac patient, also with no clinical signs of TSE, was probably infected through injections of human plasma–derived clotting factors.

Incubation Period

Iatrogenic CJD varies by route of exposure (range, 14 months–>30 years).

Diagnostic Tests

The diagnosis of human prion diseases can be made with certainty only by neuropathologic examination of affected brain tissue, usually obtained at autopsy. In most patients with classic CJD, a characteristic 1 to 2 cycles per second triphasic sharp-wave discharge on EEG tracing is regarded as indicative of CJD. The likelihood of finding this abnormality is enhanced when serial EEG recordings are obtained. A protein assay that detects the 14-3-3 protein in cerebrospinal fluid (CSF) has been reported to be reasonably sensitive, although not specific, as a marker for CJD. Measurement of the tau protein level in addition to the detection of 14-3-3 protein in CSF has been reported to increase the specificity of CSF testing for CJD. Specific disease marker PrP^{TSE} was demonstrated in CSF of 80% of CJD cases, but, currently, testing for this marker can be performed only on an investigational basis in a few laboratories using sophisticated techniques for detecting minute amounts of the protein. No validated blood test is available, but a prototype test for vCJD that captures, enriches, and detects disease-associated PrP from whole blood using stainless steel powder is being investigated. A progressive neurologic syndrome in a person bearing a pathogenic mutation of the *PRNP* gene is presumed to be prion disease. Because no unique nucleic acid has been detected in prions causing TSEs, genome amplification studies, such as polymerase chain reaction, are not possible. Consideration of brain biopsies for patients with possible CJD should be given when other potentially treatable diseases remain in the differential diagnosis. Complete postmortem examination of the brain is encouraged to confirm the clinical diagnosis and to detect emerging forms of CJD, such as vCJD. State-of-the-art diagnostic testing, including assays of 14-3-3 and tau proteins in CSF, *PRNP* gene sequencing, Western blot analysis to identify and characterize PrP^{TSE}, and histologic processing of brain tissues with expert neuropathologic consultation, are offered by the National Prion Disease Pathology Surveillance Center (telephone, 216/368-0587; **www.cjdsurveillance.com**).

Treatment

No treatment in humans slows or stops the progressive neurodegeneration in prion diseases. Experimental treatments are being studied. Supportive therapy is necessary to manage dementia, spasticity, rigidity, and seizures occurring during the course of the illness. Psychological support may help families of affected people. Genetic counseling is indicated in familial disease, taking into account that penetrance has been variable in some families in which people with a *PRNP* mutation survived to an advanced age without neurodegenerative disease.

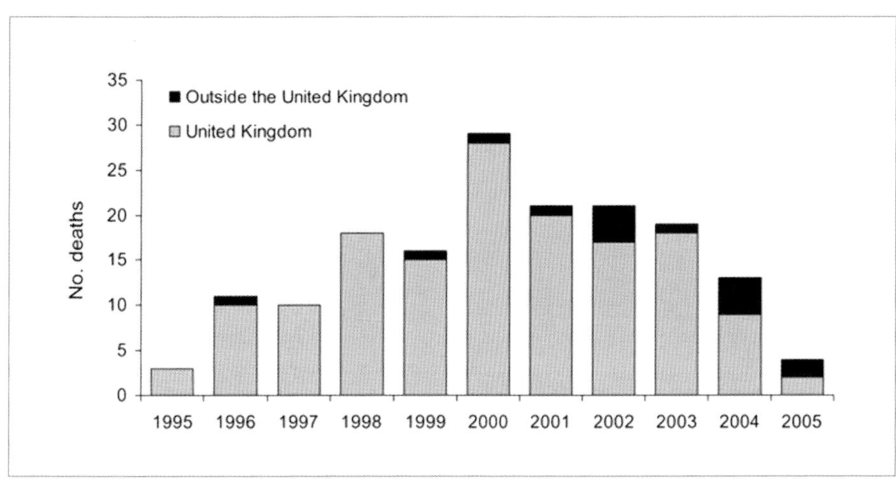

Image 110.1
Number of deceased variant Creutzfeldt-Jakob disease patients worldwide (150 from the United Kingdom and 15 outside the United Kingdom) by year of death, June 2005. Courtesy of *Emerging Infectious Diseases.*

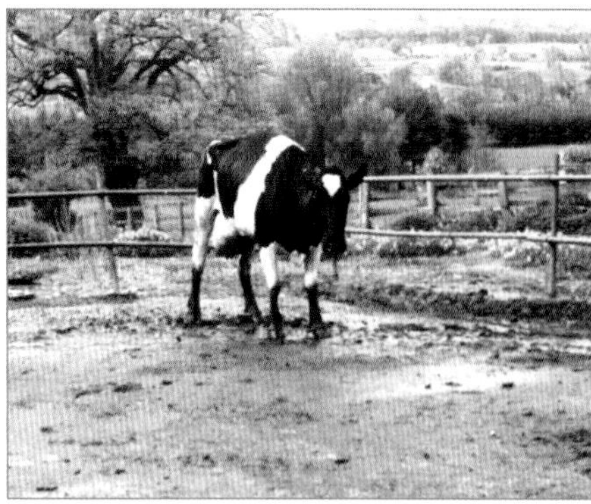

Image 110.2
Cattle, such as pictured here, which are affected by bovine spongiform encephalopathy (BSE), experience progressive degeneration of the nervous system. Behavioral changes in temperament (eg, nervousness, aggression), abnormal posture, incoordination and difficulty in rising, decreased milk production, or weight loss despite continued appetite are followed by death in cattle affected by BSE. Courtesy of Centers for Disease Control and Prevention/ US Department of Agriculture–Animal and Plant Health Inspection Service, APHIS/Dr Art Davis.

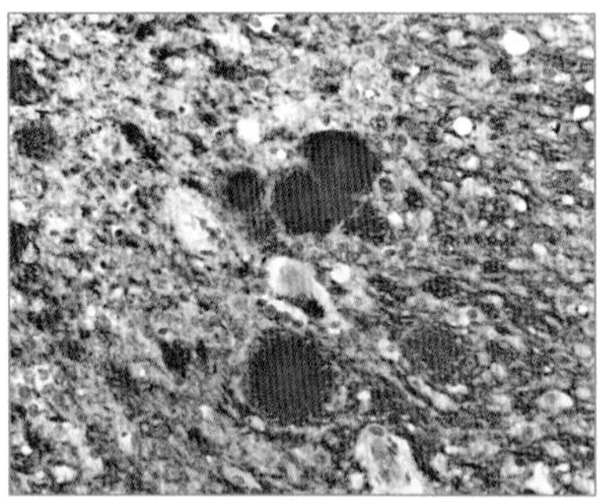

Image 110.4
Immunohistochemical staining of cerebellar tissue of the patient who died of variant Creutzfeldt-Jakob disease in the United States. Stained amyloid plaques are shown with surrounding deposits of abnormal prion protein (immunoalkaline phosphatase stain, naphthol fast red substrate with light hematoxylin counterstain; original magnification x158). Courtesy of Belay ED, Sejvar JJ, Shieh WJ, et al. Variant Creutzfeldt-Jakob disease death, United States. *Emerg Infect Dis*. 2005;11(9):1351–1354.

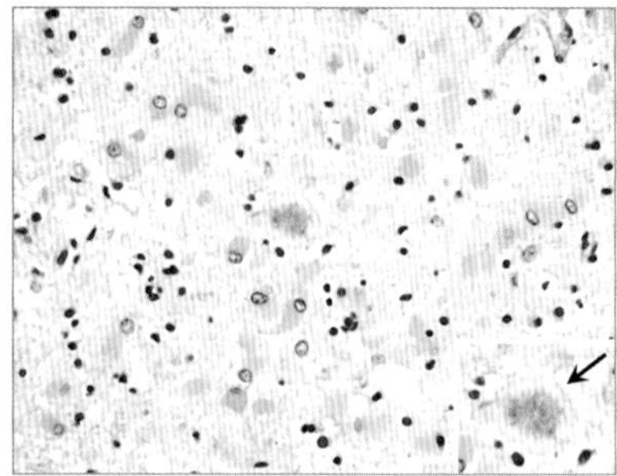

Image 110.3
Histopathologic changes in frontal cerebral cortex of the patient who died of variant Creutzfeldt-Jakob disease in the United States. Marked astroglial reaction is shown, occasionally with relatively large florid plaques surrounded by vacuoles (arrow in inset) (hematoxylin-eosin stain, original magnification x40). Courtesy of Belay ED, Sejvar JJ, Shieh WJ, et al. Variant Creutzfeldt-Jakob disease death, United States. *Emerg Infect Dis*. 2005;11(9):1351–1354.

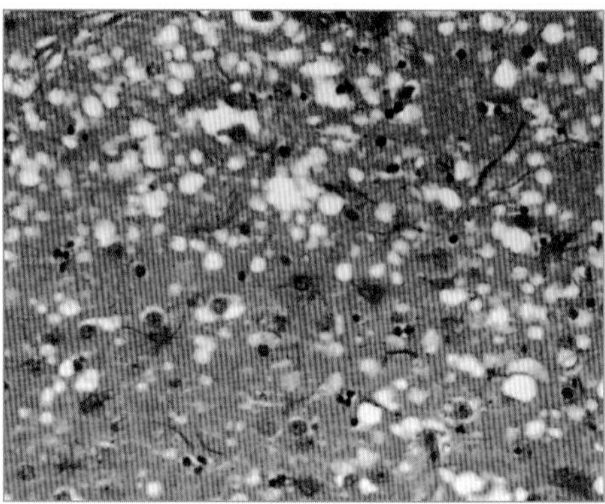

Image 110.5
This micrograph of brain tissue reveals the cytoarchitectural histopathologic changes found in bovine spongiform encephalopathy (BSE). The presence of vacuoles (ie, microscopic "holes" in the gray matter) gives the brain of BSE-affected cows a spongelike appearance when tissue sections are examined in the laboratory. Courtesy of Centers for Disease Control and Prevention/ US Department of Agriculture–Animal and Plant Health Inspection Service, APHIS/Dr Al Jenny.

111

Q Fever (*Coxiella burnetii* Infection)

Clinical Manifestations

Approximately 50% of acute Q fever infections are asymptomatic. Two types of disease, acute and chronic, exist, and both can present as fever of unknown origin. Q fever in children is typically characterized by abrupt onset of fever often accompanied by chills, headache, weakness, cough, and other nonspecific systemic symptoms. Illness is usually self-limited, although a relapsing febrile illness lasting for several months has been documented. Gastrointestinal tract symptoms, such as diarrhea, vomiting, abdominal pain, and anorexia, are reported in 50% to 80% of children. Rash has also been observed in some patients with Q fever. Q fever pneumonia usually manifests as mild cough, respiratory distress, and chest pain. Chest radiographic patterns are variable. More severe manifestations of acute Q fever are rare but include hepatitis, hemolytic uremic syndrome, myocarditis, pericarditis, cerebellitis, encephalitis, meningitis, hemophagocytosis, lymphadenitis, acalculous cholecystitis, and rhabdomyolysis. Chronic Q fever is rare in children but can present as blood culture–negative endocarditis, chronic relapsing or multifocal osteomyelitis, or chronic hepatitis. Children who are immunocompromised or have underlying valvular heart disease may be at higher risk of chronic Q fever.

Etiology

Coxiella burnetii, the cause of Q fever, was formerly considered to be a *Rickettsia* organism but is a gram-negative intracellular bacterium that belongs to the order Legionellaceae. The infectious form of *C burnetii* is highly resistant to heat, desiccation, and disinfectant chemicals and can persist for long periods in the environment. *C burnetii* is classified as a category B bioterrorism agent.

Epidemiology

Q fever is a zoonotic infection that has been reported worldwide, including every state in the United States. *C burnetii* infection is usually asymptomatic in animals. Many different species can be infected, although cattle, sheep, and goats are the primary reservoirs for human infection. Tick vectors may be important for maintaining animal and bird reservoirs but are not thought to be important in transmission to humans. Humans typically acquire infection by inhalation of fine-particle aerosols of *C burnetii* generated from birthing fluids or other excreta of infected animals or through inhalation of dust contaminated by these materials. Infection can occur by exposure to contaminated materials, such as wool, straw, bedding, or laundry. Windborne particles containing infectious organisms can travel a half mile or more, contributing to sporadic cases for which no apparent animal contact can be demonstrated. Unpasteurized dairy products can contain the organism. Seasonal trends occur in farming areas with predictable frequency, and the disease often coincides with the livestock birthing season in spring.

Incubation Period

14 to 22 days (range, 9 to 39 days), depending on inoculum size. Chronic Q fever can develop months or years after initial infection.

Diagnostic Tests

Serologic evidence of a 4-fold increase in phase 2 immunoglobulin (Ig) G by immunofluorescent assay tests between paired sera taken 3 to 6 weeks apart is the diagnostic gold standard for diagnosis of acute Q fever. Polymerase chain reaction (PCR) testing on blood or serum may be useful within 2 weeks of symptom onset and before antibiotic administration. Although a positive PCR assay result can confirm the diagnosis, a negative PCR result does not exclude Q fever. A single high serum phase 2 IgG titer (≥1:128) by immunofluorescent assay in convalescent serum may be considered evidence of probable infection. Confirmation of chronic Q fever is based on an increasing phase 1 IgG titer (typically ≥1:1,024) that is often higher than the phase 2 IgG titer **and** an identifiable nidus of infection (eg, endocarditis, vascular infection, osteomyelitis, chronic hepatitis). Detection of *C burnetii* in tissues by immunohistochemistry or PCR assay can also confirm a diagnosis of chronic

Q fever. Isolation of *C burnetii* from blood can be performed only in special laboratories because of the potential hazard to laboratory workers.

Treatment

Acute Q fever is generally a self-limited illness, and many patients recover without antimicrobial therapy. However, early treatment is extremely effective in shortening illness duration and symptom severity and is recommended. Patients with suspected Q fever should be treated empirically because laboratory results are often negative early in illness. Doxycycline is the drug of choice for severe infections. Children younger than 8 years with mild illness, pregnant women, and patients allergic to doxycycline can be treated with trimethoprim-sulfamethoxazole.

Chronic Q fever is much more difficult to treat, and relapses can occur despite appropriate therapy, necessitating repeated courses of therapy. The recommended therapy for chronic Q fever endocarditis is a combination of doxycycline and hydroxychloroquine for a minimum of 18 months. Surgical replacement of the infected valve may be necessary in some patients.

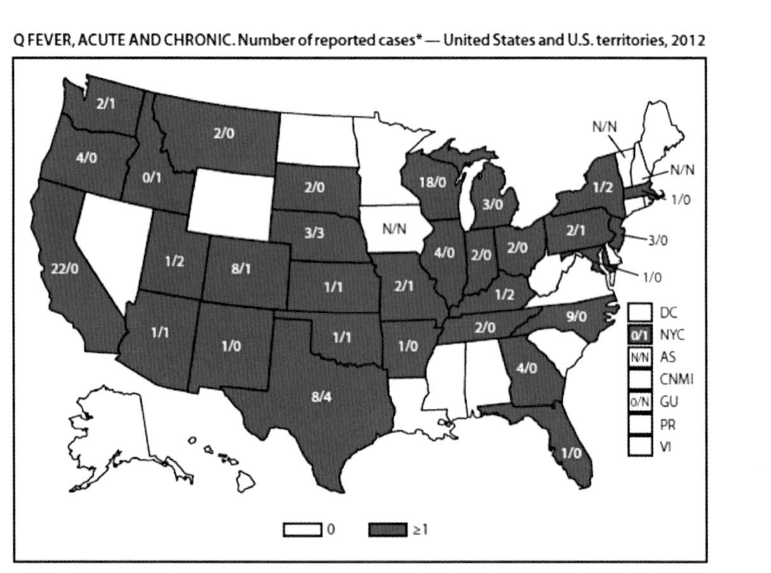

* Number of Q fever acute cases/number of Q fever chronic cases.

Q fever, caused by *Coxiella burnetii*, is reported throughout the United States. Human cases of Q fever most often result from contact with infected livestock, especially sheep, goats, and cattle.

Image 111.1
Q fever, acute and chronic. Number of reported cases—United States and US territories, 2012. Courtesy of *Morbidity and Mortality Weekly Report.*

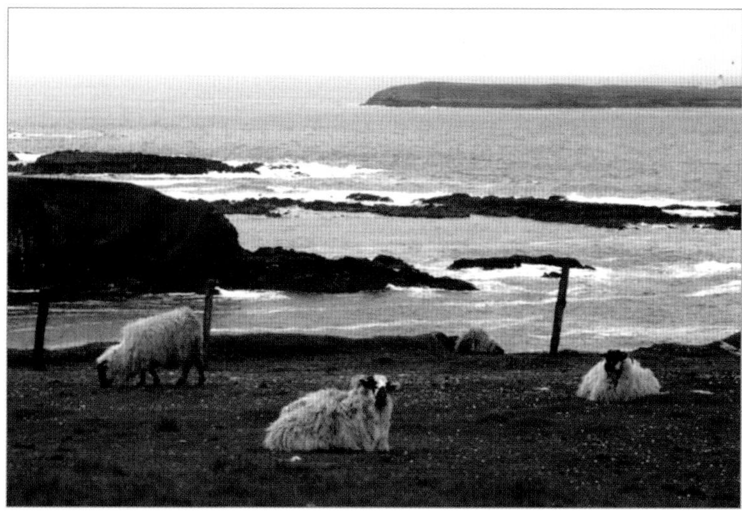

Image 111.2

These domestic sheep were lying on a hillside in Glencolmcille, County Donegal, Ireland, with the Atlantic Ocean in the background. In 2004, Ireland had almost 7 million domestic sheep. That year, the Irish state exported approximately 51,500 tons of sheep meat valued at 165 million euros. While important to national economies, livestock industries can present health hazards for producers and consumers. Diseases that can be transmitted from animals to humans are called zoonoses. Q fever, *Coxiella burnetii,* is a disease passed to humans from sheep. People working around domestic sheep should consider getting vaccinated against this disease. The disease can be acquired from the inhalation of aerosolized barnyard dust should it contain infected dried urine, manure particles, or dried fluids from the birth of calves or lambs. Domestic animals present problems not only for their handlers (ie, farmers) but also for consumers when animals are used for food. Food products made from animals include not only meat but meat derivatives that are added to sweets and other foods and, therefore, are less obvious to consumers. Courtesy of Centers for Disease Control and Prevention/Edwin P. Ewing Jr, MD.

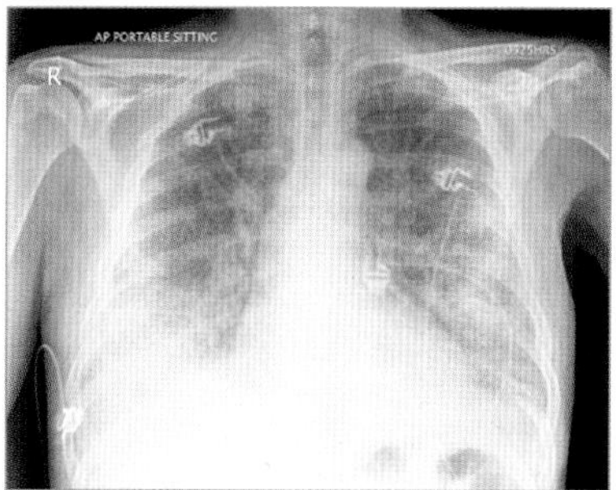

Image 111.3

Chest radiograph of patient at time of admission to hospital, before intubation, demonstrating extensive bilateral airspace disease. The first cases of Q fever in Nova Scotia were recognized in 1979 during a study of atypical pneumonia. This observation led to a series of studies that showed Q fever was common in Nova Scotia (50–60 cases per year in a population of ~950,000) and the epidemiology was unique; exposure to infected parturient cats or newborn kittens was the major risk factor for infection. At about the same time, cat-related outbreaks were noted in neighboring Prince Edward Island and New Brunswick. In the early 1990s, cases began to decline but, to our knowledge, since 1999, Q fever in this area has not been systematically studied. Courtesy of Marrie TJ, Campbell N, McNeil SA, Webster D, Hatchette TF. Q fever update, Maritime Canada. *Emerg Infect Dis.* 2008;14(1):67–69.

112

Rabies

Clinical Manifestations

Infection with rabies virus and other *Lyssavirus* species characteristically produces an acute illness with rapidly progressive central nervous system manifestations, including anxiety, radicular pain, dysesthesia or pruritus, hydrophobia, and dysautonomia. Some patients may have paralysis. Illness almost invariably progresses to death. Three unimmunized people have recovered from clinical rabies in the United States. The differential diagnosis of acute encephalitic illnesses of unknown cause or with features of Guillain-Barré syndrome should include rabies.

Etiology

Rabies virus is an RNA virus classified in the Rhabdoviridae family, *Lyssavirus* genus. The genus *Lyssavirus* currently contains 12 species with 2 additional putative species divided into 3 phylogroups.

Epidemiology

Understanding the epidemiology of rabies has been aided by viral variant identification using monoclonal antibodies and nucleotide sequencing. In the United States, human cases have decreased steadily since the 1950s, reflecting widespread immunization of dogs and the availability of effective prophylaxis after exposure to a rabid animal. From 2000 through July 2013, 31 of 43 cases of human rabies reported in the United States were acquired indigenously. Among the 31 indigenously acquired cases, all but 4 were associated with bats. Despite the large focus of rabies in raccoons in the eastern United States, only 3 human deaths have been attributed to the raccoon rabies virus variant. Historically, 2 cases of human rabies were attributable to probable aerosol exposure in laboratories, and 2 unusual cases have been attributed to possible airborne exposures in caves inhabited by millions of bats, although alternative infection routes cannot be discounted. Transmission has also occurred by transplantation of organs, corneas, and other tissues from patients dying of undiagnosed rabies. Person-to-person transmission by bite has not been documented in the United States, although the virus has been isolated from saliva of infected patients.

Wildlife rabies perpetuates throughout all 50 United States except Hawaii, which remains "rabies free." Wildlife, including bats, raccoons, skunks, foxes, coyotes, and bobcats, are the most important potential sources of infection for humans and domestic animals in the United States. Rabies in small rodents (squirrels, hamsters, guinea pigs, gerbils, chipmunks, rats, mice) and lagomorphs (rabbits, pikas, hares) is rare. Rabies may occur in woodchucks or other large rodents in areas where raccoon rabies is common. The virus is present in saliva and is transmitted by bites or, rarely, by contamination of mucosa or skin lesions by saliva or other potentially infectious material (eg, neural tissue). Worldwide, most rabies cases in humans result from dog bites in areas where canine rabies is enzootic. Most rabid dogs, cats, and ferrets shed virus for a few days before there are obvious signs of illness. No case of human rabies in the United States has been attributed to a dog, cat, or ferret that has remained healthy throughout the standard 10-day period of confinement after an exposure.

Incubation Period

In humans, average 1 to 3 months, but range from days to years.

Diagnostic Tests

Infection in animals can be diagnosed by demonstration of the presence of rabies virus antigen in brain tissue using a direct fluorescent antibody test. Suspected rabid animals should be euthanized in a manner that preserves brain tissue for appropriate laboratory diagnosis. Virus can be isolated in suckling mice or in tissue culture from saliva, brain, and other specimens and can be detected by identification of viral antigens or nucleotide sequences in affected tissues. Diagnosis in suspected human cases can be made postmortem by immunofluorescent or immunohistochemical examination of brain tissue or by detection of viral nucleotide sequences. Antemortem diagnosis can be made by direct fluorescent antibody test on skin biopsy specimens from the nape of the neck, by isolation of the virus from saliva, by detection of antibody in serum in unvaccinated people and cerebrospinal fluid in all people, and by detection of viral nucleotide sequences in saliva, skin, or other tissues. No single test is sufficiently sensitive because of the unique nature of rabies pathobiology. Laboratory personnel and state or local health departments should be consulted before submission of specimens to the Centers for Disease Control and Prevention so appropriate collection and transport of materials can be arranged.

Treatment

Once symptoms develop, neither rabies vaccine nor rabies immune globulin is useful. There is no specific treatment. Ten people have survived rabies in association with incomplete rabies vaccine schedules. Since 2004, 3 girls, each of whom had not received rabies postexposure prophylaxis, survived rabies. A combination of sedation and intensive medical intervention may be valuable adjunctive therapy.

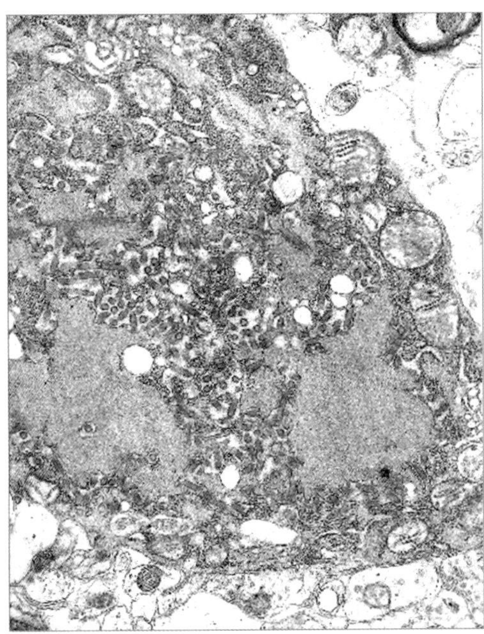

Image 112.1
Electron micrograph of the rabies virus. This electron micrograph shows the rabies virus, as well as Negri bodies or cellular inclusions. Courtesy of Centers for Disease Control and Prevention/ Dr Fred Murphy.

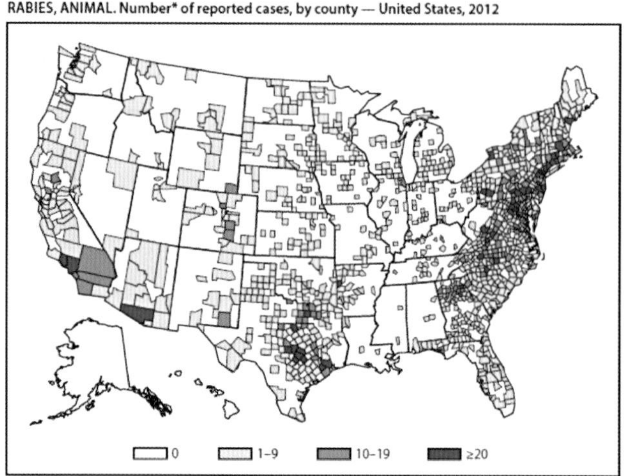

* Data from the National Center for Emerging and Zoonotic Infectious Diseases, Division of High-consequence Pathogens and Pathology.

Several rabies virus variants associated with distinct reservoir species have been identified in the United States. The circulation of rabies virus variants associated with raccoons (eastern United States), skunks (central United States and California), and foxes (Texas, Arizona, and Alaska) occur over defined geographic areas. Several distinct rabies virus variants associated with different bat species are broadly distributed across the contiguous United States. Hawaii is the only state considered free of rabies.

Image 112.2
Rabies, animal. Number of reported cases, by county—United States, 2012. Courtesy of *Morbidity and Mortality Weekly Report.*

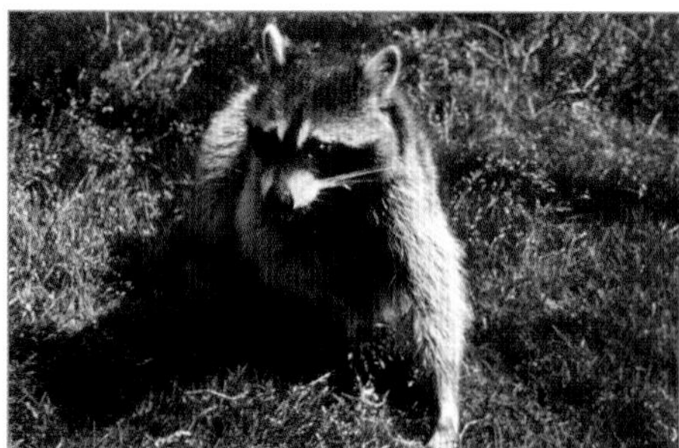

Image 112.3
Raccoons can be vectors of the rabies virus, transmitting the virus to humans and other animals. Rabies virus belongs to the order Mononegavirales. Raccoons continue to be the most frequently reported rabid wildlife species and involved 37.7% of all animal-transmitted cases during 2000. Courtesy of Centers for Disease Control and Prevention.

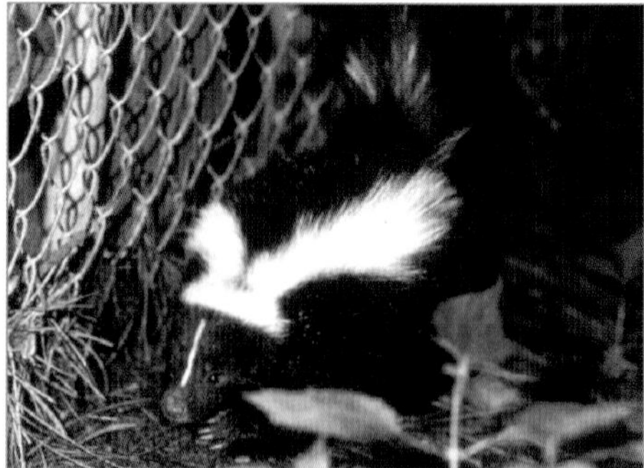

Image 112.4
Approximately one-third of reported animal rabies is attributed to the wild skunk population. Wild animals accounted for 93% of reported animal cases of rabies in 2000. Skunks were responsible for 30.1% of this number. Courtesy of Centers for Disease Control and Prevention.

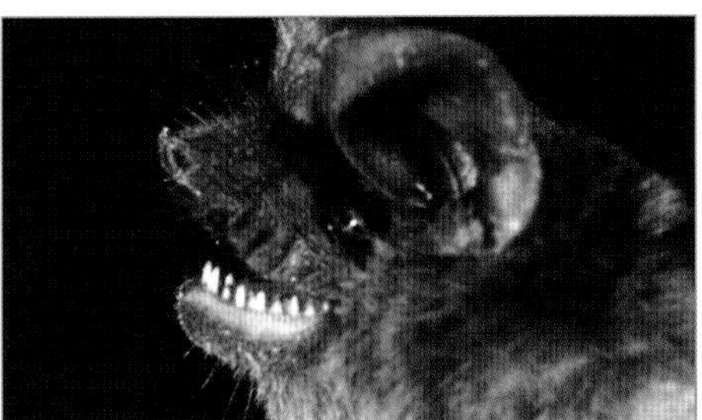

Image 112.5
This bat, *Artibeus jamaicensis*, is also known as the Jamaican fruit bat. Most of the recent human rabies cases in the United States have been caused by rabies virus that was transmitted through a bat vector. Courtesy of Centers for Disease Control and Prevention/Dr R. Keith Sikes.

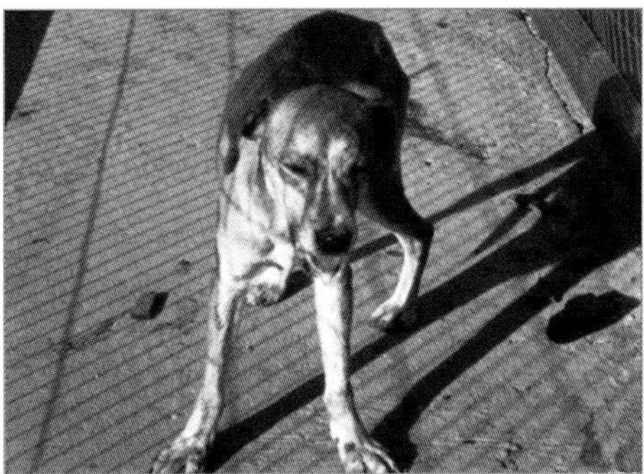

Image 112.6
This rabid dog has saliva dripping from the mouth, which is a primary indicator for the presence of rabies. Before 1960, the majority of cases were in domestic animals. In more recent years, more than 90% of all animal cases reported occur in wildlife. Courtesy of Centers for Disease Control and Prevention.

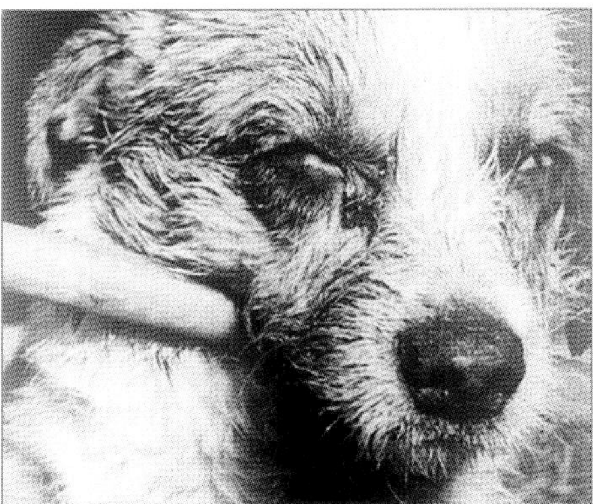

Image 112.7
Close-up of a dog's face during late-stage "dumb" paralytic rabies. Animals with dumb rabies appear depressed, lethargic, and uncoordinated. Gradually, they become completely paralyzed. When their throat and jaw muscles are paralyzed, the animals will drool and have difficulty swallowing. Courtesy of Centers for Disease Control and Prevention.

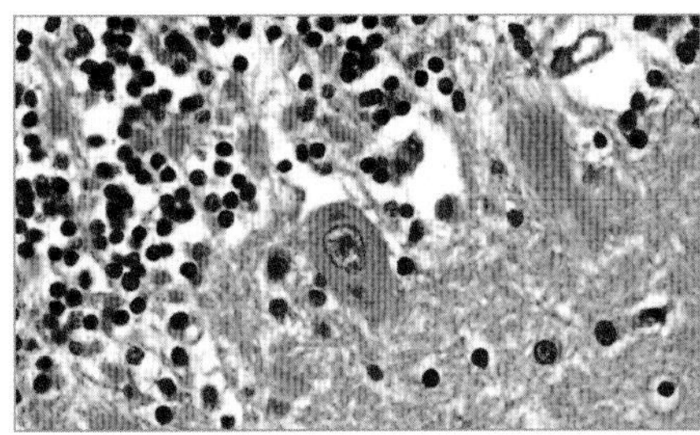

Image 112.8
Characteristic Negri bodies are present within a Purkinje cell of the cerebellum in this patient who died of rabies. Courtesy of Centers for Disease Control and Prevention/Dr Makonnen Fekadu.

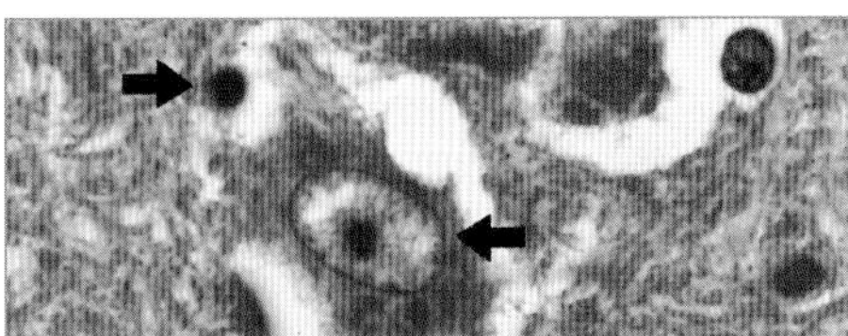

Image 112.9
Photomicrograph of brain tissue from a rabies encephalitis patient (hematoxylin-eosin stain). Histopathologic brain tissue from a rabies patient displaying the pathognomonic finding of Negri bodies within the neuronal cytoplasm (hematoxylin-eosin stain). Courtesy of Centers for Disease Control and Prevention/Dr Daniel P. Perl.

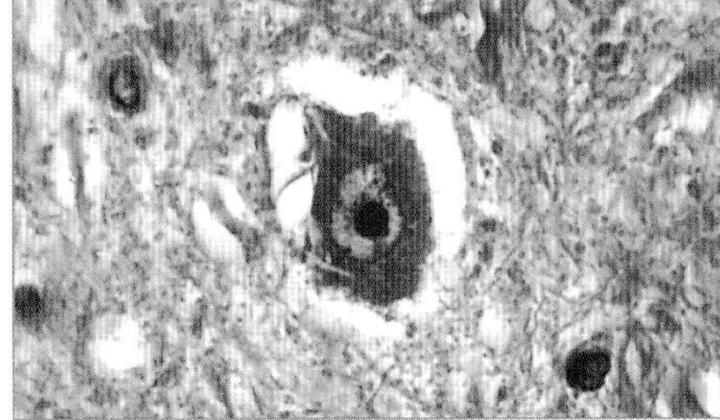

Image 112.10
This micrograph depicts the histopathologic changes associated with rabies encephalitis (hematoxylin-eosin stain). Note the Negri bodies, which are cellular inclusions found most frequently in the pyramidal cells of hippocampus proprius, and the Purkinje cells of the cerebellum. They are also found in the cells of the medulla and various other ganglia. Courtesy of Centers for Disease Control and Prevention/Dr Daniel P. Perl.

113

Rat-bite Fever

Clinical Manifestations

Rat-bite fever is caused by *Streptobacillus moniliformis* or *Spirillum minus*. *S moniliformis* infection (streptobacillary or Haverhill fever) is characterized by relapsing fever, rash, and migratory polyarthritis. There is an abrupt onset of fever, chills, muscle pain, vomiting, headache, and, rarely (unlike *S minus*), lymphadenopathy. A maculopapular, purpuric, or petechial rash develops, predominantly on the peripheral extremities, including the palms and soles, typically within a few days of fever onset. The bite site usually heals promptly and exhibits no or minimal inflammation. Nonsuppurative migratory polyarthritis or arthralgia follows in approximately 50% of patients. Symptoms of untreated infection resolve within 2 weeks, but fever can occasionally relapse for weeks or months. Complications include soft tissue and solid-organ abscesses, septic arthritis, pneumonia, endocarditis, myocarditis, and meningitis. The case-fatality rate is 7% to 13% in untreated patients, and fatal cases have been reported in young children. With *S minus* infection (sodoku), a period of initial apparent healing at the site of the bite is usually followed by fever and ulceration at the site, regional lymphangitis and lymphadenopathy, and a distinctive rash of red or purple plaques. Arthritis is rare. Infection with *S minus* is rare in the United States.

Etiology

The causes of rat-bite fever are *S moniliformis*, a microaerophilic, gram-negative, pleomorphic bacillus, and *S minus*, a small, gram-negative, spiral organism with bipolar flagellar tufts.

Epidemiology

Rat-bite fever is a zoonotic illness. The natural habitat of *S moniliformis* and *S minus* is the upper respiratory tract of rodents. *S moniliformis* is transmitted by bites or scratches from or exposure to oral secretions of infected rats (eg, kissing pet rodents); other rodents (eg, mice, gerbils, squirrels, weasels) and rodent-eating animals, including cats and dogs, can also transmit the infection. Haverhill fever refers to infection after ingestion of unpasteurized milk, water, or food contaminated with *S moniliformis* and may be associated with an outbreak of disease. *S minus* is transmitted by bites of rats and mice. *S moniliformis* infection accounts for most cases of rat-bite fever in the United States; *S minus* infections occur primarily in Asia.

Incubation Period

For *S moniliformis*, usually less than 7 days (range, 3 days–3 weeks); for *S minus*, 7 to 21 days.

Diagnostic Tests

S moniliformis is a fastidious, slow-growing organism isolated from specimens of blood, synovial fluid, aspirates from abscesses, or material from the bite lesion by inoculation into bacteriologic media enriched with blood, serum, or ascitic fluid. Cultures should be held up to 3 weeks if *S moniliformis* is suspected. Sodium polyanethol sulfonate, present in most blood culture media, is inhibitory to *S moniliformis;* therefore, sodium polyanethol sulfonate–free media should be used. *S minus* has not been recovered on artificial media but can be visualized by darkfield microscopy in wet mounts of blood, exudate of a lesion, and lymph nodes. Blood specimens should also be viewed with Giemsa or Wright stain. *S minus* can be recovered from blood, lymph nodes, or local lesions by intraperitoneal inoculation of mice or guinea pigs. *S moniliformis* has been detected using a nucleic acid amplification–based assay.

Treatment

Penicillin administered intravenously or intramuscularly for 7 to 10 days is the treatment for rat-bite fever caused by either agent. Initial intravenous penicillin for 5 to 7 days followed by oral penicillin for 7 days has also been successful. Limited experience exists for ampicillin, cefuroxime, and cefotaxime. Doxycycline or streptomycin can be substituted when a patient has a serious allergy to penicillin. Patients with endocarditis should receive intravenous high-dose penicillin G for at least 4 weeks. The addition of streptomycin or gentamicin for initial therapy may be useful.

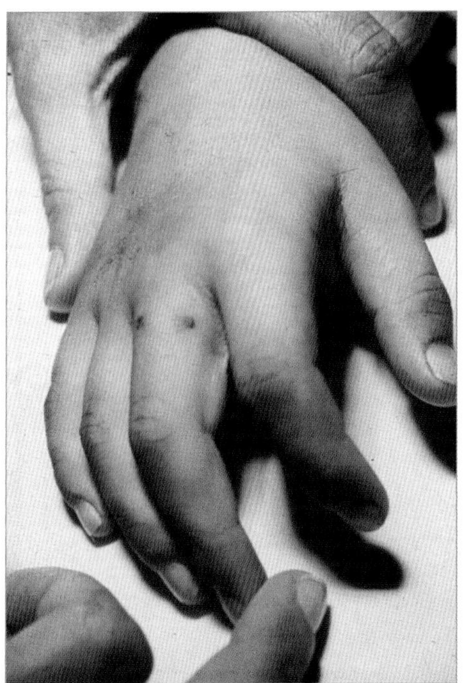

Image 113.1
Rat-bite wounds on the finger of a 5-year-old white boy 12 hours after the bite appear non-inflammatory. Because of fever, chills, headache, and rash 5 days later, blood cultures were obtained that grew *Streptobacillus moniliformis*. Courtesy of George Nankervis, MD.

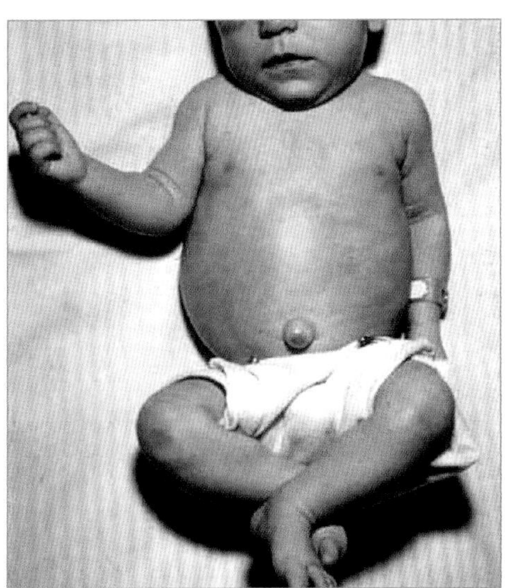

Image 113.3
The rash of rat-bite fever (*Streptobacillus moniliformis*) in an infant bitten by a rat on the right side of the face while sleeping.

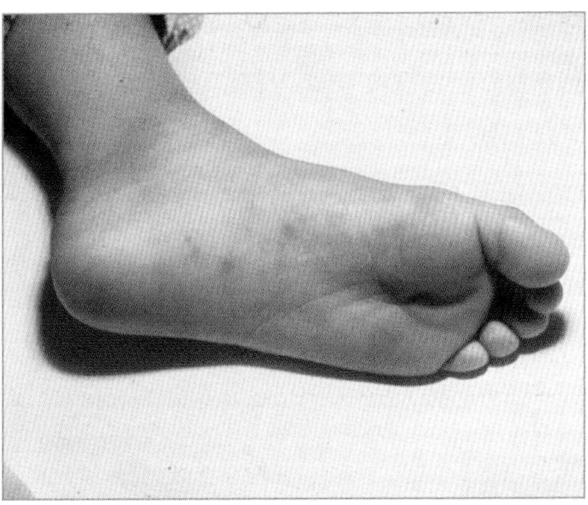

Image 113.2
Five days after being bitten by a rat, the child in Image 113.1 developed fever, chills, and headache, followed 5 days later by a papulovesicular rash on the hands and feet. *Streptobacillus moniliformis* was isolated from blood cultures, and the patient responded to intravenous penicillin therapy without complication. Courtesy of George Nankervis, MD.

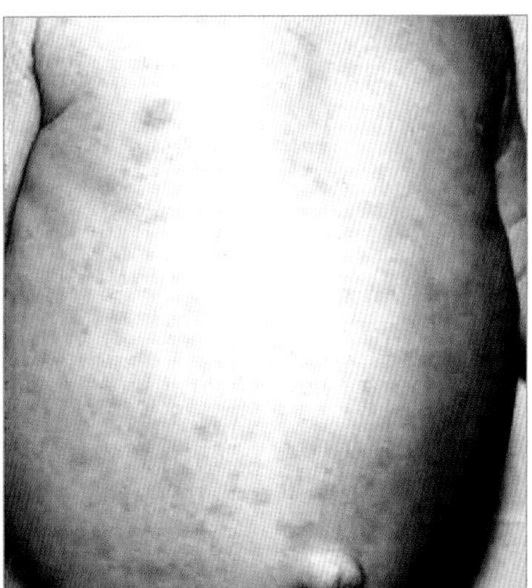

Image 113.4
Close-up view of the rash of the same infant as in Image 113.3 who was bitten on the right cheek by a rat. Sodoku, or rat-bite fever caused by *Spirillum minus*, rarely occurs in the United States.

114

Respiratory Syncytial Virus

Clinical Manifestations

Respiratory syncytial virus (RSV) causes acute respiratory tract infections in people of all ages and is one of the most common diseases of early childhood. Most patients are infected during the first year of life, with virtually all having been infected at least once by the second birthday; the majority experience upper respiratory tract symptoms, and 20% to 30% develop lower respiratory tract disease (eg, bronchiolitis, pneumonia) with the first infection. Signs and symptoms of bronchiolitis typically begin with rhinitis and cough, which progress to increased respiratory effort with tachypnea, wheezing, rales, crackles, intercostal or subcostal retractions, grunting, and nasal flaring. During the first few weeks of life, particularly among preterm neonates, infection with RSV can produce minimal respiratory tract signs; lethargy, irritability, and poor feeding, sometimes accompanied by apneic episodes, are often presenting manifestations in these neonates. Most previously healthy neonates who develop RSV bronchiolitis do not require hospitalization, and even those who are hospitalized improve with supportive care, with discharge after 2 or 3 days. Approximately 1% to 3% of all infants in the first 12 months of life will be hospitalized because of RSV lower respiratory tract disease. Most RSV hospitalizations occur in the first 3 months of life. Factors that increase the risk of severe RSV lower respiratory tract illness include extreme prematurity; cyanotic or complicated congenital heart disease, especially conditions associated with pulmonary hypertension; chronic lung disease of prematurity (formerly called bronchopulmonary dysplasia); and certain immunodeficiency states. Fewer than 100 deaths in young children are attributable to complications of RSV infection annually. The association between RSV bronchiolitis early in life and subsequent asthma remains poorly understood. Respiratory syncytial virus bronchiolitis can be associated with short-term or long-term complications that include recurrent wheezing and abnormalities in pulmonary function.

Reinfection with RSV throughout life is common. Recurrent RSV infection in older children and adults usually manifests as mild upper respiratory tract illness. Serious disease involving the lower respiratory tract can develop in older children and adults, especially in immunocompromised people, people with cardiopulmonary disease, and elderly people, particularly those with comorbidities.

Etiology

Respiratory syncytial virus is an enveloped, nonsegmented, negative-strand RNA virus of the family Paramyxoviridae. The virus uses attachment (G) and fusion (F) surface glycoproteins for virus entry; these surface proteins lack neuraminidase and hemagglutinin activities. Only one serotype is known, but variations in the surface proteins (especially attachment protein G) result in the classification of viruses in 2 major subgroups, designated A and B.

Epidemiology

Humans are the only source of infection. Respiratory syncytial virus is usually transmitted by direct or close contact with contaminated secretions, which may occur from exposure to large-particle droplets at short distances (typically <3 to 6 feet) or from fomites. Viable RSV can persist on environmental surfaces for several hours and for 30 minutes or more on hands. Infection among health care personnel and others can occur by hand-to-eye or hand-to-nasal epithelium self-inoculation with contaminated secretions. Enforcement of infection control policies is critical to decrease the risk of health care–associated transmission of RSV, especially to hematopoietic stem cell or solid organ transplant recipients or patients with cardiopulmonary abnormalities or immunocompromised conditions that can be severe and fatal. Children with HIV infection experience extended viral shedding and, sometimes, prolonged illness but usually do not exhibit enhanced disease.

Respiratory syncytial virus occurs in annual epidemics during winter and early spring in temperate climates. Spread among household and child care contacts, including adults, is common. The period of viral shedding is usually 3 to 8 days but can last longer, especially in young infants and immunosuppressed people, in whom shedding may continue for as long as 3 to 4 weeks.

Incubation Period

4 to 6 days; range, 2 to 8 days.

Diagnostic Tests

Rapid diagnostic assays, including immunofluorescent and enzyme immunoassay techniques for detection of viral antigen in nasopharyngeal specimens, are available commercially for RSV and are generally reliable in infants and young children. In children, the sensitivity of these assays in comparison with culture varies between 53% and 96%, with most in the 80% to 90% range. The sensitivity may be lower in older children and is quite poor in adults because adults typically shed low concentrations of RSV. As with all antigen detection assays, the predictive value is high during the peak season, but false-positive test results are more likely to occur when the incidence of disease is low, such as in the summer in temperate areas. Therefore, antigen detection assays should not be the only basis on which the beginning and end of monthly immunoprophylaxis is determined. In most outpatient and inpatient settings, specific viral testing has little effect on management and routine testing is not recommended.

One disadvantage of targeted antigen detection relative to comprehensive virologic assessment (culture or reverse transcriptase-polymerase chain reaction [RT-PCR] assay) is that coinfections may not be detected. Up to 30% of children with RSV bronchiolitis may be coinfected with another respiratory tract pathogen, such as human metapneumovirus, rhinovirus, bocavirus, adenovirus, coronavirus, influenza virus, or parainfluenza virus. Whether children with bronchiolitis who are coinfected with more than one virus experience more severe disease is not clear.

Molecular diagnostic tests using RT-PCR assays are available commercially and increase RSV detection rates over viral isolation or antigen detection assays, especially in older children and adults. Many commercial tests are designed as multiplex assays to facilitate testing for multiple respiratory viruses with one test. Because of the increased sensitivity of RT-PCR testing, these tests may be preferred in many clinical settings. However, these tests should be interpreted with caution, especially when a multiplex assay identifies the presence of nucleic acid from more than one virus, because genetic material from some viruses (eg, rhinovirus, adenovirus, bocavirus) may persist in the airway for many weeks after cessation of shedding of infectious virus. As many as 25% of asymptomatic children test positive for respiratory viruses using RT-PCR assays in population-based studies.

Respiratory syncytial virus isolation from respiratory tract secretions in cell culture requires 1 to 5 days (shell vial techniques can produce results within 24–48 hours), but results and sensitivity vary among laboratories. Experienced viral laboratory personnel should be consulted for optimal methods of collection and transport of specimens, which include keeping the specimen cold but unfrozen during transport, rapid specimen processing, and stabilization in virus transport media. Conventional serologic testing of acute and convalescent serum specimens cannot be relied on to confirm infection in young infants, in whom sensitivity may be low.

Treatment

Primary treatment of young children hospitalized with bronchiolitis is supportive and should include hydration, careful assessment of respiratory status, measurement of oxygen saturation, suction of the upper airway, and, if necessary, intubation and mechanical ventilation. Clinicians may choose not to administer supplemental oxygen if the oxyhemoglobin saturation exceeds 90% in infants and children hospitalized with bronchiolitis. Continuous measurement of oxygen saturation may detect transient fluctuations in oxygenation that are not clinically significant, prolong oxygen use, and delay discharge.

Ribavirin has in vitro antiviral activity against RSV, and aerosolized ribavirin therapy has been associated with a small but statistically significant increase in oxygen saturation during the acute infection in several small studies.

However, a consistent decrease in need for mechanical ventilation, decrease in length of stay in the pediatric intensive care unit, or reduction in days of hospitalization among ribavirin recipients has not been demonstrated.

- **α- and β-adrenergic agents.** β-Adrenergic agents are not recommended for care of first-time wheezing associated with RSV bronchiolitis. Evidence does not support the use of nebulized epinephrine in hospitalized children with bronchiolitis or for outpatient management of children with bronchiolitis.
- **Corticosteroid therapy.** Controlled clinical trials among children with bronchiolitis have demonstrated that corticosteroids do not reduce hospital admissions or length of stay for inpatients. Corticosteroid treatment is not recommended for infants and children with RSV bronchiolitis.
- **Antimicrobial therapy.** Antimicrobial therapy is not indicated for infants with RSV bronchiolitis or pneumonia unless there is evidence of concurrent bacterial infection.
- **Other therapies.** Chest physiotherapy should not be used in infants and children with a diagnosis of bronchiolitis. Nebulized hypertonic saline (3%) appears to be safe and effective at improving the symptoms of mild to moderate bronchiolitis after 24 hours of use and in reducing hospital length of stay in settings where the duration of stay is likely to exceed 3 days. Hypertonic saline has not been shown to be effective over the short term for patients managed in the emergency department or when length of hospitalization is brief.

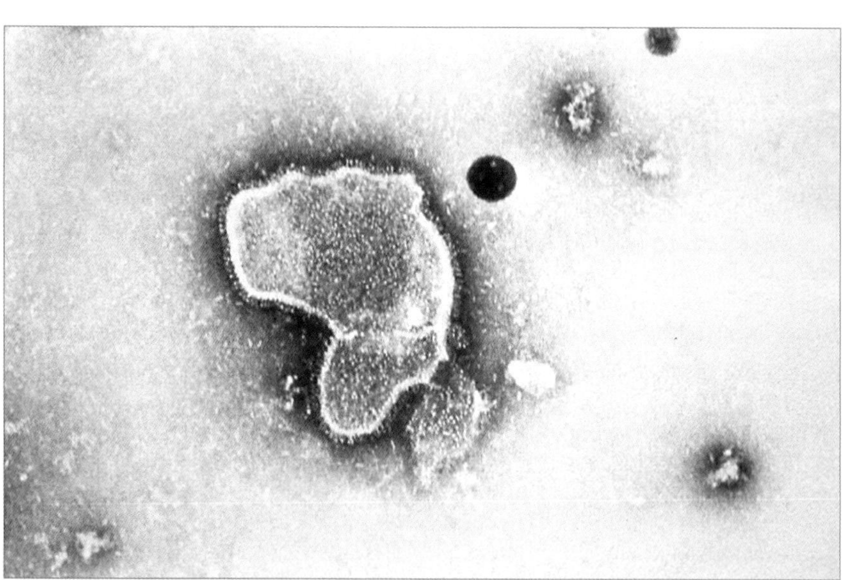

Image 114.1
Electron micrograph of a respiratory syncytial virus. The virion is variable in shape and size (average diameter between 120 and 300 nm). Respiratory syncytial virus is the most common cause of bronchiolitis and pneumonia among infants younger than 1 year. Courtesy of Centers for Disease Control and Prevention/E. L. Palmer.

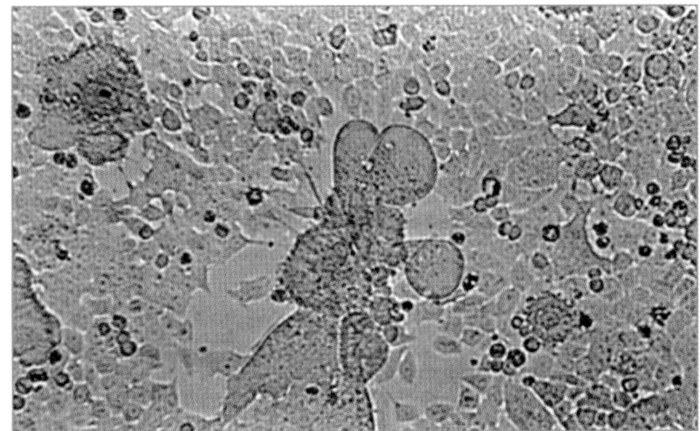

Image 114.2
The characteristic cytopathic effect of respiratory syncytial virus in tissue culture includes the formation of large multinucleated syncytial cells.

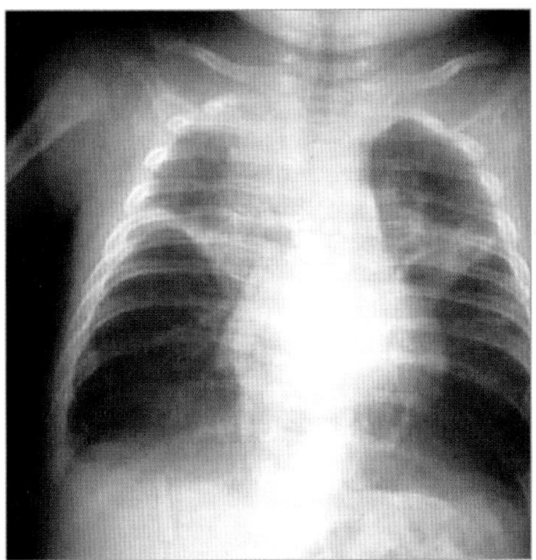

Image 114.3
Respiratory syncytial virus bronchiolitis and pneumonia. Note the bilateral infiltrates and striking hyperaeration. Copyright Martha Lepow.

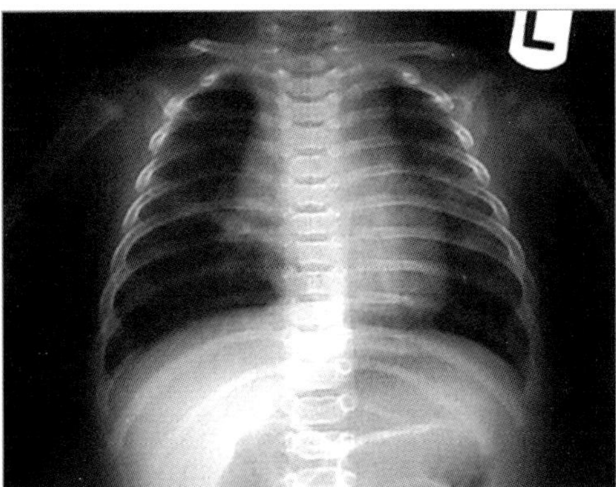

Image 114.4
An anteroposterior radiograph of a 2-month-old girl with respiratory syncytial virus bronchiolitis. Note the wide intercostal spaces, hyperaeration of the lung fields, and flattening of the diaphragm. Courtesy of Benjamin Estrada, MD.

115

Rickettsial Diseases

Clinical Manifestations

Rickettsial diseases comprise infections caused by bacterial species of the genera *Rickettsia* (endemic and epidemic typhus and spotted fever group rickettsioses), *Orientia* (scrub typhus), *Ehrlichia* (ehrlichiosis), *Anaplasma* (anaplasmosis), *Neoehrlichia,* and *Neorickettsia.*

Rickettsial infections have many features in common, including

- Fever, rash (especially in spotted fever and typhus group rickettsiae), headache, myalgia, and respiratory tract symptoms are prominent features.
- Local primary eschars occur with some rickettsial diseases, commonly with spotted fever rickettsioses, rickettsialpox, and scrub typhus.
- Systemic capillary and small vessel endothelial damage (ie, vasculitis) with increased microvascular permeability is the primary pathologic feature of most severe spotted fever and typhus group rickettsial infections.
- Rickettsial diseases can become life threatening rapidly. Risk factors for severe disease include glucose-6-phosphate dehydrogenase deficiency, male gender, and treatment with sulfonamides.

Immunity against reinfection by the same agent after natural infection is usually of long duration, except in the case of scrub typhus. Among the 4 groups of rickettsial diseases, some cross-immunity is usually conferred by infections within groups but not between groups. Reinfection of humans with *Ehrlichia* species and *Anaplasma* species has not been described.

Etiology

The rickettsiae causing human disease include *Rickettsia* species, *Orientia tsutsugamushi, Ehrlichia* species, *Anaplasma phagocytophilum, Neorickettsia sennetsu,* and *Neoehrlichia mikurensis.* Rickettsiae are small, coccobacillary gram-negative bacteria that are obligate intracellular pathogens and cannot be grown in cell-free media.

Epidemiology

Rickettsial diseases have arthropod vectors including ticks, flies, mites, and lice. The continued identification of new pathogenic rickettsial agents, such as *Rickettsia phillipi* (364D) in California in 2010 and *Rickettsia parkeri* in many states, will require ongoing research to confirm the burden of human illness. Humans are incidental hosts, except for the agent of classic epidemic typhus, for which humans are the principal reservoir and the human body louse is the vector; however, other vectors and reservoirs exist even for this disease. Rickettsial life cycles typically involve arthropod and mammalian reservoirs, and transmission occurs as a result of environmental or occupational exposure. Geographic and seasonal occurrences of rickettsial diseases are related to specific arthropod vector life cycles, activities, and distributions.

Incubation Periods

Vary according to organism.

Diagnostic Tests

Group-specific antibodies are detectable in the serum of many people 7 to 14 days after onset of illness, but slower antibody responses commonly occur in some diseases. The utility of serologic diagnoses in acute illness is limited in these infections because of their short incubations; a negative serologic test result never excludes infection in the acute phase of clinical illness. Various serologic tests for detecting antirickettsial antibodies are available. The indirect immunofluorescent antibody assay is recommended in most circumstances because of its relative sensitivity and specificity. Treatment early in the course of illness can blunt or delay serologic responses. In laboratories with experienced personnel, immunohistochemical staining and polymerase chain reaction testing of skin biopsy specimens from patients with rash or eschar can help to diagnose rickettsial infections early in the course of disease. Weil-Felix tests are not recommended. The use of tick panels is discouraged.

Treatment

Prompt and specific therapy is important for optimal outcome. The drug of choice for rickettsioses is doxycycline. The duration of treatment is 7 to 14 days. Antimicrobial treatment is most effective when individuals are treated appropriately during the first week of illness. If the disease remains untreated during the second week, therapy is less effective in preventing complications.

116

Rickettsialpox

Clinical Manifestations

Rickettsialpox is a febrile, eschar-associated illness that is characterized by generalized, relatively sparse, erythematous, papulovesicular eruptions on the trunk, face, and extremities (less often on palms and soles) or on mucous membranes of the mouth. The rash develops 1 to 4 days after onset of fever and 3 to 10 days after appearance of an eschar at the site of the bite of a house mouse mite. Regional lymph nodes in the area of the primary eschar typically become enlarged. Without specific antimicrobial therapy, systemic disease lasts approximately 7 to 10 days; manifestations include fever, headache, malaise, and myalgia. Less frequent manifestations include anorexia, vomiting, conjunctivitis, nuchal rigidity, and photophobia. The disease is mild compared with Rocky Mountain spotted fever, and no rickettsialpox-associated deaths have been described; however, disease is occasionally severe enough to warrant hospitalization.

Etiology

Rickettsialpox is caused by *Rickettsia akari,* a gram-negative intracellular bacillus, which is classified with the spotted fever group rickettsiae and related antigenically to other members of that group.

Epidemiology

The natural host for *R akari* in the United States is *Mus musculus,* the common house mouse. The disease is transmitted by the house mouse mite, *Liponyssoides sanguineus.* Disease risk is heightened in areas infested with mice and rats. The disease can occur wherever the hosts, pathogens, and humans coexist but is most frequently reported in large urban settings. In the United States, rickettsialpox has been described predominantly in northeastern metropolitan centers, especially New York. It has also been confirmed in many other countries, including Croatia, Ukraine, Turkey, Russia, South Korea, and Mexico. All age groups can be affected. No seasonal pattern of disease occurs. The disease is not communicable but occurs occasionally among families or people cohabiting a house mouse mite–infested dwelling.

Incubation Period

6 to 15 days.

Diagnostic Tests

R akari can be isolated in cell culture from blood and eschar biopsy specimens during the acute stage of disease, but culture is not attempted routinely. Because antibodies to *R akari* have extensive cross-reactivity with antibodies against *Rickettsia rickettsii* (the cause of Rocky Mountain spotted fever) and other spotted fever group rickettsiae, an indirect immunofluorescent antibody assay for *R rickettsii* can be used to demonstrate a 4-fold or greater change in antibody titers between acute and convalescent serum specimens taken 2 to 6 weeks apart. Use of *R akari* antigen is recommended for a more accurate serologic diagnosis but may only be available in specialized research laboratories. Direct fluorescent antibody or immunohistochemical testing of formalin-fixed, paraffin-embedded eschars or papulovesicle biopsy specimens can detect rickettsiae in the samples and are useful diagnostic techniques, but because of cross-reactivity, these assays are not able to confirm the etiologic agent. Use of polymerase chain reaction for detection of rickettsial DNA with subsequent sequence identification can confirm *R akari* infection.

Treatment

Doxycycline is the drug of choice in all age groups and is effective when given for 3 to 5 days. Doxycycline will shorten the course of disease; symptoms typically resolve within 12 to 48 hours after initiation of therapy. Relapse is rare. There are limited data describing the utility of other antimicrobials, including azithromycin and fluoroquinolones. Chloramphenicol is an alternative drug but is not available as an oral formulation in the United States. Untreated rickettsialpox usually will resolve within 2 to 3 weeks.

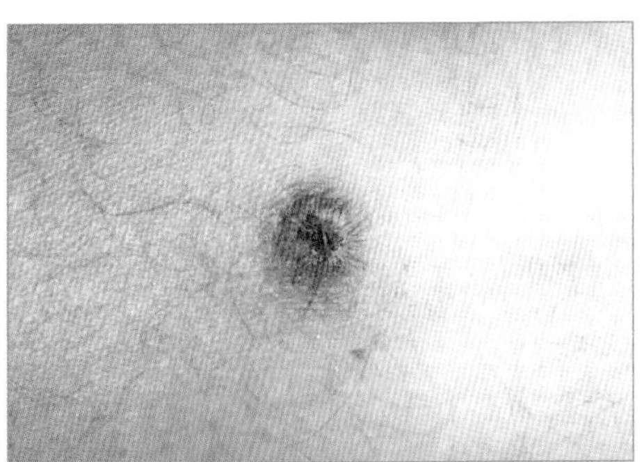

Image 116.1
Eschar on the posterior right calf of patient with rickettsialpox. This type of lesion is not seen with Rocky Mountain spotted fever. Courtesy of *Emerging Infectious Diseases.*

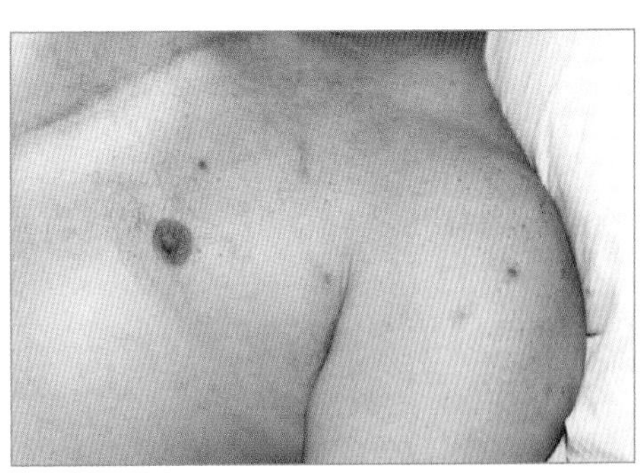

Image 116.2
Multiple papulovesicular lesions involving the upper trunk on a patient with rickettsialpox. Courtesy of *Emerging Infectious Diseases.*

117

Rocky Mountain Spotted Fever

Clinical Manifestations

Rocky Mountain spotted fever (RMSF) is a systemic, small-vessel vasculitis that often involves a characteristic rash. Fever, myalgia, severe headache, photophobia, nausea, vomiting, and anorexia are typical presenting symptoms. Abdominal pain and diarrhea are often present and can obscure the diagnosis. The rash usually begins within the first 6 days of symptoms as erythematous macules or maculopapules. The rash usually appears first on the wrists and ankles, often spreading within hours proximally to the trunk and distally to the palms and soles. Although early development of a rash is a useful diagnostic sign, the rash can be atypical or absent in up to 20% of cases. It may be difficult to visualize in patients with dark skin. A petechial rash is typically a late finding and indicates progression to severe disease. Lack of a typical rash is a risk factor for misdiagnosis and poor outcome. Hepatomegaly and splenomegaly occur in 33% of patients. Meningeal signs with a positive Kernig and Brudzinski sign can occur.

Thrombocytopenia, hyponatremia (observed in 20% of cases), and elevated liver transaminase concentrations develop in many cases, are frequently mild in the early stages of disease, and worsen as disease progresses. White blood cell count is typically normal, but leukopenia and anemia can occur. If not treated, the illness can last as long as 3 weeks and can be severe, with prominent central nervous system, cardiac, pulmonary, gastrointestinal tract, and renal involvement; disseminated intravascular coagulation; and shock leading to death. Rocky Mountain spotted fever can progress rapidly, even in previously healthy people. Delay in appropriate antimicrobial treatment beyond the fifth day of symptoms is associated with severe disease and poor outcomes. Case-fatality rates of untreated RMSF range from 20% to 80%, with a median time to death of 8 days. Significant long-term sequelae are common in patients with severe RMSF, including neurologic (paraparesis; hearing loss; peripheral neuropathy; bladder and bowel incontinence; cerebellar, vestibular, and motor dysfunction) and nonneurologic (disability from limb or digit amputation) sequelae. Patients treated early in the course of symptoms may have a mild illness, with fever resolving in the first 48 hours of treatment.

Etiology

Rickettsia rickettsii, an obligate, intracellular, gram-negative bacillus and a member of the spotted fever group of rickettsiae, is the causative agent. The primary targets of infection in mammalian hosts are endothelial cells lining the small blood vessels of all major tissues and organs.

Epidemiology

The pathogen is transmitted to humans by the bite of a tick of the Ixodidae family (hard ticks). Ticks and their small mammal hosts serve as reservoirs of the pathogen in nature. Other wild animals and dogs have been found with antibodies to *R rickettsii,* but their role as natural reservoirs is not clear. People with occupational or recreational exposure to the tick vector (eg, pet owners, animal handlers, people who spend more time outdoors) are at increased risk of acquiring the organism. People of all ages can be infected. The period of highest incidence in the United States is from April to September, although RMSF can occur year-round in certain areas with endemic disease. Laboratory-acquired infection has occasionally resulted from accidental inoculation and aerosol contamination. Transmission has occurred, on rare occasions, by blood transfusion. Mortality is highest in males, people older than 50 years, children 5 to 9 years of age, and people with no recognized tick bite or attachment. In approximately half of pediatric RMSF cases, there is no recall of a recent tick bite. Factors contributing to delayed diagnosis include absence of rash or difficulty in its recognition, especially in individuals with darker complexions; initial presentation before the fourth day of illness; and onset of illness during months of low incidence.

Rocky Mountain spotted fever is widespread in the United States, with a reported annual incidence that has increased 8-fold from

1.8 cases per 1 million people in 2000 to 14.3 cases per 1 million in 2012, or about 4,500 cases per year. Despite its name, RMSF is not common in the Rocky Mountain area. Most cases are reported in the south Atlantic, southeastern, and south central states, although most states in the contiguous United States record cases each year. The principal recognized vectors of *R rickettsii* are *Dermacentor variabilis* (the American dog tick) in the eastern and central United States and *Dermacentor andersoni* (the Rocky Mountain wood tick) in the western United States. Another common tick throughout the world that feeds on dogs, *Rhipicephalus sanguineus* (the brown dog tick), has been confirmed as a vector of *R rickettsii* in Arizona and Mexico and may play a role in other regions. Transmission parallels the tick season in a given geographic area. Rocky Mountain spotted fever also occurs in Canada, Mexico, Central America, and South America.

Incubation Period

Approximately 1 week; range, 2 to 14 days.

Diagnostic Tests

Rocky Mountain spotted fever may be diagnosed by the detection of *R rickettsii* DNA in acute whole blood and serum specimens by polymerase chain reaction assay. The specimen should preferably be obtained within the first week of symptoms and before (or within 24 hours of) initiation of antimicrobial therapy, and a negative result does not exclude RMSF infection. Diagnosis can also be confirmed by the detection of rickettsial DNA in biopsy or autopsy specimens by polymerase chain reaction assay or immunohistochemical visualization of rickettsiae in tissues. The gold standard for serologic diagnosis of RMSF is the indirect fluorescent antibody test. A negative serologic test result does not exclude a diagnosis of RMSF. Immunoglobulin (Ig) G and IgM antibodies begin to increase around day 7 to 10 after onset of symptoms; an elevated acute titer may represent past exposure rather than acute infection. Mildly elevated antibody titers can be an incidental finding in a significant proportion of the general population in some regions. IgM antibodies can remain elevated for months and are not highly specific for acute RMSF. A 4-fold or greater rise in antigen-specific IgG between acute and convalescent sera obtained 2 to 6 weeks apart confirms the diagnosis. Cross-reactivity may be observed between antibodies to other spotted fever group rickettsiae.

Treatment

Doxycycline is the treatment of choice for RMSF in patients of any age, and this drug should be initiated as soon as RMSF is suspected. Use of antibiotics other than doxycycline increases the risk of mortality. Treatment is most effective if started in the first few days of symptoms; treatment started after the fifth day of symptoms is less likely to prevent death or other adverse outcomes. Chloramphenicol is an alternative treatment but should be considered only in rare cases, such as severe doxycycline allergies or during pregnancy. Antimicrobial treatment should be continued until the patient has been afebrile for at least 3 days and has demonstrated clinical improvement; the usual duration of therapy is 7 to 10 days.

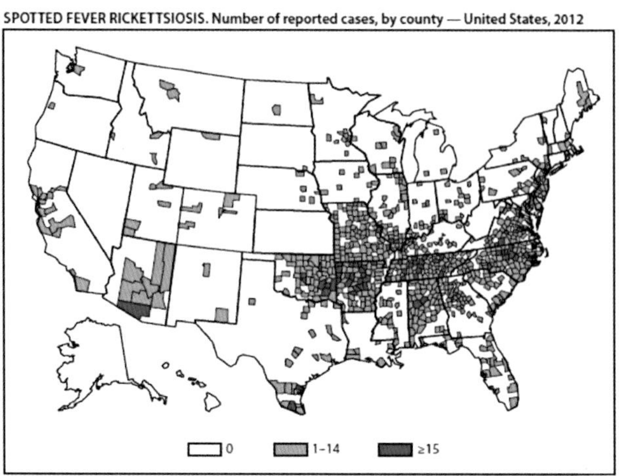

In the United States, the majority of cases of spotted fever rickettsiosis are attributed to infection with *Rickettsia rickettsii*, the causative agent of Rocky Mountain spotted fever (RMSF), but might also be from other agents such as *Rickettsia parkeri* and *Rickettsia* species 364D. RMSF is ubiquitous across the United States, which represents the widespread nature of the three tick vectors known to transmit RMSF: *Dermacentor variabilis* in the East, *Dermacentor andersoni* in the West, and *Rhipicephalus sanguineus*, recently recognized as a new tick vector in parts of Arizona. Historically, much of the incidence of RMSF has been in the Central Atlantic region and parts of the Midwest; however, endemic transmission of RMSF in Arizona communities has led to a substantial reported incidence rate.

Image 117.1
Spotted fever rickettsiosis. Number of reported cases, by county—United States, 2012. Courtesy of *Morbidity and Mortality Weekly Report.*

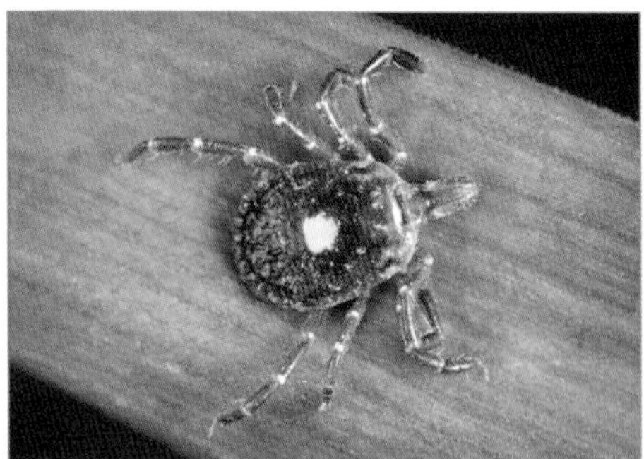

Image 117.2
This is a female lone star tick, *Amblyomma americanum*, which is found in the southeastern and mid-Atlantic United States. This tick is a vector of several zoonotic diseases, including human monocytic ehrlichiosis and Rocky Mountain spotted fever. Courtesy of Centers for Disease Control and Prevention.

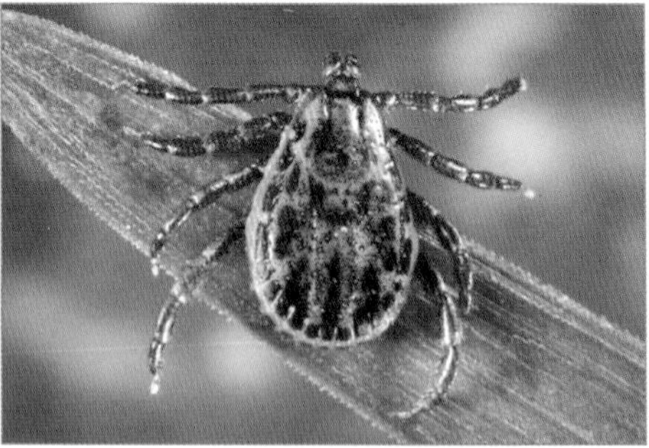

Image 117.3
This photograph depicts a dorsal view of a male Rocky Mountain wood tick, *Dermacentor andersoni*. This tick species is a known North American vector of *Rickettsia rickettsii*, which is the etiologic agent of Rocky Mountain spotted fever. Courtesy of Centers for Disease Control and Prevention/Christopher Paddock, MD.

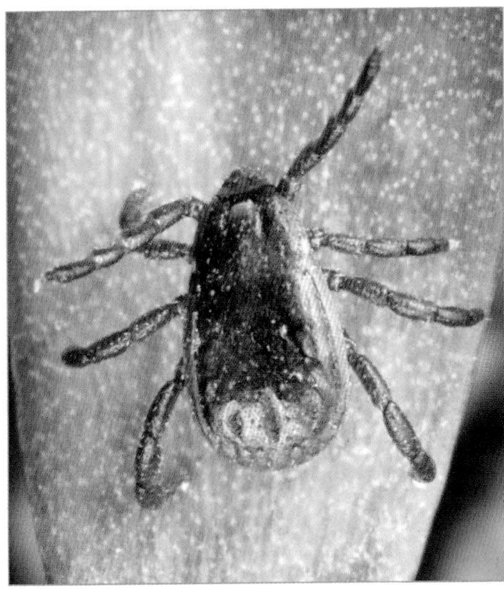

Image 117.4
This image depicts a male brown dog tick, *Rhipicephalus sanguineus*, from a superior, or dorsal, view looking down on this hard tick's scutum, which entirely covers its back, identifying it as a male. In the female, the dorsal abdomen is only partially covered, thereby offering room for abdominal expansion when she becomes engorged with blood while ingesting her blood meal obtained from her host. Courtesy of Centers for Disease Control and Prevention/James Gathany; William Nicholson.

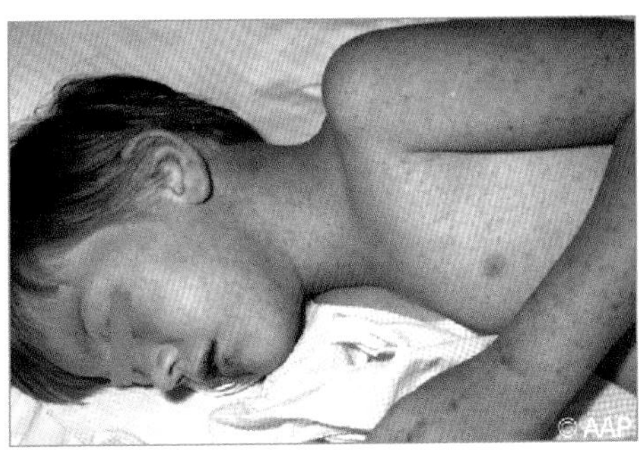

Image 117.5
Rocky Mountain spotted fever in an 8-year-old boy. Sixth day of rash without treatment.

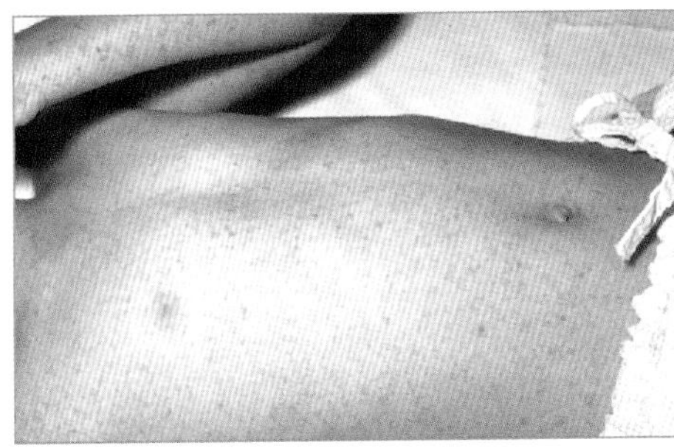

Image 117.6
Rocky Mountain spotted fever. Sixth day of rash without treatment. This is the same patient as in Image 117.5.

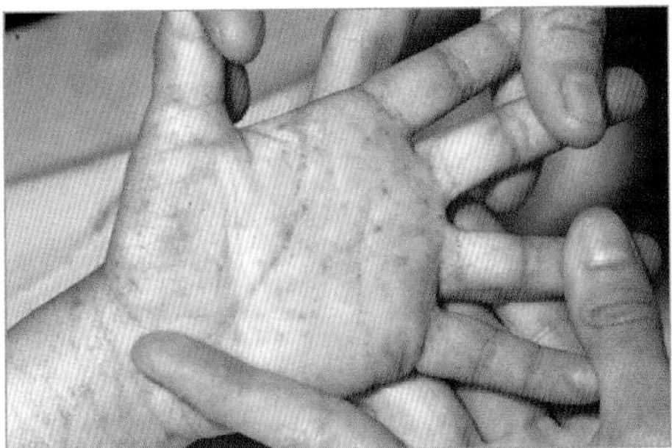

Image 117.7
Rocky Mountain spotted fever. Sixth day of rash without treatment. This is the same patient as in images 117.5 and 117.6.

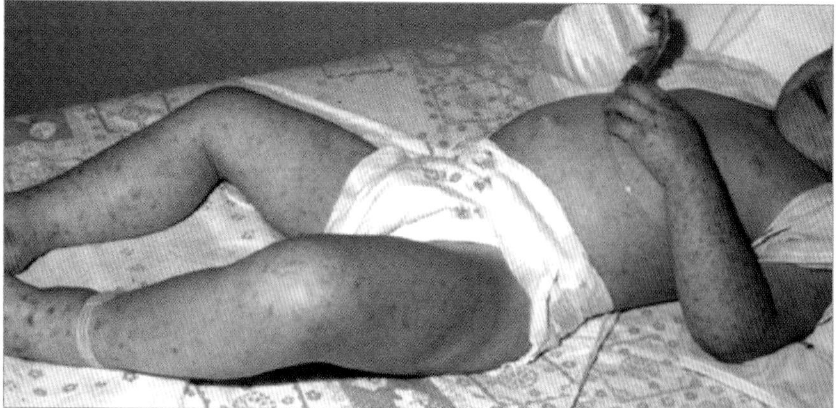

Image 117.8
A 2-year-old boy with obtundation, disorientation, and petechial rash of Rocky Mountain spotted fever, with facial and generalized edema secondary to generalized vasculitis. Rocky Mountain spotted fever is the most severe and frequently reported rickettsial illness in the United States.

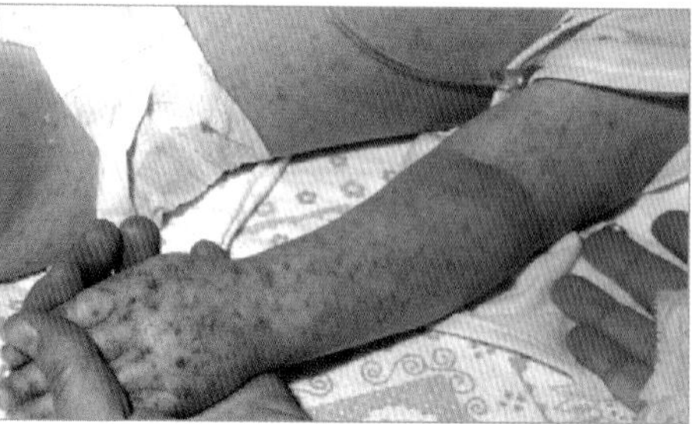

Image 117.9
This is the same patient as in Image 117.8 showing petechial rash and edema of the upper extremity. The rickettsiae multiply in the endothelial cells of small blood vessels, resulting in vasculitis.

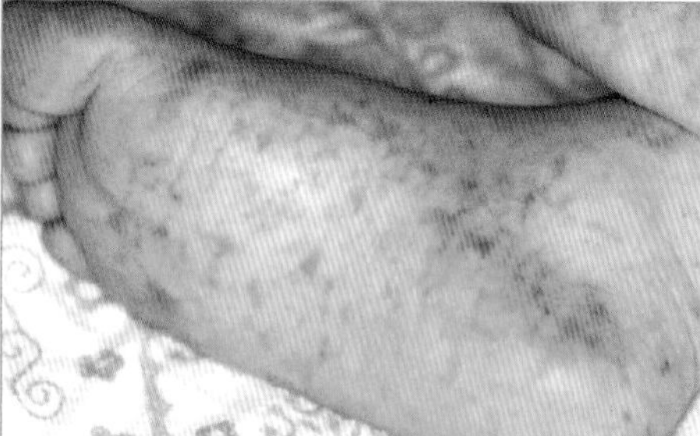

Image 117.10
This is the same patient as in images 117.8 and 117.9 showing petechiae and edema of foot.

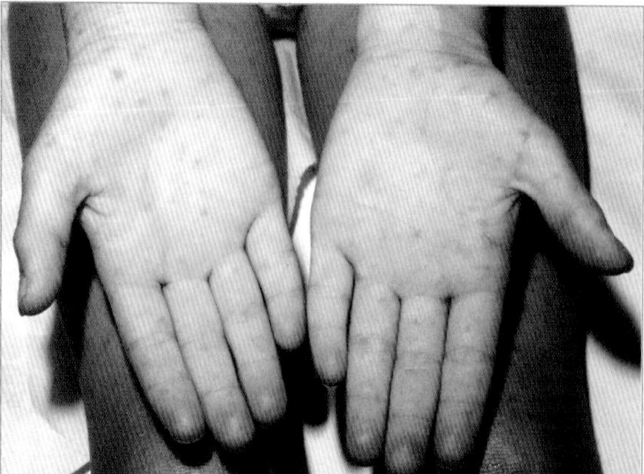

Image 117.11
This 8-year-old girl presented with a history of "chickenpox" for 11 days. She had numerous lesions on her chest, face, arms, and proximal legs. There were subcutaneous erythematous lesions on the hands, and she had 5 or 6 lesions on her feet. The diagnosis of Rocky Mountain spotted fever was confirmed serologically, and she was treated without any complications. Courtesy of Neal Halsey, MD.

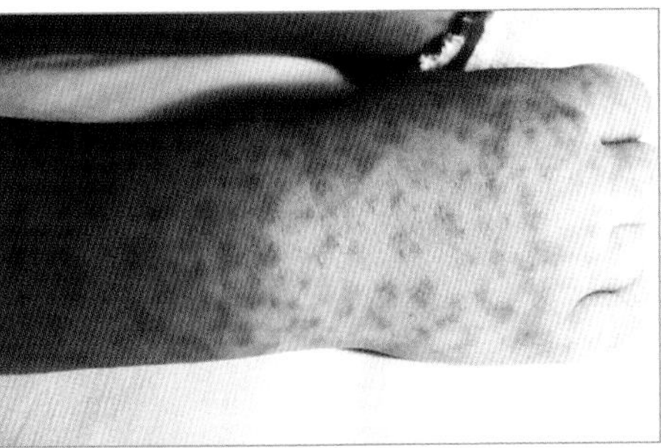

Image 117.12
A child's right hand and wrist displaying the spotted rash and edema of Rocky Mountain spotted fever. Courtesy of Centers for Disease Control and Prevention.

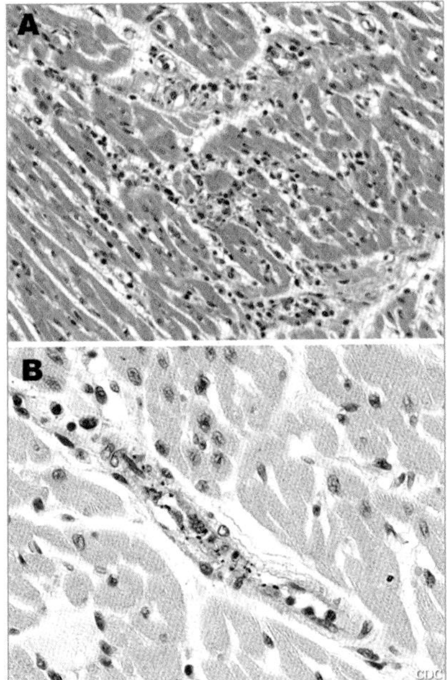

Image 117.14
A 4-year-old girl with Rocky Mountain spotted fever acquired in Panama that was misdiagnosed as meningococcemia. Autopsy findings included myocarditis, interstitial nephritis, pneumonitis, and encephalitis. Histologic and immunohistochemical evaluation of heart tissue. A, Lymphohistiocytic inflammatory cell infiltrates in the myocardium (hematoxylin-eosin stain, original magnification x25). B, Immunohistochemical detection of spotted fever group rickettsiae (red) in perivascular infiltrates of heart (immunoalkaline phosphatase with naphthol-fast red substrate and hematoxylin counterstain, original magnification x250). Courtesy of Centers for Disease Control and Prevention/*Emerging Infectious Diseases* and Dora Estripeaut.

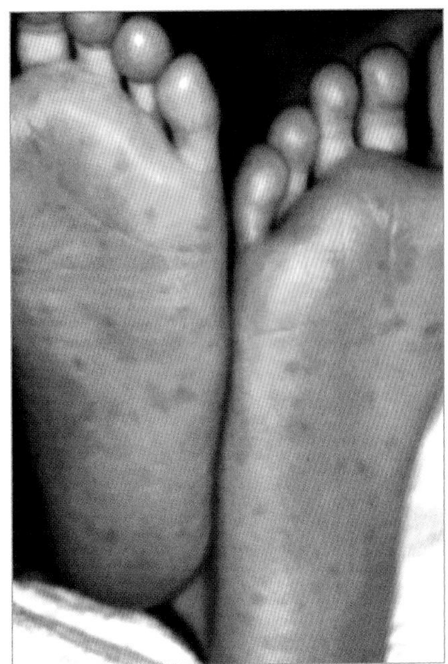

Image 117.13
The soles of the feet as well as the palms of the hands are typically involved in patients with Rocky Mountain spotted fever.

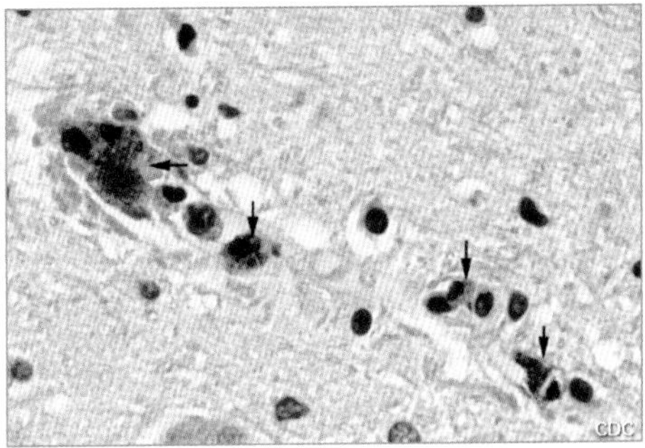

Image 117.15
Immunohistochemical analysis shows the presence of spotted fever group rickettsiae (brown) in vessels of the brain of a patient with fatal Rocky Mountain spotted fever (magnification x400). Courtesy of Centers for Disease Control and Prevention/*Emerging Infectious Diseases* and Marylin Hidalgo.

118

Rotavirus Infections

Clinical Manifestations

Infection begins with acute onset of fever and vomiting followed 24 to 48 hours later by watery diarrhea. Symptoms generally persist for 3 to 8 days. In moderate to severe cases, dehydration, electrolyte abnormalities, and acidosis can occur. In certain immunocompromised children, including children with congenital cellular immunodeficiencies or severe combined immunodeficiency and children who are hematopoietic stem cell or solid organ transplant recipients, persistent infection and diarrhea can develop.

Etiology

Rotaviruses are segmented, double-stranded RNA viruses belonging to the family Reoviridae, with at least 7 distinct antigenic groups (A–G). Group A viruses are the major causes of rotavirus diarrhea worldwide. Serotyping is based on the 2 surface proteins, VP7 glycoprotein (G) and VP4 protease-cleaved hemagglutinin (P). Prior to introduction of the rotavirus vaccine, G types 1 through 4 and 9 and P types 1A[8] and 1B[4] were most common in the United States.

Epidemiology

The epidemiology of rotavirus disease in the United States has changed following the introduction of rotavirus vaccines. Prior to widespread vaccine use, rotavirus was the most common cause of acute gastroenteritis in young children, an important cause of acute gastroenteritis in children attending child care, and the most common cause of health care–associated diarrhea in young children. Rotavirus is present in high titer in stools of infected patients several days before and several days after onset of clinical disease. Transmission is by the fecal-oral route. Rotavirus can be found on toys and hard surfaces in child care centers, indicating fomites may serve as a mechanism of transmission. Respiratory transmission likely plays a minor role in disease transmission. Spread within families and institutions is common. Rarely, common-source outbreaks from contaminated water or food have been reported.

In temperate climates, rotavirus disease is most prevalent during the cooler months. Before licensure of rotavirus vaccines in North America in 2006 and 2008, the annual rotavirus epidemic usually started during the autumn in Mexico and the southwest United States and moved eastward, reaching the northeast United States and Maritime provinces by spring. The seasonal pattern of disease is less pronounced in tropical climates, with rotavirus infection being more common during the cooler, drier months.

The epidemiology of rotavirus disease in the United States has changed dramatically since rotavirus vaccines became available. A biennial pattern has emerged, with small, short seasons beginning in late winter or early spring (eg, 2009, 2011, 2013) alternating with years with extremely low circulation (eg, 2008, 2010, 2012). The overall burden of rotavirus disease has declined dramatically. Beginning in 2008, annual hospitalizations for rotavirus disease among US children younger than 5 years declined by approximately 75%, with an estimated 40,000 to 50,000 fewer rotavirus hospitalizations nationally each year. In the United States, a full series of vaccine has been found to be approximately 85% to 90% effective against rotavirus disease resulting in hospitalization. The vaccines are also highly effective against rotavirus disease resulting in emergency department care and in office visits attributable to rotavirus.

Incubation Period

1 to 3 days.

Diagnostic Tests

It is not possible to diagnose rotavirus infection by clinical presentation or nonspecific laboratory tests. Enzyme immunoassays, immunochromatography, and latex agglutination assays for group A rotavirus antigen detection in stool are available commercially. Enzyme immunoassays are used most widely because of their high sensitivity and specificity.

Rotavirus can also be identified in stool by electron microscopy, by electrophoresis and silver staining, by standard or real-time reverse transcriptase-polymerase chain reaction assay for detection of viral genomic RNA, and by viral culture.

Treatment

No specific antiviral therapy is available. Oral or parenteral fluids and electrolytes are given to prevent or correct dehydration.

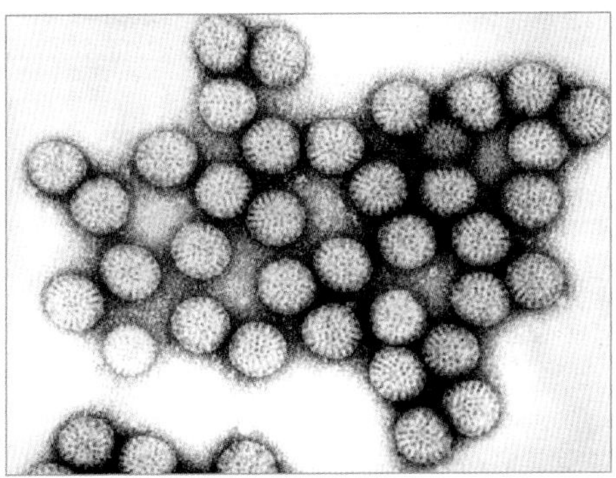

Image 118.1
Transmission electron micrograph of intact rotavirus particles, double-shelled. Distinctive rim of radiating capsomeres. Courtesy of Centers for Disease Control and Prevention/Dr Erskine Palmer.

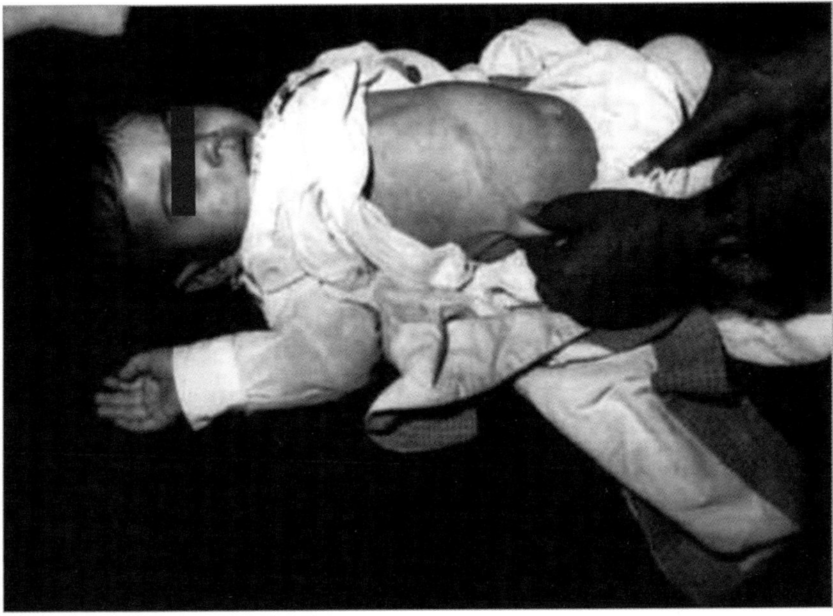

Image 118.2
Doctor examining a child dehydrated from rotavirus infection. In developing countries, rotavirus causes approximately 600,000 deaths each year in children younger than 5 years. Courtesy of World Health Organization.

119

Rubella

Clinical Manifestations

- **Postnatal rubella.** Many cases of postnatal rubella are subclinical. Clinical disease is usually mild and characterized by a generalized erythematous maculopapular rash, lymphadenopathy, and slight fever. The rash starts on the face, becomes generalized in 24 hours, and lasts a median of 3 days. Lymphadenopathy, which can precede rash, often involves posterior auricular or suboccipital lymph nodes, can be generalized, and lasts between 5 and 8 days. Conjunctivitis and palatal enanthema have been noted. Transient polyarthralgia and polyarthritis rarely occur in children but are common in adolescents and adults, especially females. Encephalitis (1 in 6,000 cases) and thrombocytopenia (1 in 3,000 cases) are complications.
- **Congenital rubella syndrome.** Maternal rubella during pregnancy can result in miscarriage, fetal death, or a constellation of congenital anomalies (congenital rubella syndrome [CRS]). The most commonly described anomalies or manifestations associated with CRS are ophthalmologic (cataracts, pigmentary retinopathy, microphthalmos, congenital glaucoma), cardiac (patent ductus arteriosus, peripheral pulmonary artery stenosis), auditory (sensorineural hearing impairment), or neurologic (behavioral disorders, meningoencephalitis, microcephaly, cognitive impairments). Neonatal manifestations of CRS include intrauterine growth restriction, interstitial pneumonitis, radiolucent bone disease, hepatosplenomegaly, thrombocytopenia, and dermal erythropoiesis (so-called blueberry muffin lesions). Mild forms of the disease can be associated with few or no obvious clinical manifestations at birth. Congenital defects occur in up to 85% of cases if maternal infection occurs during the first 12 weeks of gestation, 50% if infection occurs during 13 to 16 weeks of gestation, and 25% if infection occurs during the end of the second trimester. Natural rubella infection in pregnancy can cause autism spectrum disorder in the neonate.

Etiology

Rubella virus is an enveloped, positive-stranded RNA virus classified as a *Rubivirus* in the Togaviridae family.

Epidemiology

Humans are the only source of infection. Postnatal rubella is transmitted primarily through direct or droplet contact from nasopharyngeal secretions. The peak incidence of infection is during late winter and early spring. Approximately 25% to 50% of infections are asymptomatic. Immunity from wild-type or vaccine virus is usually prolonged, but reinfection on rare occasions has been demonstrated and, rarely, has resulted in CRS. Although volunteer studies have demonstrated rubella virus in nasopharyngeal secretions from 7 days before to a maximum of 14 days after onset of rash, the period of maximal communicability extends from a few days before to 7 days after onset of rash. A small number of infants with congenital rubella continue to shed virus in nasopharyngeal secretions and urine for 1 year or more and can transmit infection to susceptible contacts. Rubella virus has been recovered in high titer from lens aspirates in children with congenital cataracts for several years.

Before widespread use of rubella vaccine, rubella was an epidemic disease, occurring in 6- to 9-year cycles, with most cases occurring in children. In the postvaccine era, most cases in the mid-1970s and 1980s occurred in young unimmunized adults in outbreaks on college campuses and in occupational settings. More recent outbreaks have occurred in people born outside the United States or among underimmunized populations. The incidence of rubella in the United States has decreased by more than 99% from the prevaccine era.

The United States was determined to no longer have endemic rubella in 2004, and from 2004 through 2012, 79 cases of rubella and 6 cases of CRS, including 3 cases in 2012, were reported in the United States; all of the cases were import associated or from unknown sources. A national serologic survey from 1999 to 2004 indicated that among children and adolescents 6 through 19 years of age, seroprevalence was approximately 95%. Studies of rubella and CRS in the United States have identified that seronegativity is higher among people born outside the United States or from areas with poor vaccine coverage; the risk of CRS is highest among these populations.

In 2003, the Pan American Health Organization (PAHO) adopted a resolution calling for elimination of rubella and CRS in the Americas by 2010. All countries with endemic rubella in the Americas implemented the recommended PAHO strategy by the end of 2008. The strategy consists of achieving high levels of measles-rubella vaccination coverage in the routine immunization program. The last confirmed endemic case in the Americas was diagnosed in Argentina in February 2009. In September 2010, PAHO announced that the region of the Americas had achieved the rubella and CRS elimination goals on the basis of surveillance data, but documentation of elimination is ongoing.

Incubation Period

Usually 16 to 18 days; range, 14 to 21 days.

Diagnostic Tests

Detection of rubella-specific immunoglobulin (Ig) M antibody usually indicates recent postnatal infection or congenital infection in a newborn, but false-negative and false-positive results occur. Most postnatal cases are IgM-positive by 5 days after symptom onset, and most congenital cases are IgM-positive at birth and up to 3 months later. For diagnosis of postnatally acquired rubella, a 4-fold or greater increase in antibody titer between acute and convalescent periods indicates infection. Congenital infection can also be confirmed by stable or increasing serum concentrations of rubella-specific IgG over the first 7 to 11 months of life. The hemagglutination-inhibition rubella antibody test, which was previously the most commonly used method of serologic screening for rubella infection, has generally been supplanted by a number of equally or more sensitive assays for determining rubella immunity, including enzyme immunoassays and latex agglutination tests. Diagnosis of congenital rubella infection in children older than 1 year is difficult; serologic testing is usually not diagnostic, and viral isolation, although confirmatory, is possible in only a small proportion of congenitally infected children of this age.

A false-positive IgM test result may be caused by a number of factors, including rheumatoid factor, parvovirus IgM, and heterophile antibodies. The presence of high-avidity IgG or lack of increase in IgG titers can be useful in identifying false-positive rubella IgM results. Low-avidity IgG is associated with recent primary rubella infection, whereas high-avidity IgG is associated with past infection or reinfection. The avidity assay is only performed at reference laboratories.

Rubella virus can be isolated most consistently from throat or nasal specimens (and less consistently, urine) by inoculation of appropriate cell culture. Detection of rubella virus RNA by real time reverse-transcriptase polymerase chain reaction from a throat or nasal swab or urine sample with subsequent genotyping of strains may be valuable for diagnosis and molecular epidemiology. Most postnatal cases are positive virologically on the day of symptom onset, and most congenital cases are positive virologically at birth

Treatment

Supportive.

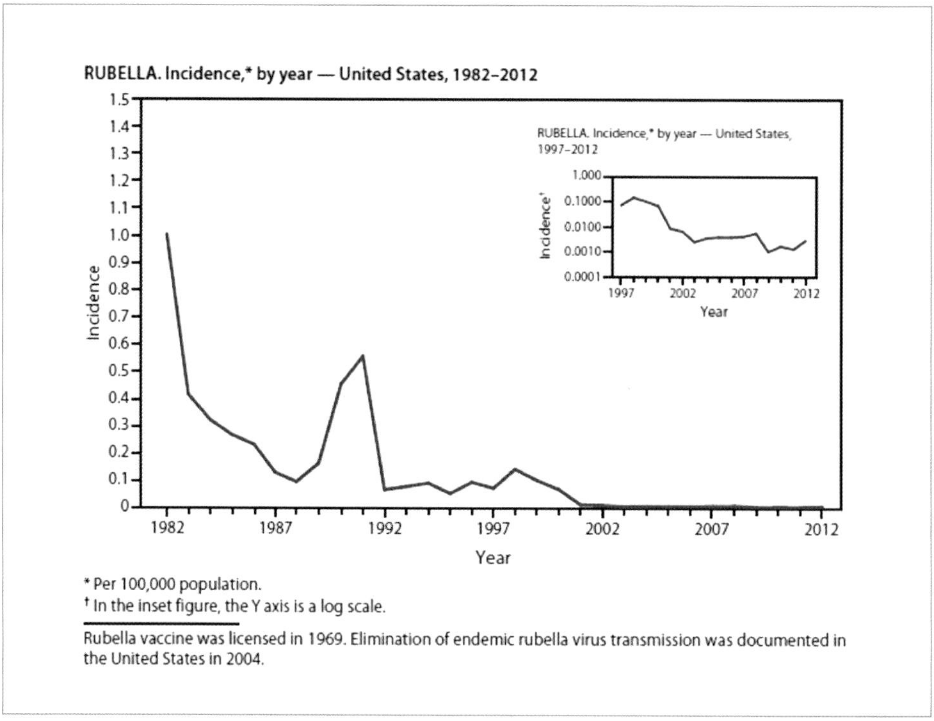

RUBELLA. Incidence,* by year — United States, 1982–2012
Incidence
Year
RUBELLA. Incidence,* by year — United States, 1997–2012
Incidence†
Year
* Per 100,000 population.
† In the inset figure, the Y axis is a log scale.
Rubella vaccine was licensed in 1969. Elimination of endemic rubella virus transmission was documented in the United States in 2004.

Image 119.1
Rubella. Incidence, by year—United States, 1982–2012. Courtesy of *Morbidity and Mortality Weekly Report.*

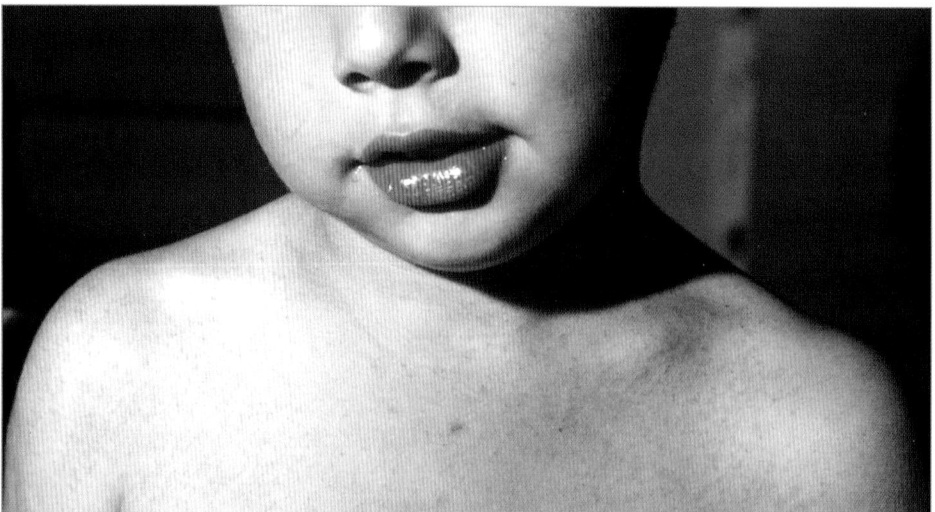

Image 119.2
This 5-year-old Hawaiian boy developed the fine macular rash noted on his face and chest. He had serologically confirmed rubella. Courtesy of Neal Halsey, MD.

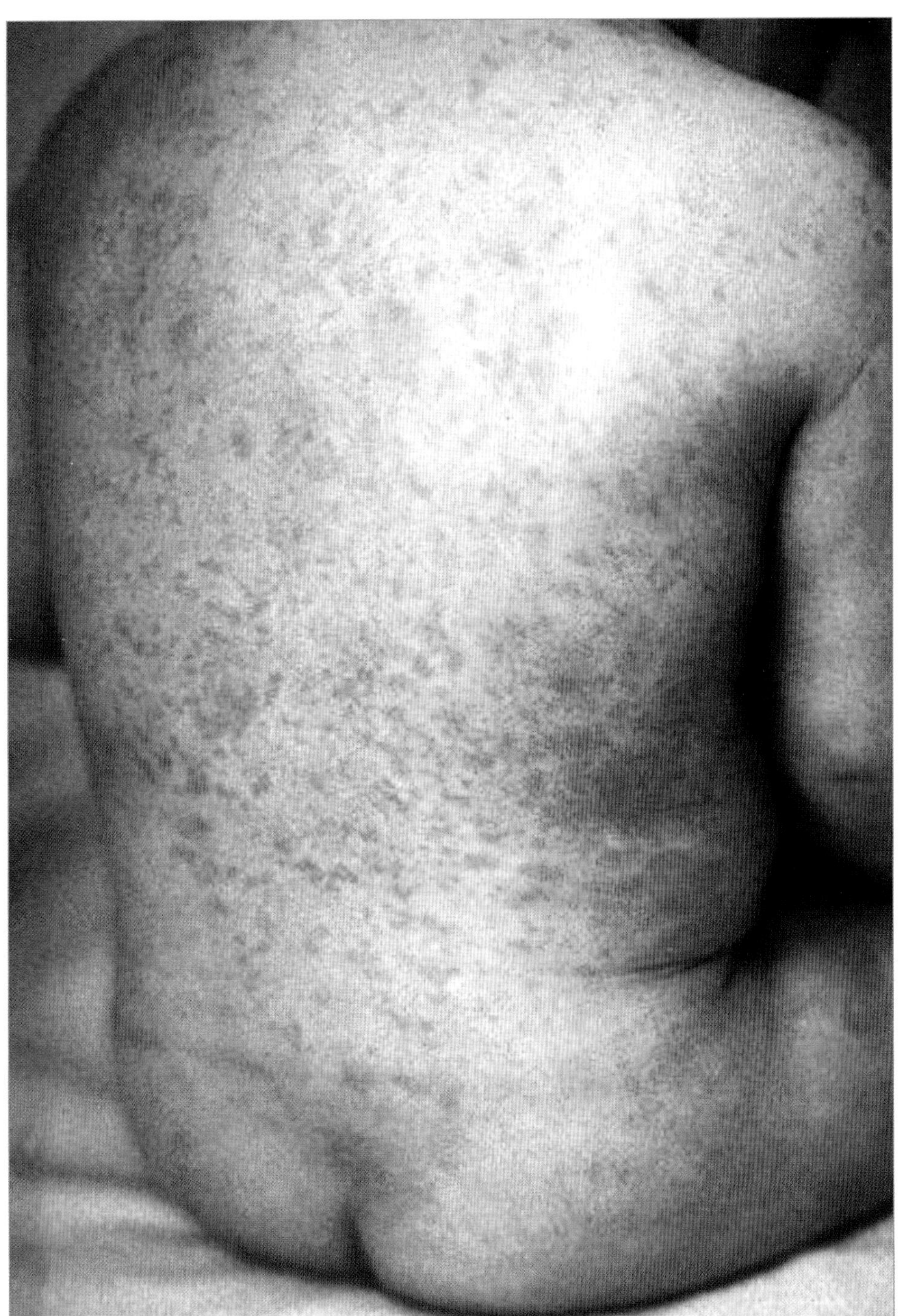

Image 119.3
Rubella rash on a child's back (1978). The distribution is similar to that of measles, although the lesions are less intensely red. Courtesy of Centers for Disease Control and Prevention.

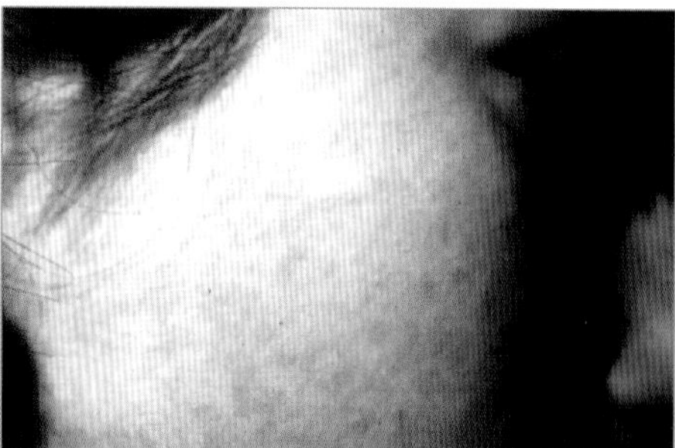

Image 119.4
Rubella rash (face) in a previously unimmunized female. Adenovirus and enterovirus infections can cause exanthema that mimics rubella. Serologic testing is important if the patient is pregnant.

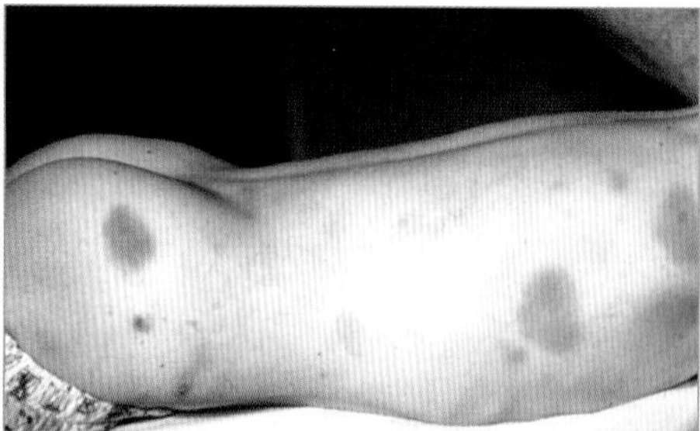

Image 119.6
Young adult male with postrubella thrombocytopenic purpura with large blueberry muffin skin lesions.

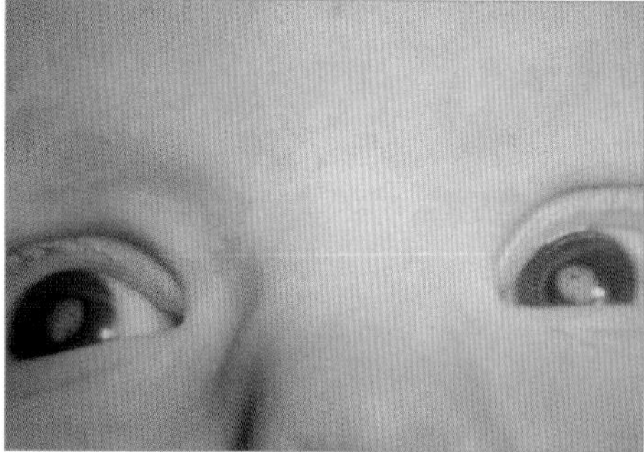

Image 119.8
This photograph shows the cataracts in an infant's eyes due to congenital rubella syndrome. Rubella is a viral disease that can affect susceptible persons of any age. Although generally a mild rash, if contracted in early pregnancy, there can be a high rate of fetal wastage or birth defects, known as congenital rubella syndrome. Courtesy of Centers for Disease Control and Prevention.

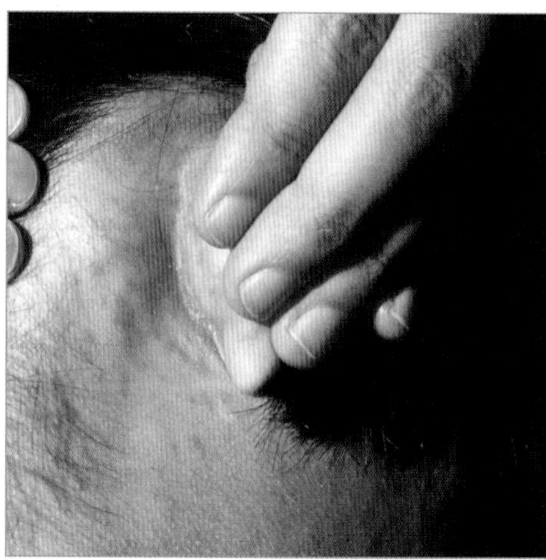

Image 119.5
During a rubella outbreak in Hawaii, this adolescent presented with a 2-day history of fever, malaise, rash, and lymphadenopathy, including these postauricular lymph nodes. Courtesy of Neal Halsey, MD.

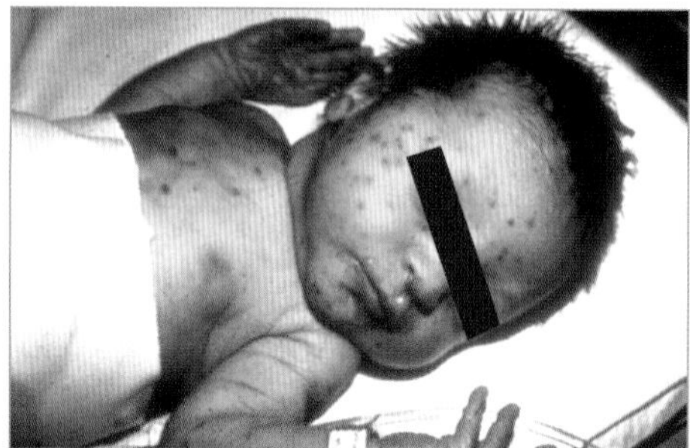

Image 119.7
Newborn with congenital rubella rash. Courtesy of Immunization Action Coalition.

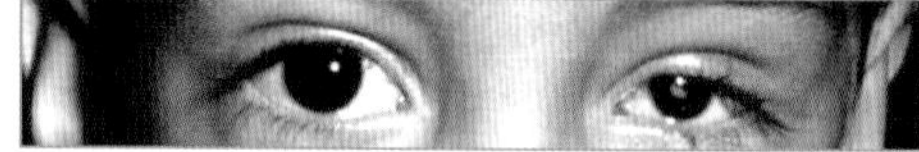

Image 119.9
A 4-year-old boy with congenital rubella syndrome with unilateral microphthalmos and cataract formation in the left eye.

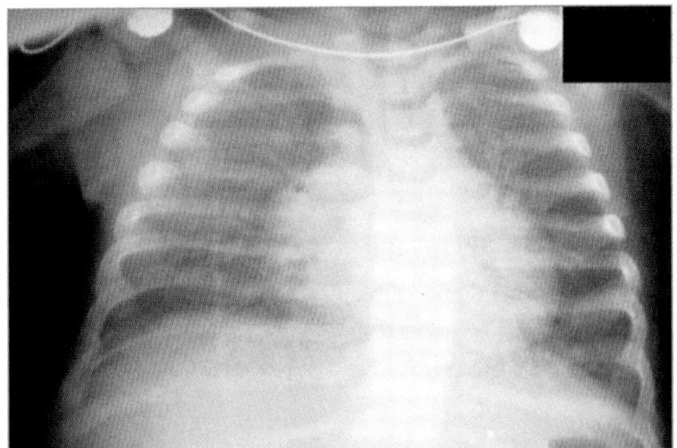

Image 119.10
Radiograph of the chest and upper abdomen of an infant with congenital rubella pneumonia with hepatosplenomegaly.

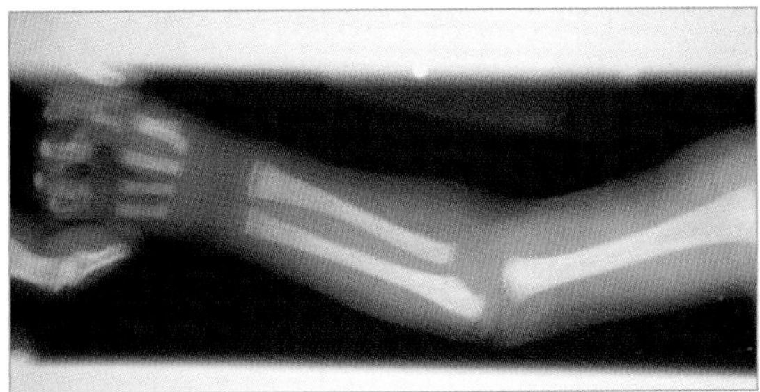

Image 119.11
Radiolucent changes in the metaphyses of the long bones of the upper extremity of an infant with congenital rubella.

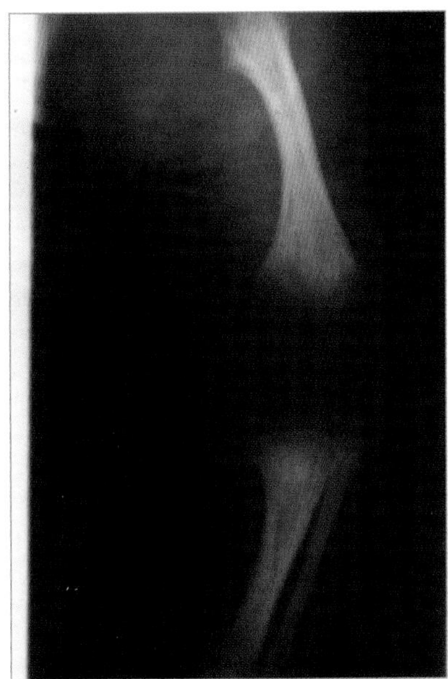

Image 119.12
Radiograph of the lower extremity of the same patient as in Image 119.11 with metaphyseal radiolucent changes, which are found in 10% to 20% of infants with congenital rubella.

120

Salmonella Infections

Clinical Manifestations

Nontyphoidal *Salmonella* organisms cause a spectrum of illness ranging from asymptomatic gastrointestinal tract carriage to gastroenteritis, bacteremia, and focal infections, including meningitis, brain abscess, and osteomyelitis. The most common illness associated with nontyphoidal *Salmonella* infection is gastroenteritis, in which diarrhea, abdominal cramps, and fever are common manifestations. The site of infection is usually the distal small intestine as well as the colon. Sustained or intermittent bacteremia can occur, and focal infections are recognized in as many as 10% of patients with nontyphoidal *Salmonella* bacteremia.

In the United States, the incidence of invasive *Salmonella* infection is highest among infants. Certain *Salmonella* serovars (eg, Dublin, Typhi, Choleraesuis), although rare, are more likely to result in invasive infection than gastroenteritis. However, in recent years in sub-Saharan Africa, certain serovars of nontyphoidal *Salmonella* have been reported to be common. Notably, these highly lethal African nontyphoidal *Salmonella* organisms are genetically distinct from their serovar counterparts causing pediatric disease in industrialized countries and exhibit a very high lethality (an estimate mortality of 20%); two-thirds of patients present without gastroenteritis or a history of antecedent diarrhea.

Salmonella enterica serovars Typhi, Paratyphi A, Paratyphi B, and Paratyphi C can cause a protracted bacteremic illness referred to, respectively, as typhoid and paratyphoid fever and, collectively, as enteric fevers. In older children, the onset of enteric fever is typically gradual, with manifestations such as fever, constitutional symptoms (eg, headache, malaise, anorexia, lethargy), abdominal discomfort and tenderness, hepatomegaly, splenomegaly, dactylitis, rose spots, and change in mental status. In infants and toddlers, invasive infection with enteric fever serovars can manifest as a mild, nondescript febrile illness accompanied by self-limited bacteremia, or invasive infection can occur in association with more severe clinical symptoms and signs, sustained bacteremia, and meningitis. Diarrhea (resembling pea soup) or constipation can be early features. Relative bradycardia (pulse rate slower than would be expected for a given body temperature) has been considered a common feature of typhoid fever in adults, but in children, this is rare.

Etiology

Salmonella organisms are gram-negative bacilli that belong to the family Enterobacteriaceae. More than 2,500 *Salmonella* serovars have been described; most serovars causing human disease are classified within O serogroups A through E. *Salmonella* ser Typhi is classified in O serogroup D, along with many other common serovars, including Enteritidis and Dublin. In 2011, the most commonly reported human isolates in the United States were *Salmonella* serovars Enteritidis, Typhimurium, Newport, Javiana, and Heidelberg; these 5 serovars generally account for nearly half of all *Salmonella* infections in the United States.

The relative prevalence of other serovars varies by country. Approximately 75% to 95% of the serovars associated with invasive pediatric disease in sub-Saharan Africa are *S* Typhimurium (Table 120.1).

Epidemiology

The principal reservoirs for nontyphoidal *Salmonella* organisms include birds, mammals, reptiles, and amphibians. However, it is believed that some of the African serotypes associated with invasive human disease have a human, rather than animal, reservoir. The major food vehicles of transmission to humans in industrialized countries include food of animal origin, such as poultry, beef, eggs, and dairy products. Multiple other food vehicles (eg, fruits, vegetables, peanut butter, frozen potpies, powdered infant formula, cereal, bakery products) have been implicated in outbreaks in the United States and Europe, presumably when the food was contaminated by contact with an infected animal product or a human carrier. Other modes of transmission include ingestion of contaminated water or contact with infected animals, mainly poultry (eg, chicks, chickens,

Table 120.1
Nomenclature for Salmonella Organisms

Complete Name[a]	Serotype[b]	Antigenic Formula
S enterica[a] subsp *enterica* ser Typhi	Typhi	9,12,[Vi]:d:-
S enterica subsp *enterica* ser Typhimurium	Typhimurium	[1],4,[5],12:i:1,2
S enterica subsp *enterica* ser Newport	Newport	6,8,[20]:e,h:1,2
S enterica subsp *enterica* ser Paratyphi A	Paratyphi A	[1],2,12:a:[1,5]
S enterica subsp *enterica* ser Enteritidis	Enteritidis	[1],9,12:g,m:-

[a] Species and subspecies are determined by biochemical reactions. Serotype is determined based on antigenic make-up. In the current taxonomy, only 2 species are recognized, *Salmonella enterica* and *Salmonella bongori*. *S enterica* has 6 subspecies, of which subspecies I (*enterica*) contains the overwhelming majority of all *Salmonella* pathogens that affect humans, other mammals, and birds.

[b] Many *Salmonella* pathogens that previously were considered species (and, therefore, were written italicized with a small case first letter) now are considered serotypes (also called serovars). Serotypes are now written nonitalicized with a capital first letter (eg, Typhi, Typhimurium, Enteritidis). The serotype of *Salmonella* is determined by its O (somatic) and H (flagellar) antigens and whether Vi is expressed.

ducks), reptiles or amphibians (eg, pet turtles, iguanas, lizards, snakes, frogs, toads, newts, salamanders), and rodents (eg, hamsters, mice) or other mammals (eg, hedgehogs). Reptiles and amphibians that live in tanks or aquariums can contaminate the water. Small turtles with a shell length of less than 4 inches are a well-known source of human *Salmonella* infections. Because of this risk, the US Food and Drug Administration has banned the interstate sale and distribution of these turtles since 1975. Animal-derived pet foods and treats have also been linked to *Salmonella* infections, especially among young children.

Unlike nontyphoidal *Salmonella* serovars, the enteric fever serovars (*Salmonella* Typhi, Paratyphi A, Paratyphi B [*sensu stricto*]) are restricted to human hosts, in whom they cause clinical and subclinical infections. Chronic human carriers (mostly involving chronic infection of the gallbladder but occasionally involving infection of the urinary tract) constitute the reservoir in areas with endemic infection. Infection with enteric fever serovars implies ingestion of a food or water vehicle contaminated by a chronic carrier or person with acute infection. Although typhoid fever (300–400 cases annually) and paratyphoid fever (~150 cases annually) are uncommon in the United States, these infections are highly endemic in many resource-limited countries, particularly in Asia. Consequently, most typhoid fever and paratyphoid fever infections in residents of the United States are usually acquired during international travel.

Age-specific incidences for nontyphoidal *Salmonella* infection are highest in children younger than 4 years. In the United States, rates of invasive infections and mortality are higher in infants, elderly people, and people with hemoglobinopathies (including sickle cell disease) and immunocompromising conditions (eg, malignant neoplasms). Most reported cases are sporadic, but widespread outbreaks, including health care–associated and institutional outbreaks, have been reported. The incidence of foodborne cases of nontyphoidal *Salmonella* gastroenteritis has diminished little in recent years.

Every year, nontyphoidal *Salmonella* organisms are one of the most common causes of laboratory-confirmed cases of enteric disease reported by the Foodborne Diseases Active Surveillance Network.

A risk of transmission of infection to others persists for as long as an infected person excretes nontyphoidal *Salmonella* organisms. Twelve weeks after infection with the most common nontyphoidal *Salmonella* serovars, approximately 45% of children younger than 5 years excrete organisms, compared with 5% of older children and adults; antimicrobial therapy can prolong excretion. Approximately 1% of adults continue to excrete nontyphoidal *Salmonella* organisms for more than 1 year.

Incubation Period

For nontyphoidal *Salmonella* gastroenteritis, 12 to 36 hours (range, 6–72 hours). For enteric fever, 7 to 14 days (range, 3–60 days).

Diagnostic Tests

Isolation of *Salmonella* organisms from cultures of stool, blood, urine, bile (including duodenal fluid–containing bile), and material from foci of infection is diagnostic. Gastroenteritis is diagnosed by stool culture. Diagnostic tests to detect *Salmonella* antigens by enzyme immunoassay, latex agglutination, and monoclonal antibodies have been developed, as have commercial immunoassays that detect antibodies to antigens of enteric fever serovars. Gene-based polymerase chain reaction diagnostic tests are also available in research laboratories. Multiplex polymerase chain reaction platforms for detection of multiple viral, parasitic, and bacterial pathogens, including *Salmonella*, have been licensed for diagnostic use.

If enteric fever is suspected, blood, bone marrow, or bile culture is diagnostic because organisms are often absent from stool. The sensitivity of blood culture and bone marrow culture in children with enteric fever is approximately 60% and 90%, respectively. The combination of a single blood culture plus culture of bile (collected from a bile-stained duodenal string) is 90% sensitive in detecting *Salmonella* Typhi infection in children with clinical enteric fever.

Treatment

Antimicrobial therapy is usually not indicated for patients with asymptomatic infection or uncomplicated (noninvasive) gastroenteritis caused by nontyphoidal *Salmonella* serovars because therapy does not shorten the duration of diarrheal disease and can prolong duration of fecal excretion. Although of unproven benefit, antimicrobial therapy is recommended for gastroenteritis caused by nontyphoidal *Salmonella* serovars in people at increased risk of invasive disease, including infants younger than 3 months and people with chronic gastrointestinal tract disease, malignant neoplasms, hemoglobinopathies, HIV infection, or other immunosuppressive illnesses or therapies.

If antimicrobial therapy is initiated in patients with gastroenteritis, amoxicillin or trimethoprim-sulfamethoxazole is recommended for susceptible strains. Resistance to these antimicrobial agents is becoming more common, especially in resource-limited countries. In areas where ampicillin and trimethoprim-sulfamethoxazole resistance is common, a fluoroquinolone or azithromycin is usually effective. For patients with localized invasive disease (eg, osteomyelitis, abscess, meningitis) or bacteremia in people infected with HIV, empirical therapy with ceftriaxone is recommended. Once antimicrobial susceptibility test results are available, ampicillin or ceftriaxone for susceptible strains is recommended.

For invasive, nonfocal infections, such as bacteremia or septicemia, caused by nontyphoidal *Salmonella* or for enteric fever caused by *Salmonella* Typhi, Paratyphi A, and Paratyphi B, 14 days of therapy is recommended, although shorter courses (7–10 days) have been effective. Therapy with a fluoroquinolone or azithromycin orally can be considered in patients with uncomplicated infections for nontyphoidal *Salmonella*. For enteric fever caused by *Salmonella* Typhi, therapy should be administered parenterally for 14 days. For localized invasive disease (eg, osteomyelitis, meningitis), at least 4 to 6 weeks of therapy is recommended. Drugs of choice, route of administration, and duration of therapy are based on susceptibility of the organism, site of infection, host, and clinical response. Multidrug-resistant isolates of *Salmonella* Typhi and Paratyphi A (exhibiting resistance to ampicillin, chloramphenicol, and trimethoprim-sulfamethoxazole) and strains with decreased susceptibility to fluoroquinolones are common in South and Southeast Asia and are increasingly found in travelers to areas with endemic infection. Invasive salmonellosis attributable to strains with decreased fluoroquinolone susceptibility is associated with greater risk for treatment failure. Azithromycin is an effective alternative for people with uncomplicated infections. Relapse of nontyphoidal *Salmonella* infection can occur, particularly in immunocompromised patients, who may require longer duration of treatment and retreatment.

The propensity to become a chronic *Salmonella* Typhi carrier (excretion >1 year) following acute typhoid infection correlates with prevalence of cholelithiasis, increases with age, and is greater in females than males. Chronic carriage in children is uncommon. The chronic carrier state may be eradicated by 4 weeks of oral therapy with ciprofloxacin or norfloxacin, antimicrobial agents that are highly concentrated in bile. High-dose parenteral ampicillin can also be used if 4 weeks of oral fluoroquinolone therapy is not well tolerated.

Corticosteroids may be beneficial in patients with severe enteric fever, which is characterized by delirium, obtundation, stupor, coma, or shock. These drugs should be reserved for critically ill patients in whom relief of manifestations of toxemia may be lifesaving. The usual regimen is high-dose dexamethasone given intravenously.

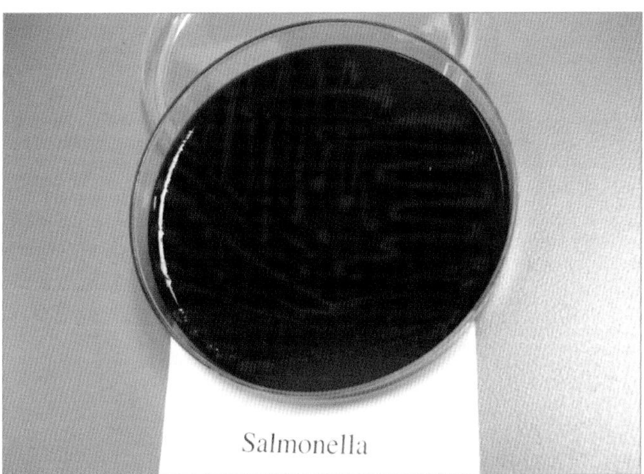

Image 120.1
Salmonella species grown on blood agar plate. Courtesy of Rita Yee, MT(ASCP) SM.

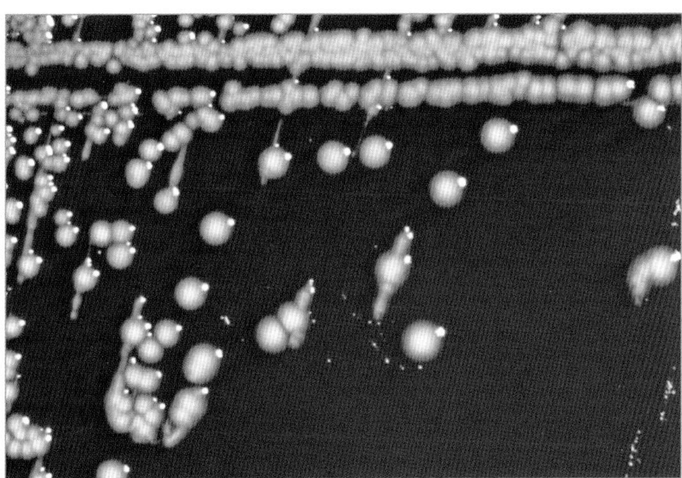

Image 120.2
This image depicts the colonial growth pattern displayed by *Salmonella enterica* subsp *arizonae* grown on blood agar, also known as *S arizonae* or *Arizona hinshawii*. *Salmonella* species are gram-negative, aerobic, rod-shaped, zoonotic bacteria that can infect people, birds, reptiles, and other animals. Courtesy of Centers for Disease Control and Prevention.

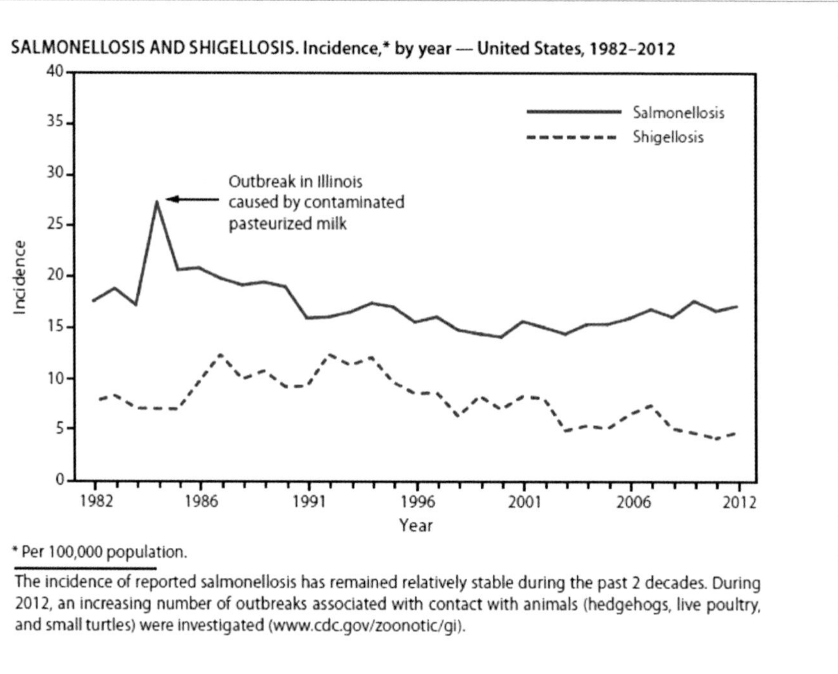

Image 120.3

Salmonellosis and shigellosis. Incidence, by year—United States, 1982–2012. Courtesy of *Morbidity and Mortality Weekly Report.*

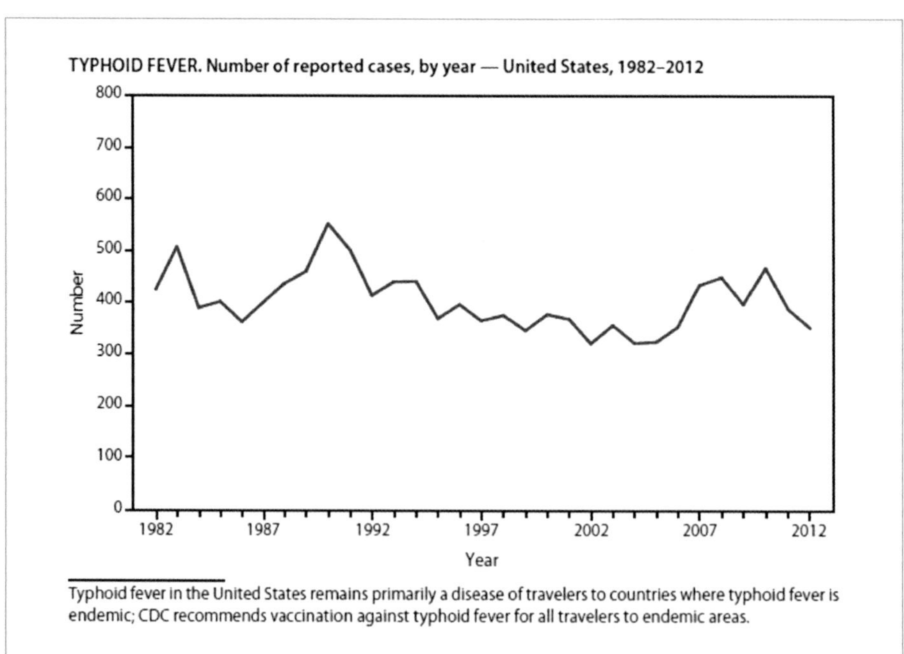

Image 120.4

Typhoid fever. Number of reported cases, by year, 1982–2012. Courtesy of *Morbidity and Mortality Weekly Report.*

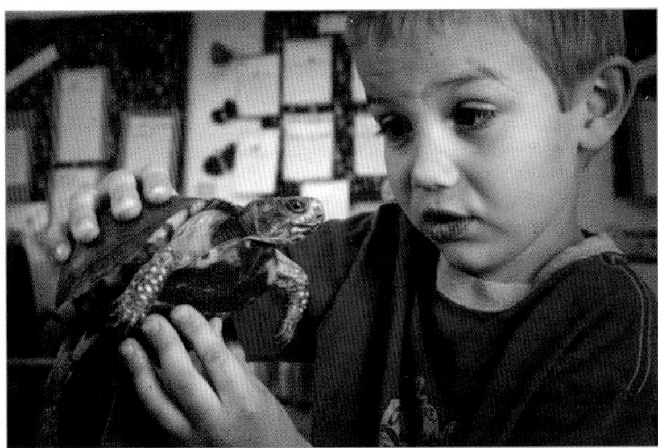

Image 120.5
This 2005 photograph depicts a young boy holding a box turtle, portraying a look of wonderment mixed with curiosity, as the turtle looks on with almost a sense of nonchalance. The importance of this image lies in the reality that turtles carry *Salmonella*. The sale of turtles less than 4 inches in length has been banned in the United States since 1975. The ban by the US Food and Drug Administration has prevented an estimated 100,000 cases of salmonellosis annually in children. Courtesy of Centers for Disease Control and Prevention/James Gathan.

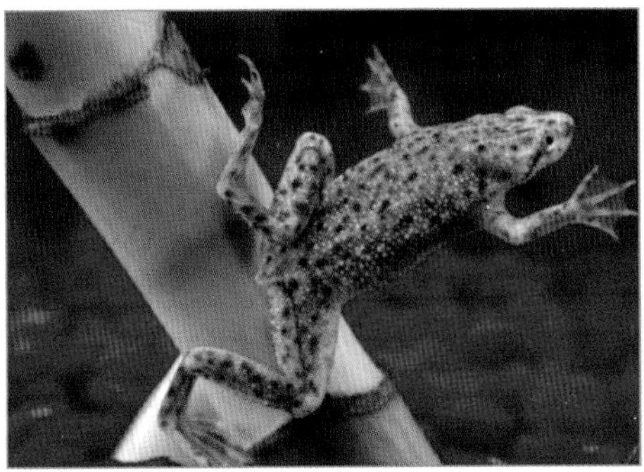

Image 120.6
African dwarf frog. *Salmonella* infection can be acquired through contact with reptiles and amphibians in homes, petting zoos, parks, child care facilities, and other locations. Courtesy of Centers for Disease Control and Prevention.

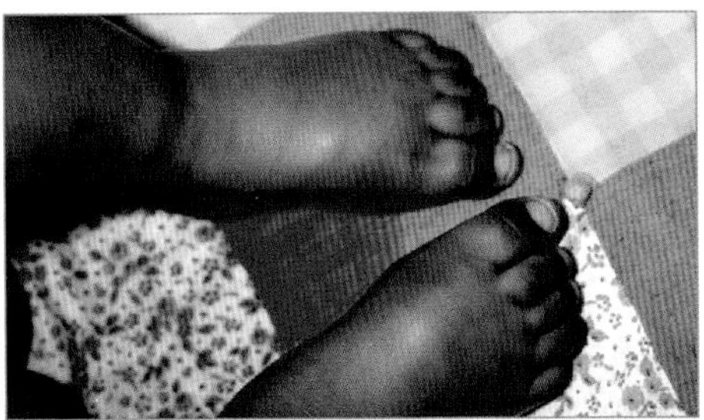

Image 120.8
A young child with sickle cell dactylitis of the foot and *Salmonella* sepsis. This is the same patient as in Image 120.7. Copyright Martin G. Myers, MD.

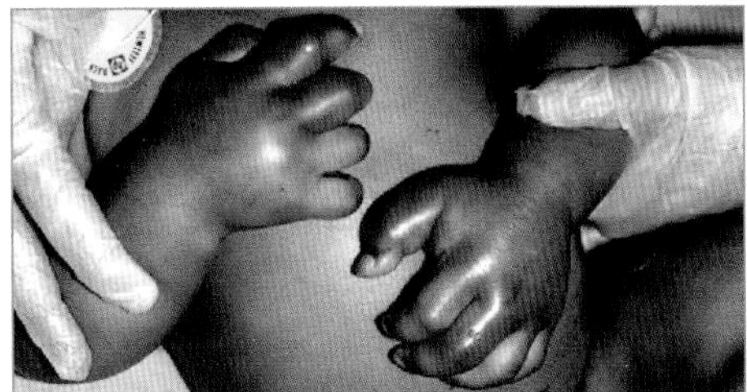

Image 120.7
A young African American child with sickle cell disease and *Salmonella* sepsis with swelling of the hands. Probable diagnosis: acute sickle cell dactylitis with septicemia. Copyright Martin G. Myers, MD.

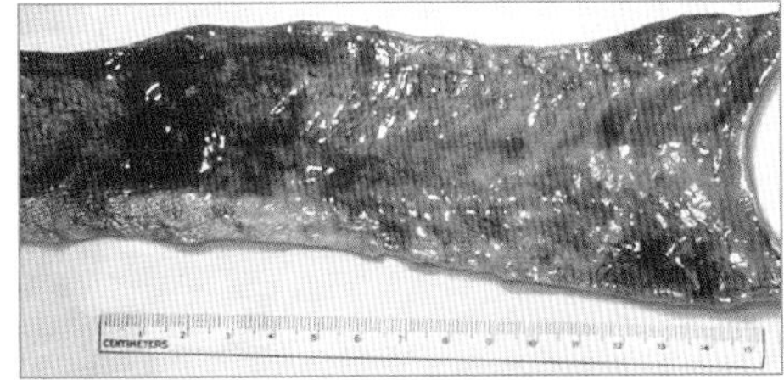

Image 120.9
Typhoid fever cholecystitis with an ulceration and perforation of the gallbladder into the jejunum. *Salmonella* ser Typhi, the bacterium responsible for causing typhoid fever, has a preference for the gallbladder and, if present, will colonize the surface of gallstones, which is how people become long-term carriers of the disease. Courtesy of Centers for Disease Control and Prevention/Armed Forces Institute of Pathology, Charles N. Farmer.

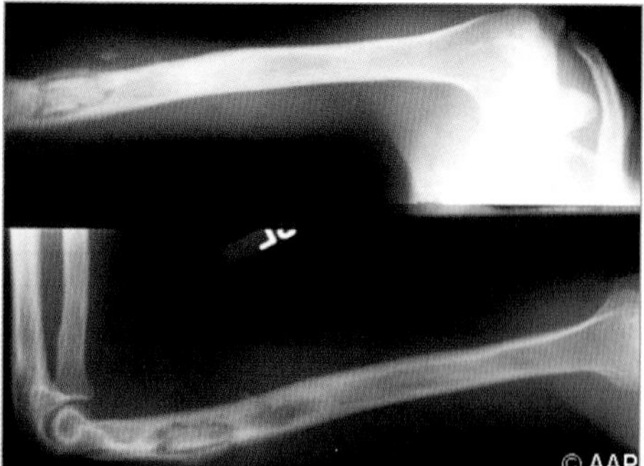

Image 120.10
Osteomyelitis due to *Salmonella* infection of the humeral shaft (diaphysis) in a 14-year-old African American boy with sickle cell disease.

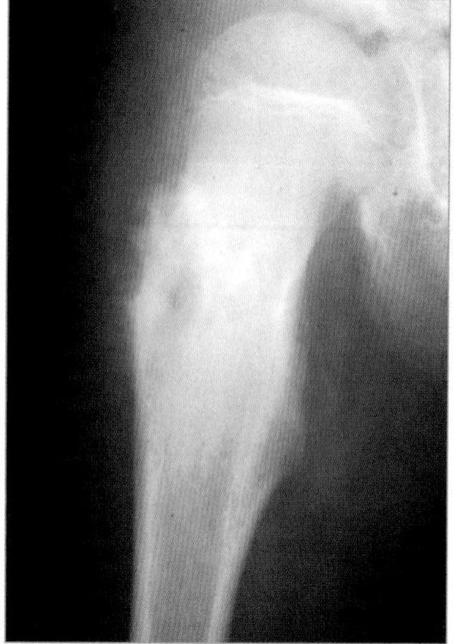

Image 120.11
Osteomyelitis (chronic) due to *Salmonella* infection of the proximal femur.

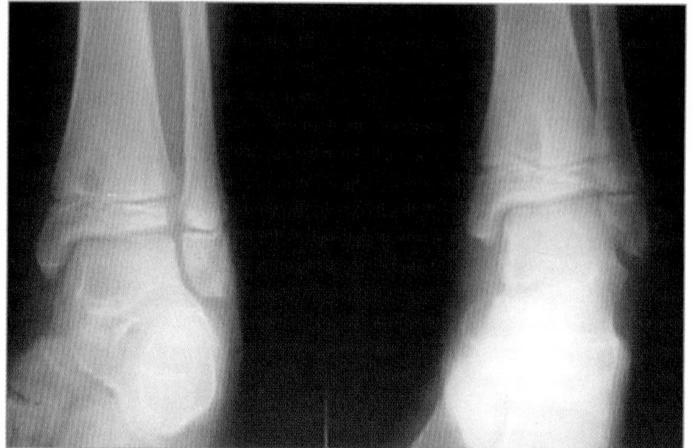

Image 120.12
Osteomyelitis due to *Salmonella* infection of the distal tibia.

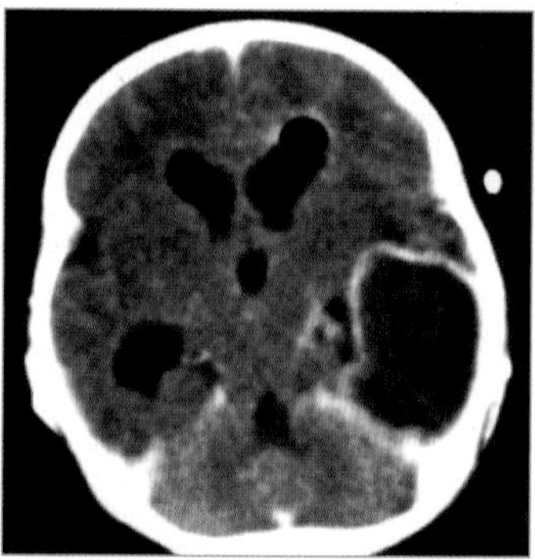

Image 120.13
A computed tomography scan showing a large brain abscess in the posterior parietal region as a complication of *Salmonella* meningitis in a neonate.

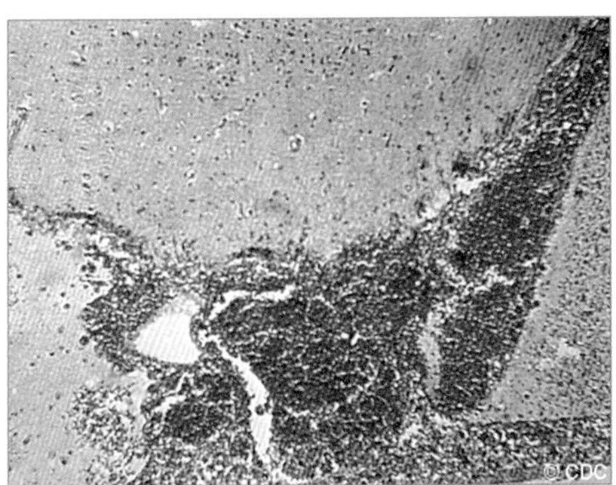

Image 120.14
Histopathologic changes in brain tissue due to *Salmonella* ser Typhi meningitis. *Salmonella* septicemia has been associated with subsequent infection of virtually every organ system, and the nervous system is no exception. Courtesy of Centers for Disease Control and Prevention/Armed Forces Institute of Pathology, Charles N. Farmer.

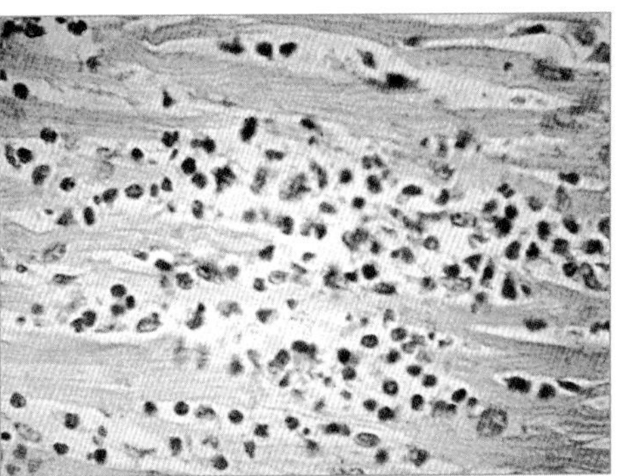

Image 120.15
A photomicrograph demonstrating the histopathologic changes in brain tissue due to *Salmonella* ser Typhi bacteria. *Salmonella* septicemia has been associated with subsequent infection of virtually every organ system, and the nervous system is no exception. Here we see an acute inflammatory encephalitis due to *S* Typhi bacteria. Courtesy of Centers for Disease Control and Prevention.

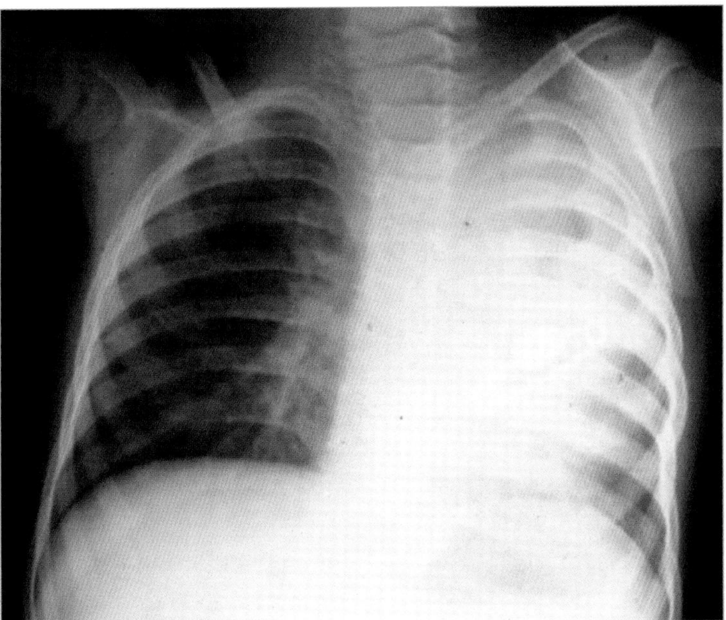

Image 120.16
Salmonella pneumonia with empyema in a 3-year-old girl with congenital neutropenia who required chest tube drainage and prolonged antibiotic treatment to control extensive pneumonia due to a nontyphoidal *Salmonella* species. Courtesy of Edgar O. Ledbetter, MD, FAAP.

121

Scabies

Clinical Manifestations

Scabies is characterized by an intensely pruritic, erythematous, papular eruption caused by burrowing of adult female mites in upper layers of the epidermis, creating serpiginous burrows. Itching is most intense at night. In older children and adults, the sites of predilection are interdigital folds, flexor aspects of wrists, extensor surfaces of elbows, anterior axillary folds, waistline, thighs, navel, genitalia, areolae, abdomen, intergluteal cleft, and buttocks. In children younger than 2 years, the eruption is generally vesicular and often occurs in areas usually spared in older children and adults, such as the scalp, face, neck, palms, and soles. The eruption is caused by a hypersensitivity reaction to the proteins of the parasite.

Characteristic scabietic burrows appear as gray or white, tortuous, threadlike lines. Excoriations are common, and most burrows are obliterated by scratching before a patient seeks medical attention. Occasionally, 2- to 5-mm red-brown nodules are present, particularly on covered parts of the body, such as the genitalia, groin, and axilla. These scabies nodules are a granulomatous response to dead mite antigens and feces; the nodules can persist for weeks and even months after effective treatment. Cutaneous secondary bacterial infection can occur and is usually caused by *Streptococcus pyogenes* or *Staphylococcus aureus*.

Crusted (Norwegian) scabies is an uncommon clinical syndrome characterized by a large number of mites and widespread, crusted, hyperkeratotic lesions. Crusted scabies usually occurs in people with debilitating conditions or developmental disabilities or who are immunocompromised. Crusted scabies can also occur in otherwise healthy children after long-term use of topical corticosteroid therapy.

Postscabetic pustulosis is a reactive phenomenon that may follow successful treatment of primary infestation with scabies. Affected infants and young children manifest episodic crops of sterile, pruritic papules and pustules predominantly in an acral distribution, but lesions can extend, to a lesser degree, onto the torso.

Etiology

The mite *Sarcoptes scabiei* subsp *hominis* is the cause of scabies. The adult female burrows in the stratum corneum of the skin and lays eggs. Larvae emerge from the eggs in 2 to 4 days and molt to nymphs and then to adults, which mate and produce new eggs. The entire cycle takes approximately 10 to 17 days. *S scabiei* subsp *canis,* acquired from dogs (with clinical mange), can cause a self-limited and mild infestation in humans usually involving the area in direct contact with the infested animal that will resolve without specific treatment.

Epidemiology

Humans are the source of infestation. Transmission usually occurs through prolonged close, personal contact. Because of the large number of mites in exfoliating scales, even minimal contact with a patient with crusted scabies can result in transmission; transmission from a patient with crusted scabies can also occur through contamination of items such as clothing, bedding, and furniture. Infestation acquired from dogs and other animals is uncommon, and these mites do not replicate in humans. Scabies of human origin can be transmitted as long as the patient remains infested and untreated, including during the interval before symptoms develop. Scabies is endemic in many countries and occurs worldwide in cycles thought to be 15 to 30 years long. Scabies affects people from all socioeconomic levels without regard to age, gender, or standards of personal hygiene. Scabies in adults often is acquired sexually.

Incubation Period

Without previous exposure, 4 to 6 weeks; if previously infested, 1 to 4 days.

Diagnostic Tests

Diagnosis is typically made by clinical examination. Diagnosis can be confirmed by identification of the mite or mite eggs or scybala (feces) from scrapings of papules or intact burrows, preferably from the terminal portion where the mite is generally found. Mineral oil, microscope immersion oil, or water applied to skin facilitates collection of scrapings. A broad-blade scalpel is used to scrape the burrow. Scrapings and oil can be placed on a slide under cover glass and examined microscopically under low power. Adult female mites average 330 to 450 μm in length. Skin scrapings provide definitive evidence of infection but have low sensitivity. Handheld dermoscopy (epiluminescence microscopy) has been used to identify in vivo the pigmented mite parts or air bubbles corresponding to infesting mites within the stratum corneum.

Treatment

Topical permethrin 5% cream or oral ivermectin are effective agents for treatment of scabies. Most experts recommend starting with topical 5% permethrin cream, particularly for infants, young children (not approved for children younger than 2 months), and pregnant or nursing women. Permethrin cream should be removed by bathing after 8 to 14 hours. Children and adults with infestation should apply lotion or cream containing this scabicide over their entire body below the head. Because scabies can affect the face, scalp, and neck in infants and young children, treatment of the entire head, neck, and body in this age group is required. Special attention should be given to trimming fingernails and ensuring application of medication to these areas. A Cochrane review found oral ivermectin is effective for treating scabies but less effective than topical permethrin. Because ivermectin is not ovicidal, it is given as 2 doses, 1 week apart. Alternative drugs include 10% crotamiton cream or lotion or unapproved 5% to 10% precipitated sulfur compounded into petrolatum. Because scabietic lesions are the result of a hypersensitivity reaction to the mite, itching may not subside for several weeks despite successful treatment. The use of oral antihistamines and topical corticosteroids can help relieve this itching. Topical or systemic antimicrobial therapy is indicated for secondary bacterial infections of the excoriated lesions. Because of safety concerns and availability of other treatments, lindane lotion should not be used as a first-line agent in the treatment of scabies.

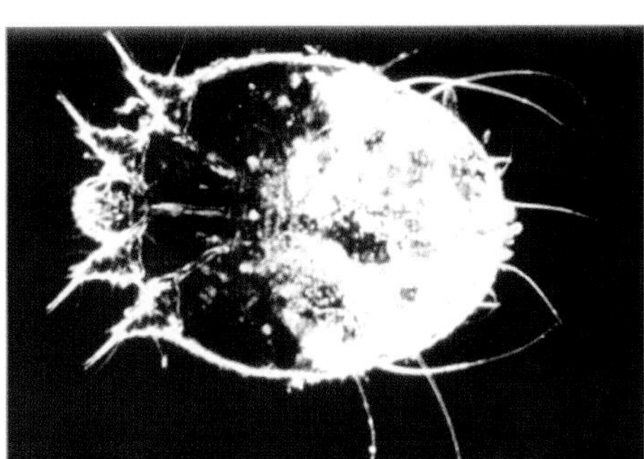

Image 121.1
This is a *Sarcoptes scabiei* subsp *hominis,* or itch mite, which is the cause of scabies. Females are 0.3- to 0.4-mm long and 0.25- to 0.35-mm wide. Male mites are slightly more than half that size. Scabies is a highly contagious infestation of the skin caused by a mite affecting humans and animals. Scabies is usually transmitted by intimate interpersonal contact, often sexual in nature, but transmission through casual contact can occur. Courtesy of Centers for Disease Control and Prevention/Reed & Carnrick Pharmaceuticals.

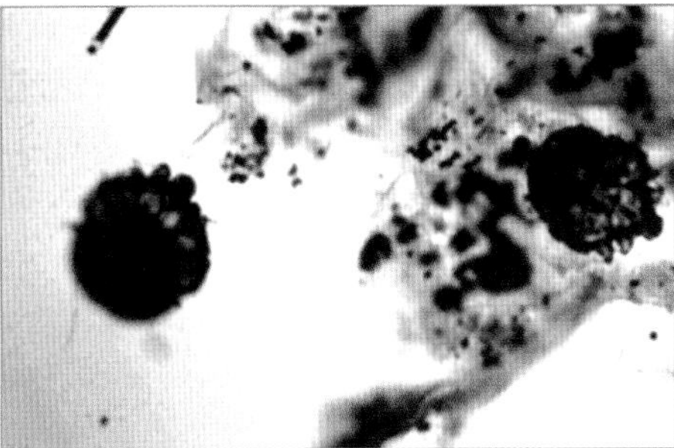

Image 121.2
Linear papulovesicular burrows often contain female scabies mites when examined in mineral oil, which confirms the diagnosis of scabies, as shown here.

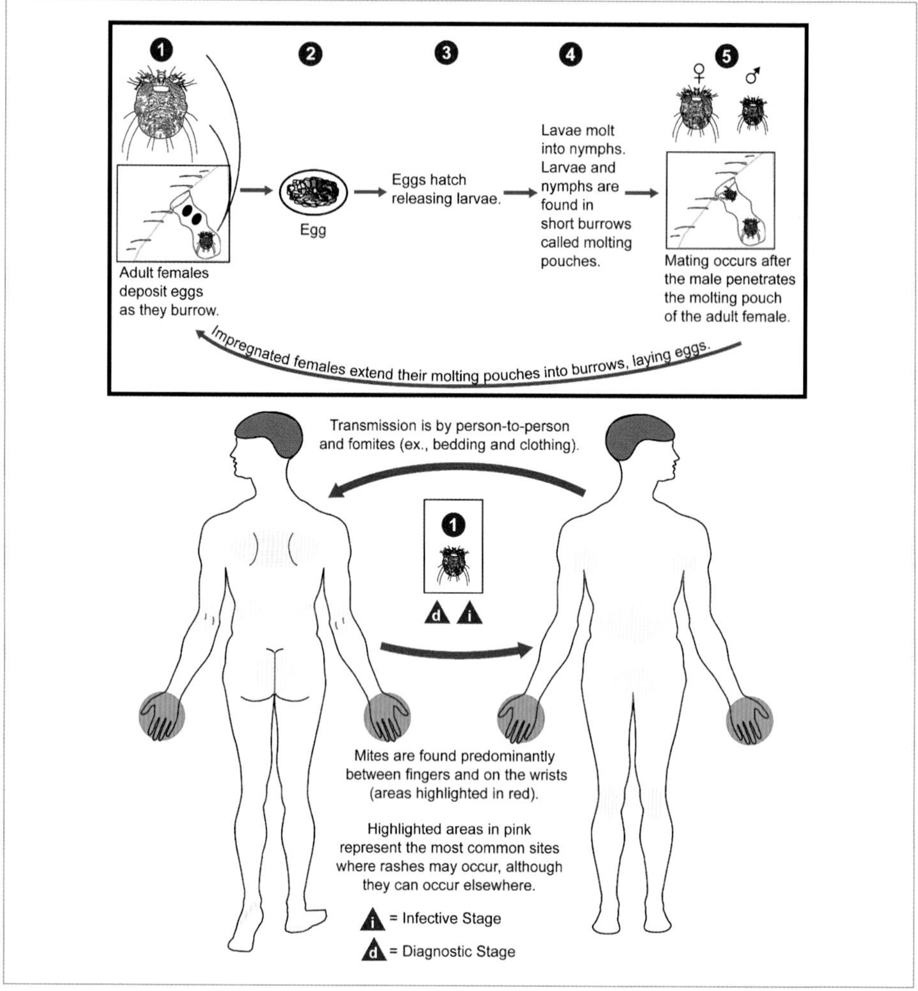

Image 121.3

Life cycle. *Sarcoptes scabiei* undergoes 4 stages in its life cycle: egg, larva, nymph, and adult. Females deposit eggs at 2- to 3-day intervals as they burrow through the skin (1). Eggs are oval and 0.1 to 0.15 mm in length (2) and incubation time is 3 to 8 days. After the eggs hatch, the larvae migrate to the skin surface and burrow into the intact stratum corneum to construct almost invisible, short burrows called molting pouches. The larval stage, which emerges from the eggs, has only 3 pairs of legs (3), and this form lasts 2 to 3 days. After larvae molt, the resulting nymphs have 4 pairs of legs (4). This form molts into slightly larger nymphs before molting into adults. Larvae and nymphs may often be found in molting pouches or in hair follicles and look similar to adults, only smaller. Adults are round, saclike, eyeless mites. Females are 0.3- to 0.4-mm long and 0.25- to 0.35-mm wide, and males are slightly more than half that size. Mating occurs after the nomadic male penetrates the molting pouch of the adult female (5). Impregnated females extend their molting pouches into the characteristic serpentine burrows, laying eggs in the process. The impregnated females burrow into the skin and spend the remaining 2 months of their lives in tunnels under the surface of the skin. Males are rarely seen. They make a temporary gallery in the skin before mating. Transmission occurs by the transfer of ovigerous females during personal contact. Mode of transmission is primarily person-to-person contact, but transmission may also occur via fomites (eg, bedding, clothing). Mites are found predominantly between the fingers and on the wrists. The mites hold onto the skin using suckers attached to the 2 most anterior pairs of legs. Courtesy of Centers for Disease Control and Prevention/Alexander J. da Silva, PhD/Melanie Moser.

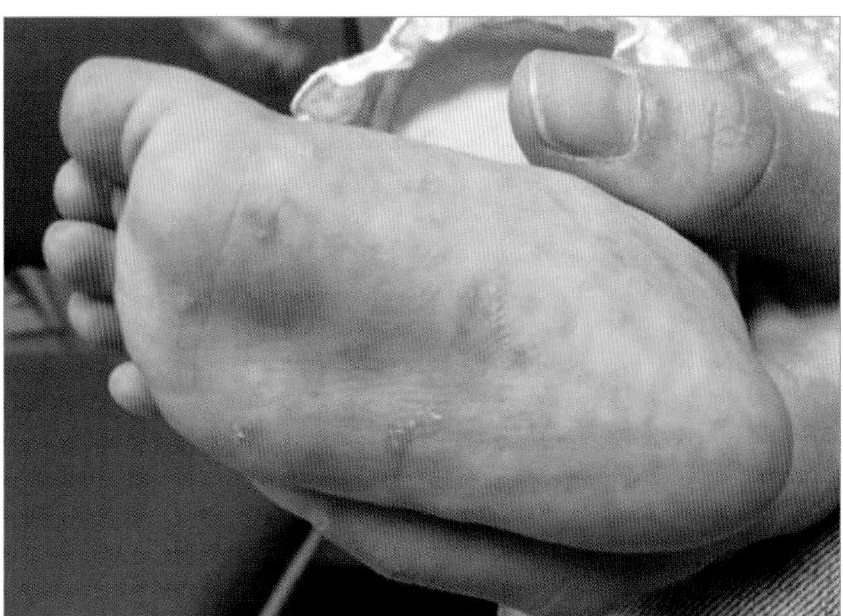

Image 121.4
A 2-year-old girl with scabies who was adopted from an orphanage in Eastern Europe. Courtesy of Daniel P. Krowchuk, MD, FAAP.

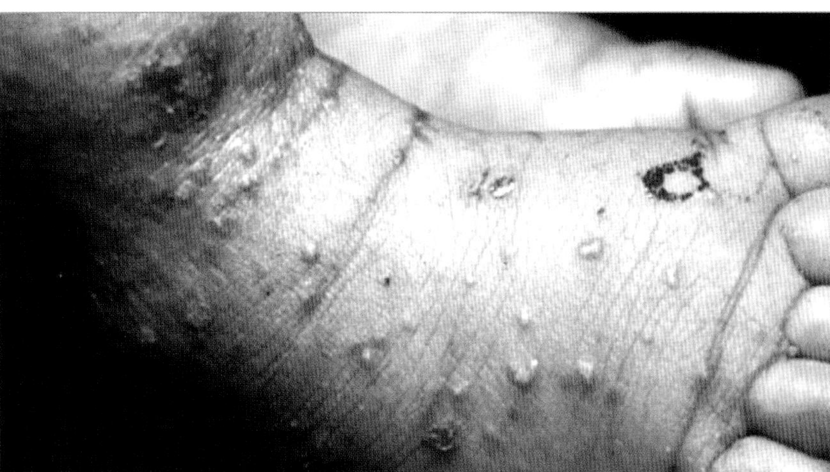

Image 121.5
Papulopustules and a widespread eczematous eruption, which represents a hypersensitivity reaction to a scabies infestation.

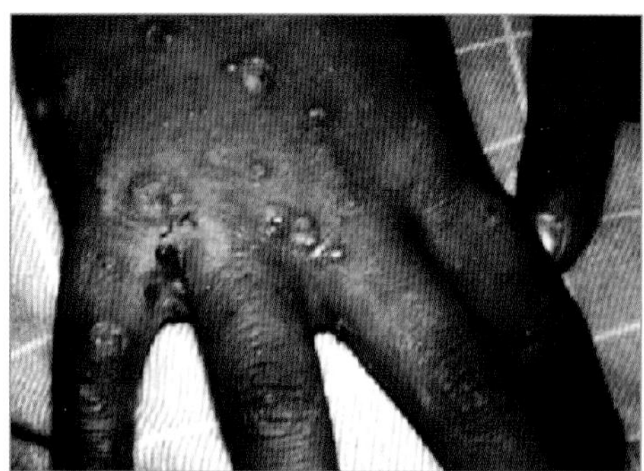

Image 121.6
Older children, adolescents, and adults with scabies exhibit erythematous papules, nodules, or burrows in the interdigital webs, as in this patient.

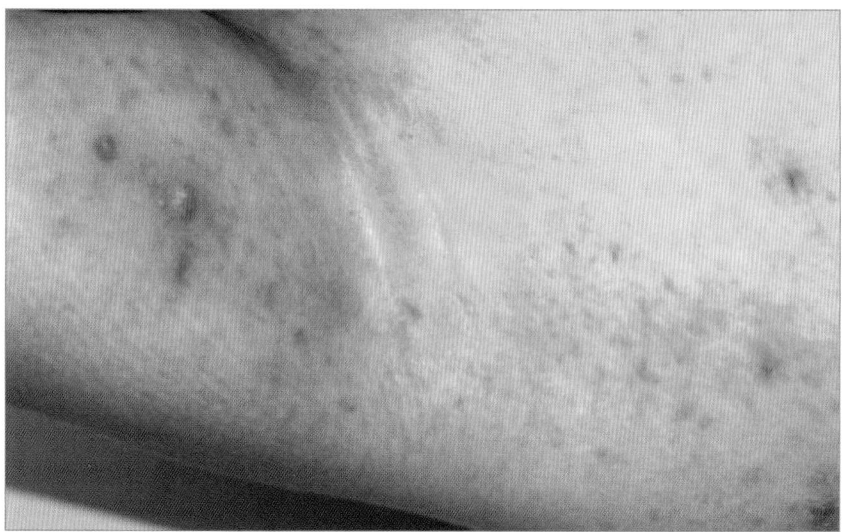

Image 121.7
A 12-year-old with itching in the axillae and groin for 2 weeks. She recently returned from a family camping trip, where she shared a tent with "dozens of cousins." Since returning home, she has had itching in the armpits and in her pubic area. She now has papules and pustules on the fingers, toes, and her gluteal furrow. The family is reluctant to inquire about relatives with similar lesions. Examination of scrapings of the lesions indicated a few oval structures suggestive of scabies eggs. She responded to treatment with topical sulfur and oil in lieu of pesticide-based therapy. Courtesy of Will Sorey, MD.

122

Schistosomiasis

Clinical Manifestations

Infections are established by skin penetration of infecting larvae (cercariae, shed by freshwater snails), which can be accompanied by a transient, pruritic, papular rash (cercarial dermatitis). After penetration, the parasites enter the bloodstream, migrate through the lungs, and eventually mature into adult worms that reside in the venous plexus that drains the intestines or, in the case of *Schistosoma haematobium,* the urogenital tract. Four to 8 weeks after exposure, an acute serum sicknesslike illness (Katayama fever) can develop that manifests as fever, malaise, cough, rash, abdominal pain, hepatosplenomegaly, diarrhea, nausea, lymphadenopathy, and eosinophilia. The severity of symptoms associated with infection is related to the worm burden. People with low to moderate worm burdens may have only subclinical disease or relatively mild manifestations, such as growth stunting or anemia. Higher worm burdens are associated with a range of symptoms caused primarily by inflammation and fibrosis triggered by the immune response to eggs produced by adult worms. Severe forms of intestinal schistosomiasis (*Schistosoma mansoni* and *Schistosoma japonicum* infections) can result in hepatosplenomegaly, abdominal pain, bloody diarrhea, portal hypertension, ascites, esophageal varices, and hematemesis. Urogenital schistosomiasis (*S haematobium* infections) can result in the bladder becoming inflamed and fibrotic. Urinary tract symptoms and signs include dysuria, urgency, terminal microscopic and gross hematuria, secondary urinary tract infections, hydronephrosis, and nonspecific pelvic pain. *S haematobium* is associated with lesions of the lower genital tract (vulva, vagina, and cervix) in women, prostatitis and hematospermia in men, and certain forms of bladder cancer. Other organ systems can be involved; for example, eggs can embolize in the lungs, causing pulmonary hypertension. Less commonly, eggs can lodge in the central nervous system, causing severe neurologic complications.

Cercarial dermatitis (swimmer's itch) is often caused by larvae of schistosome parasites of birds or other wildlife. These larvae can penetrate human skin but eventually die in the dermis and do not cause systemic disease. Skin manifestations include pruritus at the penetration site a few hours after water exposure, followed in 5 to 14 days by an intermittent pruritic, sometimes papular, eruption. In previously sensitized people, more intense papular eruptions may occur for 7 to 10 days after exposure.

Etiology

The trematodes (flukes) *S mansoni, S japonicum, Schistosoma mekongi,* and *Schistosoma intercalatum* cause intestinal schistosomiasis, and *S haematobium* causes urogenital disease. All species have similar life cycles. Swimmer's itch is typically caused by various schistosome species that are parasitic only for birds and wild mammals.

Epidemiology

Persistence of schistosomiasis depends on the presence of an appropriate snail as an intermediate host. Eggs excreted in stool (*S mansoni, S japonicum, S mekongi,* and *S intercalatum*) or urine (*S haematobium*) into freshwater hatch into motile miracidia, which infect snails. After development and asexual replication in snails, cercariae emerge and penetrate the skin of humans in contact with water. Children are commonly first infected when they accompany their mothers to lakes, ponds, and other open freshwater sources. School-aged children are typically the most heavily infected people in the community because of prolonged wading and swimming in infected waters. They are also important in maintaining transmission through behaviors such as uncontrolled defecation and urination. Communicability lasts as long as infected snails are in the environment or live eggs are excreted in the urine and feces of humans into freshwater sources with appropriate snails. In the case of *S japonicum,* animals play an important zoonotic role (as a source of eggs) in maintaining the life cycle. Infection is not transmissible by person-to-person contact or blood transfusion.

The distribution of schistosomiasis is focal and limited by the presence of appropriate snail vectors, infected human reservoirs, and freshwater sources. *S mansoni* occurs throughout tropical Africa, in parts of several Caribbean islands, and in areas of Venezuela, Brazil, Suriname, and the Arabian Peninsula. *S japonicum* is found in China, the Philippines, and Indonesia. *S haematobium* occurs in Africa and the Middle East. *S mekongi* is found in Cambodia and Laos. *S intercalatum* is found in West and Central Africa. Adult worms of *S mansoni* can live as long as 30 years in the human host. Thus, schistosomiasis can be diagnosed in patients many years after they have left an area with endemic infection. Immunity is incomplete, and reinfection occurs commonly. Swimmer's itch can occur in all regions of the world after exposure to freshwater, brackish water, or salt water.

Incubation Period

Approximately 4 to 6 weeks for *S japonicum,* 6 to 8 weeks for *S mansoni,* and 10 to 12 weeks for *S haematobium.*

Diagnostic Tests

Eosinophilia is common and may be intense in Katayama fever (acute schistosomiasis). Infection with *S mansoni* and other species (except *S haematobium*) is determined by microscopic examination of stool specimens to detect characteristic eggs, but results may be negative if performed too early in the course of infection. In light infections, several stool specimens examined by a concentration technique may be needed before eggs are found, or eggs may be seen in a biopsy of the rectal mucosa. *S haematobium* is diagnosed by examining urine for eggs. Egg excretion in urine often peaks between 12:00 noon and 3:00 pm. Biopsy of the bladder mucosa can be used to diagnose this infection. Serologic tests, available through the Centers for Disease Control and Prevention and some commercial laboratories, can be helpful for detecting light infections. However, results of these antibody-based tests remain positive for many years and are not useful in differentiating ongoing infection from past infection or reinfection.

Swimmer's itch can be difficult to differentiate from other causes of dermatitis. A skin biopsy may demonstrate larvae, but their absence does not exclude the diagnosis.

Treatment

The drug of choice for schistosomiasis caused by any species is praziquantel; the alternative drug for *S mansoni* is oxamniquine, although this drug is not available in the United States (it is used in some areas of Brazil). Praziquantel does not kill developing worms; therapy given within 4 to 8 weeks of exposure should be repeated 1 to 2 months later to improve the rate of parasitologic cure. Swimmer's itch is a self-limited disease that may require symptomatic treatment of the rash. More intense reactions may require a course of oral corticosteroids.

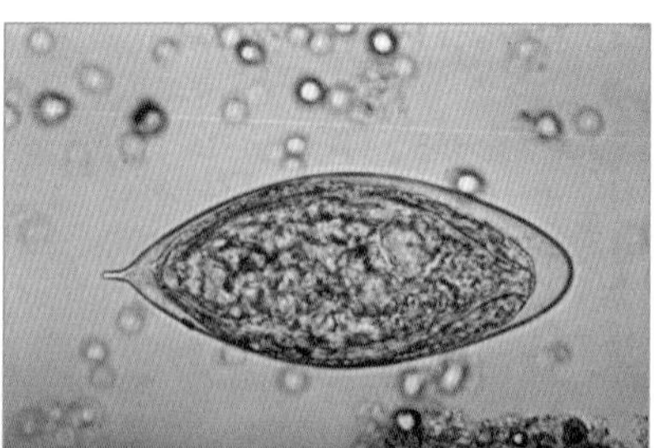

Image 122.1
This micrograph depicts an egg from a *Schistosoma haematobium* trematode parasite (magnification x500). Note the egg's posteriorly protruding terminal spine, unlike the spinal remnant, which protrudes from the lateral wall of the *Schistosoma japonicum* egg. These eggs are eliminated in an infected human's feces or urine and, under optimal conditions in a watery environment, the eggs hatch and release miracidia, which then penetrate a specific snail intermediate host. Once inside the host, the *S haematobium* parasite passes through 2 developmental generations of sporocysts and Is released by the snail into its environment as cercariae. Courtesy of Centers for Disease Control and Prevention.

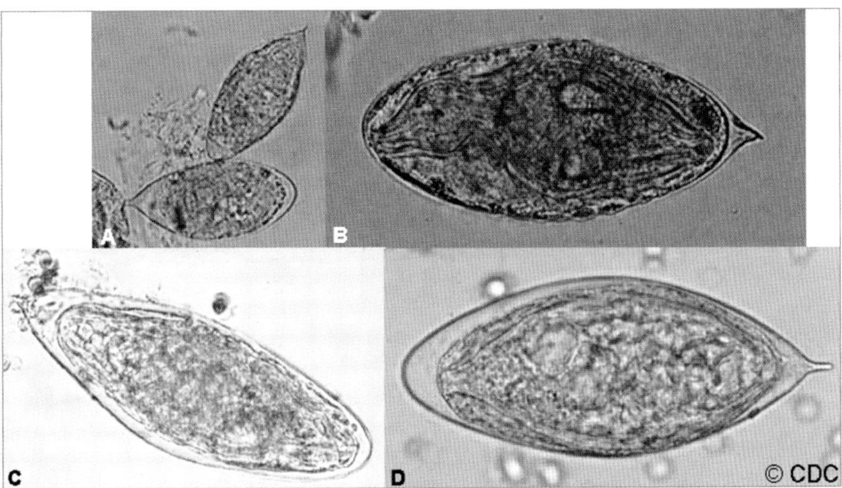

Image 122.2
A–D, *Schistosoma haematobium* eggs. In this species, the eggs are large and have a prominent terminal spine at the posterior end (length, 112–170 μm). B, The miracidium is shown inside the egg. Courtesy of Centers for Disease Control and Prevention.

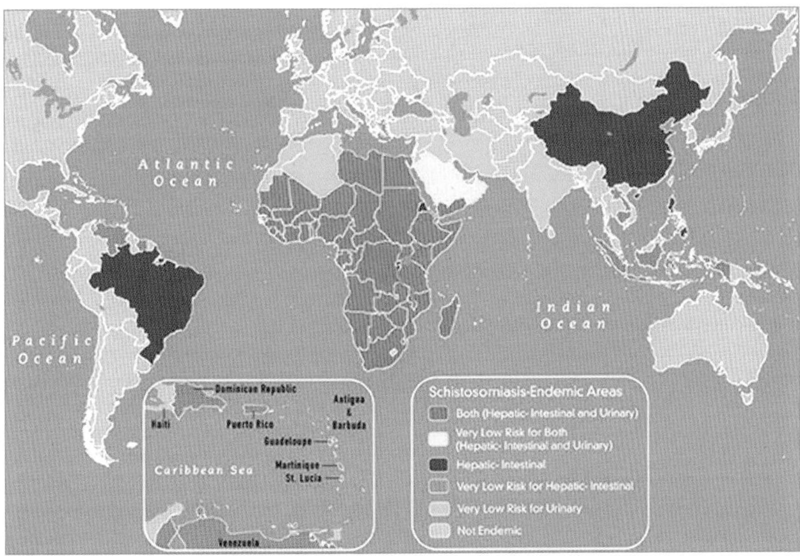

Image 122.3
Geographic distribution of schistosomiasis. Centers for Disease Control and Prevention National Center for Emerging and Zoonotic Infectious Diseases (NCEZID) Division of Global Migration and Quarantine (DGMQ).

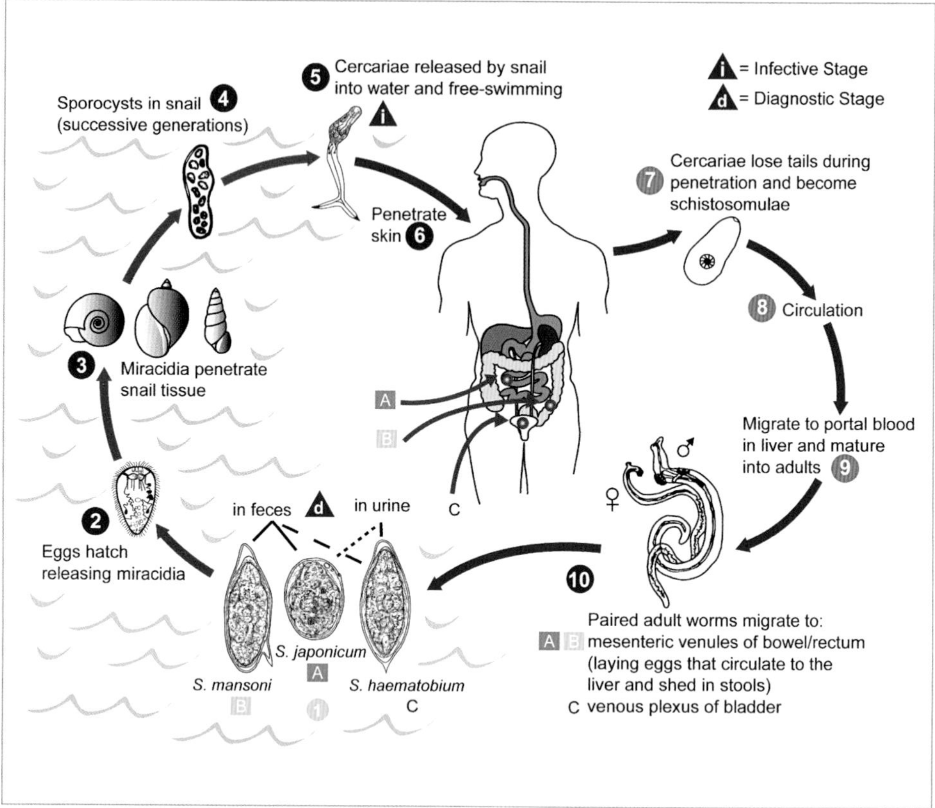

Image 122.4

Life cycle. Eggs are eliminated with feces or urine (1). Under optimal conditions, the eggs hatch and release miracidia (2), which swim and penetrate specific snail intermediate hosts (3). The stages in the snail include 2 generations of sporocysts (4) and the production of cercariae (5). On release from the snail, the infective cercariae swim, penetrate the skin of the human host (6), and shed their forked tail, becoming schistosomulae (7). The schistosomulae migrate through several tissues and stages to their residence in the veins (10). Adult worms in humans reside in the mesenteric venules in various locations, which, at times, seem to be specific for each species (10). For instance, *Schistosoma japonicum* is more frequently found in the superior mesenteric veins draining the small intestine (A), and *Schistosoma mansoni* occurs more often in the superior mesenteric veins draining the large intestine (B). However, both species can occupy either location, and they are capable of moving between sites, so it is not possible to state unequivocally that one species only occurs in one location. *Schistosoma haematobium* most often occurs in the venous plexus of the bladder (C), but it can also be found in the rectal venules. The females (size 7–20 mm; males slightly smaller) deposit eggs in the small venules of the portal and perivesical systems. The eggs are moved progressively toward the lumen of the intestine (*S mansoni* and *S japonicum*) and of the bladder and ureters (*S haematobium*) and are eliminated with feces or urine, respectively (1). Pathology of *S mansoni* and *S japonicum* schistosomiasis includes Katayama fever, presinusoidal egg granulomas, Symmers pipestem periportal fibrosis, portal hypertension, and occasional embolic egg granulomas in the brain or spinal cord. Pathology of *S haematobium* schistosomiasis includes hematuria, scarring, calcification, squamous cell carcinoma, and occasional embolic egg granulomas in the brain or spinal cord. Human contact with water is, thus, necessary for infection by schistosomes. Various animals, such as dogs, cats, rodents, pigs, horses, and goats, serve as reservoirs for *S japonicum*, and dogs for *S mekongi*. Courtesy of Centers for Disease Control and Prevention.

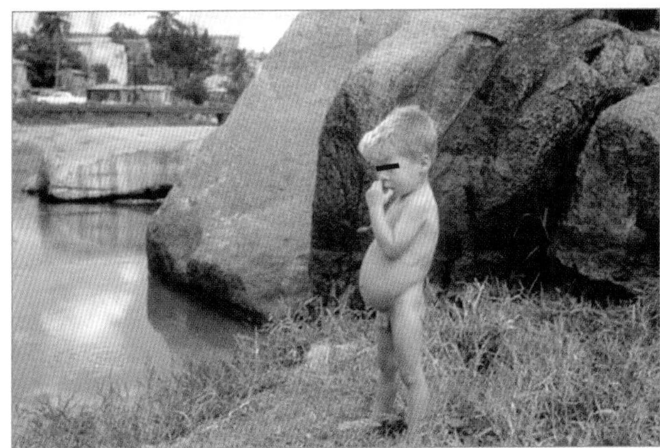

Image 122.5
A boy with swollen abdomen due to schistosomiasis with hepatosplenomegaly. Courtesy of Immunization Action Coalition.

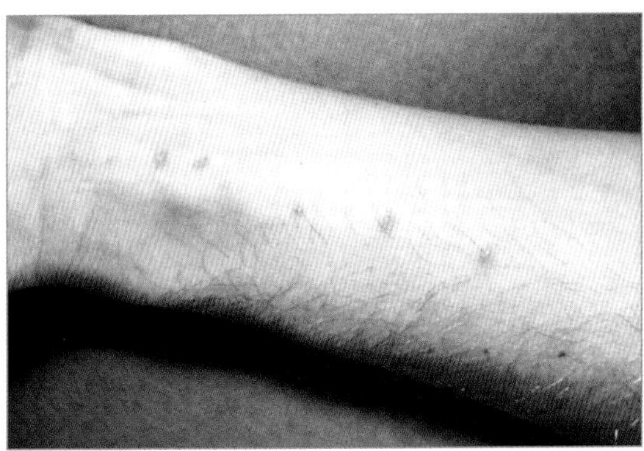

Image 122.6
Schistosome dermatitis, or swimmer's itch, occurs when skin is penetrated by a free-swimming, fork-tailed infective cercaria. On release from the snail host, the infective cercariae swim, penetrate the skin of the human host, and shed their forked tail, becoming schistosomulae. The schistosomulae migrate through several tissues and stages to their residence in the veins. Courtesy of Centers for Disease Control and Prevention.

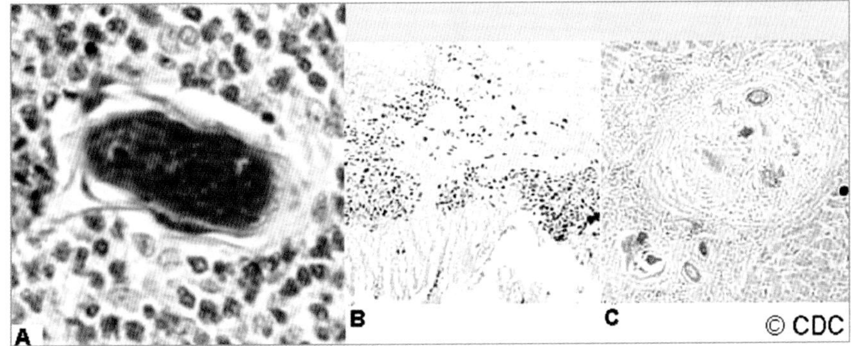

Image 122.7
A–C, Cross-section of different human tissues showing *Schistosoma* species eggs. A, *Schistosoma mansoni* eggs in intestinal wall. B, *Schistosoma japonicum* eggs in colon. C, *S japonicum* eggs in liver. Courtesy of Centers for Disease Control and Prevention.

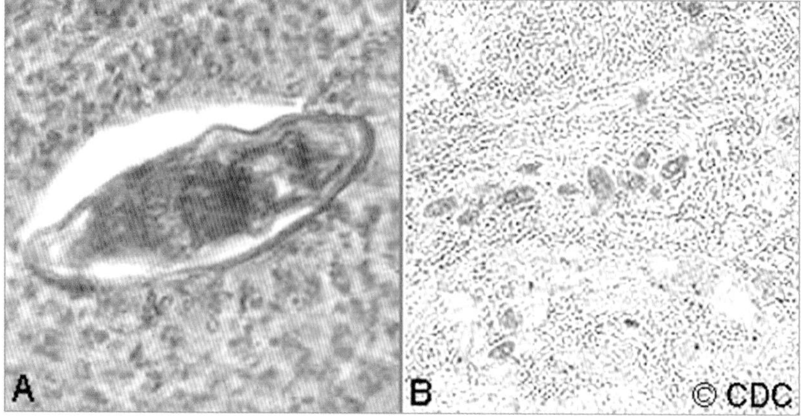

Image 122.8
A–B, Cross-section of different human tissues showing *Schistosoma* species eggs. *Schistosoma* species in liver and bladder, respectively. Courtesy of Centers for Disease Control and Prevention.

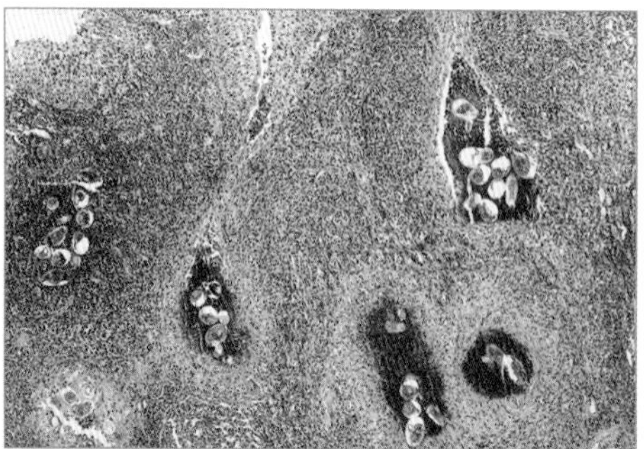

Image 122.9
Histopathology of the bladder shows eggs of *Schistosoma haematobium* surrounded by intense infiltrates of eosinophils and other inflammatory cells. Courtesy of Centers for Disease Control and Prevention/Edwin P. Ewing Jr, MD.

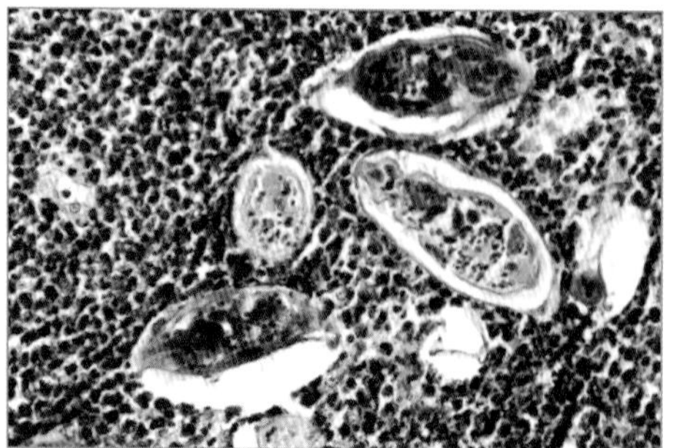

Image 122.11
Histopathology of *Schistosomiasis haematobia*, bladder. Histopathology of the bladder shows eggs of *S haematobium* surrounded by intense infiltrates of eosinophils. Courtesy of Centers for Disease Control and Prevention/Edwin P. Ewing Jr, MD.

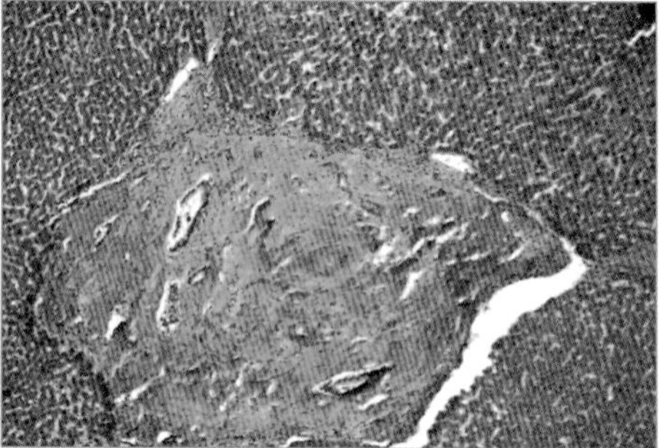

Image 122.10
This micrograph reveals signs of schistosomiasis infection of the liver, also known as pipestem cirrhosis (magnification x500). Pipestem cirrhosis occurs when schistosomes infect the liver (ie, hepatic schistosomiasis), which causes scarring to occur, thereby entrapping parasites and their ova in and around the hepatic portal circulatory vessels. Courtesy of Centers for Disease Control and Prevention.

123

Shigella Infections

Clinical Manifestations

Shigella species primarily infect the large intestine, causing clinical manifestations that range from watery or loose stools with minimal or no constitutional symptoms to more severe symptoms, including high fever, abdominal cramps or tenderness, tenesmus, and mucoid stools with or without blood. *Shigella dysenteriae* serotype 1 often causes a more severe illness than other shigellae with a higher risk of complications, including septicemia, pseudomembranous colitis, toxic megacolon, intestinal perforation, hemolysis, and hemolytic uremic syndrome. Infection attributable to *S dysenteriae* 1 has become rare in industrialized countries. Generalized seizures have been reported among young children with shigellosis attributable to any serotype; although the pathophysiology and incidence are poorly understood, such seizures are usually self-limited and associated with high fever or electrolyte abnormalities. Septicemia is rare during the course of illness and is caused by *Shigella* organisms or by other gut flora that gain access to the bloodstream through intestinal mucosa damaged during shigellosis. Septicemia occurs most often in neonates, malnourished children, and people with *S dysenteriae* 1 infection. Reactive arthritis with possible extraarticular manifestations is a rare complication that can develop weeks or months after shigellosis, especially in patients expressing HLA-B27.

Etiology

Shigella species are facultative aerobic, gram-negative bacilli in the family Enterobacteriaceae. Four species (with more than 40 serotypes) have been identified. Among *Shigella* isolates reported in the United States in 2012, approximately 81% were *Shigella sonnei,* 17% were *Shigella flexneri,* 1% was *Shigella boydii,* and less than 1% was other species. In resource-limited countries, especially in Africa and Asia, *S flexneri* predominates, and *S dysenteriae* often causes outbreaks. Shiga toxin is produced by *S dysenteriae* 1, which enhances virulence at the colonic mucosa and can cause small blood vessel and renal damage, leading to hemolytic uremic syndrome.

Epidemiology

Humans are the natural host for *Shigella* organisms, although other primates can be infected. The primary mode of transmission is fecal-oral, although transmission can also occur via contact with a contaminated inanimate object, ingestion of contaminated food or water, or sexual contact. Houseflies may also be vectors through physical transport of infected feces. Ingestion of as few as 10 organisms, depending on the species, is sufficient for infection to occur. Prolonged organism survival in water (up to 6 months) and food (up to 30 days) can occur with *Shigella.* Children 5 years or younger in child care settings and their caregivers, people living in crowded conditions, and men who have sex with men are at increased risk of infection. Infections attributable to *S flexneri, S boydii,* and *S dysenteriae* are more common in older children and adults than are infections attributable to *S sonnei* in the United States; nonetheless, more than 25% of cases caused by each species are reported among children younger than 5 years. Travel to resource-limited countries with inadequate sanitation can place travelers at risk of infection. Even without antimicrobial therapy, the carrier state usually ceases within 1 to 4 weeks after onset of illness; long-term carriage is uncommon and does not correlate with underlying intestinal dysfunction.

Incubation Period

1 to 3 days; range, 1 to 7 days.

Diagnostic Tests

Isolation of *Shigella* organisms from feces or rectal swab specimens containing feces is diagnostic; sensitivity is improved by testing stool as soon as possible after it is passed. The presence of fecal lactoferrin (or fecal leukocytes) demonstrated on a methylene-blue–stained stool smear is fairly sensitive for the diagnosis of colitis but is not specific for shigellosis. Although bacteremia is rare, blood should be cultured in children who are severely ill, immunocompromised, or malnourished. Multiplex polymerase chain reaction platforms for detection of multiple bacterial, viral, and parasitic pathogens, including *Shigella*, are commercially available.

Treatment

Although severe dehydration is rare with shigellosis, correction of fluid and electrolyte losses, preferably by oral rehydration solutions, is the mainstay of treatment. Most clinical infections with *S sonnei* are self-limited (48–72 hours), and mild episodes do not require antimicrobial therapy. Available evidence suggests antimicrobial therapy is somewhat effective in shortening duration of diarrhea and hastening eradication of organisms from feces. Treatment is recommended for patients with severe disease or with underlying immunosuppressive conditions; in these patients, empiric therapy should be given while awaiting culture and susceptibility results. Antimicrobial susceptibility testing of clinical isolates is indicated because resistance to antimicrobial agents is common and susceptibility data can guide appropriate therapy. In 2012 in the United States, approximately 25% of *Shigella* species were resistant to ampicillin, 43% were resistant to trimethoprim-sulfamethoxazole, 4% were resistant to azithromycin, 2% were resistant to ciprofloxacin, and 1.1% was resistant to ceftriaxone. Ciprofloxacin and ceftriaxone resistance is increasing around the world.

For cases in which treatment is required and susceptibilities are unknown or an ampicillin- and trimethoprim-sulfamethoxazole–resistant strain is isolated, parenteral ceftriaxone for 2 to 5 days, a fluoroquinolone (eg, ciprofloxacin) for 3 days, or azithromycin for 3 days should be administered. Oral cephalosporins (eg, cefixime) have been used successfully in treating shigellosis in adults. For susceptible strains, ampicillin or trimethoprim-sulfamethoxazole for 5 days is effective; amoxicillin is not effective because of its rapid absorption from the gastrointestinal tract. The oral route of therapy is recommended except for seriously ill patients.

Antidiarrheal compounds that inhibit intestinal peristalsis are contraindicated because they can prolong the clinical and bacteriologic course of disease and can increase the rate of complications.

Nutritional supplementation, including vitamin A and zinc orally daily, can be given to hasten clinical resolution in geographic areas where children are at risk of malnutrition.

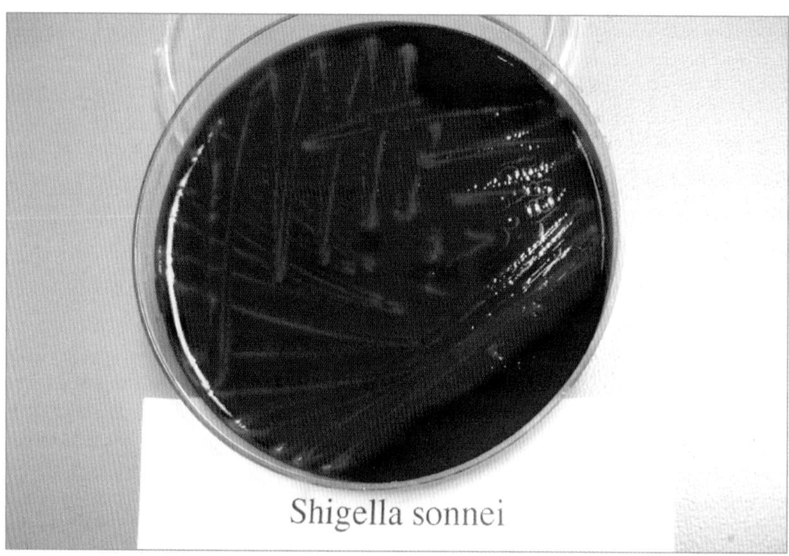

Image 123.1
Culture of *Shigella sonnei* grown on a blood agar plate. Courtesy of Rita Yee, MT(ASCP) SM.

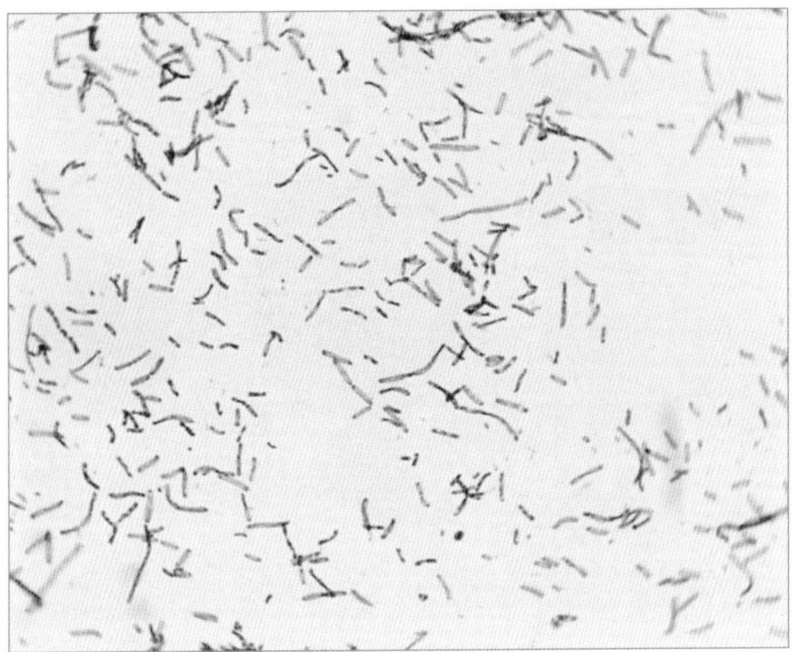

Image 123.2
Gram stain of *Shigella sonnei* from Image 123.1 (magnification x100). Courtesy of Rita Yee, MT(ASCP) SM.

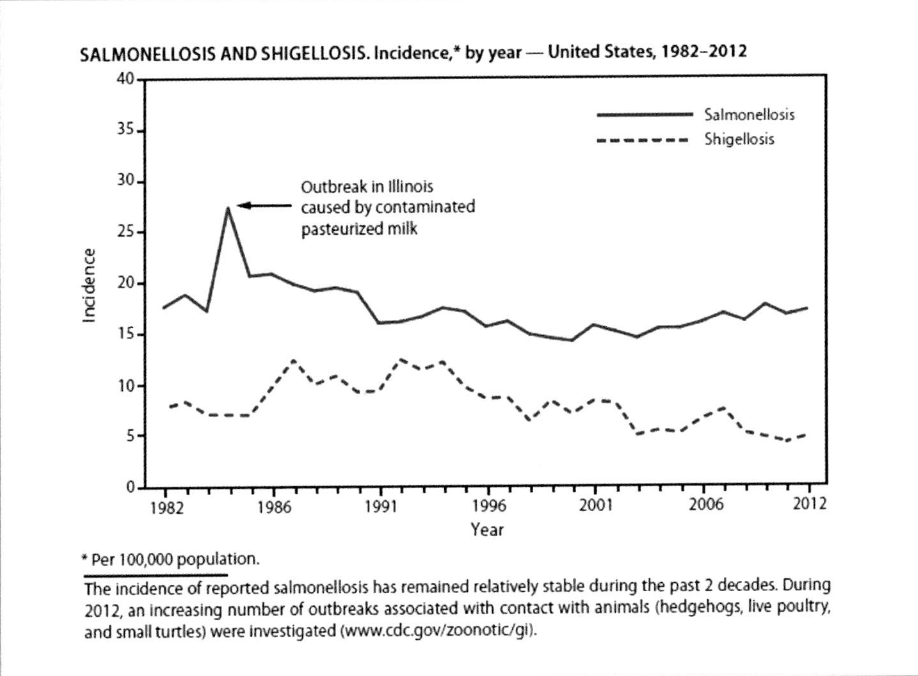

Image 123.3
Salmonellosis and shigellosis. Incidence, by year—United States, 1982–2012. Courtesy of *Morbidity and Mortality Weekly Report.*

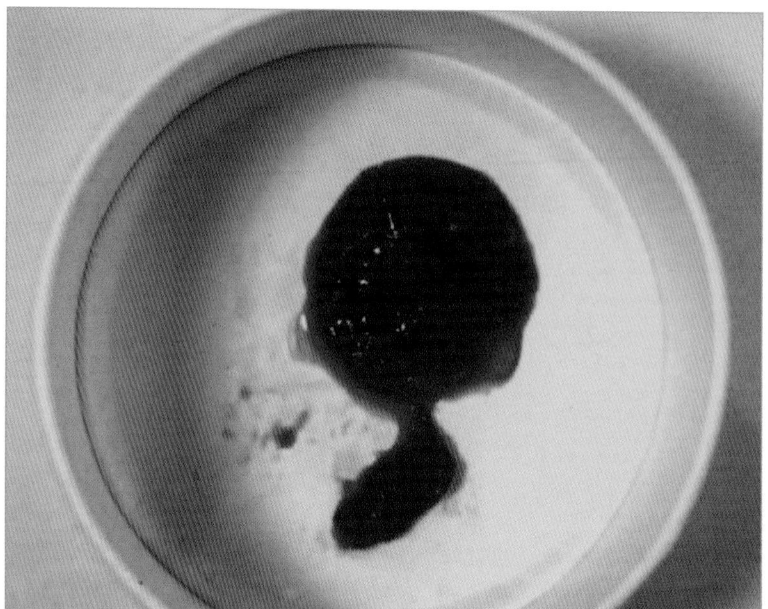

Image 123.4
Characteristic bloody mucoid stool of a child with shigellosis.

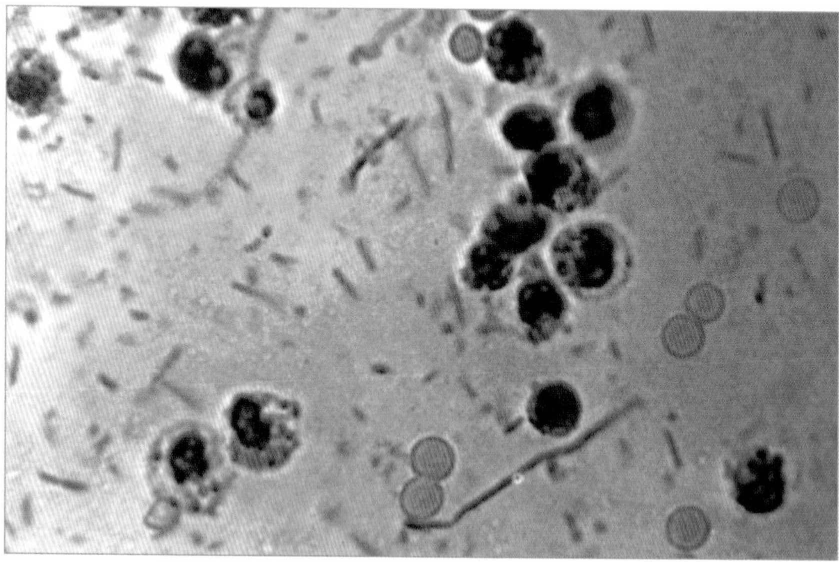

Image 123.5
Fecal leukocytes (shigellosis) (methylene-blue stain). The presence of fecal leukocytes suggests a bacterial diarrhea, although not specific for *Shigella* infection. Courtesy of Edgar O. Ledbetter, MD, FAAP.

124

Smallpox (Variola)

The last naturally occurring case of smallpox occurred in Somalia in 1977, followed by 2 cases in 1978 after a photographer was infected during a laboratory exposure and later transmitted smallpox to her mother in the United Kingdom. In 1980, the World Health Assembly declared that smallpox (variola virus) had been eradicated successfully worldwide. The United States discontinued routine childhood immunization against smallpox in 1972 and routine immunization of health care professionals in 1976. Immunization of US military personnel continued until 1990. Following eradication, 2 World Health Organization reference laboratories were authorized to maintain stocks of variola virus. As a result of terrorism events on September 11, 2001, and concern that the virus and the expertise to use it as a weapon of bioterrorism may have been misappropriated, the smallpox immunization policy was revisited. In 2002, the United States resumed immunization of military personnel deployed to certain areas of the world, and in 2003, the United States initiated a civilian smallpox immunization program for first responders to facilitate preparedness and response to a possible smallpox bioterrorism event.

Clinical Manifestations

People infected with variola major strains develop a severe prodromal illness characterized by high fever (38.9°C–40.0°C [102°F–104°F]) and constitutional symptoms, including malaise, severe headache, backache, abdominal pain, and prostration, lasting for 2 to 5 days. Infected children can suffer from vomiting and seizures during this prodromal period. Most patients with smallpox are severely ill and bedridden during the febrile prodrome. The prodromal period is followed by development of lesions on mucosa of the mouth or pharynx, which may not be noticed by the patient. This stage occurs less than 24 hours before onset of rash, which is usually the first recognized manifestation of infectiousness. With onset of oral lesions, the patient becomes infectious and remains so until all skin crust lesions have separated. The rash typically begins on the face and rapidly progresses to involve the forearms, trunk, and legs, with the greatest concentration of lesions on the face and distal extremities. Most patients will have lesions on the palms and soles. With rash onset, fever decreases but does not resolve. Lesions begin as macules that progress to papules, followed by firm vesicles and then deep-seated, hard pustules described as "pearls of pus." Each stage lasts 1 to 2 days. By the sixth or seventh day of rash, lesions may begin to umbilicate or become confluent. Lesions increase in size for approximately 8 to 10 days, after which they begin to crust. Once all the crusts have separated, 3 to 4 weeks after the onset of rash, the patient is no longer infectious. Variola minor strains cause a disease that is indistinguishable clinically from variola major, except it causes less severe systemic symptoms, more rapid rash evolution, reduced scarring, and fewer fatalities.

Varicella (chickenpox) is the condition most likely to be mistaken for smallpox. Generally, children with varicella do not have a febrile prodrome, but adults can have a brief, mild prodrome. Although the 2 diseases are confused easily in the first few days of the rash, smallpox lesions develop into pustules that are firm and deeply embedded in the dermis, whereas varicella lesions develop into superficial vesicles. Because varicella erupts in crops of lesions that evolve quickly, lesions on any one part of the body will be in different stages of evolution (papules, vesicles, and crusts), whereas all smallpox lesions on any one part of the body are in the same stage of development. The rash distribution of the 2 diseases differs; varicella most commonly affects the face and trunk, with relative sparing of the extremities, and lesions on the palms or soles are rare.

Variola major in unimmunized people is associated with case-fatality rates of 30% during epidemics of smallpox. The mortality rate is highest in pregnant women, children younger than 1 year, and adults older than 30 years.

In addition to the typical presentation of smallpox (≥90% of cases), there are 2 uncommon forms of variola major: hemorrhagic (characterized by a hemorrhagic diathesis prior to onset of the typical smallpox rash [early hemorrhagic smallpox] or by hemorrhage into skin lesions and disseminated intravascular coagulation [late hemorrhagic smallpox]) and malignant or flat type (in which the skin lesions do not progress to the pustular stage but remain flat and soft). Each variant occurs in approximately 5% of cases and is associated with a 95% to 100% mortality rate.

Etiology

Variola is a member of the Poxviridae family (genus *Orthopoxvirus*). Other members of this genus that can infect humans include monkeypox virus, cowpox virus, and vaccinia virus. In 2003, an outbreak of monkeypox linked to prairie dogs exposed to rodents imported from Ghana occurred in the United States.

Epidemiology

Humans are the only natural reservoir for variola virus (smallpox). Smallpox is spread most commonly in droplets from the oropharynx of infected people, although rare transmission from aerosol spread has been reported. Infection from direct contact with lesion material or indirectly via fomites, such as clothing and bedding, has also been reported. Because most patients with smallpox are extremely ill and bedridden, spread is generally limited to household contacts and health care professionals. Secondary household attack rates for smallpox were considerably lower than for measles and similar to or lower than rates for varicella.

Incubation Period

7 to 17 days; mean, 12 days.

Diagnostic Tests

Variola virus can be detected in vesicular or pustular fluid by a number of different methods, including electron microscopy, immunohistochemistry, culture, or polymerase chain reaction assay. Only polymerase chain reaction assay can diagnose infection with variola virus definitively; all other methods simply screen for orthopoxviruses. Diagnostic evaluation includes exclusion of varicella-zoster virus or other common conditions that cause a vesicular or pustular rash illness.

Treatment

There is no known effective antiviral therapy available to treat smallpox. Infected patients should receive supportive care. Cidofovir, a nucleotide analogue of cytosine, has demonstrated antiviral activity against certain orthopoxviruses in vitro and in animal models. Its effectiveness in treatment of variola in humans is unknown.

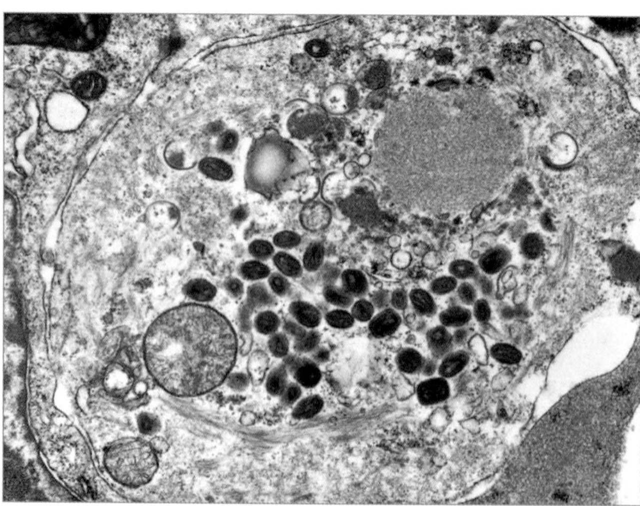

Image 124.1
A transmission electron micrograph of a tissue section containing variola virus. Smallpox is a serious, highly contagious, and, sometimes, fatal infectious disease. There is no specific treatment for smallpox disease, and the only prevention is vaccination. Courtesy of Centers for Disease Control and Prevention/Fred Murphy; Sylvia Whitfield.

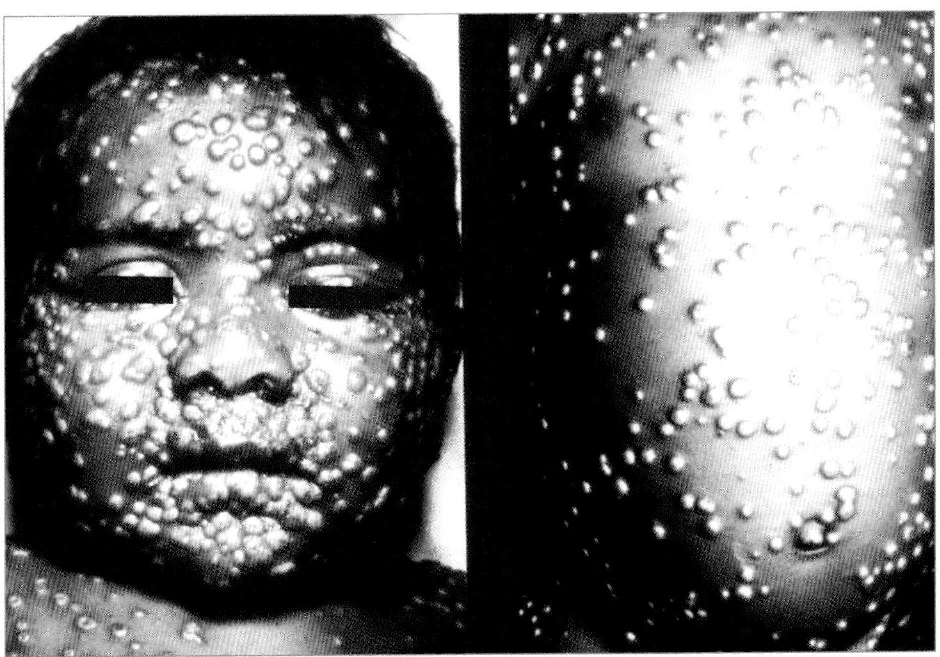

Image 124.2
Smallpox in a 2-year-old boy demonstrating commonplace greater density of lesions on the face as compared with the child's body. Courtesy of Paul Wehrle, MD.

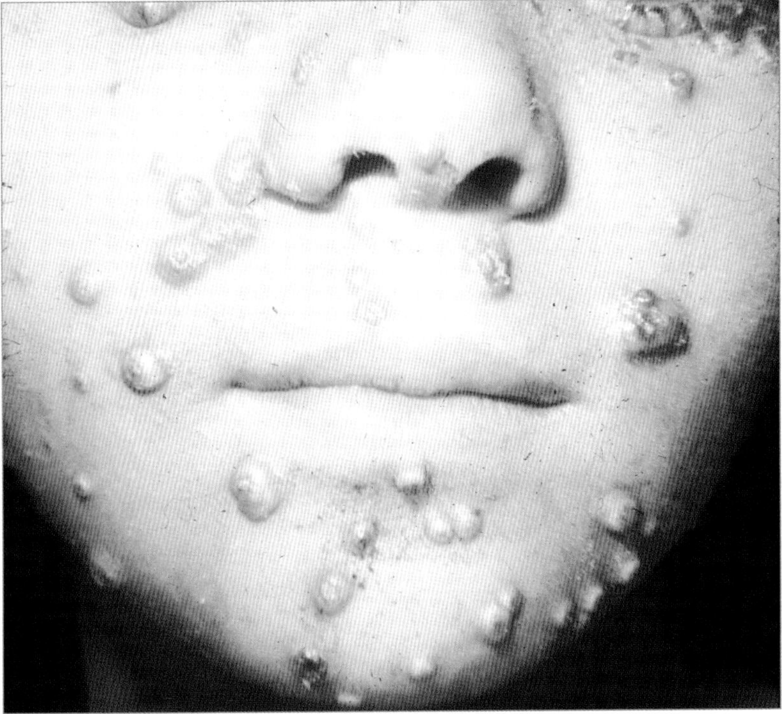

Image 124.3
Variola minor lesions on the face of a 2-year-old Latin American boy. Courtesy of Paul Wehrle, MD.

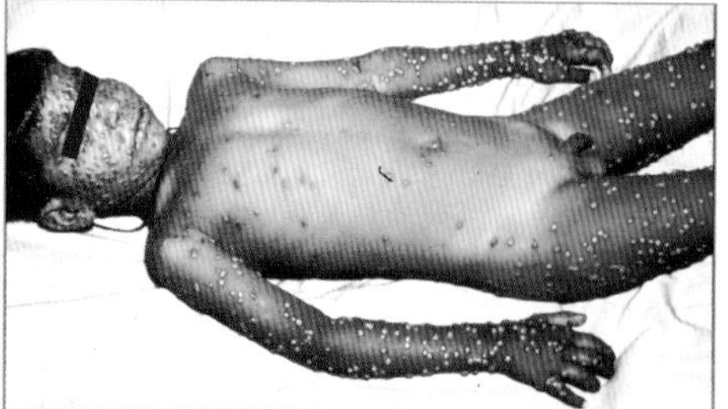

Image 124.4
A 7-year-old boy residing in India with smallpox lesions in a typical centripetal distribution. Courtesy of Paul Wehrle, MD.

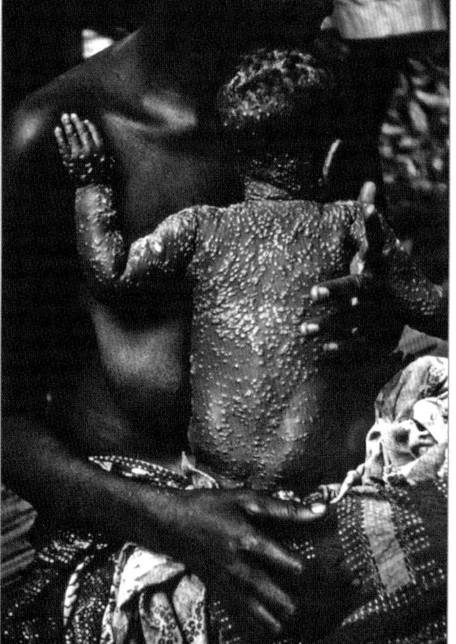

Image 124.6
This photograph reveals the back of a Nigerian child with smallpox. Note the pustules are centripetal in distribution, radiating from their densest area of eruption on the upper back and outward along the extremities. All the skin lesions are at the same stage of development. Courtesy of Centers for Disease Control and Prevention/ Dr Lyle Conrad.

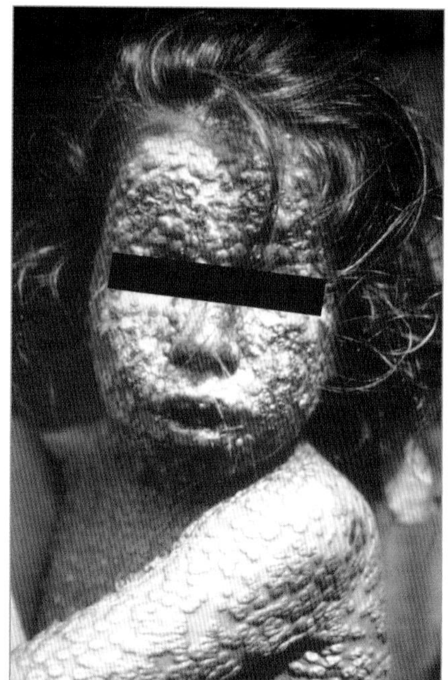

Image 124.5
This young girl in Bangladesh was infected with smallpox in 1973. Freedom from smallpox was declared in Bangladesh in December 1977 when a World Health Organization International Commission officially certified that smallpox had been eradicated from that country. Courtesy of Centers for Disease Control and Prevention/ James Hicks.

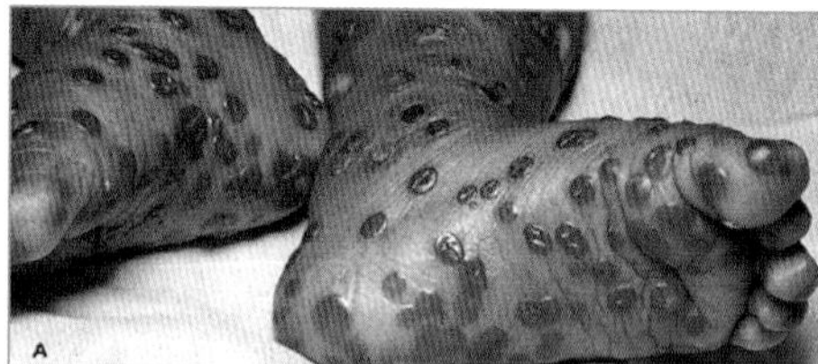

Image 124.7
Numerous healing smallpox lesions on the feet of a young child. Courtesy of Edgar O. Ledbetter, MD, FAAP.

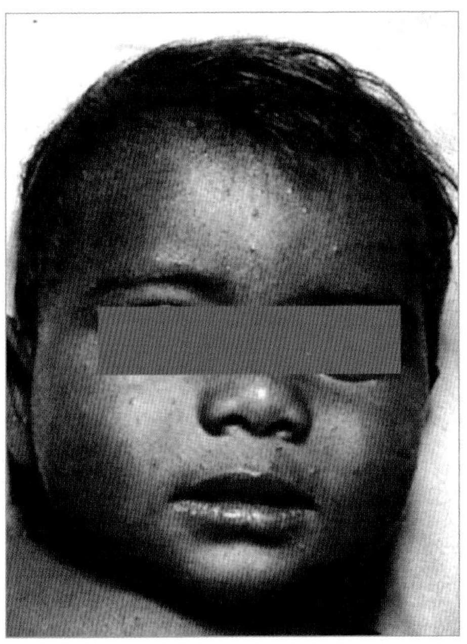

Image 124.8
Day 2 of smallpox eruption in a young child. Courtesy of Centers for Disease Control and Prevention.

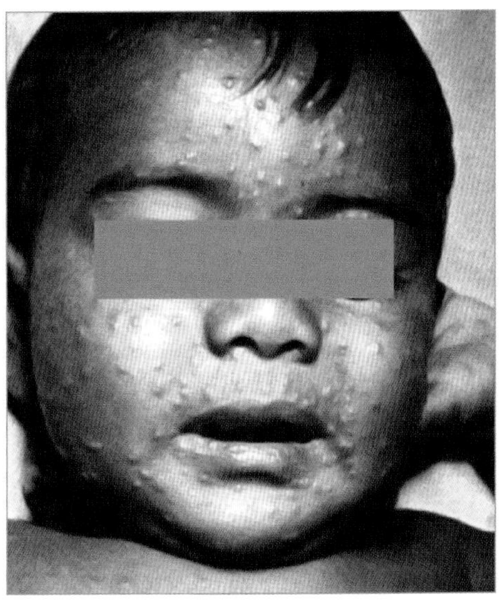

Image 124.9
Day 4 of smallpox eruption in a young child. People with smallpox become infectious with the onset of exanthema and remain most infectious throughout the initial 7 to 10 days of the rash. Courtesy of Centers for Disease Control and Prevention.

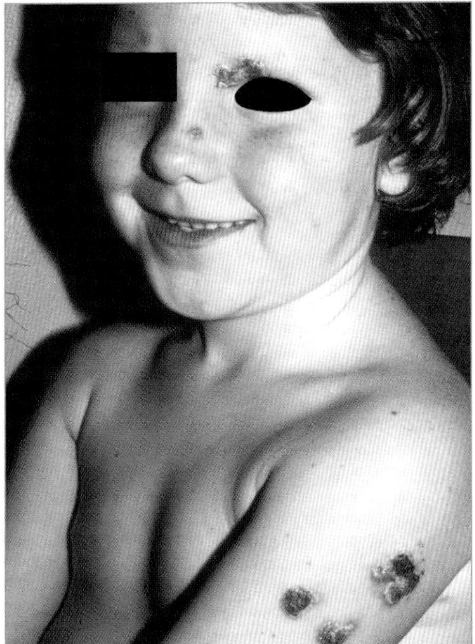

Image 124.10
Multiple secondary vaccinia lesions from autoinoculation in a 5-year-old white girl, one of the more common complications of smallpox vaccination. Courtesy of George Nankervis, MD.

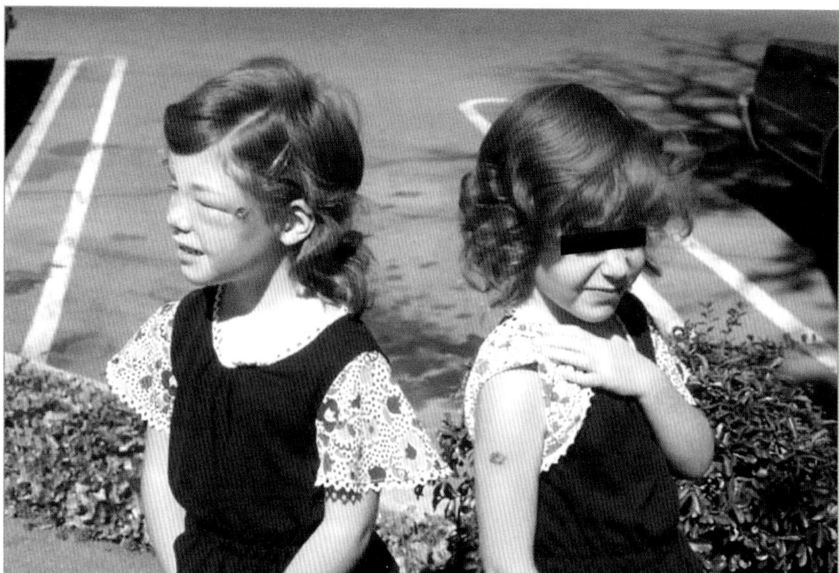

Image 124.11
The child on the left has a contact vaccinia lesion next to her left eye from her twin sister (August 24, 1974; photographed August 31, 1974). After receiving a smallpox vaccination, it is imperative the recipient take precautions to avoid transmitting the virus to another person, called contact vaccinia, or to other regions of his or her own body, called autoinoculation. Courtesy of Centers for Disease Control and Prevention/James Mitchell, MD/California Emergency Preparedness Office (Calif/EPO).

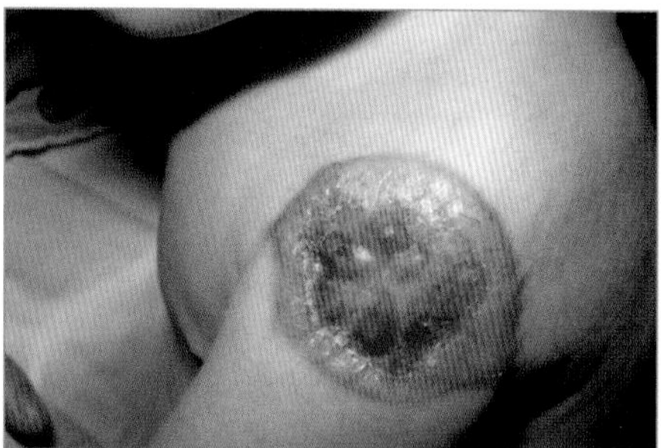

Image 124.12
Due to progressive vaccinia, this patient required a graft to correct the necrotic vaccination site. Progressive vaccinia (formerly called vaccinia gangrenosum) is one of the most severe complications of smallpox vaccination, and it is almost always life-threatening. Those who are most susceptible to this condition are the immunosuppressed. Courtesy of Centers for Disease Control and Prevention/Allen W. Mathies, MD/California Emergency Preparedness Office (Calif/EPO), Immunization Branch.

125

Sporotrichosis

Clinical Manifestations

There are 3 cutaneous patterns described for sporotrichosis. The classic lymphocutaneous process with multiple nodules is most commonly seen in adults. Inoculation occurs at a site of minor trauma, causing a painless papule that enlarges slowly to become a nodular lesion that can develop a violaceous hue or can ulcerate. Secondary lesions follow the same evolution and develop along the lymphatic distribution proximal to the initial lesion. A localized cutaneous form of sporotrichosis, also called fixed cutaneous form, is most commonly seen in children and presents as a solitary crusted papule or papuloulcerative or nodular lesion in which lymphatic spread is not observed. The extremities and face are the most common sites of infection. A disseminated cutaneous form with multiple lesions is rare, usually occurring in children who are immunocompromised.

Extracutaneous sporotrichosis is uncommon, with cases occurring primarily in immunocompromised patients or, in adults, those who are alcoholic or have chronic obstructive pulmonary disease. Osteoarticular infection results from hematogenous spread or local inoculation. The most commonly affected joints are the knee, elbow, wrist, and ankle. Pulmonary sporotrichosis clinically resembles tuberculosis and occurs after inhalation or aspiration of aerosolized conidia. Disseminated disease generally occurs after hematogenous spread from primary skin or lung infection. Disseminated sporotrichosis can involve multiple foci (eg, eyes, pericardium, genitourinary tract, central nervous system) and occurs predominantly in immunocompromised patients. Pulmonary and disseminated forms of sporotrichosis are uncommon in children.

Etiology

Sporothrix schenckii is a thermally dimorphic fungus that grows as a mold or mycelial form at room temperature and as a yeast at 35°C to 37°C (95°F–99°F) and in host tissues. *S schenckii* is a complex of at least 6 species. The related species *Sporothrix brasiliensis*, *Sporothrix globosa*, and *Sporothrix mexicana* also cause human infection.

Epidemiology

S schenckii is a ubiquitous organism that has worldwide distribution but is most common in tropical and subtropical regions of Central and South America and parts of North America and Japan. The fungus is isolated from soil and plant material, including hay, straw, sphagnum moss, and decaying vegetation. Thorny plants, such as roses and Christmas trees, are commonly implicated because pricks from their thorns or needles inoculate the organism from the soil or moss around the bush or tree. People engaging in gardening or farming are at risk of infection. Inhalation of conidia can lead to pulmonary disease. Zoonotic spread from infected cats or scratches from digging animals, such as armadillos, has led to cutaneous disease.

Incubation Period

7 to 30 days after cutaneous inoculation, but can be as long as 3 months.

Diagnostic Tests

Culture of *Sporothrix* species from a tissue, wound drainage, or sputum specimen is diagnostic. Culture of *Sporothrix* species from a blood specimen is definite evidence for the disseminated form of infection associated with immunodeficiency. Histopathologic examination of tissue may not be helpful because the organism seldom is abundant. Special fungal stains to visualize the oval or cigar-shaped organism are required. Serologic testing and polymerase chain reaction assay show promise for accurate and specific diagnosis but are available only in research laboratories.

Treatment

Sporotrichosis does not usually resolve without treatment. Itraconazole is the drug of choice for children with lymphocutaneous and localized cutaneous disease. The duration of therapy is 2 to 4 weeks after all lesions have resolved. Saturated solution of potassium iodide is an alternative therapy. Oral fluconazole should be used only if the patient cannot tolerate other agents.

Amphotericin B is recommended as the initial therapy for visceral or disseminated sporotrichosis in children. After clinical response to amphotericin B therapy is documented, itraconazole can be substituted and should be continued for at least 12 months. Itraconazole may be required for lifelong therapy in children with HIV infection. Pulmonary and disseminated infections respond less well than cutaneous infection, despite prolonged therapy. Surgical debridement or excision may be necessary to resolve cavitary pulmonary disease.

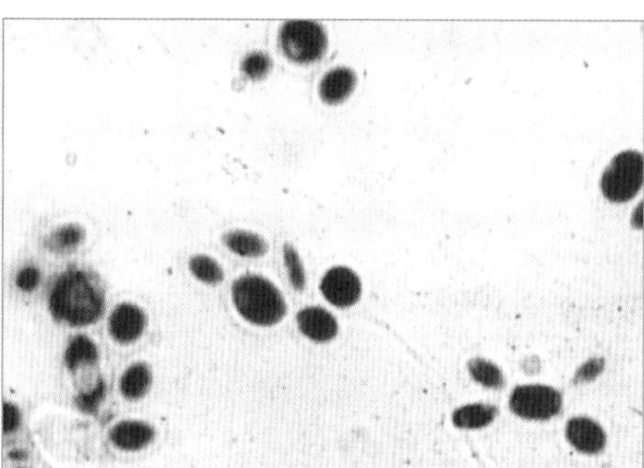

Image 125.1
This micrograph is taken from a slant culture of *Sporothrix schenckii* during its yeast phase. Courtesy of Centers for Disease Control and Prevention/Dr Lucille K. Georg.

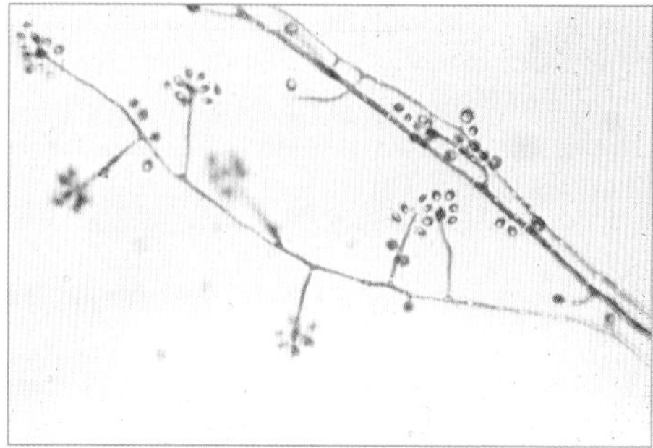

Image 125.2
Sporothrix schenckii, mold phase (48-hour potato dextrose agar, lactophenol cotton blue preparation); small tear-shaped conidia forming rosette-like clusters. Courtesy of Centers for Disease Control and Prevention.

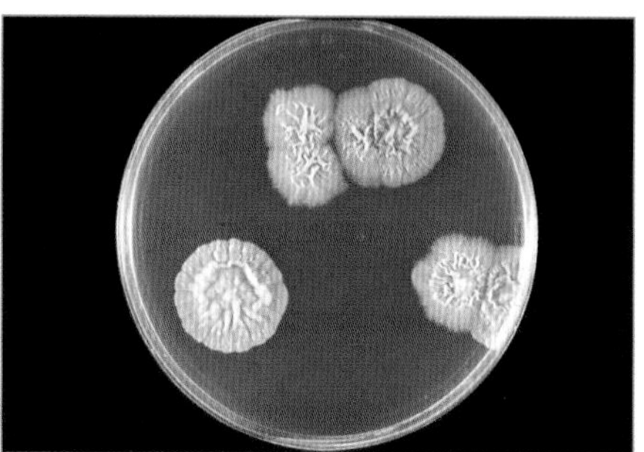

Image 125.3
This is an image of a Sabhi agar plate culture of *Sporothrix schenckii* grown at 20°C (68°F). *S schenckii* is the causative agent for the fungal infection sporotrichosis, also known as "rose handler's disease," which affects individuals who handle thorny plants, sphagnum moss, or baled hay. Courtesy of Centers for Disease Control and Prevention.

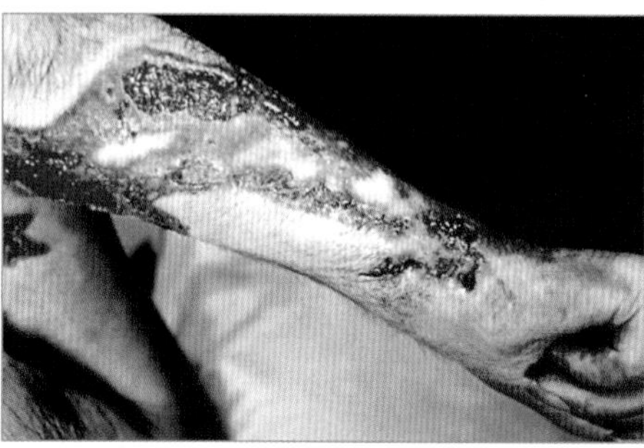

Image 125.4
This patient's arm shows the effects of the fungal disease sporotrichosis, caused by the fungus *Sporothrix schenckii*. Courtesy of Centers for Disease Control and Prevention/Dr Lucille K. Georg.

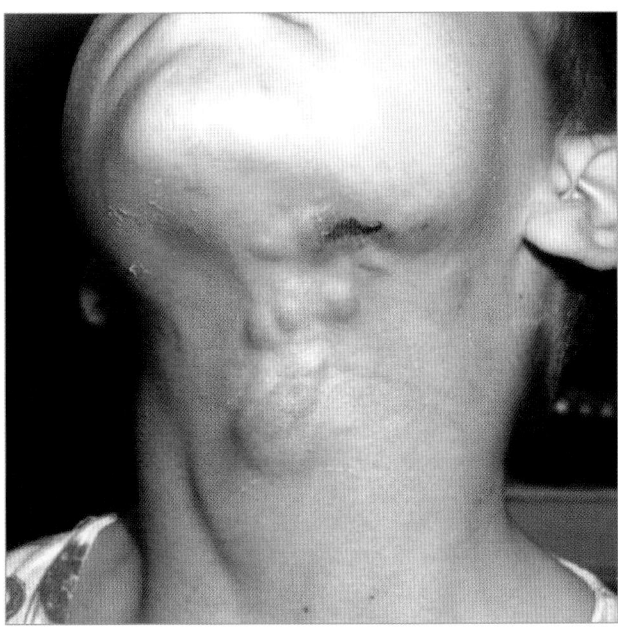

Image 125.5
Sporothrix schenckii was cultured from the biopsy specimen from an abscessed cervical lymph node of this 10-year-old boy. Test results on stained smears of purulent material aspirated from a cervical lymph node were negative.

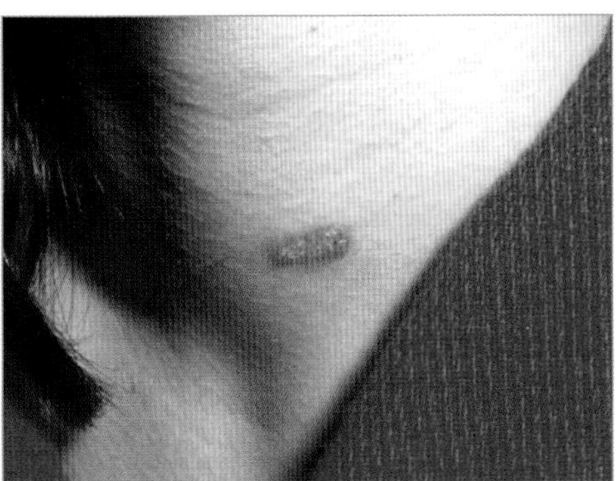

Image 125.6
Anterior cervical sporotrichosis lesions of an adolescent sister of the patient in Image 125.5.

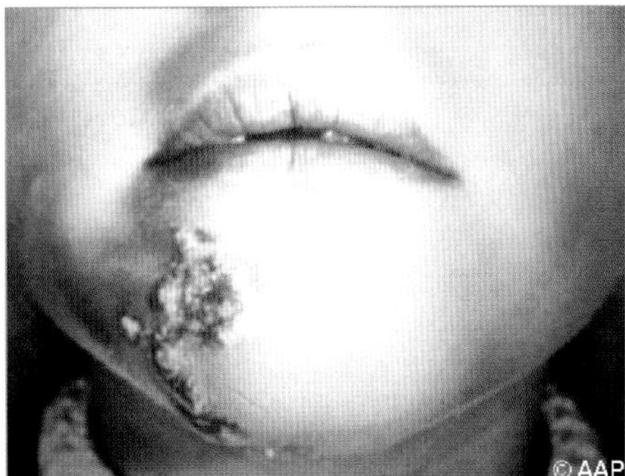

Image 125.7
Cutaneous sporotrichosis of the face in a preschool-aged child. Courtesy of Edgar O. Ledbetter, MD, FAAP.

126

Staphylococcal Infections

Clinical Manifestations

Staphylococcus aureus

Staphylococcus aureus causes a variety of localized and invasive suppurative infections and 3 toxin-mediated syndromes: toxic shock syndrome (TSS), scalded skin syndrome, and food poisoning. Localized infections include cellulitis, skin and soft tissue abscesses, pustulosis, impetigo (bullous and nonbullous), paronychia, mastitis, ecthyma, erythroderma, hordeola, furuncles, carbuncles, peritonsillar abscesses (quinsy), omphalitis, parotitis, lymphadenitis, and wound infections. *S aureus* also causes invasive infections with bacteremia associated with foreign bodies, including intravascular catheters or grafts, peritoneal catheters, cerebrospinal fluid (CSF) shunts, spinal instrumentation or intramedullary rods, pressure equalization tubes, pacemakers and other intracardiac devices, and prosthetic joints. Bacteremia can be complicated by septicemia; osteomyelitis; arthritis; endocarditis; pneumonia; pleural empyema; pericarditis; soft tissue, muscle, or visceral abscesses; septic thrombophlebitis of small and large vessels; and other foci of infection. Primary *S aureus* pneumonia can also occur after aspiration of organisms from the upper respiratory tract and is typically associated with mechanical ventilation or viral infections in the community (eg, influenza). Meningitis is rare unless accompanied by an intradermal foreign body (eg, ventriculoperitoneal shunt) or a congenital or acquired defect in the dura. *S aureus* infections can be fulminant and are often associated with metastatic foci and abscess formation, requiring drainage, foreign body removal, and prolonged antimicrobial therapy to achieve cure. Certain chronic diseases, such as diabetes mellitus, malignancy, prematurity, immunodeficiency, nutritional disorders, surgery, and transplantation, increase the risk for severe *S aureus* infections.

Staphylococcal TSS, a toxin-mediated disease, is caused by strains producing TSS toxin-1 or possibly other related staphylococcal enterotoxins. Toxic shock syndrome toxin-1 acts as a superantigen that stimulates production of tumor necrosis factor and other mediators that cause capillary leak, leading to hypotension and multiorgan failure. Staphylococcal TSS is characterized by acute onset of fever, generalized erythroderma, rapid-onset hypotension, and signs of multisystem organ involvement, including profuse watery diarrhea, vomiting, conjunctival injection, and severe myalgia (Box 126.1). Although approximately 50% of reported cases of staphylococcal TSS occur in menstruating females using tampons, nonmenstrual TSS cases occur after childbirth or abortion, after surgical procedures, and in association with cutaneous lesions. Toxic shock syndrome can also occur in males and females without a readily identifiable focus of infection. Prevailing clones (eg, USA300) of community-associated methicillin-resistant *S aureus* (MRSA) rarely produce TSS toxin. People with TSS, especially menses-associated illness, are at risk of a recurrent episode.

Staphylococcal scalded skin syndrome (SSSS) is a toxin-mediated disease caused by circulation of exfoliative toxins A and B. Manifestations of SSSS are age related and include Ritter disease (generalized exfoliation) in the neonate, a tender scarlatiniform eruption and localized bullous impetigo in older children, or a combination of these with thick white/brown flaky desquamation of the entire skin, especially on the face and neck, in older infants and toddlers. The hallmark of SSSS is the toxin-mediated cleavage of the stratum granulosum layer of the epidermis (ie, Nikolsky sign). Healing occurs without scarring. Bacteremia is rare, but dehydration and superinfection can occur with extensive exfoliation.

Coagulase-Negative Staphylococci

Most coagulase-negative staphylococci (CoNS) isolates from patient specimens represent contamination of culture material. Of the isolates that do not represent contamination, most come from infections associated with health care, such as patients with obvious disruptions of host defenses caused by surgery, medical device insertion, immunosuppression, or developmental maturity (eg, very low birth weight neonates). Coagulase-negative staphylococci are the most common cause of late-onset

Box 126.1
Staphylococcus aureus Toxic Shock Syndrome: Clinical Case Definition

Clinical Findings

- Fever: temperature 38.9°C (102.0°F) or greater
- Rash: diffuse macular erythroderma
- Desquamation: 1–2 wk after onset, particularly on palms, soles, fingers, and toes
- Hypotension: systolic pressure 90 mm Hg or less for adults; lower than fifth percentile for age for children younger than 16 y; orthostatic drop in diastolic pressure of 15 mm Hg or greater from lying to sitting; orthostatic syncope or orthostatic dizziness
- Multisystem organ involvement: 3 or more of
  1. Gastrointestinal tract: vomiting or diarrhea at onset of illness
  2. Muscular: severe myalgia or creatinine phosphokinase concentration greater than twice the upper limit of reference range
  3. Mucous membrane: vaginal, oropharyngeal, or conjunctival hyperemia
  4. Renal: serum urea nitrogen or serum creatinine concentration greater than twice the upper limit of reference range or urinary sediment with 5 white blood cells/high-power field or greater in the absence of urinary tract infection
  5. Hepatic: total bilirubin, aspartate transaminase, or alanine transaminase concentration greater than twice the upper limit of reference range
  6. Hematologic: platelet count 100,000/mm^3 or less
  7. Central nervous system: disorientation or alterations in consciousness without focal neurologic signs when fever and hypotension are absent

Laboratory Criteria

- **Negative** results on the following tests, if obtained:
  1. Blood, throat, or cerebrospinal fluid cultures; blood culture may be positive for *Staphylococcus aureus*
  2. Serologic tests for Rocky Mountain spotted fever, leptospirosis, or measles

Case Classification

- **Probable:** a case that meets the laboratory criteria and in which 4 of 5 clinical findings are present
- **Confirmed:** a case that meets laboratory criteria and all 5 of the clinical findings, including desquamation, unless the patient dies before desquamation occurs

Adapted from Wharton M, Chorba TL, Vogt RL, Morse DL, Buehler JW. Case definitions for public health surveillance. *MMWR Recomm Rep.* 1990;39(RR-13):1–43.

bacteremia and septicemia among preterm neonates, typically neonates weighing less than 1,500 g at birth, and of episodes of health care–associated bacteremia in all age groups. Coagulase-negative staphylococci are responsible for bacteremia in children with intravascular catheters or those with vascular grafts or intracardiac patches, prosthetic cardiac valves, or pacemaker wires. Infection may also occur associated with other indwelling foreign bodies, including CSF shunts, peritoneal catheters, or prosthetic joints. Mediastinitis after open-heart surgery, endophthalmitis after intraocular trauma, and omphalitis and scalp abscesses in preterm neonates have been described. Coagulase-negative staphylococci can also enter the bloodstream from the respiratory tract of mechanically ventilated preterm neonates or from the gastrointestinal tract of neonates with necrotizing enterocolitis. Some species of CoNS are associated with urinary tract infection, including *Staphylococcus saprophyticus* in adolescent females and young adult women, often after sexual intercourse, and *Staphylococcus epidermidis* and *Staphylococcus haemolyticus* in hospitalized patients with urinary tract catheters. In general, CoNS infections have an indolent clinical course in children with intact immune function, even in children who are immunocompromised.

Etiology

Staphylococci are catalase-positive, gram-positive cocci that appear microscopically as grapelike clusters. There are 32 species that are related closely on the basis of DNA base composition, but only 17 species are indigenous to humans. *S aureus* is the only species that produces coagulase, although not all *S aureus* produce coagulase. Of the 16 CoNS species, *S epidermidis, S haemolyticus, S saprophyticus, Staphylococcus schleiferi,* and *Staphylococcus lugdunensis* are most often associated with human infections. Staphylococci are ubiquitous and can survive extreme conditions of drying, heat, and low-oxygen and high-salt environments. *S aureus* has many surface proteins, including the microbial surface components recognizing adhesive matrix molecule receptors, which allow the organism to bind to tissues and foreign bodies coated with fibronectin, fibrinogen, and collagen. This permits a low inoculum of organisms to adhere to sutures, catheters, prosthetic valves, and other devices. Many CoNS produce an exopolysaccharide slime biofilm that makes these organisms, as they bind to medical devices (eg, catheters), relatively inaccessible to host defenses and antimicrobial agents.

Epidemiology

Staphylococcus aureus

S aureus, which is second only to CoNS as a cause of health care–associated bacteremia, is one of the most common causes of health care–associated pneumonia and is responsible for most health care–associated surgical site infections. *S aureus* colonizes the skin and mucous membranes of 30% to 50% of healthy adults and children. The anterior nares, throat, axilla, perineum, vagina, and rectum are usual sites of colonization. Rates of carriage of more than 50% occur in children with desquamating skin disorders or burns and in people with frequent needle use (eg, diabetes mellitus, hemodialysis, illicit drug use, allergy shots).

S aureus–mediated TSS was recognized in 1978, and many early cases were associated with tampon use. Although changes in tampon composition and use have resulted in a decreased proportion of cases associated with menses, menstrual and nonmenstrual cases of TSS continue to occur and are reported with similar frequency. Risk factors for TSS include absence of antibody to TSS toxin-1 and focal *S aureus* infection with a TSS toxin-1–producing strain. Toxic shock syndrome toxin-1–producing strains can be part of normal flora of the anterior nares or vagina, and colonization at these sites is believed to result in protective antibody in more than 90% of adults. Health care–associated TSS can occur and most often follows surgical procedures. In postoperative cases, the organism generally originates from the patient's own flora.

Transmission of *S aureus*

S aureus is most often transmitted by direct contact in community settings and indirectly from patient to patient via transiently colonized hands of health care professionals in health care settings. Health care professionals and family members who are colonized with *S aureus* in the nares or on skin can also serve as a reservoir for transmission. Contaminated environmental surfaces and objects can also play a role in transmission of *S aureus*, although their contribution for spread is probably minor. Although not routinely transmitted by the droplet route, *S aureus* can be dispersed into the air over short distances. Dissemination of *S aureus* from people with nasal carriage, including infants, is related to density of colonization, and increased dissemination occurs during viral upper respiratory tract infections. Additional risk factors for health care–associated acquisition of *S aureus* include illness requiring care in neonatal or pediatric intensive care or burn units, surgical procedures, prolonged hospitalization, local epidemic of *S aureus* infection, and the presence of indwelling catheters or prosthetic devices.

S aureus Colonization and Disease

Nasal, skin, vaginal, and rectal carriage are the primary reservoirs for *S aureus*. Although domestic animals can be colonized, data suggest colonization is acquired from humans. Adults who carry MRSA in the nose preoperatively are more likely to develop surgical site infections after general, cardiac, orthopedic, or solid organ transplant surgery than are patients who are not carriers. Heavy cutaneous colonization at an insertion site is the single most important predictor of intravenous catheter-related infections for short-term percutaneously inserted catheters. For hemodialysis patients with *S aureus* skin colonization, the incidence of central line–associated bloodstream infection is 6-fold higher than for patients without skin colonization. After head trauma, adults who are nasal carriers of *S aureus* are more likely to develop *S aureus* pneumonia than are noncolonized patients.

Health Care–Associated Methicillin-Resistant *S aureus* (MRSA)

Methicillin-resistant *S aureus* has been endemic in most US hospitals since the 1980s, recently accounting for more than 60% of health care–associated *S aureus* infections in intensive care units reported to the Centers for Disease Control and Prevention (CDC). Health care–associated MRSA strains are resistant to β-lactamase–resistant (BLR) β-lactam antimicrobial agents and cephalosporins (except the fifth-generation cephalosporin, ceftaroline), as well as to antimicrobial agents of several other classes (multidrug resistance). Methicillin-susceptible *S aureus* (MSSA) strains can be heterogeneous for methicillin resistance.

Risk factors for nasal carriage of health care–associated MRSA include hospitalization within the previous year, recent (within the previous 60 days) antimicrobial use, prolonged hospital stay, frequent contact with a health care environment, presence of an intravascular or peritoneal catheter or tracheal tube, increased number of surgical procedures, or frequent contact with a person with one or more of the preceding risk factors. A discharged patient known to have had colonization with MRSA should be assumed to have continued colonization when rehospitalized because carriage can persist for years.

Methicillin-resistant *S aureus,* health care– and community-associated strains, and methicillin-resistant CoNS are responsible for a large portion of infections acquired in health care settings. A review of 25 pediatric hospitals demonstrated a 10-fold increase in MRSA infections since 1999 without change in the frequency of MSSA infections. Health care–associated MRSA strains are difficult to treat because they are usually multidrug resistant and are predictably susceptible only to vancomycin, linezolid, and agents not approved by the US Food and Drug Administration for use in children.

Community-Associated MRSA

Unique clones of MRSA are responsible for community-associated infections in healthy children and adults without typical risk factors for health care–associated MRSA infections. The most frequent manifestation of community-associated MRSA infections is skin and soft tissue infection, but invasive disease also occurs. Antimicrobial susceptibility patterns of these strains differ from those of health care–associated MRSA strains. Although community-associated MRSA are resistant to all β-lactam antimicrobial agents except ceftaroline, they are typically susceptible to multiple other antimicrobial agents, including trimethoprim-sulfamethoxazole, gentamicin, and doxycycline; clindamycin susceptibility is variable. A review of prescribing patterns among 25 pediatric hospitals has demonstrated clindamycin to be the most commonly prescribed antimicrobial agent for non–life-threatening MRSA infections. However, attention to local resistance rates of *S aureus* to clindamycin is imperative because community-associated MRSA and MSSA isolates with intrinsic or inducible resistance to clindamycin exceeding 20% have been reported by some institutions. Community-associated MRSA infections have occurred in settings where there is crowding; frequent skin-to-skin contact; body piercing; sharing of personal items, such as towels and clothing; and poor personal hygiene, such as occurs among athletic teams, in correctional facilities, and in military training facilities. However, most community-associated MRSA infections occur in people without direct links to those settings, including healthy term neonates. Transmission of community-associated MRSA from an infected classmate or teammate has been described in child care centers and among sports teams, respectively. Although community-associated

MRSA arose from the community, in many health care settings, these clones are overtaking health care–associated MRSA strains as a cause of health care–associated MRSA infections, making usefulness of the epidemiologic terms "health care–associated" and "community-associated" of less value.

Vancomycin-Intermediate *S aureus*

Strains of MRSA with intermediate susceptibility to vancomycin (minimum inhibitory concentration [MIC], 4–8 mcg/mL) have been isolated from people (historically, dialysis patients) who had received multiple courses of vancomycin for a MRSA infection. Extensive vancomycin use allows vancomycin-intermediate *S aureus* (VISA) strains to develop. These strains may emerge during therapy. Control measures recommended by the CDC have included using proper methods to detect VISA, using appropriate infection-control measures, and adopting measures to ensure appropriate vancomycin use. Although rare, outbreaks of VISA and heteroresistant VISA have been reported in France, Spain, and Japan.

Vancomycin-Resistant *S aureus*

In 2002, two isolates of vancomycin-resistant *S aureus* (VRSA [MIC, ≥16 mcg/mL]) were identified in adults from 2 different states. As of May 2014, VRSA had been isolated in 13 adults from 4 states. Each of these adults with VRSA infections had underlying medical conditions, a history of MRSA infections, and prolonged exposure to vancomycin. No spread of VRSA beyond case patients has been documented. A concern is that most automated antimicrobial susceptibility testing methods commonly used in the United States were unable to detect vancomycin resistance in these isolates.

Coagulase-Negative Staphylococci

Coagulase-negative staphylococci are common inhabitants of the skin and mucous membranes. Virtually all neonates have colonization at multiple sites by 2 to 4 days of age. The most frequently isolated CoNS organism is *S epidermidis*. Different species colonize specific areas of the body. *S haemolyticus* is found on areas of skin with numerous apocrine glands. The frequency of health care–associated CoNS infections increased steadily until 2000, when these infections seem to have plateaued. Newborns, infants, and children in intensive care units, including neonatal intensive care units, have the highest incidence of CoNS bloodstream infections. Coagulase-negative staphylococci can be introduced at the time of medical device placement, through mucous membrane or skin breaks, through loss of bowel wall integrity (eg, necrotizing enterocolitis in very low birth weight neonates), or during catheter manipulation. Less often, health care professionals with environmental CoNS colonization on hands transmit the organism. The roles of the environment or fomites in CoNS transmission are not known.

Most CoNS strains are methicillin resistant and account for health care–associated infections associated with indwelling foreign bodies and in the neonatal population. Methicillin-resistant strains are resistant to all β-lactam drugs, including cephalosporins (except ceftaroline), and, usually, several other drug classes. Once these strains become endemic in a hospital, eradication is difficult, even when strict infection-prevention practices are followed.

Incubation Period

Variable. For toxin-mediated SSSS, 1 to 10 days; for postoperative TSS, as short as 12 hours. Menstrual-related cases can develop at any time during menses.

Diagnostic Tests

Gram-stained smears of material from skin lesions or pyogenic foci showing gram-positive cocci in clusters can provide presumptive evidence of infection. Isolation of organisms from culture of otherwise sterile body fluid is the method for definitive diagnosis. Newer molecular assays are available for direct detection of *S aureus* from blood culture bottles. Non-amplified molecular assays, such as peptide nucleic acid fluorescent in situ hybridization, and nucleic acid amplification tests, such as BD GeneOhm Staph SR (BD Molecular Diagnostics) and Xpert MRSA/SA BC (Cepheid), are approved for detection and identification of *S aureus*, including MRSA, in positive blood cultures. *S aureus* is almost never a contaminant when isolated from a blood culture. Coagulase-negative staphylococci isolated from a single blood culture are commonly dismissed as "contaminants." In a very preterm neonate (ie, <32 weeks' gestation), an immunocompromised person, or a patient with an indwelling catheter or prosthetic device, repeated isolation of the same strain of CoNS (by antimicrobial susceptibility results or molecular techniques) from blood cultures or another normally sterile body fluid suggests true infection, but genotyping more strongly supports the diagnosis. For central line–associated bloodstream infection, quantitative blood cultures from the catheter will have 5 to 10 times more organisms than cultures from a peripheral blood vessel. Criteria that suggest CoNS as pathogens rather than contaminants include

- Two or more positive blood cultures from different collection sites
- A single positive culture from blood and another sterile site (eg, CSF, joint) with identical antimicrobial susceptibility patterns for each isolate
- Growth in a continuously monitored blood culture system within 15 hours of incubation
- Clinical findings of infection
- An intravascular catheter that has been in place for 3 days or more
- Similar or identical genotypes among all isolates

S aureus–mediated TSS is a clinical diagnosis. *S aureus* grows in culture of blood specimens from fewer than 5% of patients with TSS. Specimens for culture should be obtained from an identified focal site of infection because these sites will usually yield the organism. Because approximately one-third of isolates of *S aureus* from nonmenstrual cases produce toxins other than TSS toxin-1, and TSS toxin-1–producing organisms can be present as normal flora, TSS-1 production by an isolate is not useful diagnostically.

Quantitative antimicrobial susceptibility testing should be performed for all staphylococci, including CoNS, isolated from normally sterile sites. Health care–associated MRSA heterogeneous or heterotypic strains appear susceptible by disk testing. However, when a parent strain is cultured on methicillin-containing media, resistant subpopulations are apparent.

A large proportion of community-associated *S aureus* strains are methicillin resistant, and a high percentage (>90% in some centers) of health care–associated *S aureus* from children are methicillin and multidrug resistant. More than 90% of health care–associated CoNS strains are methicillin-resistant. Because of the high rates of community-associated MRSA infections in the United States, clindamycin has become an often-used drug for treatment of nonlife-threatening presumed *S aureus* infections. Routine antimicrobial susceptibility testing of *S aureus* strains historically did not include a method to detect strains susceptible to clindamycin that rapidly become clindamycin-resistant when exposed to this agent. This clindamycin-inducible resistance can be detected by the D zone test. When a MRSA isolate is determined to be erythromycin resistant and clindamycin susceptible by routine methods, the D zone test is performed. Many automated platforms for susceptibility testing now include testing for inducible clindamycin resistance. Methicillin-resistant *S aureus* isolates that demonstrate clindamycin-inducible resistance will be reported by the laboratory as clindamycin resistant, and the patient should not be treated with clindamycin. All *S aureus* strains with an MIC to vancomycin of 4 mcg/mL or greater should be confirmed and further characterized. Early detection of VISA is critical to trigger aggressive infection-control measures (Box 126.2).

S aureus and CoNS strain genotyping has become a necessary adjunct for determining whether several isolates from one patient or from different patients are the same. Typing, in conjunction with epidemiologic information, can facilitate identification of the source, extent, and mechanism of transmission in an outbreak. Antimicrobial susceptibility testing is the most readily available method for typing by a phenotypic characteristic. A number of

Box 126.2
Recommendations for Detecting *Staphylococcus aureus* With Decreased Susceptibility to Vancomycin

Definitions

- **Vancomycin-susceptible *S aureus***
  MIC ≤2 mcg/mL
- **VISA**
  MIC 4–8 mcg/mL
  Not transferable to susceptible strains
- **VRSA**
  MIC ≥16 mcg/mL
  Potentially transferable to susceptible strains
- **Confirmation of VISA and VRSA**
  Possible VISA and VRSA isolates should be retested using vancomycin screen plates or a validated MIC method.
  VISA and VRSA isolates should be reported to the local health department or CDC.

Abbreviations: CDC, Centers for Disease Control and Prevention; MIC, minimum inhibitory concentration; VISA, vancomycin-intermediate *Staphylococcus aureus;* VRSA, vancomycin-resistant *Staphylococcus aureus.*

For information on control of spread of VISA and VRSA, e-mail **SEARCH@cdc.gov** or visit **www.cdc.gov/hai**.

molecular typing methods are available for *S aureus.* The primary method currently used by the CDC is pulsed-field gel electrophoresis.

Treatment

Skin and Soft Tissue Infection

Skin and soft tissue infections, such as diffuse impetigo or cellulitis attributable to MSSA, can be treated with oral penicillinase-resistant β-lactam drugs, such as a first- or second-generation cephalosporin. However, the continued increase in prevalence of community-associated MRSA throughout the United States limits the utility of β-lactams as empirical agents. For the penicillin-allergic patient and in cases in which MRSA is considered, trimethoprim-sulfamethoxazole, doxycycline in children 8 years and older, or clindamycin can be used if the isolate is susceptible. Trimethoprim-sulfamethoxazole should not be used as a single agent in the initial treatment of cellulitis. Topical mupirocin is recommended for localized impetigo.

The most frequent manifestation of community-associated MRSA infection is skin and soft tissue infection. Image 126.1 shows the initial management of skin and soft tissue infections suspected to be caused by community-associated MRSA. For patients with complicated skin and soft tissue infection with abscess, drainage or debridement and systemic antibiotic therapy are warranted; therapy should be focused on the pathogen identified.

Invasive Staphylococcal Infections

Empirical therapy for serious suspected staphylococcal infection is vancomycin plus a semisynthetic β-lactam (eg, nafcillin). Clindamycin is bacteriostatic and should not be used for initial treatment of endovascular infection. Serious MSSA infections require intravenous therapy with a BLR β-lactam antimicrobial agent, such as nafcillin or oxacillin, because most *S aureus* strains produce β-lactamase enzymes and are resistant to penicillin and ampicillin (Table 126.1). Vancomycin is not recommended for treatment of serious MSSA infections because outcomes are inferior compared with cases in which antistaphylococcal β-lactams are used and to minimize emergence of vancomycin resistance. First- or second-generation cephalosporins (eg, cefazolin) or vancomycin are less effective than nafcillin or oxacillin for treatment of MSSA endocarditis or meningitis. A patient with MSSA infection (and no evidence of endocarditis or central nervous system [CNS] infection) who has a nonserious allergy to

Table 126.1

Parenteral Antimicrobial Agent(s) for Treatment of Bacteremia and Other Serious *Staphylococcus aureus* Infections

Susceptibility	Antimicrobial Agents	Comments
I. Initial empiric therapy (organism of unknown susceptibility)		
Drugs of choice	Vancomycin (15 mg/kg, every 6 h) + nafcillin or oxacillin	For life-threatening infections (ie, septicemia, endocarditis, CNS infection); linezolid could be substituted for vancomycin if the patient has received several recent courses of vancomycin.
	Vancomycin (15 mg/kg, every 6–8 h)	For nonlife-threatening infection without signs of sepsis (eg, skin infection, cellulitis, osteomyelitis, pyarthrosis) when rates of MRSA colonization and infection in the community are substantial
	Clindamycin	For nonlife-threatening infection without signs of sepsis when rates of MRSA colonization and infection in the community are substantial and prevalence of clindamycin resistance is low
II. Methicillin-susceptible, penicillin-resistant *S aureus*		
Drugs of choice	Nafcillin or oxacillin[a]	
	Cefazolin	
Alternatives	Clindamycin	Only for patients with a serious penicillin allergy and clindamycin-susceptible strain
	Vancomycin	Only for patients with a serious penicillin and cephalosporin allergy
	Ampicillin + sulbactam	For patients with polymicrobial infections caused by susceptible isolates
III. MRSA (oxacillin MIC, ≥4 mcg/mL)		
A. Health care–associated (multidrug resistant)		
Drugs of choice	Vancomycin ± gentamicin[a]	
Alternatives: susceptibility testing results available before alternative drugs are used	Trimethoprim-sulfamethoxazole Linezolid[b] Quinupristin-dalfopristin[b]	

Table 126.1
Parenteral Antimicrobial Agent(s) for Treatment of Bacteremia and Other Serious *Staphylococcus aureus* Infections (*continued*)

Susceptibility	Antimicrobial Agents	Comments
III. MRSA (oxacillin MIC, ≥4 mcg/mL) (*continued*)		
B. Community-associated (not multidrug resistant)		
Drugs of choice	Vancomycin ± gentamicin[a]	For life-threatening infections or endovascular infections, including those complicated by venous thrombosis
	Clindamycin (if strain susceptible)	For pneumonia, septic arthritis, osteomyelitis, skin or soft tissue infections
	Trimethoprim-sulfamethoxazole	For skin or soft tissue infections
Alternatives	Vancomycin	For serious infections
	Linezolid	For serious infections caused by clindamycin-resistant isolates in patients with renal dysfunction or those intolerant of vancomycin
IV. Vancomycin-intermediate *S aureus* (MIC, 4–16 mcg/mL)[b]		
Drugs of choice	Optimal therapy is not known.	Dependent on in vitro susceptibility test results
	Linezolid[b]	
	Ceftaroline Daptomycin[c]	
	Quinupristin-dalfopristin[b]	
	Tigecycline	
Alternatives	Vancomycin + linezolid ± gentamicin	
	Vancomycin + trimethoprim-sulfamethoxazole[a]	

Abbreviations: CNS, central nervous system; MIC, minimum inhibitory concentration; MRSA, methicillin-resistant *Staphylococcus aureus*.

[a] Gentamicin should be considered for addition to the therapeutic regimen for endocarditis without prosthetic devices or CNS infection; gentamicin and rifampin should be added for endocarditis of a prosthetic device or infections with a vancomycin-intermediate *S aureus* strain. Addition of rifampin is recommended for other device-related infections (eg, spinal instrumentation, prosthetic joint). Some experts recommend achieving vancomycin trough concentrations between 15 and 20 mcg/mL for serious MRSA infections until the patient has improved and blood cultures are sterile. Consultation with an infectious diseases specialist should be considered to determine which agent to use and duration of use.

[b] Linezolid, ceftaroline, quinupristin-dalfopristin, and tigecycline are agents with activity in vitro and efficacy in adults with multidrug-resistant, gram-positive organisms, including *S aureus*. Because experience with these agents in children is limited, consultation with an infectious diseases specialist should be considered before use.

[c] Daptomycin is active in vitro against multidrug-resistant, gram-positive organisms, including *S aureus*, but has not been evaluated in children. Daptomycin is approved by the US Food and Drug Administration only for treatment of complicated skin and skin structure infections and for *S aureus* bloodstream infections. Daptomycin is ineffective for treatment of pneumonia and is not indicated in patients 18 years and older.

penicillin can be treated with a first- or second-generation cephalosporin or with clindamycin, if the *S aureus* strain is susceptible.

Intravenous vancomycin is recommended for treatment of serious infections caused by staphylococcal strains resistant to BLR β-lactam antimicrobial agents (eg, MRSA, all CoNS). For life-threatening *S aureus* infections, initial therapy should include vancomycin and a BLR β-lactam antimicrobial agent (eg, nafcillin). For hospital-acquired CoNS infections, vancomycin is the drug of choice. Subsequent therapy should be determined by antimicrobial susceptibility results. Guidelines for management of serious skin or soft tissue infection, complicated pneumonia or empyema, CNS infection, osteomyelitis, and endocarditis caused by MRSA are available **(www.idsociety.org/IDSA_Practice_Guidelines)**.

Vancomycin Treatment Failure and Vancomycin-Intermediate *S aureus* Infection

Vancomycin-intermediate *S aureus* infection is rare in children. For seriously ill patients with a history of recurrent MRSA infections or for patients failing vancomycin therapy in whom VISA strains are a consideration, initial therapy could include linezolid or trimethoprim-sulfamethoxazole, with or without gentamicin. If antimicrobial susceptibility results document multidrug resistance, alternative agents, such as quinupristin-dalfopristin, daptomycin (not approved for pneumonia), ceftaroline, or tigecycline, could be considered.

Duration of Therapy for Invasive Infections

Duration of therapy for serious MSSA or MRSA infections depends on the site and severity of infection but is usually 4 weeks or more for endocarditis, osteomyelitis, necrotizing pneumonia, or disseminated infection, assuming a documented clinical and microbiologic response. The duration of bacteremia for patients with staphylococcal infection can typically be 3 to 4 days for MSSA and 7 to 9 days for MRSA. In assessing whether modification of therapy is necessary, clinicians should consider whether the patient is clinically improving, should identify and drain sequestered foci of infection, and, for MRSA strains, should consider the vancomycin MIC and the achievable vancomycin trough concentrations.

Completion of the course with an oral drug can be considered if adherence can be ensured and endocarditis or CNS infection is not a consideration. For endocarditis and CNS infection, parenteral therapy is recommended for the entire treatment. Drainage of abscesses and removal of foreign bodies are desirable and are almost always required for medical treatment to be effective. In some cases, multiple debridement procedures are necessary for children with MRSA osteoarticular infection.

Duration of therapy for central line–associated bloodstream infections is controversial and depends on consideration of a number of factors, including the organism (*S aureus* vs CoNS), the type and location of the catheter, the site of infection (exit site vs tunnel vs line), the feasibility of using an alternative vascular access site at a later date, and the presence or absence of a catheter-related thrombus. Infections are more difficult to treat when associated with a thrombus, thrombophlebitis, or intra-atrial thrombus. Data detailing outcomes of treatment of serious MRSA infections in adults does not support the addition of gentamicin or rifampin to vancomycin because of an increase in adverse effects and lack of greater efficacy of the combination versus monotherapy, but the addition of rifampin can be considered in the setting of a foreign body–associated infection. If a central line can be removed, there is no demonstrable thrombus, and bacteremia resolves promptly, a 5-day course of therapy seems appropriate for CoNS infections in the immunocompetent host.

A longer course is suggested if the patient is immunocompromised or the organism is *S aureus;* experts differ on recommended duration, but many suggest a minimum of 14 days provided there is no evidence of a metastatic focus. If the patient needs a new central line, waiting 48 to 72 hours after bacteremia has apparently resolved before insertion is optimal. If a tunneled catheter is needed for ongoing care, in situ treatment of the infection can be attempted. If the patient responds to antimicrobial therapy with immediate resolution of the *S aureus* bacteremia, treatment should be continued for 10 to 14 days parenterally. Antimicrobial lock therapy of tunneled central lines may result in a higher rate of catheter salvage in adults with CoNS infections, but experience with this approach is limited in children. If blood culture results remain positive for more than 2 days for *S aureus* or 3 to 5 days for CoNS or if the clinical illness fails to improve, the central line should be removed, parenteral therapy should be continued, and the patient should be evaluated for metastatic foci of infection. Vegetations or a thrombus in the heart or great vessels should always be considered when a central line becomes infected and should be suspected more strongly if blood cultures remain positive for more than 2 days or if there are other clinical manifestations associated with endocarditis. Transesophageal echocardiography, if feasible, is the most sensitive technique for identifying vegetations, but transthoracic echocardiography is generally adequate for children younger than 10 years and those weighing less than 60 kg.

Management of *S aureus* Toxin-Mediated Diseases

As summarized in Box 126.3, the first priority in management of *S aureus* TSS is aggressive fluid management as well as management of respiratory or cardiac failure, if present. Initial antimicrobial therapy should include a parentally administered β-lactam antistaphylococcal antimicrobial agent and a protein synthesis-inhibiting drug, such as clindamycin, at maximum dosages. Vancomycin should be substituted for BLR penicillins or cephalosporins in regions where community-associated MRSA infections are common. Once the organism is identified and susceptibilities are known, therapy for *S aureus* should be modified, but an active antimicrobial agent should be continued for 10 to 14 days. Administration of antimicrobial agents can be changed to the oral route once the patient is tolerating oral alimentation. Total duration of therapy is based on the usual duration of established foci of infection (eg, osteomyelitis). Aggressive drainage and irrigation of accessible sites of purulent infection should be performed as soon as possible. All foreign bodies, including those recently inserted during surgery, should be removed if possible. Intravenous immunoglobulin (IVIG) can be considered in patients with severe staphylococcal TSS unresponsive to other therapeutic measures because IVIG may neutralize circulating toxin. The optimal IVIG regimen is unknown. Staphylococcal scalded skin syndrome in infants should be treated with a parenteral BLR β-lactam antimicrobial agent or, if MRSA is a consideration, vancomycin. Transition to an oral agent can be considered in non-neonates who have demonstrated excellent clinical and microbiologic response to parenteral therapy.

Box 126.3

Management of Staphylococcal Toxic Shock Syndrome

- Fluid management to maintain adequate venous return and cardiac filling pressures to prevent end-organ damage
- Anticipatory management of multisystem organ failure
- Parenteral antimicrobial therapy at maximum doses
  - Kill organism with bactericidal cell wall inhibitor (eg, β-lactamase–resistant antistaphylococcal antimicrobial agent).
  - Reduce enzyme or toxin production with protein synthesis inhibitor (eg, clindamycin).
- Intravenous immunoglobulin therapy may be considered for infection refractory to several hours of aggressive therapy or in the presence of an undrainable focus or persistent oliguria with pulmonary edema.

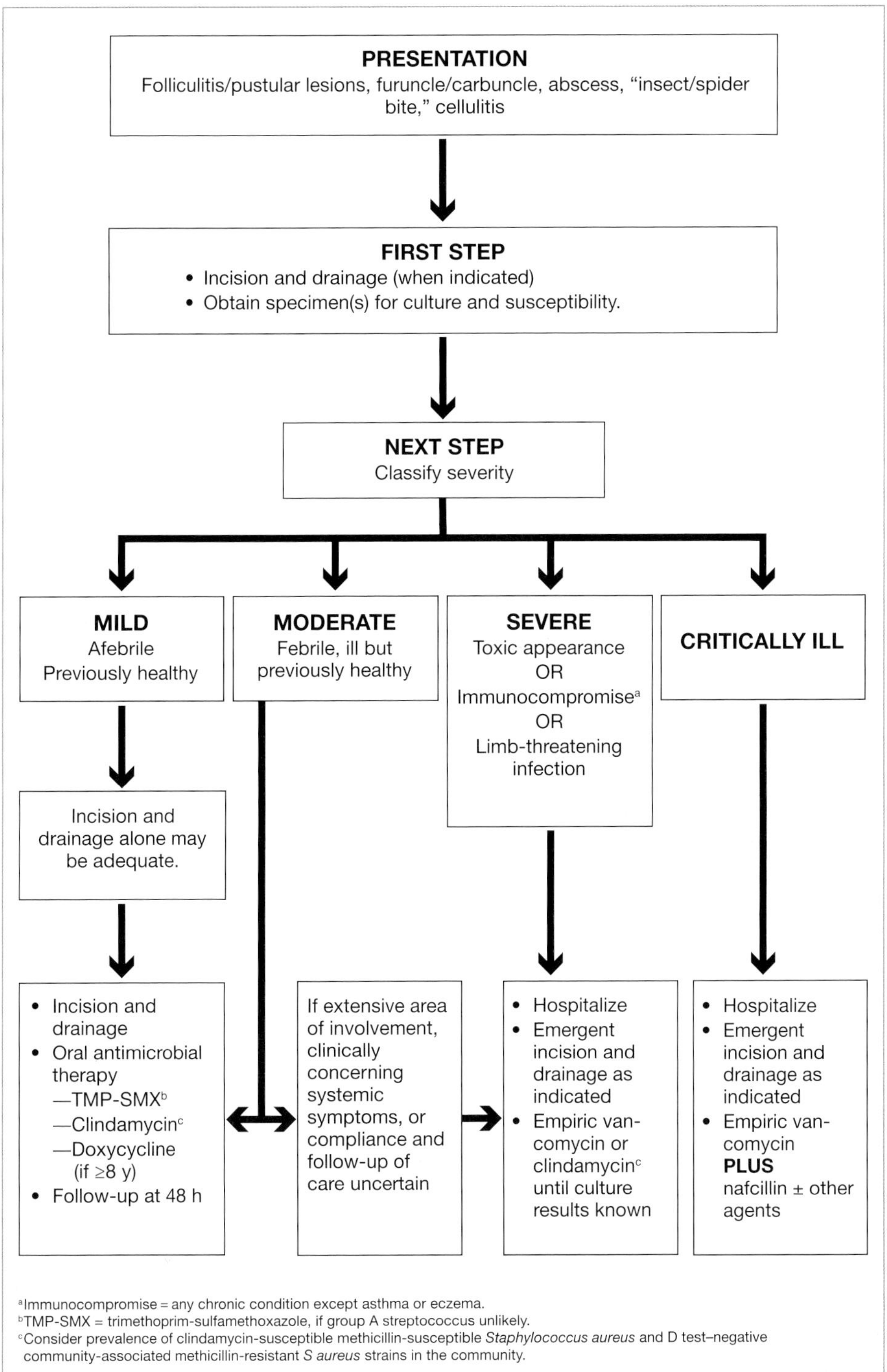

Image 126.1

Algorithm for initial management of skin and soft tissue infections caused by community-associated *Staphylococcus aureus*.

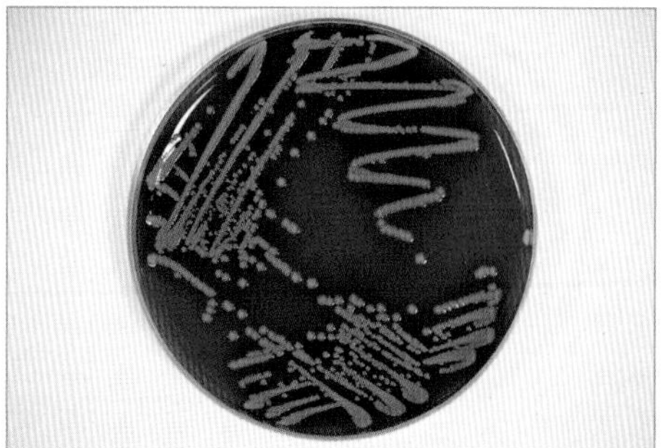

Image 126.2
Staphylococcus aureus on blood agar. Colonies have a golden or cream-colored appearance, are opaque, and produce β-hemolysis on blood agar. Courtesy of Julia Rosebush, DO; Robert Jerris, PhD; and Theresa Stanley, M(ASCP).

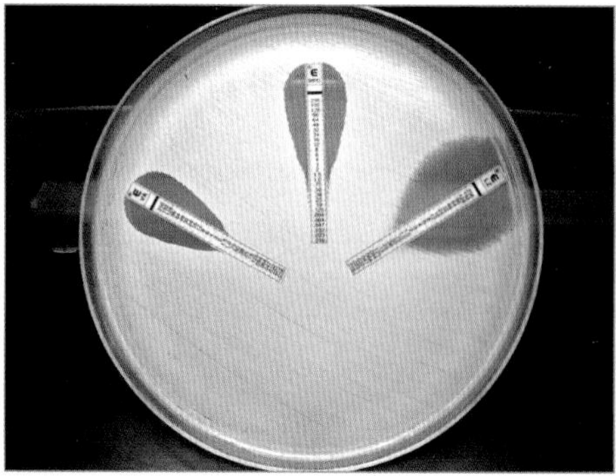

Image 126.4
A *Staphylococcus aureus* isolate tested by the Etest gradient diffusion method with vancomycin, daptomycin, and linezolid on Mueller-Hinton-IH agar. The minimum inhibitory concentration of each agent is determined by the intersection of the organism growth with the strip as measured using the scale inscribed on the strip. Used with permission from *Clinical Infectious Diseases.*

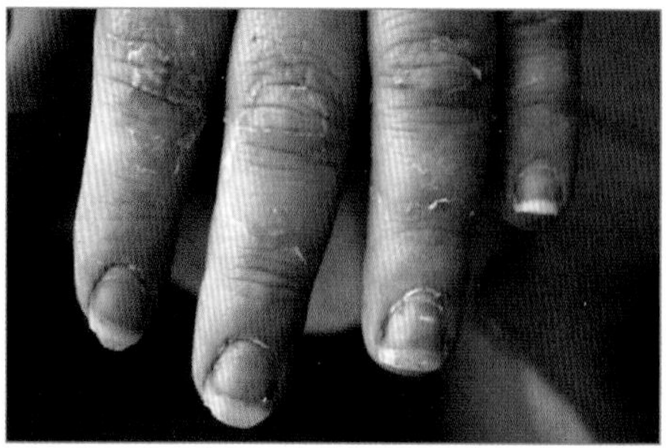

Image 126.6
Skin desquamation in a 7-year-old boy with staphylococcal scalded skin syndrome. Courtesy of Benjamin Estrada, MD.

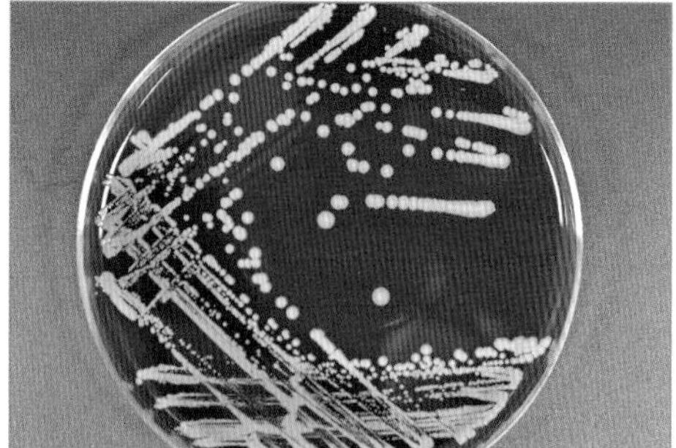

Image 126.3
Staphylococcus epidermidis on blood agar. In contrast to *Staphylococcus aureus* and other coagulase-negative *Staphylococcus* species, this organism produces a white colony with little or no pigmentation. Courtesy of Julia Rosebush, DO; Robert Jerris, PhD; and Theresa Stanley, M(ASCP).

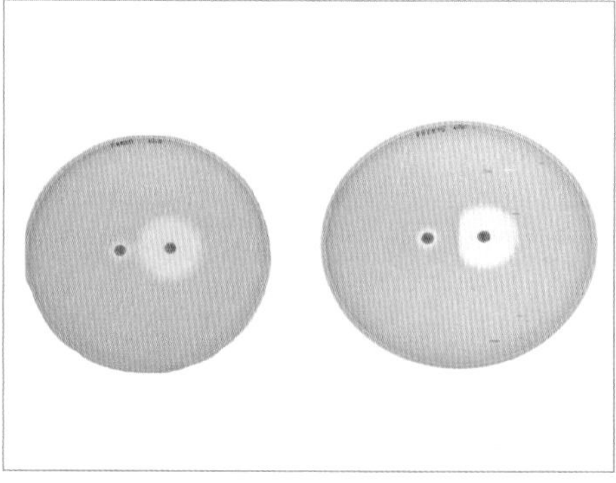

Image 126.5
D zone test for clindamycin-induced resistance by *Staphylococcus aureus*. The left shows a negative result and the right shows a positive one. Courtesy of Sarah Long, MD, FAAP.

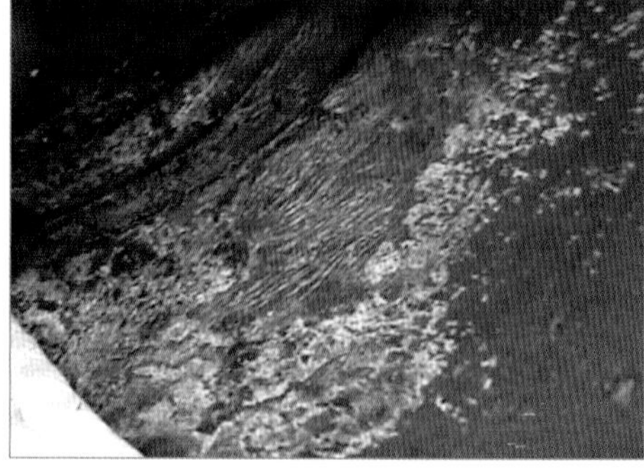

Image 126.7
Skin desquamation in a 7-year-old black boy with staphylococcal scarlatiniform eruption. Courtesy of Benjamin Estrada, MD.

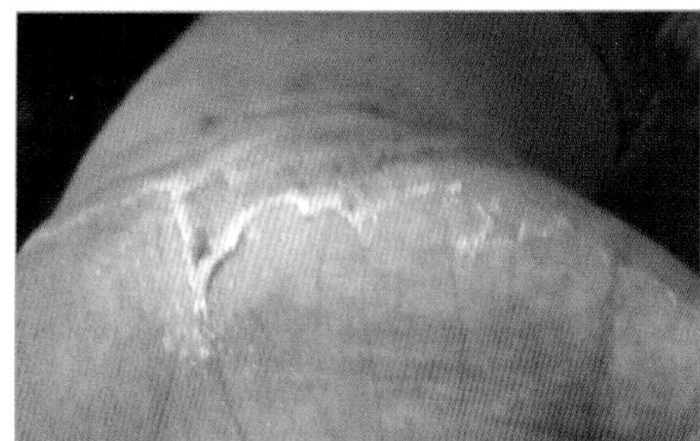

Image 126.8
Skin desquamation of the hand in a 7-year-old boy with staphylococcal scalded skin syndrome. Courtesy of Benjamin Estrada, MD.

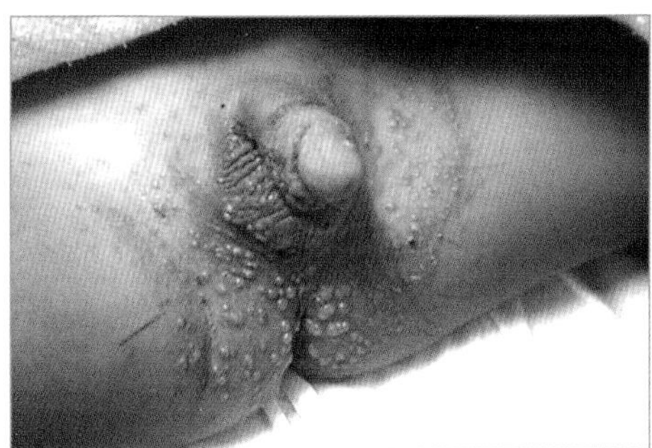

Image 126.9
Newborn with pustulosis of the perineum and genitalia due to *Staphylococcus aureus*. Copyright Michael Rajnik, MD, FAAP.

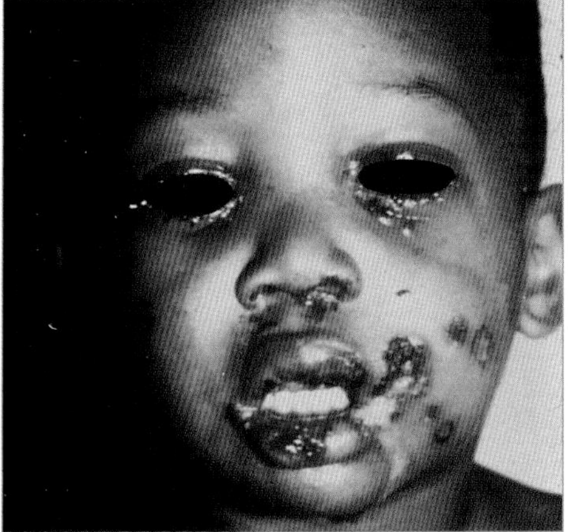

Image 126.10
Staphylococcal bullous impetigo lesions about the eyes, nose, and mouth in a 6-year-old black boy. Also note the secondary anterior cervical lymphadenopathy. Courtesy of George Nankervis, MD.

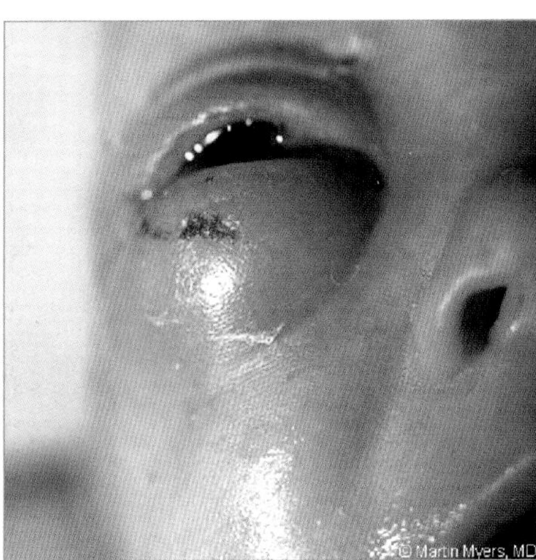

Image 126.11
An infant with orbital cellulitis and ethmoid sinusitis due to *Staphylococcus aureus*. Copyright Martin G. Myers, MD.

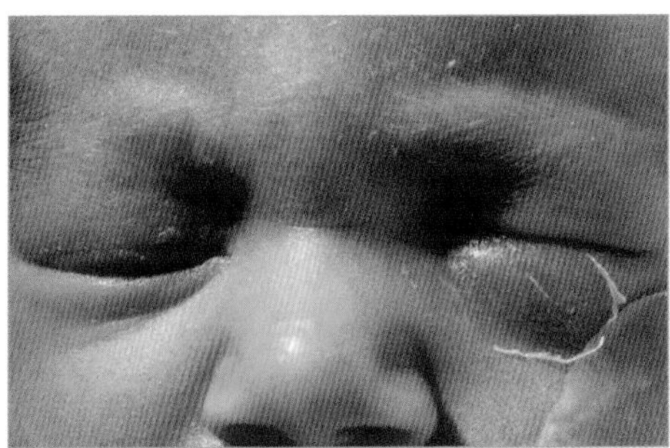

Image 126.12
A 3-week-old with an orbital abscess and bacteremia caused by methicillin-resistant *Staphylococcus aureus.* Incision and drainage of the abscess and parenteral vancomycin resulted in full recovery.

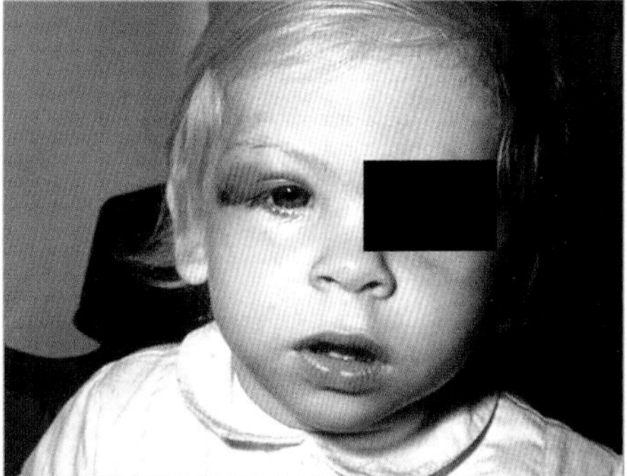

Image 126.13
Periorbital cellulitis due to *Staphylococcus aureus*–infected lesion adjacent to the orbit (most likely secondary to a recent insect bite). Courtesy of Edgar O. Ledbetter, MD, FAAP.

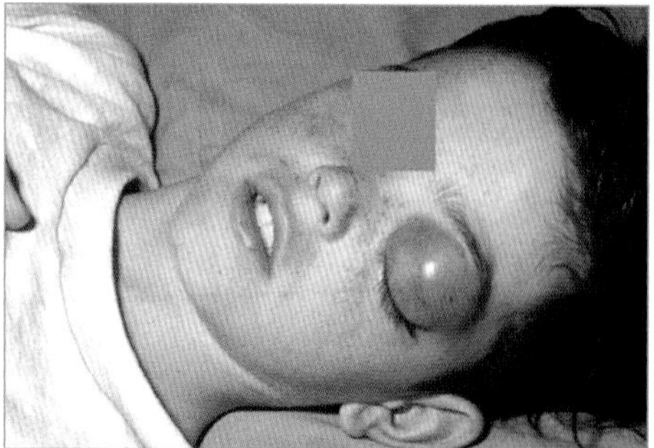

Image 126.14
Orbital abscess with proptosis of the globe due to *Staphylococcus aureus* in a 12-year-old boy. Delayed surgical drainage contributed to permanent visual impairment due to central retinal vascular involvement. The patient also had left ethmoid and maxillary sinusitis.

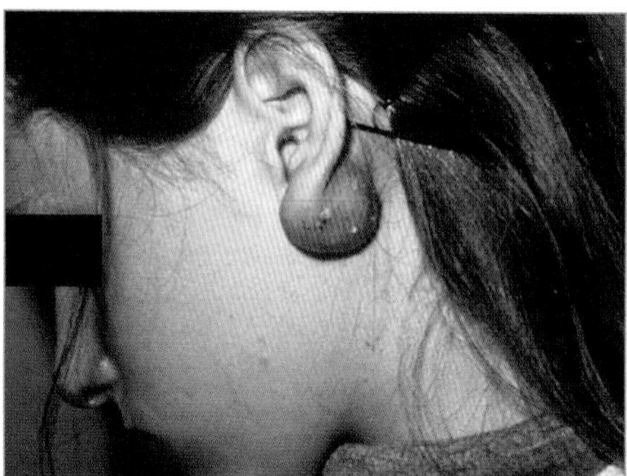

Image 126.16
Staphylococcus aureus abscess of the lobe of the left ear secondary to ear piercing in an adolescent girl. Courtesy of Edgar O. Ledbetter, MD, FAAP.

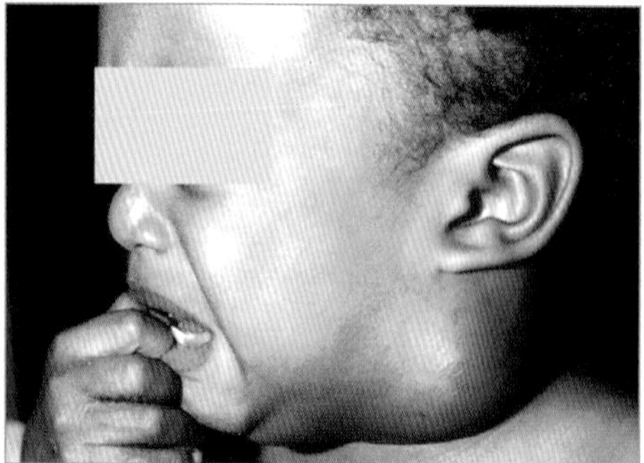

Image 126.18
Subauricular cervical adenitis *Staphylococcus aureus* in a 2-year-old boy. Courtesy of Neal Halsey, MD.

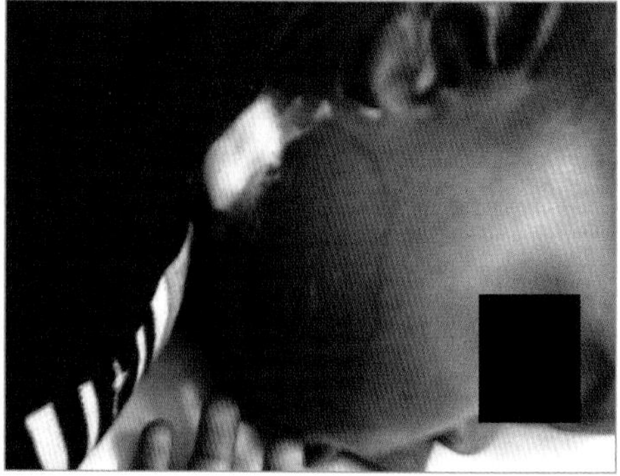

Image 126.15
Pyomyositis of the cheek of a 1-year-old girl caused by *Staphylococcus aureus*. Copyright Michael Rajnik, MD, FAAP.

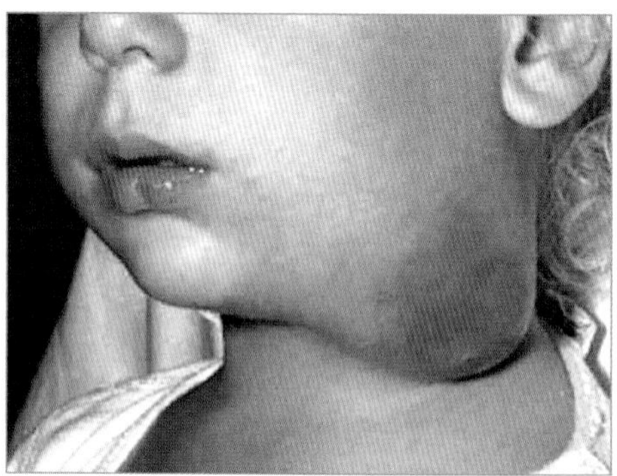

Image 126.17
Cervical adenitis with abscess formation due to *Staphylococcus aureus*. Delay in seeking medical care resulted in spontaneous drainage of the abscess.

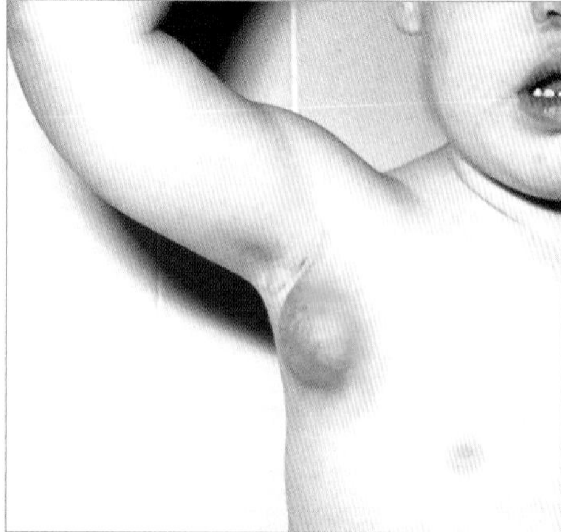

Image 126.19
Abscess of axillary lymph node due to *Staphylococcus aureus*.

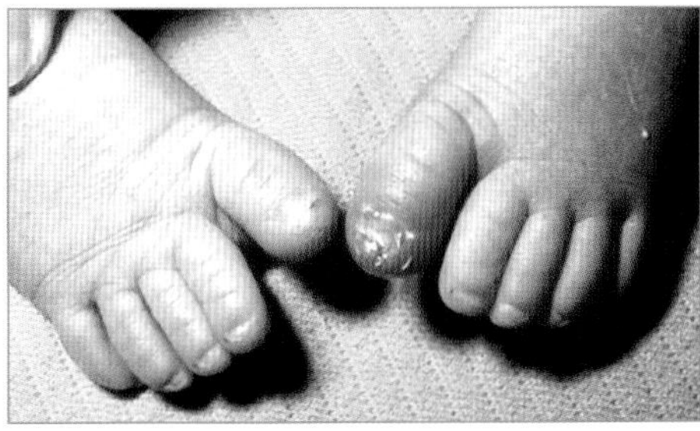

Image 126.20
Posttraumatic paronychia due to *Staphylococcus aureus* of the left great toe of an infant. Courtesy of Edgar O. Ledbetter, MD, FAAP.

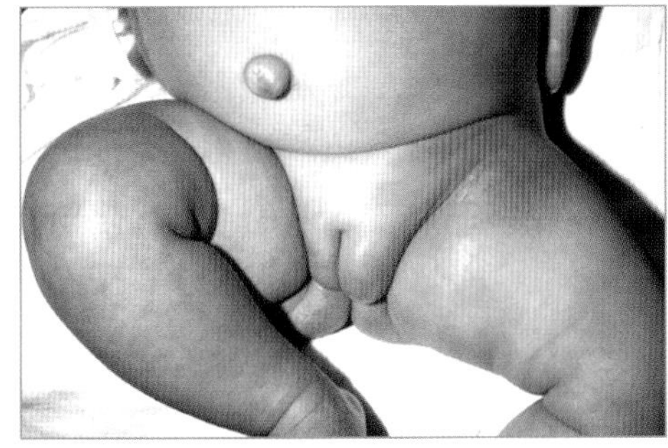

Image 126.21
Cellulitis (inguinal) due to *Staphylococcus aureus*. Courtesy of Neal Halsey, MD.

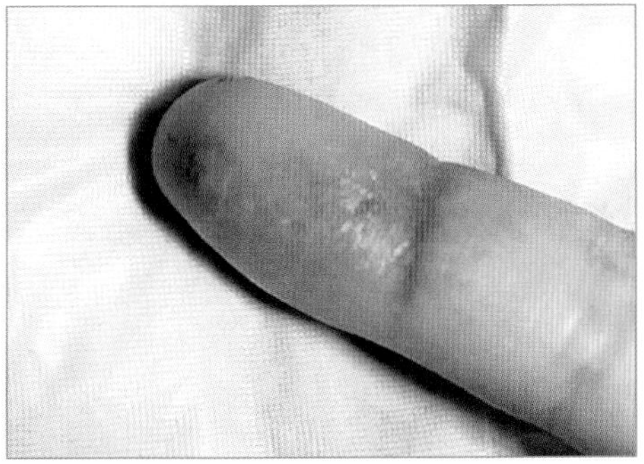

Image 126.22
A 15-year-old with Fanconi syndrome with *Staphylococcus aureus* infection at the fingerstick site. Copyright Martin G. Myers, MD.

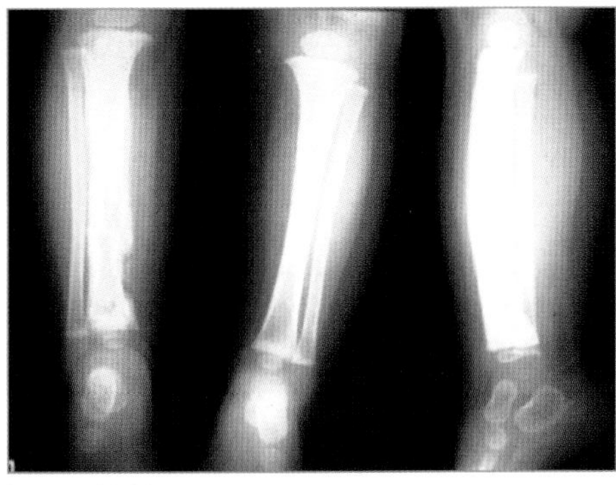

Image 126.23
Chronic osteomyelitis of the right tibia due to *Staphylococcus aureus*.

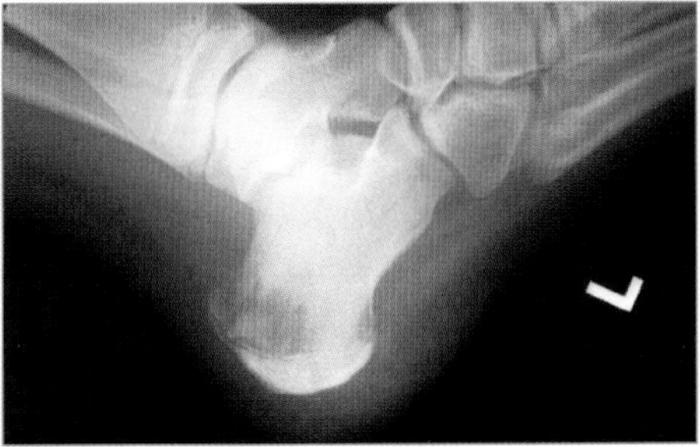

Image 126.24
Osteomyelitis of the calcaneus due to *Staphylococcus aureus* with no history of injury.

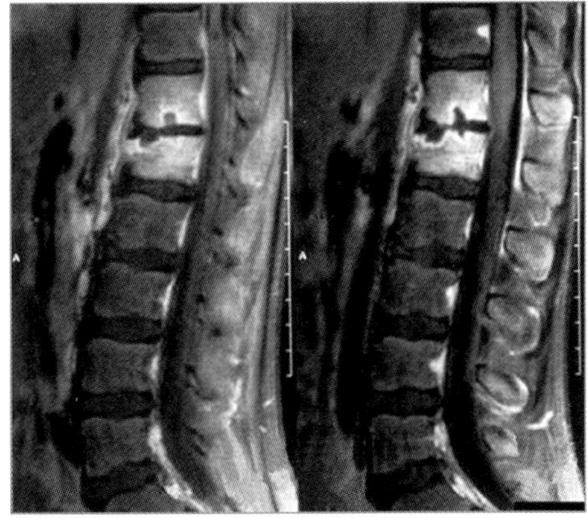

Image 126.25
Vertebral osteomyelitis in a 13-year-old with a 6-week history of back pain. Magnetic resonance imaging revealed osteolytic changes of the anterior segments of the first and second lumbar vertebrae. A culture of the biopsy specimen grew methicillin-resistant *Staphylococcus aureus*.

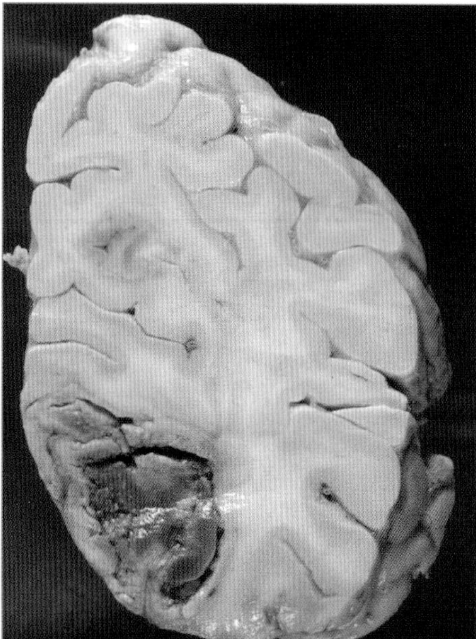

Image 126.26
Cerebral infarct in a patient with bacterial endocarditis. Courtesy of Dimitris P. Agamanolis, MD.

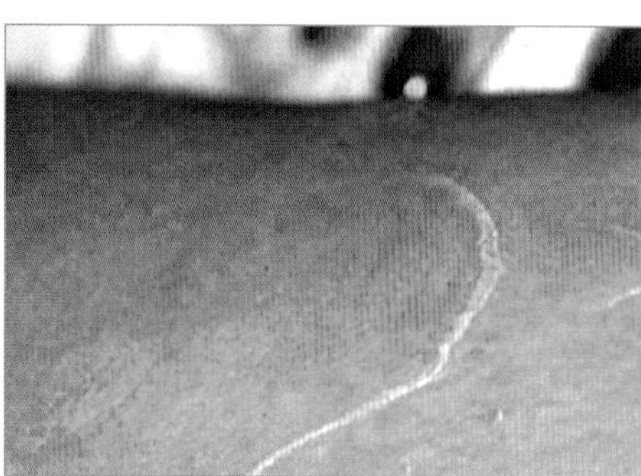

Image 126.28
Staphylococcal scalded skin syndrome with a positive Nikolsky sign.

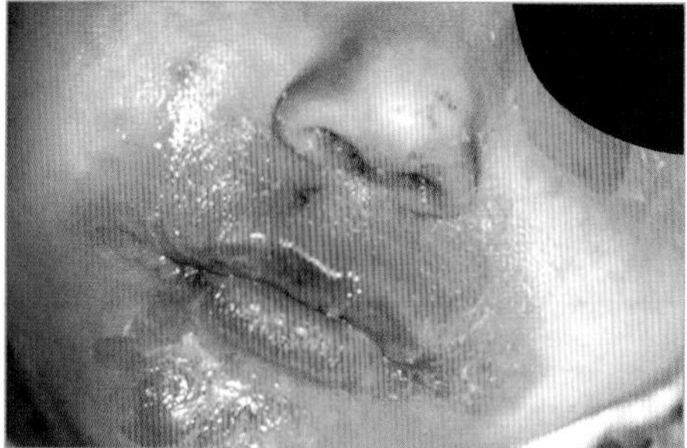

Image 126.27
Staphylococcal scalded skin syndrome. Epidermolytic toxins A and B are the components of *Staphylococcus aureus* thought to cause this syndrome.

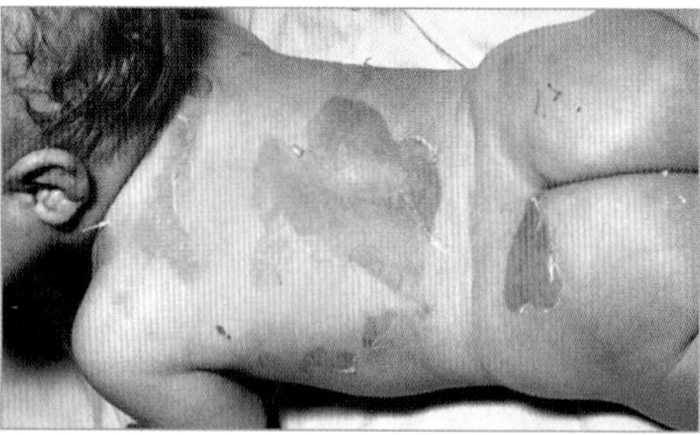

Image 126.29
Infant with staphylococcal scalded skin syndrome with sheets of skin desquamation.

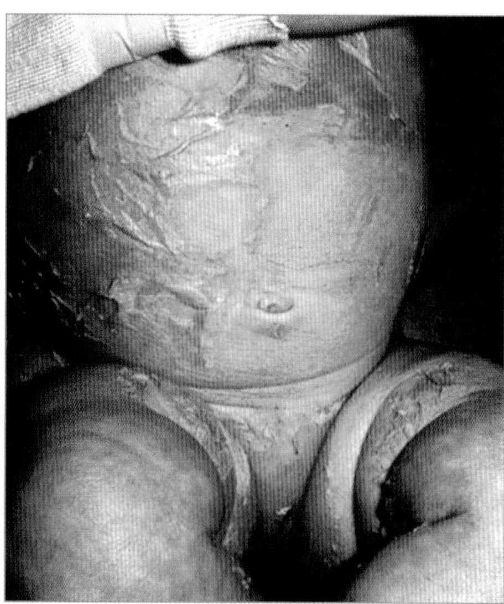

Image 126.30
Staphylococcal scalded skin syndrome. Epidermolytic exotoxin results in superficial, generalized desquamation. Courtesy of Edgar O. Ledbetter, MD, FAAP.

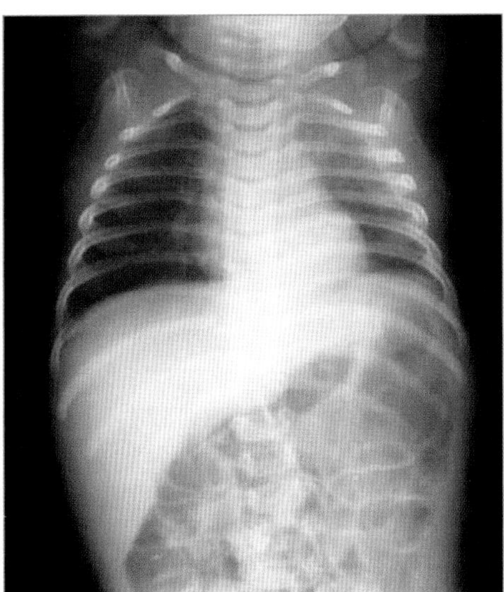

Image 126.31
Staphylococcal pneumonia, primary, with rapid progression and empyema. The infant had only mild respiratory distress and paralytic ileus without fever when first examined.

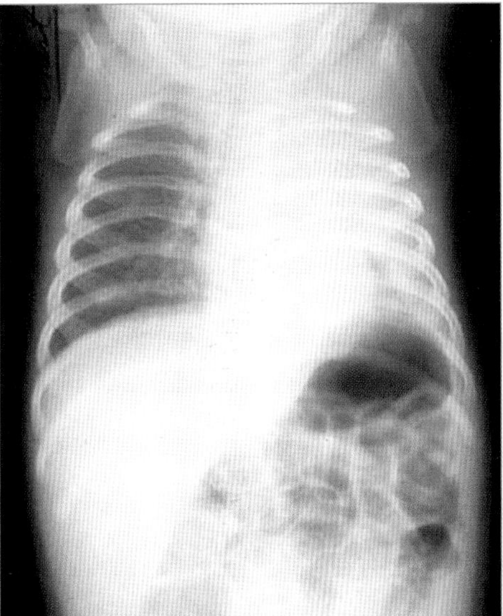

Image 126.32
Staphylococcal pneumonia, primary, with rapid progression with empyema. This is the same patient as in Image 126.30. Courtesy of Edgar O. Ledbetter, MD, FAAP.

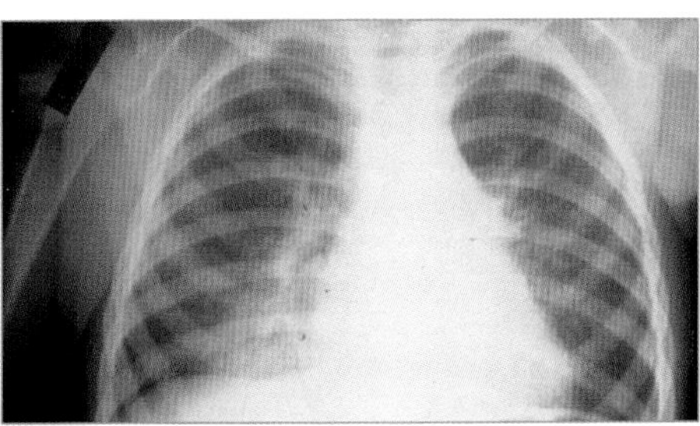

Image 126.33
Pneumonia due to *Staphylococcus aureus* with right lower lobe infiltrate in a preschool-aged child (day 1). Courtesy of Edgar O. Ledbetter, MD, FAAP.

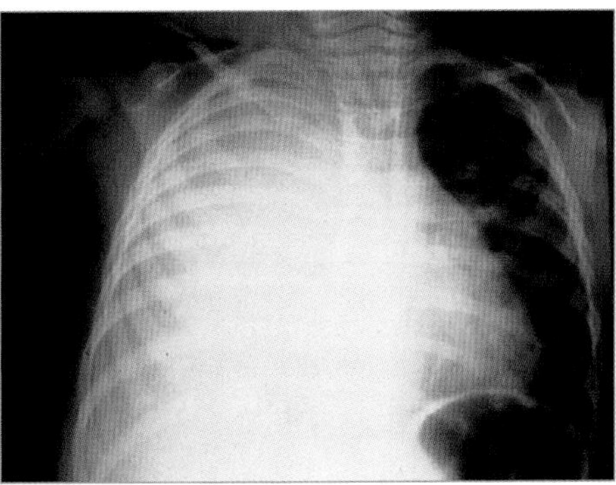

Image 126.34
Staphylococcal pneumonia with massive empyema demonstrating the rather rapid progression typical of staphylococcal infection. This is the same patient as in Image 126.32 (day 4). Courtesy of Edgar O. Ledbetter, MD, FAAP.

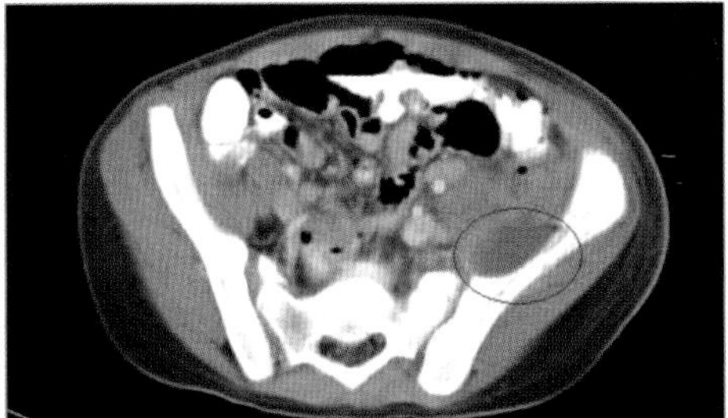

Image 126.35
Staphylococcus aureus pelvic abscess in a 14-year-old white girl demonstrated by computed tomography scan. Courtesy of Benjamin Estrada, MD.

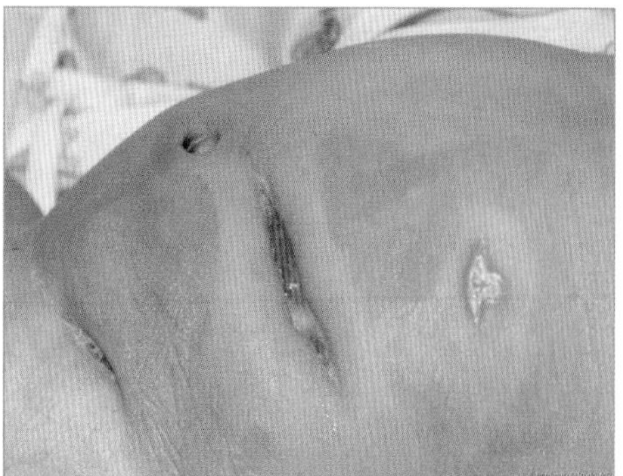

Image 126.36
Staphylococcus aureus necrotizing fasciitis in an 8-month-old girl. Courtesy of Benjamin Estrada, MD.

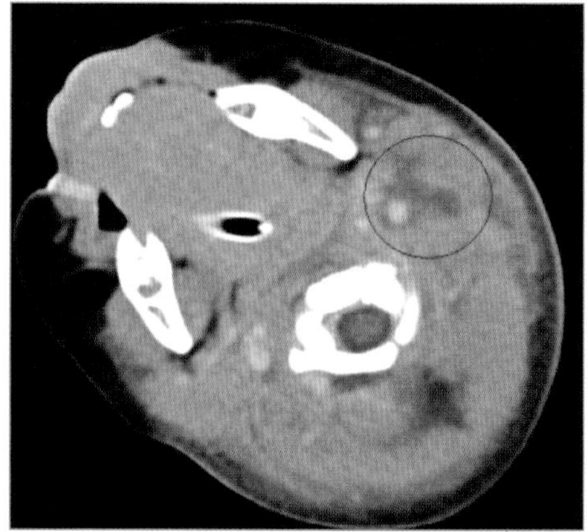

Image 126.37
Staphylococcus aureus cervical abscess in an 8-month-old girl demonstrated by computed tomography scan. Courtesy of Benjamin Estrada, MD.

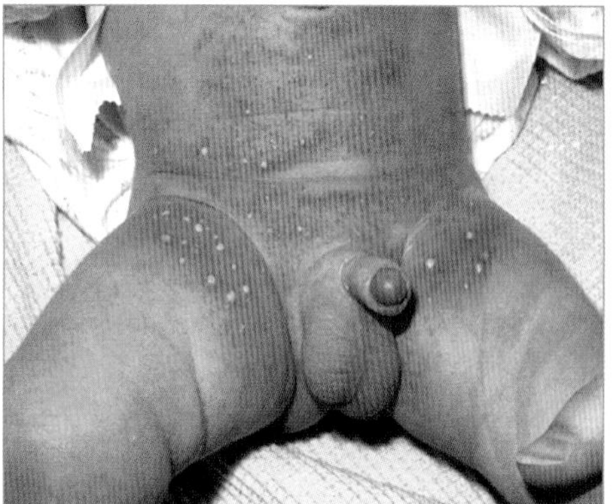

Image 126.38
Pyoderma due to *Staphylococcus aureus* in a young infant.

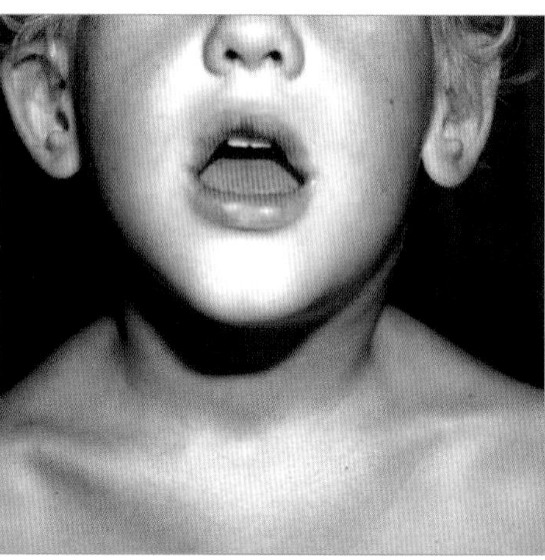

Image 126.39
A 6-year-old boy with peritonsillar abscess (quinsy) due to *Staphylococcus aureus*. Pain on swallowing and drooling are common symptoms. Copyright Martin G. Myers, MD.

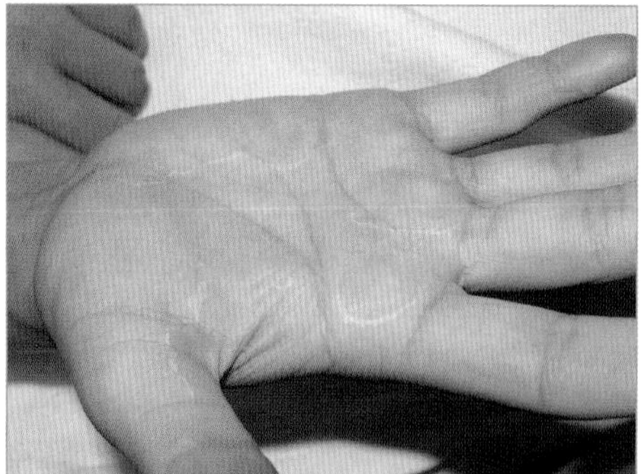

Image 126.40
Digit and palm desquamation in a 15-year-old boy during staphylococcal toxic shock syndrome convalescence. Courtesy of Benjamin Estrada, MD.

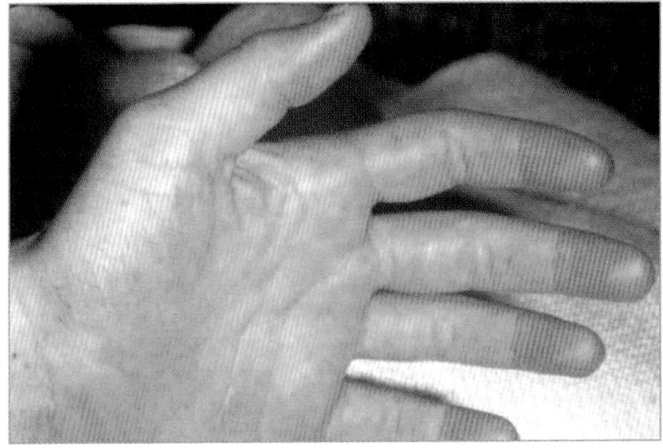

Image 126.41
Characteristic erythroderma of the hand of the patient in Image 126.40 with staphylococcal toxic shock syndrome.

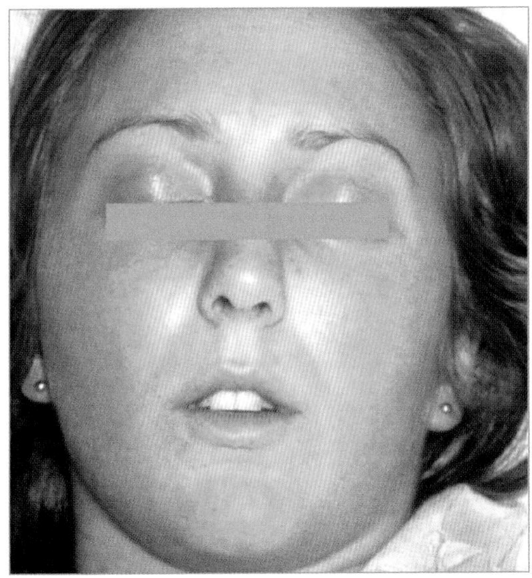

Image 126.42
Facial erythroderma secondary to *Staphylococcus aureus* toxic shock syndrome in a woman who was obtunded and hypotensive on admission.

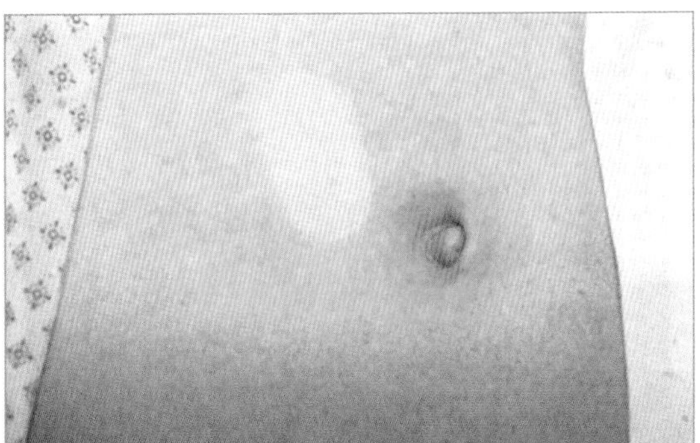

Image 126.43
Erythroderma that blanches on pressure in a patient with toxic shock syndrome. The mortality rate for staphylococcal toxic shock syndrome is lower than that of streptococcal toxic shock syndrome.

127

Group A Streptococcal Infections

Clinical Manifestations

The most common group A streptococcal (GAS) infection is acute pharyngotonsillitis (pharyngitis), which is heralded by sore throat with tonsillar inflammation and, often, tender cervical lymphadenopathy. Pharyngitis can be accompanied by palatal petechiae or a strawberry tongue. Purulent complications of pharyngitis usually occur in patients not treated with antimicrobial agents and include otitis media, sinusitis, peritonsillar or retropharyngeal abscesses, and suppurative cervical adenitis. Nonsuppurative complications include acute rheumatic fever (ARF) and acute glomerulonephritis. The goal of antimicrobial therapy for GAS pharyngitis is to reduce acute morbidity, complications, and transmission to close contacts.

Scarlet fever occurs most often in association with pharyngitis and, rarely, with pyoderma or an infected wound. Scarlet fever is usually a mild disease in the modern era and has a characteristic confluent erythematous sandpaperlike rash that is caused by one or more of several erythrogenic exotoxins produced by group A streptococci. Other than occurrence of rash, the epidemiologic features, symptoms, signs, sequelae, and treatment of scarlet fever are the same as those of streptococcal pharyngitis.

Acute streptococcal pharyngitis is uncommon in children younger than 3 years. Instead, they present with rhinitis and then develop a protracted illness with moderate fever, irritability, and anorexia (streptococcal fever or streptococcosis). The second most common site of GAS infection is skin. Streptococcal skin infections (eg, pyoderma, impetigo) can be followed by acute glomerulonephritis, which occasionally occurs in epidemics. Acute rheumatic fever is not a sequela of GAS skin infection.

Other manifestations of GAS infections include erysipelas, cellulitis (including perianal), vaginitis, bacteremia, pneumonia, endocarditis, pericarditis, septic arthritis, necrotizing fasciitis, purpura fulminans, osteomyelitis, myositis, puerperal sepsis, surgical wound infection, mastoiditis, and neonatal omphalitis. Invasive GAS infections are often associated with bacteremia with or without a local focus of infection and can present as streptococcal toxic shock syndrome (TSS) or necrotizing fasciitis. Necrotizing fasciitis can follow minor or unrecognized trauma, often involves an extremity, and presents as pain out of proportion to examination findings. An association between GAS infection and sudden onset of obsessive-compulsive behaviors, prepubertal anorexia nervosa, or tic disorders—pediatric autoimmune neuropsychiatric disorders associated with streptococcal infections, also known as pediatric acute-onset neuropsychiatric syndrome—has been proposed, but carefully performed prospective studies have not shown there is a specific relationship between these disorders and GAS infections.

Streptococcal TSS is caused by toxin-producing GAS strains and typically manifests as an acute illness characterized by fever, generalized erythroderma, rapid-onset hypotension, and signs of multiorgan involvement, including rapidly progressive renal failure (Box 127.1). Evidence of local soft tissue infection (eg, cellulitis, myositis, necrotizing fasciitis) associated with severe, rapidly increasing pain is common, but streptococcal TSS can occur without an identifiable focus of infection or with foci such as pneumonia with or without empyema, osteomyelitis, pyarthrosis, or endocarditis.

Etiology

More than 120 distinct serotypes or genotypes of group A β-hemolytic streptococci (*Streptococcus pyogenes*) have been identified based on M-protein serotype or M-protein gene sequence (*emm* types). Because of a variety of factors, including M nontypability and *emm* sequence variation within given M types, *emm* typing is generally more discriminating than M-protein serotyping. Epidemiologic studies suggest an association between certain serotypes (ie, types 1, 3, 5, 6, 18, 19, and 24) and rheumatic fever, but a specific rheumatogenic factor has not been identified. Several serotypes (ie, types 49, 55, 57, and 59) are more commonly associated with pyoderma and

Box 127.1
Streptococcal Toxic Shock Syndrome: Clinical Case Definition[a]

I. Isolation of group A streptococcus (*Streptococcus pyogenes*)
  A. From a normally sterile site (eg, blood, cerebrospinal fluid, peritoneal fluid, tissue biopsy specimen)
  B. From a nonsterile site (eg, throat, sputum, vagina, open surgical wound, superficial skin lesion)

II. Clinical signs of severity
  A. Hypotension: systolic pressure 90 mm Hg or less in adults or lower than the fifth percentile for age in children

AND

  B. Two or more of the following signs:
  - Renal impairment: creatinine concentration 177 μmol/L (2 mg/dL) or greater for adults or at least 2 times the upper limit of reference range for age[b]
  - Coagulopathy: platelet count 100,000/mm^3 or less or disseminated intravascular coagulation
  - Hepatic involvement: elevated alanine transaminase, aspartate transaminase, or total bilirubin concentrations at least 2 times the upper limit of reference range for age
  - Adult respiratory distress syndrome
  - A generalized erythematous macular rash that may desquamate
  - Soft tissue necrosis, including necrotizing fasciitis or myositis, or gangrene

[a] An illness fulfilling criteria IA and IIA and IIB can be defined as a **definite** case. An illness fulfilling criteria IB and IIA and IIB can be defined as a probable case if no other cause for the illness is identified.

[b] In patients with preexisting renal or hepatic disease, concentrations of 2-fold or greater elevation over patient's baseline.

Adapted from The Working Group on Severe Streptococcal Infections. Defining the group A streptococcal toxic shock syndrome. Rationale and consensus definition. *JAMA*. 1993;269(3):390–391.

acute glomerulonephritis. Other serotypes (ie, types 1, 6, and 12) are associated with pharyngitis and acute glomerulonephritis. Most cases of streptococcal TSS are caused by strains producing at least one of several different pyrogenic exotoxins, most commonly streptococcal pyrogenic exotoxin A. These toxins act as superantigens that stimulate production of tumor necrosis factor and other inflammatory mediators that cause capillary leak and other physiologic changes, leading to hypotension and organ damage.

Epidemiology

Pharyngitis usually results from contact with the respiratory tract secretions of a person who has GAS pharyngitis. Fomites and household pets, such as dogs, are not vectors of GAS infection. Pharyngitis and impetigo (and their nonsuppurative complications) can be associated with crowding, which is often present in socioeconomically disadvantaged populations. The close contact that occurs in schools, child care centers, contact sports (eg, wrestling), boarding schools, and military installations facilitates transmission. Foodborne outbreaks of pharyngitis occur rarely and are a consequence of human contamination of food in conjunction with improper food preparation or refrigeration procedures.

Streptococcal pharyngitis occurs at all ages but is most common among school-aged children and adolescents, peaking at 7 to 8 years of age. Group A streptococcal pharyngitis and pyoderma are substantially less common in adults than in children.

Geographically, GAS pharyngitis and pyoderma are ubiquitous. Pyoderma is more common in tropical climates and warm seasons, presumably because of antecedent insect bites and other minor skin trauma. Streptococcal pharyngitis is more common during late autumn, winter, and spring in temperate climates, in part because of close person-to-person contact in schools. Communicability of patients with streptococcal pharyngitis is highest during acute infection and, when untreated, gradually diminishes over a period of weeks. Patients are not considered to be contagious beginning 24 hours after initiation of appropriate antimicrobial therapy.

Throat culture surveys of healthy asymptomatic children during school outbreaks of pharyngitis have yielded group A streptococci prevalence rates as high as 25%. These surveys identified children who were pharyngeal carriers. Carriage of group A streptococci can persist for many months, but risk of transmission from carriers to others is low.

The incidence of ARF in the United States decreased sharply during the 20th century, and rates of this nonsuppurative sequela are low. Focal outbreaks of ARF in school-aged children occurred in several areas in the 1990s, and small clusters continue to be reported periodically. The highest rates of ARF are in Utah, Hawaii, New York, and Pennsylvania, most likely related to circulation of rheumatogenic strains. Their occurrence reemphasizes the importance of diagnosing GAS pharyngitis and treating with a recommended antimicrobial regimen.

In streptococcal impetigo, the organism is usually acquired by direct contact from another person. Group A streptococcal colonization of healthy skin usually precedes development of impetigo, but group A streptococci do not penetrate intact skin. Impetiginous lesions occur at the site of breaks in skin (eg, insect bites, burns, traumatic wounds, varicella lesions). After development of impetiginous lesions, the upper respiratory tract often becomes colonized with group A streptococci. Infection of surgical wounds and postpartum (puerperal) sepsis usually result from transmission through direct contact. Health care workers who are anal or vaginal carriers and people with skin infection can transmit GAS organisms to surgical and obstetric patients, resulting in health care–associated outbreaks. Infections in neonates result from intrapartum or contact transmission; in the latter situation, infection can begin as omphalitis, cellulitis, or necrotizing fasciitis.

In the United States, the incidence of invasive GAS infections is highest in infants and the elderly. Fatal cases in children are not common. Before use of varicella vaccine, varicella was the most commonly identified predisposing factor for invasive GAS infection. Other factors increasing risk include exposure to other children and household crowding. The portal of entry is unknown in most invasive GAS infections but is presumed to be skin or mucous membranes. Such infections rarely follow symptomatic GAS pharyngitis. An association between use of nonsteroidal anti-inflammatory drugs and invasive GAS infections in children with varicella has been described, but a causal relationship has not been established.

The incidence of streptococcal TSS is highest among young children and the elderly, although streptococcal TSS can occur at any age. Of all cases of invasive streptococcal infections in children, fewer than 5% are associated with streptococcal TSS. Among children, streptococcal TSS has been reported with focal lesions (eg, varicella, cellulitis, trauma, osteomyelitis), pneumonia, and bacteremia without a defined focus. Mortality rates are substantially lower for children than for adults with streptococcal TSS.

Incubation Period

For streptococcal pharyngitis, 2 to 5 days; for impetigo, 7 to 10 days; for streptococcal TSS, unknown, but can be as short as 14 hours in some cases (eg, childbirth, penetrating trauma).

Diagnostic Tests

Children with pharyngitis and obvious viral symptoms (eg, rhinorrhea, cough, hoarseness) should not be tested or treated for GAS infection. Laboratory confirmation is required for cases in children without viral symptoms because many will not have GAS pharyngitis. A specimen should be obtained by vigorous swabbing of a pair of swabs on tonsils and the posterior pharynx for culture or rapid antigen testing. It is recommended that a throat swab with a negative rapid antigen test result from children be submitted to the laboratory for isolation of group A streptococci; the second swab can be used for this purpose. Culture on sheep blood agar can confirm GAS infection, with latex agglutination differentiating group A streptococci from other β-hemolytic streptococci. False-negative culture results occur in fewer than 10% of symptomatic patients when an adequate throat swab specimen is obtained and cultured by trained personnel. Recovery of group A streptococci from the pharynx does not distinguish patients with true streptococcal infection (defined by a serologic response to extracellular antigens [eg, streptolysin O]) from streptococcal carriers who have an intercurrent viral pharyngitis. The number of colonies of group A streptococci on an agar culture plate also does not reliably differentiate true infection from carriage. Cultures that are negative for group A streptococci after 18 to 24 hours should be incubated for a second day to optimize recovery of organisms.

Several rapid diagnostic tests for GAS pharyngitis are available. Most are based on nitrous acid extraction of GAS carbohydrate antigen from organisms obtained by throat swab. Specificities of these tests are generally high, but the reported sensitivities vary considerably (ie, false-negative results occur). As with throat swab cultures, sensitivity of these tests is highly dependent on the quality of the throat swab specimen, experience of the person performing the test, and rigor of the culture method used for comparison. The US Food and Drug Administration has cleared a variety of rapid tests for use in home settings. Parents should be informed that their use is discouraged, and clinicians should be aware that such testing may have an even lower negative predictive value than testing performed in a clinical setting. Because of the high specificity of rapid tests, a positive test result does not require throat culture confirmation. Rapid diagnostic tests using techniques such as polymerase chain reaction and chemiluminescent DNA probes have been developed. The US Food and Drug Administration recently approved an isothermal nucleic acid amplification test for detection of group A streptococci from throat swab specimens. These tests may be as sensitive as standard throat cultures on sheep blood agar. The diagnosis of ARF is based on the Jones criteria (Box 127.2).

Indications for Group A Streptococcal Testing

Factors to be considered in the decision to obtain a throat swab specimen for testing children with pharyngitis are the patient's age, signs and symptoms, season, and family and community epidemiology, including contact with a person with GAS infection or presence in the family of a person with a history of ARF or of poststreptococcal glomerulonephritis. Group A streptococcal pharyngitis and, therefore, ARF are uncommon in children younger than 3 years, but outbreaks of GAS pharyngitis have been reported in young children in child care settings. The risk of ARF is so remote in young children in industrialized countries that diagnostic studies for GAS pharyngitis are not generally indicated. Children with manifestations highly suggestive of viral infection, such as coryza, conjunctivitis, hoarseness, cough, anterior stomatitis, discrete ulcerative oral lesions, or diarrhea, are unlikely to have GAS pharyngitis and generally should not be tested.

Box 127.2

Jones Criteria for Diagnosis of Acute Rheumatic Fever[a]

Major Criteria	Minor Criteria	Supporting Evidence
Carditis Polyarthritis Chorea Erythema marginatum Subcutaneous nodules	Clinical findings: Fever, arthralgia[b] Laboratory findings: Elevated acute phase reactants; prolonged P–R interval	Positive throat culture or rapid test for GAS antigen OR Elevated or rising streptococcal antibody test

Abbreviation: GAS, group A streptococcal.

[a] Diagnosis requires 2 major criteria or 1 major and 2 minor criteria with supporting evidence of antecedent group A streptococcal infection.

[b] Arthralgia is not a minor criterion in a patient with arthritis as a major criterion.

In contrast, children with acute onset of sore throat and clinical signs and symptoms such as pharyngeal exudate, pain on swallowing, fever, and enlarged tender anterior cervical lymph nodes or exposure to a person with GAS pharyngitis are more likely to have GAS infection and should have a rapid antigen test, and a throat culture if rapid test result is negative, performed and treatment initiated if a test result is positive.

Testing Contacts for Group A Streptococcal Infection

Indications for testing contacts for GAS infection vary according to circumstances. Testing asymptomatic household contacts for GAS infection is not recommended except when the contacts are at increased risk of developing sequelae of GAS infection, ARF, or acute glomerulonephritis; if test results are positive, contacts should be treated.

Follow-up Throat Cultures

Posttreatment throat swab cultures are indicated only for patients who are at particularly high risk of ARF or have active symptoms compatible with GAS pharyngitis. Repeated courses of antimicrobial therapy are not indicated for asymptomatic patients with cultures positive for group A streptococci; the exceptions are people who have had or whose family members have had ARF or other uncommon epidemiologic circumstances, such as a community outbreak of ARF or acute poststreptococcal glomerulonephritis.

Patients who have repeated episodes of pharyngitis at short intervals and in whom GAS infection is documented by culture or antigen detection test present a special problem. Most often, these people are chronic GAS carriers who are experiencing frequent viral illnesses and for whom repeated testing and use of antimicrobial agents are unnecessary. In assessing such patients, inadequate adherence to oral treatment should also be considered. Although relatively uncommon, macrolide and azalide resistance among GAS strains occurs, resulting in erythromycin, clarithromycin, or azithromycin treatment failures. Testing asymptomatic household contacts is usually not helpful. However, if multiple household members have pharyngitis or other GAS infections, simultaneous cultures of all household members and treatment of all people with positive cultures or rapid antigen test results may be of value.

Testing for Group A Streptococci in Nonpharyngitis Infections

Cultures of impetiginous lesions often yield streptococci and staphylococci, and determination of the primary pathogen is generally not possible. Culture is performed when it is necessary to determine susceptibility of the *Staphylococcus aureus* organisms. In suspected invasive GAS infections, cultures of blood and of focal sites of possible infection are indicated. In necrotizing fasciitis, imaging studies can delay, rather than facilitate, establishing the diagnosis. Clinical suspicion of necrotizing fasciitis should prompt surgical evaluation with intervention, including debridement of deep tissues with Gram stain and culture of surgical specimens.

Streptococcal TSS is diagnosed on the basis of clinical findings and isolation of group A streptococci (see Box 127.2). Blood culture results are positive for *S pyogenes* in approximately 50% of patients with streptococcal TSS. Culture results from a focal site of infection are also usually positive and can remain so for several days after appropriate antimicrobial agents have been initiated. *S pyogenes* species is uniformly susceptible to β-lactam antimicrobial agents (penicillins and cephalosporins), and susceptibility testing is only needed for non–β-lactam agents, such as erythromycin or clindamycin, to which *S pyogenes* can be resistant. A significant increase in antibody titers to streptolysin O, deoxyribonuclease B, or other streptococcal extracellular enzymes 4 to 6 weeks after infection can help to confirm the diagnosis if culture results are negative.

Treatment

Pharyngitis

Penicillin V is the drug of choice for treatment of GAS pharyngitis. A clinical GAS isolate resistant to penicillin or cephalosporin has never been documented. Prompt administration of penicillin shortens the clinical course, decreases risk of suppurative sequelae and transmission, and prevents ARF even when given up to 9 days after illness onset. For all patients with ARF, a complete course of penicillin or another appropriate antimicrobial agent for GAS pharyngitis should be given to eradicate group A streptococci from the throat, even if group A streptococci are not recovered in the initial throat culture. Orally administered amoxicillin as a single dose daily for 10 days is as effective as orally administered penicillin V or amoxicillin given multiple times per day for 10 days and comes as a more palatable suspension. This regimen has been endorsed by the American Heart Association in its guidelines for the treatment of GAS pharyngitis and the prevention of ARF.

Treatment failures may occur more often with oral penicillin than with intramuscular penicillin G benzathine because of inadequate adherence to oral therapy. In addition, short-course treatment (<10 days) for GAS pharyngitis, particularly with penicillin V, is associated with inferior bacteriologic eradication rates. Intramuscular penicillin G benzathine is appropriate therapy. It ensures adequate blood concentrations and avoids the problem of adherence, but administration is painful. Discomfort is less if the preparation of penicillin G benzathine is brought to room temperature before intramuscular injection. Mixtures containing shorter-acting penicillins (eg, penicillin G procaine) in addition to penicillin G benzathine have not been demonstrated to be more effective than penicillin G benzathine alone but are less painful when administered. For patients who have a history of nonanaphylactic allergy to penicillin, a 10-day course of a narrow-spectrum (first-generation) oral cephalosporin (ie, cephalexin) is indicated. Patients with immediate (anaphylactic) or type 1 hypersensitivity to penicillin should be treated with oral clindamycin (30 mg/kg per day in 3 divided doses; maximum, 900 mg/d for 10 days) rather than a cephalosporin.

An oral macrolide or azalide (eg, erythromycin, clarithromycin, azithromycin) is also acceptable for patients who are allergic to penicillins. Therapy for 10 days is indicated **except** for azithromycin, which is indicated for 5 days. Erythromycin is associated with substantially higher rates of gastrointestinal tract adverse effects compared with clarithromycin or azithromycin. Group A streptococcal strains resistant to macrolides or azalides have been highly prevalent in some areas of the world and have resulted in treatment failures. In recent years, macrolide resistance rates in most areas of the United States have been 5% to 10%, but resistance rates up to 20% have been reported, and continued monitoring is necessary. Tetracyclines, sulfonamides (including trimethoprim-sulfamethoxazole), and fluoroquinolones should not be used for treating GAS pharyngitis.

Children who have a recurrence of GAS pharyngitis shortly after completing a full course of a recommended oral antimicrobial agent can be retreated with the same antimicrobial agent, an alternative oral drug, or an intramuscular dose of penicillin G benzathine, especially if inadequate adherence to oral therapy is suspected. Alternative drugs include a narrow-spectrum cephalosporin (ie, cephalexin), amoxicillin-clavulanate, clindamycin, a macrolide, or azalide. Expert opinions differ about the most appropriate therapy in this circumstance.

Management of a patient who has repeated and frequent episodes of acute pharyngitis associated with positive laboratory tests for group A streptococci is problematic. To determine whether the patient is a long-term streptococcal pharyngeal carrier who is experiencing repeated episodes of intercurrent viral pharyngitis (which is the situation in most cases), the following should be determined: whether the clinical findings are more suggestive of group A streptococci or a virus as the cause; whether epidemiologic factors in the community support group A streptococci or a virus as the cause; the nature of the clinical response to the antimicrobial therapy (in true GAS pharyngitis, response to therapy is usually 24 hours or less); and whether laboratory test results are positive for GAS infection between episodes of acute pharyngitis (suggesting the patient is a carrier). Measurement of a serial serologic response to GAS extracellular antigens (eg, antistreptolysin O) should be discouraged.

Pharyngeal Carriers

Antimicrobial therapy is not indicated for most GAS pharyngeal carriers. The few specific situations in which eradication of carriage may be indicated include a local outbreak of ARF or poststreptococcal glomerulonephritis, an outbreak of GAS pharyngitis in a closed or semiclosed community, a family history of ARF, or multiple ("ping-pong") episodes of documented symptomatic GAS pharyngitis occurring within a family for many weeks despite appropriate therapy.

Group A streptococcal carriage can be difficult to eradicate with conventional antimicrobial therapy. A number of antimicrobial agents, including clindamycin, cephalosporins, amoxicillin-clavulanate, azithromycin, or a combination that includes penicillin V or penicillin G benzathine with rifampin for the last 4 days of treatment, have been demonstrated to be more effective than penicillin alone in eliminating chronic streptococcal carriage. Of these drugs, oral clindamycin for 10 days has been reported to be most effective. Documented eradication of the carrier state is helpful in the evaluation of subsequent episodes of acute pharyngitis; however, carriage can recur after reacquisition of GAS infection, as some individuals appear to be "carrier prone."

Nonbullous Impetigo

Local mupirocin or retapamulin ointment may be useful for limiting person-to-person spread of nonbullous impetigo and for eradicating localized disease. With multiple lesions or with nonbullous impetigo in multiple family members, child care groups, or athletic teams, impetigo should be treated with oral antimicrobials active against group A streptococci and *S aureus*.

Toxic Shock Syndrome

Most aspects of management are the same for TSS caused by group A streptococci or by *S aureus* (Box 127.3 and Box 127.4). Paramount are immediate aggressive fluid replacement management of respiratory and cardiac failure, if present, and aggressive surgical debridement of any deep-seated infection. Because *S pyogenes* and *S aureus* TSSs are difficult to distinguish clinically, initial antimicrobial therapy should include an antistaphylococcal agent and a protein synthesis–inhibiting antimicrobial agent, such as clindamycin. The addition of clindamycin to penicillin is recommended for serious GAS infections because the antimicrobial activity of clindamycin is not affected by inoculum size, has a long postantimicrobial effect, and acts on bacteria by inhibiting protein synthesis. Inhibition of protein synthesis results in suppression of synthesis of the *S pyogenes* antiphagocytic M-protein and bacterial toxins. Clindamycin should not be used **alone** as initial antimicrobial therapy in life-threatening situations because, in the United States, 1% to 2% of GAS strains are resistant to clindamycin. Higher resistance rates have been reported for strains associated with invasive infection and may be as high as 10%.

Box 127.3

Management of Streptococcal Toxic Shock Syndrome Without Necrotizing Fasciitis

- Fluid management to maintain adequate venous return and cardiac filling pressures to prevent end-organ damage
- Anticipatory management of multisystem organ failure
- Parenteral antimicrobial therapy at maximum doses with the capacity to
  - Kill organism with bactericidal cell wall inhibitor (eg, β-lactamase–resistant antimicrobial agent).
  - Decrease enzyme, toxin, or cytokine production with protein synthesis inhibitor (eg, clindamycin).
- IVIG may be considered for infection refractory to several hours of aggressive therapy or in the presence of an undrainable focus or persistent oliguria with pulmonary edema.

Abbreviation: IVIG, intravenous immunoglobulin.

Box 127.4
Management of Streptococcal Toxic Shock Syndrome With Necrotizing Fasciitis

- Immediate surgical evaluation
  - Exploration or incisional biopsy for diagnosis and culture
  - Resection of all necrotic tissue
- Repeated resection of tissue may be needed if infection persists or progresses.

Once GAS infection has been confirmed, antimicrobial therapy should be tailored to penicillin and clindamycin. Intravenous therapy should be continued until the patient is afebrile and stable hemodynamically and blood is sterile as evidenced by negative culture results. The total duration of therapy is based on duration established for the primary site of infection.

Aggressive drainage and irrigation of accessible sites of infection should be performed as soon as possible. If necrotizing fasciitis is suspected, immediate surgical exploration or biopsy is crucial to identify and debride the deep soft-tissue infection.

The use of intravenous immunoglobulin can be considered as adjunctive therapy of streptococcal TSS or necrotizing fasciitis if the patient is severely ill.

Other Infections

Parenteral antimicrobial therapy is required for severe infections, such as endocarditis, pneumonia, empyema, abscess, septicemia, meningitis, arthritis, osteomyelitis, erysipelas, necrotizing fasciitis, and neonatal omphalitis. Treatment is often prolonged.

Prevention of Sequelae

Acute rheumatic fever and acute glomerulonephritis are serious nonsuppurative sequelae of GAS infections. During epidemics of GAS infections on military bases in the 1950s, rheumatic fever developed in 3% of untreated patients with acute GAS pharyngitis. The current incidence after endemic infections is not known but is believed to be substantially less than 1%. The risk of ARF can be eliminated almost completely by adequate treatment of the antecedent GAS infection; however, rare cases have occurred even after apparently appropriate therapy. The effectiveness of antimicrobial therapy for preventing acute poststreptococcal glomerulonephritis after pyoderma or pharyngitis has not been established. Suppurative sequelae, such as peritonsillar abscesses and cervical adenitis, are usually prevented by treatment of the primary infection.

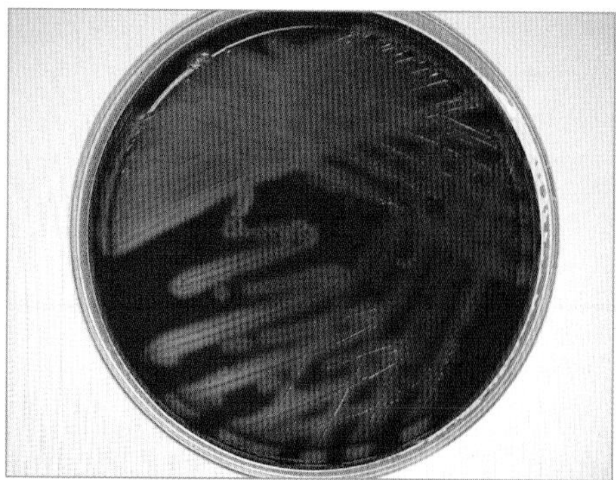

Image 127.1
Streptococcus pyogenes, 24-hour sheep blood agar plate showing β hemolysis. Courtesy of Robert Jerris, MD.

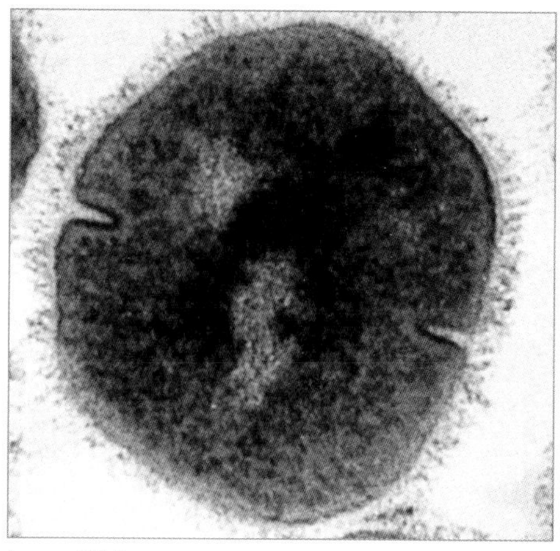

Image 127.2
Electron micrograph (magnification x70,000) of an ultrathin section of *Streptococcus pyogenes*. Courtesy of Centers for Disease Control and Prevention/Dr Vincent A. Fischetti, Rockefeller University.

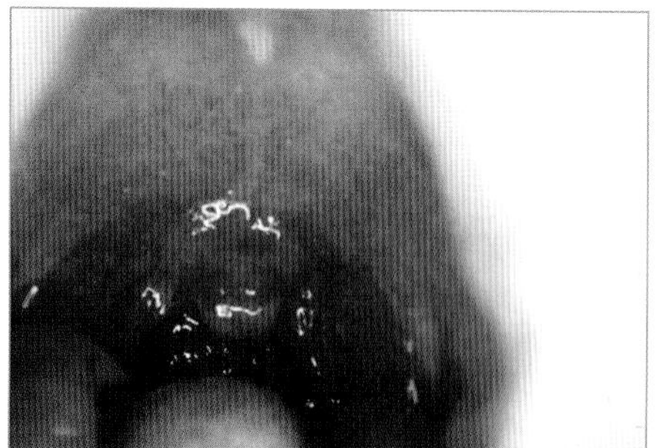

Image 127.3
Group A streptococcal pharyngitis with inflammation of the tonsils and uvula. Courtesy of Centers for Disease Control and Prevention.

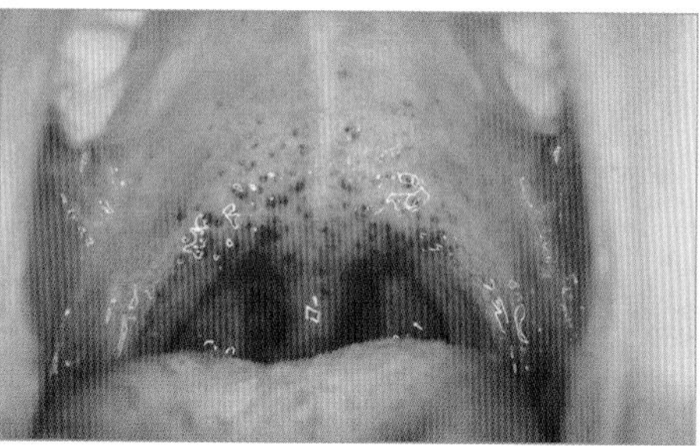

Image 127.4
Note inflammation of the oropharynx with petechiae on the soft palate, small red spots caused by group A streptococcal pharyngitis. Courtesy of Centers for Disease Control and Prevention.

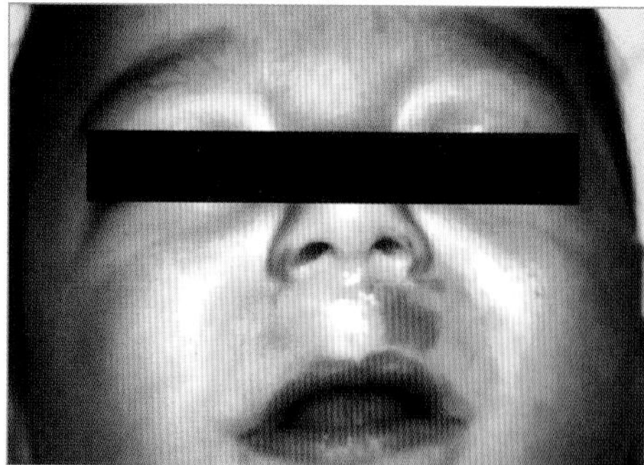

Image 127.5
Protracted nasopharyngitis is the most common presentation of group A streptococcal infection in toddlers. Inflammation of the skin beneath the nares is often present, as in this child.

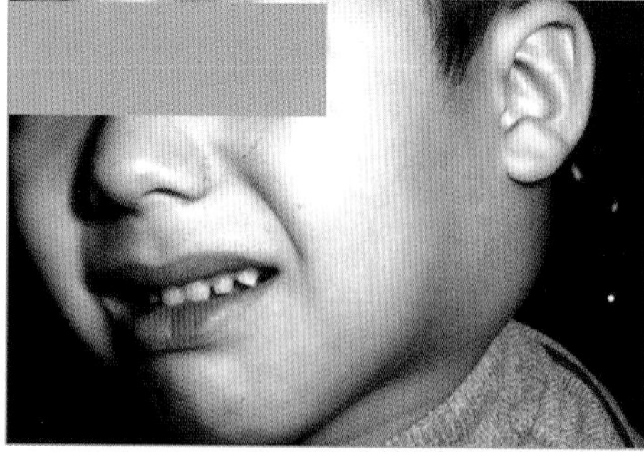

Image 127.6
Cervical lymphadenitis, unilateral, in a 6-year-old boy. The lymph node aspirate culture result was positive for group A streptococci, while the throat culture result was negative.

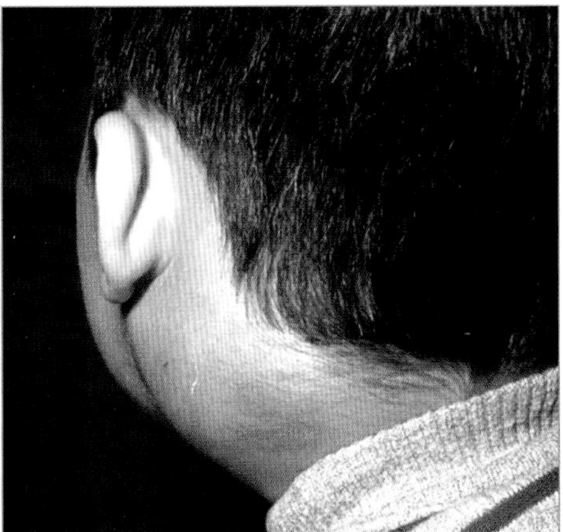

Image 127.7
Cervical lymphadenitis, unilateral. This is the same patient as in Image 127.6.

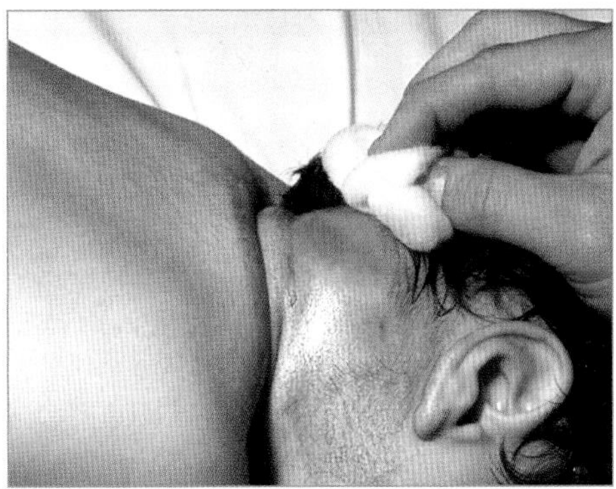

Image 127.8
Fluctuant, abscessed posterior cervical lymph node in a 4-year-old boy with impetigo of the scalp, prepped with povidone-iodine for needle aspiration for drainage and culture. Aspirate culture result was positive for group A streptococci. Courtesy of Edgar O. Ledbetter, MD, FAAP.

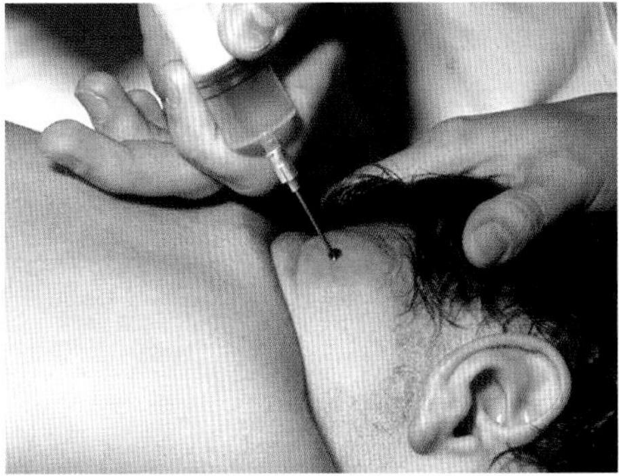

Image 127.9
Posterior cervical lymph node aspiration in the same patient as in Image 127.8. Culture result was positive for group A streptococci. Courtesy of Edgar O. Ledbetter, MD, FAAP.

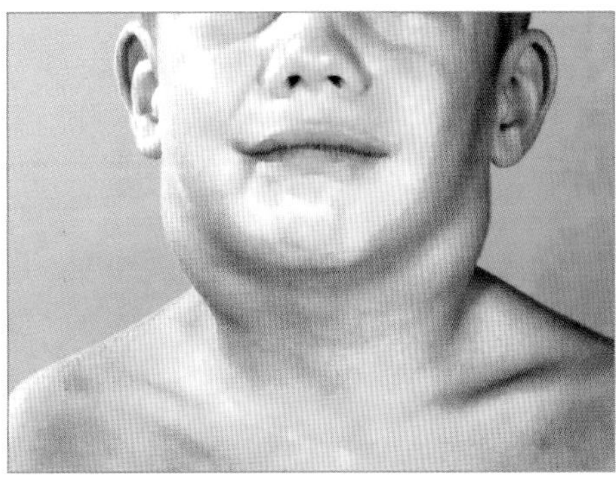

Image 127.10
Bilateral cervical lymphadenitis. The throat culture result was negative, but a lymph node aspirate culture result was positive for group A streptococci, which obviated the need for further diagnostic studies.

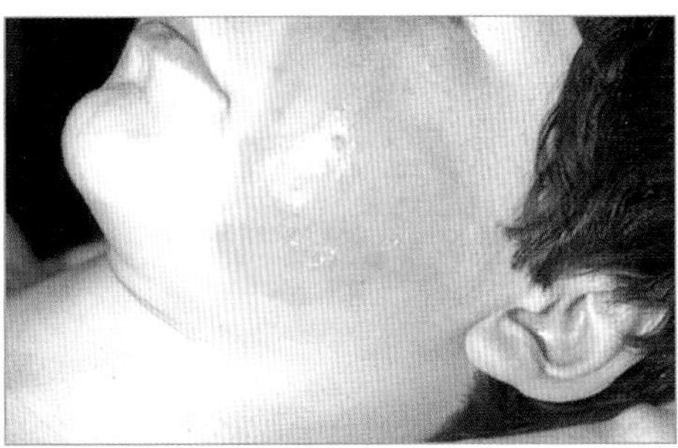

Image 127.11
A 13-year-old white boy with group A streptococcal erysipelas of the left cheek. Copyright Martin G. Myers, MD.

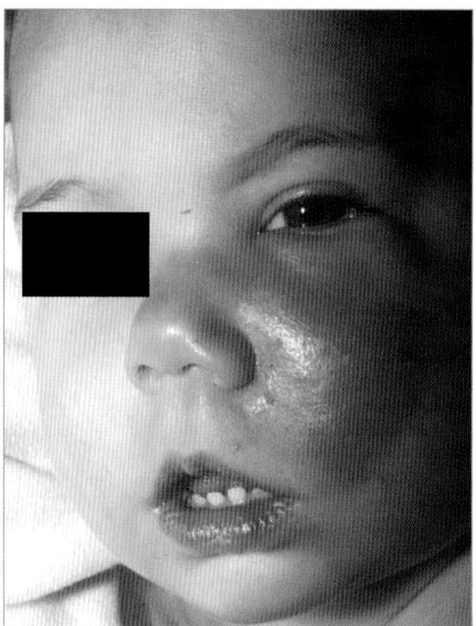

Image 127.12
Facial erysipelas in a 1-year-old white boy. Courtesy of George Nankervis, MD.

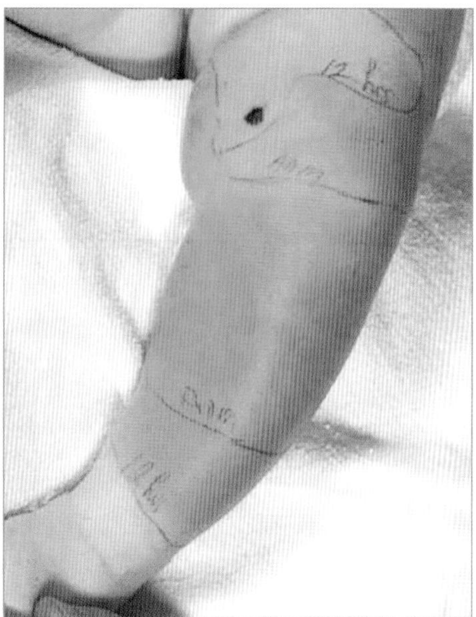

Image 127.13
Group A streptococcal cellulitis. Ink marks show the progression of cellulitis during the early hours of penicillin treatment.

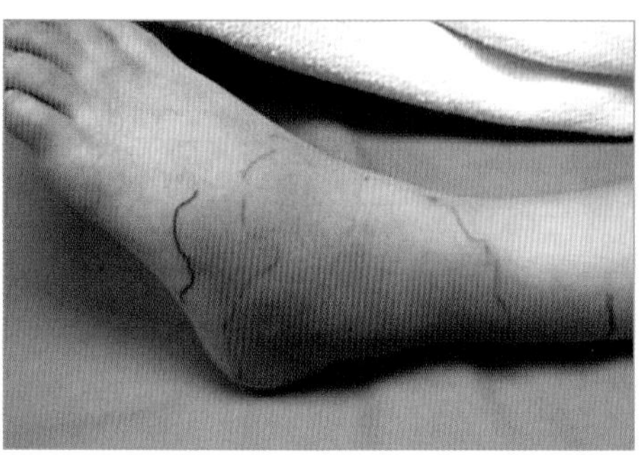

Image 127.14
Group A streptococcal cellulitis and arthritis of the left ankle in a 4-year-old white girl. Copyright Michael Rajnik, MD, FAAP.

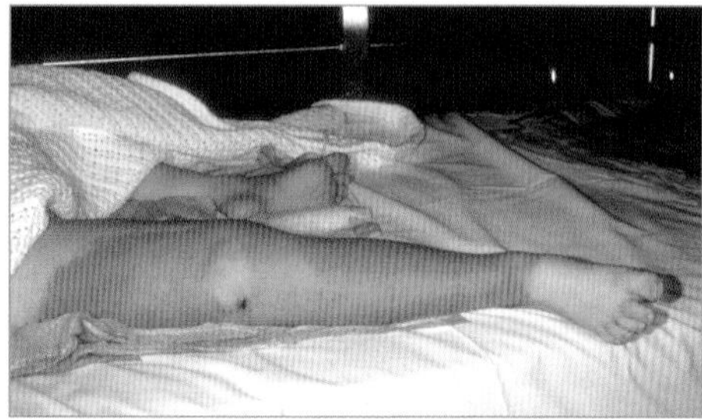

Image 127.15
Group A streptococcal cellulitis (erysipelas) of the right leg in a school-aged child secondary to impetigo. Courtesy of George Nankervis, MD.

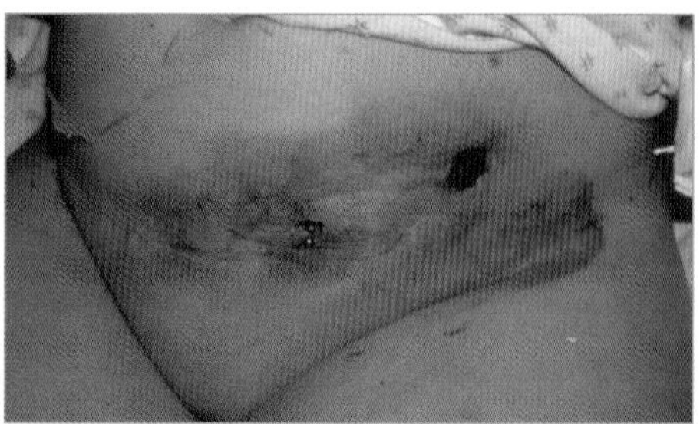

Image 127.16
Group A streptococcal necrotizing fasciitis complicating varicella in a 3-year-old white girl. Courtesy of George Nankervis, MD.

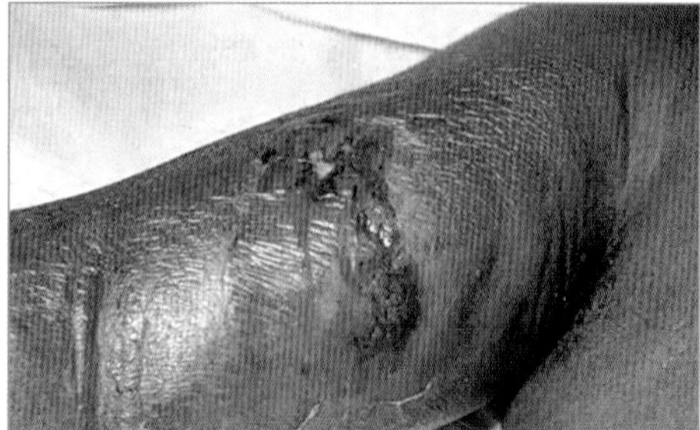

Image 127.17
Necrotizing fasciitis of the left upper arm and shoulder secondary to group A streptococcus. Courtesy of Charles Prober.

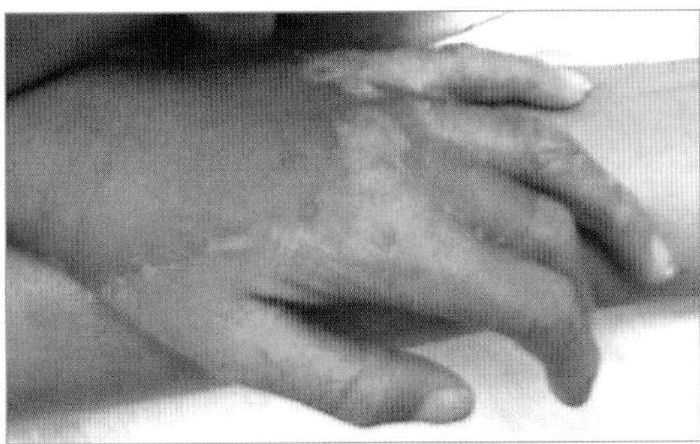

Image 127.18
Desquamation of the skin of the hand following a group A streptococcal infection (pharyngitis) in a 13-year-old black girl. Copyright Michael Rajnik, MD, FAAP.

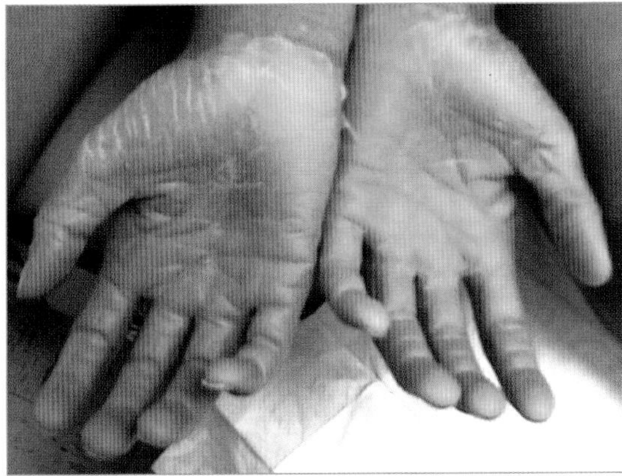

Image 127.19
Desquamation of the hands of the patient in Image 127.18. Copyright Michael Rajnik, MD, FAAP.

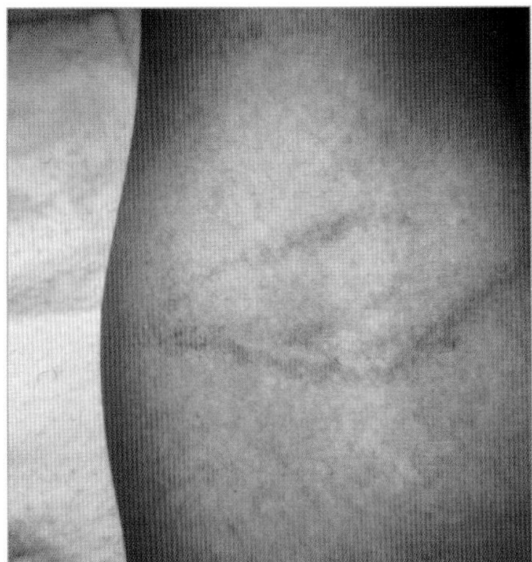

Image 127.20
Pastia lines in the antecubital space of a 12-year-old white boy with scarlet fever. Courtesy of George Nankervis, MD.

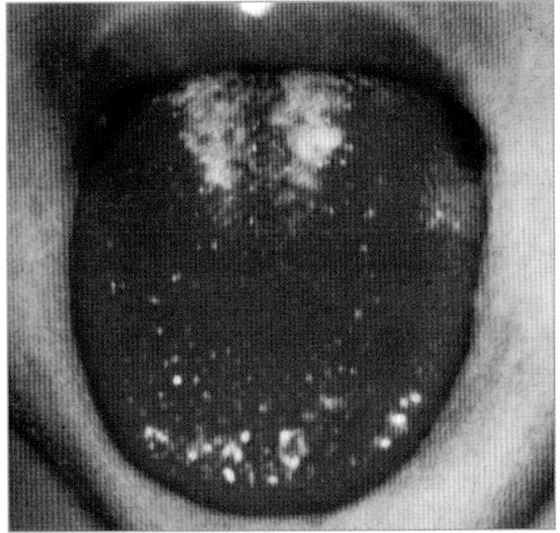

Image 127.21
The characteristic inflammatory changes in the tongue (ie, the strawberry tongue) of scarlet fever. Courtesy of Paul Wehrle, MD.

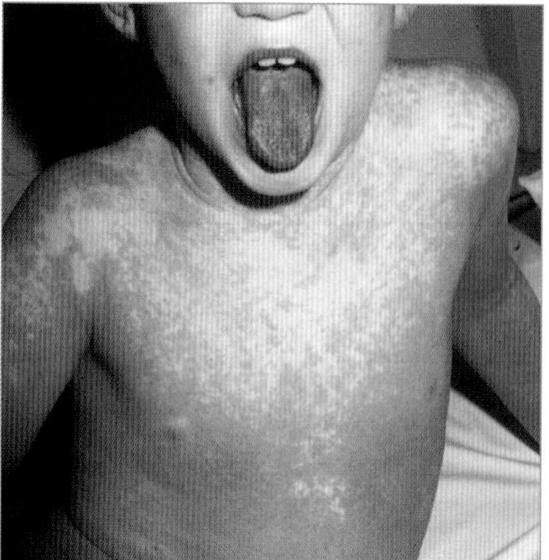

Image 127.22
A 4½-year-old white boy with the rash and strawberry tongue of scarlet fever. Courtesy of George Nankervis, MD.

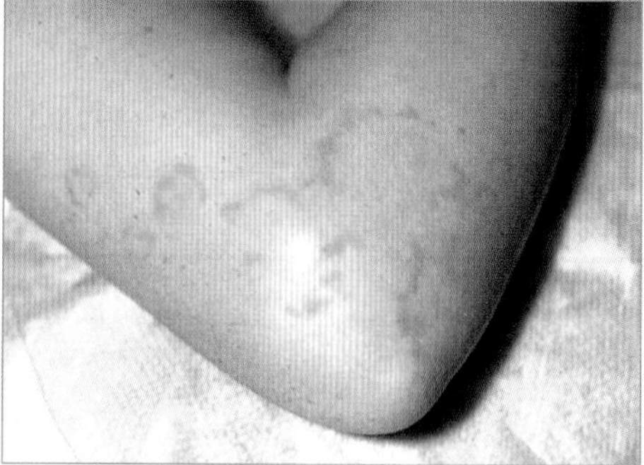

Image 127.23
Erythema marginatum in a 12-year-old white girl. Although a characteristic rash of rheumatic fever, it is noted in fewer than 3% of cases. Its serpiginous border and evanescent nature serve to distinguish it from erythema migrans lesions of Lyme disease. Copyright Martin G. Myers, MD.

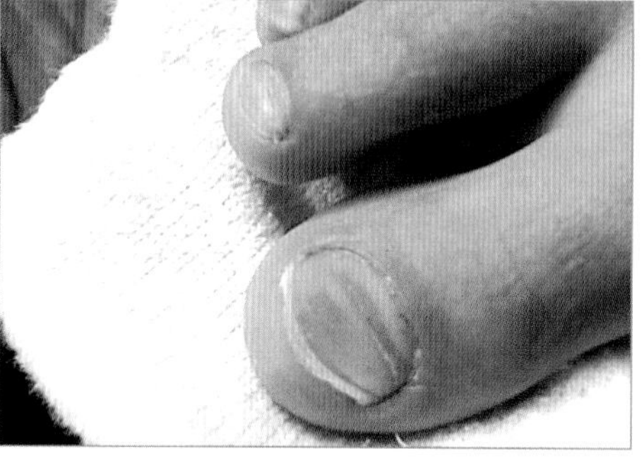

Image 127.24
Beau lines in the toenails of a child following a severe, protracted group A streptococcal illness. Copyright Michael Rajnik, MD, FAAP.

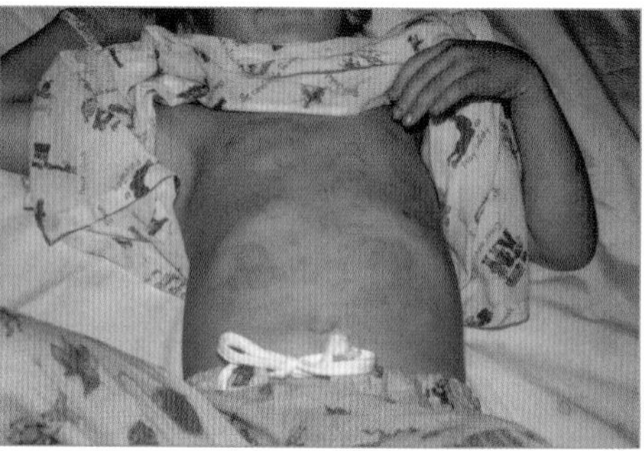

Image 127.25
Erythema marginatum lesions on the anterior trunk of a 5-year-old white boy with acute poststreptococcal rheumatic fever. Courtesy of George Nankervis, MD.

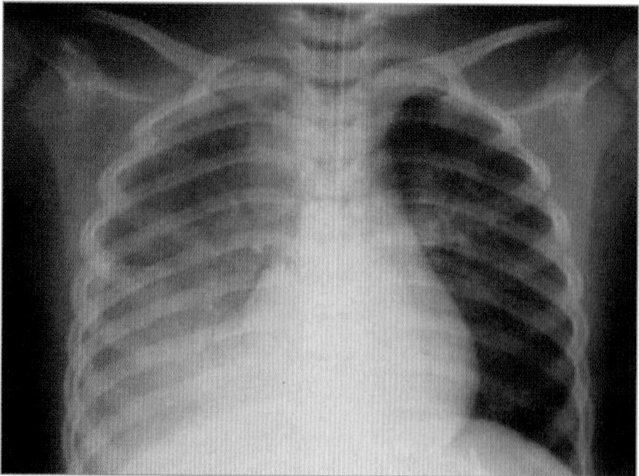

Image 127.26
Streptococcus pyogenes pneumonia in a 3-year-old girl. Courtesy of Benjamin Estrada, MD.

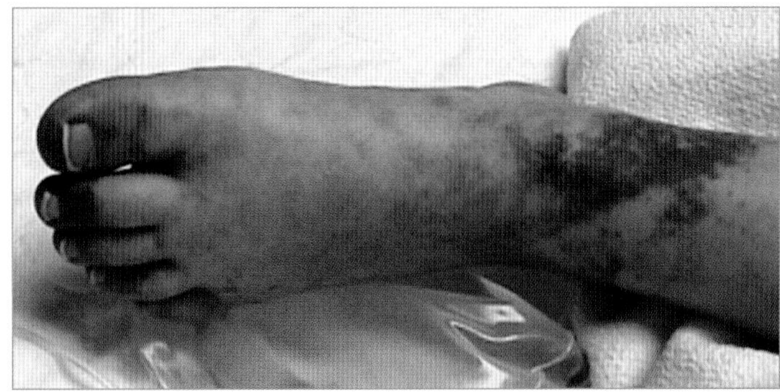

Image 127. 27
Purpura fulminans in a 6-year-old girl with *Streptococcus pyogenes* septicemia. Courtesy of Benjamin Estrada, MD.

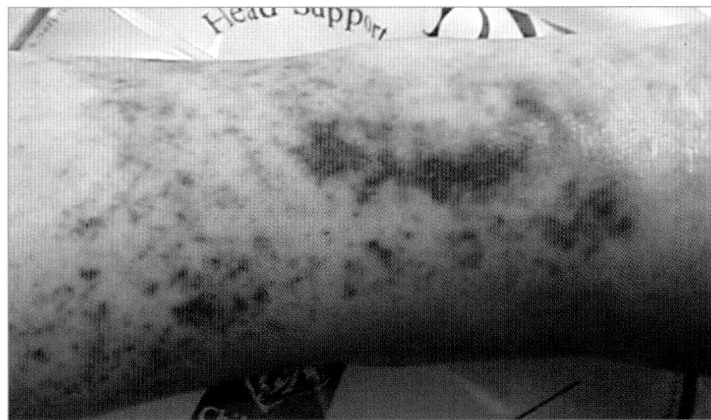

Image 127.28
Purpura fulminans in a 6-year-old girl with *Streptococcus pyogenes* septicemia. Courtesy of Benjamin Estrada, MD.

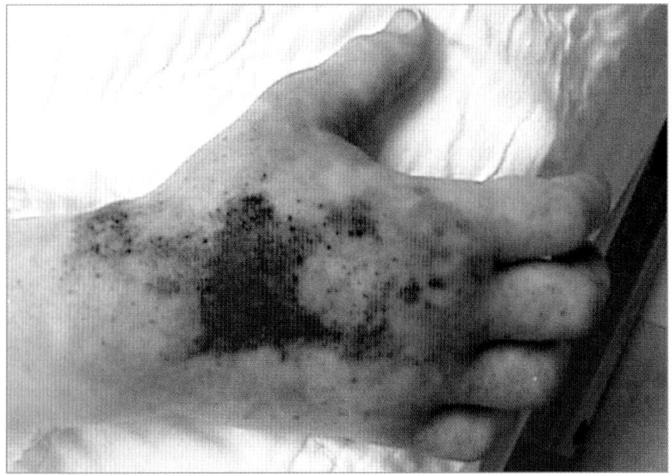

Image 127.29
Purpura fulminans in a 6-year-old girl with *Streptococcus pyogenes* septicemia. Courtesy of Benjamin Estrada, MD.

128

Group B Streptococcal Infections

Clinical Manifestations

Group B streptococci are a major cause of perinatal infections, including bacteremia, endometritis, chorioamnionitis, and urinary tract infections in pregnant women, and systemic and focal infections in neonates and young infants. Invasive disease in neonates is categorized on the basis of chronologic age at onset. Early-onset disease usually occurs within the first 24 to 36 hours of life (range, 0–6 days) and is characterized by signs of systemic infection, respiratory distress, apnea, shock, pneumonia, and, less often, meningitis (5%–10% of cases). Late-onset disease, which typically occurs at 3 to 4 weeks of age (range, 7–89 days), commonly manifests as occult bacteremia or meningitis (approximately 30% of cases); other focal infections, such as osteomyelitis, septic arthritis, necrotizing fasciitis, pneumonia, adenitis, and cellulitis, occur less commonly. Approximately 50% of survivors of early- or late-onset meningitis have long-term neurologic sequelae (encephalomalacia, cortical blindness, cerebral palsy, visual impairment, hearing deficits, or learning disabilities). Late, late-onset disease occurs beyond 89 days of age, usually in very preterm infants requiring prolonged hospitalization. Group B streptococci also cause systemic infections in nonpregnant adults with one or more underlying medical conditions, such as diabetes mellitus, chronic liver or renal disease, malignancy, or other immunocompromising conditions and in adults 65 years and older.

Etiology

Group B streptococci (*Streptococcus agalactiae*) are gram-positive, aerobic diplococci that typically produce a narrow zone of β hemolysis on 5% sheep blood agar. These organisms are divided into 10 types on the basis of capsular polysaccharides (Ia, Ib, II, and III–IX). Types Ia, Ib, II, III, and V account for approximately 95% of cases in neonates and infants in the United States. Type III is the predominant cause of early-onset meningitis and most late-onset infections in neonates and infants. Capsular polysaccharides and surface pilus islands are important virulence factors and are potential vaccine candidates.

Epidemiology

Group B streptococci are common inhabitants of the human gastrointestinal and genitourinary tracts. Less commonly, they colonize the pharynx. The colonization rate in pregnant women ranges from 15% to 35%. Colonization during pregnancy can be constant or intermittent. Before recommendations were made for prevention of early-onset group B streptococcal (GBS) disease through maternal intrapartum antimicrobial prophylaxis, the incidence was 1 to 4 cases per 1,000 live births; early-onset disease accounted for approximately 75% of cases in neonates and occurred in approximately 1 to 2 neonates per 100 colonized women. Following widespread implementation of maternal intrapartum antimicrobial prophylaxis, the incidence of early-onset disease has decreased by approximately 80% to an estimated 0.24 cases per 1,000 live births in 2012. The use of intrapartum chemoprophylaxis has had no measurable effect on late-onset GBS disease (0.32 cases per 1,000 live births in 2012). The case-fatality ratio in term neonates ranges from 1% to 3% but is higher in preterm neonates (estimated at 20% for early-onset disease and 5% for late-onset disease). Approximately 70% of early-onset and 50% of late-onset cases still afflict term neonates.

Transmission from mother to neonate occurs shortly before or during delivery. After delivery, person-to-person transmission can occur. Although uncommon, GBS infection can be acquired in the nursery from health care professionals (probably via breaks in hand hygiene) or visitors and, more commonly, in the community (colonized family members or caregivers). The risk of early-onset disease is increased in preterm neonates (<37 weeks' gestation), neonates born after the amniotic membranes have been ruptured 18 hours or more, and neonates born to women with high genital GBS inoculum, intrapartum fever (temperature ≥38°C [100.4°F]), chorioamnionitis, GBS bacteriuria during the current pregnancy, or a previous newborn with invasive GBS disease. A low or an undetectable maternal concentration of capsular type-specific serum antibody of the infecting strain is also a predisposing factor for neonatal infection. Other risk factors are intrauterine fetal monitoring and maternal age younger than 20 years. Black race is an independent risk factor for early-onset and late-onset disease. Although the incidence of early-onset disease has declined in all racial groups since the 1990s, rates have consistently been higher among black neonates (0.38 cases per 1,000 live births in 2012) compared with white neonates (0.19 cases per 1,000 live births in 2012), with the highest incidence observed among preterm black neonates. The reason for this racial/ethnic disparity is not known. The period of communicability is unknown but can extend throughout the duration of colonization or disease. Infants can remain colonized for several months after birth and after treatment for systemic infection. Recurrent GBS disease affects an estimated 1% to 3% of appropriately treated infants.

Incubation Period

Early-onset disease, fewer than 7 days (typically <24 hours); for late-onset and late, late-onset disease, unknown.

Diagnostic Tests

Gram-positive cocci in pairs or short chains by Gram stain of body fluids that are typically sterile (eg, cerebrospinal fluid [CSF], pleural fluid, joint fluid) provide presumptive evidence of infection. Growth of the organism from cultures of blood, CSF, or, if present, a suppurative focus is necessary to establish the diagnosis.

Treatment

Ampicillin plus an aminoglycoside is the empirical treatment of choice for a newborn with presumptive early-onset GBS infection. For initial treatment of late-onset disease, ampicillin and an aminoglycoside or cefotaxime are recommended. Penicillin G alone is the drug of choice when group B streptococcus has been identified as the cause of the infection and when clinical and microbiologic responses have been documented. Ampicillin is an acceptable alternative therapy. Except for meningitis or bone/joint infection, the duration of treatment is 10 days. Septic arthritis or osteomyelitis requires treatment for 3 to 4 weeks; endocarditis or ventriculitis requires treatment for at least 4 weeks.

For neonates and infants with meningitis attributable to group B streptococcus, high-dose penicillin G is the drug of choice, and ampicillin is an acceptable alternative. The duration of therapy is 2 to 3 weeks. Some experts believe a second lumbar puncture approximately 24 to 48 hours after initiation of therapy assists in management and prognosis. If CSF sterility is not achieved, a complicated course (eg, cerebral infarcts, encephalomalacia) can be expected; also, an increasing protein concentration suggests an intracranial complication (eg, infarction, ventricular obstruction). Additional lumbar punctures are indicated if response to therapy is in doubt, neurologic abnormalities persist, or focal neurologic deficits occur. Failed hearing screen, abnormal neurologic examination, and certain cranial imaging abnormalities at discharge predict an adverse long-term outcome. Consultation with a specialist in pediatric infectious diseases is often useful.

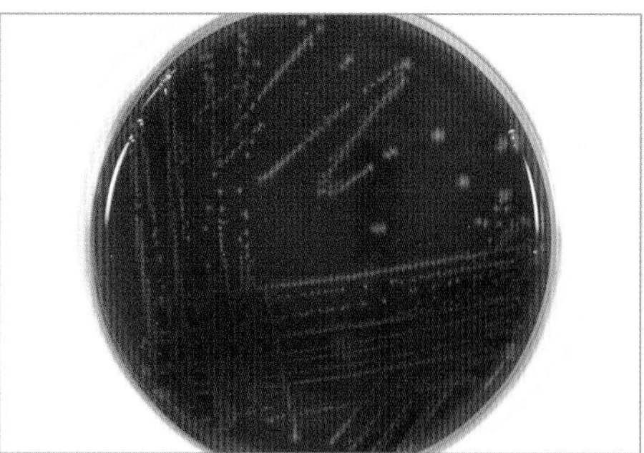

Image 128.1
Streptococcus agalactiae on blood agar. Courtesy of Julia Rosebush, DO; Robert Jerris, PhD; and Theresa Stanley, M(ASCP).

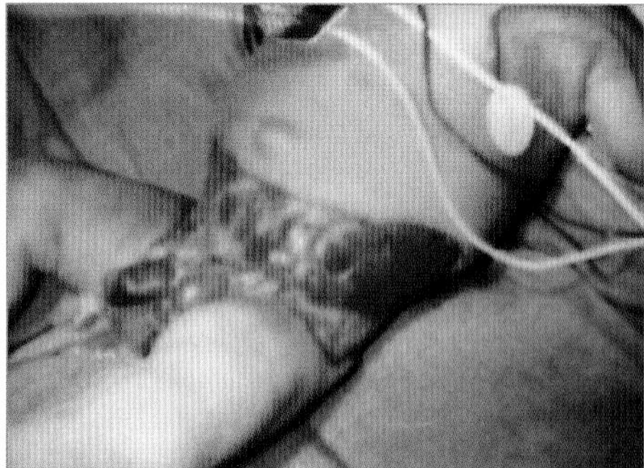

Image 128.3
Streptococcus agalactiae necrotizing fasciitis in a 3-month-old. Courtesy of Benjamin Estrada, MD.

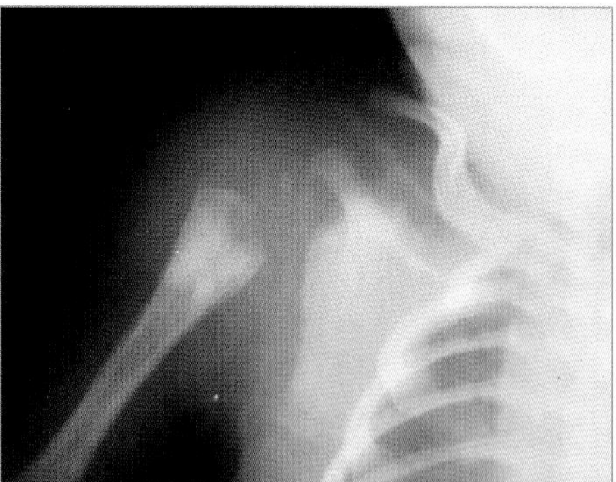

Image 128.5
Neonatal group B streptococcal septic arthritis of the right shoulder joint and osteomyelitis of the right proximal humerus. Courtesy of Neal Halsey, MD.

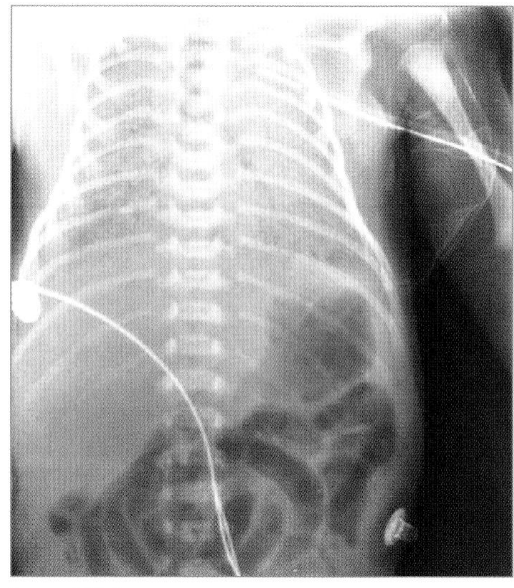

Image 128.2
Bilateral, severe group B streptococcal pneumonia in a neonate. Courtesy of David Clark, MD.

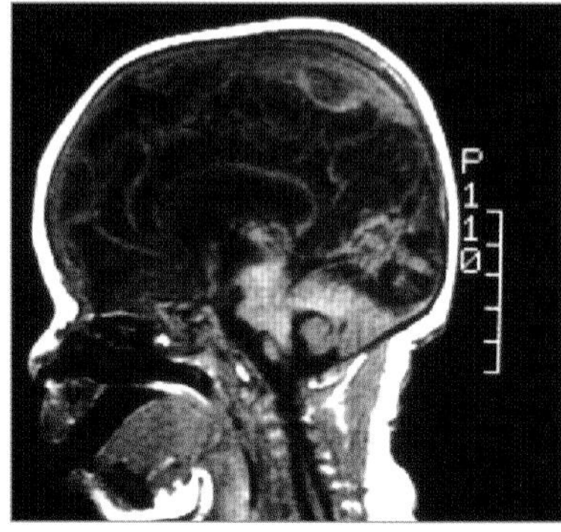

Image 128.4
Magnetic resonance imaging after group B streptococcal meningitis.

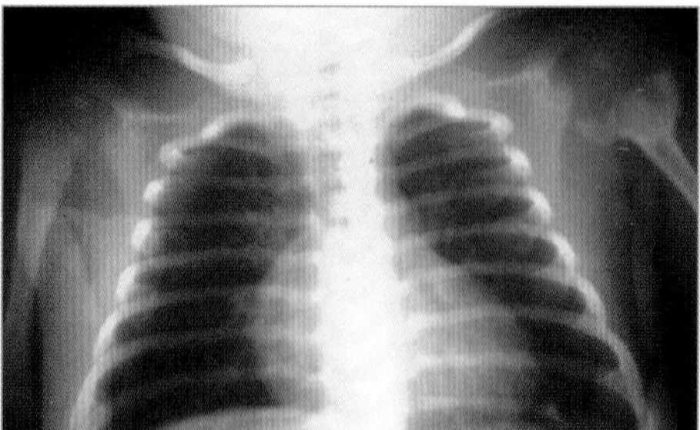

Image 128.6
Neonatal group B streptococcal septic arthritis (left shoulder joint) and osteomyelitis of the left proximal humerus. Courtesy of Edgar O. Ledbetter, MD, FAAP.

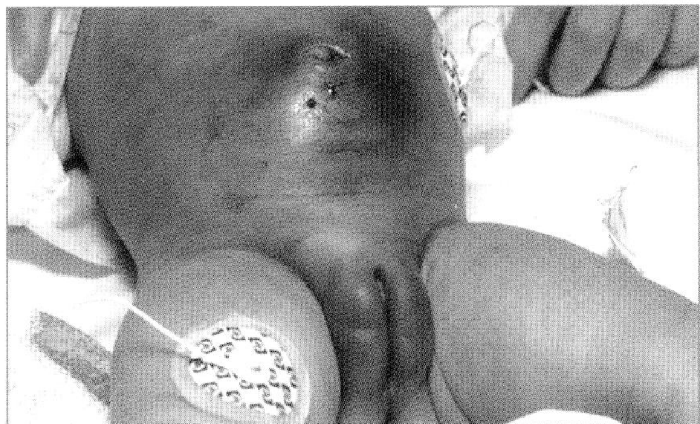

Image 128.7
Necrotizing fasciitis of the periumbilical area. Group B streptococcus, *Staphylococcus aureus*, and anaerobic streptococci were isolated at the time of surgical debridement. Courtesy of Edgar O. Ledbetter, MD, FAAP.

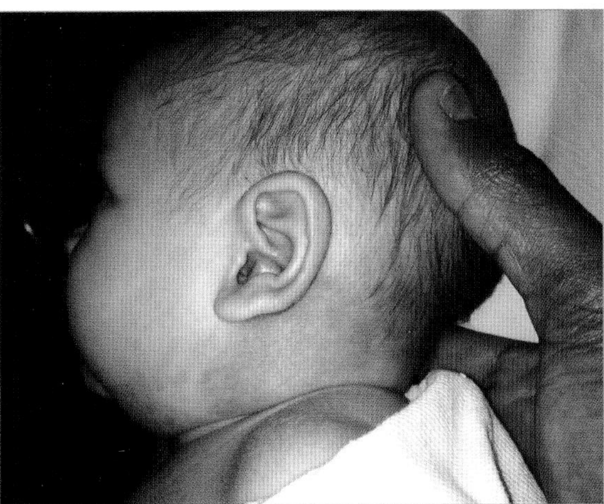

Image 128.8
A term 3-week-old who had poor feeding and irritability followed 2 hours later by fever to 38.1°C (100.6°F). On admission to the hospital 3 hours later, he required fluid resuscitation and intravenous antibiotic therapy. His spinal fluid was within normal limits, but the blood culture grew group B streptococcus. At admission, the physical examination revealed the classic facial and submandibular erythema, tenderness, and swelling characteristic of group B streptococcal cellulitis. Courtesy of Nate Serazin, MD, and C. Mary Healy, MD.

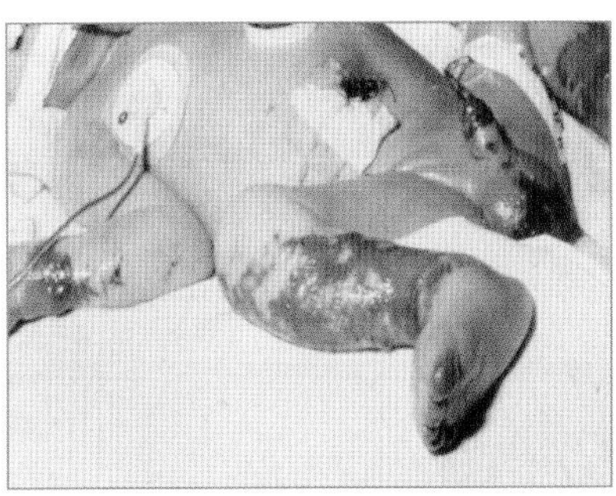

Image 128.9
A term 3-day-old neonate with fatal group B streptococcus sepsis and peripheral gangrene. Courtesy of Carol J. Baker, MD, FAAP.

129

Non–Group A or B Streptococcal and Enterococcal Infections

Clinical Manifestations

Streptococci other than Lancefield groups A or B can be associated with invasive disease in infants, children, adolescents, and adults. The principal clinical syndromes of groups C and G streptococci are septicemia, upper and lower respiratory tract infections, skin and soft tissue infections, septic arthritis, meningitis with a parameningeal focus, brain abscess, and endocarditis with various clinical manifestations. Group F streptococcus is an infrequent cause of invasive infection. Viridans streptococci are the most common cause of bacterial endocarditis in children, especially children with congenital or valvular heart disease, and these organisms have become a common cause of bacteremia in neutropenic patients with cancer and in the first 2 weeks after bone marrow transplantation. Among the viridans streptococci, organisms from the *Streptococcus anginosus* group often cause localized infections, such as brain or dental abscesses or abscesses in other sites, including lymph nodes, liver, and lung. Enterococci are associated with bacteremia in neonates and bacteremia, device-associated infections, intra-abdominal abscesses, and urinary tract infections in older children and adults.

Etiology

Changes in taxonomy and nomenclature of the *Streptococcus* genus have evolved with advances in molecular technology. Among gram-positive organisms that are catalase negative and display chains by Gram stain, the genera associated most often with human disease are *Streptococcus* and *Enterococcus*. The genus *Streptococcus* has been subdivided into 7 species groups on the basis of 16S rRNA gene sequencing. Members of the genus that are β-hemolytic on blood agar plates include *Streptococcus pyogenes, Streptococcus agalactiae* and groups C and G streptococci, all in the *Streptococcus pyogenes* species group. *Streptococcus dysgalactiae* subsp *equisimilis* is the group C subspecies most often associated with human infections. Streptococci that are non–β-hemolytic (α-hemolytic or nonhemolytic) on blood agar plates include *Streptococcus pneumoniae,* a member of the *Streptococcus mitis* group; the *Streptococcus bovis* group; and viridans streptococci clinically relevant in humans, which include 5 *Streptococcus* species groups (the *anginosus* group, the *mitis* group, the *sanguinis* group, the *salivarius* group, and the *mutans* group). The *anginosus* group includes *S anginosus, Streptococcus constellatus,* and *Streptococcus intermedius.* This group can have variable hemolysis, and approximately one-third possess group A, C, F, or G antigens. Nutritionally variant streptococci, once thought to be viridans streptococci, now are classified in the genera *Abiotrophia* and *Granulicatella.*

The genus *Enterococcus* (previously included with Lancefield group D streptococci) contains at least 18 species, with *Enterococcus faecalis* and *Enterococcus faecium* accounting for most human enterococcal infections. Outbreaks and health care–associated spread with *Enterococcus gallinarum* have also occurred occasionally. Nonenterococcal group D streptococci include *S bovis* and *Streptococcus equinus,* both members of the *bovis* group.

Epidemiology

The habitats that non-group A and B streptococci and enterococci occupy in humans include the skin (groups C and G), oropharynx (groups C and G and the *mutans* group), gastrointestinal tract (groups C and G, the *bovis* group, and *Enterococcus* species), and vagina (groups C, D, and G and *Enterococcus* species). Typical human habitats of different species of viridans streptococci are the oropharynx, epithelial surfaces of the oral cavity, teeth, skin, and gastrointestinal and genitourinary tracts. Intrapartum transmission is responsible for most cases of early-onset neonatal infection caused by non-group A and B streptococci and enterococci. Environmental contamination or transmission via hands of health care professionals can lead to colonization of patients. Groups C and G streptococci have been known to cause foodborne outbreaks of pharyngitis.

Incubation Period

Unknown.

Diagnostic Tests

Diagnosis is established by culture of usually sterile body fluids with appropriate biochemical testing and serologic analysis for definitive identification. Antimicrobial susceptibility testing of isolates from usually sterile sites should be performed to guide treatment of infections caused by viridans streptococci or enterococci. The proportion of vancomycin-resistant enterococci among hospitalized patients can be as high as 30%.

Treatment

Penicillin G is the drug of choice for groups C and G streptococci. Other agents with good activity include ampicillin, cefotaxime, vancomycin, and linezolid. The combination of gentamicin with a β-lactam antimicrobial agent (eg, penicillin, ampicillin) or vancomycin may enhance bactericidal activity needed for treatment of life-threatening infections (eg, endocarditis, meningitis).

Many viridans streptococci remain highly susceptible to penicillin. Strains with a minimum inhibitory concentration greater than 0.12 mcg/mL and less than or equal to 0.5 mcg/mL are considered relatively resistant by criteria in the American Heart Association guidelines for determining treatment of streptococcal endocarditis. Strains with a penicillin minimum inhibitory concentration greater than 0.5 mcg/mL are considered resistant. Nonpenicillin antimicrobial agents with good activity against viridans streptococci include cephalosporins (especially ceftriaxone), vancomycin, linezolid, daptomycin, and tigecycline, although pediatric experience with daptomycin and tigecycline is limited. *Abiotrophia* and *Granulicatella* organisms can exhibit relative or high-level resistance to penicillin. The combination of high-dose penicillin or vancomycin and an aminoglycoside can enhance bactericidal activity.

Enterococci exhibit uniform resistance to cephalosporins, and isolates resistant to vancomycin, especially *E faecium*, are increasing in prevalence. In general, children with a central line–associated bloodstream infection caused by enterococci should have the device removed promptly.

Systemic enterococcal infections, such as endocarditis or meningitis, should be treated with ampicillin (if the isolate is susceptible) or vancomycin in combination with an aminoglycoside. Gentamicin is the aminoglycoside recommended for achieving synergy. Gentamicin should be discontinued if in vitro susceptibility testing demonstrates high-level resistance, in which case synergy cannot be achieved. The role of combination therapy for treating central line–associated bloodstream infections is uncertain. Linezolid or daptomycin are options for treatment of infections caused by vancomycin-resistant *E faecium*. Isolates of vancomycin-resistant enterococci that are also resistant to linezolid have been described. Resistance to linezolid among vancomycin-resistant enterococci isolates can also develop during prolonged treatment. Although most vancomycin-resistant isolates of *E faecalis* and *E faecium* are daptomycin susceptible, daptomycin is only approved for use in adults and experience in children is limited. Daptomycin should not be used to treat pneumonia, as tissue levels are poor and daptomycin is inactivated by surfactants.

- **Endocarditis.** Guidelines for antimicrobial therapy in adults have been formulated by the American Heart Association and should be consulted for regimens that are appropriate for children and adolescents.

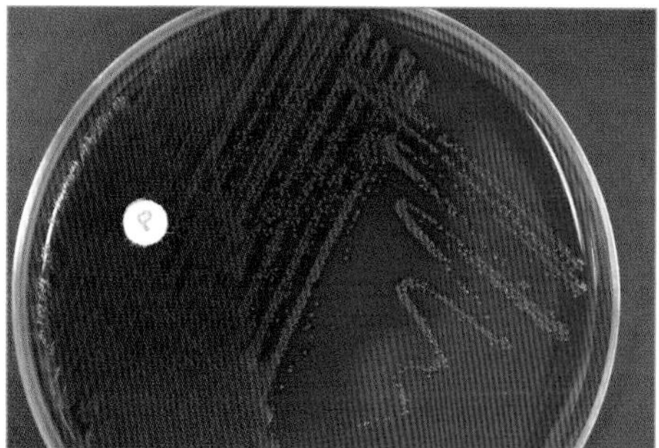

Image 129.1
Viridans streptococcus group on blood agar. This organism produces a zone of a hemolysis, rendering the colonies greenish in color. No zone of inhibition is seen surrounding the P disc, distinguishing it from *Streptococcus pneumoniae*. Courtesy of Julia Rosebush, DO; Robert Jerris, PhD; and Theresa Stanley, M(ASCP).

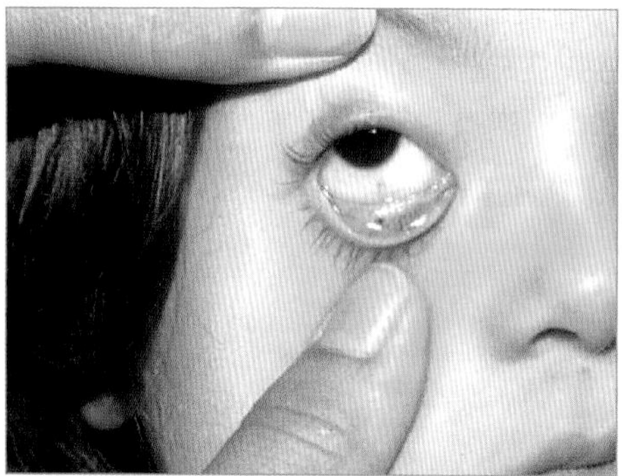

Image 129.3
Conjunctival (palpebral) petechiae in an adolescent girl with *Streptococcus viridans* subacute bacterial endocarditis.

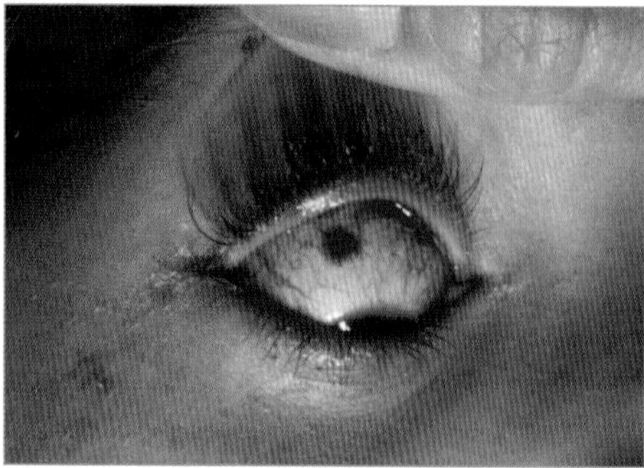

Image 129.5
A conjunctival hemorrhage in an adolescent female with enterococcal endocarditis. Courtesy of George Nankervis, MD.

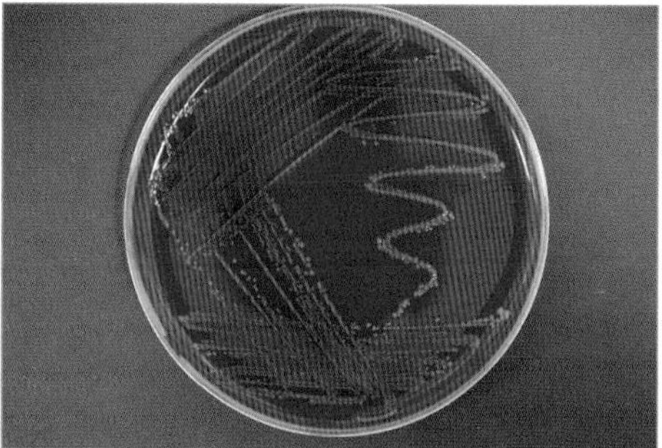

Image 129.2
Enterococcus faecalis on sheep blood agar. Small, gray, flat nonhemolytic colonies with smooth edges are seen. Courtesy of Julia Rosebush, DO; Robert Jerris, PhD; and Theresa Stanley, M(ASCP).

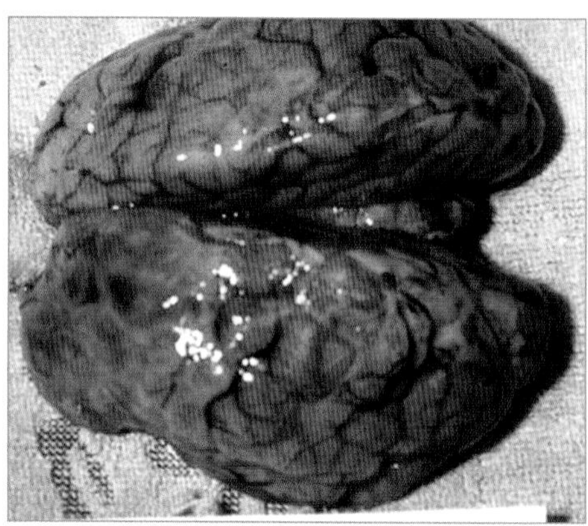

Image 129.4
Brain from a neonate with *Enterococcus faecalis* meningitis showing copious purulent exudate covering the meninges. Courtesy of Edgar O. Ledbetter MD, FAAP.

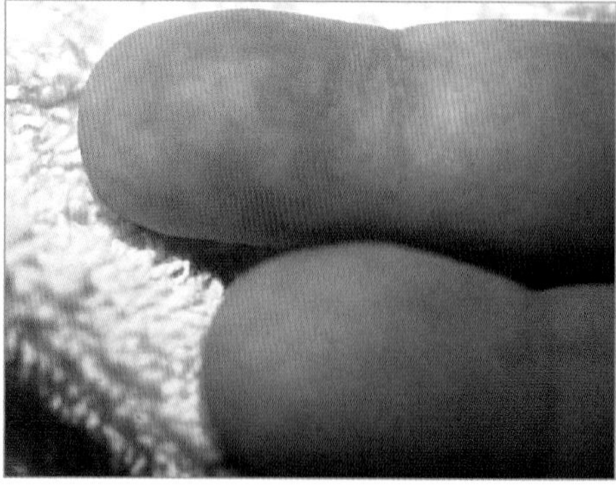

Image 129.6
A patient with Osler nodes from viridans *streptococcus* bacterial endocarditis. Copyright Martin G. Myers, MD.

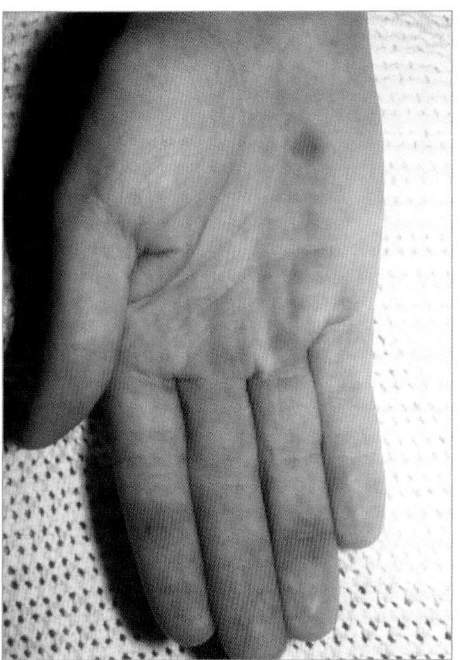

Image 129.7
Osler nodes on the fingers and a Janeway lesion in the palm of the same patient as in Image 129.5 with enterococcal endocarditis. Courtesy of George Nankervis, MD.

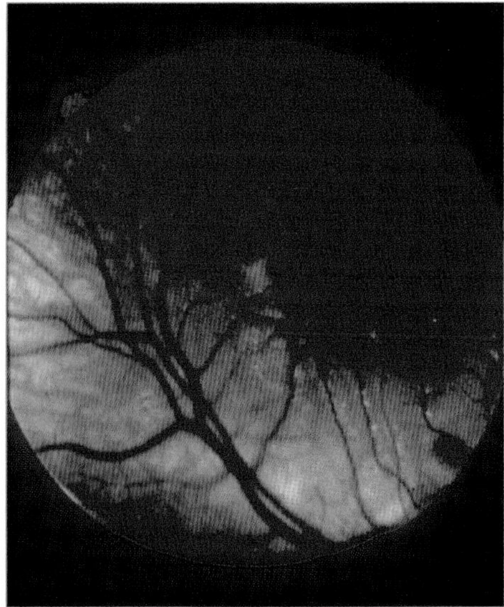

Image 129.9
Hemorrhagic retinitis with Roth spots in the adolescent female in Image 129.5 with enterococcal endocarditis. Courtesy of George Nankervis, MD.

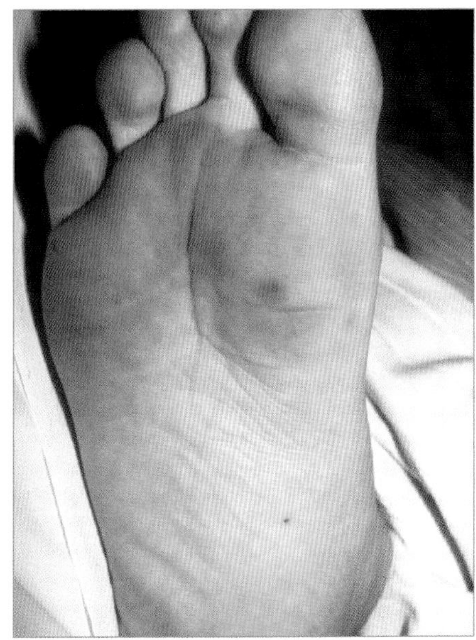

Image 129.8
A Janeway lesion on the sole of the same patient as in Image 129.5 with enterococcal endocarditis. Courtesy of George Nankervis, MD.

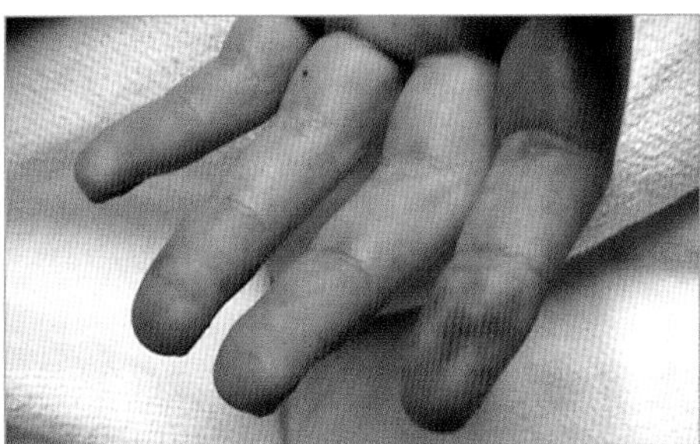

Image 129.10
Janeway lesions in a 13-year-old girl with viridans streptococcus endocarditis. Courtesy of Benjamin Estrada, MD.

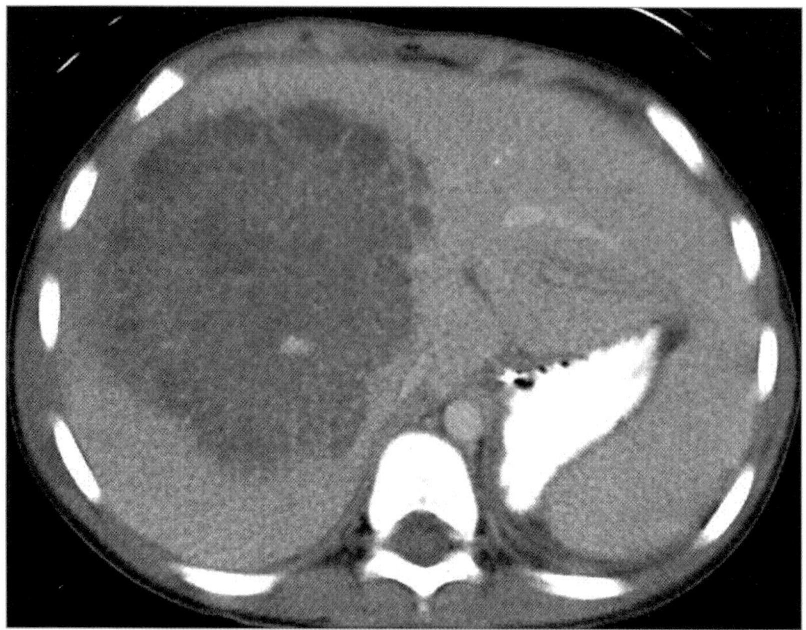

Image 129.11
Computed tomography scan showing a large liver abscess in a previously healthy 5-year-old white girl with abdominal pain and nausea. Cultures were positive for *Milleri* group streptococci. Courtesy of Preeti Jaggi, MD.

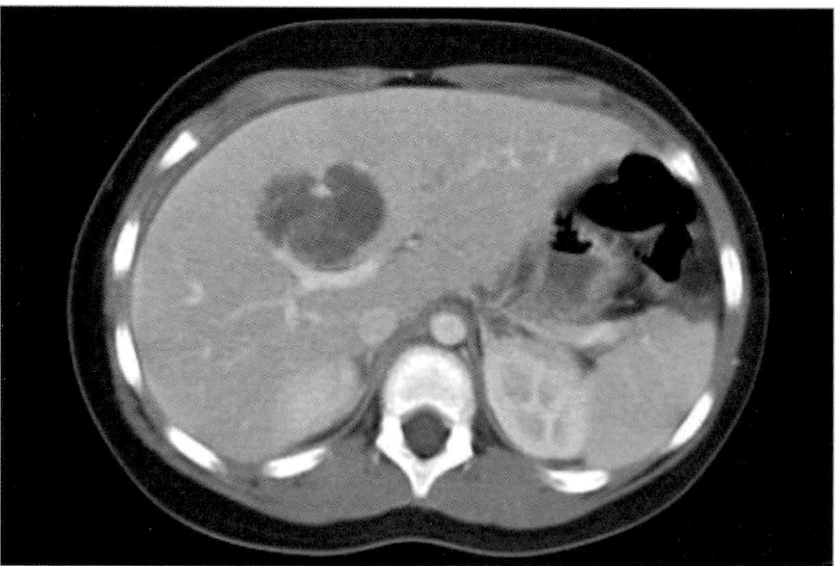

Image 129.12
A liver abscess in a 7-year-old boy from which viridans streptococci were isolated. Courtesy of Benjamin Estrada, MD.

130

Strongyloidiasis

(*Strongyloides stercoralis*)

Clinical Manifestations

Most infections with *Strongyloides stercoralis* are asymptomatic. When symptoms occur, they are most often related to larval skin invasion, tissue migration, or the presence of adult worms in the intestine. Infective (filariform) larvae are acquired from skin contact with contaminated soil, producing transient pruritic papules at the site of penetration. Larvae migrate to the lungs and can cause a transient pneumonitis or Löffler-like syndrome. After ascending the tracheobronchial tree, larvae are swallowed and mature into adults within the gastrointestinal tract. Symptoms of intestinal infection include nonspecific abdominal pain, malabsorption, vomiting, and diarrhea. Larval migration from defecated stool can result in migratory pruritic skin lesions in the perianal area, buttocks, and upper thighs, which may present as serpiginous, erythematous tracks called larva currens. Immunocompromised people, most often those receiving glucocorticoids for underlying malignancy or autoimmune disease, people receiving biologic response modifiers, and people infected with human T-lymphotropic virus 1, are at risk of *Strongyloides* hyperinfection syndrome and disseminated disease, in which larvae migrate via the systemic circulation to distant organs, including the brain, liver, kidney, heart, and skin. This condition, which is frequently fatal, is characterized by fever, abdominal pain, diffuse pulmonary infiltrates, and septicemia or meningitis caused by enteric gram-negative bacilli.

Etiology

S stercoralis is a nematode (roundworm).

Epidemiology

Strongyloidiasis is endemic in the tropics and subtropics, including the southeastern United States, wherever suitable moist soil and improper disposal of human waste coexist. Humans are the principal hosts, but dogs, cats, and other animals can serve as reservoirs. Transmission involves penetration of skin by filariform larvae from contact with contaminated soil. Infections rarely can be acquired from intimate skin contact or from inadvertent coprophagy, such as from ingestion of contaminated food or within institutional settings. Adult females release eggs in the small intestine, where they hatch as first-stage (rhabditiform) larvae that are excreted in feces. A small percentage of larvae molt to the infective (filariform) stage during intestinal transit, at which point they can penetrate the bowel mucosa or perianal skin, thus maintaining the life cycle within a single person (autoinfection). Because of this capacity for autoinfection, people can remain infected for decades after leaving an area with endemic infection.

Incubation Period

Unknown.

Diagnostic Tests

Strongyloidiasis can be difficult to diagnose in immunocompetent people because excretion of larvae in feces is highly variable and often of low intensity. At least 3 consecutive stool specimens should be examined microscopically for characteristic larvae (not eggs), but stool concentration techniques may be required to establish the diagnosis. The use of agar plate culture methods can have greater sensitivity than fecal microscopy, and examination of duodenal contents obtained using the string test (Entero-Test) or a direct aspirate through a flexible endoscope may also demonstrate larvae. Eosinophilia (blood eosinophil count >500/µL) is common in chronic infection but can be absent in hyperinfection syndrome. Serodiagnosis is sensitive and should be considered in all people with unexplained eosinophilia, especially if immunomodulatory therapy is being considered.

In disseminated strongyloidiasis, filariform larvae can be isolated from sputum or bronchoalveolar lavage fluid as well as spinal fluid. Gram-negative bacillary meningitis is a common associated finding in disseminated disease and carries a high mortality rate.

Treatment

Ivermectin is the treatment of choice for chronic (asymptomatic) strongyloidiasis and hyperinfection with disseminated disease. An alternative agent is albendazole, although it is associated with lower cure rates. Prolonged or repeated treatment may be necessary in people with hyperinfection and disseminated strongyloidiasis, and relapse can occur.

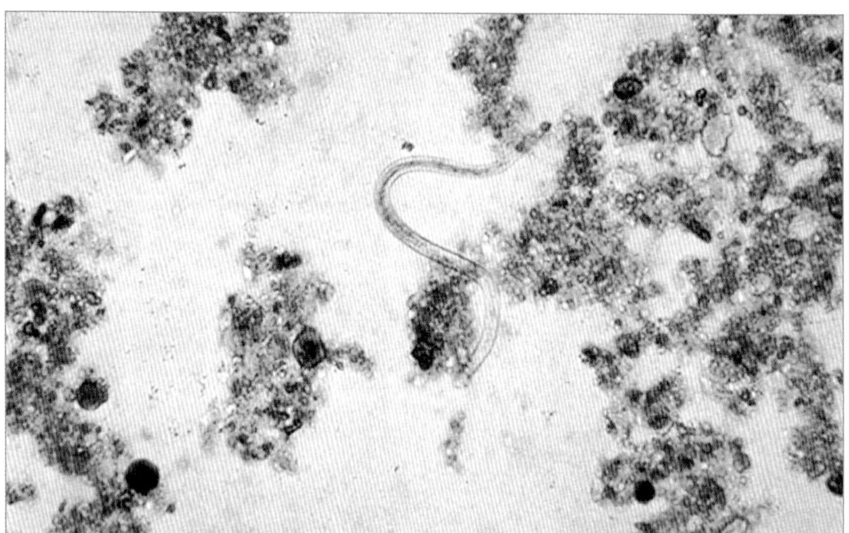

Image 130.1
Strongyloides stercoralis larvae (low-power magnification).

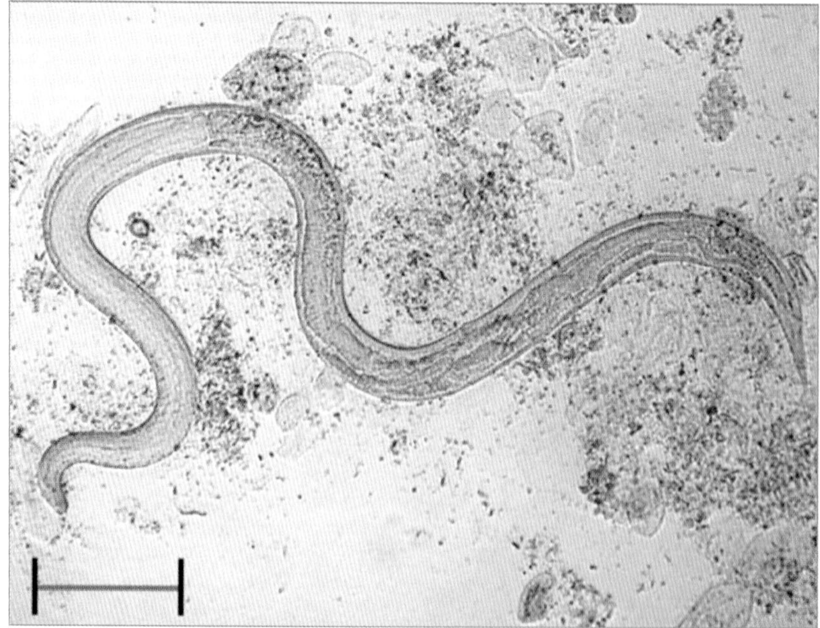

Image 130.2
Adult female of *Strongyloides stercoralis* collected in bronchial fluid of a patient with disseminated disease (scale bar = 400 µm). Courtesy of Centers for Disease Control and Prevention/*Emerging Infectious Diseases.*

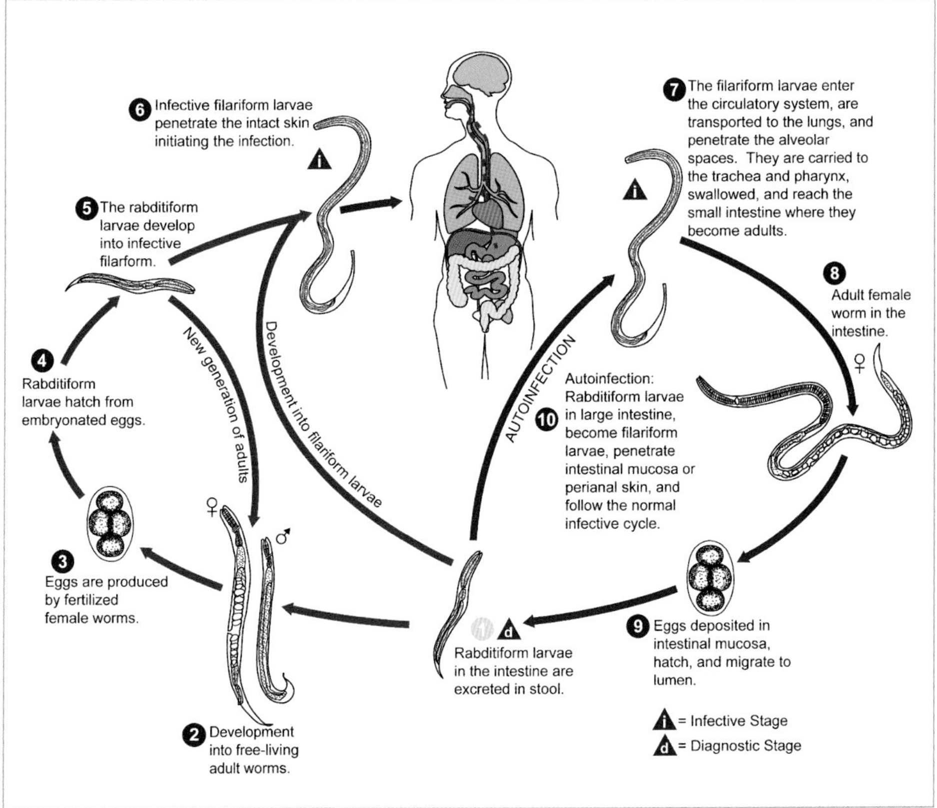

Image 130.3

The *Strongyloides* life cycle is complex among helminths with its alternation between free-living and parasitic cycles and its potential for autoinfection and multiplication within the host. Two types of cycles exist. **Free-living cycle:** The rhabditiform larvae passed in the stool (1) (see Parasitic cycle) can molt twice and become infective filariform larvae (direct development) (6) or molt 4 times and become free-living adult males and females (2) that mate and produce eggs (3), from which rhabditiform larvae hatch (4). The latter, in turn, can develop (5) into a new generation of free-living adults (as represented in 2) or into infective filariform larvae (6). The filariform larvae penetrate the human host skin to initiate the parasitic cycle. **Parasitic cycle:** Filariform larvae in contaminated soil penetrate human skin (6) and are transported to the lungs, where they penetrate the alveolar spaces; they are carried through the bronchial tree to the pharynx, are swallowed, and then reach the small intestine (7). In the small intestine they molt twice and become adult female worms (8). The females live threaded in the epithelium of the small intestine and by parthenogenesis produce eggs (9), which yield rhabditiform larvae. The rhabditiform larvae can be passed in the stool (1) (see Free-living cycle) or can cause autoinfection (10). In autoinfection, the rhabditiform larvae become infective filariform larvae, which can penetrate the intestinal mucosa (internal autoinfection) or the skin of the perianal area (external autoinfection); in either case, the filariform larvae may follow the previously described route, being carried successively to the lungs, bronchial tree, pharynx, and small intestine, where they mature into adults; or they may disseminate widely in the body. To date, occurrence of autoinfection in humans with helminthic infections is recognized only in *Strongyloides stercoralis* and *Capillaria philippinensis* infections. In the case of *Strongyloides,* autoinfection may explain the possibility of persistent infections for many years in persons who have not been in an endemic area and of hyperinfections in immunodepressed individuals. Courtesy of Centers for Disease Control and Prevention/Alexander J. da Silva, PhD/Melanie Moser.

131

Syphilis

Clinical Manifestations

Congenital Syphilis

Intrauterine infection with *Treponema pallidum* can result in stillbirth, hydrops fetalis, or preterm birth or can be asymptomatic at birth. Infected neonates and infants can have hepatosplenomegaly, snuffles (copious nasal secretions), lymphadenopathy, mucocutaneous lesions, pneumonia, osteochondritis and pseudoparalysis, edema, rash, hemolytic anemia, or thrombocytopenia at birth or within the first 4 to 8 weeks of age. Skin lesions or moist nasal secretions of congenital syphilis are highly infectious. However, organisms are rarely found in lesions more than 24 hours after treatment has begun. Untreated infants, regardless of whether they have manifestations in early infancy, can develop late manifestations, which usually appear after 2 years of age and involve the central nervous system, bones and joints, teeth, eyes, and skin. Some consequences of intrauterine infection may not become apparent until many years after birth, such as interstitial keratitis (5–20 years of age), eighth cranial nerve deafness (10–40 years of age), Hutchinson teeth (peg-shaped, notched central incisors), anterior bowing of the shins, frontal bossing, mulberry molars, saddle nose, rhagades (perioral fissures), and Clutton joints (symmetric, painless swelling of the knees). The first 3 manifestations are referred to as the Hutchinson triad. Late manifestations can be prevented by treatment of early infection.

Acquired Syphilis

Infection with *T pallidum* in childhood or adulthood can be divided into 3 stages. The **primary stage** (or "**primary syphilis**") appears as one or more painless indurated ulcers (chancres) of the skin or mucous membranes at the site of inoculation. Lesions most commonly appear on the genitalia but can appear elsewhere, depending on the sexual contact responsible for transmission (eg, oral). These lesions appear, on average, 3 weeks after exposure (10–90 days) and heal spontaneously in a few weeks. Chancres are sometimes not recognized clinically and are sometimes still present during the secondary stage of syphilis. The **secondary stage** (or "**secondary syphilis**"), beginning 1 to 2 months later, is characterized by rash, mucocutaneous lesions, and lymphadenopathy. The polymorphic maculopapular rash is generalized and typically includes the palms and soles. In moist areas around the vulva or anus, hypertrophic papular lesions (condyloma lata) can occur and can be confused with condyloma acuminata secondary to human papillomavirus infection. Generalized lymphadenopathy, fever, malaise, splenomegaly, sore throat, headache, alopecia, and arthralgia can be present. Secondary syphilis can be mistaken for other conditions because its signs and symptoms are nonspecific. This stage also resolves spontaneously without treatment in approximately 3 to 12 weeks, leaving the infected person completely asymptomatic. A variable latent period follows but is sometimes interrupted during the first few years by recurrences of symptoms of secondary syphilis. **Latent syphilis** is defined as the period after infection when patients are seroreactive but demonstrate no clinical manifestations of disease. Latent syphilis acquired within the preceding year is referred to as **early latent syphilis;** all other cases of latent syphilis are **late latent syphilis** (>1 year's duration). Patients who have latent syphilis of unknown duration should be managed clinically as if they have late latent syphilis. The **tertiary stage** of infection occurs 15 to 30 years after the initial infection and can include gumma formation (soft, noncancerous growths that can destroy tissue), cardiovascular involvement (including aortitis), or neurosyphilis. Neurosyphilis is defined as infection of the central nervous system with *T pallidum*. Manifestations of neurosyphilis can include syphilitic meningitis, uveitis, and (typically years after infection) dementia and posterior spinal cord degeneration (tabes dorsalis). Neurosyphilis can occur at any stage of infection, especially in people infected with HIV and neonates with congenital syphilis.

Etiology

T pallidum is a thin, motile spirochete that is extremely fastidious, surviving only briefly outside the host. The organism has not been successfully cultivated on artificial media.

Epidemiology

Syphilis, which is rare in much of the industrialized world, persists in the United States and in resource-limited countries. The incidence of acquired and congenital syphilis increased dramatically in the United States during the late 1980s and early 1990s but decreased subsequently; in 2000, the incidence was the lowest since reporting began in 1941. Since 2001, however, the rate of primary and secondary syphilis has increased, primarily among men who have sex with men. Among women, the rate of primary and secondary syphilis increased during 2005–2008, with a concomitant increase in cases of congenital syphilis; rates of primary and secondary syphilis among women and congenital syphilis have since decreased. The highest rates of primary and secondary syphilis and congenital syphilis are in the Southern United States. Late or limited prenatal care and failure of health care professionals to follow maternal syphilis screening recommendations have been shown to contribute to the incidence of congenital syphilis. In adults, infection with HIV is common among individuals with syphilis, particularly among men who have sex with men. Primary and secondary rates of syphilis are highest in black, non-Hispanic people and in males compared with females.

Congenital syphilis is contracted from an infected mother via transplacental transmission of *T pallidum* at any time during pregnancy or, possibly, at birth from contact with maternal lesions. Among women with untreated early syphilis, as many as 40% of pregnancies result in spontaneous abortion, stillbirth, or perinatal death. Infection can be transmitted to the fetus at any stage of maternal disease. The rate of transmission is 60% to 100% during primary and secondary syphilis and slowly decreases with later stages of maternal infection (approximately 40% with early latent infection and 8% with late latent infection). In 2008, approximately 520,900 adverse outcomes were estimated to be caused by maternal syphilis worldwide, including approximately 212,300 stillbirths (gestational age >28 weeks) or early fetal deaths (gestational age 22–28 weeks), 91,800 neonatal deaths, 65,300 neonates born preterm or with low birth weight, and 151,500 infected newborns.

Acquired syphilis is almost always contracted through direct sexual contact with ulcerative lesions of the skin or mucous membranes of infected people. Open, moist lesions of the primary or secondary stages are highly infectious. Relapses of secondary syphilis with infectious mucocutaneous lesions have been observed 4 years after primary infection.

Sexual abuse must be suspected in any young child with acquired syphilis. In most cases, identification of acquired syphilis in children must be reported to state child protective service agencies. Physical examination for signs of sexual abuse and forensic interviews may be conducted under the auspices of a pediatrician with expertise in child abuse or at a local child advocacy center.

Incubation Period

For primary syphilis, 3 weeks (range, 10–90 days).

Diagnostic Tests

Definitive diagnosis is made when spirochetes are identified by microscopic darkfield examination of lesion exudate, nasal discharge, or tissue, such as placenta, umbilical cord, or autopsy specimens. Specimens should be scraped from moist mucocutaneous lesions or aspirated from a regional lymph node. Specimens from mouth lesions can contain nonpathogenic treponemes that can be difficult to distinguish from *T pallidum* by darkfield microscopy. Although such testing can provide a definitive diagnosis, serologic testing is also necessary.

Presumptive diagnosis is possible using nontreponemal and treponemal serologic tests. Use of only one type of test is insufficient for diagnosis because false-positive nontreponemal test results occur with various medical conditions, and treponemal test results remain positive long after syphilis has been treated adequately (making the diagnosis of reinfection difficult) and can be falsely positive with other spirochetal diseases.

Standard nontreponemal tests for syphilis include the Venereal Disease Research Laboratory (VDRL) slide test and the rapid plasma reagin (RPR) test. These tests measure antibody directed against lipoidal antigen from *T pallidum,* antibody interaction with host tissues, or both. These tests are inexpensive and performed rapidly and provide semiquantitative results. Quantitative results help define disease activity and monitor response to therapy. Nontreponemal test results (eg, VDRL, RPR) can be falsely negative (ie, nonreactive) in early primary syphilis, latent acquired syphilis of long duration, and late congenital syphilis. Occasionally, a nontreponemal test performed on serum samples containing high concentrations of antibody against *T pallidum* will be weakly reactive or falsely negative, a reaction termed the **prozone** phenomenon. Diluting serum results in a positive test. Rapid plasma reagin titers are generally higher than VDRL titers; thus, when nontreponemal tests are used to monitor treatment response, the same specific test (eg, VDRL, RPR) must be used throughout the follow-up period, preferably performed by the same laboratory, to ensure comparability of results.

A reactive nontreponemal test result from a patient with typical lesions indicates a presumptive diagnosis of syphilis and the need for treatment. However, any reactive nontreponemal test result must be confirmed by one of the specific treponemal tests to exclude a false-positive test result. False-positive results can be caused by certain viral infections (eg, Epstein-Barr virus infection, hepatitis, varicella, measles), lymphoma, tuberculosis, malaria, endocarditis, connective tissue disease, pregnancy, abuse of injection drugs, laboratory or technical error, or Wharton jelly contamination when umbilical cord blood specimens are used. Treatment should not be delayed while awaiting the results of the treponemal test results if the patient is symptomatic or at high risk of infection. A sustained 4-fold decrease in titer, equivalent to a change of 2 dilutions (eg, from 1:32 to 1:8), of the nontreponemal test result after treatment usually demonstrates adequate therapy, whereas a sustained 4-fold increase in titer (eg, from 1:8 to 1:32) after treatment suggests reinfection or relapse. The nontreponemal test titer usually decreases 4-fold within 6 to 12 months after therapy for primary or secondary syphilis and usually becomes nonreactive within 1 year after successful therapy if the infection (primary or secondary syphilis) was treated early. The patient usually becomes seronegative within 2 years even if the initial titer was high or the infection was congenital. Some people will continue to have low stable nontreponemal antibody titers despite effective therapy. This serofast state is more common in patients treated for latent or tertiary syphilis.

Treponemal tests in use include the *T pallidum* particle agglutination (TP-PA) test, *T pallidum* enzyme immunoassay (TP-EIA), *T pallidum* chemiluminescent assay (TP-CIA), and fluorescent treponemal antibody absorption (FTA-ABS) test. People who have reactive treponemal test results usually remain reactive for life, even after successful therapy. However, 15% to 25% of patients treated during the primary stage revert to being serologically nonreactive after 2 to 3 years. Treponemal test antibody titers correlate poorly with disease activity and should not be used to assess response to therapy.

Treponemal tests are also not 100% specific for syphilis; positive reactions occur variably in patients with other spirochetal diseases, such as yaws, pinta, leptospirosis, rat-bite fever, relapsing fever, and Lyme disease. Nontreponemal tests can be used to differentiate Lyme disease from syphilis because the VDRL test is nonreactive in Lyme disease.

The Centers for Disease Control and Prevention recommends syphilis serologic screening with a nontreponemal test, such as the RPR or VDRL test, to identify people with possible untreated infection; this screening is followed by confirmation using one of several available treponemal tests. Some clinical laboratories and blood banks have begun to screen samples using treponemal EIA tests rather than beginning with a nontreponemal test; the reasons for this change in sequence of the screening relate to cost. However, this "reverse-sequence screening" approach is associated with high rates of false-positive results, and in 2011, the Centers for Disease Control and Prevention reaffirmed its long-standing recommendation that nontreponemal tests be used to screen for syphilis and treponemal testing be used to confirm syphilis as the cause of nontreponemal reactivity. The traditional algorithm performs well in identifying people with active infection who require further evaluation and treatment while minimizing false-positive results in low-prevalence populations. All patients who have syphilis should be tested for HIV infection and other sexually transmitted infections.

Cerebrospinal Fluid Tests

Cerebrospinal fluid (CSF) abnormalities in patients with neurosyphilis include increased protein concentration, increased white blood cell (WBC) count, or a reactive CSF-VDRL test result. The CSF-VDRL is highly specific but is insensitive. Thus, the CSF-VDRL test results should be interpreted cautiously because a negative result on a VDRL test of CSF does not exclude a diagnosis of neurosyphilis. Alternatively, a reactive CSF-VDRL test in the CSF of neonates can be the result of non-treponemal immunoglobulin G antibodies that cross the blood-brain barrier. The CSF leukocyte count is usually elevated in neurosyphilis (>5 WBCs/mm^3) in a non-neonate. Cerebrospinal fluid test results obtained during the neonatal period can be difficult to interpret; normal values differ by gestational age and are higher in preterm neonates. Values as high as 21 WBCs/mm^3 or protein up to 130 mg/dL can occur in term neonates. Although the FTA-ABS test of CSF is less specific than the CSF-VDRL test, some experts recommend using the FTA-ABS test, believing it to be more sensitive than the CSF-VDRL test. A positive CSF FTA-ABS result can support the diagnosis of neurosyphilis but, by itself, cannot establish the diagnosis. Fewer data exist for the TP-PA test for CSF, and none exist for the RPR test; these tests should not be used for CSF evaluation.

Testing During Pregnancy

All women should be screened serologically for syphilis early in pregnancy with a nontreponemal test (RPR or VDRL) and preferably again at delivery. In areas of high prevalence of syphilis and in patients considered at high risk of syphilis, a nontreponemal serum test at the beginning of the third trimester (28 weeks of gestation) and at delivery is indicated. For women treated for syphilis during pregnancy, follow-up nontreponemal serologic testing is necessary to assess the efficacy of therapy. Low-titer false-positive nontreponemal antibody test results occasionally occur in pregnancy. A positive nontreponemal antibody test result should be confirmed with a treponemal antibody test (eg, TP-PA, TP-EIA, TP-CIA, FTA-ABS). In most cases, if the treponemal antibody test result is negative, the nontreponemal test result is falsely positive, and no further evaluation is necessary. However, in patients with early syphilis, the nontreponemal test result can be positive before the treponemal test result. Therefore, retesting in 2 to 4 weeks and later, if clinically indicated, should be considered for high-risk pregnant women with a positive nontreponemal test and a negative treponemal test. Some laboratories are screening pregnant women using an EIA treponemal test, but this **"reverse-sequence" screening approach is not recommended.** Pregnant women with reactive treponemal EIA screening tests should have confirmatory testing with a nontreponemal test. Subsequent evaluation and possible treatment of the neonate should follow the mother's RPR or VDRL result and her management, as outlined in Image 131.1. Any woman who delivers a stillborn neonate after 20 weeks' gestation should be tested for syphilis.

Evaluation of Neonates and Infants for Congenital Infection During the Newborn Period and First Months of Life

No newborn should be discharged from the hospital without determination of the mother's serologic status for syphilis at least once during pregnancy and also at delivery. All neonates born to seropositive mothers require a careful examination and a nontreponemal syphilis test obtained from the neonate. The test performed on the neonate should be the same as that performed on the mother to enable comparison of titer results. A negative maternal RPR or VDRL test result at delivery does not exclude congenital syphilis, although such a situation is uncommon. The diagnostic and therapeutic approach to neonates being evaluated for congenital syphilis is summarized in Image 131.1 and depends on identification of maternal syphilis, adequacy of maternal therapy, maternal serologic response to therapy, comparison of maternal and neonatal serologic titers, and the findings on the neonate's physical examination. On the basis of maternal history and initial findings, the evaluation includes laboratory tests (liver function tests, complete blood cell and platelet counts, a CSF-VDRL, and CSF cell count and protein concentration), long-bone and chest radiography, and an ophthalmologic examination. Neonates with an abnormal physical examination consistent with congenital syphilis, born to mothers with no or inadequate therapy, and whose mothers received therapy less than 4 weeks before delivery will need CSF evaluation to establish the diagnosis of neurosyphilis and aid in planning follow-up evaluations. Additional recommendations for neonate evaluation are found in Image 131.1. Other causes of elevated CSF values should be considered when a neonate is being evaluated for congenital syphilis. Neonates born to mothers who are coinfected with syphilis and HIV do not require different evaluation, therapy, or follow-up for syphilis than is recommended for all neonates.

Evaluation and Treatment of Older Infants and Children

Children who are identified as having reactive serologic tests for syphilis should have maternal serologic test results and records reviewed to assess whether they have congenital or acquired syphilis. The recommended evaluation includes CSF analysis for CSF-VDRL testing, cell count, and protein concentration; complete blood cell count, differential, and platelet count; and other tests as indicated clinically (eg, long-bone or chest radiography, liver function tests, abdominal ultrasonography, ophthalmologic examination, auditory brainstem response testing, neuroimaging studies).

Cerebrospinal Fluid Testing

Cerebrospinal fluid should be examined in all patients with neurologic or ophthalmic signs or symptoms, evidence of active tertiary syphilis (eg, aortitis and gumma), treatment failure, or HIV infection with late latent syphilis.

Treatment

Parenteral penicillin G remains the preferred drug for treatment of syphilis at any stage. Recommendations for penicillin G use and duration of therapy vary, depending on the stage of disease and clinical manifestations. Parenteral penicillin G is the only documented effective therapy for patients who have neurosyphilis, congenital syphilis, or syphilis during pregnancy and is recommended for HIV-infected patients. Such patients should always be treated with penicillin, even if desensitization for penicillin allergy is necessary.

Congenital Syphilis: Neonates in the First Month of Life

The diagnostic and therapeutic approach to neonates delivered to mothers with syphilis is outlined in Image 131.1. For proven or probable congenital syphilis (on the basis of the neonate's physical examination and radiographic and laboratory test results), the preferred treatment is aqueous crystalline penicillin G, administered intravenously for 10 days. The dosage should be based on chronologic age rather than gestational age. Alternatively, procaine penicillin G, intramuscularly, can be administered as a single daily dose for 10 days; no treatment failures have occurred with this formulation despite its low CSF concentrations. When the neonate is at risk of congenital syphilis because of inadequate maternal treatment or response to treatment (or reinfection) during pregnancy but the neonate's physical examination, radiographic imaging, and laboratory analyses are normal (including neonate RPR/VDRL titer the same as or less than 4-fold the maternal RPR/VDRL), some experts would treat with a single dose of penicillin G benzathine intramuscularly, but most would still prefer 10 days of treatment. If more than 1 day of therapy is missed, the entire course should be restarted. Data supporting use of other antimicrobial agents (eg, ampicillin) for treatment of congenital syphilis are not available. When possible, a full 10-day course of penicillin is preferred, even if ampicillin was initially provided for possible sepsis.

Neonates who have a normal physical examination and a serum quantitative nontreponemal serologic titer less than 4-fold higher than the maternal titer (eg, 1:16 is 4-fold higher than 1:4) are at minimal risk of syphilis if they are born to mothers who completed appropriate penicillin treatment for syphilis during pregnancy and more than 4 weeks before delivery and the mother had no evidence of reinfection or relapse. Although a full evaluation may be unnecessary, these neonates should be treated with a single intramuscular injection of penicillin G benzathine because fetal treatment failure can occur despite adequate maternal treatment during pregnancy. Alternatively, these neonates can be examined carefully, preferably monthly, until their nontreponemal serologic test results are negative.

Neonates who have a normal physical examination and a serum quantitative nontreponemal serologic titer the same as or lower than the maternal titer and whose mother's treatment was adequate before pregnancy and whose mother's nontreponemal serologic titer remained low and stable before and during pregnancy and at delivery (VDRL <1:2; RPR <1:4) require no evaluation. Some experts, however, would treat with penicillin G benzathine as a single intramuscular injection if follow-up is uncertain.

Congenital Syphilis: Older Infants and Children

Because establishing the diagnosis of neurosyphilis is difficult, infants older than 1 month who possibly have congenital syphilis or who have neurologic involvement should be treated with intravenous aqueous crystalline penicillin for 10 days (Table 131.1). This regimen should also be used to treat children older than 2 years who have late and previously untreated congenital syphilis. If the patient has no clinical manifestations of disease, the CSF examination is normal, and the result of the CSF-VDRL test is negative, some experts would treat with 3 weekly doses of penicillin G benzathine.

Syphilis in Pregnancy

Regardless of stage of pregnancy, women should be treated with penicillin according to the dosage schedules appropriate for the stage of syphilis as recommended for nonpregnant patients. For penicillin-allergic patients, no proven alternative therapy has been established. A pregnant woman with a history of penicillin allergy should be treated with penicillin after desensitization. Desensitization should be performed in consultation with a specialist and only in facilities in which emergency assistance is available.

Early Acquired Syphilis (Primary, Secondary, Early Latent Syphilis)

A single intramuscular dose of penicillin G benzathine is the preferred treatment for children and adults. All children should have a CSF examination before treatment to exclude a diagnosis of neurosyphilis. Evaluation of CSF in adolescents and adults is necessary only if clinical signs or symptoms of neurologic or ophthalmic involvement are present. Neurosyphilis should be considered in the differential diagnosis of neurologic disease in HIV-infected people.

For nonpregnant adults and adolescents who are allergic to penicillin, doxycycline or tetracycline should be given for 14 days. Clinical studies (along with biologic and pharmacologic considerations) suggest ceftriaxone once daily, intramuscularly or intravenously, for 10 to 14 days (for adolescents and adults) is effective for early-acquired syphilis, but the optimal dose and duration of therapy have not been defined. Single-dose therapy with ceftriaxone is not effective, as has been documented in several geographic areas.

Close follow-up of people receiving any alternative therapy is essential. When follow-up cannot be ensured, especially for children younger than 8 years, consideration must be given to hospitalization and desensitization followed by administration of penicillin G.

Syphilis of More Than 1 Year's Duration (Late Latent Syphilis and Late Syphilis)

Penicillin G benzathine should be given intramuscularly, weekly, for 3 successive weeks. In patients who are allergic to penicillin,

Table 131.1
Recommended Treatment for Syphilis in People Older Than 1 Month

Status	Children	Adults
Congenital syphilis	Aqueous crystalline penicillin G, 200,000–300,000 U/kg/d, IV, administered as 50,000 U/kg, every 4–6 h for 10 d[a]	
Primary, secondary, and early latent syphilis[b]	Penicillin G benzathine,[c] 50,000 U/kg, IM, up to the adult dose of 2.4 million U in a single dose	Penicillin G benzathine, 2.4 million U, IM, in a single dose **OR** *If allergic to penicillin and not pregnant,* doxycycline, 100 mg, orally, twice a day for 14 d **OR** Tetracycline, 500 mg, orally, 4 times/d for 14 d
Late latent syphilis[d]	Penicillin G benzathine, 50,000 U/kg, IM, up to the adult dose of 2.4 million U, administered as 3 single doses at 1-wk intervals (total 150,000 U/kg, up to the adult dose of 7.2 million U)	Penicillin G benzathine, 7.2 million U total, administered as 3 doses of 2.4 million U, IM, each at 1-wk intervals **OR** *If allergic to penicillin and not pregnant,* doxycycline, 100 mg, orally, twice a day for 4 wk **OR** Tetracycline, 500 mg, orally, 4 times/d for 4 wk
Tertiary	…	Penicillin G benzathine 7.2 million U total, administered as 3 doses of 2.4 million U, IM, at 1-wk intervals *If allergic to penicillin and not pregnant, consult an infectious diseases expert.*
Neurosyphilis[e]	Aqueous crystalline penicillin G, 200,000–300,000 U/kg/d, IV, every 4–6 h for 10–14 d, in doses not to exceed the adult dose	Aqueous crystalline penicillin G, 18–24 million U per day, administered as 3–4 million U, IV, every 4 h for 10–14 d[f] **OR** Penicillin G procaine,[c] 2.4 million U, IM, once daily **PLUS** probenecid, 500 mg, orally, 4 times/d, both for 10–14 d[f]

Abbreviations: IM, intramuscularly; IV, intravenously.

[a] If the patient has no clinical manifestations of disease, the cerebrospinal fluid (CSF) examination is normal, and the CSF Venereal Disease Research Laboratory test result is negative, some experts would treat with up to 3 weekly doses of penicillin G benzathine, 50,000 U/kg, IM. Some experts also suggest giving these patients a single dose of penicillin G benzathine, 50,000 U/kg, IM, after the 10-day course of intravenous aqueous penicillin.

[b] Early latent syphilis is defined as being acquired within the preceding year.

[c] Penicillin G benzathine and penicillin G procaine are approved for intramuscular administration only.

[d] Late latent syphilis is defined as syphilis beyond 1 year's duration.

[e] Patients who are allergic to penicillin should be desensitized.

[f] Some experts administer penicillin G benzathine, 2.4 million U, IM, once per week for up to 3 weeks after completion of these neurosyphilis treatment regimens.

doxycycline or tetracycline for 4 weeks should be given only with close serologic and clinical follow-up. Limited clinical studies suggest ceftriaxone might be effective, but the optimal dose and duration have not been defined. Patients who have syphilis and who demonstrate any of the following criteria should have a prompt CSF examination:

1. Neurologic or ophthalmic signs or symptoms
2. Evidence of active tertiary syphilis (eg, aortitis, gumma, iritis, uveitis)
3. Serologic treatment failure

If dictated by circumstances and patient or parent preferences, a CSF examination may be performed for patients who do not meet these criteria. Some experts recommend performing a CSF examination on all patients who have latent syphilis and a nontreponemal serologic test result of 1:32 or greater or if the patient is HIV infected and has a serum $CD4^+$ T-lymphocyte count of 350 or less. The risk of asymptomatic neurosyphilis in these circumstances is increased approximately 3-fold. If a CSF examination is performed and the results indicate abnormalities consistent with neurosyphilis, the patient should be treated for neurosyphilis.

Neurosyphilis

The recommended regimen for adults is aqueous crystalline penicillin G, intravenously, for 10 to 14 days. If adherence to therapy can be ensured, patients may be treated with an alternative regimen of daily intramuscular penicillin G procaine plus oral probenecid for 10 to 14 days. Some experts recommend following both of these regimens with penicillin G benzathine intramuscularly, weekly, for 1 to 3 doses. For children, intravenous aqueous crystalline penicillin G for 10 to 14 days is recommended.

If the patient has a history of allergy to penicillin, consideration should be given to desensitization, and the patient should be managed in consultation with an allergy specialist.

Other Considerations

Mothers of neonates with congenital syphilis should be tested for other sexually transmitted infections, including *Neisseria gonorrhoeae*, *Chlamydia trachomatis*, HIV, and hepatitis B. If injection drug use is suspected, the mother may also be at risk of hepatitis C virus infection. All recent sexual contacts of people with acquired syphilis should be evaluated for other sexually transmitted infections as well as syphilis. Partners who were exposed within 90 days preceding the diagnosis of primary, secondary, or early latent syphilis in the index patient should be treated presumptively for syphilis, even if they are seronegative.

All patients with syphilis should be tested for other sexually transmitted infections, including *N gonorrhoeae*, *C trachomatis*, HIV, and hepatitis B. Patients who have primary syphilis should be retested for HIV after 3 months if the first HIV test result is negative. For HIV-infected patients with syphilis, careful follow-up is essential. Patients infected with HIV who have early syphilis may be at increased risk of neurologic complications and higher rates of treatment failure with currently recommended regimens. Children with acquired primary, secondary, or latent syphilis should be evaluated for possible sexual assault or abuse.

Follow-up and Management

Congenital Syphilis

All neonates and infants who have reactive serologic tests for syphilis or were born to mothers who were seroreactive at delivery should receive careful follow-up evaluations during regularly scheduled well-child care visits at 2, 4, 6, and 12 months of age. Serologic nontreponemal tests should be performed every 2 to 3 months until the nontreponemal test becomes nonreactive or the titer has decreased at least 4-fold (ie, 1:16 to 1:4). Nontreponemal antibody titers should decrease by 3 months of age and should be nonreactive by 6 months of age if the infant was infected and adequately treated or was not infected and initially seropositive because of transplacentally acquired maternal antibody. The serologic response after therapy may be slower for infants treated after the neonatal period. Patients with increasing titers or with persistent stable titers 6 to 12 months after initial treatment should be reevaluated, including a CSF examination, and treated with a 10-day course of parenteral penicillin G, even if they were treated previously.

Treponemal tests should not be used to evaluate treatment response because results for an infected child can remain positive despite effective therapy. Passively transferred maternal treponemal antibodies can persist in a child until 15 months of age. A reactive treponemal test after 18 months of age is diagnostic of congenital syphilis. If the nontreponemal test is nonreactive at this time, no further evaluation or treatment is necessary. If the nontreponemal test is reactive at 18 months of age, the child should be evaluated (or reevaluated) fully and treated for congenital syphilis.

Treated infants with congenital neurosyphilis and initially positive results of CSF-VDRL tests or abnormal CSF cell counts or protein concentrations should undergo repeated clinical evaluation and CSF examination at 6-month intervals until their CSF examination is normal. A reactive CSF-VDRL test or abnormal CSF indices that cannot be attributed to another ongoing illness at the 6-month interval are indications for retreatment. Neuroimaging studies, such as magnetic resonance imaging, should be considered in these children.

Acquired Syphilis

Treated pregnant women with syphilis should have quantitative nontreponemal serologic tests repeated at 28 to 32 weeks of gestation, at delivery, and according to recommendations for the stage of disease. Serologic titers may be repeated monthly in women at high risk of reinfection or in geographic areas where the prevalence of syphilis is high. The clinical and antibody response should be appropriate for stage of disease, but most women will deliver before their serologic response to treatment can be assessed definitively. Inadequate maternal treatment is likely if clinical signs of infection are present at delivery or if maternal antibody titer is 4-fold higher than the pretreatment titer. Fetal treatment is considered inadequate if delivery occurs within 28 days of maternal therapy.

Indications for Retreatment

Primary/Secondary Syphilis

If clinical signs or symptoms persist or recur or if a 4-fold increase in titer of a nontreponemal test occurs, evaluate CSF and HIV status and repeat therapy. If the nontreponemal titer fails to decrease 4-fold within 6 months after therapy, evaluate for HIV; repeat therapy unless follow-up for continued clinical and serologic assessment can be ensured. Some experts recommend CSF evaluation.

Latent Syphilis

In the following situations, CSF examination should be performed and retreatment should be provided:

- Titers increase at least 4-fold (ie, 1:4 to 1:16).
- An initially high titer (>1:32) fails to decrease at least 4-fold (ie, 1:32 to 1:8) within 12 to 24 months.
- Signs or symptoms attributable to syphilis develop.

In all these instances, retreatment should be performed with 3 weekly injections of penicillin G benzathine, intramuscularly, unless CSF examination indicates neurosyphilis is present, at which time treatment for neurosyphilis should be initiated. Retreated patients should be treated with the schedules recommended for patients with syphilis for more than 1 year. In general, only one retreatment course is indicated. The possibility of reinfection or concurrent HIV infection should always be considered when retreating patients with early syphilis, and repeat HIV testing should be performed in such cases.

Patients with neurosyphilis associated with acquired syphilis must have periodic serologic testing, clinical evaluation at 6-month intervals, and repeat CSF examinations. If the CSF white blood cell count has not decreased after 6 months or if the CSF white blood cell count or protein are not within reference range after 2 years, retreatment should be considered. Cerebrospinal fluid abnormalities may persist for extended periods in HIV-infected people with neurosyphilis. Close follow-up is warranted.

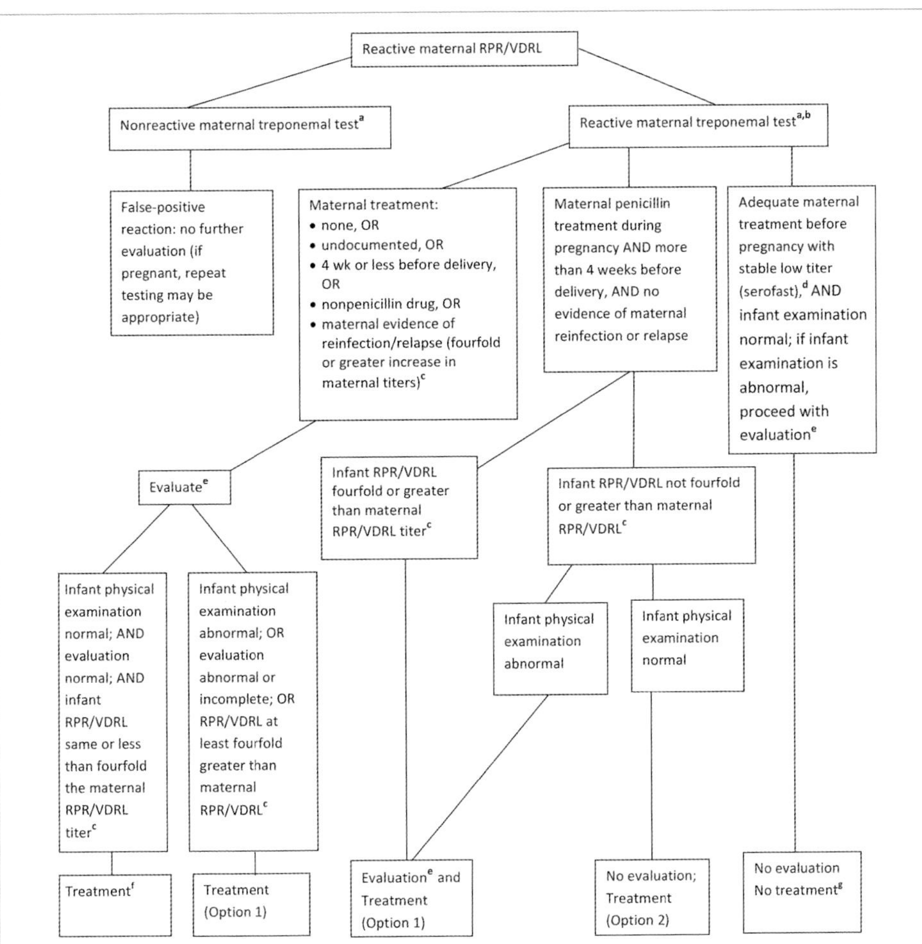

Abbreviations: RPR, rapid plasma reagin; VDRL, Venereal Disease Research Laboratory.

[a] *Treponema pallidum* particle agglutination (TP-PA), fluorescent treponemal antibody absorption (FTA-ABS), *T pallidum* enzyme immunoassay (TP-EIA), or microhemagglutination test for antibodies to *T pallidum* (MHA-TP).

[b] Test for HIV antibody. Neonates of HIV-infected mothers do not require different evaluation or treatment for syphilis.

[c] A 4-fold change in titer is the same as a change of 2 dilutions. For example, a titer of 1:64 is 4-fold greater than a titer of 1:16, and a titer of 1:4 is 4-fold lower than a titer of 1:16. When comparing titers, the same type of nontreponemal test should be used (eg, if the initial test was an RPR, the follow-up test should also be an RPR).

[d] Women who maintain a VDRL titer 1:2 or less or an RPR 1:4 or less beyond 1 year after successful treatment are considered serofast.

[e] Complete blood cell and platelet count; cerebrospinal fluid examination for cell count, protein, and quantitative VDRL; other tests as clinically indicated (eg, chest radiographs, long-bone radiographs, eye examination, liver function tests, neuroimaging, auditory brainstem response).

[f] Treatment (option 1 or option 2, below), with most experts recommending treatment option 1. If a single dose of benzathine penicillin G is used, the neonate must be fully evaluated, full evaluation must be normal, and follow-up must be certain. If any part of the neonate's evaluation is abnormal or not performed, or if the CSF analysis is rendered uninterpretable, a 10-day course of penicillin is required.

[g] Some experts would consider a single intramuscular injection of benzathine penicillin (treatment option 2), particularly if follow-up is not certain.

Treatment Options

1. Aqueous penicillin G, 50,000 U/kg, intravenously, every 12 hours (1 week of age or younger) or every 8 hours (older than 1 week); or procaine penicillin G, 50,000 U/kg, intramuscularly, as a single daily dose for 10 days. If 24 or more hours of therapy is missed, the entire course must be restarted.
2. Benzathine penicillin G, 50,000 U/kg, intramuscularly, single dose.

Image 131.1

Algorithm for evaluation and treatment of neonates born to mothers with reactive serologic tests for syphilis.

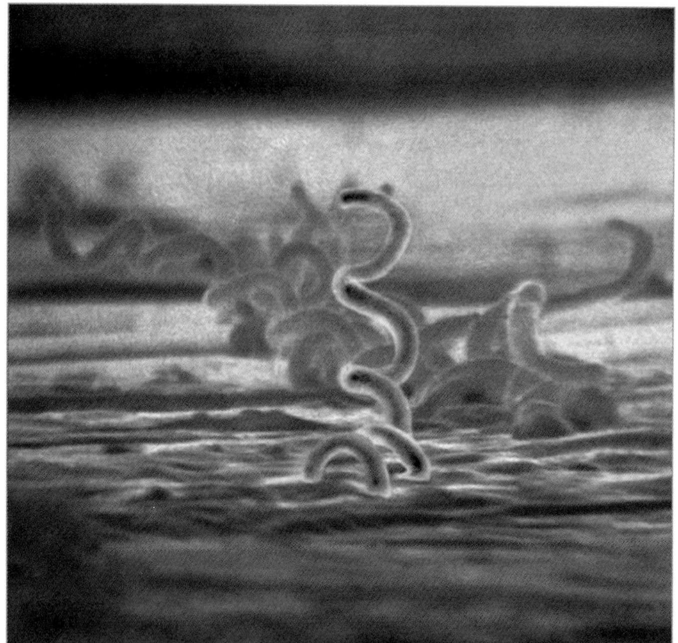

Image 131.2
This electron micrograph shows *Treponema pallidum* on cultures of cotton-tail rabbit epithelium cells. Courtesy of Centers for Disease Control and Prevention.

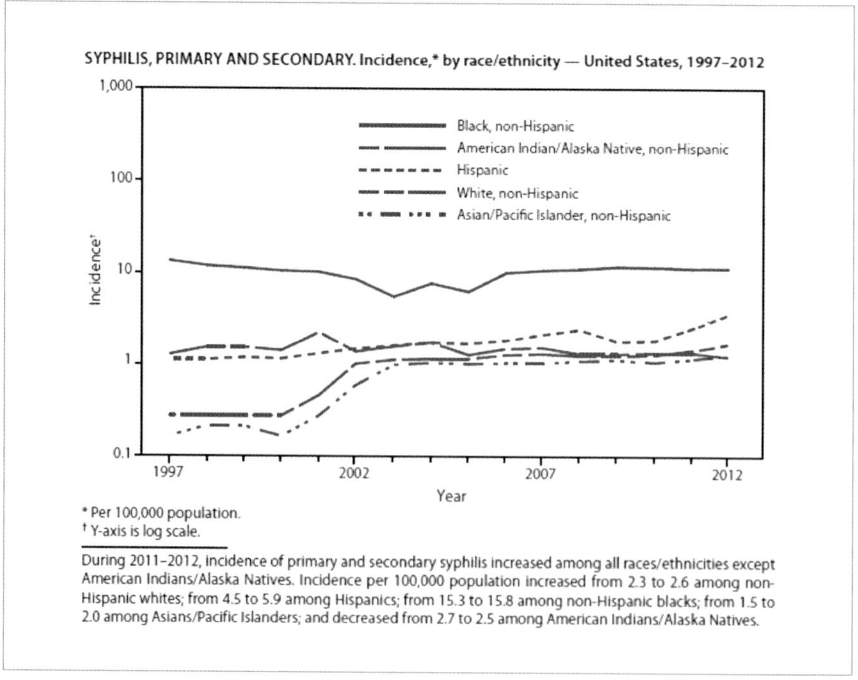

Image 131.3
Syphilis, primary and secondary. Incidence, by race/ethnicity—United States, 1997–2012. Courtesy of *Morbidity and Mortality Weekly Report.*

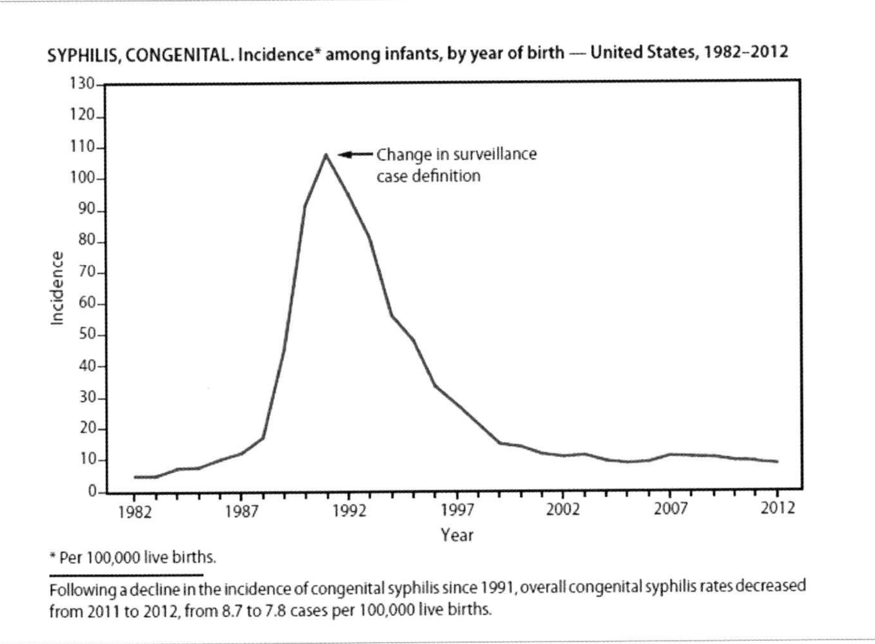

Image 131.4
Syphilis, congenital. Incidence among infants, by year of birth—United States, 1982–2012. Courtesy of *Morbidity and Mortality Weekly Report.*

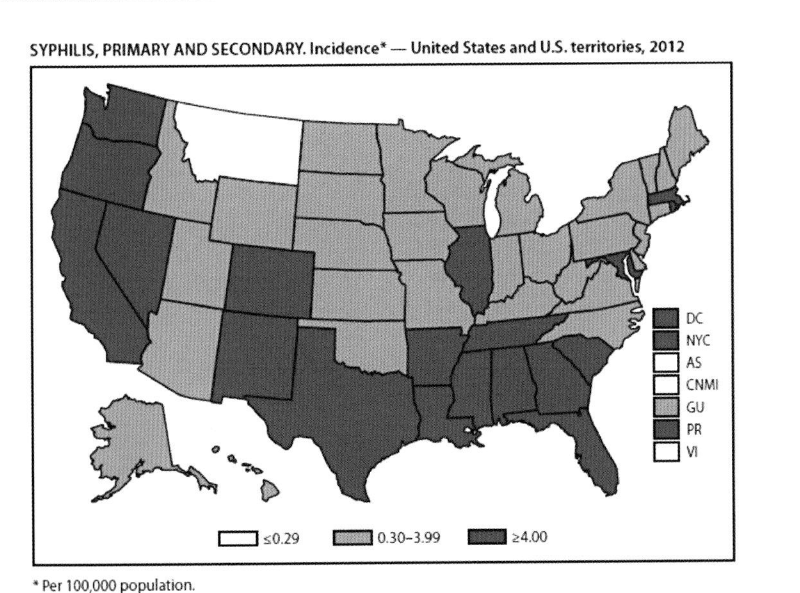

Image 131.5
Syphilis, primary and secondary. Incidence—United States and US territories, 2012. Courtesy of *Morbidity and Mortality Weekly Report.*

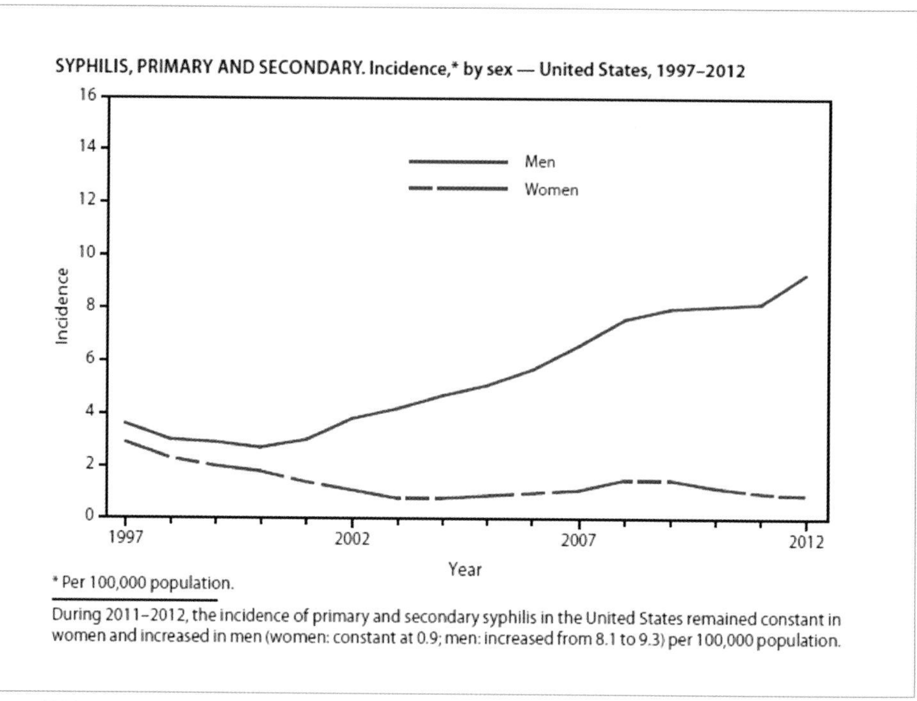

Image 131.6
Syphilis, primary and secondary. Incidence, by sex—United States, 1997–2012. Courtesy of *Morbidity and Mortality Weekly Report.*

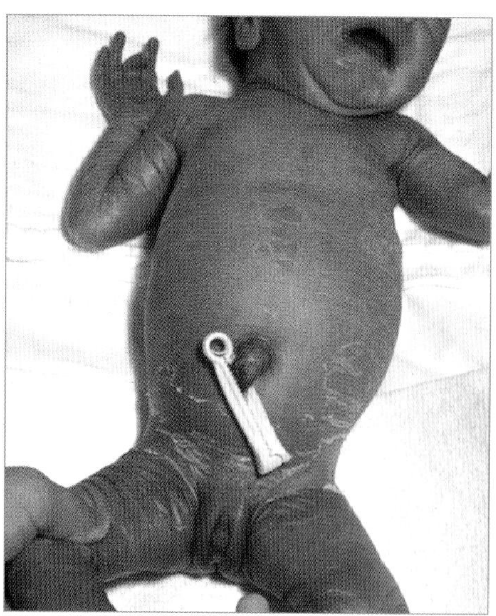

Image 131.7
A newborn with congenital syphilis. Note the marked generalized desquamation.

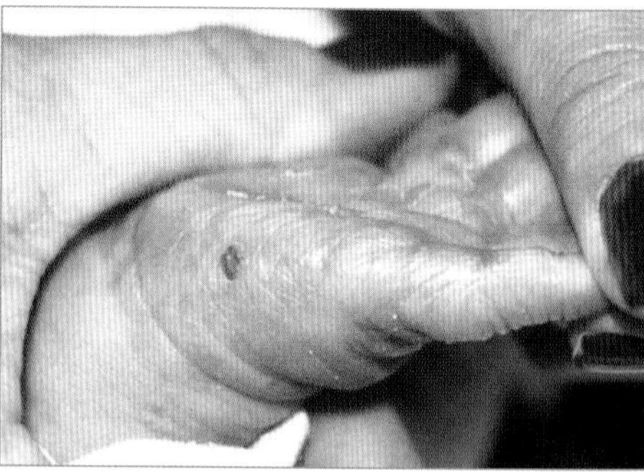

Image 131.8
Congenital syphilis with desquamation over the hand. Courtesy of Charles Prober.

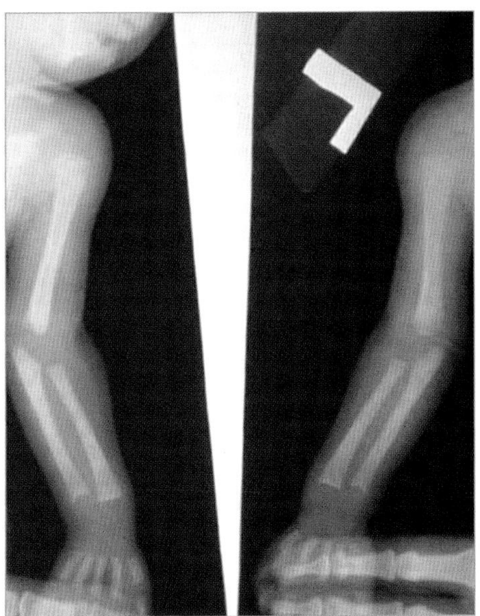

Image 131.9
Upper extremities of a patient with early periostitis and radiolucency of the distal radius and ulna bilaterally. Courtesy of Edgar O. Ledbetter, MD, FAAP.

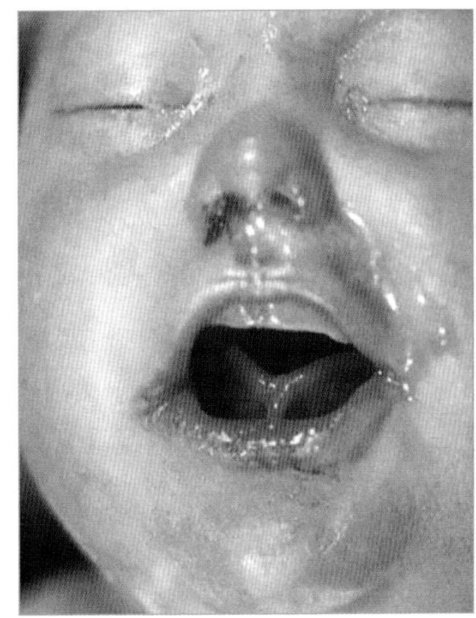

Image 131.10
The face of a newborn displaying pathologic morphology indicative of congenital syphilis with striking mucous membrane involvement. Courtesy of Centers for Disease Control and Prevention/Dr Norman Cole.

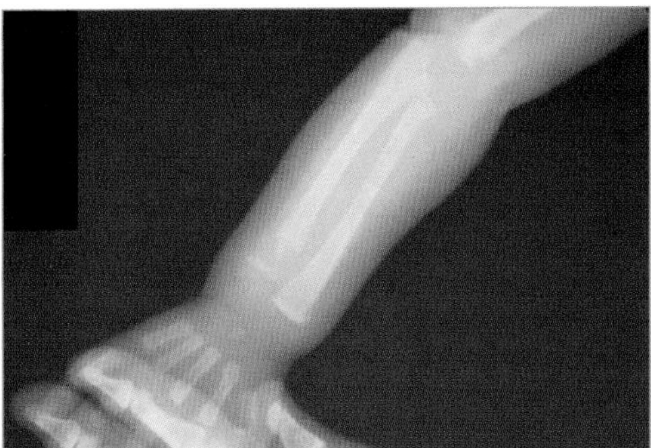

Image 131.11
Congenital syphilis with metaphyseal destruction of distal humerus, radius, and ulna.

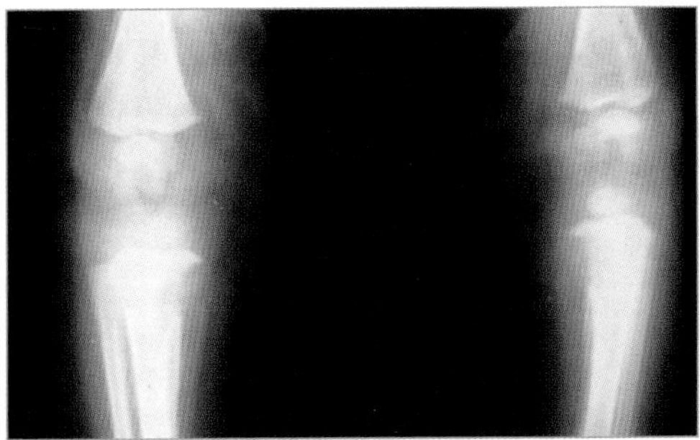

Image 131.12
Congenital syphilis with proximal tibial metaphysitis (Wimberger sign).

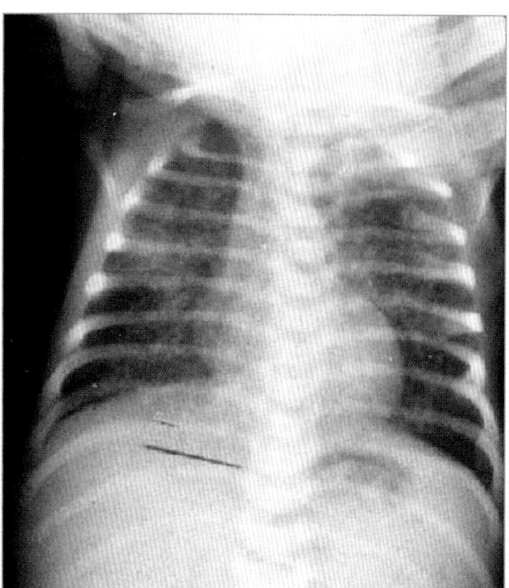

Image 131.13
Congenital syphilis with pneumonia alba. The infant survived with penicillin treatment.

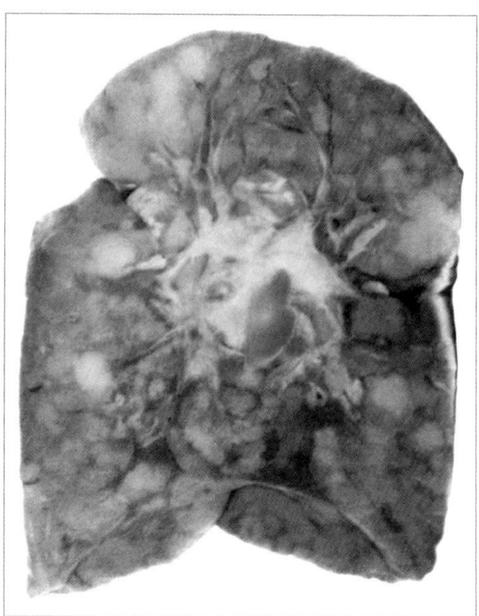

Image 131.14
This pathologic condition of the lungs, know as pneumonia alba, is caused by congenital syphilis. The lungs are enlarged, heavy, uniformly firm, and yellow-white in color. Seventy percent of all pregnant women with untreated primary syphilis may transmit the infection to their fetuses. Courtesy of Centers for Disease Control and Prevention/Susan Lindsley.

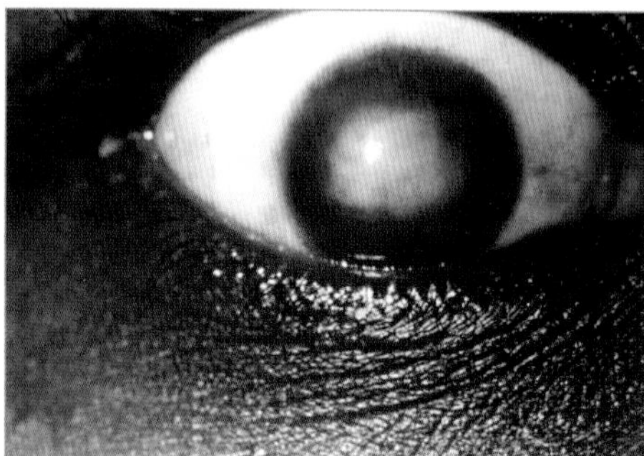

Image 131.15
This photograph depicts the presence of a diffuse stromal haze in the cornea of a female patient, known as interstitial keratitis, which was due to her late-staged congenital syphilitic condition. Interstitial keratitis, which is an inflammation of the cornea's connective tissue elements and usually affects both eyes, can occur as a complication brought on by congenital or acquired syphilis. Interstitial keratitis usually occurs in children older than 2 years. Courtesy of Centers for Disease Control and Prevention.

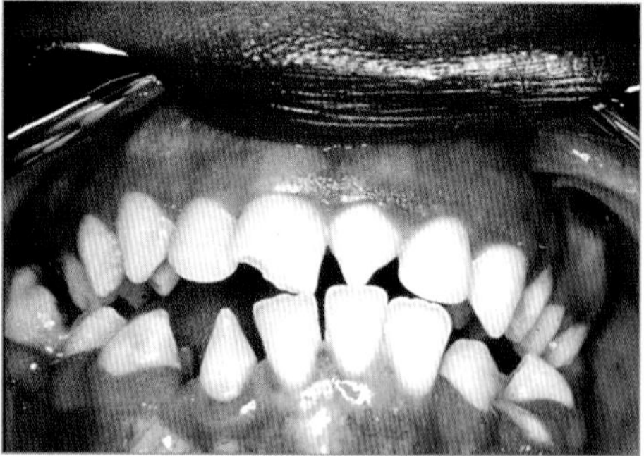

Image 131.16
Hutchinson teeth, a late manifestation of congenital syphilis. Changes occur in secondary dentition. The central incisors are smaller than normal and have sloping sides. Courtesy of Edgar O. Ledbetter, MD, FAAP.

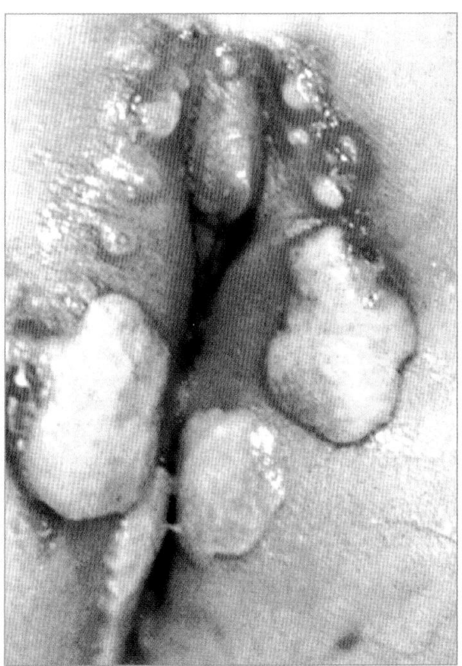

Image 131.17
Condyloma latum in a 7-year-old girl who has been sexually abused. These whitish gray, moist lesions are caused by *Treponema pallidum* and are highly contagious.

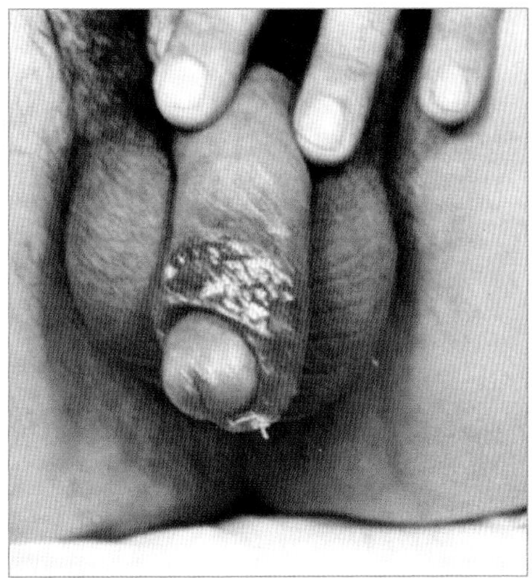

Image 131.18
This image shows an extensive chancre located on the penile shaft due to a primary syphilitic infection caused by *Treponema pallidum.* The primary stage of syphilis is usually marked by the appearance of a single lesion, called a chancre. The chancre is usually firm, round, small, and painless. It appears at the spot where *T pallidum* entered the body and lasts 3 to 6 weeks, healing on its own. Courtesy of Centers for Disease Control and Prevention/Susan Lindsley.

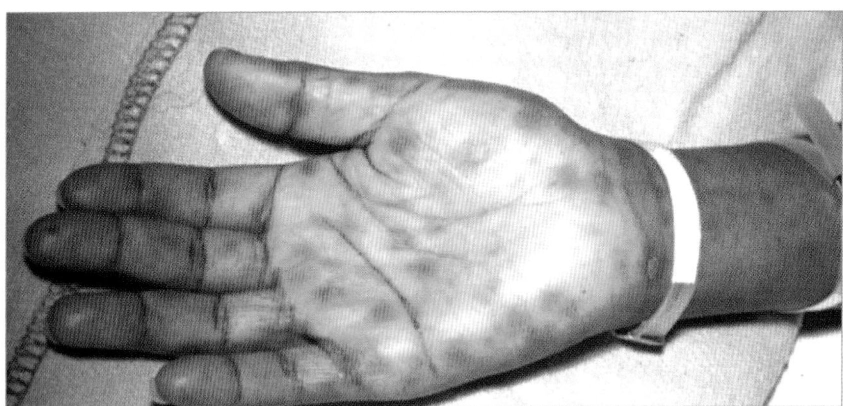

Image 131.19
A 16-year-old girl with rash of secondary syphilis noticed at 3 months' gestation of her pregnancy. The sign and symptoms of secondary syphilis generally occur 6 to 8 weeks after the primary infection when primary lesions have usually healed.

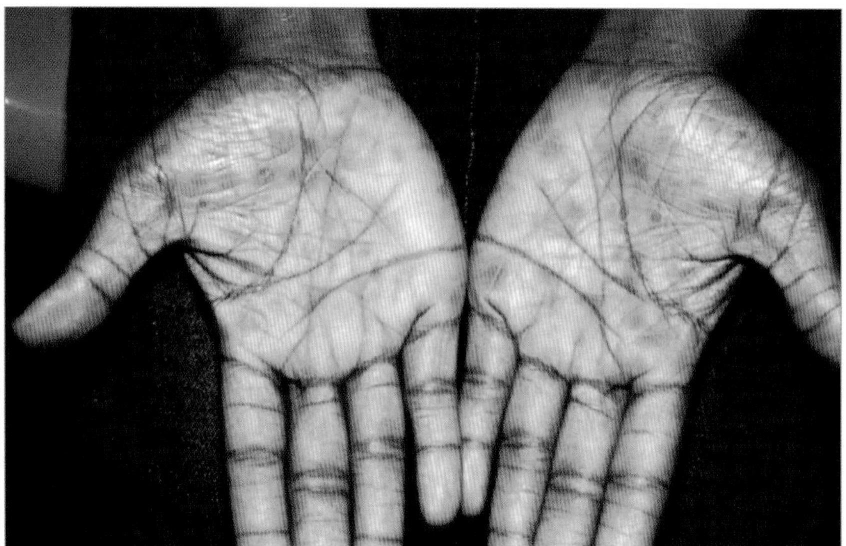

Image 131.20
Secondary syphilis in a different patient than Image 131.20 with discrete palmar lesions. The diagnosis was suspected because of the palmar lesions.

132

Tapeworm Diseases

(Taeniasis and Cysticercosis)

Clinical Manifestations

- **Taeniasis.** Infection with adult tapeworms is often asymptomatic; however, mild gastrointestinal tract symptoms, such as nausea, diarrhea, and pain, can occur. Tapeworm segments can be seen migrating from the anus or in feces.
- **Cysticercosis.** Manifestations depend on the location and number of pork tapeworm larval cysts (cysticerci) and the host response. Cysticerci can be found anywhere in the body. The most common and serious manifestations are caused by cysticerci in the central nervous system (CNS). Larval cysts of *Taenia solium* in the brain (neurocysticercosis) can cause seizures, behavioral disturbances, obstructive hydrocephalus, and other neurologic signs and symptoms. Neurocysticercosis is the leading infectious cause of epilepsy in the developing world. The host reaction to degenerating cysticerci can produce signs and symptoms of meningitis. Cysts in the spinal column can cause gait disturbance, pain, or transverse myelitis. Subcutaneous cysticerci produce palpable nodules, and ocular involvement can cause visual impairment.

Etiology

Taeniasis is caused by intestinal infection by the adult tapeworm, *Taenia saginata* (beef tapeworm) or *T solium* (pork tapeworm). *Taenia saginata asiatica* causes taeniasis in Asia. Human cysticercosis is caused only by the larvae of *T solium* (*Cysticercus cellulosae*).

Epidemiology

These tapeworm diseases have worldwide distribution. Prevalence is high in areas with poor sanitation and human fecal contamination in areas where cattle graze or swine are fed. Most cases of *T solium* infection in the United States are imported from Latin America or Asia, although the disease is prevalent in sub-Saharan Africa as well. High rates of *T saginata* infection occur in Mexico, parts of South America, East Africa, and central Europe. *T saginata asiatica* is common in China, Taiwan, and Southeast Asia. Taeniasis is acquired by eating undercooked beef (*T saginata*) or pork (*T solium*). *T saginata asiatica* is acquired by eating viscera of infected pigs that contain encysted larvae. Infection is often asymptomatic.

Cysticercosis in humans is acquired by ingesting eggs of the pork tapeworm (*T solium*), through direct fecal-oral contact with a person harboring the adult tapeworm, or through ingestion of fecally contaminated food. Autoinfection is possible. Eggs are only found in human feces because humans are the obligate definitive host. Eggs liberate oncospheres in the intestine that migrate through the blood and lymphatics to tissues throughout the body, including the CNS, where the oncospheres develop into cysticerci. Although most cases of cysticercosis in the United States have been imported, cysticercosis can be acquired in the United States from tapeworm carriers who emigrated from an area with endemic infection and still have *T solium* intestinal-stage infection. *T saginata* and *T saginata asiatica* do not cause cysticercosis.

Incubation Period

For taeniasis (time from ingestion of the larvae until segments are passed in the feces), 2 to 3 months; for cysticercosis, several years.

Diagnosis

Diagnosis of taeniasis (adult tapeworm infection) is based on demonstration of the proglottids or ova in feces or the perianal region. However, these techniques are insensitive. Species identification of the parasite is based on the different structures of gravid proglottids and scolex. Diagnosis of neurocysticercosis typically requires imaging of the CNS and serologic testing. Computed tomography scanning or magnetic resonance imaging of the brain or spinal cord is used to demonstrate lesions compatible with cysticerci. Antibody assays that detect specific antibodies to larval *T solium* in serum and cerebrospinal fluid are useful to confirm the diagnosis but can have limited sensitivity if few cysticerci are present. In the United States, antibody tests are available through the Centers for Disease Control and Prevention and a few commercial laboratories. In general, antibody tests are more sensitive with serum specimens than with cerebrospinal fluid specimens. Serum antibody assay results are often negative in children with solitary parenchymal lesions but usually are positive in patients with multiple lesions.

Treatment

- **Taeniasis.** Praziquantel is highly effective for eradicating infection with the adult tapeworm, and niclosamide is an alternative. Niclosamide is not approved for treatment of *T solium* infection but is approved for treatment of *T saginata* infection. However, niclosamide is not available in the United States.
- **Cysticercosis.** Neurocysticercosis treatment should be individualized on the basis of the number, location, and viability of cysticerci as assessed by neuroimaging studies (magnetic resonance imaging or computed tomography scan) and the clinical manifestations. Management is generally aimed at symptoms and should include anticonvulsants for patients with seizures and insertion of shunts for patients with hydrocephalus. Two antiparasitic drugs—albendazole and praziquantel—are available. Although both drugs are cysticercidal and hasten radiologic resolution of cysts, most symptoms result from the host inflammatory response and can be exacerbated by treatment. Most experts recommend therapy with albendazole or praziquantel for patients with nonenhancing or multiple cysticerci. Albendazole is preferred over praziquantel because it has fewer drug-drug interactions with anticonvulsants. Coadministration of corticosteroids during antiparasitic therapy may decrease adverse effects if more extensive viable CNS cysticerci are suspected, and a prolonged course may be required for some forms of the disease (eg, basal, subarachnoid). Corticosteroids can affect the tissue concentrations of albendazole. Arachnoiditis, vasculitis, or diffuse cerebral edema (cysticercal encephalitis) is treated with corticosteroid therapy until the cerebral edema is controlled.

The medical and surgical management of cysticercosis can be highly complex and often needs to be conducted in consultation with a neurologist or neurosurgeon. Seizures may recur for months or years. Anticonvulsant therapy is recommended until there is neuroradiologic evidence of resolution and seizures have not occurred for 1 to 2 years. Calcification of cysts may require prolonged or indefinite use of anticonvulsants. Intraventricular cysticerci and hydrocephalus usually require surgical therapy. Intraventricular cysticerci can often be removed by endoscopic surgery, which is the treatment of choice. If cysticerci cannot be removed easily, hydrocephalus should be corrected with placement of intraventricular shunts. Ocular cysticercosis is treated by surgical excision of the cysticerci. Ocular and spinal cysticerci generally are not treated with anthelmintic drugs, which can exacerbate inflammation. An ophthalmic examination should be performed before treatment to rule out intraocular cysticerci.

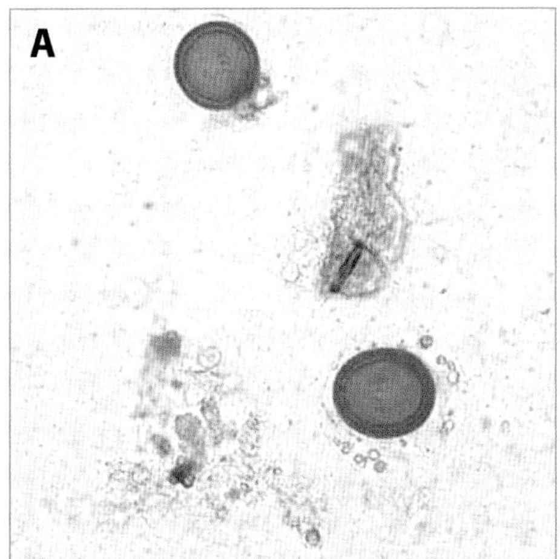

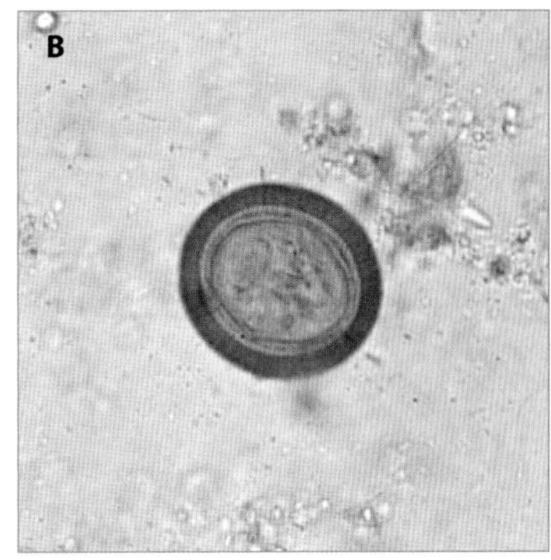

Image 132.1

The eggs of *Taenia solium* and *Taenia saginata* are indistinguishable from each other, as well as from other members of the Taeniidae family. The eggs measure 30 to 35 µm in diameter and are radially striated. The internal oncosphere contains 6 refractile hooks. *Taenia* species eggs in unstained wet mounts. Courtesy of Centers for Disease Control and Prevention.

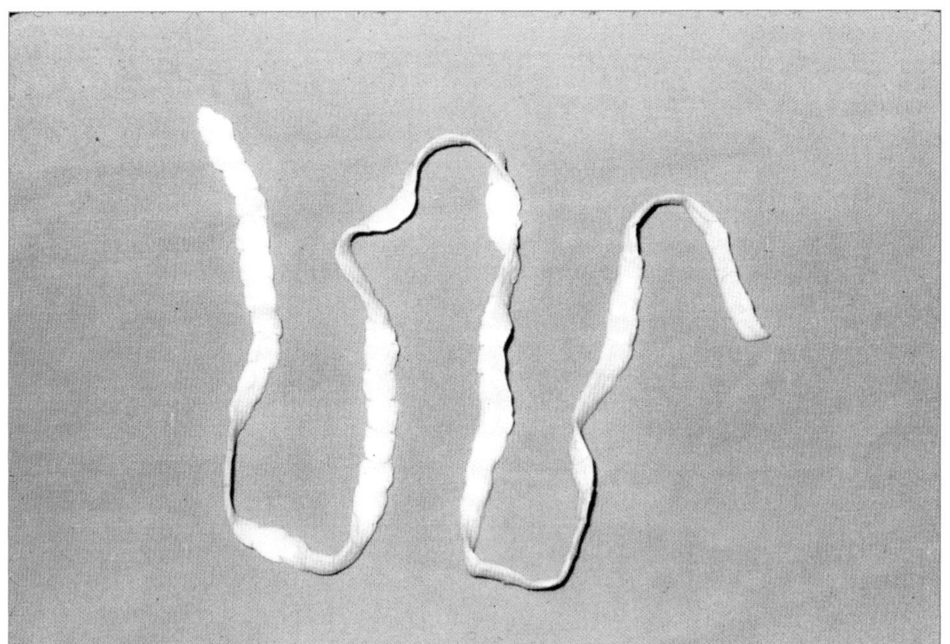

Image 132.2

Taenia saginata. Courtesy of Gary Overturf, MD.

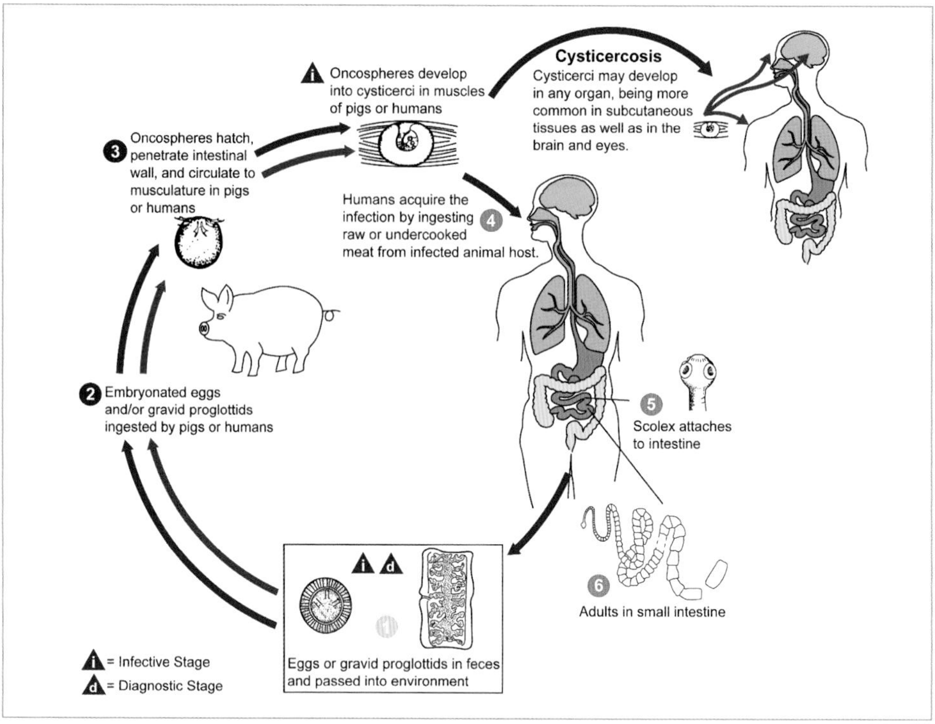

Image 132.3

Cysticercosis is an infection of humans and pigs with the larval stages of the parasitic cestode, *Taenia solium*. This infection is caused by ingestion of eggs shed in the feces of a human tapeworm carrier (1). Pigs and humans become infected by ingesting eggs or gravid proglottids (2). Humans are infected by ingestion of food contaminated with feces or by autoinfection. In the latter case, a human infected with adult *T solium* can ingest eggs produced by that tapeworm through fecal contamination or, possibly, from proglottids carried into the stomach by reverse peristalsis. Once eggs are ingested, oncospheres hatch in the intestine (3), invade the intestinal wall, and migrate to striated muscles, as well as the brain, liver, and other tissues, where they develop into cysticerci. In humans, cysts can cause serious sequelae if they localize in the brain, resulting in neurocysticercosis. The parasite life cycle is completed, resulting in human tapeworm infection when humans ingest undercooked pork containing cysticerci (4). Cysts evaginate and attach to the small intestine by their scolex (5). Adult tapeworms develop (up to 2–7 m in length and produce <1,000 proglottids, each with ~50,000 eggs) and reside in the small intestine for years (6). Courtesy of Centers for Disease Control and Prevention/Alexander J. da Silva, PhD/Melanie Moser.

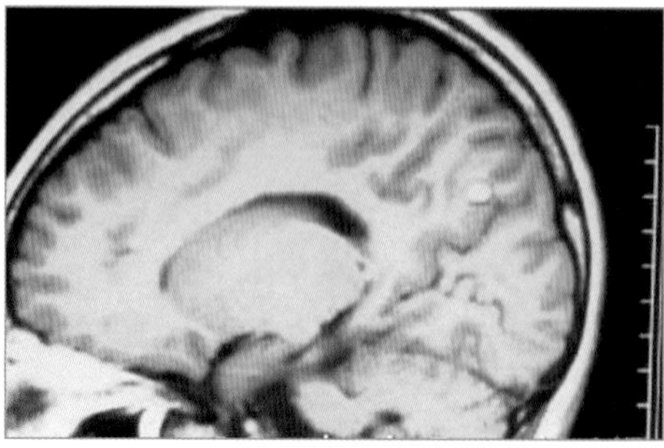

Image 132.4

Neurocysticercosis in an 11-year-old Asian girl apparent on computed tomography scan. Courtesy of Benjamin Estrada, MD.

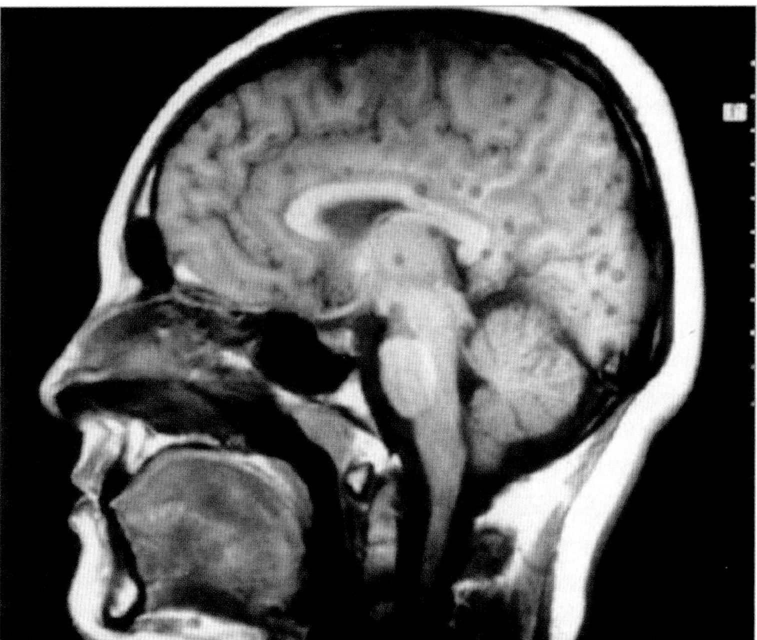

Image 132.5
Cerebral neurocysticercosis with diffuse, scattered, ring-enhancing lesions throughout the brain parenchyma with focal edema evident on computed tomography scan. Courtesy of David Waagner.

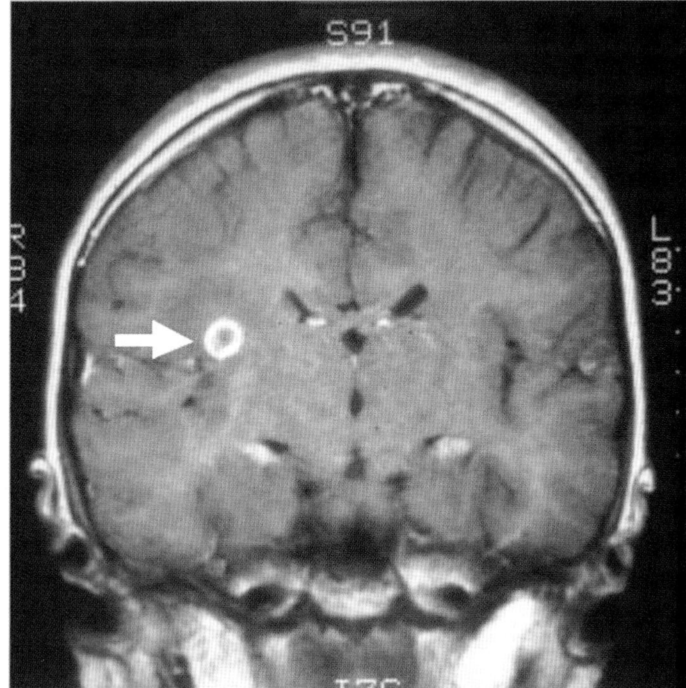

Image 132.6
A young boy with a seizure. Magnetic resonance imaging of the brain revealed a ringlike lesion characteristic of neurocysticercosis. Copyright Barbara Ann Jantausch, MD, FAAP.

133

Other Tapeworm Infections

(Including Hydatid Disease)

Most tapeworm infections are asymptomatic, but nausea, abdominal pain, and diarrhea have been observed in people who are heavily infected.

Etiologies, Diagnosis, and Treatment

Hymenolepis nana

This tapeworm, also called the dwarf tapeworm because it is the smallest of the adult human tapeworms, can complete its entire life cycle within humans. New infection can be acquired by ingestion of eggs passed in feces of infected people or of infected arthropods (fleas). More problematic is autoinfection, which perpetuates infection in the host, because eggs can hatch within the intestine and reinitiate the life cycle, leading to development of new worms and a large worm burden. Diagnosis is made by recognition of the characteristic eggs passed in stool. Praziquantel is the treatment of choice, with nitazoxanide as an alternative drug. If infection persists after treatment, retreatment with praziquantel is indicated.

Dipylidium caninum

This tapeworm is the most common and widespread adult tapeworm of dogs and cats. *Dipylidium caninum* infects children when they inadvertently swallow a dog or cat flea, which serves as the intermediate host. Diagnosis is made by finding the characteristic eggs or motile proglottids in stool. Proglottids resemble rice kernels. Therapy with praziquantel is effective. Niclosamide is an alternative therapeutic option but is not available in the United States.

Diphyllobothrium latum (and related species)

Fish are one of the intermediate hosts of the *Diphyllobothrium latum* tapeworm, also called fish tapeworm. Consumption of infected, raw freshwater fish (including trout and pike) leads to infection. Three to 5 weeks are needed for the adult tapeworm to mature and begin to lay eggs. The worm sometimes causes mechanical obstruction of the bowel or diarrhea, abdominal pain, or, rarely, megaloblastic anemia secondary to vitamin B_{12} deficiency. Infection with other related species of fish tapeworm are associated with consumption of anadromous or saltwater fish, such as salmon. Diagnosis is made by recognition of the characteristic proglottids or eggs passed in stool. Therapy with praziquantel is effective; niclosamide is an alternative but is not available in the United States.

Echinococcus granulosus and *Echinococcus multilocularis*

The larval forms of these tapeworms cause cystic echinococcosis, also known as hydatid disease, and alveolar echinococcosis, respectively. The distribution of *Echinococcus granulosus* is related to sheep or cattle herding. Areas of high prevalence include parts of Central and South America, East Africa, Eastern Europe, the Middle East, the Mediterranean region, China, and Central Asia. The parasite is also endemic in Australia and New Zealand. In the United States, small foci of endemic transmission have been reported in Arizona, California, New Mexico, and Utah, and a strain of the parasite is adapted to wolves, moose, and caribou in Alaska and Canada. Dogs, coyotes, wolves, dingoes, and jackals can become infected by swallowing protoscolices of the parasite within hydatid cysts in the organs of sheep or other intermediate hosts. Dogs pass embryonated eggs in their stools, and sheep become infected by swallowing the eggs. If humans swallow *Echinococcus* eggs, they can become inadvertent intermediate hosts, and cysts can develop in various organs, such as the liver, lungs, kidneys, and spleen. Cysts caused by larvae of *E granulosus* usually grow slowly (1 cm in diameter per year) and eventually can contain several liters of fluid. If a cyst ruptures, anaphylaxis and multiple secondary cysts from seeding of protoscolices can result. Clinical diagnosis is often difficult. A history of contact with dogs in an area with endemic infection is helpful. Cystic lesions can be demonstrated by radiography, ultrasonography, or computed tomography of various organs. Serologic testing, available at the Centers for Disease Control and Prevention, is helpful, but false-negative results occur; conversely, tests at commercial laboratories may provide false-positive results. Treatment depends on ultrasonographic staging and may include watchful waiting, antiparasitic therapy, PAIR (**p**uncture **a**spiration, **i**njection of protoscolicidal agents, and **r**easpiration), surgical excision, or no treatment. In uncomplicated cases, treatment of choice is PAIR. Contraindications to PAIR include communication of the cyst with the biliary tract (eg, bile staining after initial aspiration), superficial cysts, and heavily septated cysts. Surgical therapy is indicated for complicated cases and requires meticulous care to prevent spillage, including preparations such as soaking of surgical drapes in hypertonic saline. In general, the cyst should be removed intact because leakage of contents is associated with a higher rate of complications. Patients are at risk of anaphylactic reactions to cyst contents. Treatment with albendazole generally should be initiated days to weeks before surgery or PAIR and continued for several weeks to months afterward.

Echinococcus multilocularis, a species for which the life cycle involves foxes, dogs, and rodents, causes alveolar echinococcosis, which is characterized by invasive growth of the larvae in the liver with occasional metastatic spread. Alveolar echinococcosis is limited to the northern hemisphere and usually is diagnosed in people 50 years or older. The disease has been reported frequently from Western China. The preferred treatment is surgical removal of the entire larval mass. In nonresectable cases, continuous treatment with albendazole has been associated with clinical improvement.

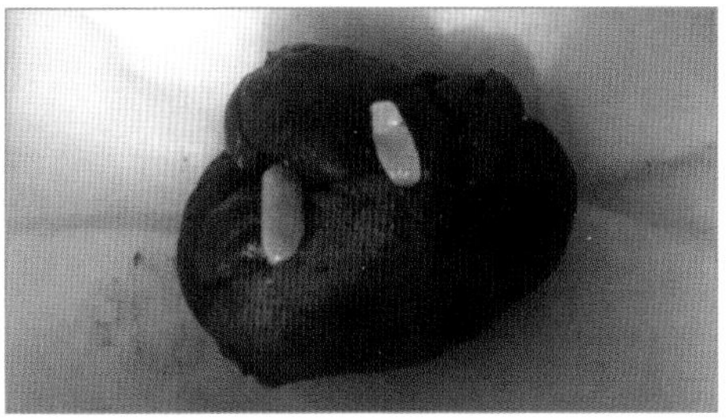

Image 133.1
Dog tapeworm, *Dipylidium caninum*, in the stool of a healthy 7-month-old boy. Courtesy of Carol J. Baker, MD, FAAP.

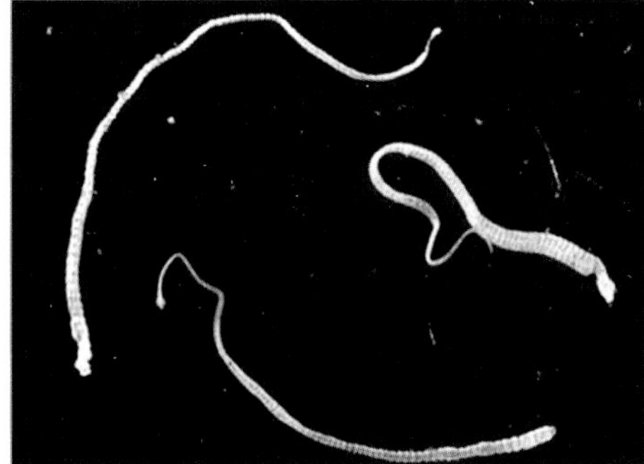

Image 133.3
Three adult *Hymenolepis nana* tapeworms. Each tapeworm (length, 15–40 mm) has a small, rounded scolex at the anterior end, and proglottids can be distinguished at the posterior, wider end. Courtesy of Centers for Disease Control and Prevention.

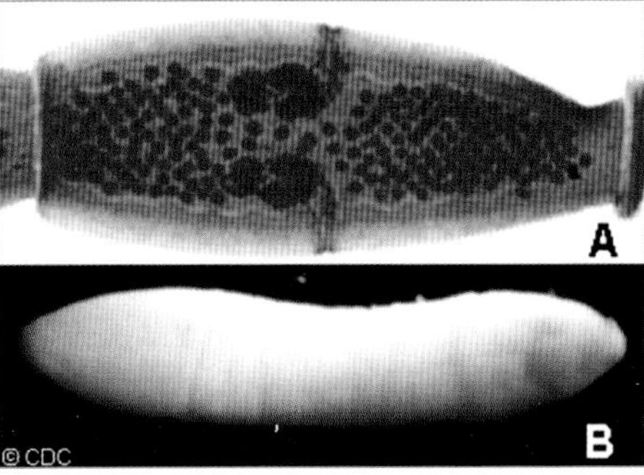

Image 133.2
Proglottids of *Dipylidium caninum.* Such proglottids (average mature size, 12 x 3 mm) have 2 genital pores, one in the middle of each lateral margin. Proglottids may be passed singly or in chains and, occasionally, may be seen dangling from the anus. They are pumpkin seed–shaped when passed and often resemble rice grains when dried. Courtesy of Centers for Disease Control and Prevention.

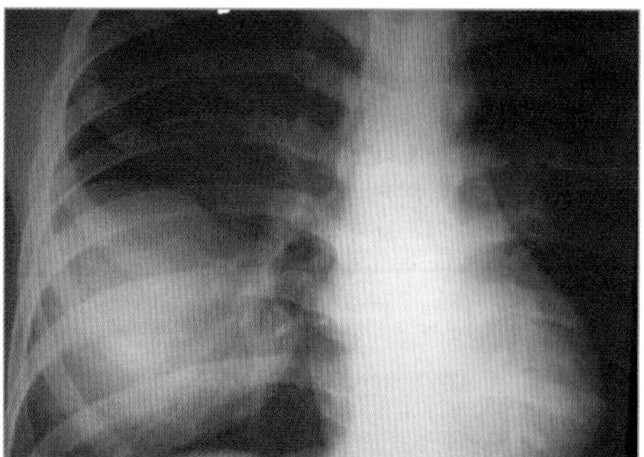

Image 133.4
Fluid-filled echinococcus cyst in the lungs of an adolescent male. Courtesy of Edgar O. Ledbetter, MD, FAAP.

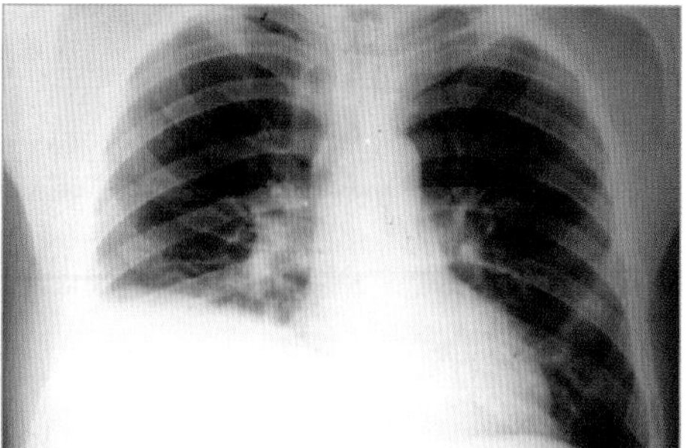

Image 133.5
Echinococcus cyst in the right lobe of the liver in a 27-year-old man. Note the striking elevation of the right hemidiaphragm. Courtesy of Edgar O. Ledbetter, MD, FAAP.

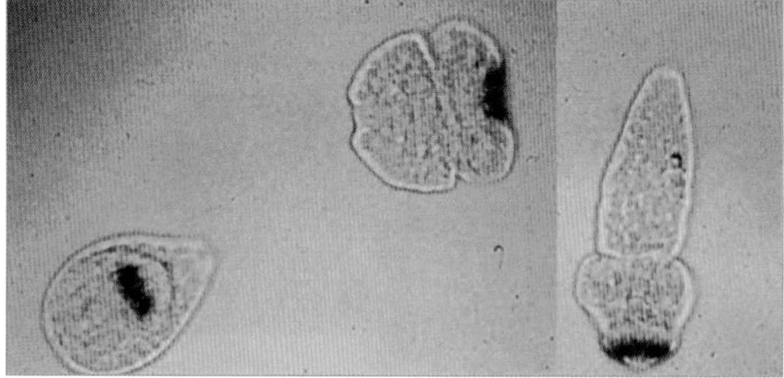

Image 133.6
Hydatid sand. Fluid aspirated from a hydatid cyst will show multiple protoscolices (size, approximately 100 µm), each of which has typical hooklets. The protoscolices are normally invaginated (left), and evaginate (middle, then right) when put in saline. Courtesy of Centers for Disease Control and Prevention.

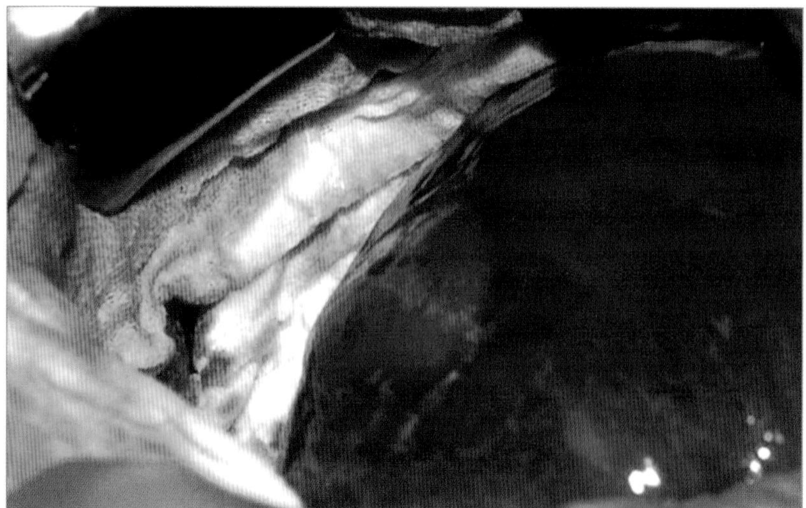

Image 133.7
Echinococcus abscess of liver in an adult, the most common site of abscess formation.

134

Tetanus

(Lockjaw)

Clinical Manifestations

Tetanus can manifest in 4 overlapping clinical forms: generalized, neonatal, local, and cephalic.

- **Generalized tetanus (lockjaw)** is a neurologic disease manifesting as trismus and severe muscular spasms, including risus sardonicus. Onset is gradual, occurring over 1 to 7 days, and symptoms progress to severe, painful generalized muscle spasms, which are often aggravated by any external stimulus. Autonomic dysfunction, manifesting as diaphoresis, tachycardia, labile blood pressure, and arrhythmias, is often present. Severe spasms persist for 1 week or more and subside over several weeks in people who recover.
- **Neonatal tetanus** is a form of generalized tetanus occurring in newborns lacking protective passive immunity because their mothers are not immune.
- **Local tetanus** manifests as local muscle spasms in areas contiguous to a wound.
- **Cephalic tetanus** is a dysfunction of cranial nerves associated with infected wounds on the head and neck. Local and cephalic tetanus can precede generalized tetanus.

Etiology

Clostridium tetani is a spore-forming, obligate anaerobic, gram-positive bacillus. This organism is a wound contaminant that causes neither tissue destruction nor an inflammatory response. The vegetative form of *C tetani* produces a potent plasmid-encoded exotoxin (tetanospasmin), which binds to gangliosides at the myoneural junction of skeletal muscle and on neuronal membranes in the spinal cord, blocking inhibitory impulses to motor neurons. The action of tetanus toxin on the brain and sympathetic nervous system is less well documented.

Epidemiology

Tetanus occurs worldwide and is more common in warmer climates and during warmer months, in part because of higher frequency of contaminated wounds associated with those locations and seasons. The organism, a normal inhabitant of soil and animal and human intestines, is ubiquitous in the environment, especially where contamination by excreta is common. Organisms multiply in wounds, recognized or unrecognized, and elaborate toxins in the presence of anaerobic conditions. Contaminated wounds, especially wounds with devitalized tissue and deep-puncture trauma, are at greatest risk. Neonatal tetanus is common in many developing countries where pregnant women are not immunized appropriately against tetanus and nonsterile umbilical cord care practices are followed. More than 250,000 deaths from neonatal tetanus were estimated to have occurred worldwide each year between 2000 and 2003. Widespread active immunization against tetanus has modified the epidemiology of disease in the United States, where 40 or fewer cases have been reported annually since 1999. Tetanus is not transmissible from person to person.

Incubation Period

Usually within 8 days (range, 3–21 days); neonatal tetanus, usually 7 days (range, 4–14 days).

Diagnostic Tests

The diagnosis of tetanus is made clinically by excluding other causes of tetanic spasms, such as hypocalcemic tetany, phenothiazine reaction, strychnine poisoning, and conversion disorder. Attempts to culture *C tetani* are associated with poor yield, and a negative culture does exclude disease. A protective serum antitoxin concentration should not be used to exclude the diagnosis of tetanus.

Treatment

Human tetanus immune globulin (TIG), given in a single dose, is recommended for treatment. Available preparations must be given intramuscularly. Infiltration of part of the dose locally around the wound is recommended, although the efficacy of this approach has not been proven. In countries where human TIG is not available, equine tetanus antitoxin may be available. Equine antitoxin is administered after appropriate testing for sensitivity and desensitization if necessary. This product is no longer available in the United States. Intravenous immunoglobulin contains antibodies to tetanus and can be considered for treatment.

All wounds should be cleaned and debrided properly, especially if extensive necrosis is present. In neonatal tetanus, wide excision of the umbilical stump is not indicated.

Supportive care and pharmacotherapy to control tetanic spasms are of major importance. Oral (or intravenous) metronidazole is effective in decreasing the number of vegetative forms of *C tetani* and is the antimicrobial agent of choice. Parenteral penicillin G is an alternative treatment. Therapy for 7 to 10 days is recommended.

Active immunization against tetanus should always be undertaken during convalescence from tetanus. Because of the extreme potency of tiny amounts of toxin, tetanus disease may not result in immunity.

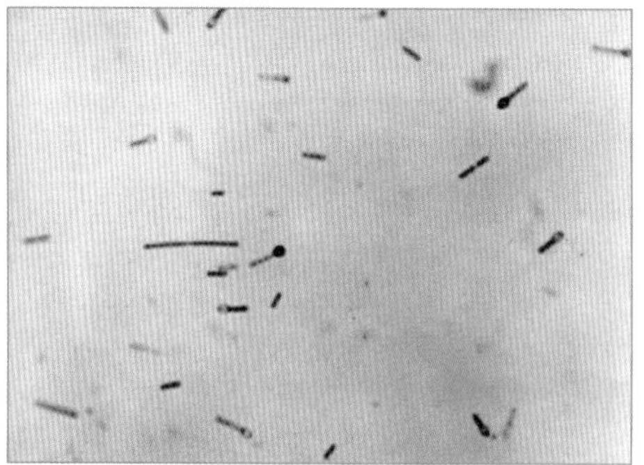

Image 134.1
This Gram-stained photomicrograph depicts gram-positive *Clostridium tetani,* which had been cultivated on a blood agar plate over 48 hours (magnification x956). Courtesy of Centers for Disease Control and Prevention/Dr Holdeman.

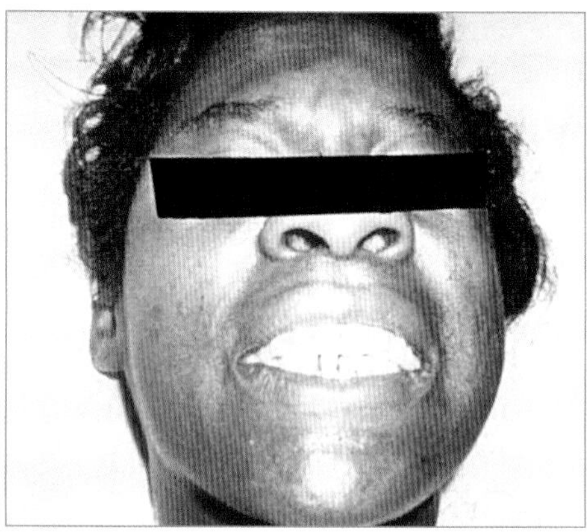

Image 134.2
Trismus in an adult with tetanus. Courtesy of Charles Prober, MD.

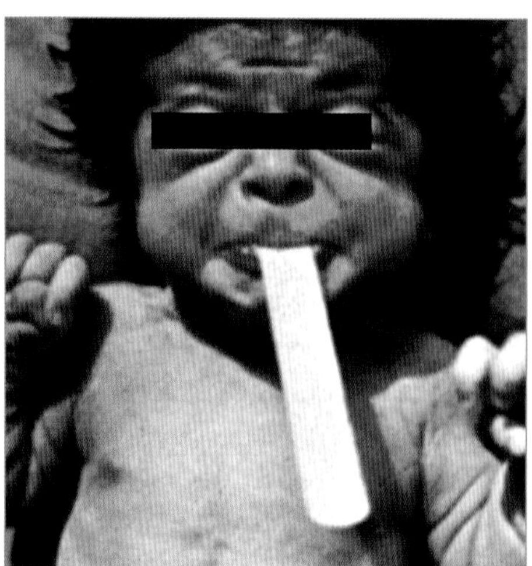

Image 134.3
Severe muscular spasms with trismus in an infant who acquired neonatal tetanus from contamination of the umbilical stump.

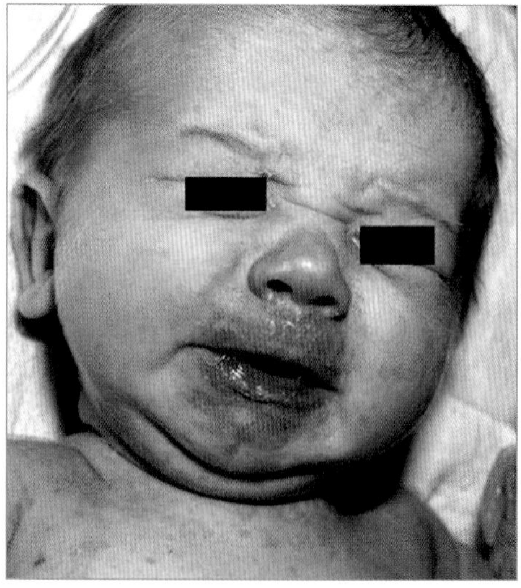

Image 134.4
The face of an infant with neonatal tetanus with risus sardonicus. Copyright Martin G. Myers, MD.

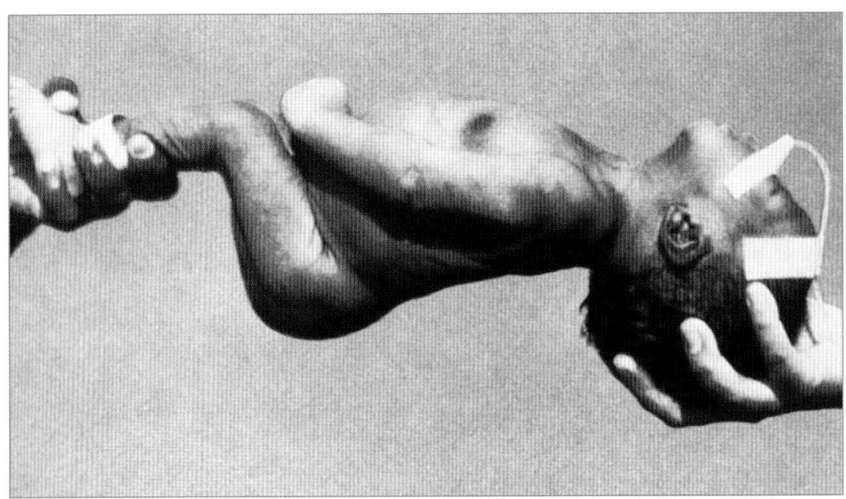

Image 134.5
This neonate is displaying a body rigidity produced by *Clostridium tetani* exotoxin. Neonatal tetanus may occur in neonates born without protective passive immunity, when the mother is not immune. It usually occurs through infection of the unhealed umbilical stump, particularly when the stump is cut with an unsterile instrument. Courtesy of Centers for Disease Control and Prevention.

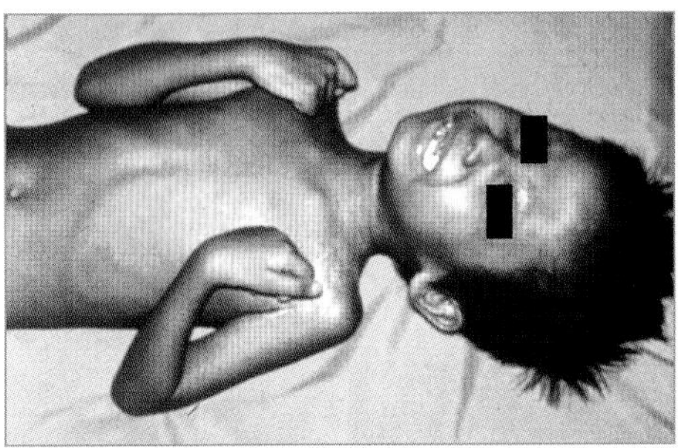

Image 134.6
A preschool-aged boy with tetanus with severe muscle contractions, generalized, caused by tetanospasmin action in the central nervous system. Courtesy of Centers for Disease Control and Prevention.

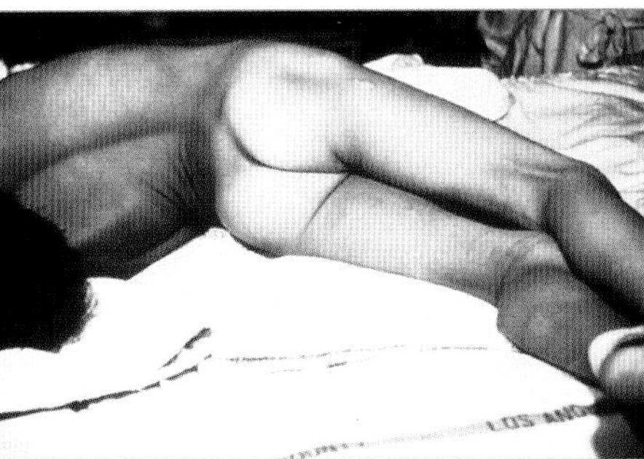

Image 134.7
This patient is displaying a body posture known as opisthotonos due to *Clostridium tetani* exotoxin. Generalized tetanus, the most common type (about 80%), usually presents with a descending pattern, starting with trismus or lockjaw, followed by stiffness of the neck, difficulty in swallowing, and rigidity of abdominal muscles. Courtesy of Centers for Disease Control and Prevention.

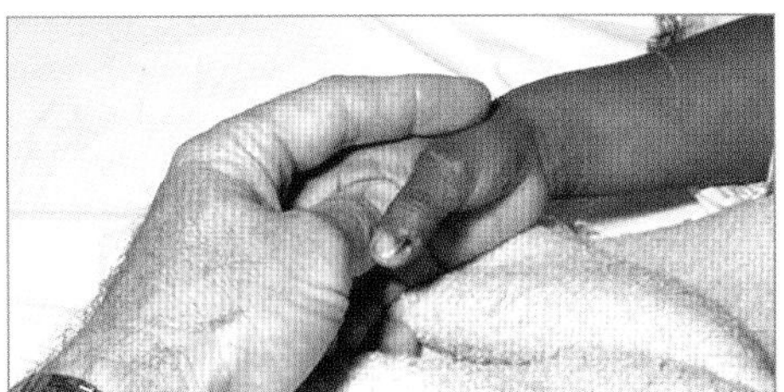

Image 134.8
A preschool-aged boy with localized tetanus secondary to the parent attempting to drain an impetigo lesion with a mesquite thorn contaminated with tetanus spores. Courtesy of Edgar O. Ledbetter, MD, FAAP.

135

Tinea Capitis

(Ringworm of the Scalp)

Clinical Manifestations

Dermatophytic fungal infections of the scalp have 3 major forms: black dot, gray patch, and favus. **Black dot** tinea capitis is the most common manifestation in the United States. It begins as an erythematous scaling patch over the scalp that slowly enlarges and is often recognized only when hair loss becomes noticeable. The name comes from the areas of alopecia in which the hair is broken off flush with the scalp, giving the appearance of black dots. Inflammation, which may be accompanied by tender lymphadenopathy, can be prominent. Scarring with permanent alopecia can occur in the absence of treatment. **Gray patch** tinea capitis also begins as a well-demarcated erythematous, scaling patch over the scalp and spreads centrifugally. Lesions can be singular or multiple and are accompanied by hair breakage a few millimeters above the scalp. **Favus (tinea favosa)** primarily manifests as a perifollicular erythema of the scalp that can progress to yellow crusting known as scutula, which can coalesce into confluent, adherent masses overlying severe hair loss.

Both black dot and gray patch tinea capitis can evolve into kerion, a boggy erythematous nodule lacking hair, which can become suppurative and drain. Kerion can be mistaken for a primary bacterial abscess or cellulitis because it represents an extreme inflammatory response to the fungus. However, secondary bacterial infection can also occur. As with other forms of tinea, a dermatophytic or id reaction can develop and can involve a papular, vesicular, or eczemalike eruption that is often pruritic and may be extensive, involving the face, trunk, or extremities. When this reaction develops following initiation of therapy, it is sometimes mistaken for a drug eruption.

Tinea capitis can be confused with atopic dermatitis, seborrheic dermatitis, psoriasis, bacterial folliculitis or abscess, trichotillomania, alopecia areata, head lice, and scarring alopecia.

Etiology

The prime causes of the disease are fungi of the genus *Trichophyton*, including *Trichophyton tonsurans* (commonly associated with black dot tinea capitis) and *Trichophyton schoenleinii* (commonly associated with favus). An endemic form of gray patch tinea capitis is caused by *Microsporum canis*.

Epidemiology

Black dot tinea capitis is predominantly a disease of young African American school-aged children but has been reported in all racial and ethnic groups as well as in infants and postmenopausal female caregivers. Gray patch tinea capitis is rare in North America, as is favus, which remains more common in areas such as Iran, China, and Nigeria. Pathogenic dermatophytes can be transmitted to affected people by other humans, animals (especially pet cats or dogs), or the environment. The organism remains viable for prolonged periods on fomites (eg, brushes, combs), and the rate of asymptomatic carriage and infected individuals among family members of index cases is high. The role of asymptomatic carriers is unclear, but they may serve as a reservoir of infection within families, schools, and communities.

Incubation Period

Unknown; thought to be 1 to 3 weeks.

Diagnostic tests

The presence of alopecia, scale, and neck lymphadenopathy makes the diagnosis of tinea capitis almost certain, and most clinicians will choose to treat empirically prior to laboratory confirmation. Dermoscopic evaluation of areas of alopecia with a lighted magnifier may show comma- or corkscrew-shaped hairs. Hairs and scale obtained by gentle scraping of a moistened area of the scalp with a blunt scalpel, toothbrush, brush, or tweezers are used for potassium hydroxide wet mount examination. The dermatophyte test medium is also a reliable, simple, and inexpensive method of diagnosing tinea capitis. Skin scrapings from lesions are inoculated directly onto culture medium and incubated at room temperature.

After 1 to 2 weeks, a phenol red indicator in the agar will turn from yellow to red in the area surrounding a dermatophyte colony. When necessary, the diagnosis can also be confirmed by culture on Sabouraud dextrose agar, although this often requires incubation for 3 to 4 weeks.

Scalp scales and hairs can be scraped or plucked from the scalp for immediate evaluation using potassium hydroxide preparation mounts. Arthroconidia can be visualized within the hair shaft in endothrix infections, such as *T tonsurans*, while ectothrix infections, such as *M canis*, exhibit conidia on the outside of the hair shaft. In both forms, septate hyphae may be visualized in scrapings from the scalp surface. Wood lamp evaluation is only useful if a *Microsporum* infection is present, in which case affected areas will fluoresce yellow-green.

Treatment

Optimal treatment of tinea capitis is controversial. Experts generally use higher doses of griseofulvin than have been approved by the US Food and Drug Administration. Griseofulvin is approved by the FDA for children 2 years or older, is available in liquid or tablet form, can be dosed on a daily basis, and should be taken with fatty foods. Although high-dose griseofulvin is considered standard of care for *M canis* infections, many experts believe that terbinafine for 6 weeks is a better choice for *T tonsurans* infections because of the shorter duration of therapy required for cure. Shorter (usually 4 weeks) courses of terbinafine are equal or superior to longer-term griseofulvin therapy for *T tonsurans* infection. Fluconazole is the only oral antifungal that is approved by the US Food and Drug Administration for children younger than 2 years, and azole agents have also been used for tinea capitis.

Topical treatment can be useful as an adjunct to systemic therapy to decrease carriage of viable conidia. Selenium sulfide, ketoconazole, or ciclopirox shampoos can be applied 2 to 3 times per week and left in place for 5 to 10 minutes; duration of therapy should continue for at least 2 weeks. Some experts recommend continuing topical treatments until clinical and mycologic cure occurs.

Kerion is managed by antifungal therapy; corticosteroid therapy (oral or intralesional) has not been shown to be superior to antifungal therapy alone. Unless secondary bacterial infection has occurred, treatment with antibiotics is generally unnecessary.

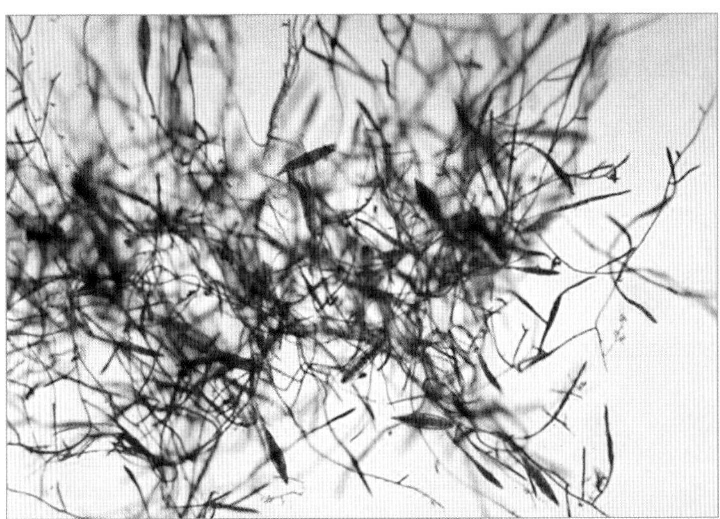

Image 135.1

Microsporum audouinii. Microsporum canis, a zoophilic dermatophyte often found in cats and dogs, is a common cause of tinea corporis and tinea capitis in humans. Other dermatophytes are included in the genera *Epidermophyton* and *Trichophyton.* Courtesy of Centers for Disease Control and Prevention.

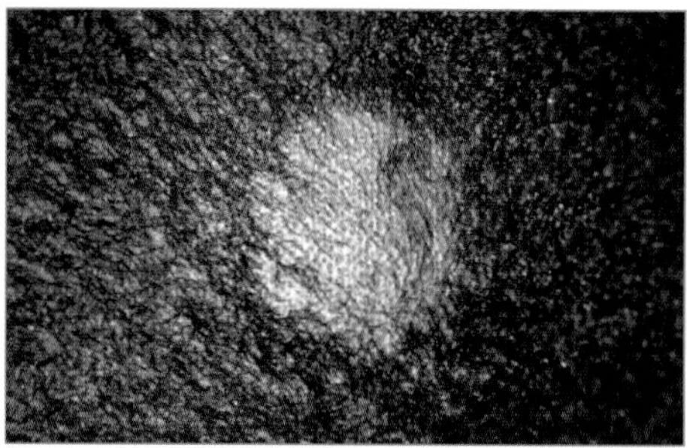

Image 135.2
A 6-year-old boy with hair loss on the top of his head for the past 2 weeks. The area is slightly pruritic and has increased in size. Mom recalls a scaly patch developing a few days after having his head shaved. Wood lamp evaluation result was negative. Culture of the area was positive for *Trichophyton tonsurans.* He responded well to 6 weeks of therapy with griseofulvin. He had no residual scarring or hair loss. Courtesy of Will Sorey, MD.

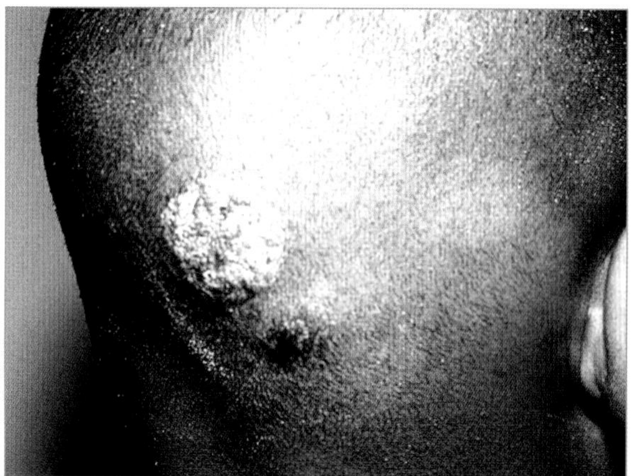

Image 135.3
A 3-year-old boy with a tinea lesion on the occiput for 1 month. The mother had been applying a topical antifungal agent, but the lesion became progressively larger. The patient was treated successfully with griseofulvin. Copyright Larry I. Corman.

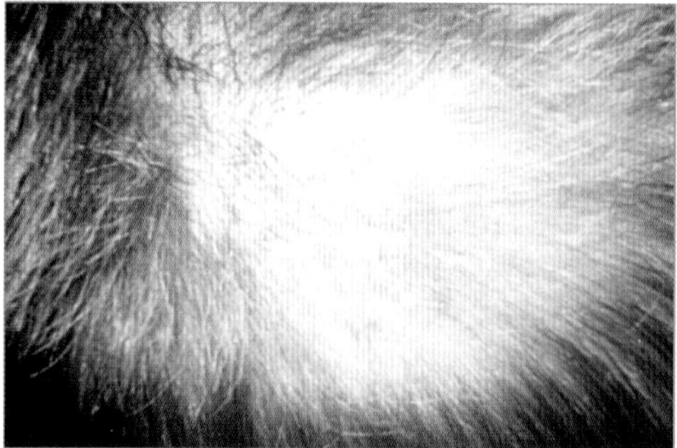

Image 135.4
This patient had ringworm of the scalp, or tinea capitis, due to *Microsporum nanum* when first examined in 1964. Tinea capitis is an infection of the scalp with mold-like fungi called dermatophytes. This type of fungus thrives in warm, moist areas. Susceptibility to tinea infection is increased by poor hygiene, prolonged moist skin, and minor skin or scalp injuries. Courtesy of Centers for Disease Control and Prevention/Dr Lucille K. Georg.

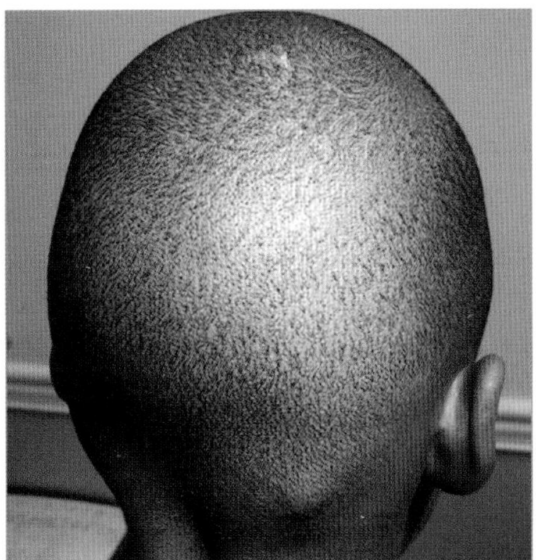

Image 135.5
An 8-year-old boy with a bald spot, hair loss, and enlarging posterior cervical lymph node for 2 weeks. The node was described as tender, not fluctuant, and without erythema of the overlying scalp. The area of hair loss was boggy and fluctuant. The patient responded well to treatment with griseofulvin. Copyright Stan Block, MD, FAAP.

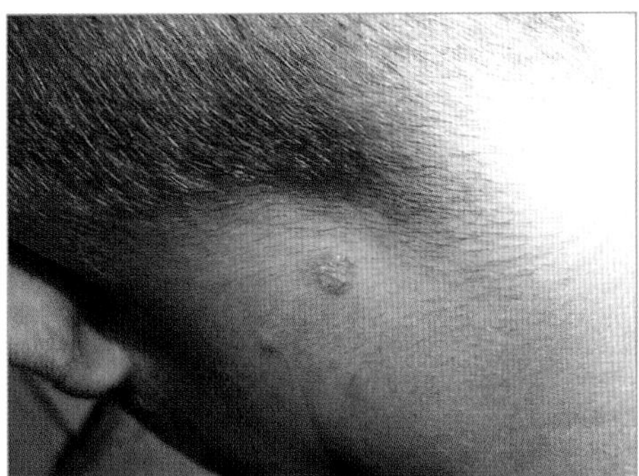

Image 135.6
Tinea capitis in the hairline of an 8-year-old boy. Copyright Stan Block, MD, FAAP.

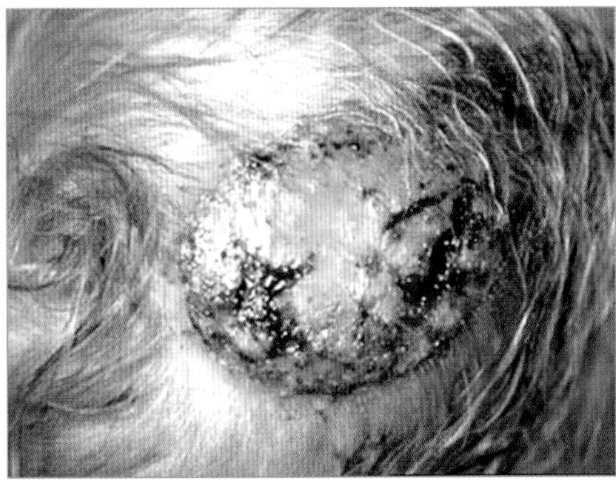

Image 135.7
A 2½-year-old boy with a kerion secondary to chronic, progressive tinea capitis. Copyright Martin G. Myers, MD.

136

Tinea Corporis

(Ringworm of the Body)

Clinical Manifestations

Superficial tinea infections of the nonhairy (glabrous) skin, termed tinea corporis, involve the face, trunk, or limbs. The lesion is often ring-shaped or circular (hence, the lay term, ringworm), slightly erythematous, and well demarcated with a scaly, vesicular, or pustular border and central clearing. Small confluent plaques or papules, as well as multiple lesions, can occur, particularly in wrestlers (tinea gladiatorum). Lesions can be mistaken for psoriasis, pityriasis rosea, nummular eczema, erythema annulare centrifugum, or atopic, seborrheic, or contact dermatitis. A frequent source of confusion is an alteration in the appearance of lesions as a result of application of a topical corticosteroid preparation, termed tinea incognito. Such patients can also develop Majocchi granuloma (trichophytic granuloma), a follicular fungal infection associated with a granulomatous dermal reaction. In patients with diminished T-lymphocyte function (eg, HIV infection), skin lesions may appear as grouped papules or pustules unaccompanied by scaling or erythema.

A pruritic, fine, papular or vesicular eruption (dermatophytic or id reaction) involving the trunk, hands, or face, caused by a hypersensitivity response to infecting fungus, can accompany skin lesions. Tinea corporis can occur in association with tinea capitis, and examination of the scalp should be performed.

Etiology

The prime causes of the disease are fungi of the genus *Trichophyton*, especially *Trichophyton tonsurans*, *Trichophyton rubrum*, and *Trichophyton mentagrophytes*; the genus *Microsporum*, especially *Microsporum canis*; and *Epidermophyton floccosum*. *Microsporum gypseum* can also occasionally cause infection.

Epidemiology

These causative fungi occur worldwide and are transmissible by direct contact with infected humans, animals, soil, or fomites. Fungi in lesions are communicable.

Incubation Period

Typically 1 to 3 weeks, but can be shorter.

Diagnostic Tests

Fungi responsible for tinea corporis can be detected by microscopic examination of a potassium hydroxide wet mount of skin scrapings. Use of dermatophyte test medium is also a reliable, simple, and inexpensive method of diagnosing tinea corporis. Skin scrapings from lesions are inoculated directly onto culture medium and incubated at room temperature. After 1 to 2 weeks, a phenol red indicator in the agar will turn from yellow to red in the area surrounding a dermatophyte colony. When necessary, the diagnosis can also be confirmed by culture on Sabouraud dextrose agar, although this often requires incubation for 3 to 4 weeks. Histopathologic diagnosis using periodic acid–Schiff reaction and polymerase chain reaction diagnostic tools are available but are expensive and, generally, unnecessary.

Treatment

Topical application of a miconazole, clotrimazole, terbinafine (12 years and older), tolnaftate, or ciclopirox (10 years and older) preparation twice a day or of a ketoconazole, econazole, naftifine, oxiconazole, sertaconazole, butenafine (12 years and older), or sulconazole preparation once a day is recommended. Although clinical resolution can be evident within 2 weeks of therapy, continuing therapy for another 2 to 4 weeks is generally recommended. If significant clinical improvement is not observed after 4 to 6 weeks of treatment, an alternate diagnosis should be considered. Topical preparations of antifungal medication mixed with high-potency corticosteroids should not be used; in addition, local and systemic adverse events from the corticosteroids can occur.

If lesions are extensive or unresponsive to topical therapy, griseofulvin can be administered orally for 6 weeks. Oral itraconazole, fluconazole, and terbinafine are alternative effective options for more severe cases. If Majocchi granulomas are present, oral antifungal therapy is recommended because topical therapy is unlikely to penetrate deeply enough to eradicate infection.

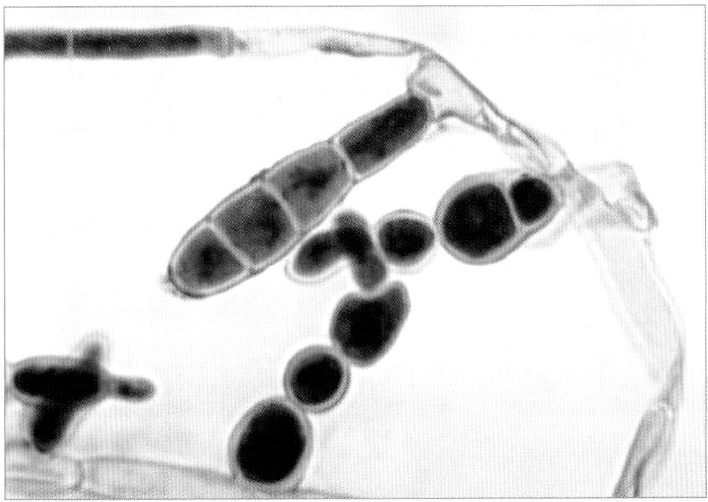

Image 136.1
This photomicrograph reveals a number of macroconidia of the dermatophytic fungus *Epidermophyton floccosum. E floccosum* is known to be a cause of dermatophytosis leading to tinea corporis (ringworm), tinea cruris (jock itch), tinea pedis (athlete's foot), and onychomycosis or tinea unguium, a fungal infection of the nail bed. Courtesy of Centers for Disease Control and Prevention/Libero Ajello, MD.

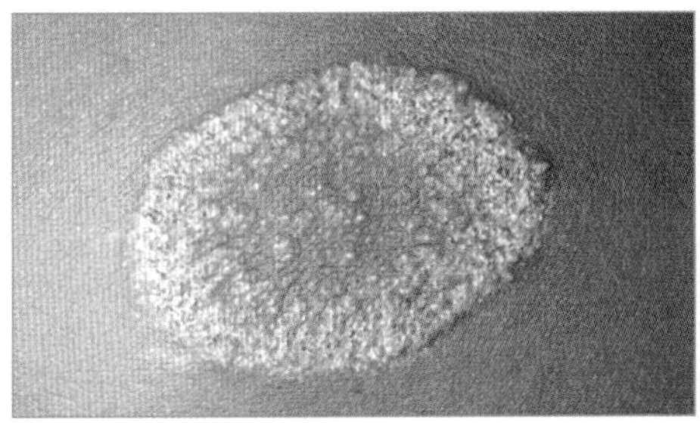

Image 136.2
Tinea corporis lesion in a 10-year-old girl. Courtesy of Gary Williams, MD.

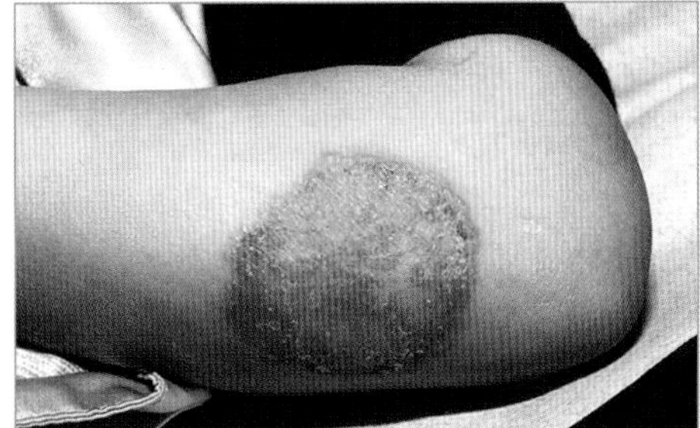

Image 136.3
Tinea corporis of the arm. This 6-year-old girl had enlarging skin lesion that had been present for a week. Copyright Larry I. Corman.

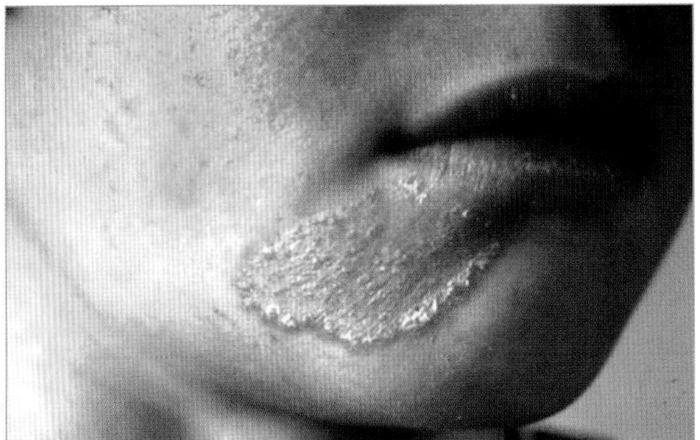

Image 136.4
Tinea corporis of the face. These annular erythematous lesions have a scaly center. Courtesy of Charles Prober, MD.

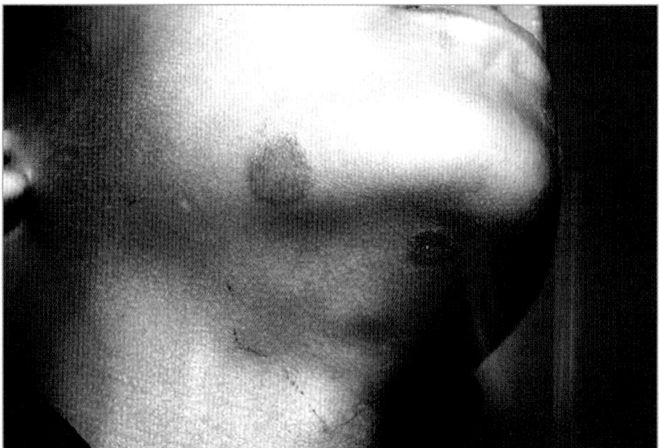

Image 136.5
Tinea corporis of the chin on a 6-year-old girl with enlarging lesions. The patient was successfully treated with clotrimazole. Copyright Larry I. Corman.

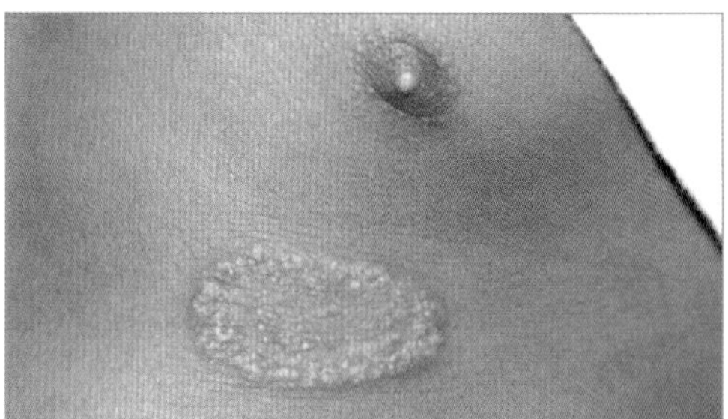

Image 136.6
A 16-month-old with a pruritic patch on his trunk. It has gotten larger over the past 3 days. He has a cat with dandruff and hair loss. The cat sleeps on his bed during the sunny part of the day. The child was treated with antifungal cream. The cat was evaluated by a veterinarian and cultured positive for *Microsporum canis.* This represents tinea corporis, commonly called ringworm. Courtesy of Will Sorey, MD.

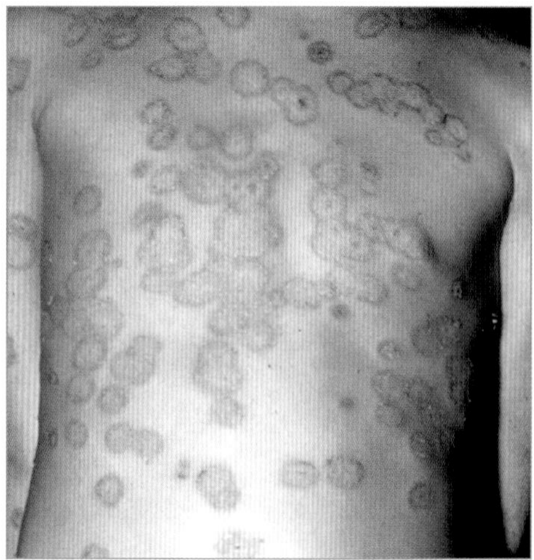

Image 136.7
Generalized tinea corporis in a 5-year-old girl.

137

Tinea Cruris

(Jock Itch)

Clinical Manifestations

Tinea cruris is a common superficial fungal disorder of the groin and upper thighs. Concomitant tinea pedis has been reported in patients with tinea cruris as well as previous episodes of tinea cruris. The eruption is usually bilaterally symmetric and sharply marginated, often with polycyclic borders. Involved skin is erythematous and scaly and varies from red to brown; occasionally, the eruption is accompanied by central clearing and can have a vesiculopapular border. In chronic infections, the margin can be subtle, and lichenification can be present. Tinea cruris skin lesions can be extremely pruritic. The appearance of tinea cruris can be altered in patients who have erroneously been treated with topical corticosteroids (tinea incognito), including diminished erythema, absence of typical scaling border, and development of folliculitis (Majocchi [trichophytic] granuloma). These lesions should be differentiated from candidiasis, intertrigo, seborrheic dermatitis, psoriasis, atopic dermatitis, irritant or allergic contact dermatitis (generally caused by therapeutic agents applied to the area), and erythrasma. The latter is a superficial bacterial infection of the skin caused by *Corynebacterium minutissimum*.

Etiology

The fungi *Epidermophyton floccosum, Trichophyton rubrum*, and *Trichophyton mentagrophytes* are the most common causes. *Trichophyton tonsurans, Trichophyton verrucosum*, and *Trichophyton interdigitale* have also been identified.

Epidemiology

Tinea cruris occurs predominantly in adolescent and adult males, mainly via indirect contact from desquamated epithelium or hair. Moisture, close-fitting garments, friction, and obesity are predisposing factors. Direct or indirect person-to-person transmission can occur. This infection commonly occurs in association with tinea pedis, and all infected patients should be evaluated for this possibility, with careful evaluation of the interdigital web spaces. Onychomycosis is also a possible association, particularly in adolescents and adults.

Incubation Period

Estimated to be 1 to 3 weeks.

Diagnostic Tests

Fungi responsible for tinea cruris may be detected by microscopic examination of a potassium hydroxide wet mount of scales. Use of dermatophyte test medium is also a reliable, simple, and inexpensive method of diagnosing tinea cruris. Skin scrapings from lesions are inoculated directly onto culture medium and incubated at room temperature. After 1 to 2 weeks, a phenol red indicator in the agar will turn from yellow to red in the area surrounding a dermatophyte colony. When necessary, the diagnosis can also be confirmed by culture on Sabouraud dextrose agar, although this often requires incubation for 3 to 4 weeks. Polymerase chain reaction assay is a more expensive diagnostic tool that generally is not required. A characteristic coral-red fluorescence under Wood light can identify the presence of erythrasma (an eruption of reddish brown patches attributable to the presence of *C minutissimum*) and, thus, exclude tinea cruris.

Treatment

Twice-daily topical application for 4 to 6 weeks of a clotrimazole, miconazole, terbinafine (12 years and older), tolnaftate, or ciclopirox (10 years and older) preparation rubbed or sprayed onto the affected areas and surrounding skin is effective. Once-daily therapy with topical econazole, ketoconazole, naftifine, oxiconazole, butenafine (12 years and older), or sulconazole preparation is also effective. Tinea pedis, if present, should be treated concurrently.

Topical preparations of antifungal medication mixed with high-potency corticosteroids should be avoided because of the potential for prolonged infections and local and systemic adverse corticosteroid-induced events. Loose-fitting, washed cotton underclothes to decrease chafing; avoidance of hot baths; and use of an absorbent powder can be helpful adjuvants to therapy. Griseofulvin, given orally for 6 weeks, may be effective in unresponsive cases. If Majocchi granulomas are present, oral antifungal therapy is recommended, as topical therapy is unlikely to penetrate deeply enough to eradicate infection. Because many conditions mimic tinea cruris, a differential diagnosis should be considered if primary treatments fail, and a fungal culture should be performed if the diagnosis is in question.

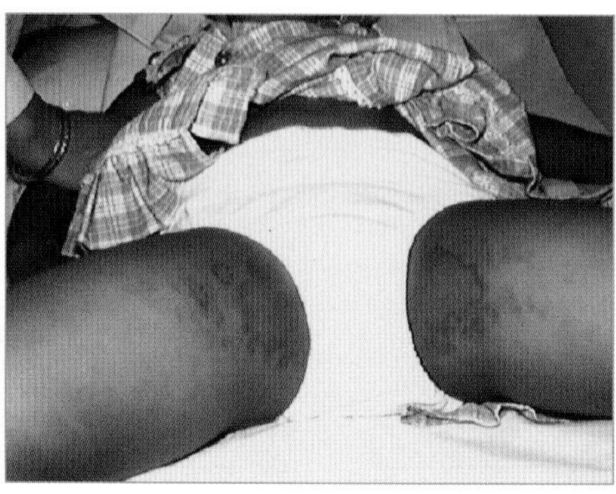

Image 137.1
Symmetric, confluent, annular, scaly red, and hyperpigmented plaques. This 10-year-old girl developed a chronic itchy eruption on the groin that spread to the anterior thighs. A potassium hydroxide preparation showed hyphae, and she was treated successfully with topical antifungal cream.

138

Tinea Pedis and Tinea Unguium

(Athlete's Foot, Ringworm of the Feet)

Clinical Manifestations

Tinea pedis manifests as a fine scaly or vesiculopustular eruption that is commonly pruritic. Lesions can involve all areas of the foot but usually are patchy in distribution, with a predisposition to fissures and scaling between toes, particularly in the third and fourth interdigital spaces or distributed around the sides of the feet. Toenails can be infected and can be thickened with subungual debris and yellow or white discoloration (tinea unguium [onychomycosis]). Toenails can be the source for recurrent tinea pedis. Tinea pedis must be differentiated from dyshidrotic eczema, atopic dermatitis, contact dermatitis, juvenile plantar dermatosis, palmoplantar keratoderma, and erythrasma (an eruption of reddish brown patches caused by *Corynebacterium minutissimum*). Tinea pedis commonly occurs in association with tinea cruris and onychomycosis (tinea unguium). Dermatophyte infections commonly affect otherwise healthy people, but immunocompromised people have increased susceptibility.

Tinea pedis and many other fungal infections can be accompanied by a hypersensitivity reaction to the fungi (the dermatophytid or id reaction), with resulting papular or papulovesicular eruptions on the palms and the sides of fingers and, occasionally, by an erythematous vesicular eruption on the extremities, trunk, and face.

Etiology

The fungi *Trichophyton rubrum*, *Trichophyton mentagrophytes*, and *Epidermophyton floccosum* are the most common causes of tinea pedis.

Epidemiology

Tinea pedis is a common infection worldwide in adolescents and adults but is less common in young children. Fungi are acquired by contact with skin scales containing fungi or with fungi in damp areas, such as swimming pools, locker rooms, and showers. Tinea pedis can spread throughout a household among family members and is communicable for as long as infection is present.

Incubation Period

Estimated to be approximately 1 to 3 weeks.

Diagnostic Tests

Tinea pedis usually is diagnosed by clinical manifestations and can be confirmed by microscopic examination of a potassium hydroxide wet mount of cutaneous scrapings. Use of dermatophyte test medium is a reliable, simple, and inexpensive method of diagnosing tinea pedis and tinea unguium. Skin scrapings from lesions are inoculated directly onto the culture medium and incubated at room temperature. After 1 to 2 weeks, a phenol red indicator in the agar will turn from yellow to red in the area surrounding a dermatophyte colony. When necessary, the diagnosis can also be confirmed by culture on Sabouraud dextrose agar, although this often requires incubation for 3 to 4 weeks. Infection of the nail can be verified by direct microscopic examination with potassium hydroxide, fungal culture of desquamated subungual material, or fungal stain of a nail clipping fixed in formalin. Periodic acid-Schiff reaction has the highest sensitivity for detecting fungus but does not identify the associated species and cannot necessarily differentiate other mold infections from dermatophyte infections.

Treatment

Topical application of terbinafine, twice daily; ciclopirox; or an azole agent (clotrimazole, miconazole, econazole, oxiconazole, sertaconazole, ketoconazole), once or twice daily, is usually adequate for milder cases of tinea pedis. Acute vesicular lesions can be treated with intermittent use of open wet compresses (eg, with Burow [aluminum acetate topical] solution, 1:80). Dermatophyte infections in other locations, if present, should be treated concurrently.

Tinea pedis that is severe, chronic, or refractory to topical treatment can be treated with oral therapy. Oral itraconazole or terbinafine is the most effective, with griseofulvin next and fluconazole least effective. Id (hypersensitivity response) reactions are treated by wet compresses, topical corticosteroids, occasionally systemic corticosteroids, and eradication of the primary source of infection.

Recurrence is prevented by proper foot hygiene, which includes keeping the feet dry and cool, gentle cleaning, drying between the toes, use of absorbent antifungal foot powder, frequent airing of affected areas, and avoidance of occlusive footwear and nylon socks or other fabrics that interfere with dissipation of moisture.

In people with onychomycosis (tinea unguium), topical therapy should only be used when the infection is confined to the distal ends of the nail; however, even topical therapy for 48 weeks typically has a cure rate less than 20%. Topical ciclopirox (8%) can be applied to affected toenail(s) once daily in combination with a comprehensive nail management program. Studies in adults have demonstrated the best cure rates after therapy with oral itraconazole or terbinafine; however, safety and effectiveness in children has not been established. Recurrences are common. Removal of the nail plate followed by use of oral therapy during the period of regrowth can help to affect a cure in resistant cases.

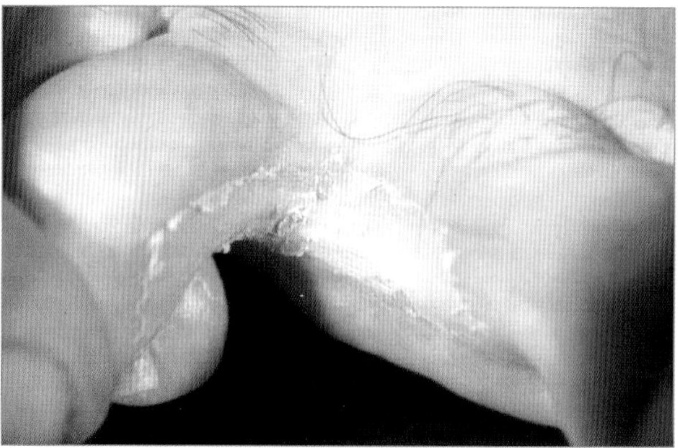

Image 138.1
This patient presented with ringworm or tinea pedis of the toes, which is also known as athlete's foot. Tinea pedis is a fungal infection of the feet, principally involving the toe webs and soles. Athlete's foot can be caused by the fungi *Epidermophyton floccosum* or by numerous members of the *Trichophyton* genus. Courtesy of Centers for Disease Control and Prevention/Dr Lucille K. Georg.

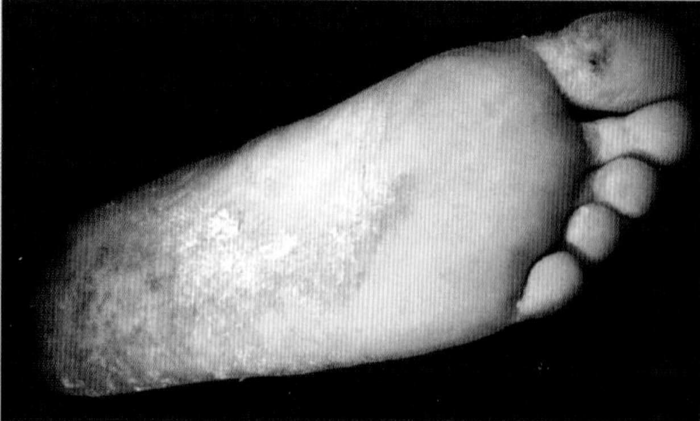

Image 138.2
This patient presented with ringworm of the foot (tinea pedis) due to the dermatophytic fungus *Trichophyton rubrum.* Individuals who practice generally poor hygiene, wear enclosed footwear such as tennis shoes, endure prolonged wetting of the skin (ie, sweating during exercise), and suffer with minor skin or nail injuries are more prone to suffer from tinea infections. Courtesy of Centers for Disease Control and Prevention.

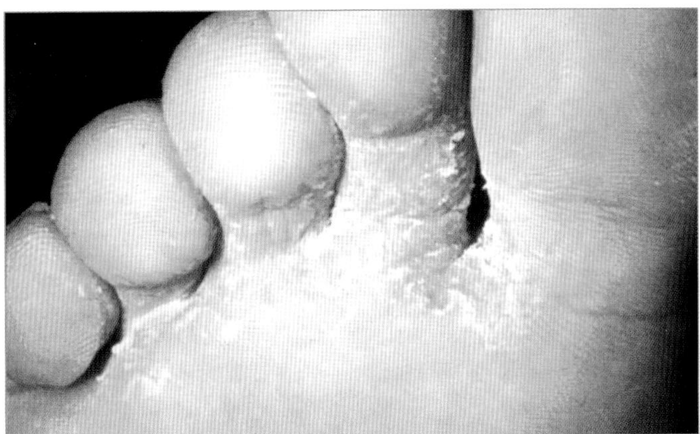

Image 138.3
Tinea pedis and tinea unguium.

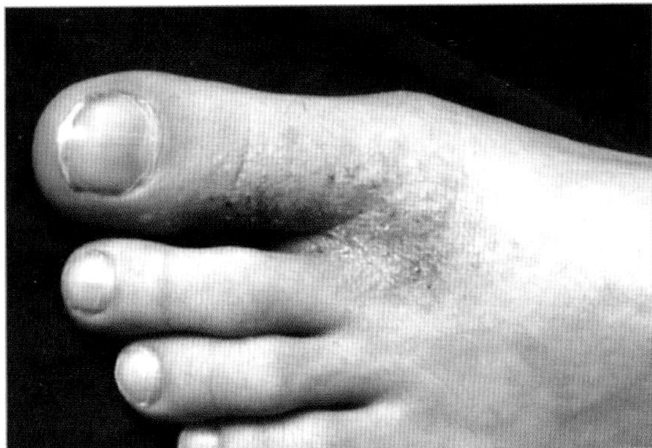

Image 138.4
Tinea pedis and tinea unguium. Courtesy of Gary Williams, MD.

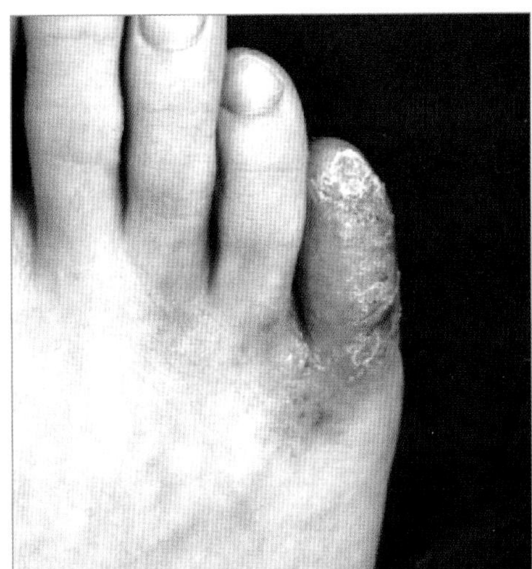

Image 138.5
Tinea pedis and tinea unguium infection. This is the same patient as in Image 138.4. Courtesy of Gary Williams, MD.

139

Toxocariasis

(Visceral Toxocariasis [previously Visceral Larva Migrans]; Ocular Toxocariasis [previously Ocular Larva Migrans])

Clinical Manifestations

The severity of symptoms depends on the number of larvae ingested and the degree of the inflammatory response. Most people who are infected are asymptomatic. Characteristic manifestations of visceral toxocariasis include fever, leukocytosis, eosinophilia, hypergammaglobulinemia, wheezing, abdominal pain, and hepatomegaly. Other manifestations include malaise, anemia, cough, and, in rare instances, pneumonia, myocarditis, and encephalitis. Atypical manifestations include hemorrhagic rash and seizures. When ocular invasion (resulting in endophthalmitis or retinal granulomas) occurs, other evidence of infection is usually lacking, suggesting the visceral and ocular manifestations are distinct syndromes.

Etiology

Toxocariasis is caused by *Toxocara* species, which are common roundworms of dogs and cats (especially puppies or kittens), specifically *Toxocara canis* and *Toxocara cati*. In the United States, most cases are caused by *T canis*. Other nematodes of animals can also cause this syndrome, although rarely.

Epidemiology

On the basis of a nationally representative survey, 14% of the US population has serologic evidence of *Toxocara* infection. Visceral toxocariasis typically occurs in children 2 to 7 years of age, often with a history of pica, but can occur in older children and adults. Ocular toxocariasis usually occurs in older children and adolescents. Humans are infected by ingestion of soil containing infective eggs of the parasite. Eggs may be found wherever dogs and cats defecate, often in sandboxes and playgrounds. Eggs become infective after 2 to 4 weeks in the environment and may persist long term in the soil. Direct contact with dogs is of secondary importance because eggs are not infective immediately when shed in the feces. Infection risk is highest in hot, humid regions where eggs persist in soil.

Incubation Period

Unknown.

Diagnostic Tests

Hypereosinophilia and hypergammaglobulinemia associated with increased titers of isohemagglutinin to the A and B blood group antigens are presumptive evidence of infection. An enzyme immunoassay for *Toxocara* antibodies in serum, available at the Centers for Disease Control and Prevention and some commercial laboratories, can provide confirmatory evidence of toxocariasis but does not distinguish between past and current, active infection. This assay is specific and sensitive for diagnosis of visceral toxocariasis but is less sensitive for diagnosis of ocular toxocariasis. Microscopic identification of larvae in a liver biopsy specimen is diagnostic, but this finding is rare. A liver biopsy negative for larvae, however, does not exclude the diagnosis.

Treatment

Albendazole is the recommended drug for treatment of toxocariasis. Alternative drugs include mebendazole and ivermectin, although mebendazole is no longer available in the United States. In severe cases with myocarditis or involvement of the central nervous system, corticosteroid therapy should be considered. Correcting the underlying causes of pica helps prevent reinfection.

Antiparasitic treatment of ocular toxocariasis may not be effective. Inflammation may be decreased by topical or systemic corticosteroids and secondary damage decreased with ophthalmologic surgery.

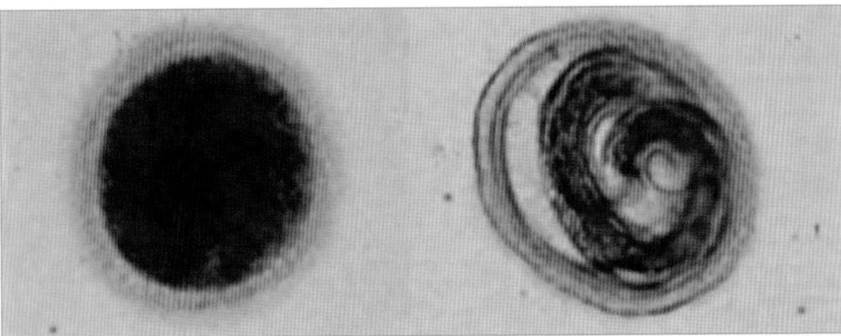

Image 139.1
Eggs of *Toxocara canis.* These eggs are passed in dog feces, especially puppy feces. Humans do not produce or excrete eggs; therefore, eggs are not a diagnostic finding in human toxocariasis. The egg to the left is fertilized but not yet embryonated, while the egg to the right contains a well-developed larva. The latter egg would be infective if ingested by a human (frequently, a child). Courtesy of Centers for Disease Control and Prevention.

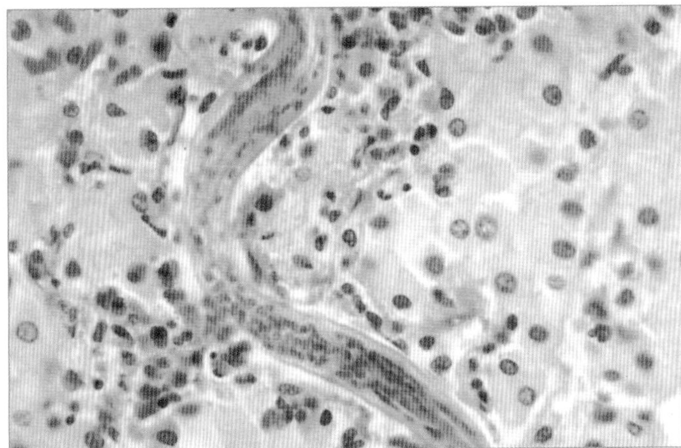

Image 139.2
Visceral toxocariasis (previously visceral larva migrans) with *Toxocara canis* larvae on liver biopsy.

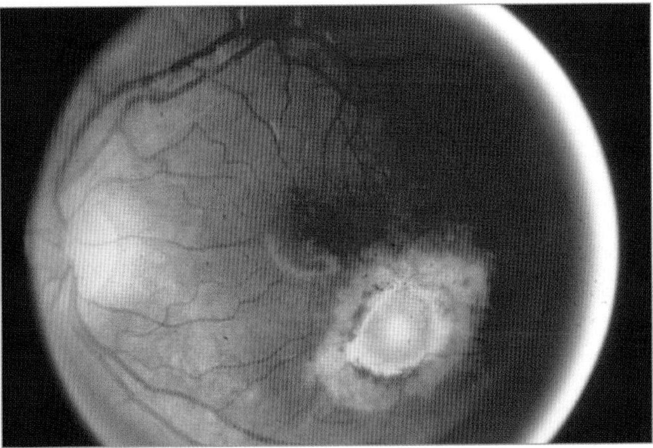

Image 139.3
Toxocara canis. Fundus damage from larval invasion. Courtesy of Hugh Moffet, MD.

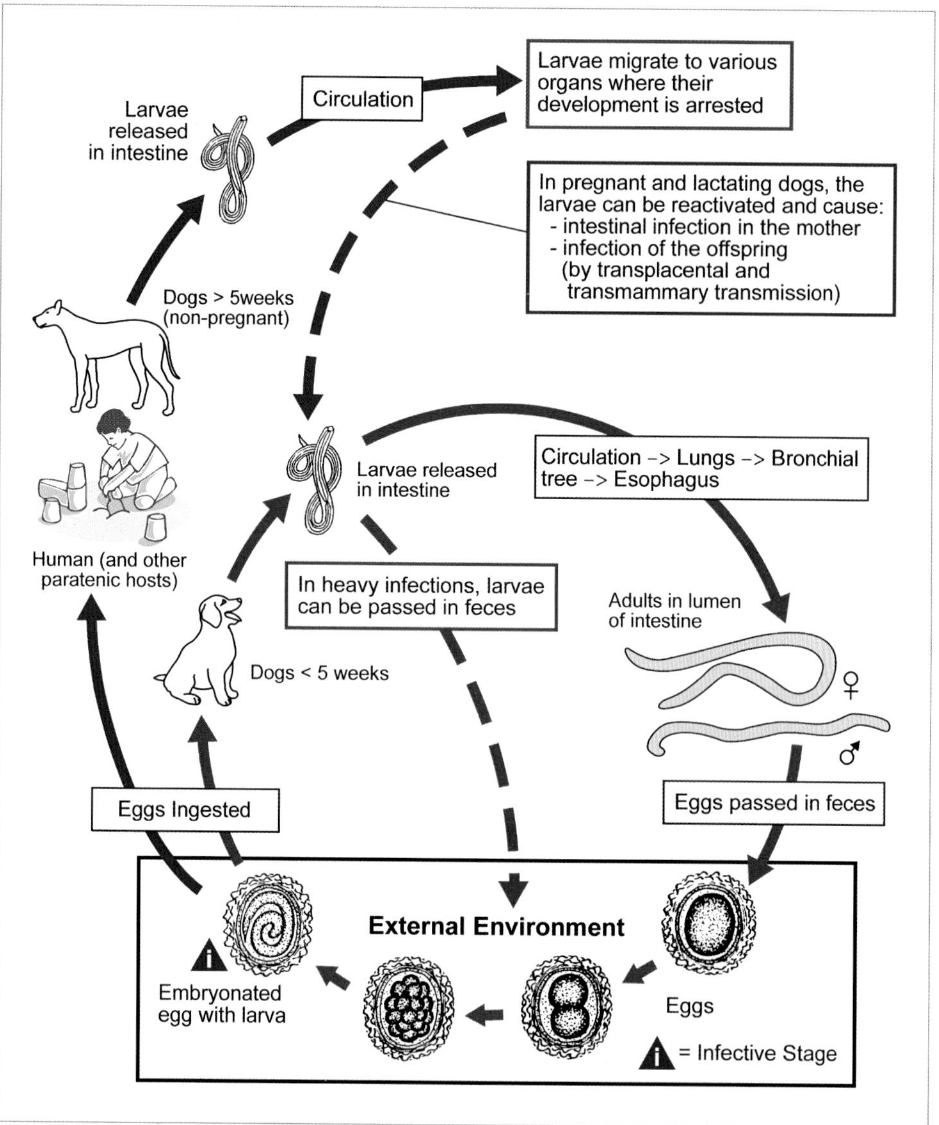

Image 139.4

Toxocara canis accomplishes its life cycle in dogs, with humans acquiring the infection as accidental hosts. Following ingestion by dogs, the infective eggs yield larvae that penetrate the gut wall and migrate into various tissues, where they encyst if the dog is older than 5 weeks. In younger dogs, the larvae migrate through the lungs, bronchial tree, and esophagus; adult worms develop and oviposit in the small intestine. In older dogs, the encysted stages are reactivated during pregnancy and infect by the transplacental and transmammary routes of the puppies, in whose small intestine adult worms become established. Thus, infective eggs are excreted by lactating adult female dogs and puppies. Humans are paratenic hosts who become infected by ingesting infective eggs in contaminated soil. After ingestion, the eggs yield larvae that penetrate the intestinal wall and are carried by the circulation to a wide variety of tissues (liver, heart, lungs, brain, muscle, eyes). While the larvae do not undergo any further development in these sites, they can cause severe local reactions that are the basis of toxocariasis. Courtesy of Centers for Disease Control and Prevention/Alexander J. da Silva, PhD/ Melanie Moser.

140

Toxoplasma gondii Infections

(Toxoplasmosis)

Clinical Manifestations

Congenital Infection

Although most children with congenital infection are born without clinical manifestations, visual or hearing impairment, learning disabilities, or intellectual disability (mental retardation) will become apparent in a large proportion several months to years later. Major clinical signs at birth include chorioretinitis cerebral calcifications and hydrocephalus; they can be present alone or in combination. The concomitant presence of these 3 signs ("classic triad") is rare but highly suggestive of congenital toxoplasmosis. More than 70% of congenitally infected children develop chorioretinitis later in life. Additional signs of congenital toxoplasmosis at birth include microcephaly, seizures, hearing loss, strabismus, a maculopapular rash, generalized lymphadenopathy, hepatomegaly, splenomegaly, jaundice, pneumonitis, diarrhea, hypothermia, anemia, petechiae, and thrombocytopenia. As a consequence of intrauterine infection, meningoencephalitis with cerebrospinal fluid (CSF) abnormalities can develop. Some severely affected fetuses and newborns die in utero or within a few days of birth. Cerebral calcifications can be demonstrated by plain radiograph, ultrasonography, or computed tomography (CT) imaging of the head. Computed tomography is the radiologic technique of choice because it is the most sensitive for calcifications and can reveal brain abnormalities when plain radiographic or ultrasonographic studies are normal.

Postnatally Acquired Primary Infection

Toxoplasma gondii infection acquired after birth is asymptomatic in most immunocompetent patients. When symptoms develop, they may be nonspecific and can include fever, malaise, headache, sore throat, arthralgia, and myalgia. Lymphadenopathy, frequently cervical, is the most common sign. Patients occasionally have a mononucleosis-like illness associated with a macular rash and hepatosplenomegaly. The clinical course is usually benign and self-limited. In a subset of immunocompetent individuals and in immunocompromised patients, primary infection presents with persistent fever, myocarditis, myositis, hepatitis, pericarditis, pneumonia, encephalitis with and without brain abscesses, and skin lesions. These manifestations and a more aggressive clinical course, including life-threatening pneumonia, have been documented in patients who acquired primary toxoplasmosis in certain tropical countries in South America, such as French Guiana, Brazil, and Colombia. Toxoplasmosis should be included in the differential diagnosis of ill travelers who return home with these unexplained syndromes.

Ocular toxoplasmosis also occurs in the setting of postnatally acquired infection. In Brazil and Canada, up to 17% of patients diagnosed with postnatally acquired toxoplasmosis have toxoplasmic chorioretinitis. Acute ocular involvement manifests as blurred vision, eye pain, decreased visual acuity, floaters, scotoma, photophobia, or epiphora. The most common late finding is chorioretinitis, which can result in vision loss. Ocular disease can become reactivated years after the initial infection in healthy and immunocompromised people.

Reactivation of Chronic Infection in Immunocompromised Patients

In chronically infected immunodeficient patients, including people with HIV infection, reactivation of *T gondii* can result in life-threatening encephalitis, pneumonitis, toxoplasmic chorioretinitis (a posterior uveitis), fever of unknown origin, or disseminated toxoplasmosis. In patients with AIDS, toxoplasmic encephalitis (TE) is the most common cause of encephalitis and typically presents with acute to subacute neurologic or psychiatric symptoms and multiple ring-enhancing brain lesions. In these patients, a clear improvement in their symptoms and signs within 7 to 10 days of beginning empiric anti-toxoplasma drugs is considered diagnostic of TE. However, immunocompromised patients without AIDS (eg, transplant or cancer patients, patients taking immunosuppressive drugs) who are chronically infected with *T gondii* and who present with multiple ring-enhancing brain lesions should undergo an immediate brain biopsy to confirm the diagnosis. Toxoplasmic encephalitis can also present as a single brain lesion by magnetic resonance imaging (MRI) or as a diffuse and rapidly progressive process in the setting of apparently negative brain MRI studies. Magnetic resonance imaging is superior to CT for the diagnosis of TE and can detect lesions not revealed by CT. Seropositive hematopoietic stem cell and solid organ transplant patients are at risk of their latent *T gondii* infection being reactivated. In these patients, toxoplasmosis may manifest as pneumonia, unexplained fever or seizures, myocarditis, hepatosplenomegaly, lymphadenopathy, or skin lesions, in addition to brain abscesses and diffuse encephalitis. *T gondii*–seropositive solid organ donors (D+) can transmit the parasite via the allograft to seronegative recipients (R–). Thirty percent of D+/R– heart transplant recipients develop toxoplasmosis in the absence of anti-*T gondii* prophylaxis.

Etiology

T gondii is a protozoan and obligate intracellular parasite. *T gondii* organisms exist in nature in 3 primary clonal lineages (types 1, 2, and 3) and several infectious forms (tachyzoite, tissue cysts containing bradyzoites, and oocysts containing sporozoites). The tachyzoite and host immune response are responsible for symptoms observed during the acute infection or during reactivation of a latent infection in immunocompromised patients. The tissue cyst is responsible for latent infection and is usually present in brain, skeletal muscle, cardiac tissue, and eyes of humans and other vertebrate animals. It is the tissue cyst form that is transmitted through ingestion of undercooked or raw meat. The oocyst is present in the small intestine of cats and other members of the feline family; it is responsible for transmission through ingestion of soil, water, or food contaminated with cat feces that contain the organism.

Epidemiology

T gondii is worldwide in distribution and infects most species of warm-blooded animals. The seroprevalence of *T gondii* infection (a reflection of the chronic infection and measured by the presence of *T gondii*–specific immunoglobulin [Ig] G antibodies) varies by geographic locale and the socioeconomic strata of the population. The age-adjusted seroprevalence of infection in the United States has been estimated at 11% among women 15 to 44 years old. Members of the feline family are definitive hosts. Cats generally acquire the infection by ingestion of infected animals (eg, mice), uncooked household meats, soil organic matter, and water or food contaminated with their own oocysts. The parasite replicates sexually in the feline small intestine. Cats may begin to excrete millions of oocysts in their stools 3 to 30 days after primary infection and may shed oocysts for 7 to 14 days. After excretion, oocysts require a maturation phase (sporulation) of 1 to 5 days in temperate climates before they are infective by the oral route. Sporulated oocysts survive for long periods under most ordinary environmental conditions, eg, surviving in moist soil for months and even years. Intermediate hosts (including sheep, pigs, and cattle) can have tissue cysts in the brain, myocardium, skeletal muscle, and other organs. These cysts remain viable for the lifetime of the host. Humans usually become infected by consumption of raw or undercooked meat that contains cysts or by accidental ingestion of sporulated oocysts from soil or in contaminated food or water. A large outbreak linked epidemiologically to contamination of a municipal water supply has also been reported. Risk factors associated with acute infection in the United States are eating raw ground beef, rare lamb, or locally produced cured, dried, or smoked meat, raw oyster, clams or mussels; working with meat; drinking unpasteurized goat milk; and owning 3 or more kittens. Drinking untreated water was also found to have a trend toward increased risk for acute infection in the United States. Up to 50% of acutely infected people do not recall identifiable risk factors or symptoms. Thus, *T gondii* infection and toxoplasmosis may occur even in patients without a suggestive epidemiologic history or illness. Only appropriate laboratory testing can establish or exclude the diagnosis of *T gondii* infection or toxoplasmosis. There is no evidence of human-to-human transmission except through vertical transmission, blood products, or organ transplantation.

Transmission of *T gondii* has been documented in the setting of solid organ (eg, heart, kidney, liver) or hematopoietic stem cell transplantation from a seropositive donor with latent infection to an R–. Infection has rarely occurred as a result of a laboratory accident or from blood or blood product transfusion. In most cases, congenital transmission occurs as a result of primary maternal infection during gestation. In utero infection rarely occurs as a result of reactivated parasitemia during pregnancy in chronically infected immunocompromised women. The incidence of congenital toxoplasmosis in the United States has been estimated to be 1 in 1,000 to 1 in 10,000 live births.

Incubation Period

Approximately 7 days; range, 4 to 21 days.

Diagnostic Tests

Serologic tests are the primary means of diagnosing primary and latent infection. Polymerase chain reaction (PCR) testing of body fluids and staining of a biopsy specimen with *T gondii*–specific immunoperoxidase are valuable for confirming the diagnosis of toxoplasmosis. Laboratories with special expertise in *Toxoplasma* serologic assays and their interpretation, such as the Palo Alto Medical Foundation Toxoplasma Serology Laboratory (PAMF-TSL, CA) are useful to clinicians and nonreference laboratories.

Immunoglobulin G–specific antibodies achieve a peak concentration 1 to 2 months after infection and remain positive indefinitely. The vast majority of patients will have low-positive IgG antibody titers 6 months after the acute infection. To determine the approximate time of infection in IgG-positive adults, specific IgM antibody determinations should be performed. The lack of *T gondii*–specific IgM antibodies in a person with low-positive titers of IgG antibodies (eg, a Sabin-Feldman dye test at PAMF-TSL ≤512) indicates infection of at least 6 months' duration. Detectable *T gondii*–specific IgM antibodies can indicate recent infection, chronic infection, or a false-positive reaction. Sera with positive *T gondii*–specific IgM test results can be sent to PAMF-TSL for confirmatory testing and to establish whether the patient has an acute or a chronic infection. Enzyme immunoassays are the most sensitive tests for IgM, and indirect fluorescent antibody tests are the least sensitive tests for detecting IgM. Immunoglobulin M–specific antibodies can be detected 2 weeks after infection (IgG-specific antibodies are usually negative during this period), achieve peak concentrations in 1 month, decrease thereafter, and usually become undetectable within 6 to 9 months. However, in some people, a positive IgM test result may persist for years without apparent clinical significance. In adults, a positive IgM test should be followed by confirmatory testing at a laboratory with special expertise in *Toxoplasma* serology when determining the timing of infection is important clinically (eg, in a pregnant woman).

Laboratory tests that have been found to be helpful in determining timing of infection in patients with positive IgM test results include an IgG avidity test, the differential agglutination (AC/HS) test, and IgA- and IgE-specific antibody tests. The presence of high-avidity IgG antibodies indicates infection occurred at least 12 to 16 weeks prior. The presence of low-avidity antibodies is not a reliable indication of more recent infection, and treatment may affect the maturation of IgG avidity and prolong the presence of low-avidity antibodies. A nonacute pattern in the AC/HS test is usually indicative of an infection that was acquired at least 12 months before the serum was obtained. Tests to detect IgA and IgE antibodies, which decrease to undetectable concentrations sooner than IgM antibodies do, are also useful for diagnosis of congenital infections and infections in pregnant women, for whom more precise information about the duration of infection is needed. *T gondii*–specific IgA and IgE antibody tests are available in *Toxoplasma* reference laboratories but, generally, not in other laboratories. Diagnosis of

Toxoplasma infection during pregnancy should be made on the basis of results of serologic assays performed in a reference laboratory.

Polymerase chain reaction assay and *T gondii*–specific immunoperoxidase staining can be attempted with virtually any body fluid or tissue, depending on the clinical scenario. Specimens on which PCR assay can be performed include amniotic fluid, CSF, whole blood, bronchoalveolar lavage fluid, vitreous fluid, aqueous humor, peritoneal fluid, ascitic fluid, pleural fluid, bone marrow, and urine. Essentially any tissue can be stained with *T gondii*–specific immunoperoxidase; the presence of extracellular antigens and a surrounding inflammatory response are also diagnostic of toxoplasmosis. A positive PCR test result in tissue must be interpreted with caution because it does not distinguish reactivation from inactive chronic latent infection.

Special Situations

Prenatal

A definitive diagnosis of congenital toxoplasmosis can be made prenatally by detecting parasite DNA in amniotic fluid by PCR assay. Isolation of the parasite by mouse or tissue culture inoculation can also be attempted from amniotic fluid. Serial fetal ultrasonographic examinations can be performed in cases of suspected congenital infection to detect any increase in size of the lateral ventricles of the central nervous system or other signs of fetal infection, such as brain, hepatic, or splenic calcifications. Some states routinely screen all newborns for the presence of antibody to *T gondii*.

Postnatal

Congenital toxoplasmosis should be considered in neonates born to women suspected of having or who have been diagnosed with primary *T gondii* infection during gestation, women infected shortly before conception (eg, within 3 months of conception), immunocompromised women with serologic evidence of past infection with *T gondii*, or any neonate with clinical signs or laboratory abnormalities suggestive of congenital infection. *Toxoplasma*-specific IgG, IgM (by the immunosorbent agglutination assay [ISAGA] method), and IgA tests should be performed for all newborns suspected of having congenital toxoplasmosis. Infected newborns can have any combination of positive or negative IgM and IgA antibodies. Although placental leak can occasionally lead to false-positive IgM or IgA reactions in the newborn, repeat testing at approximately age 10 days can help confirm the diagnosis because the half-life of these immunoglobulins is short and the titers in a neonate who is not infected should decrease rapidly. The sensitivity of *T gondii*–specific IgM as determined by an immunosorbent agglutination assay is 87% in newborns born to mothers not treated during gestation; sensitivity for IgA antibodies is 77%; and when both are taken into consideration, the sensitivity increases to 93%. The indirect fluorescent assay or enzyme immunoassay for IgM should not be relied on to diagnose congenital infection.

If the mother was not tested during pregnancy, a maternal serum sample should also be tested for IgG and IgM, and the AC/HS test should be performed as soon as it is feasible. Maternal test results can help in the interpretation of newborn test results. In newborns with clinical signs, peripheral blood, CSF, and urine specimens should be assayed for *T gondii* by PCR assay in a reference laboratory. Evaluation of the newborn should include ophthalmologic, auditory, and neurologic examinations; lumbar puncture; and CT of the head. An attempt may be made to isolate *T gondii* by mouse inoculation from placenta, umbilical cord blood, CSF, urine, or peripheral blood specimens. Examination of the placenta by histologic tools and PCR assay can be helpful, but a positive result does not necessarily indicate the newborn is infected.

Congenital infection is confirmed serologically by persistently positive IgG titers beyond the first 12 months of life. Conversely, in an uninfected infant, a continuous decrease in IgG titer before 12 months without detection of IgM or IgA antibodies will occur. Transplacentally transmitted IgG antibody usually becomes undetectable by 6 to 12 months of age. Congenital toxoplasmosis can be confirmed before 12 months of age in infants with the following laboratory test results: a persistently positive or increasing IgG antibody concentration compared with the mother; a positive *Toxoplasma*-specific IgM (after 5 days of life) or IgA assay (after 10 days of life); a positive PCR test result in CSF, peripheral blood, or urine; or a positive IgG antibody test accompanied by clinical signs in a newborn born to a mother who was infected during gestation.

Immunocompromised Patients

Immunocompromised patients (eg, patients with AIDS, solid organ transplant recipients, patients with cancer, people taking immunosuppressive drugs) who are infected latently with *T gondii* have variable titers of IgG antibody to *T gondii* but rarely have IgM antibody. Immunocompromised patients should be tested for *T gondii*–specific IgG before commencing immunosuppressive therapy or as soon as their status of immunosuppression is diagnosed to determine whether they are chronically infected with *T gondii* and at risk of reactivation of latent infection. Active disease in immunosuppressed patients may or may not result in seroconversion and a 4-fold increase in IgG antibody titers; consequently, serologic diagnosis in these patients is often difficult. Previously seropositive patients may have changes in their IgG titers in any direction (increase, decrease, or no change) without any clinical relevance. In these patients, PCR testing, histologic examination, and attempts to isolate the parasite become the laboratory methods of choice to diagnose toxoplasmosis.

In HIV-infected patients who are seropositive for *T gondii* IgG, reactivation of their latent infection is usually manifested by TE. Toxoplasmic encephalitis can be diagnosed presumptively on the basis of characteristic clinical and radiographic findings. Magnetic resonance imaging usually reveals the presence of multiple brain-occupying and ring-enhancing lesions. If there is no clinical response within 10 days to an empiric trial of anti-*T gondii* therapy, demonstration of *T gondii* organisms, antigen, or DNA in specimens such as blood, CSF, or bronchoalveolar fluid may be necessary to confirm the diagnosis. Toxoplasmic encephalitis can also present as diffuse encephalitis without space-occupying lesions on brain MRI. Prompt recognition of this syndrome and confirmation of the diagnosis by PCR testing in CSF is crucial because these patients usually exhibit a rapidly progressive and fatal clinical course.

Diagnosis of TE in immunocompromised patients other than HIV-infected people requires confirmation by brain biopsy or PCR testing of CSF. In these patients, other organisms, such as invasive mold infections and nocardiosis, should be considered before beginning an empiric anti-*T gondii* therapy.

Neonates born to women who are infected simultaneously with HIV and *T gondii* should be evaluated for congenital toxoplasmosis because of an increased likelihood of maternal reactivation and congenital transmission in this setting. Expert advice is available at the PAMF-TSL (**www.pamf.org/serology**; telephone 650/853-4828; e-mail **toxolab@pamf.org**) and the National Collaborative Chicago-Based Congenital Toxoplasmosis Study, IL; **www.uchospitals.edu/specialties/infectious-diseases/toxoplasmosis;** telephone 773/834-4131; e-mail **rmcleod@midway.uchicago.edu**).

Ocular Toxoplasmosis

Toxoplasmic chorioretinitis is usually diagnosed on the basis of characteristic retinal lesions in conjunction with a positive serum *T gondii*–specific IgG test result. All patients with eye disease should have an IgM test performed; if a positive IgM test result is confirmed at a reference laboratory and eye lesions are consistent with toxoplasmic chorioretinitis, ocular disease is the result of an acute *T gondii* infection rather than reactivation of a chronic infection. Patients who have atypical retinal lesions or who fail to respond to anti-*T gondii* therapy should undergo examination of vitreous fluid or aqueous humor by PCR, and antibody testing (by using the Goldmann-Witmer coefficient, which compares the levels of intraocular antibody production to that of serum, as measured by enzyme-linked immunosorbent assay or radioimmunoassay) should be considered.

Treatment

Most cases of acquired infection in an immunocompetent host do not require specific antimicrobial therapy unless infection occurs during pregnancy or symptoms are severe or persistent. When indicated (eg, chorioretinitis, significant organ damage), the combination of pyrimethamine and sulfadiazine, with supplemental leucovorin (folinic acid) to minimize pyrimethamine-associated hematologic toxicity, is the regimen most widely accepted for children and adults with acute symptomatic disease. Trimethoprim-sulfamethoxazole (TMP-SMX) has been reported to be equivalent to pyrimethamine and sulfadiazine in the treatment of patients with toxoplasmic chorioretinitis. In addition, pyrimethamine can be used in combination with clindamycin, atovaquone, or azithromycin if the patient does not tolerate sulfonamide compounds. Corticosteroids appear to be useful in management of ocular complications, central nervous system disease (CSF protein >1,000 mg/dL), and focal lesions with substantial mass effects in certain patients.

HIV-infected adolescents and children 6 years or older who have completed initial therapy (at least 6 weeks and clinical response) for TE should receive suppressive therapy to prevent recurrence until their CD4+ T-lymphocyte count recovers above 200 cells/µL and their HIV viral load is nondetectable for at least 6 months. HIV-infected children 1 through 5 years of age should also receive suppressive therapy after completion of initial therapy; discontinuation may be considered after they have been on stable antiretroviral therapy for longer than 6 months, are asymptomatic, and have demonstrated an increase in CD4+ T-lymphocyte percentage above 15% for more than 3 consecutive months. Prophylaxis should be reinstituted whenever these parameters are not met. Regimens for primary treatment are also effective for suppressive therapy.

Primary prophylaxis to prevent the first episode of toxoplasmosis is generally recommended for HIV-infected adolescents and children 6 years or older who are *T gondii*–seropositive and have CD4+ T-lymphocyte counts less than 100/µL. HIV-infected children 1 through 5 years of age should have initiation of primary prophylaxis when CD4+ T-lymphocyte percentage falls below 15%. Alternative regimens and recommendations for discontinuation of prophylaxis after the CD4+ T-lymphocyte count recovers in association with antiretroviral therapy are available. Trimethoprim-sulfamethoxazole, when administered for *Pneumocystis jiroveci* pneumonia (PCP) prophylaxis, also provides prophylaxis against toxoplasmosis. Dapsone plus pyrimethamine or atovaquone may also provide protection. Children older than 12 months who need PCP prophylaxis and who are receiving an agent other than TMP-SMX or atovaquone should have serologic testing for *Toxoplasma* antibodies because alternative drugs for PCP prophylaxis, such as pentamidine, are not effective against *T gondii*. Severely immunosuppressed children who are not receiving TMP-SMX or atovaquone and who are found to be seropositive for *Toxoplasma* infection should receive prophylaxis for PCP and toxoplasmosis (ie, dapsone plus pyrimethamine).

Primary prophylaxis with TMP-SMX or atovaquone is also recommended for previously seropositive patients who undergo allogeneic hematopoietic stem cell or bone marrow transplantation. In addition, D+/R– heart transplant recipients must also receive primary prophylaxis with TMP-SMX, atovaquone, or pyrimethamine. For immunocompromised patients without HIV infection, suppressive therapy should be continued for life or until the patient is no longer significantly immunosuppressed.

For symptomatic and silent congenital infections, pyrimethamine combined with sulfadiazine (supplemented with folinic acid) is recommended as initial therapy. Duration of therapy is prolonged and often is 1 year. However, the optimal dosage and duration are not established definitively and should be determined in consultation with an infectious diseases specialist.

Treatment of primary *T gondii* infection in pregnant women, including women with HIV infection, is recommended. Appropriate specialists should be consulted for management.

Spiramycin treatment of primary infection during gestation is used in an attempt to prevent transmission of *T gondii* from the mother to the fetus but does not treat the fetus if in utero infection has already occurred because spiramycin does not cross the placenta. Maternal therapy may decrease the severity of sequelae in the fetus once congenital toxoplasmosis has occurred. Spiramycin is available only as an investigational drug in the United States but may be obtained from the manufacturer following the advice of PAMF-TSL. If fetal infection is confirmed at or after 18 weeks of gestation or if the mother acquires infection during the third trimester, consideration should be given to starting therapy with pyrimethamine and sulfadiazine.

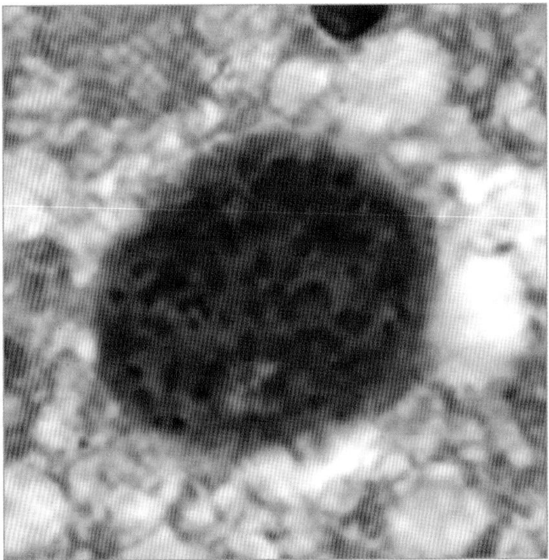

Image 140.1
Cysts of *Toxoplasma gondii* usually range in size from 5 to 50 µm in diameter. Cysts are usually spherical in the brain but more elongated in cardiac and skeletal muscles. They may be found in various sites throughout the body of the host but are most common in the brain and skeletal and cardiac muscles. *T gondii* cyst in brain tissue (hematoxylin-eosin stain). Courtesy of Centers for Disease Control and Prevention.

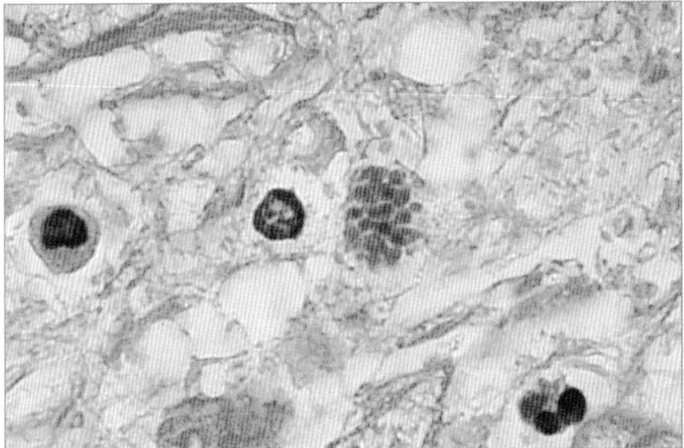

Image 140.2
Histopathology of toxoplasmosis of the brain in fatal AIDS. Pseudocyst contains numerous tachyzoites of *Toxoplasma gondii*. Courtesy of Centers for Disease Control and Prevention.

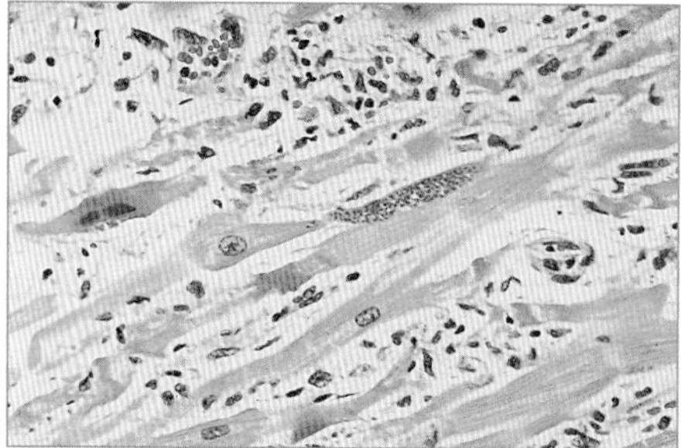

Image 140.3
Histopathology of toxoplasmosis of the heart in fatal AIDS. Within a myocyte is a pseudocyst containing numerous tachyzoites of *Toxoplasma gondii.* Several myocardial contraction bands and scattered inflammatory cells are visible. Courtesy of Centers for Disease Control and Prevention.

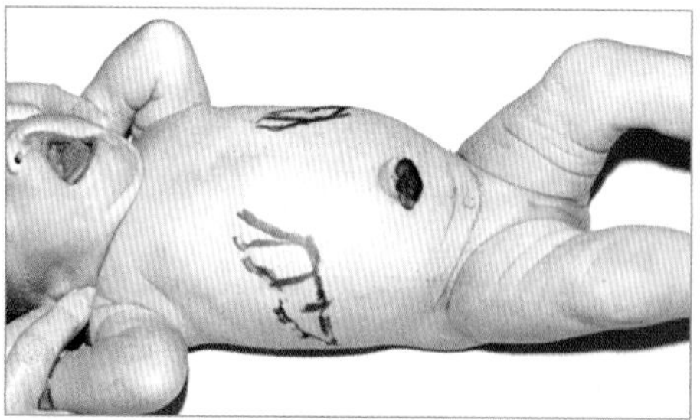

Image 140.5
Infant girl with congenital toxoplasmosis with hepatosplenomegaly. Courtesy of Edgar O. Ledbetter, MD, FAAP.

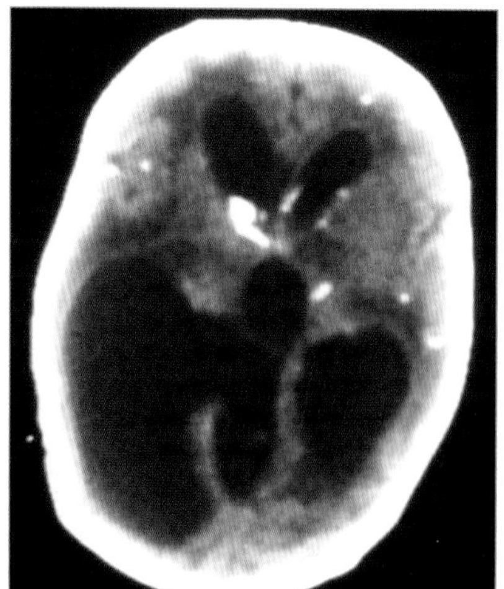

Image 140.7
Congenital infection evident on a computed tomography scan of the head that shows diffuse calcifications and hydrocephaly. Courtesy of Charles Prober, MD.

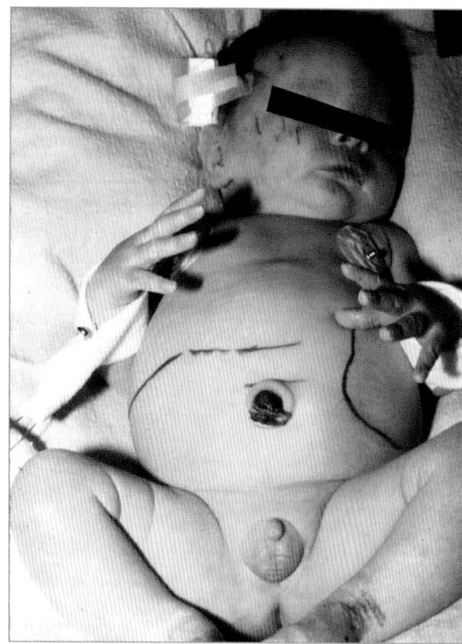

Image 140.4
A 12-day-old white boy with congenital toxoplasmosis with marked hepatosplenomegaly. Courtesy of George Nankervis, MD.

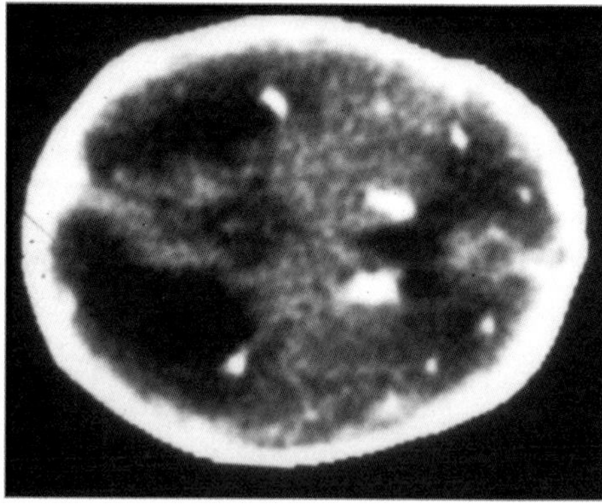

Image 140.6
A computed tomography scan of an infant with congenital toxoplasmosis demonstrating multiple intracranial calcifications. Courtesy of Larry Frenkel, MD.

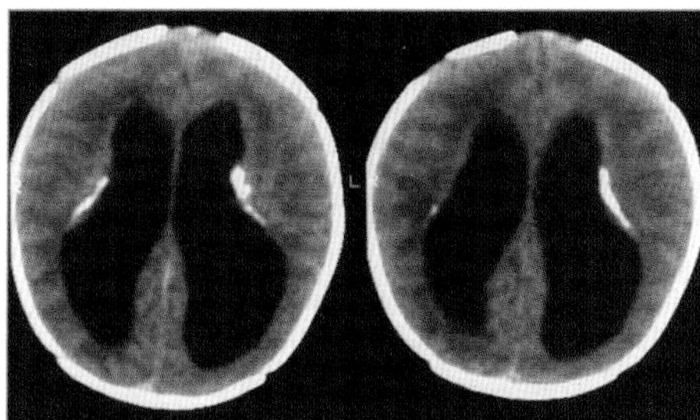

Image 140.8
A 3-day-old boy presented with a seizure. His computed tomography scan demonstrated hydrocephalus and periventricular calcification, suggestive of congenital infection, such as toxoplasmosis, rubella, cytomegalovirus, or herpes simplex. *Toxoplasma* serology was positive and the neonate was treated for congenital toxoplasmosis with pyrimethamine, sulfadiazine, and folinic acid. Copyright Barbara Jantausch, MD, FAAP.

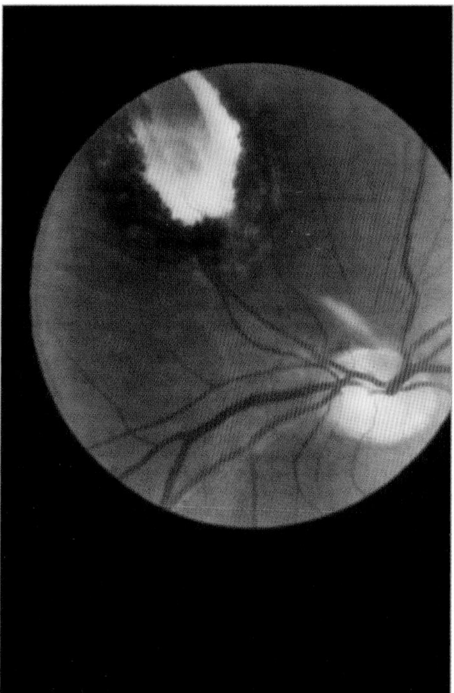

Image 140.10
Peripheral chorioretinitis in an infant with congenital toxoplasmosis. Courtesy of George Nankervis, MD.

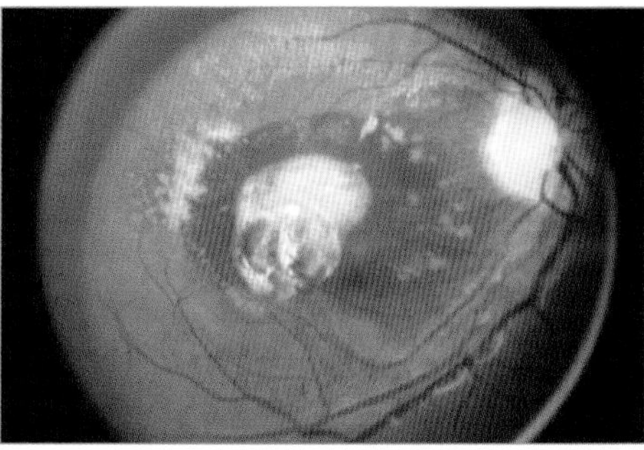

Image 140.9
Toxoplasma gondii retinitis. Note well-defined areas of choroidoretinitis with pigmentation and irregular scarring.

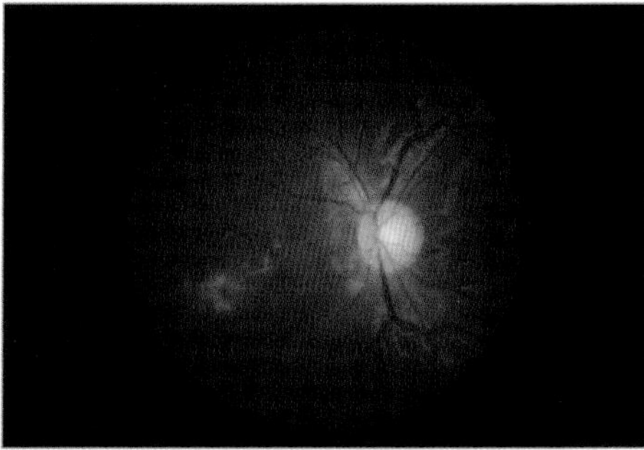

Image 140.11
A 12-year-old boy with chorioretinal scar with surrounding retinitis in the left eye nasal to the disk measuring a one-quarter disc diameter adjacent to the scar with mild overlying mild vitritis. No lesions in the macula. Findings typical of toxoplasmosis. Courtesy of Vicki Chen, MD.

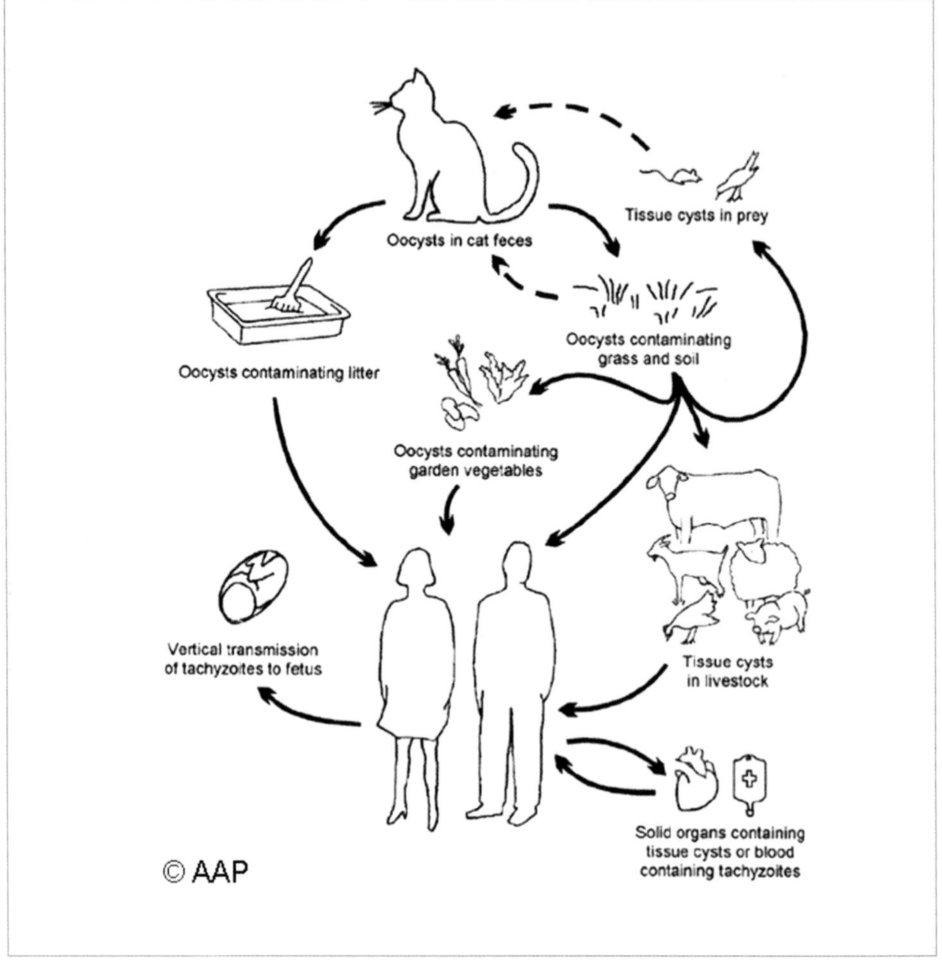

Image 140.12

Pathways for infection with *Toxoplasma gondii.* The only source for the production of *T gondii* oocysts is the feline intestinal tract. Humans usually acquire the disease by direct ingestion of oocysts from contaminated sources (eg, soil, cat litter, garden vegetables) or the ingestion of tissue cysts present in undercooked tissues from infected animals. Fetal infection occurs most commonly following acute maternal infection in pregnancy, but it can also occur following reactivation of latent infection in immunocompromised women. Pathways leading to human disease (solid arrow); pathways leading to feline infection (dashed arrow).

141

Trichinellosis

(*Trichinella spiralis* and Other Species)

Clinical Manifestations

The clinical spectrum of infection ranges from inapparent to fulminant and fatal illness, but most infections are asymptomatic. The severity of disease is proportional to the infective dose. During the first week after ingesting infected meat, a person may experience abdominal discomfort, nausea, vomiting, or diarrhea as excysted larvae infect the intestine. Two to 8 weeks later, as progeny larvae migrate into tissues, fever, myalgia, periorbital edema, urticarial rash, and conjunctival and subungual hemorrhages can develop. In severe infections, myocarditis, neurologic involvement, and pneumonitis can occur in 1 or 2 months. Larvae may remain viable in tissues for years; calcification of some larvae in skeletal muscle usually occurs within 6 to 24 months and may be detected on radiographs.

Etiology

Infection is caused by nematodes (roundworms) of the genus *Trichinella*. At least 5 species capable of infecting only warm-blooded animals have been identified. Worldwide, *Trichinella spiralis* is the most common cause of human infection.

Epidemiology

Infection is enzootic worldwide in carnivores and omnivores, especially scavengers. Infection occurs as a result of ingestion of raw or insufficiently cooked meat containing encysted larvae of *Trichinella* species. Commercial and home-raised pork remain a source of human infections, but meats other than pork, such as venison, horse meat, and, particularly, meats from wild carnivorous or omnivorous game (especially bear, boar, seal, and walrus) are now the most common sources of infection. The disease is not transmitted from person to person.

Incubation Period

Usually less than 1 month.

Diagnostic Tests

Eosinophilia up to 70%, in conjunction with compatible symptoms and dietary history, suggests the diagnosis. Increases in concentrations of muscle enzymes, such as creatinine phosphokinase and lactic dehydrogenase, occur. Identification of larvae in suspect meat can be the most rapid source of diagnostic information. Encapsulated larvae in a skeletal muscle biopsy specimen (particularly deltoid and gastrocnemius) can be visualized microscopically beginning 2 weeks after infection by examining hematoxylin-eosin–stained slides or sediment from digested muscle tissue. Serologic tests are available through commercial and state laboratories and the Centers for Disease Control and Prevention. Serum antibody titers generally take 3 or more weeks to become positive and can remain positive for years. Testing paired acute and convalescent serum specimens is usually diagnostic.

Treatment

Albendazole and mebendazole have comparable efficacy for treatment of trichinellosis (trichinosis). However, albendazole and mebendazole are less effective for *Trichinella* larvae already in the muscles. Mebendazole is no longer available in the United States. Coadministration of corticosteroids with mebendazole or albendazole is often recommended when systemic symptoms are severe. Corticosteroids can be lifesaving when the central nervous system or heart is involved.

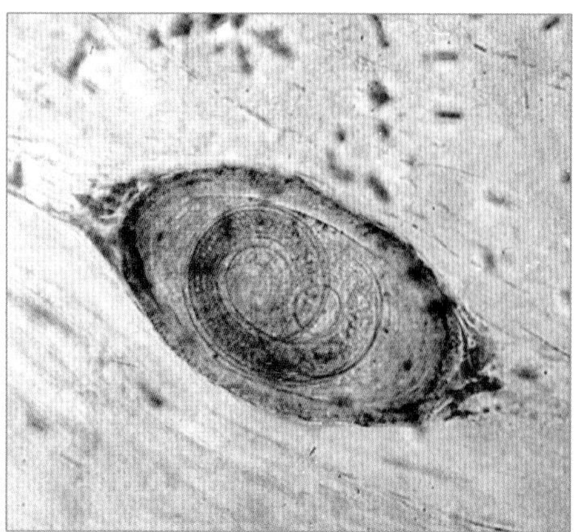

Image 141.1
Trichinella larvae in a sample of infected meat (light microscopy, magnification x100). Courtesy of *Emerging Infectious Diseases.*

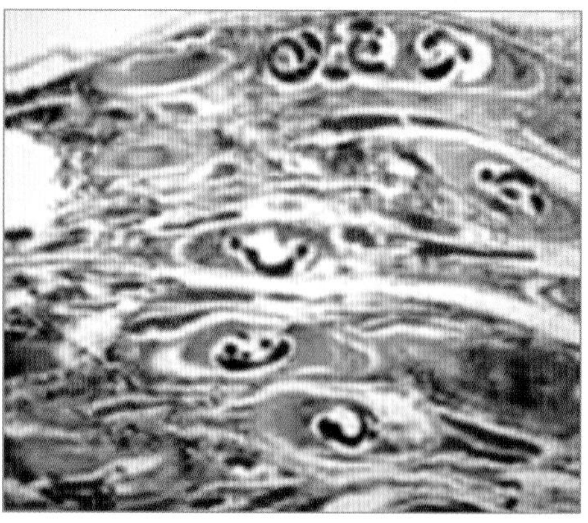

Image 141.2
Adult *Trichinella* species reside in the intestinal tract of the mammalian host; larvae can be found encapsulated in muscle tissue. Diagnosis is usually made serologically or based on observation of the larvae in muscle tissue following biopsies or autopsies. *Trichinella spiralis* larvae in muscle tissue. Courtesy of Centers for Disease Control and Prevention.

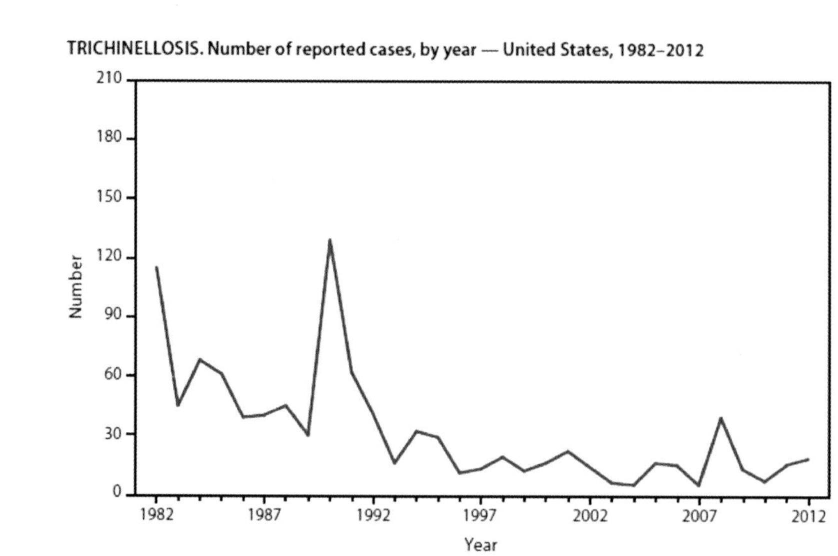

Image 141.3
Trichinellosis. Number of reported cases, by year—United States, 1982–2012. Courtesy of *Morbidity and Mortality Weekly Report.*

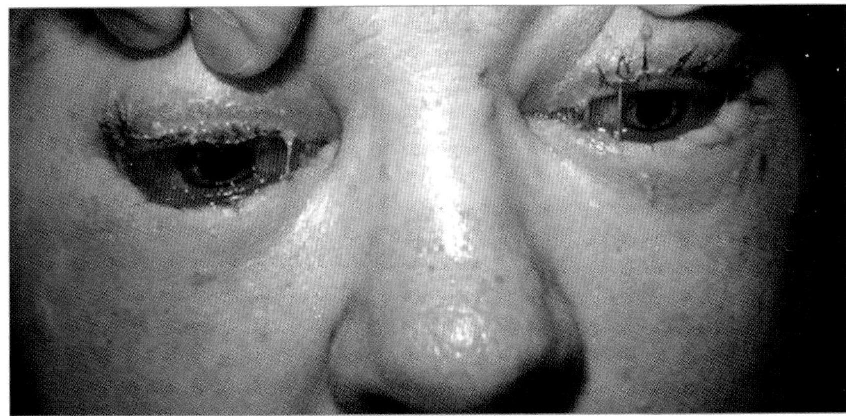

Image 141.4
This patient with trichinellosis (trichinosis) had periorbital swelling, muscle pain, diarrhea, and 28% (0.28) eosinophils. Courtesy of Centers for Disease Control and Prevention/Dr Thomas F. Sellers, Emory University.

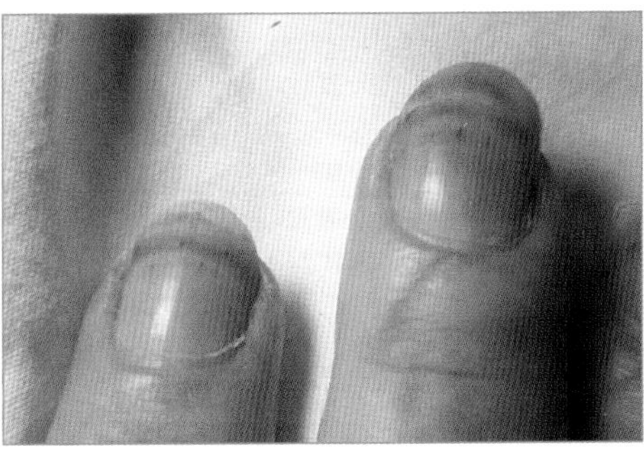

Image 141.5
Here the parasitic disease trichinellosis (trichinosis) is manifested by splinter hemorrhages under the fingernails. Trichinellosis is caused by eating raw or undercooked pork infected with the larvae of a species of worm called *Trichinella.* Initial symptoms include nausea, diarrhea, vomiting, fatigue, fever, and abdominal discomfort. Courtesy of Centers for Disease Control and Prevention/Dr Thomas F. Sellers, Emory University.

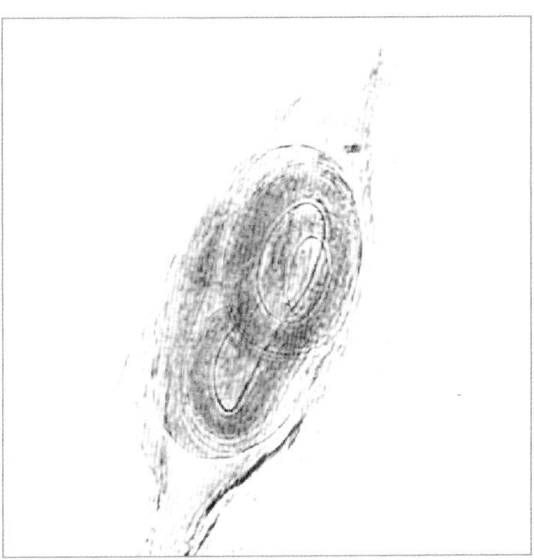

Image 141.6
Larvae of *Trichinella spiralis* in skeletal muscle biopsy.

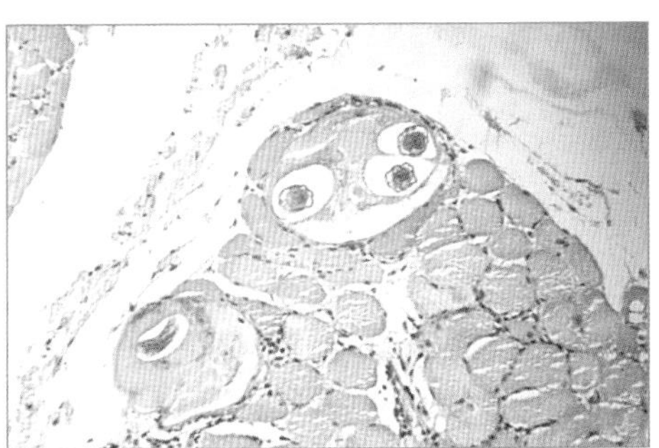

Image 141.7
Trichinella spiralis organisms on cross-section of muscle biopsy of the patient in images 141.4 and 141.5. Courtesy of Edgar O. Ledbetter, MD, FAAP.

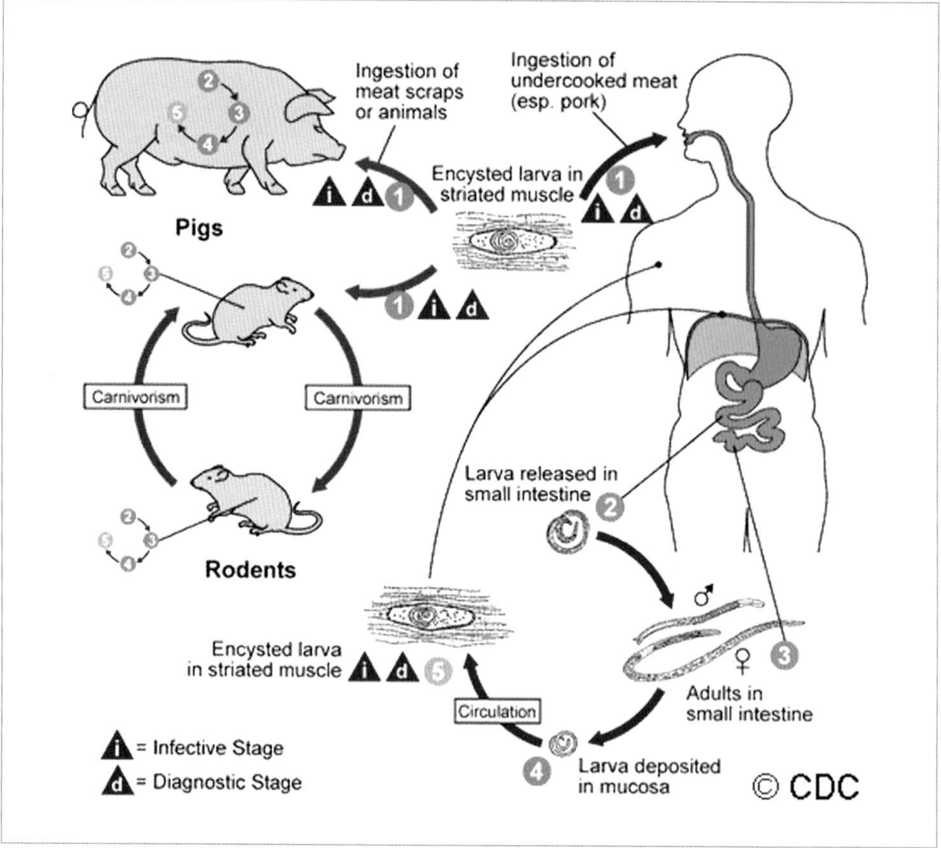

Image 141.8
Trichinellosis (trichinosis) is acquired by ingesting meat containing cysts (encysted larvae) (1) of *Trichinella.* After exposure to gastric acid and pepsin, the larvae are released (2) from the cysts and invade the small bowel mucosa, where they develop into adult worms (3) (female, 2.2 mm in length; males, 1.2 mm in length; life span in the small bowel, 4 weeks). After 1 week, the females release larvae (4) that migrate to the striated muscles, where they encyst (5). *Trichinella pseudospiralis,* however, do not encyst. Encystment is completed in 4 to 5 weeks and the encysted larvae may remain viable for several years. Ingestion of the encysted larvae perpetuates the cycle. Rats and rodents are primarily responsible for maintaining the endemicity of this infection. Carnivorous or omnivorous animals, such as pigs or bears, feed on infected rodents or meat from other animals. Different animal hosts are implicated in the life cycle of the different species of *Trichinella.* Humans are accidentally infected when eating improperly processed meat of these carnivorous animals (or eating food contaminated with such meat). Courtesy of Centers for Disease Control and Prevention.

142

Trichomonas vaginalis Infections

(Trichomoniasis)

Clinical Manifestations

Trichomonas vaginalis infection is asymptomatic in 70% to 85% of infected people. Clinical manifestations in symptomatic pubertal or postpubertal females consist of a diffuse vaginal discharge, odor, and vulvovaginal pruritus and irritation. Dysuria and, less often, lower abdominal pain can occur. Vaginal discharge may be any color but is classically yellow-green, frothy, and malodorous. The vulva and vaginal mucosa can be erythematous and edematous. The cervix can be inflamed and is sometimes covered with numerous punctate cervical hemorrhages and swollen papillae, referred to as strawberry cervix (colpitis macularis). This finding occurs in fewer than 5% of infected females but is highly suggestive of trichomoniasis. Clinical manifestations in symptomatic men include urethritis and, rarely, epididymitis or prostatitis. Reinfection is common, and resistance to treatment is rare but increasing. Rectal infections are uncommon, and oral infections have not been described.

T vaginalis infections in pregnant women have been associated with premature rupture of the membranes and preterm delivery. Perinatal infection can occur in up to 5% of neonates of infected mothers. *T vaginalis* infection in female newborns may cause vaginal discharge during the first weeks of life but is usually self-limited, resolving as maternal hormones are metabolized.

Etiology

T vaginalis is a flagellated protozoan approximately the size of a leukocyte. It requires adherence to host cells for survival.

Epidemiology

Although formal surveillance programs are not in place, several studies suggest that *T vaginalis* infection is the most common curable sexually transmitted infection in the United States and globally. Prevalence in a nationally representative sample of sexually experienced 14- to 19-year-old girls in the United States was 3.6%. It commonly coexists with other conditions, particularly with *Neisseria gonorrhoeae* and *Chlamydia trachomatis* infections and bacterial vaginosis. Transmission results almost exclusively from sexual contact, and the presence of *T vaginalis* in a child or preadolescent beyond the perinatal period is considered highly suspicious for sexual abuse. *T vaginalis* infection can increase the acquisition and transmission of HIV.

Incubation Period

Typically 1 week (range, 5–28 days).

Diagnostic Tests

Diagnosis in a symptomatic female is typically established by careful and immediate examination of a wet-mount preparation of vaginal discharge. The jerky motility of the protozoan and the movement of the flagella are distinctive. Microscopy has 50% to 65% sensitivity for *T vaginalis* diagnosis in females and is less sensitive in males; test sensitivity declines if the evaluation is delayed. The presence of symptoms and the identification of the organism are related directly to the number of organisms present. The nucleic acid amplification test is the most sensitive means of diagnosing *T vaginalis* infection and is encouraged for detection in females and males. The Aptima *T vaginalis* assay (Hologic, Inc, Marlborough, MA) is commercially available for testing vaginal specimens, endocervical specimens, female urine, and liquid cytology specimens. The BD ProbeTec T vaginalis Q^X Amplified DNA Assay (BD Diagnostics, Baltimore, MD) can detect *T vaginalis* from endocervical, vaginal, or female urine specimens. Culture of *T vaginalis* in diamond media or other trichomoniasis-specific culture systems (eg, InPouch, Biomed Diagnostics, White City, OR) is a sensitive and specific method of diagnosis in females but has lower sensitivity in males.

Two point-of-care tests are available for testing female vaginal swab specimens in settings where no microscope is available and rapid results are desirable. The OSOM *Trichomonas* Test (Sekisui Diagnostics, LLC, Lexington, MA) is a Clinical Laboratory Improvement Amendments–waived, antigen-detection, point-of-care test that uses immunochromatographic capillary flow dipstick technology. Results are available within 10 minutes. The BD Affirm VPIII (Becton, Dickinson and Company, Franklin Lakes, NJ) is a nucleic acid probe test for *T vaginalis, Gardnerella vaginalis,* and *Candida albicans.* Although the Affirm VPIII is considered a point-of-care diagnostic tool, test results are available in 45 minutes. Vaginal specimens can also be sent to a clinical laboratory for Affirm VPIII testing. Both of these vaginitis tests are reported to be more sensitive than microscopy (63% when compared with culture) and to have a specificity of 99%. False-positive results may occur in populations with a low prevalence of disease.

Treatment

Treatment of adults with metronidazole, in a single dose, results in cure rates of approximately 90% to 95%. Treatment with tinidazole in a single dose appears to be similar or even superior to metronidazole. Topical vaginal preparations should not be used because they do not achieve therapeutic concentrations in the urethra or perivaginal glands. Sexual partners should be treated, even if asymptomatic, because reinfection is a major factor in treatment failures. *T vaginalis* strains with decreased susceptibility to metronidazole have been reported; most of these infections respond to tinidazole or higher doses of metronidazole. If treatment failure occurs and reinfection is excluded, metronidazole twice daily for 7 days should be used. If treatment failure occurs following this regimen, a course of metronidazole or tinidazole may be used. If several 1-week regimens have failed in a person who is unlikely to have nonadherence or reinfection, testing of the organism for metronidazole and tinidazole susceptibility is recommended.

People infected with *T vaginalis* should be evaluated for other sexually transmitted infections, including syphilis, gonorrhea, chlamydia, HIV, and hepatitis B. For newborns, infection with *T vaginalis* acquired maternally is self-limited, and treatment is generally not recommended.

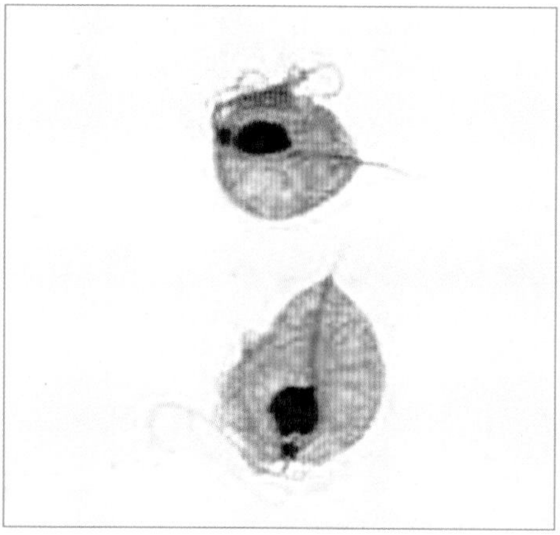

Image 142.1
Two trophozoites of *Trichomonas vaginalis* obtained from in vitro culture (Giemsa stain). Courtesy of Centers for Disease Control and Prevention.

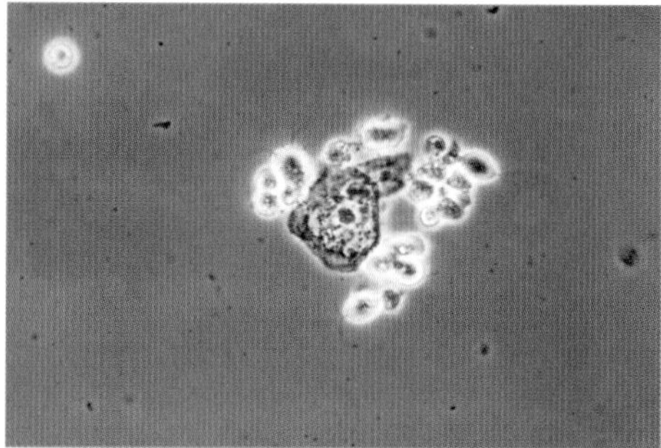

Image 142.2
This phase contrast wet mount micrograph of a vaginal discharge revealed the presence of *Trichomonas vaginalis* protozoa. *T vaginalis,* a flagellate, is the most common pathogenic protozoan of humans in industrialized countries. This protozoan resides in the female lower genital tract and the male urethra and prostate, where it replicates by binary fission. Courtesy of Centers for Disease Control and Prevention.

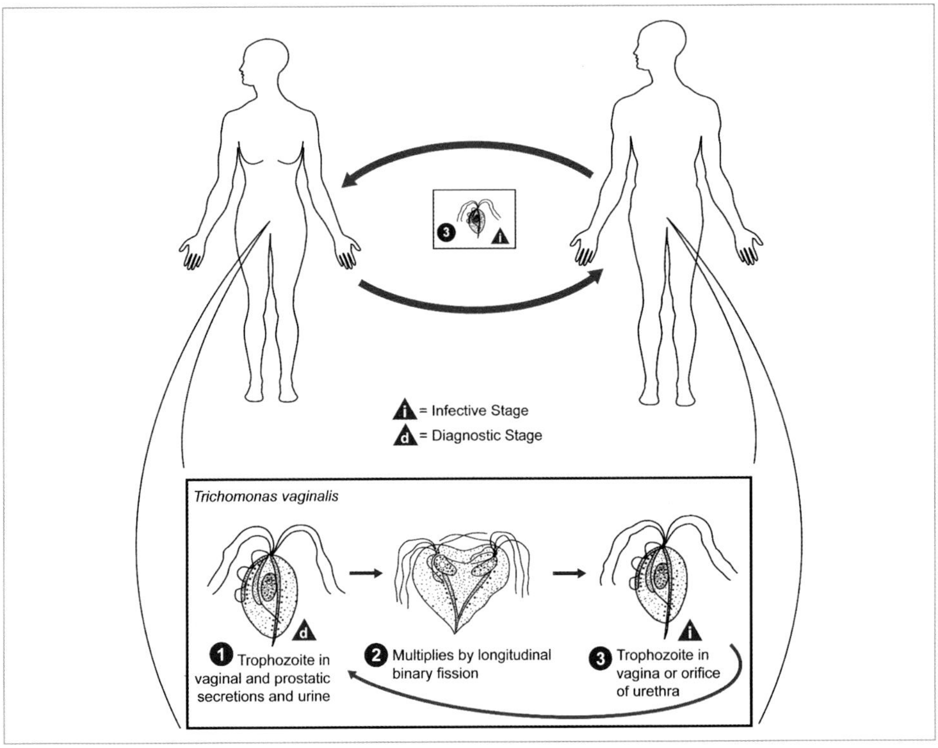

= Infective Stage
= Diagnostic Stage

Trichomonas vaginalis

1 Trophozoite in vaginal and prostatic secretions and urine

2 Multiplies by longitudinal binary fission

3 Trophozoite in vagina or orifice of urethra

Image 142.3
Trichomonas vaginalis resides in the female lower genital tract and the male urethra and prostate (1), where it replicates by binary fission (2). The parasite does not appear to have a cyst form and does not survive well in the external environment. *T vaginalis* is transmitted among humans, its only known host, primarily by sexual intercourse (3). Courtesy of Centers for Disease Control and Prevention/Alexander J. da Silva, PhD/Melanie Moser.

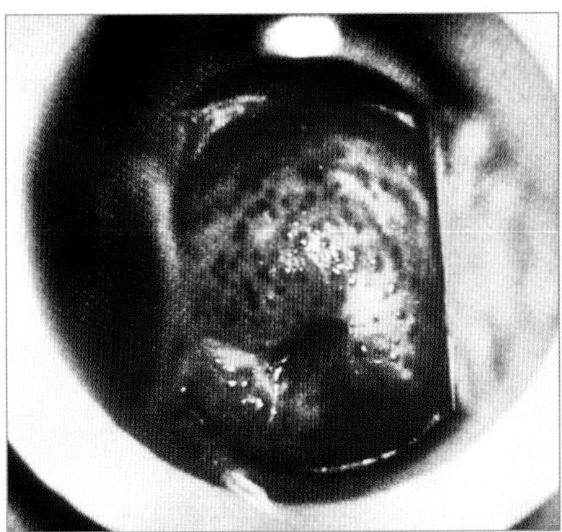

Image 142.4
This patient presented with a strawberry cervix (colpitis macularis) due to a *Trichomonas vaginalis* infection, or trichomoniasis. The term strawberry cervix is used to describe the appearance of the cervix due to the presence of *T vaginalis* protozoa. The cervical mucosa reveals punctate hemorrhages along with accompanying vesicles or papules. Courtesy of Centers for Disease Control and Prevention.

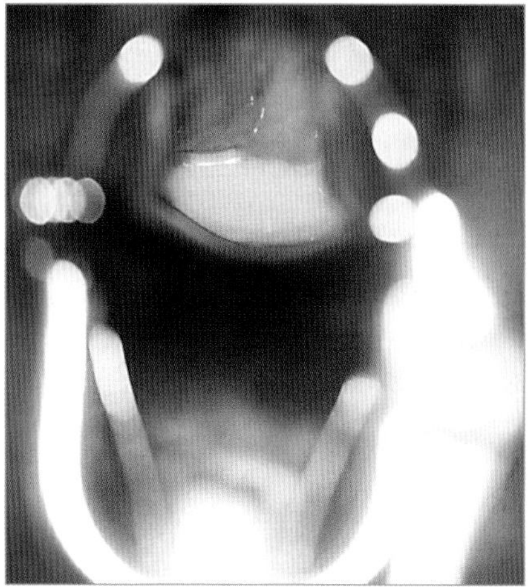

Image 142.5
This was a case of *Trichomonas* vaginitis revealing a copious purulent discharge emanating from the cervical os. *Trichomonas vaginalis,* a flagellate, is the most common pathogenic protozoan of humans in industrialized countries. This protozoan resides in the female lower genital tract and the male urethra and prostate, where it replicates by binary fission. Courtesy of Centers for Disease Control and Prevention.

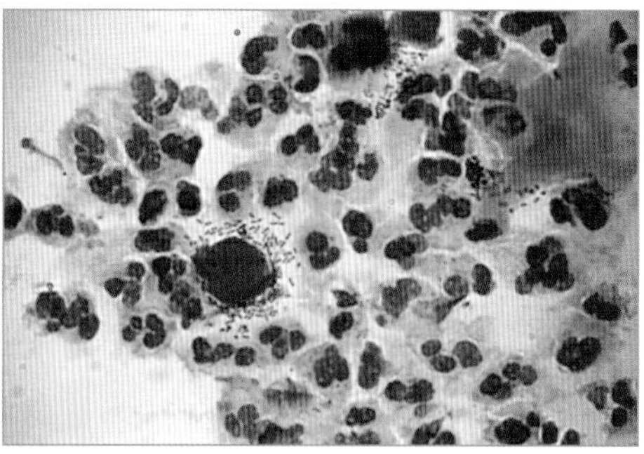

Image 142.6
This Gram-stained micrograph of a urethral discharge revealed the presence of trichomonads and gram-negative rods. *Trichomonas vaginalis,* a flagellate, is the most common pathogenic protozoan of humans in industrialized countries. This protozoan resides in the female lower genital tract and the male urethra and prostate, where it replicates by binary fission. Courtesy of Centers for Disease Control and Prevention.

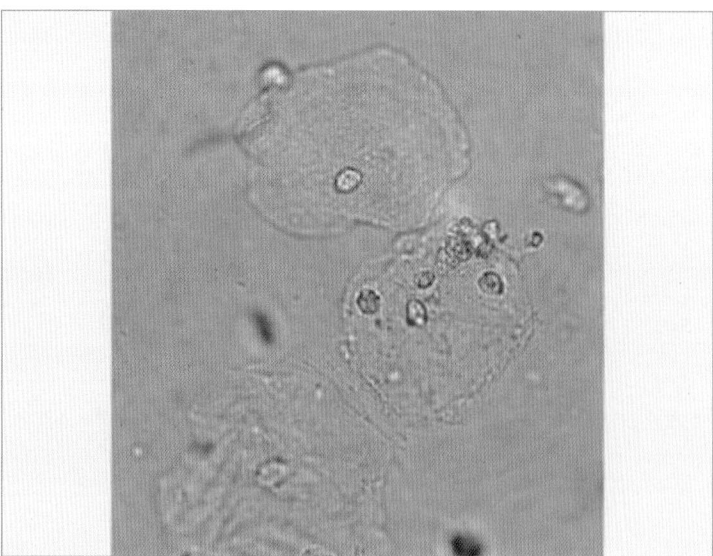

Image 142.7
An asymptomatic vaginal discharge in a premenarcheal girl who has other signs of the effects of estrogen is most likely due to physiological leukorrhea. The discharge is caused by the desquamation of vaginal epithelial cells in response to the effect of estrogen on the vaginal mucosa. Prior to puberty, the vaginal mucosa is atrophic, the pH of vaginal secretions is 6.5 to 7.5, and the bacterial flora are mixed. Following the onset of puberty, *Lactobacillus* becomes the predominant organism in the vagina. These gram-positive bacilli metabolize sloughed epithelial cells, producing lactic acid and decreasing the pH of the vagina to less than 4.5. Courtesy of H. Cody Meissner, MD, FAAP.

143

Trichuriasis

(Whipworm Infection)

Clinical Manifestations

Disease caused by the whipworm *Trichuris trichiura* is generally proportional to the intensity of the infection. Although most infected children are asymptomatic, those with heavy infestations can develop a colitis that mimics inflammatory bowel disease and can lead to anemia, physical growth restriction, and clubbing. *T trichiura* dysentery syndrome is more intense and characterized by abdominal pain, tenesmus, and bloody diarrhea with mucus; it can be associated with rectal prolapse.

Etiology

T trichiura, the human whipworm, is the causative agent. Adult worms are 30 to 50 mm long with a large, threadlike anterior end that embeds in the mucosa of the large intestine.

Epidemiology

The parasite is the second most common soil-transmitted helminth in the world, occurring mainly in tropical regions with poor sanitation. It is coendemic with *Ascaris* and hookworm species. Humans are the natural reservoir. Eggs require a minimum of 10 days of incubation in the soil before they are infectious. The disease is not communicable from person to person.

Incubation Period

Approximately 12 weeks.

Diagnostic Tests

Eggs may be found on direct examination of stool, although diagnosis of light to moderate infections may require concentration techniques.

Treatment

Albendazole, ivermectin, or mebendazole administered for 3 days provides only moderate rates of cure. Albendazole is considered the treatment of choice in the United States because mebendazole is no longer available. Reexamination of stool specimens 2 weeks after therapy to determine whether the worms have been eliminated is helpful for assessing the effectiveness of therapy. A recent study suggests combination therapy with mebendazole and ivermectin is associated with a higher cure rate than any currently available monotherapy.

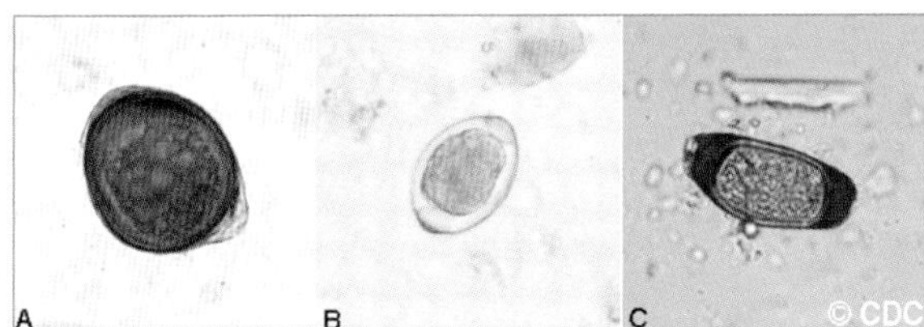

Image 143.1
Trichuris trichiura ova. A–C, Atypical *Trichuris* species eggs. Courtesy of Centers for Disease Control and Prevention.

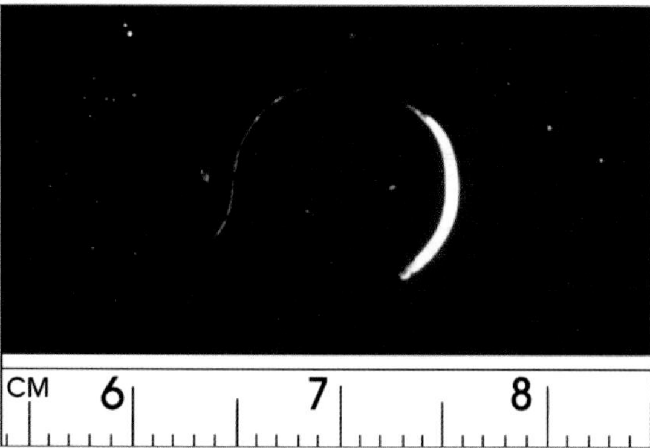

Image 143.2
This micrograph of an adult *Trichuris* female human whipworm reveals that its size in centimeters is approximately 4 cm. The female *Trichuris trichiura* worms begin to oviposit in the cecum and ascending colon 60 to 70 days after infection. Female worms in the cecum shed between 3,000 and 20,000 eggs per day. The life span of the adults is about 1 year. Courtesy of Centers for Disease Control and Prevention.

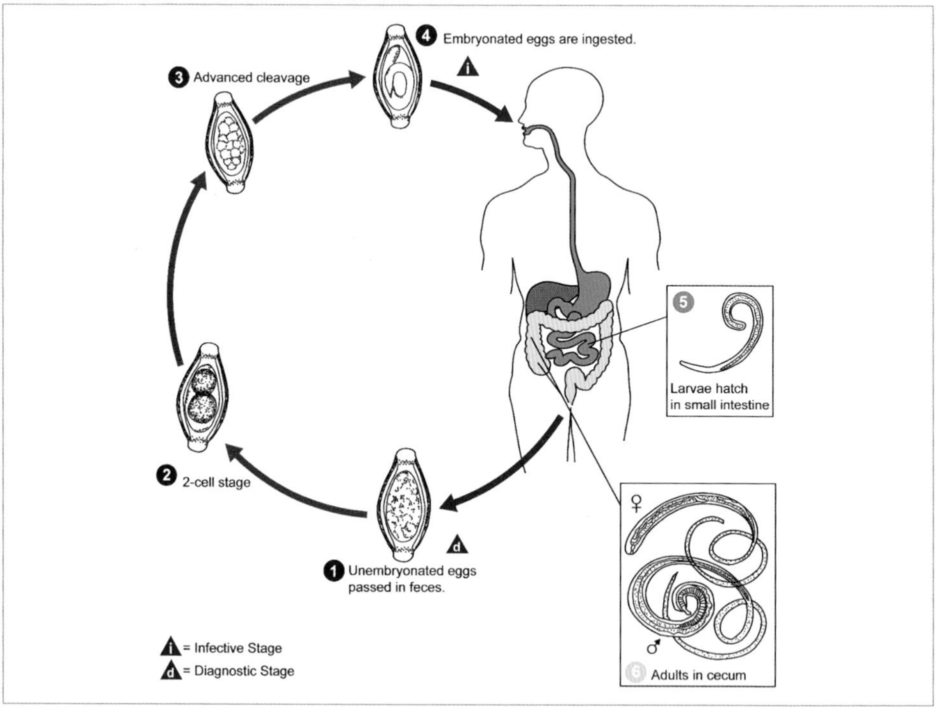

Image 143.3
Trichuris trichiura life cycle. The unembryonated eggs are passed with the stool (1). In the soil, the eggs develop into a 2-cell stage (2) and an advanced cleavage stage (3) and then they embryonate (4); eggs become infective in 15 to 30 days. After ingestion (soil-contaminated hands or food), the eggs hatch in the small intestine and release larvae (5) that mature and establish themselves as adults in the colon (6). The adult worms (~4 cm in length) live in the cecum and ascending colon. The adult worms are fixed in that location, with the anterior portions threaded into the mucosa. The females begin to oviposit 60 to 70 days after infection. Female worms in the cecum shed between 3,000 and 20,000 eggs per day. The life span of the adults is about 1 year. Courtesy of Centers for Disease Control and Prevention.

144

African Trypanosomiasis

(African Sleeping Sickness)

Clinical Manifestations

The clinical course of human African trypanosomiasis (sleeping sickness) has 2 stages: the first is the hemolymphatic stage, in which the parasite multiplies in subcutaneous tissues, lymph, and blood; once the parasite crosses the blood-brain barrier and infects the central nervous system (CNS), the disease enters the second stage, known as the neurologic stage. The rapidity of disease progression and clinical manifestations vary with the infecting subspecies. With *Trypanosoma brucei gambiense* infection (West African sleeping sickness), initial symptoms can be mild, with fever, muscle aches, and malaise. Pruritus, rash, weight loss, and generalized lymphadenopathy can occur. Posterior cervical lymphadenopathy (Winterbottom sign) may be present. Central nervous system involvement typically develops 1 to 2 years later with development of behavioral changes, cachexia, headache, hallucinations, delusions, and daytime somnolence followed by nighttime insomnia. In contrast, *Trypanosoma brucei rhodesiense* infection (East African sleeping sickness) is an acute, generalized illness that develops days to weeks after parasite inoculation, with manifestations including high fever, lymphadenopathy, rash, muscle and joint aches, thrombocytopenia, hepatitis, anemia, myocarditis, and, rarely, laboratory evidence of disseminated intravascular coagulopathy. A chancre may develop at the site of the tsetse fly bite. Clinical meningoencephalitis can develop as early as 3 weeks after onset of the untreated systemic illness. Both forms of African trypanosomiasis have high fatality rates; without treatment, infected patients usually die within weeks to months after clinical onset of disease caused by *T brucei rhodesiense* and within a few years from disease caused by *T brucei gambiense.*

Etiology

Human African trypanosomiasis occurs in sub-Saharan Africa. It is caused by the protozoan parasite *T brucei,* transmitted by blood-feeding tsetse flies. The west and central African (Gambian) form progresses more slowly and is caused by *T brucei gambiense.* The east and southern African (Rhodesian) form is more acute and is caused by *T brucei rhodesiense.* Both are extracellular protozoan hemoflagellates that live in blood and tissue of the human host.

Epidemiology

Approximately 7,000 human cases are reported annually worldwide, although only a few cases, which are acquired in Africa, are reported every year in the United States. Transmission is confined to an area in Africa between the latitudes of 15° north and 20° south, corresponding precisely with the distribution of the tsetse fly vector (*Glossina* species). In West and Central Africa, humans are the main reservoir of *T brucei gambiense,* although the parasite can sometimes be found in domestic animals, such as dogs and pigs. In East Africa, wild animals, such as antelope, bushbuck, and hartebeest, constitute the major reservoirs for sporadic infections with *T brucei rhodesiense,* although cattle serve as reservoir hosts in local outbreaks. In addition to the bite of the tsetse fly, *T brucei* can also be transmitted congenitally and through blood transfusions or organ transplantation, although these modes are uncommon.

Incubation Period

For *T brucei rhodesiense* infection, 3 to 21 days; for *T brucei gambiense* infection, 5 to 14 days.

Diagnostic Tests

Diagnosis is made by identification of trypanosomes in specimens of blood, cerebrospinal fluid (CSF), or fluid aspirated from a chancre or lymph node or by inoculation of susceptible laboratory animals (mice) with heparinized blood. Examination of CSF is critical to management and should be performed using the double-centrifugation technique. Concentration and Giemsa staining of the buffy coat layer of peripheral blood can also be helpful and is easier for *T brucei rhodesiense* because the density of organisms in circulating blood is higher than for *T brucei gambiense. T brucei gambiense* is more likely to be found in lymph node aspirates. Identification of trypanosomes or a white blood cell count of 6 or higher in the

CSF is the most widely used criteria for CNS involvement; elevated protein and an increase in immunoglobulin M also suggest second stage disease. Serologic testing is available outside the United States for *T brucei gambiense;* there is no serologic screening test for *T brucei rhodesiense.*

Treatment

The choice of drug used for treatment will be dependent on the type and stage of African trypanosomiasis. When no evidence of CNS involvement is present, the drug of choice for the acute hemolymphatic stage of infection is pentamidine for *T brucei gambiense* infection and suramin for *T brucei rhodesiense* infection. For treatment of infection with CNS involvement, the drug of choice is eflornithine for *T brucei gambiense* infection and melarsoprol for *T brucei rhodesiense* infection. Suramin, eflornithine, and melarsoprol can be obtained from the Centers for Disease Control and Prevention.

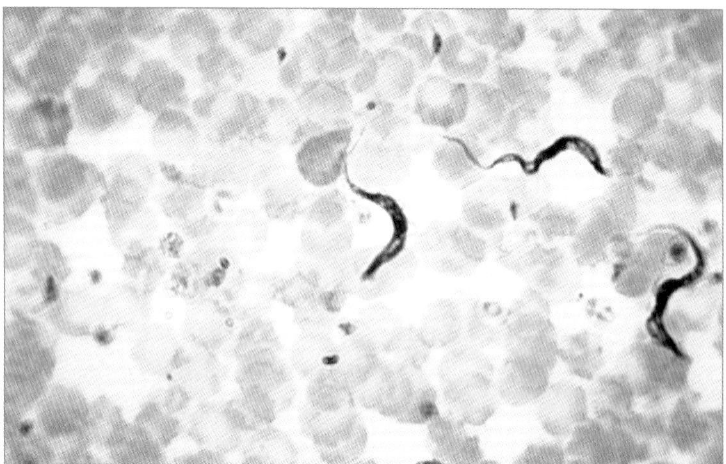

Image 144.1
Trypanosoma brucei gambiense in blood smear (Giemsa stain).

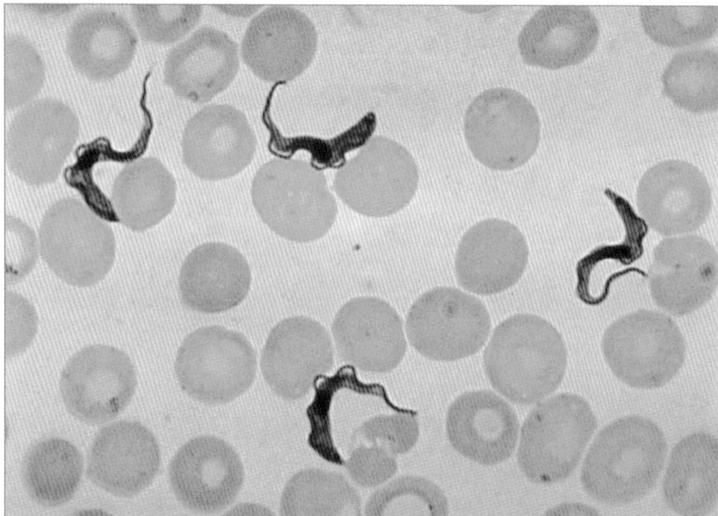

Image 144.2
Trypanosoma forms in blood smear from a patient with African trypanosomiasis (hematoxylin-eosin stain).

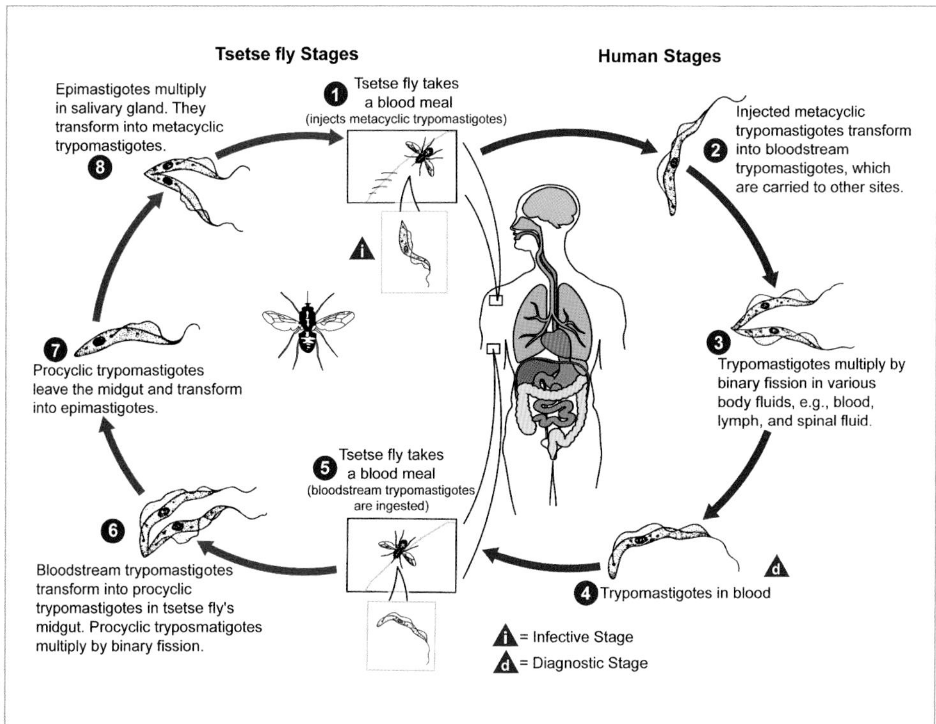

Image 144.3

During a blood meal on the mammalian host, an infected tsetse fly (genus *Glossina*) injects metacyclic trypomastigotes into skin tissue. The parasites enter the lymphatic system and pass into the bloodstream (1). Inside the host, they transform into bloodstream trypomastigotes (2), are carried to other sites throughout the body, reach other body fluids (eg, lymph, spinal fluid), and continue the replication by binary fission (3). The entire life cycle of African trypanosomes is represented by extracellular stages. The tsetse fly becomes infected with bloodstream trypomastigotes when taking a blood meal on an infected mammalian host (4, 5). In the fly's midgut, the parasites transform into procyclic trypomastigotes, multiply by binary fission (6), leave the midgut, and transform into epimastigotes (7). The epimastigotes reach the fly's salivary glands and continue multiplication by binary fission (8). The cycle in the fly takes approximately 3 weeks. Humans are the main reservoir for *Trypanosoma brucei gambiense,* but this species can also be found in animals. Wild game animals are the main reservoir of *Trypanosoma brucei rhodesiense.* Courtesy of Centers for Disease Control and Prevention/ Alexander J. da Silva, PhD/Melanie Moser.

145

American Trypanosomiasis

(Chagas Disease)

Clinical Manifestations

The acute phase of *Trypanosoma cruzi* infection lasts 2 to 3 months, followed by the chronic phase that, in the absence of successful antiparasitic treatment, is lifelong. The acute phase, when parasites circulate in the blood, is commonly asymptomatic or characterized by mild, nonspecific symptoms. Young children are more likely to exhibit symptoms than are adults. In some patients, a red, indurated nodule known as a **chagoma** develops at the site of the original inoculation, usually on the face or arms. Unilateral edema of the eyelids, known as the Romaña sign, may occur if the portal of entry was the conjunctiva; it usually is not present. The edematous skin may be violaceous and associated with conjunctivitis and enlargement of the ipsilateral preauricular lymph node. Fever, malaise, generalized lymphadenopathy, and hepatosplenomegaly can develop. In rare instances, acute myocarditis or meningoencephalitis can occur. The symptoms of acute Chagas disease resolve without treatment within 3 months, and patients pass into the chronic phase of the infection, during which few or no parasites are found in the blood. Most people with chronic *T cruzi* infection have no signs or symptoms and are said to have the indeterminate form of chronic Chagas disease. In 20% to 30% of cases, serious progressive sequelae affecting the heart or gastrointestinal tract develop years to decades after the initial infection (called determinate forms of chronic Chagas disease). Chagas cardiomyopathy is characterized by conduction system abnormalities, especially right bundle branch block, and ventricular arrhythmias and can progress to dilated cardiomyopathy and congestive heart failure. Patients with Chagas cardiomyopathy may die suddenly from ventricular arrhythmias, complete heart block, or emboli phenomena; death may also occur from intractable congestive heart failure. Although cardiac manifestations are more common, some patients with chronic Chagas disease develop digestive disease with dilatation of the colon or esophagus with swallowing difficulties accompanied by severe weight loss. Congenital Chagas disease occurs in 1% to 10% of neonates born to infected mothers and is characterized by low birth weight, hepatosplenomegaly, myocarditis, or meningoencephalitis with seizures and tremors. However, most neonates with congenital *T cruzi* infection have no signs or symptoms of disease. Reactivation of chronic *T cruzi* infection with parasites found in the circulating blood, which can be life threatening, may occur in immunocompromised people, including people infected with HIV and those who are immunosuppressed after transplantation.

Etiology

T cruzi, a protozoan hemoflagellate, is the cause.

Epidemiology

Parasites are transmitted in feces of infected triatomine insects (sometimes called "kissing bugs"; local Spanish/Portuguese names include vinchuca, chinche picuda, or barbeiro). The bugs defecate during or after taking blood. The bitten person is inoculated through inadvertent rubbing of insect feces containing the parasite into the site of the bite or mucous membranes of the eye or mouth. The parasite can also be transmitted congenitally, during solid organ transplantation, through blood transfusion, and by ingestion of food or drink contaminated by the vector's excreta. Accidental laboratory infections can result from handling parasite cultures or blood from infected people or laboratory animals, usually through needlestick injuries. Vectorborne transmission of the disease is limited to the Western hemisphere, predominantly Mexico and Central and South America. The southern United States has established enzootic cycles of *T cruzi* involving several triatomine vector species and mammalian hosts, such as raccoons, opossums, rodents, and domestic dogs. Nevertheless, most *T cruzi*–infected individuals in the United States are immigrants from areas of Latin America with endemic infection. There are an estimated 300,000 individuals with *T cruzi* infection in the United States. Assuming a 1% to 5% risk of congenital transmission, based on estimates of maternal infection, approximately 63 to 315 neonates are born with Chagas disease in the United States every year. Several transfusion- and transplantation-associated cases have been documented in the United States.

The disease is an important cause of morbidity and death in Latin America, where an estimated 8 million people are infected, of whom approximately 30% to 40% have or will develop cardiomyopathy or gastrointestinal tract disorders.

Incubation Period

Acute phase, 1 to 2 weeks or longer; chronic manifestations do not appear for years to decades.

Diagnostic Tests

During the acute phase of disease, the parasite is demonstrable in blood specimens by Giemsa staining after a concentration technique or in direct wet-mount or buffy coat preparations. Molecular techniques and hemoculture in special media (available at the Centers for Disease Control and Prevention) also have high sensitivity in the acute phase. The chronic phase of *T cruzi* infection is characterized by low-level parasitemia; the sensitivity of culture and polymerase chain reaction assay is generally less than 50%. Diagnosis in the chronic phase relies on serologic tests to demonstrate immunoglobulin (Ig) G antibodies against *T cruzi*. Serologic tests include indirect immunofluorescent and enzyme immunosorbent assays; however, no single serologic test is sufficiently sensitive or specific for confirmed diagnosis of chronic *T cruzi* infection. The Pan American Health Organization and World Health Organization recommend that samples be tested using 2 assays of different formats before diagnostic decisions are made.

The diagnosis of congenital Chagas disease can be made during the first 3 months of life by identification of motile trypomastigotes by direct microscopy of fresh anticoagulated blood specimens. Polymerase chain reaction testing has higher sensitivity than microscopy. All infants born to seropositive mothers should be screened using conventional serologic testing after 9 months of age, when IgG measurements reflect infant response rather than maternal antibody.

Treatment

Antitrypanosomal treatment is recommended for all cases of acute and congenital Chagas disease, reactivated infection attributable to immunosuppression, and chronic *T cruzi* infection in children younger than 18 years. Treatment of chronic *T cruzi* infection in adults without advanced cardiomyopathy is also generally recommended. The only drugs with proven efficacy are benznidazole and nifurtimox; neither drug is approved by the US Food and Drug Administration for use in the United States, but both drugs can be obtained from the Centers for Disease Control and Prevention under compassionate use protocols.

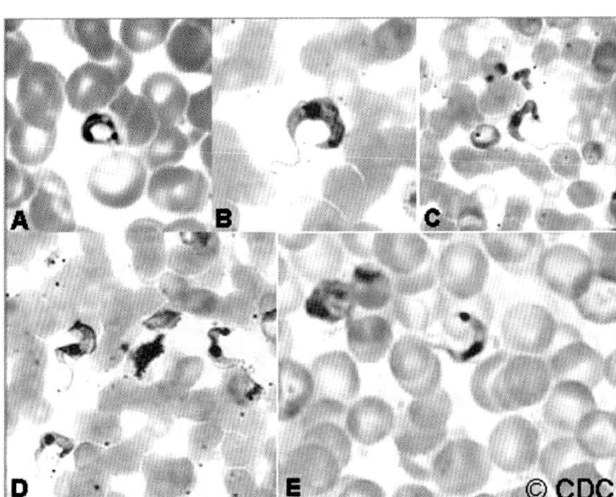

Image 145.1

A–E, *Trypanosoma cruzi* in blood smears (Giemsa stain). Courtesy of Centers for Disease Control and Prevention.

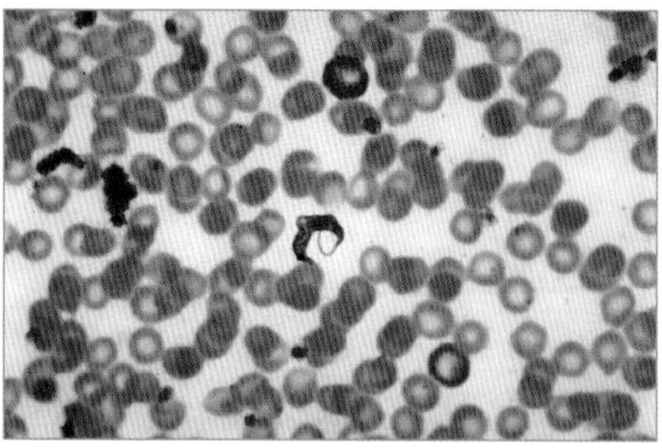

Image 145.2
This is a photomicrograph of *Trypanosoma cruzi* in a blood smear using Giemsa staining technique. This protozoan parasite, *T cruzi,* is the causative agent for Chagas disease, also known as American trypanosomiasis. It is estimated that 16 to 18 million people are infected with Chagas disease and, of those infected, 50,000 will die each year. Courtesy of Centers for Disease Control and Prevention.

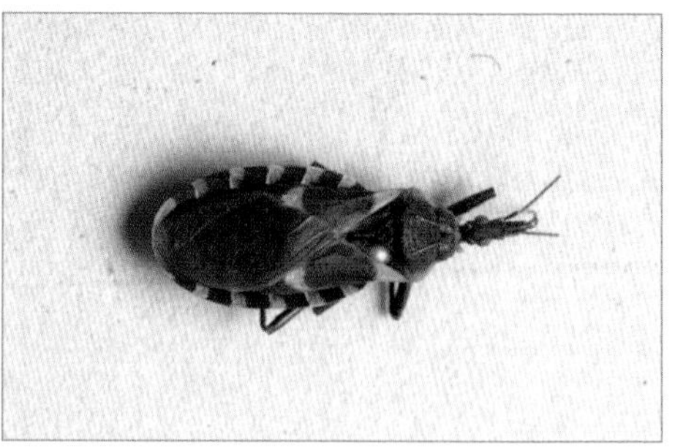

Image 145.3
Dorsal view of a male triatomine bug, *Triatoma sanguisuga,* one of the most important species in the United States for Chagas disease transmission. Courtesy of Centers for Disease Control and Prevention/*Emerging Infectious Diseases* and Patricia L. Dorn.

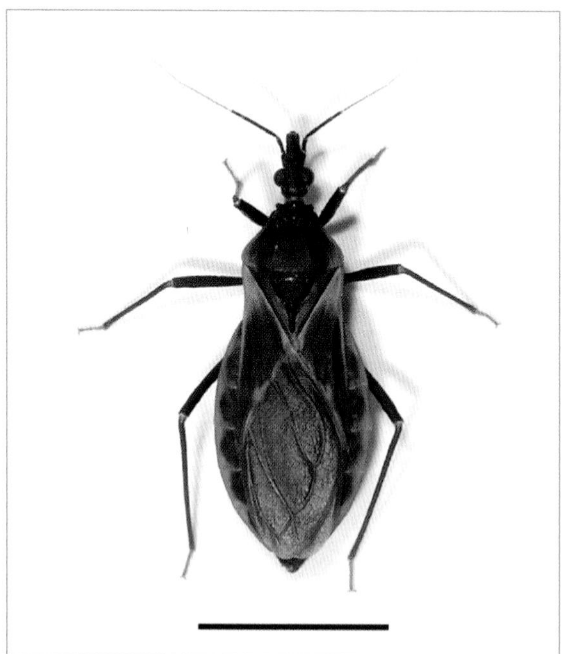

Image 145.4
Adult female "kissing bug" of the species *Triatoma rubida,* the most abundant triatomine species in southern Arizona (scale bar = 1 cm). Chagas disease is endemic throughout Mexico and Central and South America, with 7.7 million persons infected, 108.6 million persons considered at risk, 33.3 million symptomatic cases, an annual incidence of 42,500 cases (through vectorial transmission), and 21,000 deaths every year. This disease is caused by the protozoan parasite *Trypanosoma cruzi,* which is transmitted to humans by bloodsucking insects of the family Reduviidae (Triatominae). Although mainly a vectorborne disease, Chagas disease can also be acquired by humans through blood transfusions and organ transplantation, congenitally (from a pregnant woman to her baby), and through oral contamination (eg, foodborne). Courtesy of *Emerging Infectious Diseases*/C. Hedgecock.

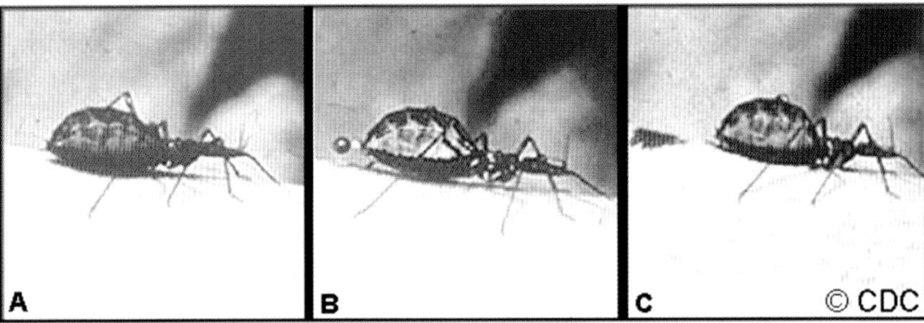

Image 145.5

A–C, Triatomine bug, *Trypanosoma cruzi* vector, defecating on the wound after taking a blood meal. Courtesy of Centers for Disease Control and Prevention.

Triatomine Bug Stages

Human Stages

1 Triatomine bug takes a blood meal (passes metacyclic trypomastigotes in feces, trypomastigotes enter bite wound or mucosal membranes, such as the conjunctiva)

2 Metacyclic trypomastigotes penetrate various cells at bite wound site. Inside cells they transform into amastigotes.

3 Amastigotes multiply by binary fission in cells of infected tissues.

Trypomastigotes can infect other cells and transform into intracellular amastigotes in new infection sites. Clinical manifestations can result from this infective cycle.

4 Intracellular amastigotes transform into trypomastigotes, then burst out of the cell and enter the bloodstream.

5 Triatomine bug takes a blood meal (trypomastigotes ingested)

6 Epimastigotes in midgut

7 Multiply in midgut

8 Metacyclic trypomastigotes in hindgut

i = Infective Stage

d = Diagnostic Stage

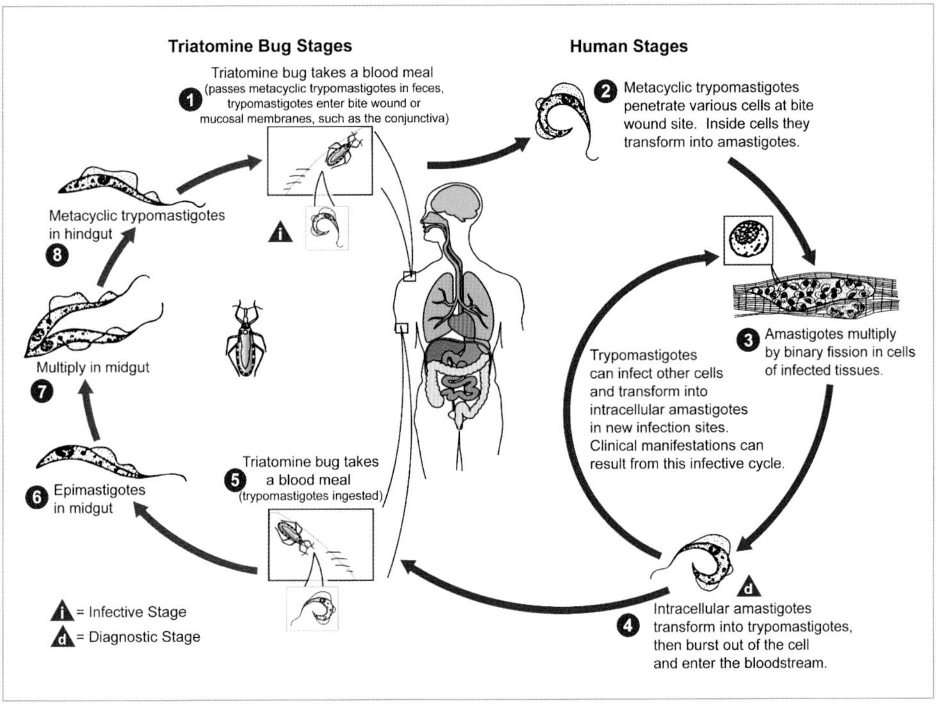

Image 145.6

An infected triatomine insect vector (or "kissing bug") takes a blood meal and releases trypomastigotes in its feces near the site of the bite wound. Trypomastigotes enter the host through the wound or through intact mucosal membranes, such as the conjunctiva (1). Common triatomine vector species for trypanosomiasis belong to the genera *Triatoma, Rhodnius,* and *Panstrongylus.* Inside the host, the trypomastigotes invade cells, where they differentiate into intracellular amastigotes (2). The amastigotes multiply by binary fission (3), differentiate into trypomastigotes, and then are released into the circulation as bloodstream trypomastigotes (4). Trypomastigotes infect cells from a variety of tissues and transform into intracellular amastigotes in new infection sites. Clinical manifestations can result from this infective cycle. The bloodstream trypomastigotes do not replicate (different from African trypanosomes). Replication resumes only when the parasites enter human or animal blood that contains circulating parasites (5). The ingested trypomastigotes transform into epimastigotes in the vector's midgut (6). The parasites multiply and differentiate in the midgut (7) and differentiate into infective metacyclic trypomastigotes in the hindgut (8). *Trypanosoma cruzi* can also be transmitted through blood transfusions, organ transplantation, transplacentally, and in laboratory accidents. Courtesy of Centers for Disease Control and Prevention/Alexander J. da Silva, PhD/Melanie Moser.

146

Tuberculosis

Clinical Manifestations

Tuberculosis disease is caused by infection with organisms of the *Mycobacterium tuberculosis* complex. Most infections caused by *M tuberculosis* complex in children and adolescents are asymptomatic. When tuberculosis disease occurs, clinical manifestations most often appear 1 to 6 months after infection (up to 18 months for osteoarticular disease) and include fever, weight loss or poor weight gain, growth delay, cough, night sweats, and chills. Chest radiographic findings after infection are rarely specific for tuberculosis and range from normal to diverse abnormalities, such as lymphadenopathy of the hilar, subcarinal, paratracheal, or mediastinal nodes; atelectasis or infiltrate of a segment or lobe; pleural effusion that can conceal small interstitial lesions; interstitial cavities; or miliary-pattern infiltrates. In selected instances, computed tomography or magnetic resonance imaging of the chest can resolve indistinct radiographic findings, but these methods are not necessary for routine diagnosis. Although cavitation is common in reactivation "adult" tuberculosis, cavitation is uncommon in childhood tuberculosis. Necrosis and cavitation can result from a progressive primary focus in very young or immunocompromised patients and in the setting of lymphobronchial disease. Extrapulmonary manifestations include meningitis and granulomatous inflammation of the lymph nodes, bones, joints, skin, and middle ear and mastoid. Gastrointestinal tuberculosis can mimic inflammatory bowel disease. Renal tuberculosis and progression to disease from latent *M tuberculosis* infection (LTBI) ("adult-type pulmonary tuberculosis") are unusual in younger children but can occur in adolescents. In addition, chronic abdominal pain with peritonitis and intermittent partial intestinal obstruction can be present in disease caused by *Mycobacterium bovis*. Congenital tuberculosis can mimic neonatal sepsis, or the infant may come to medical attention in the first 90 days of life with bronchopneumonia and hepatosplenomegaly. Clinical findings in patients with drug-resistant tuberculosis disease are indistinguishable from manifestations in patients with drug-susceptible disease.

Etiology

The causative agent is *M tuberculosis* complex, a group of closely related acid-fast bacilli (AFB), which routinely includes the human pathogens *M tuberculosis, M bovis,* and *Mycobacterium africanum*. *M africanum* is rare in the United States, so clinical laboratories do not distinguish it routinely. *M bovis* can be distinguished from *M tuberculosis* in reference laboratories, and although the spectrum of illness caused by *M bovis* is similar to that of *M tuberculosis,* the epidemiology, and treatment are different.

Definitions

- **Positive tuberculin skin test (TST) result.** A positive TST result (Box 146.1) indicates possible infection with *M tuberculosis* complex. Tuberculin reactivity appears 2 to 10 weeks after initial infection; the median interval is 3 to 4 weeks. Bacille Calmette-Guérin (BCG) immunization can produce a positive TST result.
- **Positive interferon-gamma release assay (IGRA) result.** A positive IGRA result indicates probable infection with *M tuberculosis* complex.
- **Exposed person** is a person who has had recent (ie, within 3 months) contact with another person with suspected or confirmed contagious tuberculosis disease and who has a negative TST or IGRA result, normal physical examination, and chest radiographic findings that are normal or not compatible with tuberculosis. Some exposed people are or become infected (and, subsequently, develop a positive TST or IGRA result), while others do not; the 2 groups cannot be distinguished initially.
- **Source case** is the person who has transmitted infection with *M tuberculosis* complex to another person who subsequently develops LTBI or tuberculosis disease.

Box 146.1
Definitions of Positive Tuberculin Skin Test Results in Infants, Children, and Adolescents[a]

Induration ≥5 mm

Children in close contact with known or suspected contagious people with tuberculosis disease

Children suspected to have tuberculosis disease
- Findings on chest radiograph consistent with active or previous tuberculosis disease
- Clinical evidence of tuberculosis disease[b]

Children receiving immunosuppressive therapy[c] or with immunosuppressive conditions, including HIV infection

Induration ≥10 mm

Children at increased risk of disseminated tuberculosis disease
- Children younger than 4 years
- Children with other medical conditions, including Hodgkin disease, lymphoma, diabetes mellitus, chronic renal failure, or malnutrition

Children with likelihood of increased exposure to tuberculosis disease
- Children born in high-prevalence regions of the world
- Children who travel to high-prevalence regions of the world
- Children frequently exposed to adults who are HIV infected, homeless, users of illicit drugs, residents of nursing homes, incarcerated, or institutionalized

Induration ≥15 mm

Children 4 years or older without any risk factors

Abbreviations: BCG, bacille Calmette-Guérin; HIV, human immunodeficiency virus; TST, tuberculin skin test.

[a] These definitions apply regardless of previous BCG immunization; erythema alone at TST site does not indicate a positive test result. Tests should be read at 48 to 72 hours after placement.

[b] Evidence by physical examination or laboratory assessment that would include tuberculosis in the working differential diagnosis (eg, meningitis).

[c] Including immunosuppressive doses of corticosteroids or tumor necrosis factor α antagonists or blockers.

- **Latent *M tuberculosis* infection** is *M tuberculosis* complex infection in a person who has a positive TST or IGRA result, no physical findings of disease, and chest radiograph findings that are normal or reveal evidence of healed infection (ie, calcification in the lung, hilar lymph nodes, or both).
- **Tuberculosis disease** is an infection in a person in whom symptoms, signs, or radiographic manifestations caused by *M tuberculosis* complex are apparent; disease can be pulmonary, extrapulmonary, or both.
- **Contagious tuberculosis** refers to tuberculosis disease typical of the lungs or airway in a person when there is the potential to transmit *M tuberculosis* to other people.
- **Directly observed therapy** (DOT) is an intervention by which medications are administered directly to the patient by a health care professional or trained third party (not a relative or friend) who observes and documents that the patient ingests each dose of medication.
- **Multidrug-resistant (MDR) tuberculosis** is infection or disease caused by a strain of *M tuberculosis* complex that is resistant to at least isoniazid and rifampin, the 2 first-line drugs with greatest efficacy.
- **Extensively drug-resistant tuberculosis** is an infection or disease caused by a strain of *M tuberculosis* complex that is resistant to isoniazid and rifampin, at least one fluoroquinolone, and at least one of the following parenteral drugs: amikacin, kanamycin, or capreomycin.

- **Bacille Calmette-Guérin** is a live-attenuated vaccine strain of *M bovis*. BCG vaccine is rarely administered to children in the United States but is one of the most widely used vaccines in the world. An isolate of BCG can be distinguished from wildtype *M bovis* only in a reference laboratory.

Epidemiology

Case rates of tuberculosis in all ages are higher in urban, low-income areas and in nonwhite racial and ethnic groups; more than 80% of reported cases in the United States occur in Hispanic and nonwhite people. In recent years, 60% of all US cases have been in people born outside the United States. Almost 75% of all childhood tuberculosis is associated with some form of foreign contact of the child, parent, or a household member. Specific groups with greater LTBI and disease rates include immigrants, international adoptees, refugees from or travelers to high-prevalence regions (eg, Asia, Africa, Latin America, countries of the former Soviet Union), homeless people, people who use alcohol excessively or illicit drugs, and residents of correctional facilities and other congregate settings. Increased risk of infection also occurs in children with exposure to secondhand smoke.

Infants and postpubertal adolescents are at increased risk of progression of LTBI to tuberculosis disease. Other predictive factors for development of disease include recent infection (within the past 2 years); immunodeficiency, especially from HIV infection; use of immunosuppressive drugs, such as prolonged or high-dose corticosteroid therapy or chemotherapy; intravenous drug use; and certain diseases or medical conditions, including Hodgkin disease, lymphoma, diabetes mellitus, chronic renal failure, and malnutrition. There have been reports of tuberculosis disease in adolescents and adults being treated for arthritis, inflammatory bowel disease, and other conditions with tumor necrosis factor α antagonists or blockers, such as infliximab and etanercept. A positive TST or IGRA result should be accepted as indicative of infection in individuals receiving or about to receive these medications.

A diagnosis of LTBI or tuberculosis disease in a young child is a public health sentinel event often representing recent transmission. Transmission of *M tuberculosis* complex is airborne, with inhalation of droplet nuclei usually produced by an adult or adolescent with contagious pulmonary, endobronchial, or laryngeal tuberculosis disease. *M bovis* is most often transmitted by unpasteurized dairy products, but airborne human-to-human transmission can occur. The duration of contagiousness of an adult receiving effective treatment depends on drug susceptibilities of the organism, adherence to an appropriate drug regimen by the patient, the number of organisms in sputum, and frequency of cough. Although contagiousness usually lasts only a few days to weeks after initiation of effective drug therapy, it can last longer, especially when the adult patient has pulmonary cavities, does not adhere to medical therapy, or is infected with a drug-resistant strain. If the sputum smear result is negative for AFB on 3 separate specimens at least 8 hours apart and the patient has improved clinically with resolution of cough, the treated person can be considered at low risk of transmitting *M tuberculosis*. Children younger than 10 years with small pulmonary lesions (paucibacillary disease) and nonproductive cough are rarely contagious. Unusual cases of adult-form pulmonary disease in young children, particularly with lung cavities and positive sputum-smear microscopy result for AFB, and cases of congenital tuberculosis can be highly contagious.

Incubation Period

Latent *M tuberculosis* infection, 2 to 10 weeks after exposure; tuberculosis disease, 6 to 24 months after exposure, but can be years between initial *M tuberculosis* infection and subsequent disease.

Diagnostic Tests

Assessing for *Mycobacterium tuberculosis* Disease

Patients testing positive for *M tuberculosis* infection should have a chest radiograph and physical examination to assess for tuberculosis disease. Most experts recommend that infants younger than 12 months who are suspected of having pulmonary or extrapulmonary tuberculosis disease (ie, have a positive TST **and** clinical history, physical examination signs, or chest radiograph abnormalities consistent with tuberculosis disease), with or without neurologic signs, should have a lumbar puncture to evaluate for tuberculous meningitis. Some experts also recommend performing a lumbar puncture in children 12 through 23 months of age with tuberculosis disease, with or without neurologic findings. Children 24 months and older with tuberculosis disease require a lumbar puncture only if they have neurologic signs or symptoms.

Laboratory isolation of *M tuberculosis* complex by culture from specimens of sputum, gastric aspirates, bronchial washings, pleural fluid, cerebrospinal fluid (CSF), urine, or other body fluids or a tissue biopsy specimen establishes the diagnosis. Children older than 5 years and adolescents can frequently produce sputum spontaneously or by induction with aerosolized hypertonic saline. Successful collections of induced sputum from infants with pulmonary tuberculosis are theoretically possible, but this requires special expertise. The best specimen for diagnosis of pulmonary tuberculosis in any child or adolescent in whom cough is absent or nonproductive and sputum cannot be induced is an early-morning gastric aspirate. Gastric aspirate specimens should be obtained with a nasogastric tube on awakening the child and before ambulation or feeding, and the acid pH of the gastric secretions should be neutralized as soon as possible. Aspirates collected on 3 separate mornings should be submitted for testing by staining and culture. Fluorescent staining methods for specimen smears are more sensitive than AFB smears and are preferred. The overall diagnostic yield of microscopy of gastric aspirates and induced sputum is low in children with clinically suspected pulmonary tuberculosis, and false-positive smear results caused by the presence of nontuberculous mycobacteria can occur. Histologic examination for and demonstration of AFB and granulomas in biopsy specimens from lymph node, pleura, mesentery, liver, bone marrow, or other tissues can be useful, but *M tuberculosis* complex organisms cannot be reliably distinguished from other mycobacteria in stained specimens. Regardless of results of the AFB smears, each specimen should be cultured.

Because *M tuberculosis* complex organisms are slow growing, detection of these organisms may take as long as 10 weeks using solid media; use of liquid media allows detection within 1 to 6 weeks and usually within 3 weeks. Even with optimal culture techniques, *M tuberculosis* complex organisms are isolated from fewer than 50% of children and 75% of infants with pulmonary tuberculosis diagnosed by other clinical criteria. Current methods for species identification of isolates from culture include molecular probes, genetic sequencing, mass spectroscopy, and biochemical tests. *M bovis* is usually suspected because of pyrazinamide resistance, which is characteristic of almost all *M bovis* isolates, but further biochemical or molecular testing is required to distinguish *M bovis* from *M tuberculosis*.

Several nucleic acid amplification tests for rapid diagnosis of tuberculosis are available. Nucleic acid amplification tests have varying sensitivity and specificity for sputum, gastric aspirate, CSF, and tissue specimens, with false-negative and false-positive results reported. Further research is needed before nucleic acid amplification tests can be routinely recommended for the diagnosis of tuberculosis in children when specimens other than sputum are submitted to the laboratory.

For a child with clinically suspected tuberculosis disease, finding the culture-positive source case supports the child's presumptive diagnosis and provides the likely drug susceptibility of the child's organism. Culture material should be collected from children with evidence of tuberculosis disease, especially when an isolate from a source case is not available, the presumed source case has drug-resistant tuberculosis, the child is immunocompromised or ill enough to require hospital admission, or the child has extrapulmonary disease. Traditional methods of determining drug susceptibility require bacterial isolation. Several new molecular methods of rapidly determining drug resistance directly from clinical samples are available in reference laboratories and are expected to be used in hospital laboratories in the near future.

Testing for *M tuberculosis* Infection

Tuberculin Skin Test

The TST is an indirect method for detecting *M tuberculosis* infection. It is one of 2 methods for diagnosing LTBI in asymptomatic people, the other method being IGRA. Both methods rely on specific cellular sensitization after infection. Conditions that decrease lymphocyte numbers or functionality can reduce the sensitivity of these tests. The routine (ie, Mantoux) technique of administering the skin test consists of 5 tuberculin units of purified protein derivative (0.1 mL) injected intradermally using a 27-gauge needle and a 1.0-mL syringe into the volar aspect of the forearm. Creation of a palpable wheal 6 to 10 mm in diameter is crucial to accurate testing. Administration of TSTs and interpretation of results should be performed by trained and experienced health care personnel because administration and interpretation by unskilled people and family members are unreliable. The recommended time for assessing the TST result is 48 to 72 hours after administration. The diameter of induration in millimeters is measured transversely to the long axis of the forearm. Positive TST results are defined in Box 146.1, and induration can persist for several weeks in some patients.

Lack of reaction to a TST does not exclude LTBI or tuberculosis disease. Approximately 10% to 40% of immunocompetent children with culture-documented tuberculosis disease do not initially react to a TST. Host factors, such as young age, poor nutrition, immunosuppression, viral infections (especially measles, varicella, and influenza), recent *M tuberculosis* infection, and disseminated tuberculosis disease can decrease TST reactivity. Many children and adults coinfected with HIV and *M tuberculosis* complex do not react to a TST. **Control skin tests to assess cutaneous energy are not recommended routinely** because the diagnostic significance of sensitivity and anergy to the control antigens is unknown.

Classification of TST results is based on epidemiologic and clinical factors. Interpretation of the size of induration (mm) as a positive result varies with the person's risk of LTBI and likelihood of progression to tuberculosis disease. Current guidelines from the Centers for Disease Control and Prevention (CDC), American Thoracic Society, and American Academy of Pediatrics, which recommend interpretation of TST findings on the basis of an individual's risk stratification, are summarized in Box 146.1. Prompt clinical and radiographic evaluation of all children and adolescents with a positive TST result is recommended.

Generally, interpretation of TST results in BCG vaccine recipients who are known contacts of a person with tuberculosis disease or who are at high risk of tuberculosis disease is the same as for people who have not received BCG vaccine. After BCG immunization, distinguishing between a positive TST result caused by pathogenic *M tuberculosis* complex infection and that caused by BCG is difficult. Reactivity of the TST after receipt of BCG vaccine does not occur in some patients. The size of the TST reaction attributable to BCG immunization depends on many factors, including age at BCG immunization, quality and strain of BCG vaccine used, number of doses of BCG vaccine received, nutritional and immunologic status of the vaccine recipient, frequency of TST administration, and time lapse between immunization and TST. Evidence that increases the probability that a positive TST result is attributable to LTBI includes known contact with a person with contagious tuberculosis, a family history of tuberculosis disease, a long interval (>5 years) since neonatal BCG immunization, and a TST reaction of 15 mm or greater.

Blood-Based Testing with Interferon-Gamma Release Assays

QuantiFERON-TB Gold In-Tube and T-SPOT.*TB* are IGRAs and are the preferred tests for tuberculosis infection in asymptomatic children 5 years and older who have been vaccinated with BCG. These tests measure ex vivo interferon-gamma production from T lymphocytes in response to stimulation with antigens specific to *M tuberculosis* complex, which includes *M tuberculosis* and *M bovis*. However, the IGRA antigens used are not found in BCG. As with TSTs, IGRAs cannot distinguish between latent infection and disease, and a negative result from these tests cannot exclude the possibility of tuberculosis disease in a patient with suggestive findings. The sensitivity of IGRA tests is similar to that of TSTs for detecting infection in adults and older children who have untreated culture-confirmed tuberculosis. In many clinical settings, the specificity of IGRAs is higher than that for the TST because the antigens used are not found in BCG or most pathogenic nontuberculous mycobacteria (ie, are not found in *Mycobacterium avium* complex but are found in *Mycobacterium kansasii, Mycobacterium szulgai,* and *Mycobacterium marinum*). Interferon-gamma release assays are recommended by the CDC for all indications in which TST would be used, and some experts prefer IGRAs for use in adults. The published experience testing children with IGRAs demonstrates that IGRAs consistently perform well in children 5 years and older, and some data support their use for children as young as 3 years. The negative predictive value of IGRAs is not known, but if the IGRA result is negative and the TST result is positive in an asymptomatic child, the diagnosis of LTBI is unlikely. A negative result for a TST or an IGRA should be considered as especially unreliable in infants younger than 3 months.

At this time, neither an IGRA nor the TST can be considered the gold standard for diagnosis of LTBI. Current recommendations for use of IGRAs in children for LTBI are shown in Box 146.2 and Image 146.1.

Box 146.2

Tuberculin Skin Test and Interferon-Gamma Release Assay Recommendations for Infants, Children, and Adolescents[a]

Children for whom immediate TST or IGRA is indicated[b]

- Contacts of people with confirmed or suspected contagious tuberculosis (contact investigation)
- Children with radiographic or clinical findings suggesting tuberculosis disease
- Children immigrating from countries with endemic infection (eg, Asia, Middle East, Africa, Latin America, countries of the former Soviet Union), including international adoptees
- Children with travel histories to countries with endemic infection and substantial contact with indigenous people from such countries[c]

Children who should have annual TST or IGRA

- Children infected with HIV infection (TST only)

Children at increased risk of progression of LTBI to tuberculosis disease

Children with other medical conditions, including diabetes mellitus, chronic renal failure, malnutrition, or congenital or acquired immunodeficiencies, and children receiving TNF antagonists deserve special consideration. Without recent exposure, these people are not at increased risk of acquiring *Mycobacterium tuberculosis* infection. Underlying immune deficiencies associated with these conditions would theoretically enhance the possibility for progression to severe disease. Initial histories of potential exposure to tuberculosis should be included for all of these patients. If these histories or local epidemiologic factors suggest a possibility of exposure, immediate and periodic TST or IGRA should be considered. **A TST or IGRA should be performed before initiation of immunosuppressive therapy, including prolonged systemic corticosteroid administration, organ transplantation, use of TNF-α antagonists or blockers, or other immunosuppressive therapy in any child requiring these treatments.**

Abbreviations: BCG, Bacille Calmette-Guérin; HIV, human immunodeficiency virus; IGRA, interferon-gamma release assay; LTBI, latent *Mycobacterium tuberculosis* infection; TNF, tumor necrosis factor; TST, tuberculin skin test.

[a] BCG immunization is not a contraindication to a TST.

[b] Beginning as early as 3 months of age for TST and 3 years of age for IGRAs for LTBI and disease.

[c] If the child is well and has no history of exposure, the TST or IGRA should be delayed for up to 10 weeks after return.

- Children with a positive result from an IGRA should be considered infected with *M tuberculosis* complex. A negative IGRA result cannot be interpreted universally as absence of infection.
- Indeterminate IGRA results have several possible causes that could be related to the patient, assay, or assay performance. Indeterminate results do not exclude *M tuberculosis* infection and may necessitate repeat testing, possibly with a different test. Indeterminate IGRA results should not be used to make clinical decisions.

Use of Tests for *M tuberculosis* Infection

A TST or IGRA should be performed in children who are at increased risk of infection with *M tuberculosis*. Universal testing with TST or IGRA, including programs based at schools, child care centers, and camps that include populations at low risk, is discouraged because it results in a low yield of positive results or a large proportion of false-positive results, leading to an inefficient use of health care resources. However, using a questionnaire to determine risk factors for LTBI can be effective in health care settings. Simple questionnaires can identify children with risk factors for LTBI (Box 146.3) who should then have a TST or IGRA performed. Risk assessment for tuberculosis should be performed at the first health care encounter with a child and every 6 months thereafter for the first year of life (eg, 2 weeks and 6 and 12 months of age). After 1 year of age, risk assessment for tuberculosis should be performed at the time of routine care, annually if possible. The most reliable strategies for identifying LTBI and preventing tuberculosis disease in children are based on thorough and expedient contact investigations rather than nonselective skin testing of large populations. Contact investigations are public health interventions that should be coordinated through the local public health department. Only children deemed to have increased risk of contact with people with contagious tuberculosis or children with suspected tuberculosis disease should be considered for a TST or IGRA. Household investigation of children for tuberculosis is indicated whenever a TST or IGRA result of a household member converts from negative to positive (indicating recent infection).

HIV Infection

Children with HIV infection are considered at high risk of tuberculosis, and an annual TST beginning at 3 through 12 months of age is recommended, or, if older, when HIV infection is diagnosed. Children who have tuberculosis disease should be tested for HIV infection. The clinical manifestations and radiographic appearance of tuberculosis disease in children with HIV infection tend to be similar to those in immunocompetent children, but manifestations in these children can be more severe and unusual and can include extrapulmonary involvement of multiple organs. In HIV-infected patients, a TST induration of 5 mm or greater is considered a positive result; however, a negative TST result attributable to HIV-related immunosuppression can also occur. An IGRA test can also be used, but a negative result does not exclude tuberculosis. Specimens for culture should be obtained from all HIV-infected children with suspected tuberculosis.

Box 146.3

Validated Questions for Determining Risk of Latent *Mycobacterium tuberculosis* Infection in Children in the United States

Has a family member or contact had tuberculosis disease?
Has a family member had a positive tuberculin skin test result?
Was your child born in a high-risk country (countries other than the United States, Canada, Australia, New Zealand, or Western and North European countries)?
Has your child traveled (had contact with resident populations) to a high-risk country for longer than 1 week?

Organ Transplant Patients

The risk of tuberculosis in organ transplant patients is several-fold greater than in the general population. A careful history of previous exposure to tuberculosis should be taken from all transplant candidates, including details about previous TST results and exposure to individuals with active tuberculosis. All transplant candidates should undergo evaluation by TST or IGRA for LTBI. A positive result of either test should be taken as evidence of *M tuberculosis* infection.

Patients Receiving Immunosuppressive Therapies, Including Tumor Necrosis Factor Antagonists or Blockers

Patients should be screened for risk factors for *M tuberculosis* complex infection and have a TST or IGRA performed before the initiation therapy of systemic corticosteroids, antimetabolite agents, and tumor necrosis factor antagonists or blockers (ie, infliximab and etanercept). A positive result of either test should be taken as evidence of *M tuberculosis* infection.

Other Considerations

Testing for tuberculosis at any age is not required before administration of live virus vaccines. Measles vaccine can temporarily suppress tuberculin reactivity for at least 4 to 6 weeks. If indicated, a TST can be applied at the same visit during which these vaccines are administered. The effects of vaccination on IGRA characteristics have not been determined; the same precautions as for TST should be followed. The effect of live virus varicella, yellow fever, and live-attenuated influenza vaccines on TST reactivity and IGRA results is not known. In the absence of data, the same spacing recommendation should be applied to these vaccines as described for measles-mumps-rubella vaccine. There is no evidence that inactivated vaccines, polysaccharide-protein conjugate vaccines, or recombinant or subunit vaccines or toxoids interfere with clinical interpretation of TST or IGRAs.

Chest radiographic findings of a granuloma, calcification, or adenopathy can be caused by infection with *M tuberculosis* complex but not by BCG immunization. Bacille Calmette-Guérin can cause suppurative lymphadenitis in the regional lymph node drainage of the inoculation site of a healthy child and can cause disseminated disease in children with severe forms of immunodeficiency.

Sensitivity to purified protein derivative tuberculin antigen persists for years in most instances, even after effective treatment. The durability of positive IGRA results has not been determined. Studies seeking to show reversion of TST or IGRA results after treatment of LTBI or tuberculosis disease have had inconclusive findings. Currently, repeat testing with TST or IGRA has no known clinical utility for assessing the effectiveness of treatment or for diagnosing new infection in patients who were previously infected with *M tuberculosis* and who are reexposed.

Treatment

Specific Drugs

Antituberculosis drugs kill or inhibit multiplication of *M tuberculosis* complex organisms, thereby arresting progression of infection and preventing most complications. Chemotherapy does not cause rapid disappearance of already caseous or granulomatous lesions (eg, mediastinal lymphadenitis). Recommendations and the more commonly reported adverse reactions of major antituberculosis drugs are summarized in Table 146.1 and Box 146.4. For treatment of tuberculosis disease, these drugs must always be used in recommended combination and dosage to minimize emergence of drug-resistant strains. Use of nonstandard regimens for any reason (eg, drug allergy, drug resistance) should be undertaken only in consultation with an expert in treating tuberculosis.

- **Isoniazid** is bactericidal, rapidly absorbed, and well tolerated and penetrates into body fluids, including CSF. Isoniazid is metabolized in the liver and excreted primarily through the kidneys. Hepatotoxic effects are rare in children but can be life threatening. Caution should be used in storing and administering isoniazid because accidental or deliberate overdose is dangerous. In children and adolescents given recommended doses, peripheral neuritis or seizures caused by inhibition of pyridoxine metabolism are

Table 146.1
Recommended Usual Treatment Regimens for Drug-Susceptible Tuberculosis in Infants, Children, and Adolescents

Infection or Disease Category	Regimen	Remarks
Latent *Mycobacterium tuberculosis* infection (positive TST or IGRA result, no disease)[a]		
• Isoniazid susceptible	9 mo of isoniazid, once a day	If daily therapy is not possible, DOT twice a week can be used for 9 mo.
• Isoniazid resistant	4 mo of rifampin, once a day	If daily therapy is not possible, DOT twice a week can be used for 4 mo.
• Isoniazid-rifampin resistant	Consult a tuberculosis specialist	
Pulmonary and extrapulmonary (except meningitis)[b]	2 mo of isoniazid, rifampin, pyrazinamide, and ethambutol daily or twice weekly, followed by 4 mo of isoniazid and rifampin[c] by DOT[d] for drug-susceptible *M tuberculosis* 9–12 mo of isoniazid and rifampin for drug-susceptible *Mycobacterium bovis*	Some experts recommend a 3-drug initial regimen (isoniazid, rifampin, and pyrazinamide) if the risk of drug resistance is low. DOT is highly desirable. If hilar adenopathy only and the risk of drug resistance is low, a 6-mo course of isoniazid and rifampin is sufficient. Drugs can be given 2 or 3 times/wk under DOT.
Meningitis	2 mo of isoniazid, rifampin, pyrazinamide, and an aminoglycoside or ethionamide, once a day, followed by 7–10 mo of isoniazid and rifampin, once a day or twice a week (9–12 mo total) for drug-susceptible *M tuberculosis* At least 12 mo of therapy without pyrazinamide for drug-susceptible *M bovis*	For patients who may have acquired tuberculosis in geographic areas where resistance to streptomycin is common, kanamycin, amikacin, or capreomycin can be used instead of streptomycin.

Abbreviations: DOT, directly observed therapy; HIV, human immunodeficiency virus; IGRA, interferon-gamma release assay; TST, tuberculin skin test.

[a] See text for additional acceptable or alternative regimens.

[b] Duration of therapy may be longer for HIV-infected people, and additional drugs and dosing intervals may be indicated.

[c] Medications should be administered daily for the first 2 weeks to 2 months of treatment and then can be administered 2 to 3 times per week by DOT. (Twice-weekly therapy is not recommended for HIV-infected people).

[d] If initial chest radiograph shows pulmonary cavities and sputum culture after 2 months of therapy remains positive, the continuation phase is extended to 7 months, for a total treatment duration of 9 months.

Box 146.4
People at Increased Risk of Drug-Resistant Tuberculosis Infection or Disease

People with a history of treatment for tuberculosis disease (or whose source case for the contact received such treatment)
Contacts of a patient with drug-resistant contagious tuberculosis disease
People from countries with high prevalence of drug-resistant tuberculosis
Infected people whose source case has positive smears for acid-fast bacilli or cultures after 2 months of appropriate antituberculosis therapy and patients who do not respond to a standard treatment regimen
Residence in geographic area with a high percentage of drug-resistant isolates

rare, and most do not need pyridoxine supplements. Pyridoxine supplementation is recommended for exclusively breastfed infants and for children and adolescents on meat- and milk-deficient diets; children with nutritional deficiencies, including all symptomatic HIV-infected children; and pregnant adolescents and women. For infants and young children, isoniazid tablets can be pulverized.

- **Rifampin** is a bactericidal agent in the rifamycin class of drugs that is absorbed rapidly and penetrates into body fluids, including CSF. Other drugs in the rifamycin class approved for treating tuberculosis are rifabutin and rifapentine. Rifampin is metabolized by the liver and can alter the pharmacokinetics and serum concentrations of many other drugs. Rare adverse effects include hepatotoxicity, influenza-like symptoms, pruritus, and thrombocytopenia. Rifampin is excreted in bile and urine and can cause orange urine, sweat, and tears, with discoloration of soft contact lenses. Rifampin can make oral contraceptives ineffective, so nonhormonal birth-control methods should be adopted when rifampin is administered to sexually active female adolescents and adults. For infants and young children, the contents of the capsules can be suspended in cherry-flavored syrup or sprinkled on semisoft foods (eg, pudding). *M tuberculosis* complex isolates that are resistant to rifampin are almost always resistant to isoniazid. Rifabutin is a suitable alternative to rifampin in HIV-infected children receiving antiretroviral therapy that restricts the use of rifampin because of drug interactions; however, experience in children is limited. Major toxicities of rifabutin include leukopenia, gastrointestinal tract upset, polyarthralgia, rash, increased transaminase concentrations, and skin and secretion discoloration (pseudojaundice). Anterior uveitis has been reported among children receiving rifabutin as prophylaxis or as part of a combination regimen for treatment, usually when administered at high doses. Rifabutin also increases hepatic metabolism of many drugs but is a less potent inducer of cytochrome P450 enzymes than rifampin and has fewer problematic drug interactions than rifampin. However, adjustments in doses of rifabutin and coadministered antiretroviral drugs may be necessary for certain combinations. Rifapentine is a long-acting rifamycin that permits weekly dosing in selected adults and adolescents, but its evaluation in younger pediatric patients has been limited.

- **Pyrazinamide** attains therapeutic CSF concentrations, is detectable in macrophages, is administered orally, and is metabolized by the liver. Administration of pyrazinamide for the first 2 months with isoniazid and rifampin allows for 6-month regimens in immunocompetent patients with drug-susceptible tuberculosis. Almost all isolates of *M bovis* are resistant to pyrazinamide, precluding therapy for this pathogen. In daily doses of 40 mg/kg per day or less, pyrazinamide seldom has hepatotoxic effects and is well tolerated by children. Some adolescents and many adults develop arthralgia and hyperuricemia because of inhibition of uric acid excretion. Pyrazinamide must be used with caution in people with underlying liver disease; when administered with rifampin, pyrazinamide is associated with somewhat higher rates of hepatotoxicity.

- **Ethambutol** is well absorbed after oral administration, diffuses well into tissues, and is excreted in urine. However, concentrations in CSF are low. At 20 mg/kg per day, ethambutol is bacteriostatic, and its primary therapeutic role is to prevent emergence of drug resistance. Ethambutol can cause reversible or irreversible optic neuritis, but reports in children with normal renal function are rare. Children who are receiving ethambutol should be monitored monthly for visual acuity and red-green color discrimination if they are old enough to cooperate. Use of ethambutol in young children whose visual acuity cannot be monitored requires consideration of risks and benefits, but it can be used routinely to treat tuberculosis disease in infants and children unless otherwise contraindicated.
- The less commonly used (ie, second-line) antituberculosis drugs have limited usefulness because of decreased effectiveness and greater toxicity and should only be used in consultation with a specialist familiar with childhood tuberculosis. **Ethionamide** is an orally administered antituberculosis drug that is well tolerated by children, achieves therapeutic CSF concentrations, and may be useful for treatment of people with meningitis or drug-resistant tuberculosis. **Fluoroquinolones** have antituberculosis activity and can be used in special circumstances, including drug-resistant organisms, but are not US Food and Drug Administration (FDA) approved for this indication. Because some fluoroquinolones are approved by the FDA for use only in people 18 years and older, their use in younger patients necessitates careful assessment of the potential risks and benefits. Occasionally, a patient cannot tolerate oral medications. Isoniazid, rifampin, **streptomycin** and related drugs, and fluoroquinolones can be administered parenterally.

Treatment Regimens for Latent *M tuberculosis* Infection (LTBI)

Isoniazid Therapy for LTBI

A 9-month course of isoniazid is the preferred regimen in the United States for treatment of LTBI in most children. Isoniazid given to adults who have LTBI (ie, no clinical or radiographic abnormalities suggesting tuberculosis disease) provides substantial protection (54%–88%) against development of tuberculosis disease for at least 20 years. Among children, efficacy approaches 100% if adherence to therapy is high. Unfortunately, many studies have shown the adherence rate to be 50% to 75% over 9 months when families give isoniazid on their own. All infants and children who have LTBI but no evidence of tuberculosis disease and who have never received antituberculosis therapy should be considered for isoniazid unless resistance to isoniazid is suspected (ie, known exposure to a person with isoniazid-resistant tuberculosis) or a specific contraindication exists. Isoniazid, in this circumstance, is therapeutic and prevents development of disease. A physical examination and chest radiograph should be performed prior to initiation of isoniazid therapy to exclude tuberculosis disease.

Duration of Isoniazid Therapy for LTBI

For infants, children, and adolescents, including those with HIV infection or other immunocompromising conditions, the recommended duration of isoniazid therapy in the United States is 9 months. Physicians who treat LTBI should educate patients and their families about the adverse effects of isoniazid, provide written information about adverse drug effects, and prescribe it in monthly allocations with clinic visits scheduled for periodic face-to-face monitoring. Successful completion of therapy is based on total number of doses taken. When adherence with daily therapy with isoniazid cannot be ensured, twice-a-week DOT can be considered. The twice-weekly regimen should not be prescribed unless each dose is documented by DOT. Routine determination of serum transaminase concentrations during the 9 months of therapy for LTBI is not indicated except for children and adolescents who have concurrent or recent liver or biliary disease, are pregnant or in the first 12 weeks' postpartum, are having clinical evidence of hepatotoxic effects, or are concurrently taking other hepatotoxic drugs (eg, anticonvulsant or HIV agents). If therapy is completed successfully, there is no need to perform additional tests or chest radiographs unless a new exposure to tuberculosis is documented or the child develops a clinical illness consistent with tuberculosis.

Isoniazid-Rifapentine Therapy for LTBI

In 2011, on the basis of a large clinical trial, the CDC recommended a 12-week, once-weekly dose of isoniazid and rifapentine, **given under DOT by a health department,** as an alternative regimen for treating LTBI in people 12 years or older. This regimen was shown to be at least as effective with fewer adverse reactions than 9 months of isoniazid given by self-supervision. Children between 2 and 11 years of age were enrolled in the trial, and the regimen was shown to be safe and well tolerated. However, efficacy of this regimen in this age group could not be determined. This regimen should not be used routinely for children younger than 12 years but can be considered when the likelihood of completing another regimen is low. This regimen should not be used in children younger than 2 years.

Additional Regimens for Treatment of LTBI

Additional possible regimens for treatment of LTBI are 3 months of daily isoniazid and rifampin or 2 months of daily rifampin and pyrazinamide when given as part of rifampin, isoniazid, pyrazinamide, and ethambutol (RIPE) therapy for suspected tuberculosis disease (which is subsequently determined to be *M tuberculosis* infection only).

Therapy for Contacts of Patients With Isoniazid-Resistant M tuberculosis *and When Isoniazid Cannot Be Given*

The incidence of isoniazid resistance among *M tuberculosis* complex isolates from US patients is approximately 9%. Risk factors for drug resistance are listed in Box 146.4. Most experts recommend isoniazid be used to treat LTBI in children unless the child has had contact with a person known to have isoniazid-resistant tuberculosis or the infection was acquired in a locale known to have a high prevalence of isoniazid resistance. If the source case is found to have isoniazid-resistant, rifampin-susceptible organisms, isoniazid should be discontinued and rifampin should be given daily for a total course of 4 months. Some experts would choose to treat children younger than 12 years with rifampin daily for 6 months. Rifampin can also be used when isoniazid cannot be given because of patient intolerance or when isoniazid is unavailable. Optimal therapy for children with LTBI caused by organisms with resistance to isoniazid and rifampin (ie, MDR) is not known. In these circumstances, fluoroquinolones alone and multidrug regimens have been used, but the safety and the efficacy of these empiric regimens have not been assessed in clinical trials. Drugs to consider include pyrazinamide, a fluoroquinolone, and ethambutol, depending on susceptibility of the isolate. Consultation with a tuberculosis specialist is indicated.

Treatment of Tuberculosis Disease

The goal of treatment is to achieve killing of replicating organisms in the tuberculous lesion in the shortest possible time. Achievement of this goal minimizes the possibility of development of resistant organisms. The major problem limiting successful treatment is poor adherence to prescribed treatment regimens. The use of DOT decreases the rates of relapse, treatment failures, and drug resistance; therefore, DOT is strongly recommended for treatment of all children and adolescents with tuberculosis disease in the United States.

For tuberculosis disease, a 6-month, 4-drug regimen consisting of RIPE for the first 2 months and isoniazid and rifampin for the remaining 4 months is recommended for treatment of pulmonary disease, pulmonary disease with hilar adenopathy, and hilar adenopathy disease in infants, children, and adolescents when an MDR case is not suspected as the source of infection or when drug-susceptibility results are available from the patient or the likely source case. Some experts would administer 3 drugs (isoniazid, rifampin, pyrazinamide) as the initial regimen if a source case has been identified with known pansusceptible *M tuberculosis* or if the presumed source case has no risk factors for drug-resistant *M tuberculosis*. For children with hilar adenopathy in whom drug resistance is not a consideration, a 6-month regimen of only isoniazid and rifampin is considered adequate by some experts. If the chest radiograph shows one or more pulmonary cavities and sputum culture result remains positive after 2 months of therapy, the duration of therapy should be extended to 9 months.

In the 6-month regimen with 4-drug therapy, RIPE is given once a day for at least the first 2 weeks by DOT daily (at least 5 days per week). An alternative to daily dosing between 2 weeks and 2 months of treatment is to give these drugs twice or 3 times a week by DOT (except in HIV-infected people, in whom twice-weekly dosing is not recommended). After the initial 2-month period, a DOT regimen of isoniazid and rifampin given 2 or 3 times a week is acceptable. Several alternative regimens with differing durations of daily therapy and total therapy have been used successfully in adults and children. These alternative regimens should be prescribed and managed by a specialist in tuberculosis.

Therapy for Drug-Resistant Tuberculosis Disease

Drug resistance is more common in the following groups: people previously treated for tuberculosis disease; people born in areas with a high prevalence of drug resistance, such as Russia and the nations of the former Soviet Union, Asia, Africa, and Latin America; and contacts, especially children, with tuberculosis disease whose source case is a person from one of these groups. When **resistance to drugs other than isoniazid** is likely, initial therapy should be adjusted by adding at least 2 drugs to match the presumed drug susceptibility pattern until drug susceptibility results are available. If an isolate from the pediatric case under treatment is not available, drug susceptibilities can be inferred by the drug susceptibility pattern of isolates from the adult source case. Data for guiding drug selection may not be available for foreign-born children or in circumstances of international travel or adoption. If this information is not available, a 4- or 5-drug initial regimen is recommended with close monitoring for clinical response.

Most cases of pulmonary tuberculosis in children that are caused by an isoniazid-resistant but rifampin- and pyrazinamide-susceptible strain of *M tuberculosis* complex can be treated with a 6-month regimen of rifampin, pyrazinamide, and ethambutol. For cases of MDR tuberculosis disease, the treatment regimen needed for cure should include at least 4 or 5 antituberculosis drugs to which the organism is susceptible. Bedaquiline was recently approved by the FDA as treatment for adults with MDR tuberculosis for whom an effective 4-drug regimen could not be instituted without the use of bedaquiline; unfortunately, currently, there are no safety, efficacy, or pharmacokinetic data for children for this drug. Therapy for MDR tuberculosis is administered for 12 to 24 months from the time of culture conversion to negativity. An injectable drug, such as kanamycin or capreomycin, should be used for the first 4 to 6 months of treatment, as tolerated. Regimens in which drugs are administered 2 or 3 times per week are not recommended for drug-resistant disease; daily DOT is critical to prevent emergence of additional resistance. An expert in drug-resistant tuberculosis should be consulted for all drug-resistant cases.

Extrapulmonary Tuberculosis Disease

In general, extrapulmonary tuberculosis—with the exception of meningitis—can be treated with the same regimens as used for pulmonary tuberculosis. For suspected drug-susceptible tuberculous meningitis, daily treatment with isoniazid, rifampin, pyrazinamide, and ethionamide, if possible, or an aminoglycoside should be initiated. When susceptibility to all drugs is established, the ethionamide or aminoglycoside can be discontinued. Pyrazinamide is given for a total of 2 months, and isoniazid and rifampin are given for a total of 9 to 12 months. Isoniazid and rifampin can be given daily or 2 or 3 times per week after the first 2 months of treatment if the child has responded well.

Other Treatment Considerations

Corticosteroids

The evidence supporting adjuvant treatment with corticosteroids for children with tuberculosis disease is incomplete. Corticosteroids are definitely indicated for children with tuberculous meningitis because corticosteroids decrease rates of mortality and long-term neurologic impairment. Corticosteroids can be considered for children with pleural and pericardial effusions (to hasten reabsorption of fluid), severe miliary disease (to mitigate alveolocapillary block), endobronchial disease (to relieve obstruction and atelectasis), and abdominal tuberculosis (to decrease the risk of strictures). Corticosteroids should be given only when accompanied by appropriate antituberculosis therapy. Most experts consider 2 mg/kg per day of prednisone (maximum, 60 mg/d) or its equivalent for 4 to 6 weeks followed by tapering.

Tuberculosis Disease and HIV Infection

Most HIV-infected adults with drug-susceptible tuberculosis respond well to standard treatment regimens when appropriate therapy is initiated early. However, optimal therapy for tuberculosis in children with HIV infection has not been established. Treating tuberculosis in an HIV-infected child is complicated by antiretroviral drug interactions with the rifamycins and overlapping toxicities. Therapy always should include at least 4 drugs initially, should be administered daily via DOT, and should be continued for at least 6 months. Isoniazid, rifampin, and pyrazinamide, usually with ethambutol or an aminoglycoside, should be given for at least the first 2 months. Ethambutol can be discontinued once drug-resistant tuberculosis disease is excluded. Rifampin may be contraindicated in people who are receiving antiretroviral therapy. Rifabutin can be substituted for rifampin in some circumstances. Consultation with a specialist who has experience in managing HIV-infected patients with tuberculosis is advised.

Evaluation and Monitoring of Therapy in Children and Adolescents

Careful monthly monitoring of clinical and bacteriologic responses to therapy is important. With DOT, clinical evaluation is an integral component of each visit for drug administration. For patients with pulmonary tuberculosis, chest radiographs should be obtained after 2 months of therapy to evaluate response. Even with successful 6-month regimens, hilar adenopathy can persist for 2 to 3 years; normal radiographic findings are not necessary to discontinue therapy. Follow-up chest radiography beyond termination of successful therapy is not usually necessary unless clinical deterioration occurs.

If therapy has been interrupted, the date of completion should be extended. Although guidelines cannot be provided for every situation, factors to consider when establishing the date of completion include length of interruption of therapy, time during therapy (early or late) when interruption occurred, and the patient's clinical, radiographic, and bacteriologic status before, during, and after interruption of therapy. The total doses administered by DOT should be calculated to guide the duration of therapy. Consultation with a specialist in tuberculosis is advised.

Untoward effects of isoniazid therapy, including severe hepatitis in otherwise healthy infants, children, and adolescents, are rare. Routine determination of serum transaminase concentrations is not recommended. However, for children with severe tuberculosis disease, especially children with meningitis or disseminated disease, transaminase concentrations should be monitored approximately monthly during the first several months of treatment. Other indications for testing include having concurrent or recent liver or biliary disease, being pregnant or in the first 12 weeks' postpartum, having clinical evidence of hepatotoxic effects, or concurrently using other hepatotoxic drugs (eg, anticonvulsant or HIV agents). In most other circumstances, monthly clinical evaluations to observe for signs or symptoms of hepatitis and other adverse effects of drug therapy without routine monitoring of transaminase concentrations is appropriate follow-up. In all cases, regular physician-patient contact to assess drug adherence, efficacy, and adverse effects is an important aspect of management. Patients should be provided with written instructions and advised to call a physician immediately if symptoms of adverse events, in particular hepatotoxicity (eg, nausea, vomiting, abdominal pain, jaundice), develop.

Immunizations

Patients who are receiving treatment for tuberculosis can be given measles and other age-appropriate, attenuated, live virus vaccines unless they are receiving high-dose systemic corticosteroids, are severely ill, or have other specific contraindications to immunization.

Tuberculosis During Pregnancy and Breastfeeding

Tuberculosis treatment during pregnancy is complex. If tuberculosis disease is diagnosed during pregnancy, a regimen of isoniazid, rifampin, and ethambutol is recommended. Pyrazinamide is commonly used in a 3- or 4-drug regimen, but safety during pregnancy has not been established. At least 6 months of therapy is indicated for drug-susceptible tuberculosis disease if pyrazinamide is used; at least 9 months of therapy is indicated if pyrazinamide is not used. Prompt initiation of therapy is mandatory to protect mother and fetus.

Asymptomatic pregnant women with a positive TST or IGRA result, normal chest radiographic findings, and recent contact with a contagious person should be considered for isoniazid therapy. The recommended duration of therapy is 9 months. Therapy in these circumstances should begin after the first trimester. Pyridoxine supplementation is indicated for all pregnant and breastfeeding women receiving isoniazid.

Isoniazid, ethambutol, and rifampin are relatively safe for the fetus. The benefit of ethambutol and rifampin for therapy of tuberculosis disease in the mother outweighs the risk to the fetus. Because streptomycin can cause ototoxic effects in the fetus, it should not be used unless administration is essential for effective treatment. The effects of other second-line drugs on the fetus are unknown, and ethionamide has been demonstrated to be teratogenic, so its use during pregnancy is contraindicated.

Although isoniazid is secreted in human milk, no adverse effects of isoniazid on nursing neonates and infants have been demonstrated. Breastfed neonates and infants do not require pyridoxine supplementation unless they are receiving isoniazid. The isoniazid dosage of a breastfed baby whose mother is taking isoniazid does not require adjustment for the small amount of drug in the milk.

Congenital Tuberculosis

Women who have only pulmonary tuberculosis are not likely to infect the fetus but can infect their newborn after delivery. Congenital tuberculosis is rare, but in utero infections can occur after maternal bacillemia.

If a newborn is suspected of having congenital tuberculosis, a TST, chest radiography, lumbar puncture, and appropriate cultures and radiography should be performed promptly. The TST result is usually negative in newborns with congenital or perinatally acquired infection. Hence, regardless of the TST result, treatment of the newborn should be initiated promptly with isoniazid, rifampin, pyrazinamide, and an aminoglycoside (eg, amikacin). The placenta should be examined histologically for granulomata and AFB, and a specimen should be cultured for *M tuberculosis* complex. The mother should be evaluated for presence of pulmonary or extrapulmonary disease, including genitourinary tuberculosis. If the physical examination and chest radiographic findings support the diagnosis of tuberculosis disease, the newborn should be treated with regimens recommended for tuberculosis disease. If meningitis is confirmed, corticosteroids should be added. Drug susceptibility testing of the organism recovered from the mother or household contact, newborn, or both should be performed.

Management of the Newborn Whose Mother (or Other Household Contact) Has LTBI or Tuberculosis Disease

Management of the newborn is based on categorization of the maternal (or household contact) infection. Although protection of the newborn from exposure and infection is of paramount importance, contact between newborn and mother should be allowed when possible. Differing circumstances and resulting recommendations are as follows:

- **Mother (or household contact) has a positive TST or IGRA result and normal chest radiographic findings.** If the mother (or household contact) is asymptomatic, no separation is required. The mother is usually a candidate for treatment of LTBI after the initial postpartum period. The newborn needs no special evaluation or therapy. Because of the newborn's exquisite susceptibility, and because the mother's positive TST result could be a marker of an unrecognized case of contagious tuberculosis within the household, other household members should have a TST or IGRA and further evaluation; this should not delay the newborn's discharge from the hospital. These mothers can breastfeed their newborns.
- **Mother (or household contact) has clinical signs and symptoms or abnormal findings on chest radiograph consistent with tuberculosis disease.** Cases of suspected or proven tuberculosis disease in mothers (or household contacts) should be reported immediately to the local health department, and investigation of all household members should start as soon as possible. If the mother has tuberculosis disease, the newborn should be evaluated for congenital tuberculosis, and the mother should be tested for HIV infection. The mother (or household contact) and newborn should be separated until the mother (or household contact) has been evaluated and, if tuberculosis disease is suspected, until the mother (or household contact) and newborn are receiving appropriate antituberculosis therapy, the mother wears a mask, and the mother understands and is willing to adhere to infection-control measures. Once the newborn is receiving isoniazid, separation is not necessary unless the mother (or household contact) has possible MDR tuberculosis disease or has poor adherence to treatment and DOT is not possible. If the mother is suspected of having MDR tuberculosis disease, an expert in tuberculosis disease treatment should be consulted. Women with drug-susceptible tuberculosis disease who have been treated appropriately for 2 or more weeks and who are not considered contagious can breastfeed.

  If congenital tuberculosis is excluded, isoniazid is given until the infant is 3 or 4 months of age, when a TST should be performed. If the TST result is positive, the infant should be reassessed for tuberculosis disease. If tuberculosis disease is excluded in an infant with a positive TST result, isoniazid alone should be continued for a total of 9 months. The infant should be evaluated monthly during treatment for signs of illness or poor growth. If the TST result is negative at 3 to 4 months of age and the mother (or household contact) has good adherence and response to treatment and is no longer contagious, isoniazid should be discontinued.
- **Mother (or household contact) has a positive TST or IGRA and abnormal findings on chest radiography but no evidence of tuberculosis disease.** If the chest radiograph of the mother (or household contact) appears abnormal but is not suggestive of tuberculosis disease and the history, physical examination, and sputum smear indicate no evidence of tuberculosis disease, the newborn can be assumed to be at low risk of *M tuberculosis* infection and need not be separated from the mother (or household contact). The mother and her newborn should receive follow-up care and the mother should be treated for LTBI. Other household members should have a TST or IGRA and further evaluation.

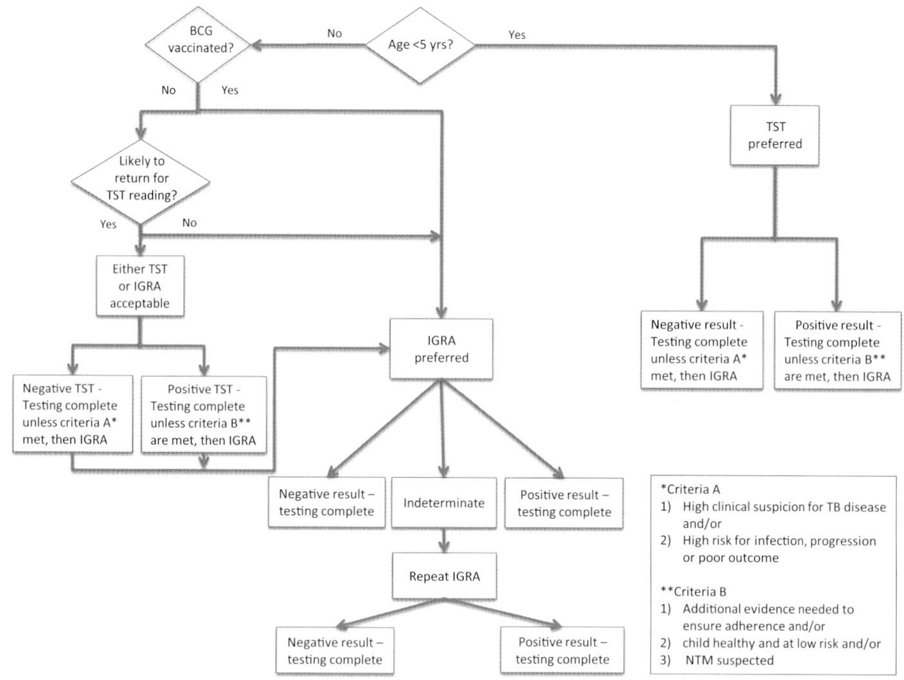

BCG vaccinated?
No
Age <5 yrs?
Yes
No
Yes
TST preferred
Likely to return for TST reading?
Yes
No
Either TST or IGRA acceptable
IGRA preferred
Negative result - Testing complete unless criteria A* met, then IGRA
Positive result - Testing complete unless criteria B** are met, then IGRA
Negative TST - Testing complete unless criteria A* met, then IGRA
Positive TST - Testing complete unless criteria B** are met, then IGRA
Negative result – testing complete
Indeterminate
Positive result – testing complete
Repeat IGRA
Negative result – testing complete
Positive result – testing complete

*Criteria A
1) High clinical suspicion for TB disease and/or
2) High risk for infection, progression or poor outcome

**Criteria B
1) Additional evidence needed to ensure adherence and/or
2) child healthy and at low risk and/or
3) NTM suspected

Abbreviations: BCG, Bacille Calmette-Guérin; IGRA, interferon-gamma release assay; NTM, nontuberculous mycobacteria; TB, tuberculosis; TST, tuberculin skin test.

Image 146.1
Guidance on strategy for use of tuberculin skin test and interferon-gamma release assay by age and bacille Calmette-Guérin immunization status.

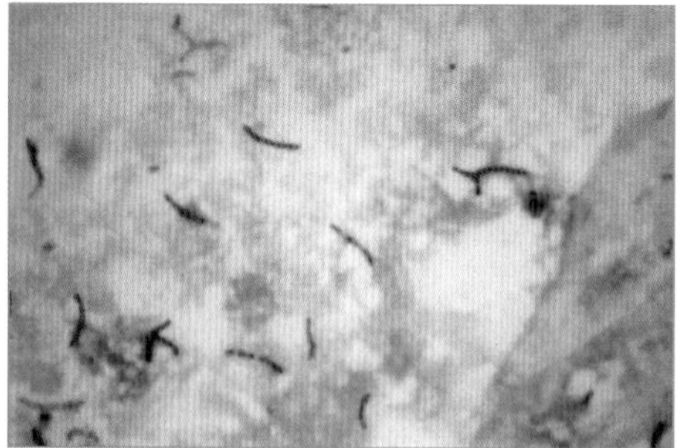

Image 146.2
This photomicrograph reveals *Mycobacterium tuberculosis* bacteria using acid-fast Ziehl-Neelsen stain (magnification x1,000). The acid-fast stains depend on the ability of mycobacteria to retain dye when treated with mineral acid or an acid-alcohol solution, such as the Ziehl-Neelsen, or the Kinyoun stains that are carbolfuchsin methods specific for *M tuberculosis*. Courtesy of Centers for Disease Control and Prevention/Dr George P. Kubica.

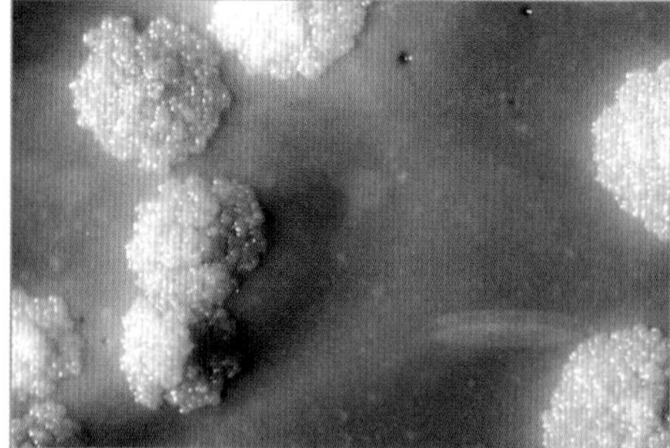

Image 146.3
This is a close-up of a *Mycobacterium tuberculosis* culture revealing this organism's colonial morphology. Courtesy of Centers for Disease Control and Prevention/Dr George P. Kubica.

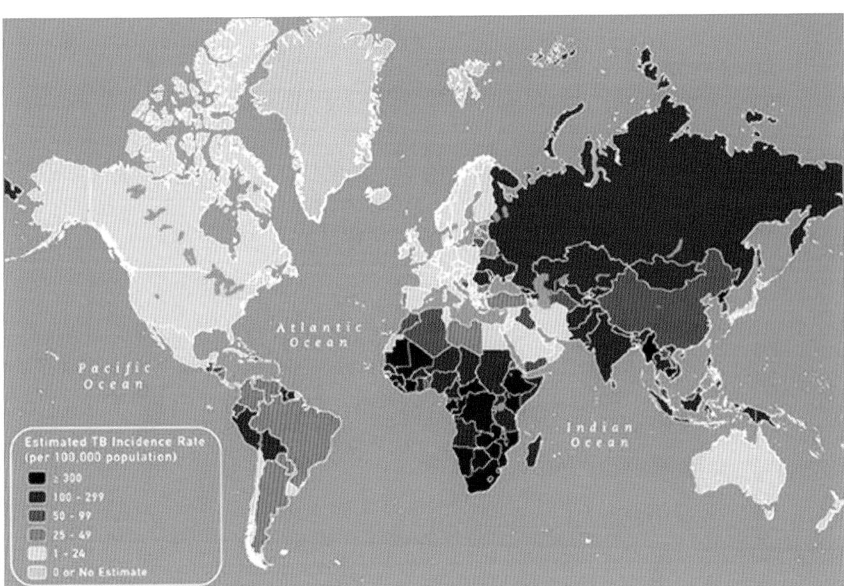

Image 146.4
Estimated tuberculosis incidence rates, 2009. Courtesy of Centers for Disease Control and Prevention.

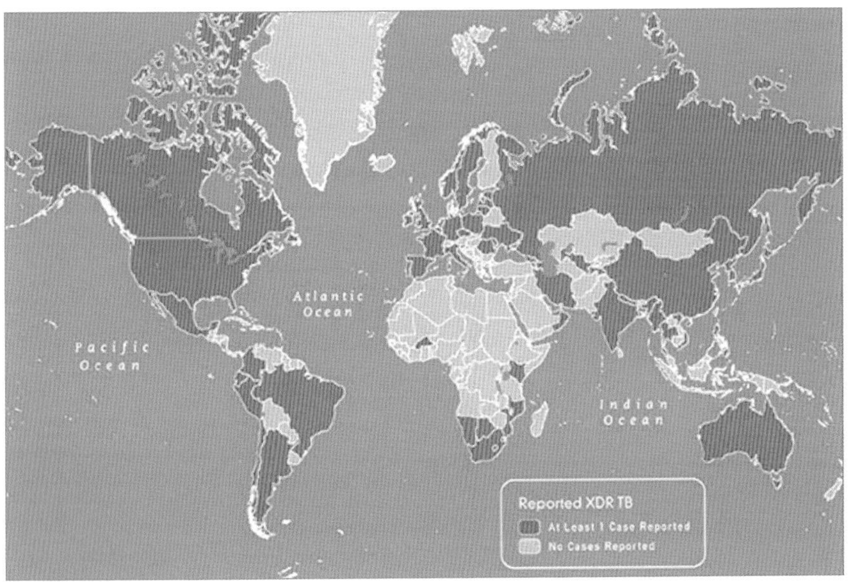

Image 146.5
Distribution of countries and territories reporting at least one case of extensively drug-resistant tuberculosis as of 2010. Courtesy of Centers for Disease Control and Prevention.

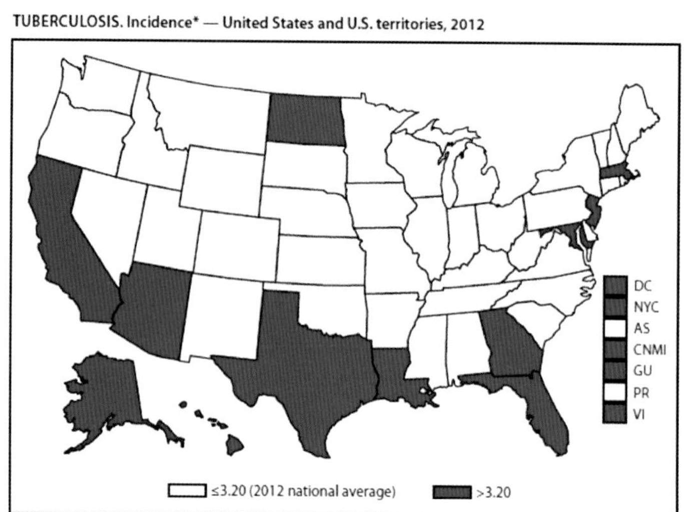

Image 146.6

Tuberculosis. Incidence—United States and US territories, 2012. Courtesy of *Morbidity and Mortality Weekly Report.*

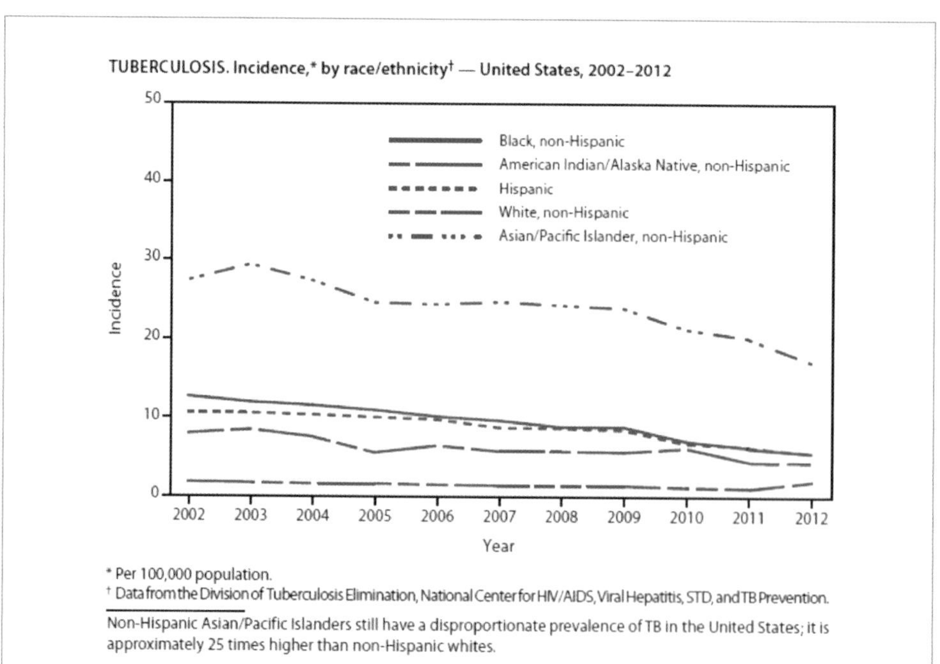

Image 146.7

Tuberculosis. Incidence, by race/ethnicity—United States, 2002–2012. Courtesy of *Morbidity and Mortality Weekly Report.*

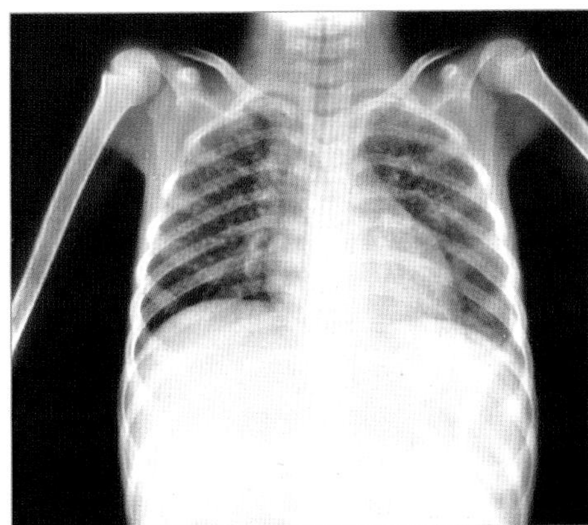

Image 146.8
Miliary tuberculosis. Courtesy of Gary Overturf, MD.

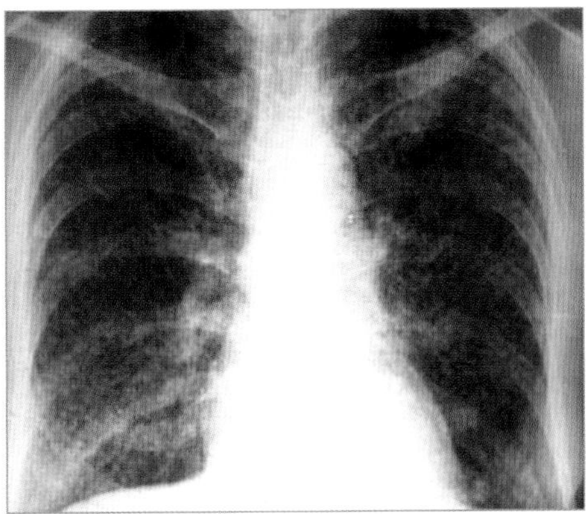

Image 146.9
Tuberculosis, miliary, in a 29-year-old woman 4 months after delivery. Tuberculosis may exacerbate during pregnancy.

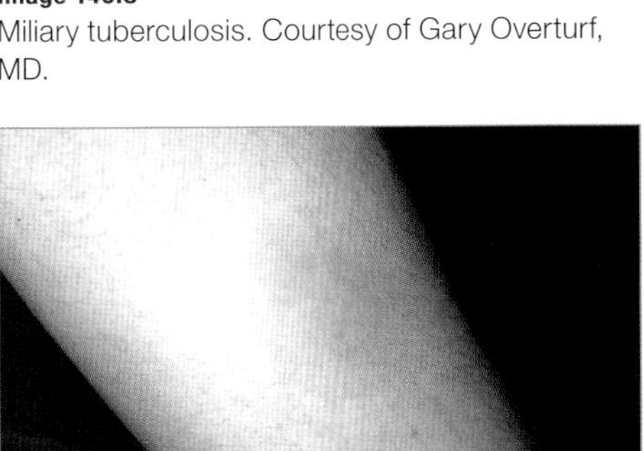

Image 146.10
A young child with a positive tuberculin skin test reaction with erythema and induration. Courtesy of Martin G. Myers, MD.

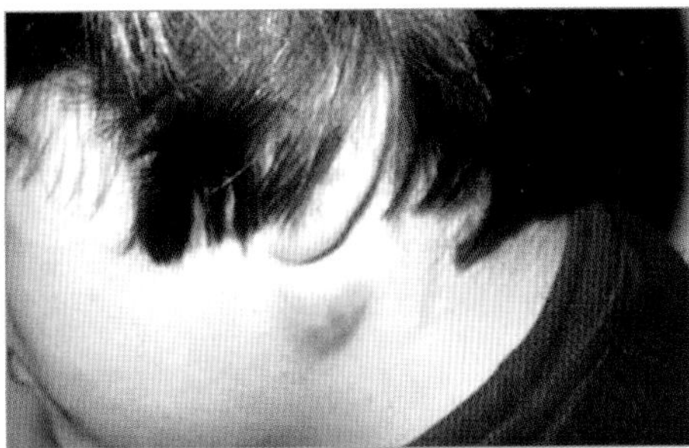

Image 146.11
Young man with *Mycobacterium tuberculosis* cervical lymphadenitis. Copyright Martin G. Myers, MD.

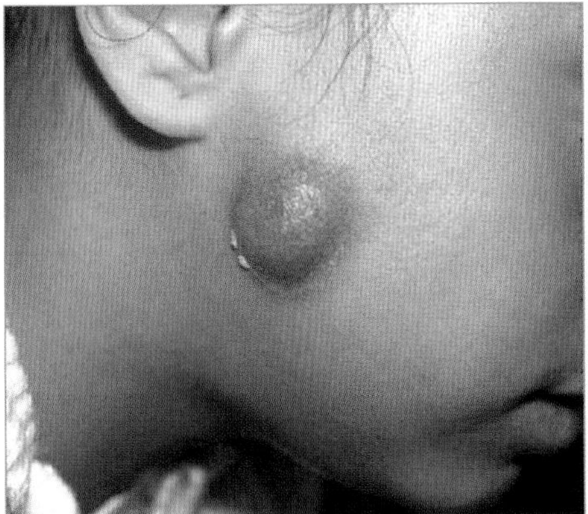

Image 146.12
Young woman with *Mycobacterium tuberculosis* cervical lymphadenitis. Copyright Martin G. Myers, MD.

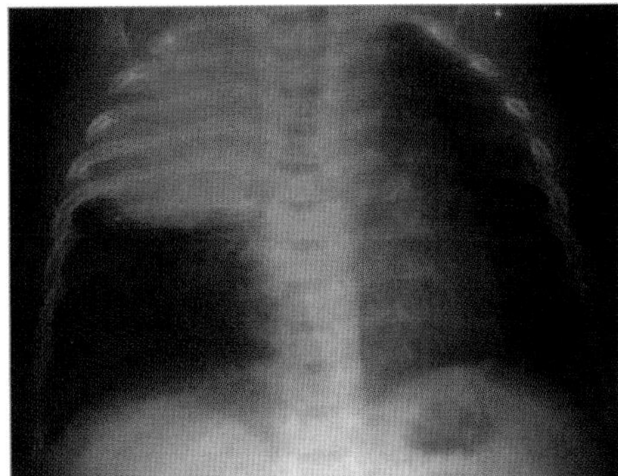

Image 146.13
A 3-month-old with tuberculosis. The child had a fever when first examined. Chest radiograph revealed right upper lobe consolidation. A purified protein derivative was placed and was positive. *Mycobacterium tuberculosis* grew from gastric aspirate culture. Copyright Barbara Jantausch, MD, FAAP.

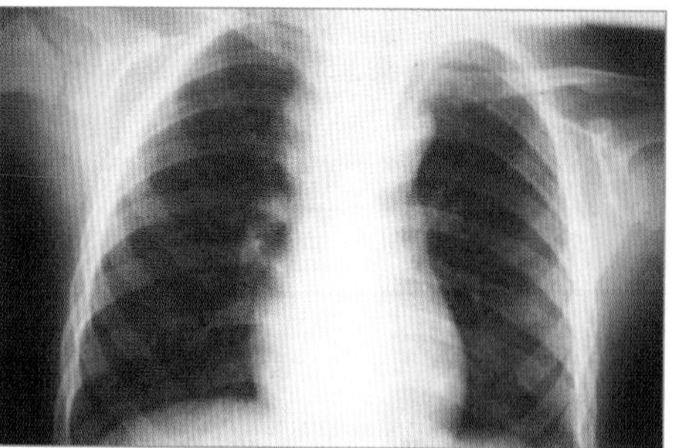

Image 146.14
Mycobacterium tuberculosis infection with paratracheal lymph nodes. Courtesy of Martha Lepow, MD.

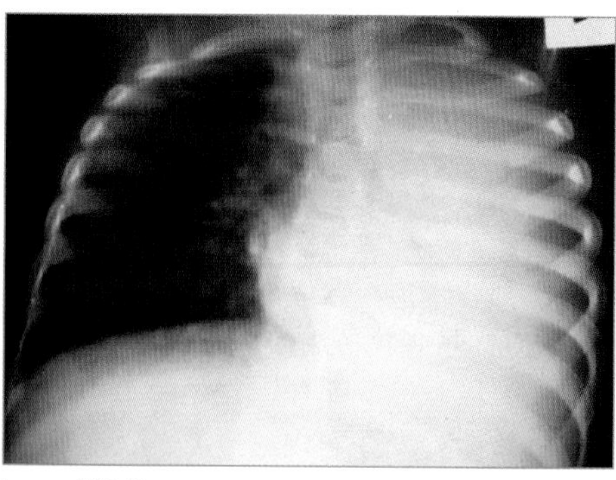

Image 146.15
A 1-year-old with endobronchial tuberculosis with pulmonary consolidation.

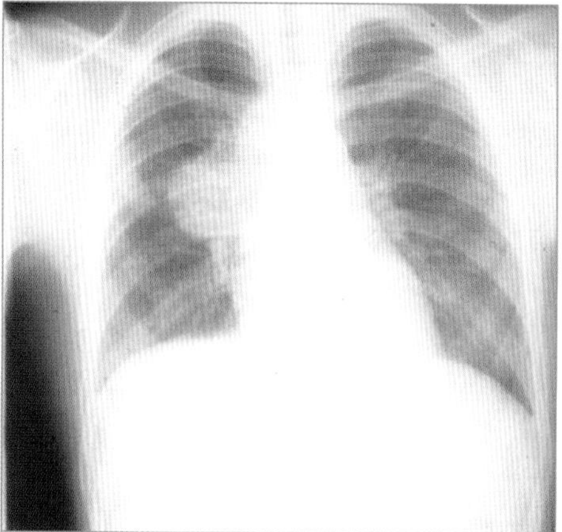

Image 146.16
A 13-year-old boy with tuberculosis. The patient had a 1-week history of shortness of breath and sharp pain on his right side while riding his bicycle. A purified protein derivative revealed 20 by 25 mm of induration at 72 hours. The chest computed tomography scan revealed right hilar adenopathy and a primary complex in the right peripheral lung field. Copyright Barbara Jantausch, MD, FAAP.

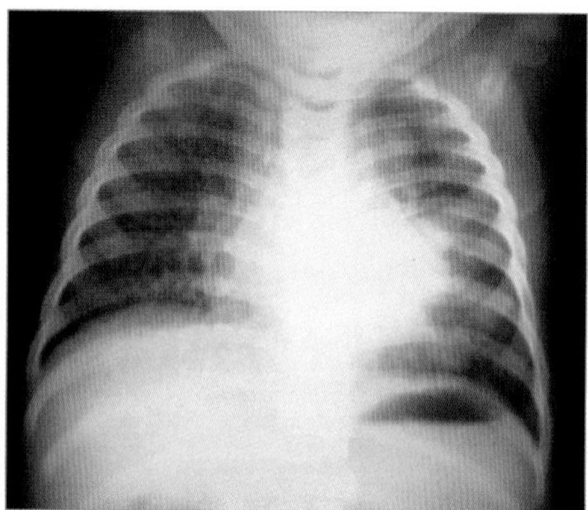

Image 146.17
A 10-month-old with radiographic changes of miliary tuberculosis.

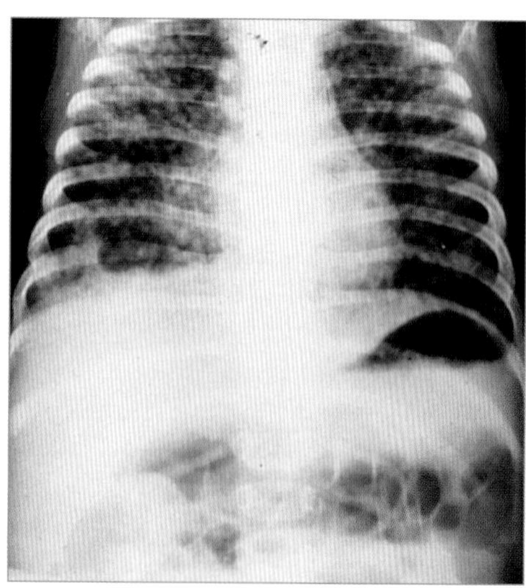

Image 146.18
Miliary tuberculosis with pulmonary cavitation (right lung).

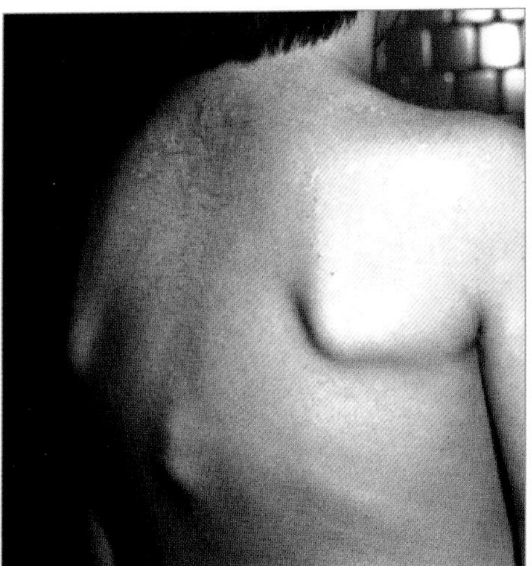

Image 146.19
Tuberculosis of the spine with paravertebral abscess (Pott disease).

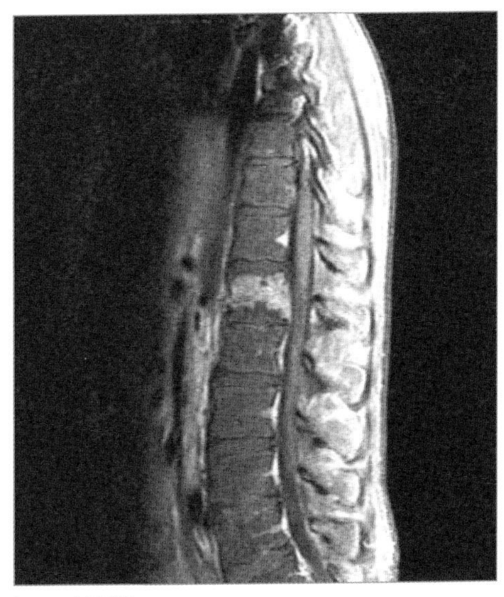

Image 146.20
Tuberculous spondylitis in a 14-year-old boy demonstrated by magnetic resonance imaging. Courtesy of Benjamin Estrada, MD.

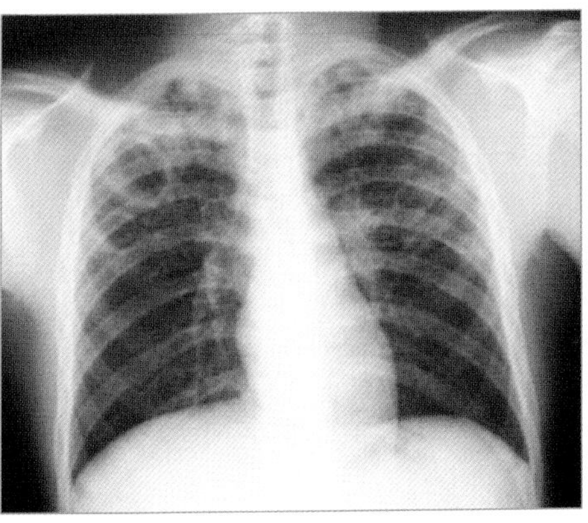

Image 146.21
Cavitary tuberculosis in a 15-year-old boy. Courtesy of Benjamin Estrada, MD.

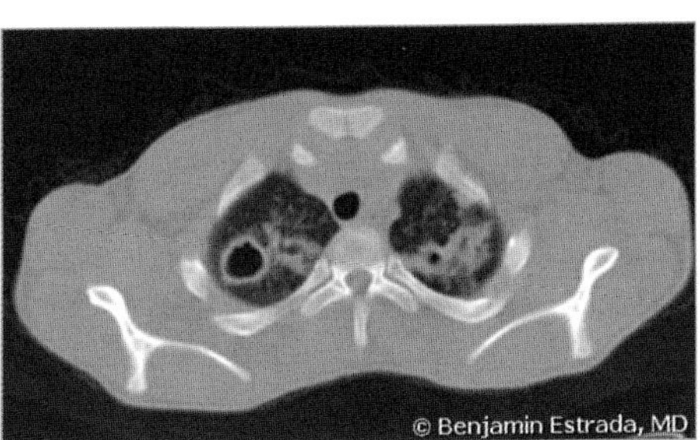

Image 146.22
Cavitary tuberculosis in a 15-year-old boy delineated by computed tomography scan. Courtesy of Benjamin Estrada, MD.

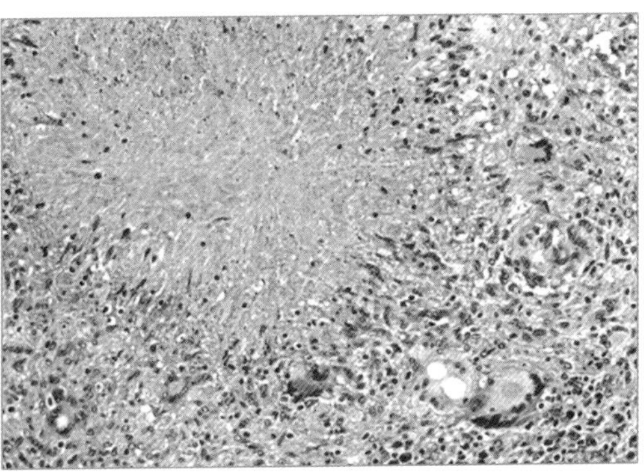

Image 146.23
Tuberculosis. Caseation and Langhans giant cells in a lymph node. Courtesy of Dimitris P. Agamanolis, MD.

147

Diseases Caused by Nontuberculous Mycobacteria

(Environmental Mycobacteria, Mycobacteria Other Than *Mycobacterium tuberculosis*)

Clinical Manifestations

Several syndromes are caused by nontuberculous mycobacteria (NTM). In children, the most common of these syndromes is cervical lymphadenitis. Cutaneous infection can follow soil- or water-contaminated traumatic wounds, surgeries, or cosmetic procedures (eg, tattoos, pedicures, body piercings). Less common syndromes include soft tissue infection, osteomyelitis, otitis media, catheter-associated bloodstream infections, and pulmonary infections, especially in adolescents with cystic fibrosis. Nontuberculous mycobacteria, especially *Mycobacterium avium* complex (MAC [including *M avium* and *Mycobacterium avium-intracellulare* complex]) and *Mycobacterium abscessus,* can be recovered from sputum in 10% to 20% of adolescents and young adults with cystic fibrosis and can be associated with fever and declining clinical status. Disseminated infections are almost always associated with impaired cell-mediated immunity, as found in children with congenital immune defects (eg, interleukin-12 deficiency, NF-kappa-B essential modulator mutation and related disorders, interferon-gamma receptor defects), hematopoietic stem cell transplants, or advanced HIV infection. Disseminated MAC is rare in HIV-infected children during the first year of life, but the frequency increases with increasing age and declining $CD4^+$ T-lymphocyte counts (<50 cells/µL, in children older than 6 years). Manifestations of disseminated NTM infections depend on the species and route of infection but include fever, night sweats, weight loss, abdominal pain, fatigue, diarrhea, and anemia. These signs and symptoms are also found in advanced immunosuppressed HIV-infected children without disseminated MAC. For HIV-infected children who have disseminated MAC, respiratory symptoms and isolated pulmonary disease are uncommon. In HIV-infected patients developing immune restoration with initiation of antiretroviral therapy, local MAC symptoms can worsen temporarily. This immune reconstitution syndrome usually occurs 2 to 4 weeks after initiation of antiretroviral therapy. Symptoms can include worsening fever, swollen lymph nodes, local pain, and laboratory abnormalities.

Etiology

Of the more than 130 species of NTM that have been identified, only a few account for most human infections. The species most commonly infecting children in the United States are MAC, *Mycobacterium fortuitum, M abscessus,* and *Mycobacterium marinum* (Table 147.1). Several new species, which can be detected by nucleic acid amplification testing but cannot be grown by routine culture methods, have been identified in lymph nodes of children with cervical adenitis. Nontuberculous mycobacteria disease in patients with HIV infection is usually caused by MAC. *M fortuitum, Mycobacterium chelonae, Mycobacterium smegmatis,* and *M abscessus* are commonly referred to as "rapidly growing" mycobacteria. The rapidly growing mycobacteria have sufficient growth within 3 to 5 days so identification can be achieved, whereas MAC, *M marinum,* and *Mycobacterium szulgai* usually require several weeks before sufficient growth occurs for identification. Rapidly growing mycobacteria have been implicated in wound, soft tissue, bone, pulmonary, central venous catheter, and middle-ear infections. Other mycobacterial species that usually are not pathogenic have caused infections in immunocompromised hosts or have been associated with the presence of a foreign body.

Epidemiology

Many NTM species are ubiquitous in nature and are found in soil, food, water, and animals. Tap water is the major reservoir for *Mycobacterium kansasii, Mycobacterium lentiflavum, Mycobacterium xenopi, Mycobacterium simiae,* and health care–associated infections attributable to the rapidly growing mycobacteria, *M abscessus* and *M fortuitum.* Outbreaks have been associated with contaminated water used for pedicures and inks used for tattooing. For *M marinum,* water in a fish tank or aquarium or an injury in a saltwater environment is the

Table 147.1
Diseases Caused by Nontuberculous *Mycobacterium* Species

Clinical Disease	Common Species	Less Common Species in the United States
Cutaneous infection	*M chelonae, M fortuitum, M abscessus, M marinum*	*M ulcerans*[a]
Lymphadenitis	MAC, *M haemophilum, M lentiflavum*	*M kansasii, M fortuitum, M malmoense*[b]
Otologic infection	*M abscessus*	*M fortuitum*
Pulmonary infection	MAC, *M kansasii, M abscessus*	*M xenopi, M malmoense,*[b] *M szulgai, M fortuitum, M simiae*
Catheter-associated infection	*M chelonae, M fortuitum*	*M abscessus*
Skeletal infection	MAC, *M kansasii, M fortuitum*	*M chelonae, M marinum, M abscessus, M ulcerans*[a]
Disseminated	MAC	*M kansasii, M genavense, M haemophilum, M chelonae*

Abbreviation: MAC, *Mycobacterium avium* complex.
[a] Not endemic in the United States.
[b] Found primarily in Northern Europe.

major source of infection. The environmental reservoir for *M abscessus* and MAC causing pulmonary infection is unknown. Although many people are exposed to NTM, it is unknown why some exposures result in acute or chronic infection. Usual portals of entry for NTM infection are believed to be abrasions in the skin (eg, cutaneous lesions caused by *M marinum*), penetrating trauma (needles and organic material most often associated with *M abscessus* and *M fortuitum*), surgical sites (especially for central vascular catheters), oropharyngeal mucosa (the presumed portal of entry for cervical lymphadenitis), gastrointestinal or respiratory tract for disseminated MAC, and respiratory tract (including tympanostomy tubes for otitis media). Pulmonary disease and rare cases of mediastinal adenitis and endobronchial disease do occur. Nontuberculous mycobacteria can be an important pathogen in patients with cystic fibrosis and is an emerging pathogen in individuals receiving biologic response modifiers, such as antitumor necrosis factor α. Most infections remain localized at the portal of entry or in regional lymph nodes. Dissemination to distal sites primarily occurs in immunocompromised hosts. No definitive evidence of person-to-person transmission of NTM exists. Outbreaks of otitis media caused by *M abscessus* have been associated with polyethylene ear tubes and use of contaminated equipment or water. A waterborne route of transmission has been implicated for MAC infection in some immunodeficient hosts. Buruli ulcer disease is a skin and bone infection caused by *Mycobacterium ulcerans,* an emerging disease causing significant morbidity and disability in tropical areas such as Africa, Asia, South America, Australia, and the western Pacific.

Incubation Period

Variable.

Diagnostic Tests

Definitive diagnosis of NTM disease requires isolation of the organism. Consultation with the laboratory should occur to ensure culture specimens are handled correctly. Because these organisms are commonly found in the environment, contamination of cultures or transient colonization can occur. Caution must be exercised in interpretation of cultures obtained from nonsterile sites, such as gastric washing specimens, endoscopy material, a single expectorated sputum sample, or urine specimens, and also when the species cultured is usually nonpathogenic (eg, *Mycobacterium terrae* complex, *Mycobacterium gordonae*). An acid-fast bacilli smear-positive sample and repeated isolation on culture media of a single species from any site are more likely to indicate disease than culture contamination or transient colonization. Diagnostic criteria for NTM lung disease in adults include 2 or more separate sputum samples that grow NTM or one bronchial alveolar lavage specimen that grows NTM. These criteria have not been validated in children and apply best to MAC, *M kansasii,* and *M abscessus.* Nontuberculous mycobacteria isolates from draining sinus tracts or wounds are almost always significant clinically. Recovery of NTM from sites that are usually sterile, such as cerebrospinal fluid, pleural fluid, bone marrow, blood, lymph node aspirates, middle ear or mastoid aspirates, or surgically excised tissue, is the most reliable diagnostic test. With radiometric or nonradiometric broth techniques, blood cultures are highly sensitive in recovery of disseminated MAC and other blood-borne NTM species. Disseminated MAC disease should prompt a search for underlying immunodeficiency.

Patients with NTM infection, such as *M marinum* or MAC cervical lymphadenitis, can have a positive tuberculin skin test result because the purified protein derivative preparation, derived from *M tuberculosis,* shares a number of antigens with NTM species. These tuberculin skin test reactions usually measure less than 10 mm of induration but can measure more than 15 mm. The interferon-gamma release assays use 2 or 3 antigens to detect infection with *M tuberculosis.* Although these antigens are not found on *M avium-intracellulare* complex and most other NTM species, cross reactions can occur with infection caused by *M kansasii, M marinum,* and *M szulgai.*

Treatment

Many NTM are relatively resistant in vitro to antituberculosis drugs. In vitro resistance to these agents, however, does not necessarily correlate with clinical response, especially with MAC infections. The approach to therapy should be directed by the species causing the infection, the results of drug-susceptibility testing, the site(s) of infection, the patient's immune status, and the need to treat a patient presumptively for tuberculosis while awaiting culture reports that subsequently reveal NTM.

For NTM lymphadenitis in otherwise healthy children, especially when the disease is caused by MAC, complete surgical excision is curative. Antimicrobial therapy has been shown to provide no additional benefit. Therapy with clarithromycin or azithromycin combined with ethambutol or rifampin or rifabutin may be beneficial for children in whom surgical excision is incomplete or for children with recurrent disease (Table 147.2).

Isolates of rapidly growing mycobacteria (*M fortuitum, M abscessus,* and *M chelonae*) should be tested in vitro against drugs to which they are commonly susceptible and that have been used with some therapeutic success (eg, amikacin, imipenem, sulfamethoxazole or trimethoprim-sulfamethoxazole, cefoxitin, ciprofloxacin, clarithromycin, linezolid, doxycycline). Clarithromycin and at least one other agent is the treatment of choice for cutaneous (disseminated) infections attributable to *M chelonae* or *M abscessus.* Indwelling foreign bodies should always be removed, and surgical debridement for serious localized disease is optimal. The choice of drugs, dosages, and duration should be reviewed with a consultant experienced in the management of NTM infections.

For patients with cystic fibrosis and isolation of MAC species, treatment is suggested only for those with clinical symptoms not attributable to other causes, worsening lung function, and chest radiographic progression. The decision to embark on therapy should take into consideration susceptibility testing results and should involve consultation with an expert in cystic fibrosis care. *M abscessus* is difficult to treat, and the role of therapy in clinical benefit is unknown.

In patients with AIDS and in other immunocompromised people with disseminated MAC infection, multidrug therapy is recommended. Clinical isolates of MAC are usually resistant to many of the approved antituberculosis drugs, including isoniazid, but are susceptible to clarithromycin and azithromycin and often

Table 147.2
Treatment of Nontuberculous Mycobacteria Infections in Children

Organism	Disease	Initial Treatment
Slowly Growing *Mycobacterium* Species		
MAC, *M haemophilum, M lentiflavum*	Lymphadenitis	Complete excision of lymph nodes; if excision incomplete or disease recurs, clarithromycin or azithromycin plus ethambutol or rifampin (or rifabutin)
	Pulmonary infection	Clarithromycin or azithromycin plus ethambutol with rifampin or rifabutin (pulmonary resection in some patients who fail to respond to drug therapy). For severe disease, an initial course of amikacin or streptomycin is often included. Clinical data in adults support that 3-times-weekly therapy is as effective as daily therapy, with less toxicity for adult patients with mild to moderate disease. For patients with advanced or cavitary disease, drugs should be given daily.
	Disseminated	See text.
M kansasii	Pulmonary infection	Rifampin plus ethambutol with isoniazid daily. If rifampin resistance is detected, a 3-drug regimen based on drug susceptibility testing should be used.
	Osteomyelitis	Surgical debridement and prolonged antimicrobial therapy using rifampin plus ethambutol with isoniazid
M marinum	Cutaneous infection	None, if minor; rifampin, trimethoprim-sulfamethoxazole, clarithromycin, or doxycycline[a] for moderate disease; extensive lesions may require surgical debridement. Susceptibility testing is not routinely required.
M ulcerans	Cutaneous and bone infections	Daily intramuscular streptomycin and oral rifampin for 8 weeks; excision to remove necrotic tissue, if present; disability prevention
Rapidly Growing *Mycobacterium* Species		
M fortuitum group	Cutaneous infection	Initial therapy for serious disease is amikacin plus meropenem, IV, followed by clarithromycin, doxycycline[a] or trimethoprim-sulfamethoxazole, or ciprofloxacin, orally, on the basis of in vitro susceptibility testing; may require surgical excision. Up to 50% of isolates are resistant to cefoxitin.
	Catheter infection	Catheter removal and amikacin plus meropenem, IV; clarithromycin, trimethoprim-sulfamethoxazole, or ciprofloxacin, orally, on the basis of in vitro susceptibility testing
M abscessus	Otitis media; cutaneous infection	There is no reliable antimicrobial regimen because of variability in drug susceptibility. Clarithromycin plus initial course of amikacin plus cefoxitin or meropenem; may require surgical debridement on the basis of in vitro susceptibility testing (50% are amikacin resistant).

Table 147.2
Treatment of Nontuberculous Mycobacteria Infections in Children (*continued*)

Organism	Disease	Initial Treatment
Rapidly Growing *Mycobacterium* Species (*continued*)		
M abscessus (*continued*)	Pulmonary infection (in cystic fibrosis)	Serious disease, clarithromycin, amikacin, and cefoxitin or meropenem on the basis of susceptibility testing; may require surgical resection.
M chelonae	Catheter infection	Catheter removal and tobramycin (initially) plus clarithromycin
	Disseminated cutaneous infection	Tobramycin and meropenem or linezolid (initially) plus clarithromycin

Abbreviations: IV, intravenously; MAC, *Mycobacterium avium* complex.

[a] Tetracycline-based antimicrobial agents, including doxycycline, may cause permanent tooth discoloration for children younger than 8 years if used for repeated treatment courses. However, doxycycline binds less readily to calcium compared with older tetracyclines, and, in some studies, doxycycline was not associated with visible teeth staining in younger children. Only 50% of isolates of *M marinum* are susceptible to doxycycline.

are susceptible to combinations of ethambutol, rifabutin or rifampin, and amikacin or streptomycin. Susceptibility testing to these other agents has not been standardized and, thus, is not recommended routinely. The optimal regimen is yet to be determined. Treatment of disseminated MAC infection should be undertaken in consultation with an infectious diseases expert.

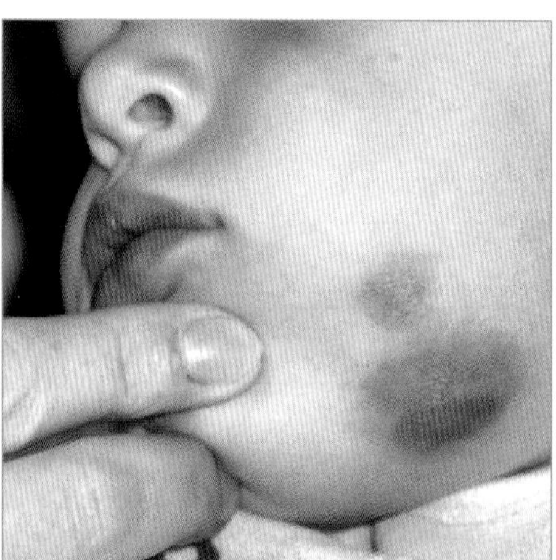

Image 147.1
Atypical mycobacterial tuberculosis (lymphadenitis) with ulceration.

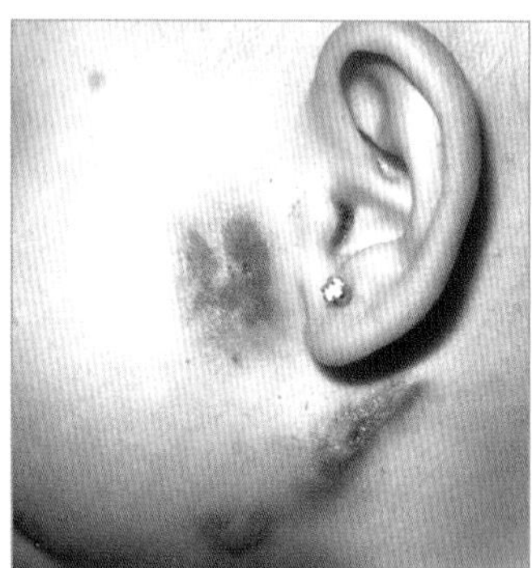

Image 147.2
Atypical mycobacterial lymphadenitis.

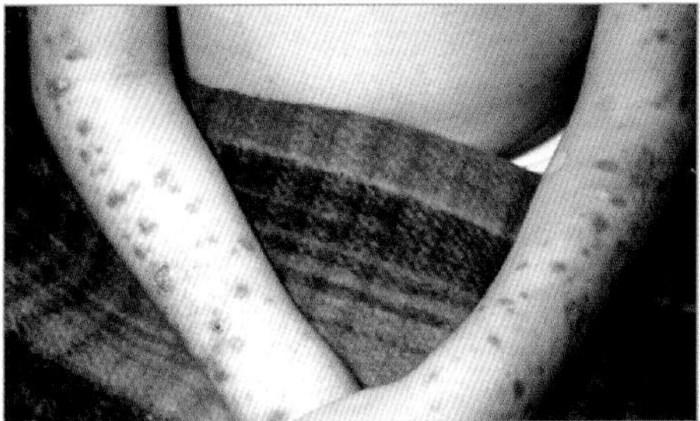

Image 147.3
Disseminated atypical mycobacterial tuberculosis with generalized cutaneous lesions in a boy with acute lymphoblastic leukemia in remission.

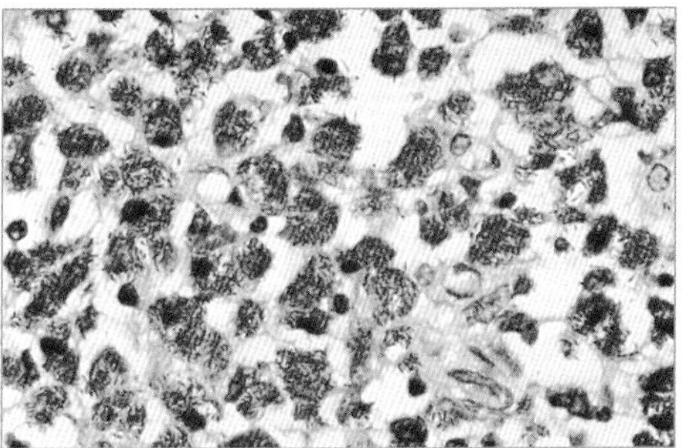

Image 147.5
Mycobacterium avium-intracellulare complex infection of the lymph node in a patient with AIDS (Ziehl-Neelsen stain). Courtesy of Centers for Disease Control and Prevention/Dr Edwin P. Ewing Jr.

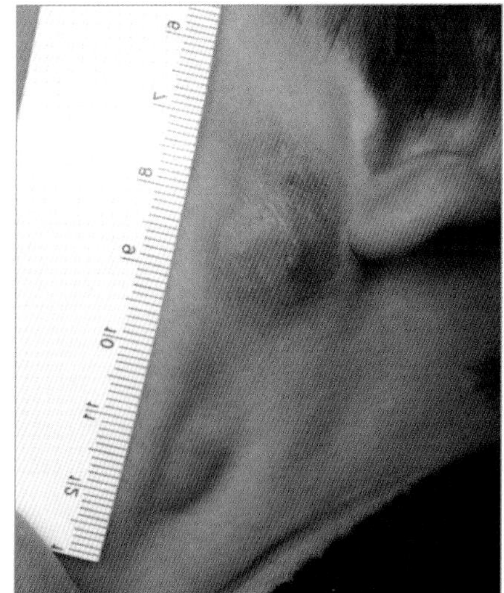

Image 147.7
A 4-year-old white boy with an atypical mycobacterial infection involving left preauricular lymph nodes. Courtesy of Ed Fajardo, MD.

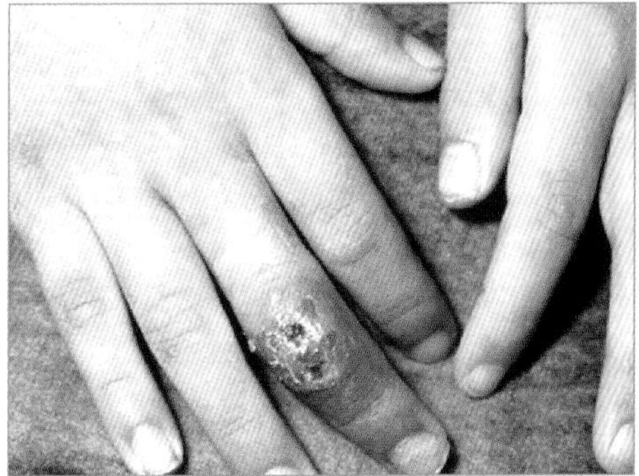

Image 147.4
The same patient as in Image 147.3 with atypical mycobacterial tuberculosis osteomyelitis of the right middle finger.

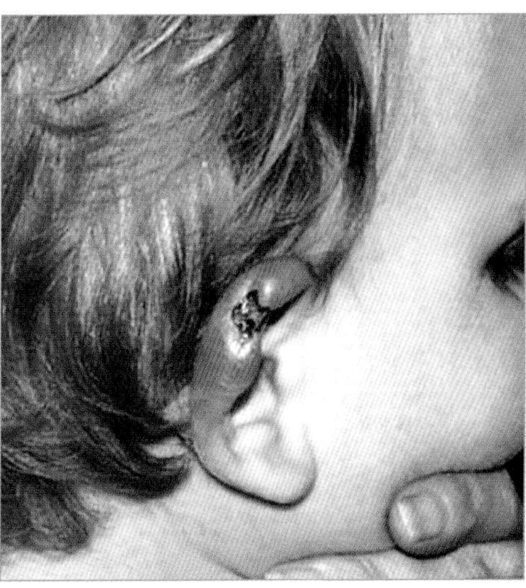

Image 147.6
An 18-month-old with culture- and polymerase chain reaction–confirmed Buruli ulcer of the right ear. She had briefly visited St Leonards, Australia, in 2001. The initial lesion resembled a mosquito or other insect bite. Courtesy of Centers for Disease Control and Prevention/*Emerging Infectious Diseases* and Paul D. R. Johnson.

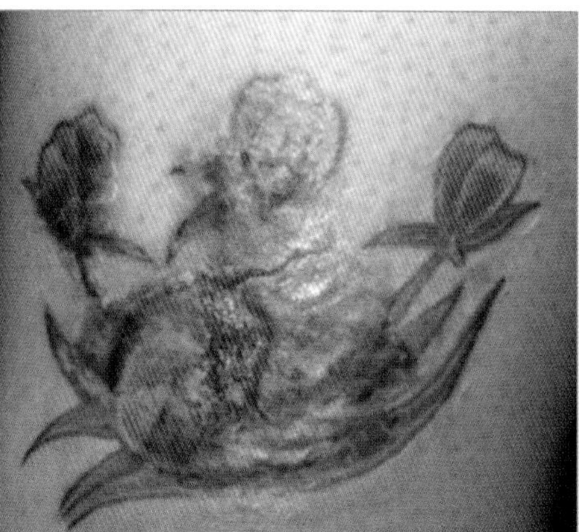

Image 147.8

Approximately 21% of adults in the United States report having at least one permanent tattoo. Outbreaks caused by nontuberculous mycobacteria (NTM) have been reported infrequently after tattooing. One such report describes characteristics of tattoo-associated NTM infection clusters in 4 states during 2011–2012. In January 2012, public health officials in New York reviewed reports of *Mycobacterium chelonae* skin infections in 14 residents who received tattoos in the last quarter of 2011. All infections were associated with use of the same nationally distributed, prediluted gray ink manufactured by Company A. In February 2012, the Centers for Disease Control and Prevention disseminated an Epi-X public health alert to identify additional tattoo-associated NTM skin infections. A confirmed case was defined as a patient with persistent inflammatory reaction localized within the margins of a new tattoo received between May 1, 2011, and February 10, 2012, and isolation of NTM from a wound or skin biopsy. Results of this study showed 22 cases were identified from 4 states: Colorado, Iowa, New York, and Washington. Nineteen of the 22 cases (86%) were caused by *M chelonae*, the others by *Mycobacterium abscessus*. Investigations found the use of ink contaminated with NTM before distribution or just before tattooing likely led to infections in each of the reported clusters. Copyright Paige Brase, used with permission.

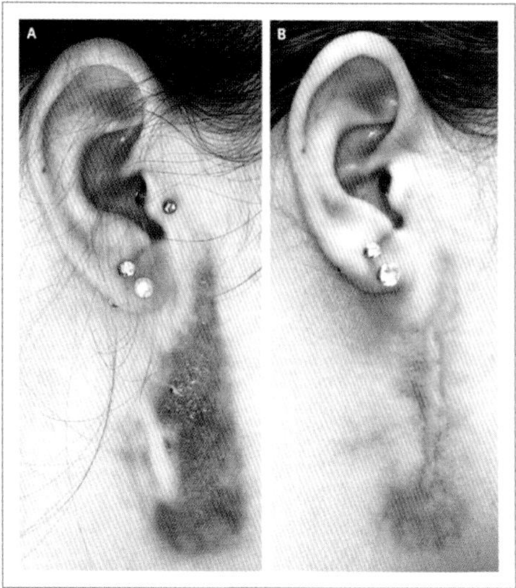

Image 147.9

An 18-year-old woman presented with a large, fluctuant, violaceous plaque on her right cheek (A). Her right tragus had been professionally pierced 6 months earlier, and streaking had developed along the angle of her jaw 1 month after the piercing. A biopsy specimen showed granulomatous inflammation. The tissue culture grew *Mycobacterium fortuitum*. From *The New England Journal of Medicine,* Piercing-Related Nontuberculous Mycobacterial Infection, 362, 2012. Copyright © 2010. Massachusetts Medical Society. Reprinted with permission from Massachusetts Medical Society.

148

Tularemia

Clinical Manifestations

Most patients with tularemia have abrupt onset of fever, chills, myalgia, and headache. Illness usually conforms to one of several tularemic syndromes. Most common is the **ulceroglandular** syndrome characterized by a maculopapular lesion at the entry site with subsequent ulceration and slow healing, associated with painful, acutely inflamed regional lymph nodes that can drain spontaneously. The **glandular** syndrome (regional lymphadenopathy with no ulcer) is also common. Less common disease syndromes are **pneumonic** (flu-like symptoms, often without chest radiograph abnormalities), **oculoglandular** (severe conjunctivitis and preauricular lymphadenopathy), **oropharyngeal** (severe exudative stomatitis, pharyngitis, or tonsillitis and cervical lymphadenopathy), **vesicular** skin lesions that can be mistaken for herpes simplex or varicella-zoster virus cutaneous infections, **typhoidal** (systemic infection, high fever, hepatomegaly, splenomegaly, and, possibly, septicemia), and **intestinal** (intestinal pain, vomiting, and diarrhea). Pneumonic tularemia, characterized by fever, dry cough, chest pain, and hilar adenopathy, is normally associated with farming or lawn maintenance activities that create aerosols and dust. This would also be the anticipated syndrome after intentional aerosol release of organisms.

Etiology

Francisella tularensis is a small, weakly staining, gram-negative pleomorphic coccobacillus. Two subspecies cause human infection in North America, *F tularensis* subsp *tularensis* (type A), and *F tularensis* subsp *holarctica* (type B). Type A is generally is considered more virulent, although either can be lethal, especially if inhaled.

Epidemiology

F tularensis can infect more than 100 animal species; vertebrates considered most important in enzootic cycles are rabbits, hares, and rodents, especially muskrats, voles, beavers, and prairie dogs. Domestic cats are another source of infection. In the United States, human infection is usually associated with direct contact with one of these species or with the bite of arthropod vectors such as ticks and deerflies. Infection has been reported in commercially traded hamsters and in a child bitten by a pet hamster. Infection can also be acquired following ingestion of contaminated water or inadequately cooked meat or inhalation of contaminated aerosols generated during lawn mowing, brush cutting, or certain farming activities, such as baling contaminated hay. At-risk people have occupational or recreational exposure to infected animals or their habitats, such as rabbit hunters and trappers, people exposed to certain ticks or biting insects, and laboratory technicians working with *F tularensis,* which is highly infectious and may be aerosolized when grown in culture. In the United States, most cases occur during May through September. Approximately two-thirds of cases occur in males, and one-quarter of cases occur in children 1 to 14 years of age. Tularemia has been reported in all US states except Hawaii. Six states accounted for 59% of reported cases: Missouri (19%), Arkansas (13%), Oklahoma (9%), Massachusetts (7%), South Dakota (5%), and Kansas (5%). During 2001–2010, 1,208 cases were reported (median, 126.5 cases per year; range, 90–154). Organisms can be present in blood during the first 2 weeks of disease and in cutaneous lesions for as long as 1 month if untreated. Person-to-person transmission has not been reported.

Incubation Period

3 to 5 days; range, 1 to 21 days.

Diagnostic Tests

Diagnosis is established most often by serologic testing. Most clinical laboratories are not equipped to perform the generally accepted diagnostic tests for tularemia, and suspect samples may need to be processed by a designated reference laboratory. Patients do not develop antibodies until the second week of illness. A single serum antibody titer of 1:128 or greater determined by microagglutination (MA) or of 1:160 or greater determined by tube agglutination (TA) is consistent with recent or past infection and constitutes a presumptive diagnosis. Confirmation by serologic testing requires a 4-fold or greater titer change between serum samples obtained at least 2 weeks apart, with one of the specimens having a minimum titer of 1:128 or greater by MA or 1:160 or greater by TA. Nonspecific cross-reactions can occur with specimens containing heterophile antibodies or antibodies to *Brucella* species, *Legionella* species, or other gram-negative bacteria. However, cross-reactions rarely result in MA or TA titers that are diagnostic. Some clinical laboratories can presumptively identify *F tularensis* in ulcer exudate or aspirate material by polymerase chain reaction assay or direct fluorescent antibody assay. Immunohistochemical staining is specific for detection of *F tularensis* in fixed tissues; however, this method is not available in most clinical laboratories. Isolation of *F tularensis* from specimens of blood, skin, ulcers, lymph node drainage, gastric washings, or respiratory tract secretions is best achieved by inoculation of cysteine-enriched media. Suspect growth on culture can be identified presumptively by polymerase chain reaction or direct fluorescent antibody assays. Because of its propensity for causing laboratory-acquired infections, laboratory personnel should be alerted when *F tularensis* infection is suspected.

Treatment

Gentamicin, intravenously or intramuscularly, is the drug of choice for the treatment of tularemia in children. Duration of therapy usually is 7 to 10 days. A 5- to 7-day course may be sufficient in mild disease, but a longer course is required for more severe illness (eg, meningitis). Ciprofloxacin is an alternative for mild disease. Doxycycline is another alternative agent but is associated with a higher rate of relapses, and longer courses (14 days) of therapy should be used. Suppuration of lymph nodes can occur despite antimicrobial therapy. *F tularensis* is resistant to β-lactam drugs and carbapenems.

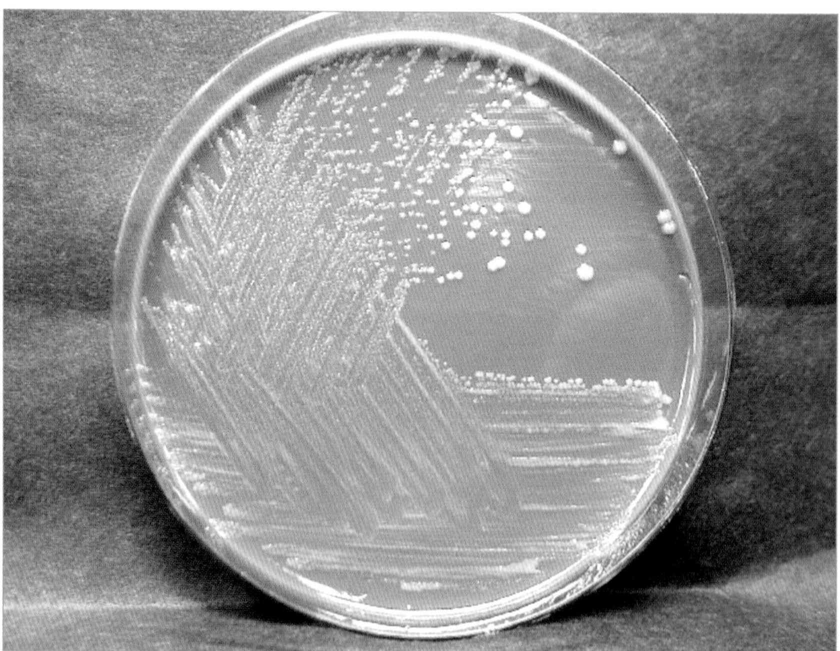

Image 148.1
Francisella tularensis. Colony characteristics when grown on chocolate agar or Martin-Lewis or Thayer-Martin medium include colony size of 1 to 3 mm, gray-white at 48 to 72 hours. Courtesy of Centers for Disease Control and Prevention/Courtesy of Larry Stauffer, Oregon State Public Health Laboratory.

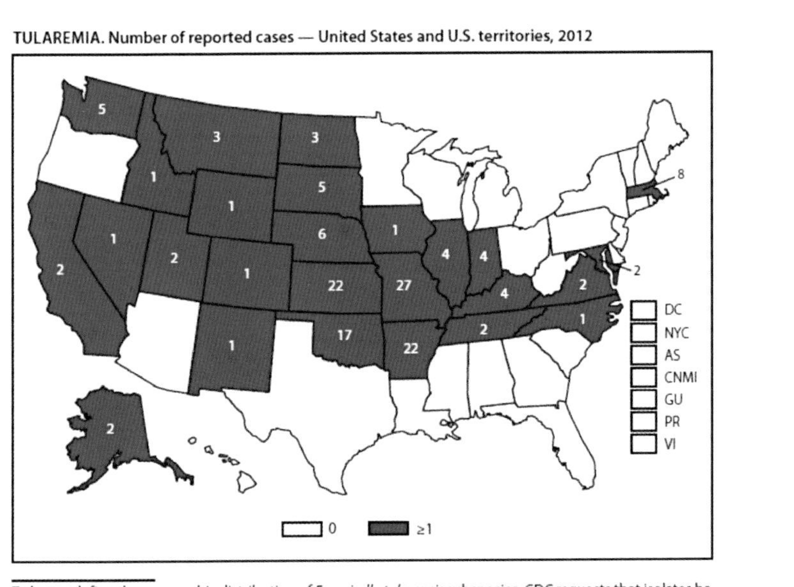

Image 148.2
Tularemia. Number of reported cases—United States and US territories, 2012. Courtesy of *Morbidity and Mortality Weekly Report.*

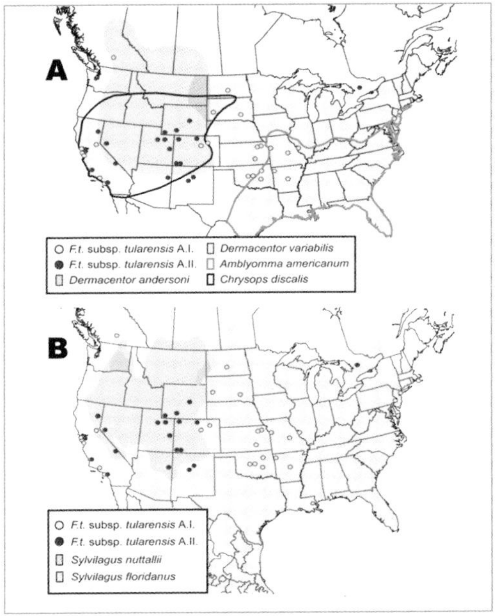

Image 148.3
Spatial distributions of isolates from the AI and AII subpopulations of *Francisella tularensis* subsp *tularensis* relative to (A) distribution of tularemia vectors *Dermacentor variabilis, Dermacentor andersoni, Amblyomma americanum*, and *Chrysops discalis* and (B) distribution of tularemia hosts *Sylvilagus nuttallii* and *S floridanus*. Courtesy of Emerging Infectious Diseases.

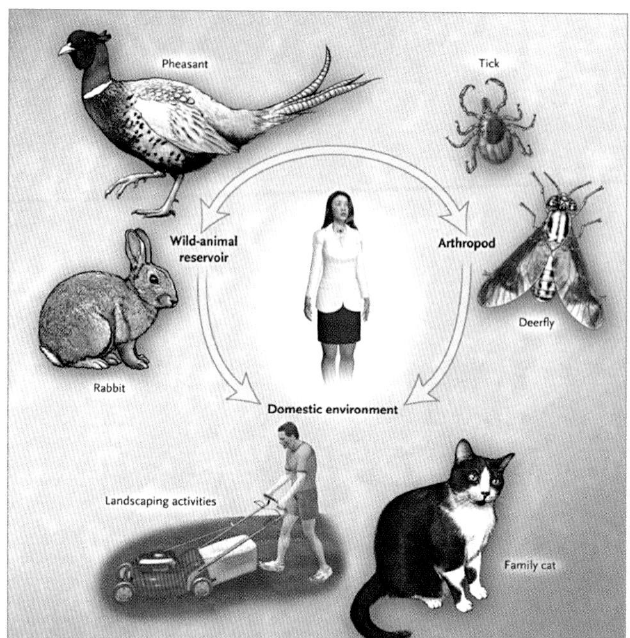

Image 148.4
Francisella tularensis is maintained in nature by interactions between animals and the ticks and flies that bite them. In recent years, more cases have been reported in humans from ticks and deerflies than from direct contact with wild animals. Spread occurs from wild-animal reservoirs to domestic animals, especially cats, and transmission to humans results from animal or insect bites, the handling of infected animal tissues, or inhalation of aerosolized organisms during activities such as landscaping or lawn mowing. From *The New England Journal of Medicine,* Case 31-2010 — A 29-Year-Old Woman with Fever after a Cat Bite, 363:1560-1568 © 2010. Massachusetts Medical Society. Reprinted with permission from Massachusetts Medical Society.

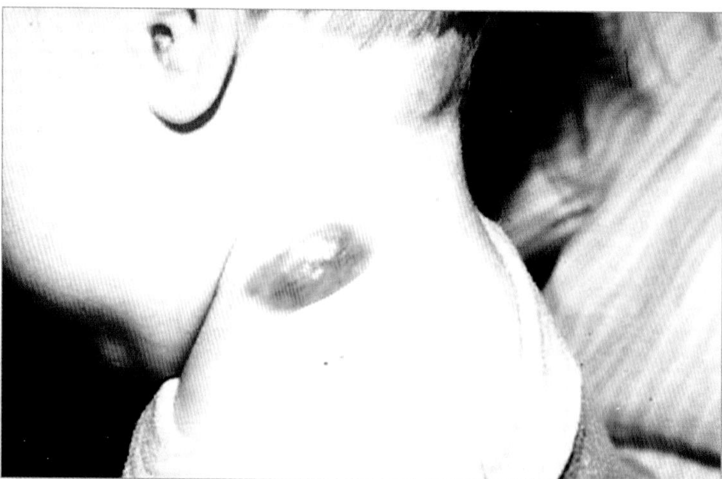

Image 148.5
An 8-year-old boy with 7 days of fever unresponsive to ceftriaxone was examined because of occipital and posterior cervical lymphadenitis. The cervical lymph node had spontaneously drained purulent material. A culture of the node aspirate was positive for *Francisella tularensis*. Courtesy of Richard Jacobs, MD.

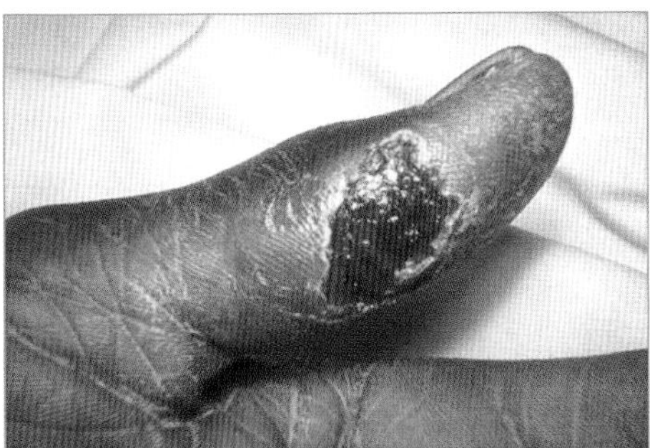

Image 148.6
Tularemic ulcer on the thumb. Irregular ulceration occurred at the site of entry of *Francisella tularensis*. Courtesy of Centers for Disease Control and Prevention/Courtesy Emory University, Dr Sellers.

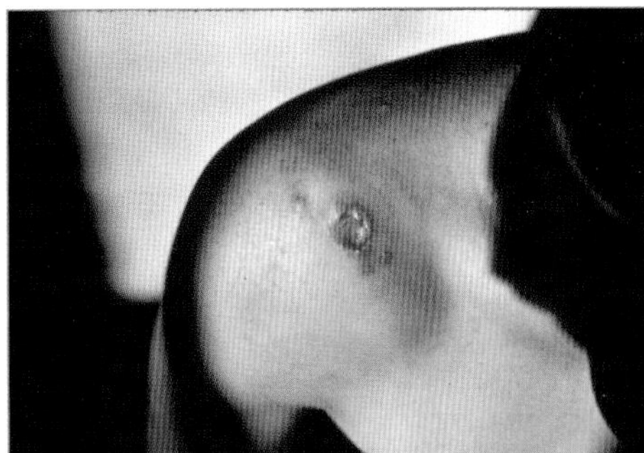

Image 148.7
Tularemic ulcer on the shoulder. Tularemia has been reported in all states except Hawaii. Courtesy of Gary Overturf, MD.

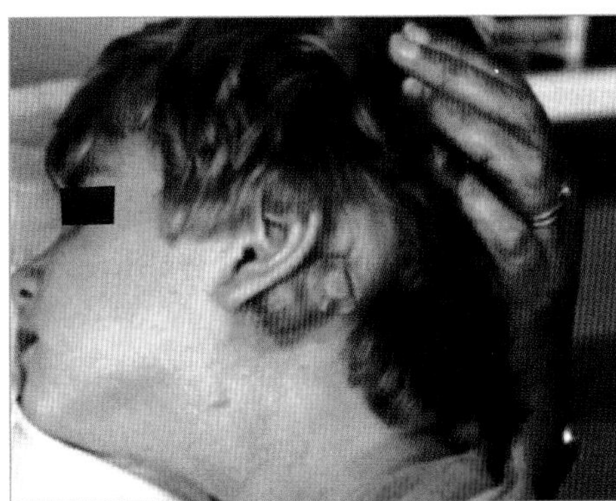

Image 148.8
Tularemia is a relatively rare infection that can manifest with painful cervical adenitis. This boy had a tick bite on his scalp that developed an ulcer followed by a large postauricular node. His tularemia titer results were positive and he responded to treatment with gentamycin.

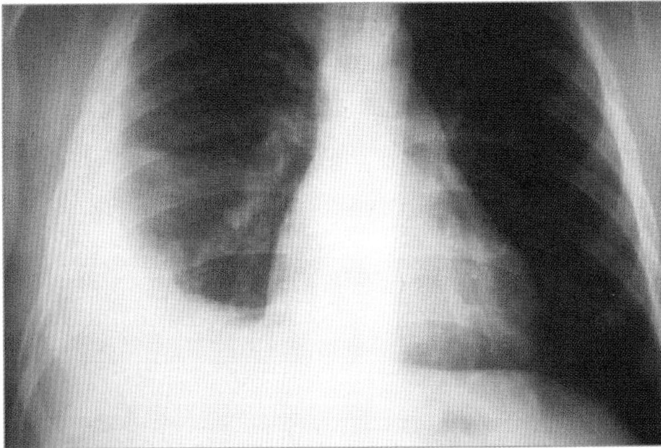

Image 148.9
Tularemia pneumonia. Posteroanterior chest radiograph showing pneumonia and pleural effusion in the lower lobe of the right lung; the pneumonia was unresponsive to ceftriaxone, azithromycin, and nafcillin. The patient had a history of tick bite and a high fever for 8 days, and his tularemia agglutinin titer was 1:2,048. An outbreak of pneumonic tularemia should prompt consideration of bioterrorism.

149

Endemic Typhus

(Murine Typhus)

Clinical Manifestations

Endemic typhus resembles epidemic (louse-borne) typhus but usually has a less abrupt onset with less severe systemic symptoms. In young children, the disease can be mild. Fever, present in almost all patients, can be accompanied by a persistent, usually severe, headache and myalgia. Nausea and vomiting also develop in approximately half of patients. A rash typically appears on day 4 to 7 of illness, is macular or maculopapular, lasts 4 to 8 days, and tends to remain discrete, with sparse lesions and no hemorrhage. Rash is present in approximately 50% of patients. Illness seldom lasts longer than 2 weeks; visceral involvement is uncommon. Laboratory findings include thrombocytopenia, elevated liver transaminases, and hyponatremia. Fatal outcome is rare except in untreated severe disease.

Etiology

Endemic typhus is caused by *Rickettsia typhi* and *Rickettsia felis.*

Epidemiology

Rats, in which infection is unapparent, are the natural reservoirs for *R typhi*. The primary vector for transmission among rats and to humans is the rat flea, *Xenopsylla cheopis,* although other fleas and mites have been implicated. Cat fleas and opossums have been implicated as the source of some cases of endemic typhus caused by *R felis*. Infected flea feces are rubbed into broken skin or mucous membranes or are inhaled. The disease is worldwide in distribution and tends to occur most commonly in adults, in males, and during the months of April to October in the United States; in children, males and females are affected equally. Exposure to rats and their fleas is the major risk factor for infection, although a history of such exposure is often absent. Endemic typhus is rare in the United States, with most cases occurring in southern California, southern Texas, the southeastern Gulf Coast, and Hawaii.

Incubation Period

6 to 14 days.

Diagnostic Tests

Antibody titers determined with *R typhi* antigen by an indirect fluorescent antibody assay, enzyme immunoassay, or latex agglutination test peak around 4 weeks after infection, but results of these tests are often negative early in the course of illness. A 4-fold immunoglobulin (Ig) G titer change between acute and convalescent serum specimens taken 2 to 3 weeks apart is diagnostic. Although more prone to false-positive results, immunoassays demonstrating increases in specific IgM antibody can aid in distinguishing clinical illness from previous exposure if interpreted with a concurrent IgG test; use of IgM assays alone is not recommended. Serologic tests may not differentiate murine typhus from epidemic (louseborne) typhus, *R felis* infection, or infection with spotted fever rickettsiosis, such as *Rickettsia rickettsii,* without antibody cross-absorption for indirect fluorescent antibody or western blotting analyses, which are not available routinely. Routine hospital blood cultures are not suitable for culture of *R typhi*. Molecular diagnostic assays on infected whole blood and skin biopsies can distinguish endemic typhus and other rickettsioses and are performed at the Centers for Disease Control and Prevention. Immunohistochemical procedures on formalin-fixed skin biopsy tissues can also be performed at the Centers for Disease Control and Prevention.

Treatment

Doxycycline is the treatment of choice for endemic typhus, regardless of patient age, administered intravenously or orally. Treatment should be continued for at least 3 days after defervescence and evidence of clinical improvement is documented, and the total treatment course is usually for 7 to 14 days. Fluoroquinolones or chloramphenicol are alternative medications but may not be as effective.

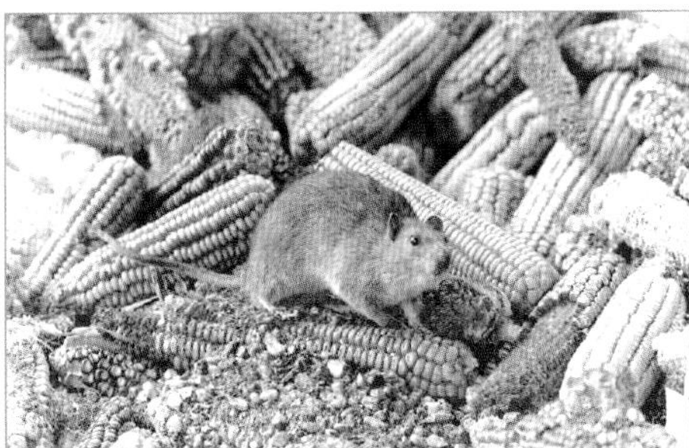

Image 149.1
A Norway rat, *Rattus norvegicus,* in a Kansas City, MO, corn storage bin. *R norvegicus* is known to be a reservoir of bubonic plague (transmitted to man by the bite of a flea or other insect), endemic typhus fever, rat-bite fever, and a few other dreaded diseases. Courtesy of Centers for Disease Control and Prevention.

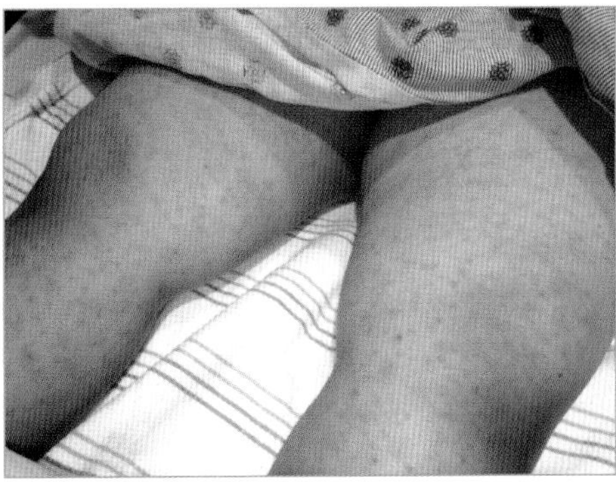

Image 149.2
A healthy 8-year-old boy had 5 days of fever, severe headache, and malaise before this rash began. He had been exposed to numerous cats with fleas before the onset of illness. Courtesy of Carol J. Baker, MD, FAAP.

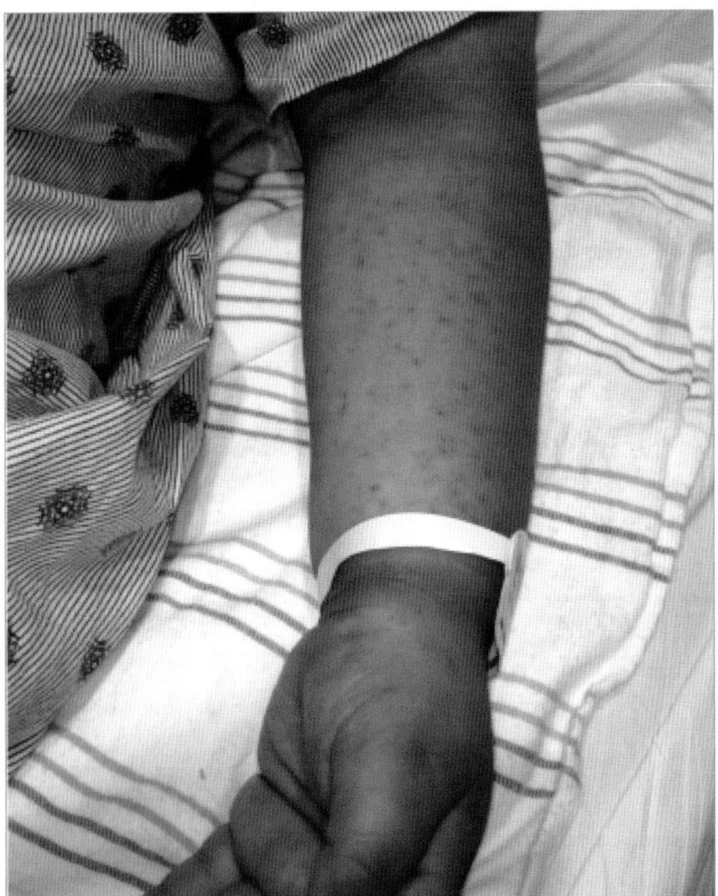

Image 149.3
The same boy as in Image 149.2 who had rash involving palms and soles as well as pancytopenia. He recovered completely with doxycycline therapy. Courtesy of Carol J. Baker, MD, FAAP.

150

Epidemic Typhus

(Louseborne or Sylvatic Typhus)

Clinical Manifestations

Clinically, epidemic typhus should be considered when people in crowded conditions develop abrupt onset of high fever, chills, and myalgia accompanied by severe headache and malaise. Although epidemic typhus patients often develop a rash by day 4 to 7 after the start of illness, rash may not always be present and should not be relied on for diagnosis. When present, the rash usually begins on the trunk, spreads to the limbs, and generally spares the face, palms, and soles. The rash is typically macular to maculopapular but, in advanced stages, can become petechial or hemorrhagic. There is no eschar, as is often present in many other rickettsial diseases. Abdominal complaints (eg, stomach pain, nausea) and changes in mental status are common, and delirium or coma can occur. Myocardial and renal failure can occur when the disease is severe. The case-fatality rate in untreated people is as high as 30%. Mortality is less common in children, and the rate increases with advancing age. Untreated patients who recover typically have an illness lasting 2 weeks. Brill-Zinsser disease is a relapse of epidemic typhus that can occur years after the initial episode. Factors that reactivate the rickettsiae are unknown, but relapse is often milder and of shorter duration.

Etiology

Epidemic typhus is caused by *Rickettsia prowazekii.*

Epidemiology

Humans are the primary reservoir of the organism, which is transmitted from person to person by the human body louse, *Pediculus humanus corporis.* Infected louse feces are rubbed into broken skin or mucous membranes or are inhaled. All ages are affected. Poverty, crowding, and poor sanitary conditions contribute to the spread of body lice and, hence, the disease. Cases of epidemic typhus are rare in the United States but have occurred throughout the world, including the colder, mountainous areas of Asia, Africa, some parts of Europe, and Central and South America, particularly in refugee camps and jails of resource-limited countries. Epidemic typhus is most common during winter, when conditions favor person-to-person transmission of the vector, the body louse. Rickettsiae are present in the blood and tissues of patients during the early febrile phase but are not found in secretions. Direct person-to-person spread of the disease does not occur in the absence of the louse vector. In the United States, sporadic human cases associated with close contact with infected flying squirrels (*Glaucomys volans*), their nests, or their ectoparasites are occasionally reported in the eastern United States. Cases have been reported in people who reside or work in flying squirrel–infested dwellings, even when direct contact is not reported. Flying squirrel–associated disease, called **sylvatic typhus,** typically presents with a similar illness to that observed with body louse–transmitted infection. Illness can be severe, although fatalities are uncommonly reported with sylvatic typhus; the later development of Brill-Zinsser disease has been confirmed in at least one case of untreated sylvatic typhus. *Amblyomma* ticks in the Americas and in Ethiopia have been shown to carry *R prowazekii,* but their vector potential is unknown.

Incubation Period

1 to 2 weeks.

Diagnostic Tests

Epidemic typhus may be diagnosed by the detection of *R prowazekii* DNA in acute blood and serum specimens by polymerase chain reaction assay. The specimen should preferably be taken within the first week of symptoms and before (or within 24 hours of) doxycycline administration; a negative result does not exclude *R prowazekii* infection. Diagnosis may also be determined by detection of rickettsial DNA in biopsy or autopsy specimens by polymerase chain reaction assay or immunohistochemical visualization of rickettsiae in tissues. The gold standard for serologic diagnosis of epidemic typhus is a 4-fold increase in immunoglobulin (Ig) G antibody titer by the indirect fluorescent antibody test. IgG and IgM antibodies begin to increase by day 7 to 10 after onset of symptoms; thus, an elevated acute titer can represent past exposure rather than acute infection. Low-level elevated antibody titers can be an incidental finding in a significant proportion of the general population in some regions. IgM antibodies may remain elevated for months and are not highly specific for acute epidemic typhus. A confirmed case, therefore, is one that shows a 4-fold or greater increase in antigen-specific IgG between acute and convalescent sera obtained 2 to 6 weeks apart. Cross-reactivity may be observed to antibodies to *Rickettsia typhi* (the agent of endemic typhus), *Rickettsia rickettsii* (the agent of Rocky Mountain spotted fever), and other spotted fever group rickettsiae. Testing of acute and convalescent sera by enzyme immunoassays or dot blot immunoassay tests can also be used for assessing presence of antibody but is less useful for quantifying changes in titer.

Treatment

Doxycycline is the drug of choice to treat epidemic typhus, regardless of patient age, administered intravenously or orally. Treatment should be continued for at least 3 days after defervescence and evidence of clinical improvement is documented, and the total treatment course is usually for 5 to 10 days. Other broad-spectrum antibiotics, including ciprofloxacin, are not recommended and may be more likely to result in fatal outcome. Chloramphenicol may be used in cases of absolute contraindication of doxycycline. To halt the spread of disease to other people, louse-infested patients should be treated with cream or gel pediculicides containing pyrethrins or permethrin; malathion is prescribed most often when pyrethroids fail. In epidemic situations in which antimicrobial agents may be limited (eg, refugee camps), a single dose of doxycycline may provide effective treatment, especially when combined with delousing efforts.

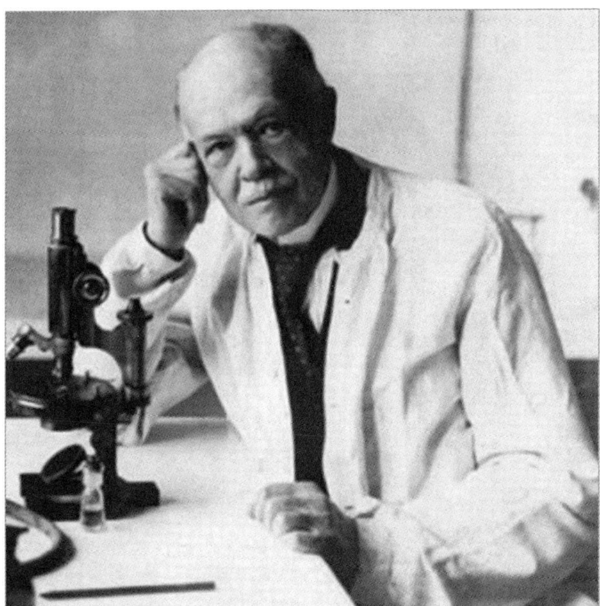

Image 150.1
Charles-Jules-Henri Nicolle (1866–1936), a physician, microbiologist, novelist, philosopher, and historian. From 1903 until his death in 1936, he was director of the Institut Pasteur in Tunis, Tunisia. Nicolle's many accomplishments include the discovery that epidemic typhus is transmitted by body lice (*Pediculus humanis corporis*), discovery of the phenomenon of inapparent infection, and, possibly, the first isolation of human influenza virus after experimental transmission. Nicolle made many other fundamental contributions to knowledge of infectious diseases. He was awarded the 1928 Nobel Prize in Physiology or Medicine for his discovery about typhus transmission, made in the summer of 1909. Courtesy of Centers for Disease Control and Prevention/*Emerging Infectious Diseases*/David M. Morens.

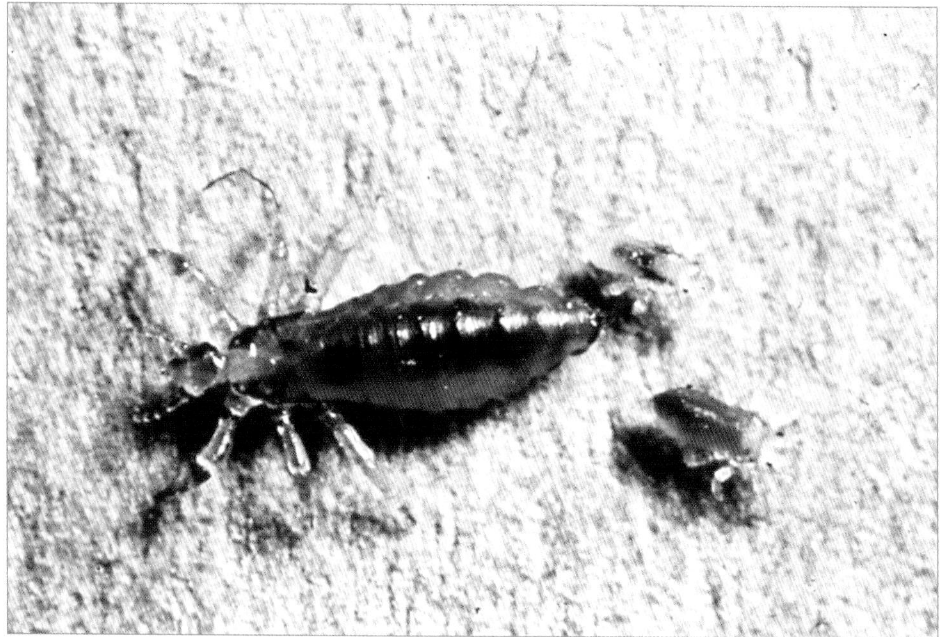

Image 150.2
This image depicts an adult female body louse, *Pediculus humanus,* and 2 larval young, which serve as the vector of epidemic typhus. Courtesy of Centers for Disease Control and Prevention/World Health Organization.

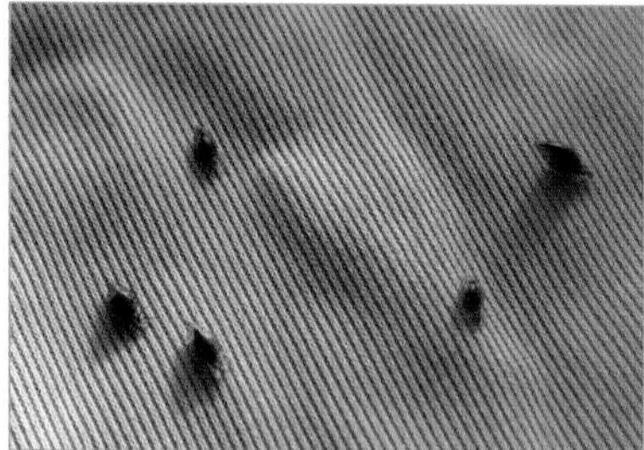

Image 150.3
Human body lice in clothes. Courtesy of Centers for Disease Control and Prevention/*Emerging Infectious Diseases* and Cédric Foucault.

151

Varicella-Zoster Virus Infections

Clinical Manifestations

Primary infection results in varicella (chickenpox), manifesting in unvaccinated people as a generalized, pruritic, vesicular rash typically consisting of 250 to 500 lesions in varying stages of development (papules, vesicles) and resolution (crusting), low-grade fever, and other systemic symptoms. Complications include bacterial superinfection of skin lesions with or without bacterial sepsis, pneumonia, central nervous system involvement (acute cerebellar ataxia, encephalitis, stroke/vasculopathy), thrombocytopenia, and other rare complications, such as glomerulonephritis, arthritis, and hepatitis. Primary viral pneumonia is not common among immunocompetent children but is the most common complication in adults. Varicella tends to be more severe in infants, adolescents, and adults than in children. Before the introduction of routine immunization against varicella in the United States, an average of 100 to 125 people died of chickenpox each year. Breakthrough varicella cases can occur in immunized children and are usually mild and clinically modified. Reye syndrome can follow cases of varicella, although this outcome has become rare since the recommendation not to use salicylate-containing compounds (eg, aspirin, bismuth-subsalicylate) for children during varicella illness. In immunocompromised children, progressive, severe varicella may occur with continuing eruption of lesions and high fever, persisting into the second week of illness, and visceral dissemination (ie, encephalitis, hepatitis, and pneumonia) can develop. Hemorrhagic varicella is more common among immunocompromised patients than among immunocompetent hosts. In children with HIV infection, recurrent varicella or disseminated herpes zoster can develop. Severe and even fatal varicella has been reported in otherwise healthy children receiving courses of high-dose corticosteroids (>2 mg/kg/d of prednisone or equivalent) for treatment of asthma and other illnesses. The risk is especially high when corticosteroids are given during the incubation period.

Varicella-zoster virus (VZV) establishes latency in sensory (dorsal root, cranial nerve, and autonomic, including enteric) ganglia during infection. Latency in sensory ganglia can occur as a result of primary infection with wild-type VZV in an unvaccinated individual or infection with wild-type VZV in a previously vaccinated individual or after vaccination with vaccine-strain VZV. Reactivation results in herpes zoster ("shingles"), characterized by grouped vesicular skin lesions in the distribution of 1 to 3 sensory dermatomes, frequently accompanied by pain or itching localized to the area. **Postherpetic neuralgia,** pain that persists after resolution of the zoster rash, can last for weeks to months. Childhood zoster tends to be milder than disease in adults and is rarely associated with postherpetic neuralgia. Zoster can occasionally become disseminated in immunocompromised patients, with lesions appearing outside the primary dermatomes and resulting in visceral complications. Varicella-zoster virus reactivation may occur less frequently in the absence of skin rash (zoster sine eruptione [or herpete]); these patients can present with aseptic meningitis or encephalitis as well as with gastrointestinal tract involvement. Visceral zoster can arise from reactivation of latent VZV in the enteric (gastrointestinal) nervous system. Some, but not all, of these patients may eventually develop a zosteriform skin rash.

The attenuated VZV in the varicella vaccine may establish latent infection and reactivate as herpes zoster. However, prelicensure data from immunocompromised children indicate risk of developing zoster is lower among vaccine recipients than among children who have experienced natural varicella. Postlicensure studies have also documented a lower risk of herpes zoster among healthy children who received varicella vaccines compared with unvaccinated children.

Fetal infection after maternal varicella during the first or early second trimester of pregnancy occasionally results in fetal death or varicella embryopathy, characterized by limb hypoplasia, cutaneous scarring, eye abnormalities, and damage to the central nervous system (congenital varicella syndrome). The incidence of congenital varicella syndrome among neonates born to mothers who experience gestational varicella is approximately 1% to 2% when infection occurs between 8 and 20 weeks of gestation. Rarely, cases of congenital varicella syndrome have been reported in neonates of women infected after 20 weeks' gestation, the latest occurring at 28 weeks. Children infected with VZV in utero can develop zoster early in life without having had extrauterine varicella. Varicella infection has a higher case-fatality rate in neonates when the mother develops varicella from 5 days before to 2 days after delivery because there is little opportunity for development and transfer of antibody from mother to neonate and the neonate's cellular immune system is immature. When varicella develops in a mother more than 5 days before delivery and gestation is 28 weeks or more, the severity of disease in the newborn is modified by transplacental transfer of VZV-specific maternal immunoglobulin (Ig) G antibody.

Etiology

Varicella-zoster virus (also known as human herpesvirus 3) is a member of the Herpesviridae family, the subfamily Alphaherpesvirinae, and the genus *Varicellovirus*.

Epidemiology

Humans are the only source of infection for this highly contagious virus. Humans are infected when the virus comes in contact with the mucosa of the upper respiratory tract or the conjunctiva of a susceptible person. Person-to-person transmission occurs by the airborne route and from direct contact with patients with vesicular VZV lesions (varicella and herpes zoster); vesicles contain infectious virus that can be aerosolized. Skin lesions appear to be the major source of transmissible VZV; transmission from infected respiratory tract secretions is possible but probably less common than from skin vesicles. There is no evidence of VZV spread from fomites; the virus is extremely labile and is unable to survive for long in the environment. In utero infection occurs as a result of transplacental passage of virus during maternal VZV viremia. Varicella-zoster virus infection in a household member usually results in infection of almost all susceptible people in that household. Children who acquire their infection at home (secondary family cases) often have more skin lesions than the index case. Health care–associated transmission is well-documented in pediatric units, but transmission is rare in newborn nurseries.

In temperate climates in the prevaccine era, varicella was a childhood disease with a marked seasonal distribution, with peak incidence during late winter and early spring and among children younger than 10 years. High rates of vaccine coverage in the United States have effectively eliminated discernible seasonality of varicella. In tropical climates, the epidemiology of varicella is different; acquisition of disease occurs at later ages, resulting in a higher proportion of adults being susceptible to varicella. Following implementation of universal immunization in the United States in 1995, varicella declined in all age groups, resulting in herd protection. In areas with active surveillance and with high vaccine coverage, the rate of varicella disease decreased by approximately 90% between 1995 and 2005. Since recommendation of a routine second dose of vaccine in 2006, the incidence of varicella has declined further. The age of peak varicella incidence is shifting from children younger than 10 years to children 10 through 14 years of age, although the incidence in this and all age groups is lower than in the prevaccine era. Immunity to varicella generally is lifelong. Cellular immunity is more important than humoral immunity for limiting the extent of primary infection with VZV and for preventing reactivation of virus with herpes zoster. Symptomatic reinfection is uncommon in immunocompetent people, in whom asymptomatic reinfection is more frequent. Asymptomatic primary infection is unusual.

Since 2007, coverage with 1 or more doses of varicella vaccine among 19- through 35-month-old children in the United States has been greater than 90%. As of 2013, more than 78% of 13- to 17-year-olds have received 2 doses of varicella vaccine. This should not be confused as evidence of an increasing rate of breakthrough disease or vaccine failure.

Immunocompromised people with primary (varicella) or recurrent (herpes zoster) infection are at increased risk of severe disease.

Severe varicella and disseminated zoster are more likely to develop in children with congenital T-lymphocyte defects or AIDS than in people with B-lymphocyte abnormalities. Other groups of pediatric patients who can experience more severe or complicated disease include infants, adolescents, patients with chronic cutaneous or pulmonary disorders, and patients receiving systemic corticosteroids, other immunosuppressive therapy, or long-term salicylate therapy.

Patients are contagious from 1 to 2 days before onset of the rash until all lesions have crusted.

Incubation Period

14 to 16 days (range, 10–21 days) after exposure to rash. The incubation period can be prolonged for up to 28 days after receipt of varicella-zoster immune globulin or intravenous immunoglobulin. Varicella can develop between 2 and 16 days after birth in neonates born to mothers with active varicella.

Diagnostic Tests

Diagnostic tests for VZV are summarized in Table 151.1. Vesicular fluid or a scab can be used to identify VZV using a polymerase chain reaction (PCR) assay test, which is currently the diagnostic method of choice. This testing can be used to distinguish between wild-type and vaccine-strain VZV (genotyping). During the acute phase of illness, VZV can also be identified by PCR assay of saliva or buccal swabs, from unimmunized and immunized patients, although VZV is more likely to be detected in vesicular fluid or scabs. Varicella-zoster virus can be demonstrated by direct fluorescent antibody assay, using scrapings of a vesicle base during the first 3 to 4 days of the eruption or by viral isolation in cell culture from vesicular fluid. Viral culture and direct fluorescent antibody assay are less sensitive than PCR assay, and neither test has the capacity to distinguish vaccine-strain from wild-type viruses. A significant increase in serum

Table 151.1
Diagnostic Tests for Varicella-Zoster Virus Infection

Test	Specimen	Comments
PCR	Vesicular swabs or scrapings, scabs from crusted lesions, biopsy tissue, CSF	Very sensitive method. Specific for VZV. Methods have been designed that distinguish vaccine strain from wild-type (see text).
DFA	Vesicle scraping, swab of lesion base (must include cells)	Specific for VZV. More rapid and more sensitive than culture, less sensitive than PCR.
Viral culture	Vesicular fluid, CSF, biopsy tissue	Distinguishes VZV from herpes simplex. Cost, limited availability, requires up to a week for result. Least sensitive method.
Tzanck test	Vesicle scraping, swab of lesion base (must include cells)	Observe multinucleated giant cells with inclusions. Not specific for VZV. Less sensitive and accurate than DFA.
Serology (IgG)	Acute and convalescent serum specimens for IgG	Specific for VZV. Commercial assays generally have low sensitivity to reliably detect vaccine-induced immunity. gpELISA and FAMA are the only IgG methods that can readily detect vaccine seroconversion, but these tests are not commercially available.
Capture IgM	Acute serum specimens for IgM	Specific for VZV. IgM inconsistently detected. Not reliable method for routine confirmation, but positive result indicates current/recent VZV activity. Requires special equipment.

Abbreviations: CSF, cerebrospinal fluid; DFA, direct fluorescent antibody; FAMA, fluorescent antibody to membrane antigen (assay); gpELISA, glycoprotein enzyme-linked immunoassay; IgG, immunoglobulin G; IgM, immunoglobulin M; PCR, polymerase chain reaction; VZV, varicella-zoster virus.

varicella IgG antibody between acute and convalescent samples by any standard serologic assay can confirm a diagnosis retrospectively. These antibody tests are reliable for diagnosing natural infection in healthy hosts but may not be reliable in immunocompromised people. However, diagnosis of VZV infection by serologic testing is seldom necessary. Commercially available enzyme immunoassay tests usually are not sufficiently sensitive to reliably demonstrate a vaccine-induced antibody response; routine postvaccination serologic testing is not recommended. IgM tests are not reliable for routine confirmation or ruling out of acute infection. All VZV IgM assays are prone to false-positive results, but in the presence of a rash, positive results can indicate current or recent VZV infection or reactivation.

Treatment

The decision to use antiviral therapy and the route and duration of therapy should be determined by specific host factors, extent of infection, and initial response to therapy. Antiviral drugs have a limited window of opportunity to affect the outcome of VZV infection. In immunocompetent hosts, most virus replication has stopped by 72 hours after onset of rash; the duration of replication may be extended in immunocompromised hosts. Oral acyclovir or valacyclovir is not recommended for routine use in otherwise healthy children with varicella. Administration within 24 hours of onset of rash in healthy children results in only a modest decrease in symptoms. Oral acyclovir or valacyclovir should be considered for otherwise healthy people at increased risk of moderate to severe varicella, such as unvaccinated people older than 12 years, people with chronic cutaneous or pulmonary disorders, people receiving long-term salicylate therapy, and people receiving short, intermittent, or aerosolized courses of corticosteroids. Some experts also recommend use of oral acyclovir or valacyclovir for secondary household cases in which the disease is usually more severe than in the primary case.

Some experts recommend oral acyclovir or valacyclovir for pregnant women with varicella, especially during the second and third trimesters. Intravenous acyclovir is recommended for the pregnant patient with serious complications of varicella.

Intravenous acyclovir therapy is recommended for immunocompromised patients, including patients being treated with high-dose corticosteroid therapy for more than 14 days. Therapy initiated early in the course of the illness, especially within 24 hours of rash onset, maximizes benefit. Oral acyclovir should not be used to treat immunocompromised children with varicella because of poor oral bioavailability. Some experts have used valacyclovir, with its improved bioavailability compared with oral acyclovir, in selected immunocompromised patients perceived to be at low to moderate risk of developing severe varicella, such as HIV-infected patients with relatively normal numbers of $CD4^+$ T lymphocytes and children with leukemia in whom careful follow-up is ensured. Famciclovir is available for treatment of VZV infections in adults, but its efficacy and safety have not been established for children. Although VariZIG or, if not available, intravenous immunoglobulin given shortly after exposure can prevent or modify the course of disease, immunoglobulin preparations are not effective treatment once disease is established.

Infections caused by acyclovir-resistant VZV strains, which are generally rare and limited to immunocompromised hosts, should be treated with parenteral foscarnet.

Children with varicella should not receive salicylates or salicylate-containing products because administration of salicylates to such children increases the risk of Reye syndrome. Salicylate therapy should be stopped in an unimmunized child who is exposed to varicella.

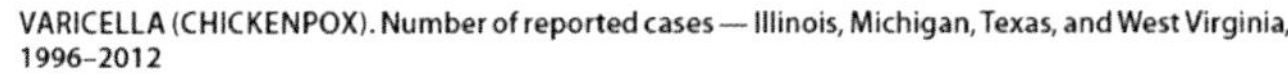
VARICELLA (CHICKENPOX). Number of reported cases — Illinois, Michigan, Texas, and West Virginia, 1996–2012

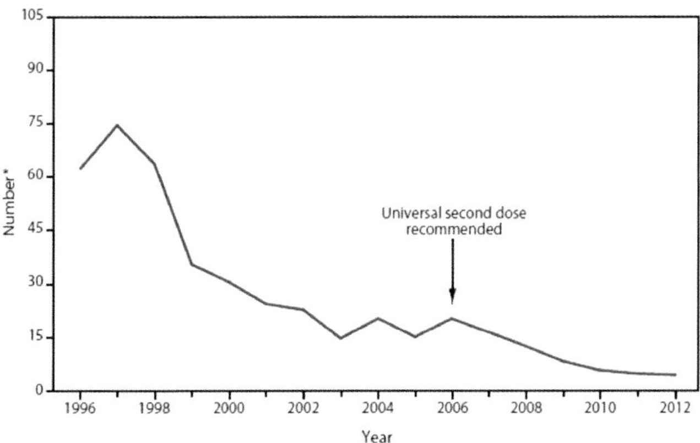

* In thousands.

Varicella was not nationally notifiable in 1996, when the first dose of the varicella vaccine was recommended in the United States. However, four states (Michigan, Illinois, Texas, and Virginia) were reporting varicella cases to CDC before the varicella vaccine was recommended and have continued reporting, providing consistent data to allow for monitoring of trends in varicella disease. In these four states, the number of cases reported in 2012 was 8% lower than 2011 and 94% less than the average number reported during the pre-vaccine years (1993–1995).

Image 151.1
Varicella (chickenpox). Number of reported cases—Illinois, Michigan, Texas, and West Virginia, 1996–2012. Courtesy of *Morbidity and Mortality Weekly Report.*

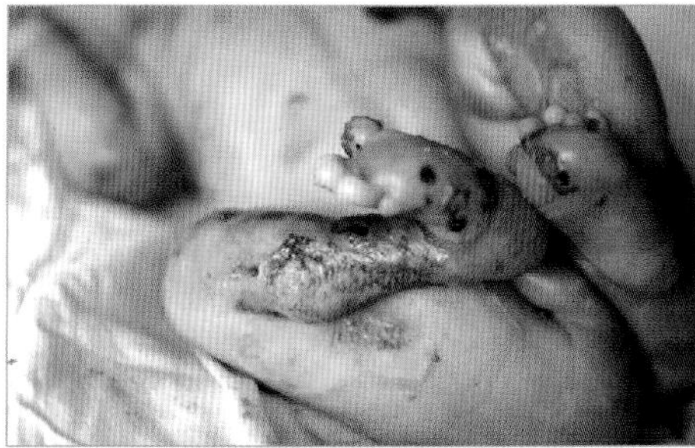

Image 151.2
Congenital varicella with short-limb syndrome and scarring of the skin. The mother had varicella during the first trimester of pregnancy. Copyright David Clark, MD.

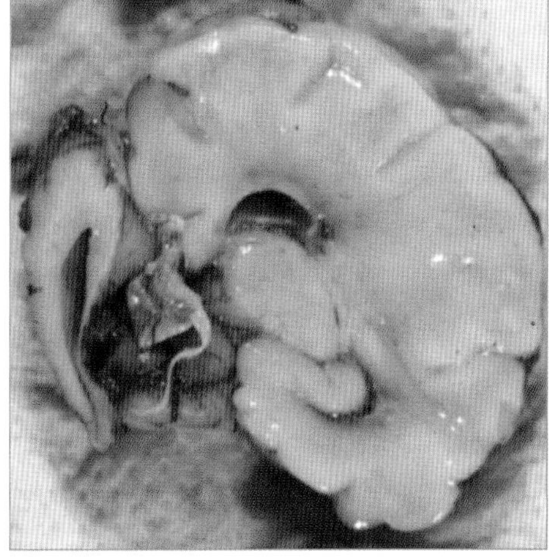

Image 151.3
Varicella embryopathy with involvement of the brain. Atrophy of the left cerebral hemisphere. Courtesy of Dimitris P. Agamanolis, MD.

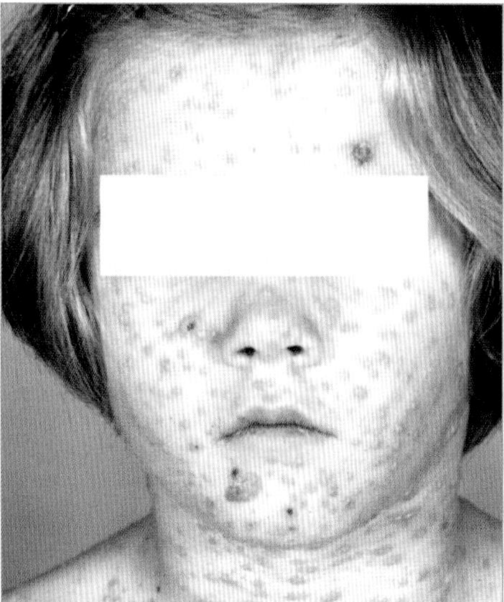

Image 151.4
School-aged girl with varicella who acquired it from a younger sibling, who had a more mild clinical course with fewer lesions.

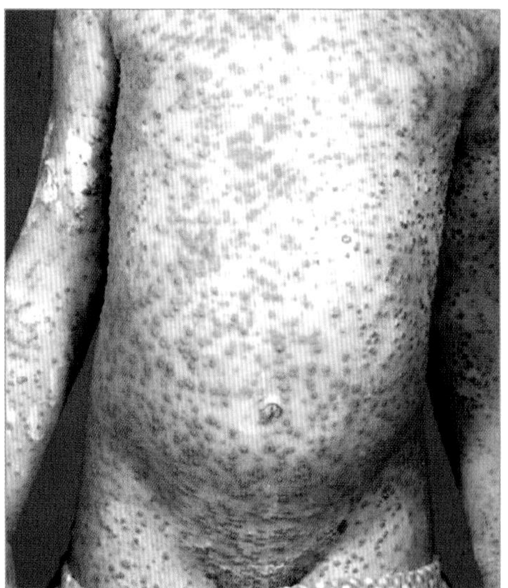

Image 151.6
School-aged child with varicella who acquired it from a younger sibling. This is the same child as in images 151.4 and 151.5 who had calamine lotion applied by the parents for itching. She recovered without incident.

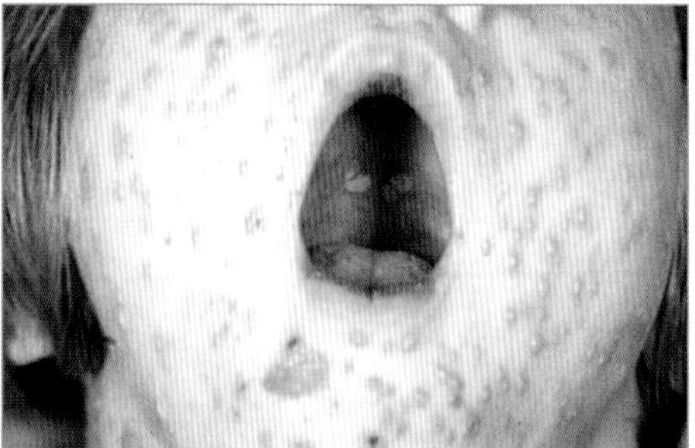

Image 151.5
This child acquired her infection from a younger sibling. Varicella lesions are apparent on the palate. This is the same child as in Image 151.4.

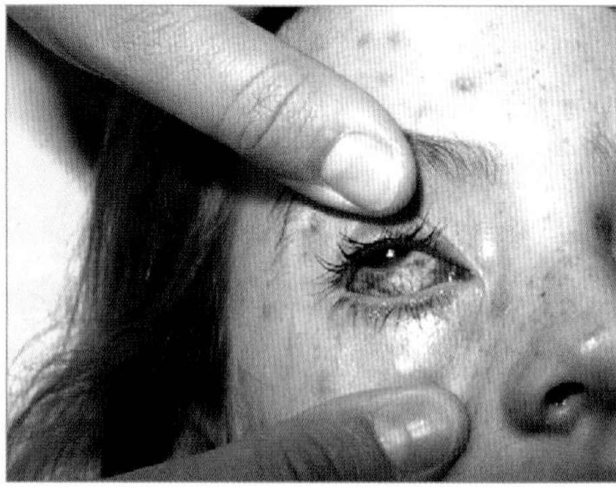

Image 151.7
Varicella with scleral lesions and bulbar conjunctivitis.

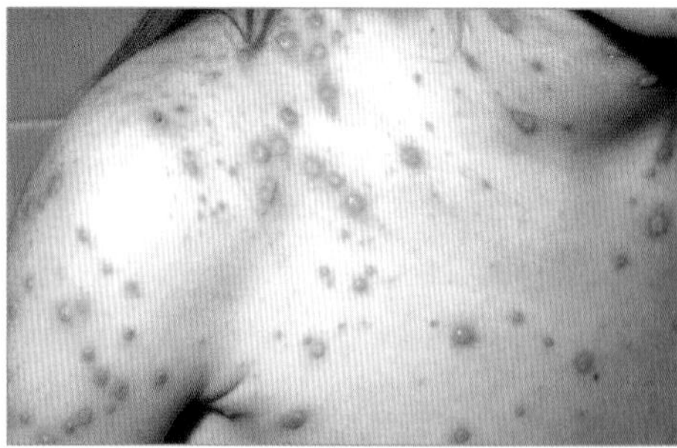

Image 151.8
An adolescent white girl with varicella lesions in various stages. This is the same patient as in Image 151.7.

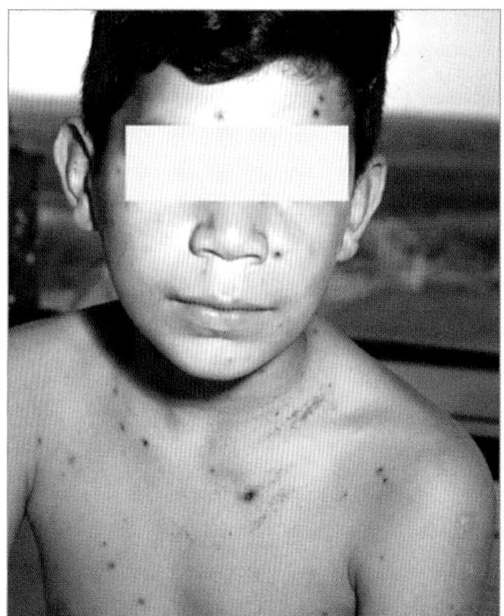

Image 151.9
Varicella with secondary thrombocytopenic purpura.

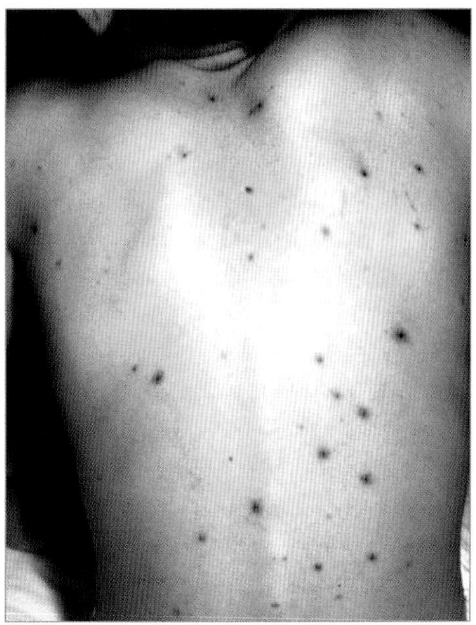

Image 151.10
Varicella with secondary thrombocytopenic purpura in the same Latin American child as in Image 151.9.

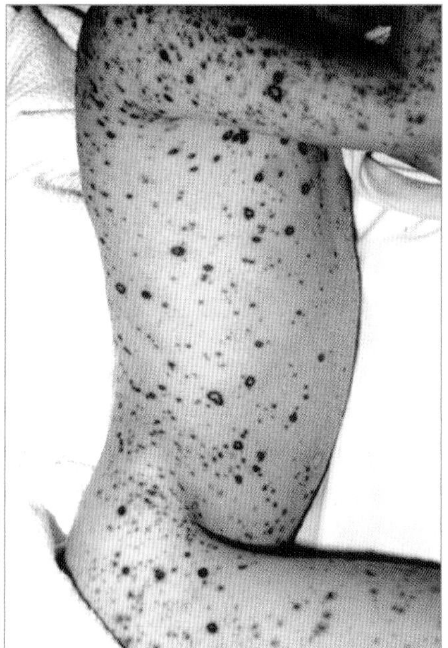

Image 151.11
Hemorrhagic varicella in a 6-year-old white boy with eczema.

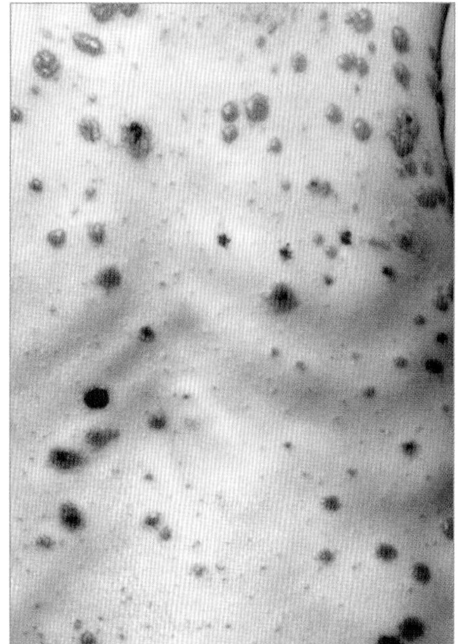

Image 151.12
Hemorrhagic, disseminated, and fatal varicella with lesions over the anterior chest of a 7-month-old. Courtesy of David Ascher, MD/Howard Johnson, MD.

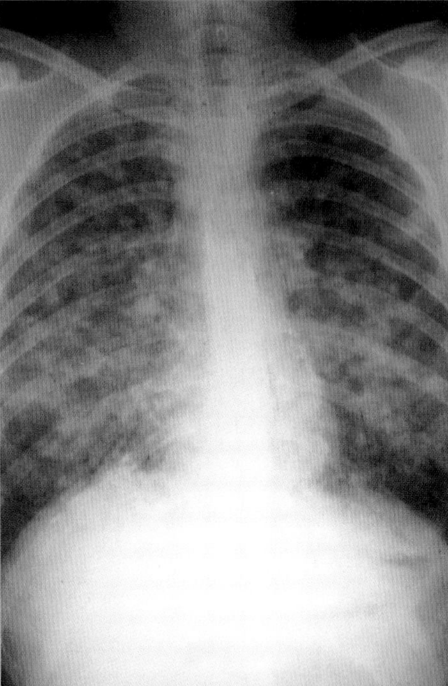

Image 151.13
Diffuse varicella pneumonia bilaterally shown in the chest radiograph of a patient with Hodgkin disease. Courtesy of George Nankervis, MD.

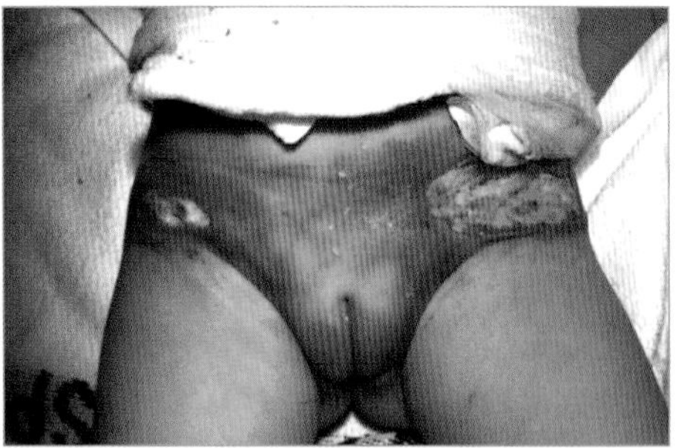

Image 151.15
Varicella and necrotizing fasciitis in a patient shortly after surgical debridement.

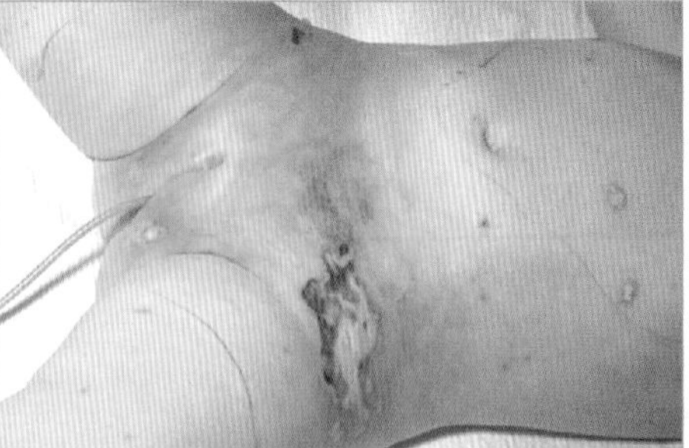

Image 151.14
Varicella complicated by necrotizing fasciitis. A blood culture result was positive for group A *Streptococcus*. The disease responded to antibiotics and surgical debridement followed by primary surgical closure.

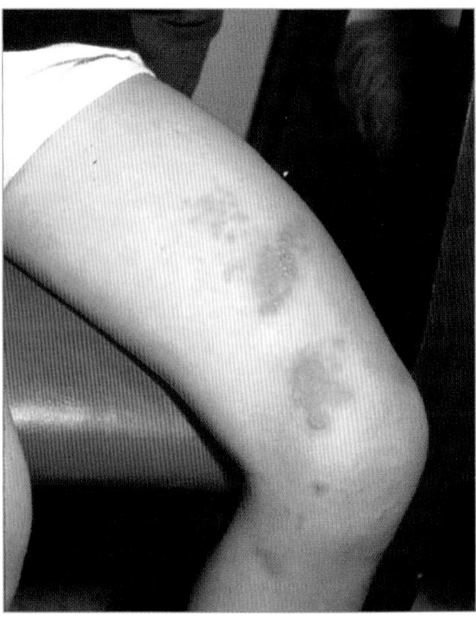

Image 151.16
Herpes zoster lesions in an otherwise healthy child. The lesions were not particularly painful, as is often the case for immunocompetent children with herpes zoster, particularly in the absence of trigeminal nerve involvement.

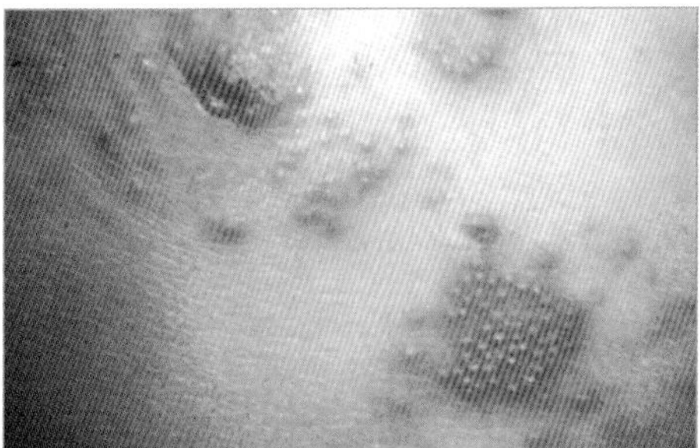

Image 151.17
Close-up of the varicella-zoster lesions of the patient in Image 151.16.

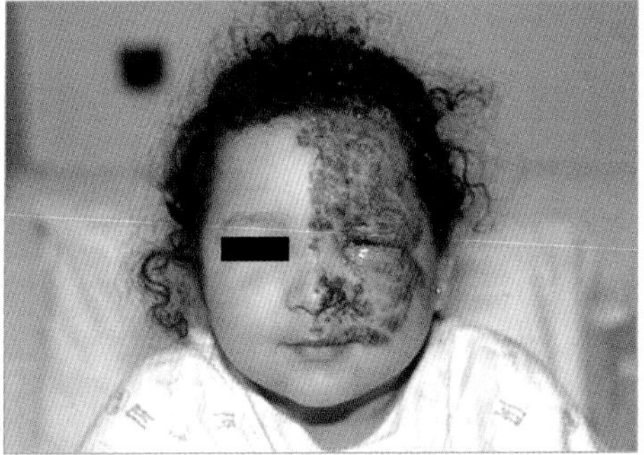

Image 151.19
Varicella zoster in a 7-year-old girl. The patient had an erythematous vesicular skin rash on the face on first examination. The dermatologic distribution suggested the diagnosis of herpes zoster. This image was taken 3 days after acyclovir therapy was initiated. The lesions were crusting. The child had no prior history of recurring infections and was growing well. Copyright Barbara Jantausch, MD, FAAP.

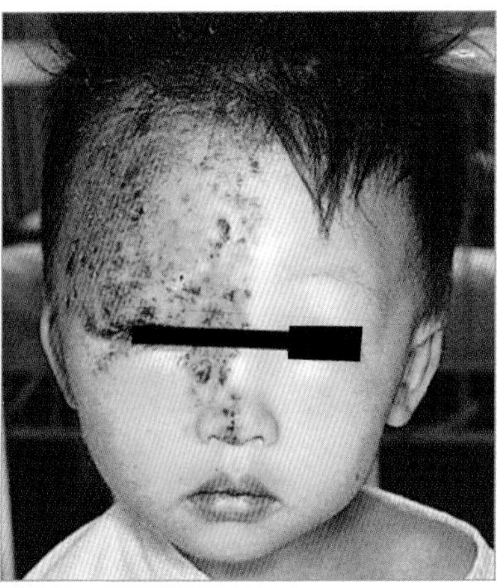

Image 151.21
Herpes zoster (shingles). Courtesy of C. W. Leung.

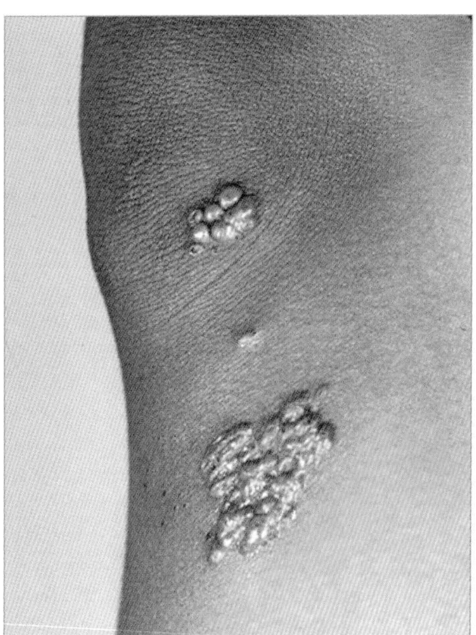

Image 151.18
Herpes zoster in an otherwise healthy child.

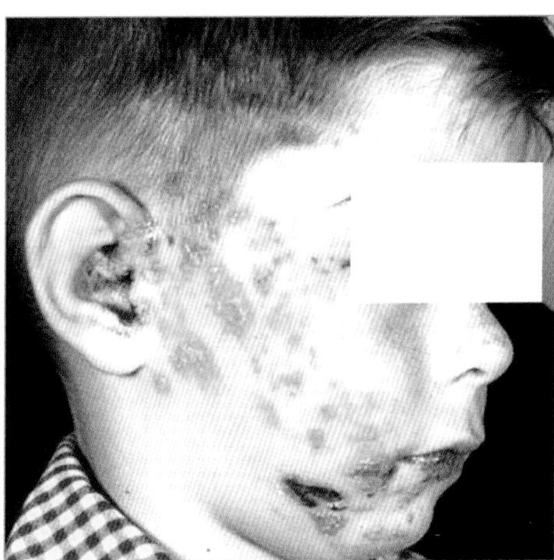

Image 151.20
Herpes zoster. Trigeminal nerve involvement. There may be significant pain associated with lesions in the trigeminal nerve distribution. Courtesy of David Ascher, MD/Howard Johnson, MD.

152

Vibrio *Infections*

Cholera

(*Vibrio cholerae*)

Clinical Manifestations

Cholera is characterized by voluminous watery diarrhea and rapid onset of life-threatening dehydration. Hypovolemic shock can occur within hours of the onset of diarrhea. Stools have a characteristic rice-water appearance, are white-tinged, and contain small flecks of mucus and high concentrations of sodium, potassium, chloride, and bicarbonate. Vomiting is a common feature of cholera. Fever and abdominal cramps are usually absent. In addition to dehydration and hypovolemia, common complications of cholera include hypokalemia, metabolic acidosis, and hypoglycemia, particularly in children. Although severe cholera is a distinctive illness characterized by profuse diarrhea and rapid dehydration, most people infected with toxigenic *Vibrio cholerae* O1 have no symptoms or mild to moderate diarrhea lasting 3 to 7 days.

Etiology

V cholerae is a curved or comma-shaped, motile, gram-negative rod. There are more than 200 *V cholerae* serogroups, some of which carry the cholera toxin gene. Although those serogroups with the cholera toxin gene and others without the cholera toxin gene can cause acute watery diarrhea, only toxin-producing serogroups O1 and O139 cause epidemic cholera, with O1 causing the vast majority of cases of cholera. *V cholerae* O1 is classified into 2 biotypes, classical and *V cholerae* biovar El Tor, and 2 major serotypes, Ogawa and Inaba. Since 1992, toxigenic *V cholerae* serogroup O139 has been recognized as a cause of epidemic cholera in Asia. Aside from the substitution of the O139 for the O1 antigen, the organism is almost identical to *V cholerae* O1 biovar El Tor. All other serogroups of *V cholerae* are collectively known as *V cholerae* non-O1/non-O139. Toxin-producing strains of *V cholerae* non-O1/non-O139 can cause sporadic cases of severe dehydrating diarrheal illness but have not caused large outbreaks of epidemic cholera. Nontoxin-producing strains of *V cholerae* non-O1/non-O139 are associated with sporadic cases of gastroenteritis, sepsis, and rare cases of wound infection.

Epidemiology

Since the early 1800s, there have been 7 cholera pandemics. The current pandemic began in 1961 and is caused by *V cholerae* O1 biovar El Tor. Molecular epidemiology shows this pandemic has occurred in 3 successive waves, with each one spreading from South Asia to other regions in Asia, Africa, and the Western Pacific Islands (Oceania). In 1991, epidemic cholera caused by toxigenic *V cholerae* O1 biovar El Tor appeared in Peru and spread to most countries in South, Central, and North America, causing more than 1 million cases of cholera before subsiding. In 2010, *V cholerae* O1 biovar El Tor was introduced into Haiti, initiating a massive epidemic of cholera. In the United States, sporadic cases resulting from travel to or ingestion of contaminated food transported from regions with endemic cholera are reported, including several cases imported from Hispaniola since 2010.

Humans are the only documented natural host, but free-living *V cholerae* organisms can persist in the aquatic environment. Infection is primarily acquired by ingestion of large numbers of organisms from contaminated water or food (particularly raw or undercooked shellfish, raw or partially dried fish, or moist grains or vegetables held at ambient temperature). People with low gastric acidity and with blood group O are at increased risk of severe cholera infection.

Incubation Period

1 to 3 days (range, few hours to 5 days).

Diagnostic Tests

V cholerae can be cultured from fecal specimens (preferred) or vomitus plated on thiosulfate citrate–bile salts–sucrose agar. Because most laboratories in the United States do not culture routinely for *V cholerae* or other *Vibrio* organisms, clinicians should request appropriate cultures for clinically suspected cases. Isolates of *V cholerae* should be sent to a state health department laboratory for confirmation and then forwarded to the Centers for Disease Control and Prevention for confirmation, serogrouping, and detection of the cholera toxin gene. Tests to detect serum antibodies to *V cholerae,* such as the vibriocidal assay and an anticholera toxin enzyme-linked immunoassay, are available at the Centers for Disease Control and Prevention. Both assays require submission of acute and convalescent serum specimens. A 4-fold increase in vibriocidal or anticholera toxin antibody titers between acute and convalescent sera suggests the diagnosis of cholera. Several commercial tests for rapid antigen detection of *V cholerae* O1 and O139 in stool specimens have been developed. These *V cholerae* O1 and O139 rapid diagnostic tests have sensitivities ranging from approximately 80% to 97% and specificities of approximately 70% to 90%. Rapid diagnostic tests are not a substitute for stool culture but potentially provide a rapid presumptive indication of a suspect cholera outbreak in regions where stool culture is not immediately available.

Treatment

Appropriate rehydration therapy is the cornerstone of management of cholera and reduces the mortality of severe cholera to less than 0.5%. Rehydration therapy should be based on World Health Organization standards, with the goal of replacing the estimated fluid deficit within 3 to 4 hours of initial presentation. In patients with severe dehydration, isotonic intravenous fluids should be used, and lactated Ringer injection is the widely preferred option. For patients without severe dehydration, oral rehydration therapy using World Health Organization reduced-osmolality oral rehydration solution (ORS) has been the standard, but data suggest rice-based ORS or amylase-resistant starch ORS is more effective.

Prompt initiation of antimicrobial therapy decreases the duration and volume of diarrhea and shedding of viable bacteria. Antimicrobial therapy should be considered for people who are moderately to severely ill. The choice of antimicrobial therapy should be made on the basis of the age of the patient as well as prevailing patterns of antimicrobial resistance. In cases in which prevailing patterns of resistance are unknown, antimicrobial susceptibility testing should be performed and monitored.

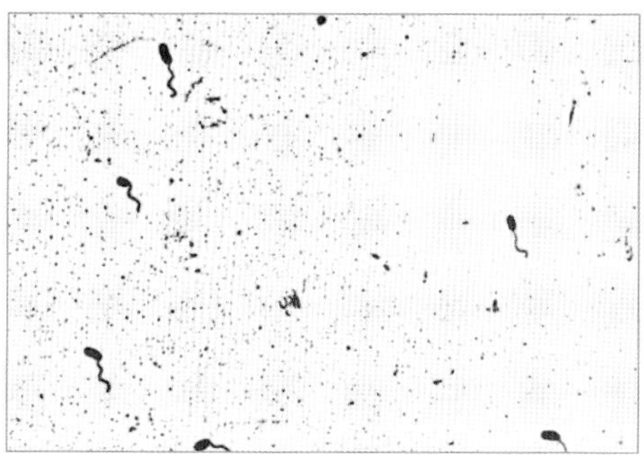

Image 152.1
Vibrio cholerae (Leifson flagella stain, digitally colorized). Courtesy of Centers for Disease Control and Prevention/Dr William A. Clark.

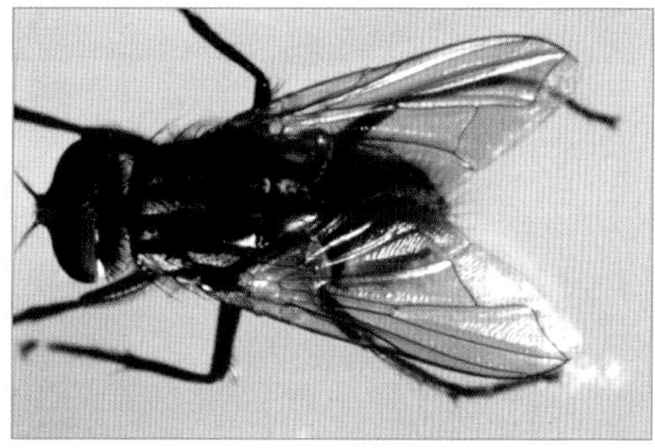

Image 152.2
This fly, *Musca domestica,* was photographed during a 1972 study of disease carriers and pests of migrant labor camps. Annoying houseflies may spread typhoid, cholera, dysentery, and diarrhea. They can carry these disease-causing organisms from garbage, sewage, and fecal matter to food or to a person's hands or lips. Courtesy of Centers for Disease Control and Prevention.

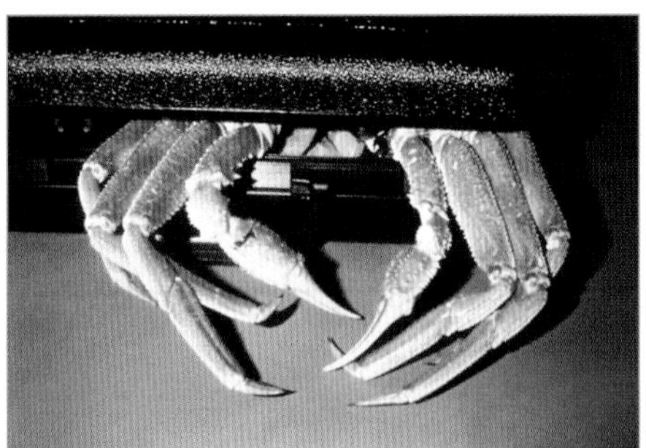

Image 152.3
In 1991, 17 persons in the United States were infected with *Vibrio cholerae* related to travel to Latin America. Of these, only 6 had actually traveled there (1 to Peru, 1 to Columbia, and 4 to Ecuador). The other 11 were family members in the United States who ate crab brought back from Latin America in the 4 travelers' suitcases. Courtesy of Centers for Disease Control and Prevention.

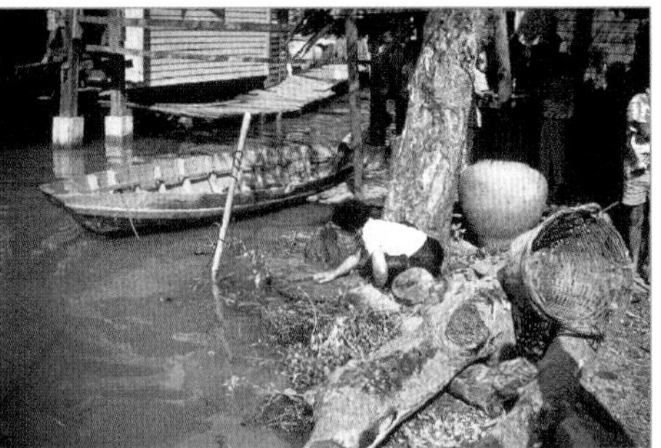

Image 152.4
Typical *Vibrio cholerae*–contaminated water supply. Ingestion of *V cholerae*–contaminated water is a typical mode of pathogen transmission. Courtesy of Centers for Disease Control and Prevention.

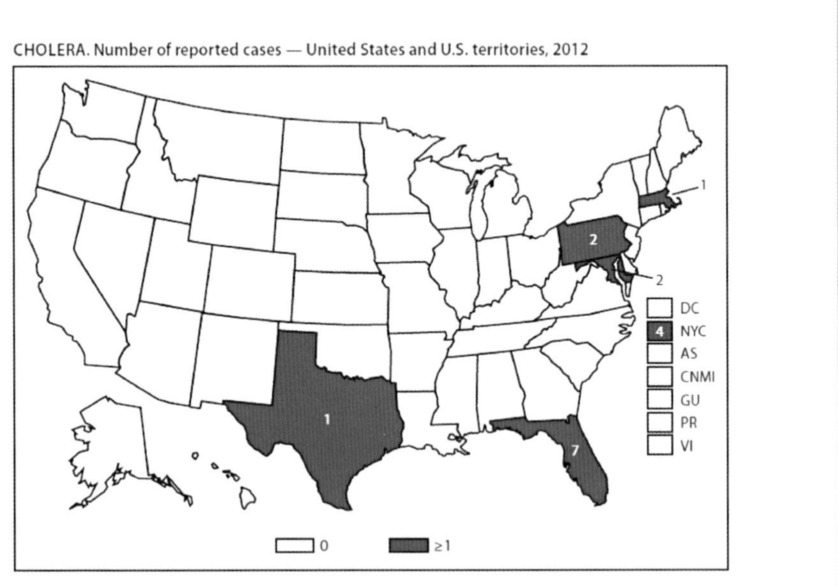

Image 152.5
Number of reported cases—United States and US territories, 2012. Courtesy of *Morbidity and Mortality Weekly Report.*

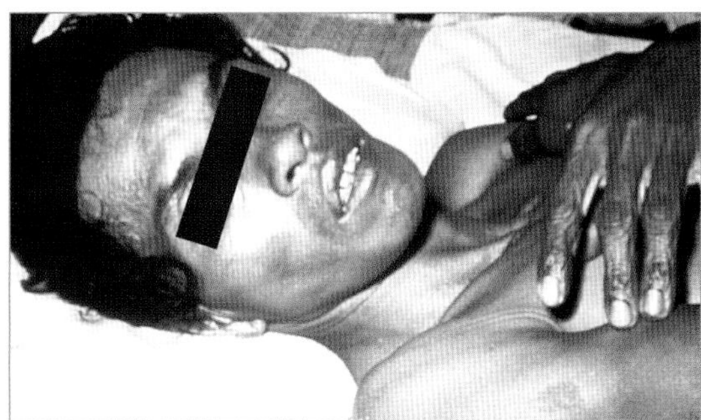

Image 152.6
An adult cholera patient with "washerwoman's hand" sign. Due to severe dehydration, cholera manifests itself in decreased skin turgor, which produces the so-called washerwoman's hand sign. Courtesy of Centers for Disease Control and Prevention.

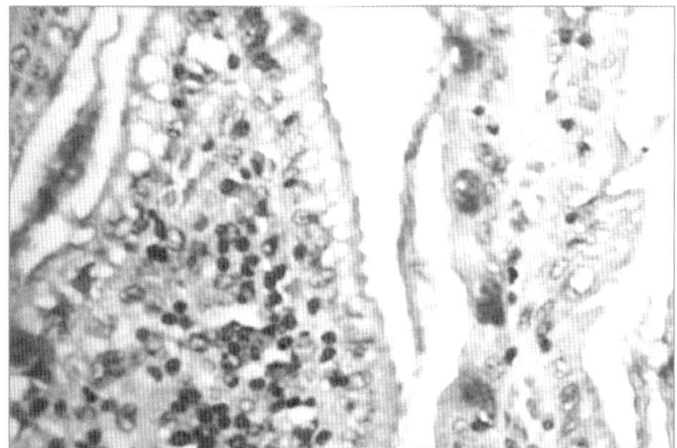

Image 152.7
Intestinal biopsy showing *Vibrio cholerae* causing increased mucus production. *V cholerae* is transmitted to humans through the ingestion of contaminated food or water and produces a cholera toxin that acts on the intestinal mucosa and causes severe diarrhea. Courtesy of Centers for Disease Control and Prevention.

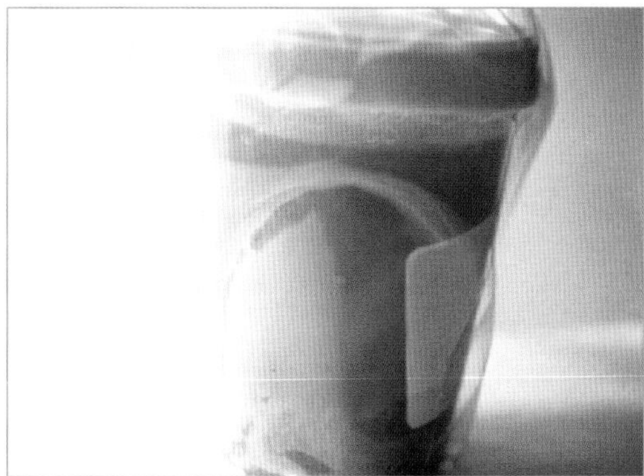

Image 152.8
Here, a cup of typical rice-water stool from a cholera patient shows flecks of mucus that have settled to the bottom. These stools are inoffensive, with a faint fishy odor. They are isotonic with plasma and contain high levels of sodium, potassium, and bicarbonate. They also contain extraordinary quantities of *Vibrio cholerae* bacterial organisms. Courtesy of Centers for Disease Control and Prevention.

153

Other *Vibrio* Infections

Clinical Manifestations

Illnesses attributable to nontoxigenic species of the Vibrionaceae family are considered vibriosis. This includes infections attributable to toxigenic *Vibrio cholerae* O75 and O141, nontoxigenic *V cholerae* O1, members of the Vibrionaceae family that are not in the genus *Vibrio* (eg, *Grimontia hollisae*), and other *Vibrio* species. Associated clinical syndromes include gastroenteritis, wound infection, and septicemia. Gastroenteritis is the most common syndrome and is characterized by acute onset of watery stools and crampy abdominal pain. Approximately half of those afflicted will have low-grade fever, headache, and chills; approximately 30% will have vomiting. Spontaneous recovery follows in 2 to 5 days. Primary septicemia is uncommon but can develop in immunocompromised people with preceding gastroenteritis or wound infection. Wound infections can be severe in people with liver disease or who are immunocompromised. Septicemia and hemorrhagic bullous or necrotic skin lesions can be seen in people with infections caused by *Vibrio vulnificus,* with associated high morbidity and mortality rates.

Etiology

Vibrio organisms are facultatively anaerobic, motile, gram-negative bacilli that are tolerant of salt. The most commonly reported nontoxigenic *Vibrio* species associated with diarrhea are *Vibrio parahaemolyticus* and *V cholerae* non-O1/non-O139. *V vulnificus* typically causes primary septicemia and severe wound infections; the other species can also cause these syndromes. *Vibrio alginolyticus* typically causes wound infections.

Epidemiology

Vibrio species are natural inhabitants of marine and estuarine environments. In temperate climates, most noncholera *Vibrio* infections occur during summer and autumn months, when *Vibrio* populations in seawater are highest. Gastroenteritis usually follows ingestion of raw or undercooked seafood, especially oysters, clams, crabs, and shrimp. Wound infections can result from exposure of a preexisting wound to contaminated seawater or from punctures resulting from handling of contaminated shellfish. Exposure to contaminated water during natural disasters, such as hurricanes, has resulted in wound infections. Person-to-person transmission of infection has not been reported. People with liver disease, low gastric acidity, and immunodeficiency have increased susceptibility to infection with *Vibrio* species. Infections associated with noncholera *Vibrio* organisms became nationally notifiable in January 2007.

Incubation Period

Gastroenteritis, typically 24 hours (range, 5–92 hours).

Diagnostic Tests

Vibrio organisms can be isolated from stool of patients with gastroenteritis, from blood specimens, and from wound exudates. Extraintestinal specimens can be cultured according to standard laboratory practice because *Vibrio* species grow well on most nonselective plating media with sodium chloride, such as blood or chocolate agar. Because identification of the organism requires special techniques, laboratory personnel should be notified when infection with *Vibrio* species is suspected.

Treatment

Most episodes of diarrhea are mild and self-limited and do not require treatment other than oral rehydration. Antimicrobial therapy can benefit people with severe diarrhea, wound infection, or septicemia. Septicemia with or without hemorrhagic bullae should be treated with a third-generation cephalosporin plus doxycycline. In children younger than 8 years, a combination of trimethoprim-sulfamethoxazole and an aminoglycoside is an alternative regimen. Wound infections require surgical debridement of necrotic tissue, if present.

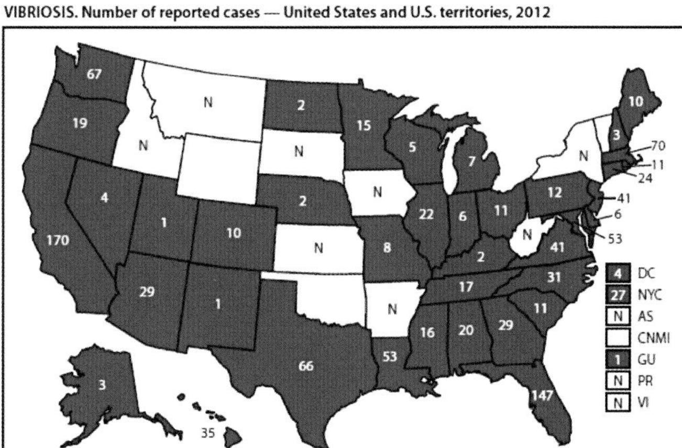

Consumption of raw or undercooked seafood, especially molluscan shellfish, remains a major risk factor for foodborne vibriosis (infection caused by a species from the family *Vibrionaceae* other than toxigenic *Vibrio cholerae* O1 or O139). In 2012, a multistate outbreak of *Vibrio parahaemolyticus* infections of a serotype previously only associated in the United States with shellfish from the Pacific Northwest was associated with consumption of shellfish harvested from Oyster Bay Harbor, New York.

Image 153.1
Vibriosis. Number of reported cases—United States and US territories, 2012. Courtesy of *Morbidity and Mortality Weekly Report.*

154

West Nile Virus

Clinical Manifestations

An estimated 70% to 80% of people infected with West Nile virus (WNV) are asymptomatic. Most symptomatic people experience an acute systemic febrile illness that often includes headache, myalgia, or arthralgia; gastrointestinal tract symptoms and a transient maculopapular rash are also commonly reported. Fewer than 1% of infected people develop neuroinvasive disease, which typically manifests as meningitis, encephalitis, or acute flaccid paralysis. West Nile virus meningitis is indistinguishable clinically from aseptic meningitis caused by most other viruses. Patients with WNV encephalitis usually present with seizures, mental status changes, focal neurologic deficits, or movement disorders. West Nile virus acute flaccid paralysis is often clinically and pathologically identical to poliovirus-associated poliomyelitis, with damage of anterior horn cells, and may progress to respiratory paralysis requiring mechanical ventilation. West Nile virus–associated Guillain-Barré syndrome has also been reported and can be distinguished from WNV acute flaccid paralysis by clinical manifestations and electrophysiologic testing. Cardiac dysrhythmias, myocarditis, rhabdomyolysis, optic neuritis, uveitis, chorioretinitis, orchitis, pancreatitis, and hepatitis have been described rarely after WNV infection.

Routine clinical laboratory results are generally nonspecific in WNV infections. In patients with neuroinvasive disease, cerebrospinal fluid (CSF) examination generally shows lymphocytic pleocytosis, but neutrophils can predominate early in the illness. Brain magnetic resonance imaging is frequently normal, but signal abnormalities may be seen in the basal ganglia, thalamus, and brainstem with WNV encephalitis and in the spinal cord with WNV acute flaccid paralysis.

Most patients with WNV nonneuroinvasive disease or meningitis recover completely, but fatigue, malaise, and weakness can linger for weeks or months. Patients who recover from WNV encephalitis or acute flaccid paralysis often have residual neurologic deficits. Among patients with neuroinvasive disease, the overall case-fatality rate is approximately 10% but is significantly higher in WNV encephalitis and myelitis than in WNV meningitis.

Most women known to have been infected with WNV during pregnancy have delivered neonates without evidence of infection or clinical abnormalities. In the single known instance of confirmed congenital WNV infection, the mother developed WNV encephalitis at 27 weeks' gestation, and the neonate was born with cystic destruction of cerebral tissue and chorioretinitis. If WNV disease is diagnosed during pregnancy, a detailed examination of the fetus and of the newborn should be performed.

Etiology

West Nile virus is an RNA virus of the Flaviviridae family (genus *Flavivirus*) that is related antigenically to St. Louis encephalitis and Japanese encephalitis viruses.

Epidemiology

West Nile virus is an arthropodborne virus (arbovirus) that is transmitted in an enzootic cycle between mosquitoes and amplifying vertebrate hosts, primarily birds. West Nile virus is transmitted to humans primarily through bites of infected *Culex* mosquitoes. Humans usually do not develop a level or duration of viremia sufficient to infect mosquitoes. Therefore, humans are dead-end hosts. However, person-to-person WNV transmission can occur through blood transfusion and solid organ transplantation. Intrauterine and probable breastfeeding transmission is rare. Transmission through percutaneous and mucosal exposure has occurred in laboratory workers and occupational settings.

West Nile virus transmission has been documented on every continent except Antarctica. Since the 1990s, the largest outbreaks of WNV neuroinvasive disease have occurred in the Middle East, Europe, and North America. West Nile virus was first detected in the western hemisphere in New York, NY, in 1999 and subsequently spread across the continental

United States and Canada. From 1999 through 2012, 16,196 cases of WNV neuroinvasive disease were reported in the United States, including 605 (4%) among children younger than 18 years. The national incidence of WNV neuroinvasive disease peaked in 2002 (1.02 per 100,000) and 2003 (0.98). During 2004 through 2011, annual incidence was relatively low (median, 0.31; range, 0.13–0.50), but in 2012, the national incidence of WNV neuroinvasive disease increased to 0.92 per 100,000. West Nile virus remains the leading cause of neuroinvasive arboviral disease in the United States; in 2013, 2,469 cases of WNV neuroinvasive disease were reported, more than 20 times the number of neuroinvasive disease cases reported than for all other domestic arboviruses combined.

In temperate and subtropical regions, most human WNV infections occur in summer or early autumn. Although all age groups and both genders are susceptible to WNV infection, the incidence of severe disease (ie, encephalitis and death) is highest among adults older than 60 years. Chronic renal failure, history of cancer, history of alcohol abuse, diabetes, and hypertension has been associated with developing severe WNV disease (eg, hospitalization) or acquiring encephalitis.

Incubation Period

2 to 6 days; range, 2 to 14 days and up to 21 days in immunocompromised people.

Diagnostic Tests

Detection of anti-WNV immunoglobulin (Ig) M antibodies in serum or CSF is the most common way to diagnose WNV infection. The presence of anti-WNV IgM is usually good evidence of recent WNV infection but can indicate infection with another closely related flavivirus. Because anti-WNV IgM can persist in the serum of some patients for longer than 1 year, a positive test result may occasionally reflect past infection. Detection of WNV IgM in CSF is generally indicative of recent neuroinvasive infection. West Nile virus IgM antibodies are detectable in most WNV-infected patients within 7 days of symptom onset. For patients in whom serum collected within 10 days of illness lacks detectable IgM, testing should be repeated on a convalescent-phase sample. IgG antibody is generally detectable shortly after IgM and can persist for years. Plaque-reduction neutralization tests can be performed to measure virus-specific neutralizing antibodies and to discriminate between cross-reacting antibodies from closely related flaviviruses. A 4-fold or greater increase in virus-specific neutralizing antibodies between acute- and convalescent-phase serum specimens collected 2 to 3 weeks apart may be used to confirm recent WNV infection.

Viral culture and WNV nucleic acid amplification tests can be performed on acute-phase serum, CSF, or tissue specimens. However, by the time most immunocompetent patients present with clinical symptoms, WNV RNA is usually no longer detectable; thus, polymerase chain reaction assay is not recommended for diagnosis in immunocompetent hosts. The sensitivity of these tests is likely higher in immunocompromised patients. Immunohistochemical staining can detect WNV antigens in fixed tissue, but negative results are not definitive.

West Nile virus disease should be considered in the differential diagnosis of febrile or acute neurologic illnesses associated with recent exposure to mosquitoes, blood transfusion, or solid organ transplantation and of illnesses in neonates whose mothers were infected with WNV during pregnancy or while breastfeeding. In addition to other, more common causes of aseptic meningitis and encephalitis, other arboviruses should also be considered in the differential diagnosis.

Treatment

Management of WNV disease is supportive. Although various therapies have been evaluated or used for WNV disease, none has shown specific benefit thus far.

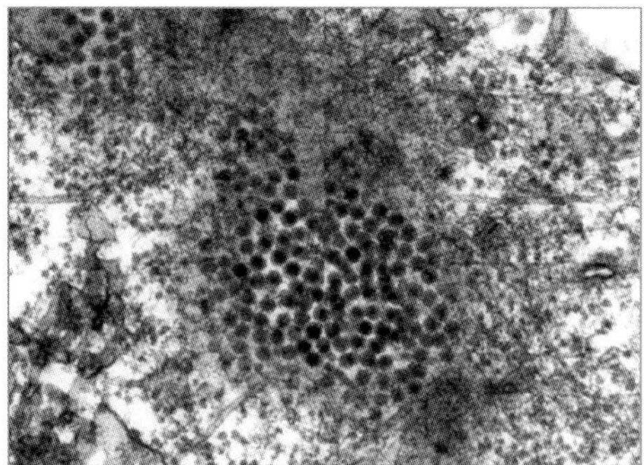

Image 154.1
Transmission electron micrograph of West Nile virus. Courtesy of Centers for Disease Control and Prevention/Institut Pasteur.

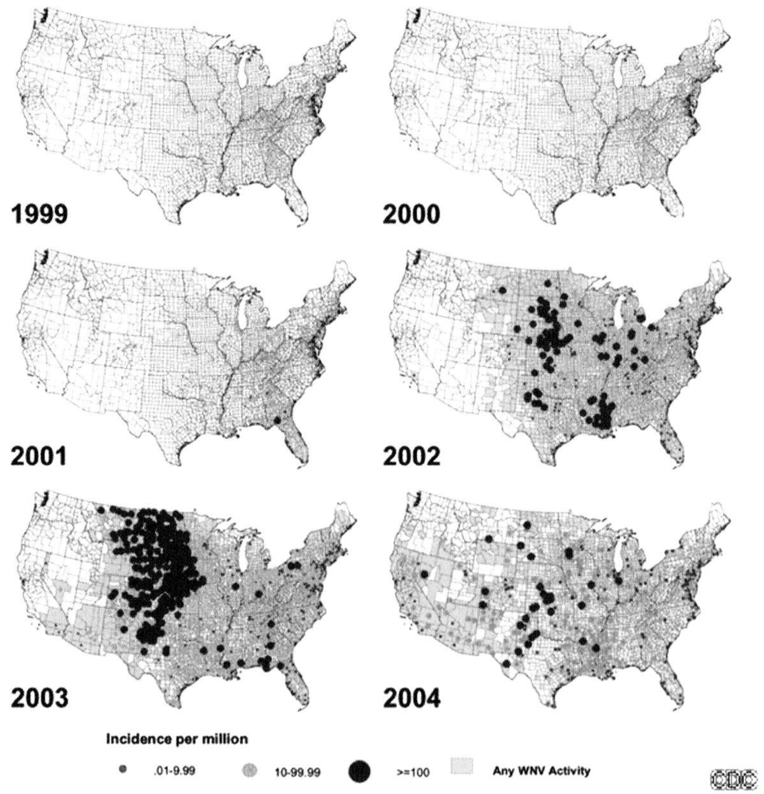

1999
2000
2001
2002
2003
2004
Incidence per million
.01-9.99
10-99.99
>=100
Any WNV Activity
CDC

Image 154.2
Reported incidence of neuroinvasive West Nile virus disease by county in the United States, 1999–2004. Reported to Centers for Disease Control and Prevention by states through April 21, 2005. Courtesy of *Emerging Infectious Diseases.*

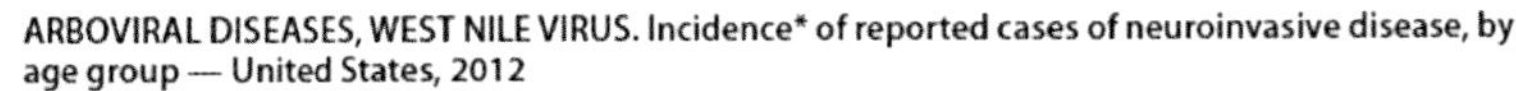

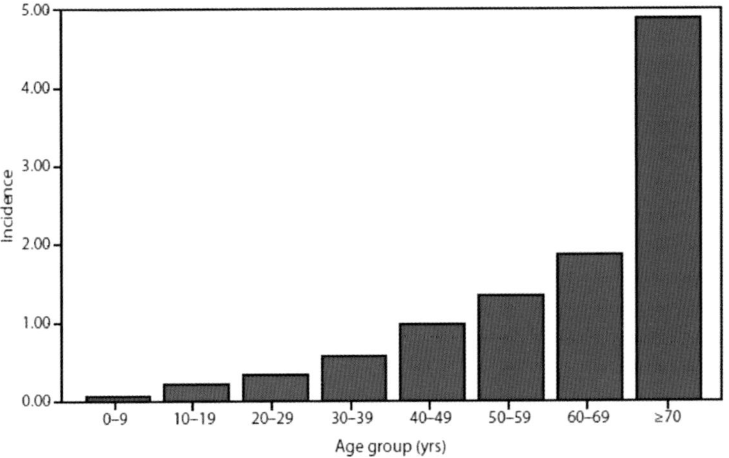

Image 154.3
Arboviral diseases, West Nile virus. Incidence of reported cases of neuroinvasive disease, by age group—United States, 2012. Courtesy of *Morbidity and Mortality Weekly Report*.

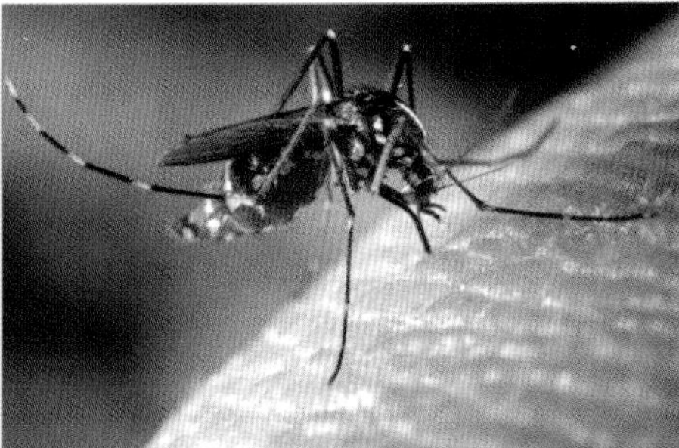

Image 154.4
A blood-engorged female *Aedes albopictus* mosquito feeding on a human host. Under experimental conditions, the *A albopictus* mosquito, also known as the Asian tiger mosquito, has been found to be a vector of West Nile virus. *Aedes* is a genus of the Culicinae family of mosquitoes. Courtesy of Centers for Disease Control and Prevention/James Gathany.

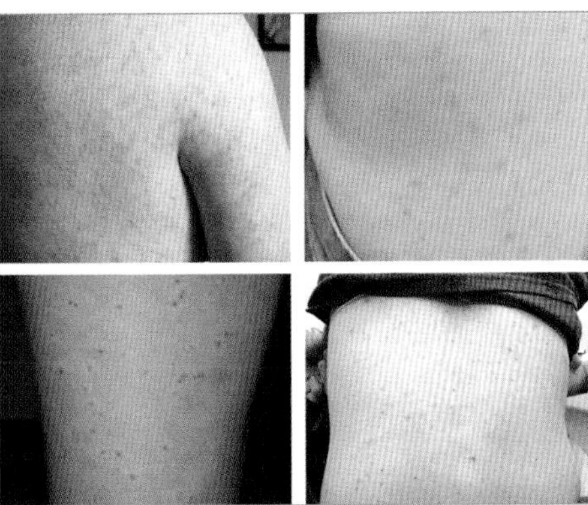

Image 154.5
Four patients with West Nile virus fever and erythematous, maculopapular rashes on the back (top left), flank (top right), posterior thigh (bottom left), and back (bottom right). Ferguson DD, Gershman K, LeBailly A, Petersen LR. Characteristics of the rash associated with West Nile virus fever. *Clin Infect Dis*. 2005;41(8):1204–1207. Reprinted with permission from Oxford University Press.

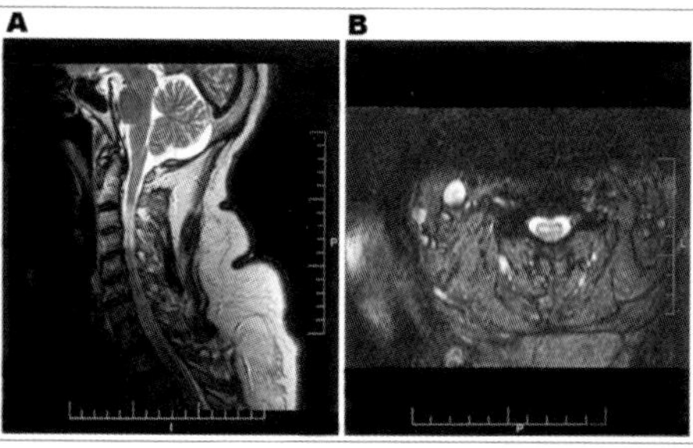

Image 154.6
West Nile virus–associated flaccid paralysis. Saggital (A) and axial (B) T2-weighted magnetic resonance images of the cervical spinal cord in a patient with acute asymmetric upper extremity weakness and subjective dyspnea. A, Diffuse cervical cord signal abnormality. B, Abnormal signal in the anterior horn region. Courtesy of *Emerging Infectious Diseases.*

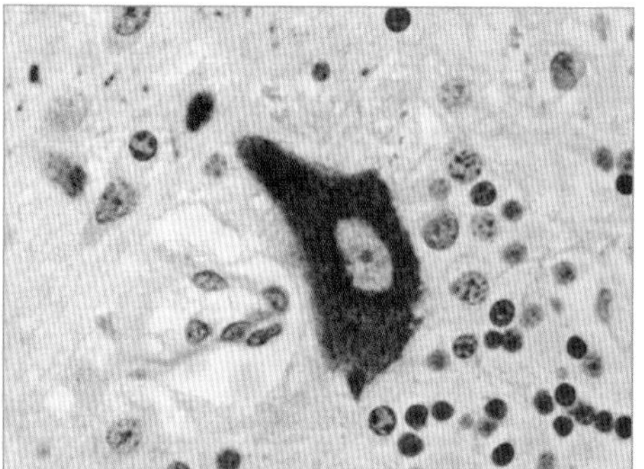

Image 154.8
Staining of West Nile virus antigen in the cytoplasm of a Purkinje cell in the cerebellum (immunohistochemistry, magnification x40). Courtesy of Centers for Disease Control and Prevention.

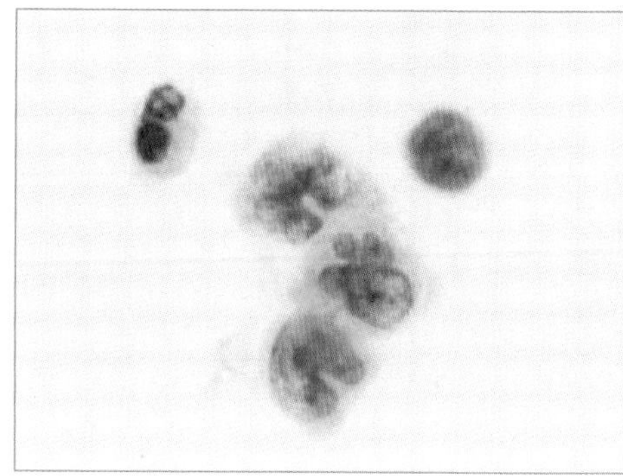

Image 154.7
Three Mollaret-like cells are present (center), with a neutrophil (upper left) and a lymphocyte (upper right) in cerebrospinal fluid from a patient with West Nile virus encephalitis, confirmed by reverse-transcription polymerase chain reaction and serologic testing (Papanicolaou stain, magnification x500). Courtesy of Centers for Disease Control and Prevention.

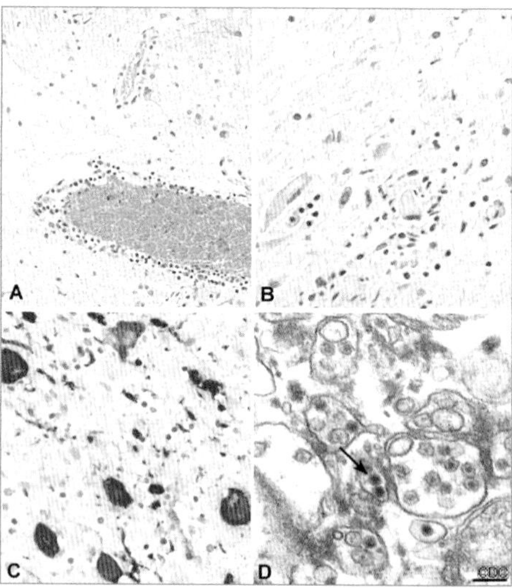

Image 154.9
Histopathologic features of West Nile virus (WNV) in human tissues. A and B show inflammation, microglial nodules, and variable necrosis that occur during WNV encephalitis; C shows WNV antigen (red) in neurons and neuronal processes using an immunohistochemical stain; D is an electron micrograph of WNV in the endoplasmic reticulum of a nerve cell (arrow) (bar = 100 nm). These 4 images are from a fatal case of WNV infection in a 39-year-old African American female. Courtesy of *Emerging Infectious Diseases.*

155

Yersinia enterocolitica and *Yersinia pseudotuberculosis* Infections

(Enteritis and Other Illnesses)

Clinical Manifestations

Yersinia enterocolitica causes several age-specific syndromes and a variety of other, less commonly reported clinical illnesses. Infection with *Y enterocolitica* typically manifests as fever and diarrhea in young children; stool often contains leukocytes, blood, and mucus. Relapsing disease and, rarely, necrotizing enterocolitis have also been described. In older children and adults, a pseudoappendicitis syndrome (ie, fever, abdominal pain, tenderness in the right lower quadrant of the abdomen, and leukocytosis) predominates. Bacteremia with *Y enterocolitica* most often occurs in infants younger than 1 year and in older children with predisposing conditions, such as excessive iron storage (eg, deferoxamine use, sickle cell disease, β-thalassemia) and immunosuppressive states. Focal manifestations of *Y enterocolitica* are uncommon and include pharyngitis, meningitis, osteomyelitis, pyomyositis, conjunctivitis, pneumonia, pleural empyema, endocarditis, acute peritonitis, abscesses of the liver and spleen, and primary cutaneous infection. Postinfectious sequelae with *Y enterocolitica* infection include erythema nodosum, reactive arthritis, and proliferative glomerulonephritis. These sequelae occur most often in older children and adults, particularly people with HLA-B27 antigen.

Major manifestations of *Yersinia pseudotuberculosis* infection include fever, scarlatiniform rash, and abdominal symptoms. Acute pseudoappendiceal abdominal pain is common, resulting from ileocecal mesenteric adenitis or terminal ileitis. Other findings include diarrhea, erythema nodosum, septicemia, and sterile pleural and joint effusions. Clinical features can mimic those of Kawasaki disease (mucocutaneous lymph node syndrome); in Hiroshima, Japan, nearly 10% of children with a diagnosis of Kawasaki disease have serologic or culture evidence of *Y pseudotuberculosis* infection.

Etiology

The genus *Yersinia* consists of 11 species of gram-negative bacilli. *Y enterocolitica*, *Y pseudotuberculosis*, and *Yersinia pestis* are the 3 most recognized human pathogens. *Y enterocolitica* bioserotypes most often associated with human illness are 1B/O:8, 2/O:5,27, 2/O:9, 3/O:3, and 4/O:3, with bioserotype 4/O:3 now predominating as the most common type in the United States. Virulence can be attributed to adhesion or invasion genes, enterotoxins, iron-scavenging genomic islands, and secretion systems. Highly pathogenic *Yersinia* are known to carry a 70 kb pYV virulence plasmid, which encodes a type 3 secretion system that is activated at human body temperatures and promotes entry into lymph tissues and subsequent evasion of host defense mechanisms.

Epidemiology

Yersinia infections are uncommonly reported in the United State. *Y enterocolitica* and *Y pseudotuberculosis* are isolated most often during the cool months of temperate climates. According to the Foodborne Disease Active Surveillance Network, during 2012, 3.3 laboratory-confirmed infections per 1 million people were reported to surveillance sites. During Foodborne Disease Active Surveillance Network surveillance from 1996 to 2009, 47% of infections were in children younger than 5 years; 28% were hospitalized, and 1% died. In contrast, the average annual incidence of *Y pseudotuberculosis* was 0.04 cases per 1 million people; the median age was 47 years, 72% were hospitalized, and 11% died. Two-thirds of *Y pseudotuberculosis* isolates were recovered from blood.

The principal reservoir of *Y enterocolitica* is swine; feral *Y pseudotuberculosis* has been isolated from ungulates (deer, elk, goats, sheep, cattle), rodents (rats, squirrels, beaver), rabbits, and many bird species. Infection with *Y enterocolitica* is believed to be transmitted by ingestion of contaminated food (raw or incompletely cooked pork products, tofu, and unpasteurized or inadequately pasteurized milk), by contaminated surface or well water, by direct or indirect contact with animals, and, rarely, by transfusion with contaminated packed red blood cells and by person-to-person transmission. Cross-contamination has been documented to lead to infection in infants if their caregivers handle raw pork intestines (ie, chitterlings) and do not cleanse their hands adequately before handling the infant or the infant's toys, bottles, or pacifiers.

Incubation Period

4 to 6 days; range, 1 to 14 days. Organisms are typically excreted for 2 to 3 weeks.

Diagnostic Tests

Y enterocolitica and *Y pseudotuberculosis* can be recovered from stool, throat swab specimens, mesenteric lymph nodes, peritoneal fluid, and blood. *Y enterocolitica* has also been isolated from synovial fluid, bile, urine, cerebrospinal fluid, sputum, pleural fluid, and wounds. Stool cultures generally yield bacteria during the first 2 weeks of illness, regardless of the nature of gastrointestinal tract manifestations. *Yersinia* organisms are not sought routinely in stool specimens by most laboratories in the United States. Consequently, laboratory personnel should be notified when *Yersinia* infection is suspected so stool can be cultured on suitable media (cefsulodin-irgasan-novobiocin agar). Infection can also be confirmed by demonstrating increases in serum antibody titer after infection, but these tests are generally available only in reference or research laboratories. Characteristic ultrasonographic features demonstrating edema of the wall of the terminal ileum and cecum help to distinguish pseudoappendicitis from appendicitis and can help avoid exploratory surgery.

Treatment

Neonates, immunocompromised hosts, and all patients with septicemia or extraintestinal disease require treatment for *Yersinia* infection. Parenteral therapy with a third-generation cephalosporin is appropriate, and evaluation of cerebrospinal fluid should be performed for infected neonates. Otherwise healthy non-neonates with enterocolitis can be treated symptomatically. Other than decreasing the duration of fecal excretion of *Y enterocolitica* and *Y pseudotuberculosis*, a clinical benefit of antimicrobial therapy for immunocompetent patients with enterocolitis, pseudoappendicitis syndrome, or mesenteric adenitis has not been established. In addition to third-generation cephalosporins, *Y enterocolitica* and *Y pseudotuberculosis* are usually susceptible to trimethoprim-sulfamethoxazole, aminoglycosides, fluoroquinolones, chloramphenicol, tetracycline, or doxycycline. *Y enterocolitica* isolates are usually resistant to first-generation cephalosporins and most penicillins.

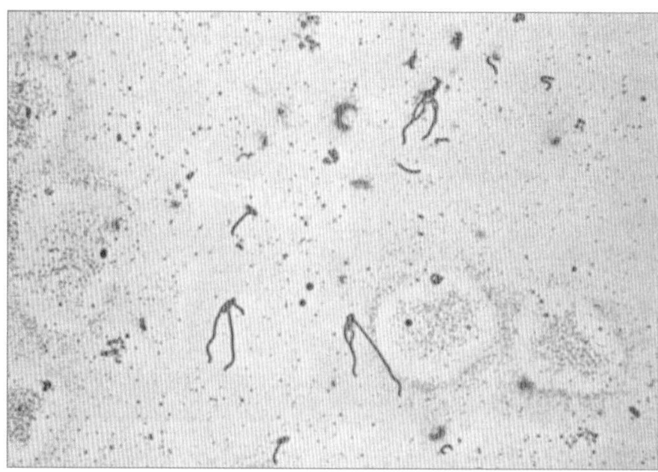

Image 155.1
A photomicrograph of *Yersinia enterocolitica* using flagella staining technique. Symptoms of yersiniosis are fever, abdominal pain, and diarrhea (often bloody), and *Y enterocolitica* is the cause of most *Yersinia*-related illnesses in the United States (mostly in children). Courtesy of Centers for Disease Control and Prevention.

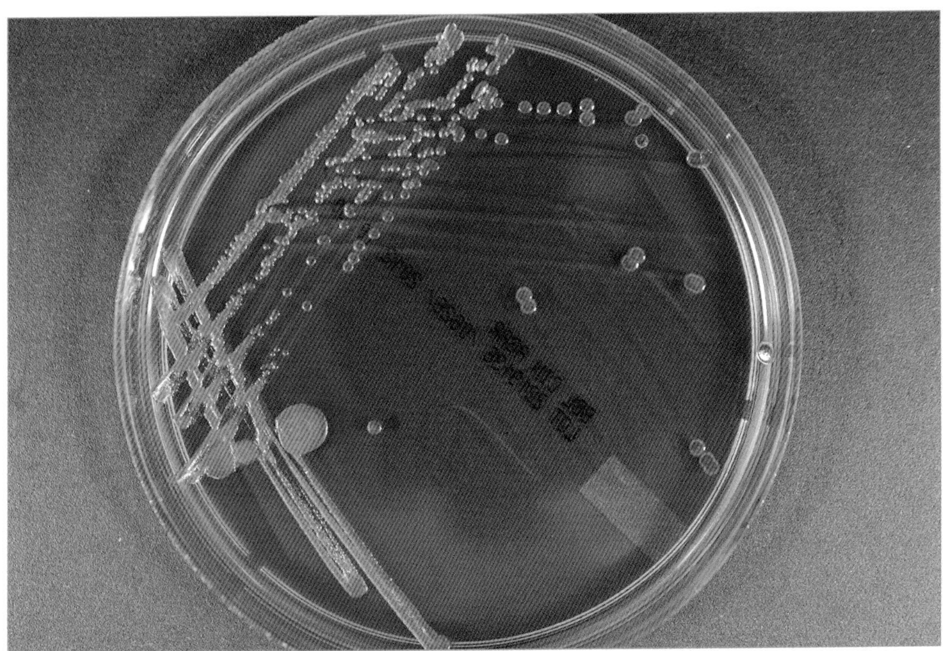

Image 155.2
Yersinia kristensenii on cefsulodin-irgasan-novobiocin agar. Colonies appear light rose in color with a darker, reddish center. Courtesy of Julia Rosebush, DO; Robert Jerris, PhD; and Theresa Stanley, M(ASCP).

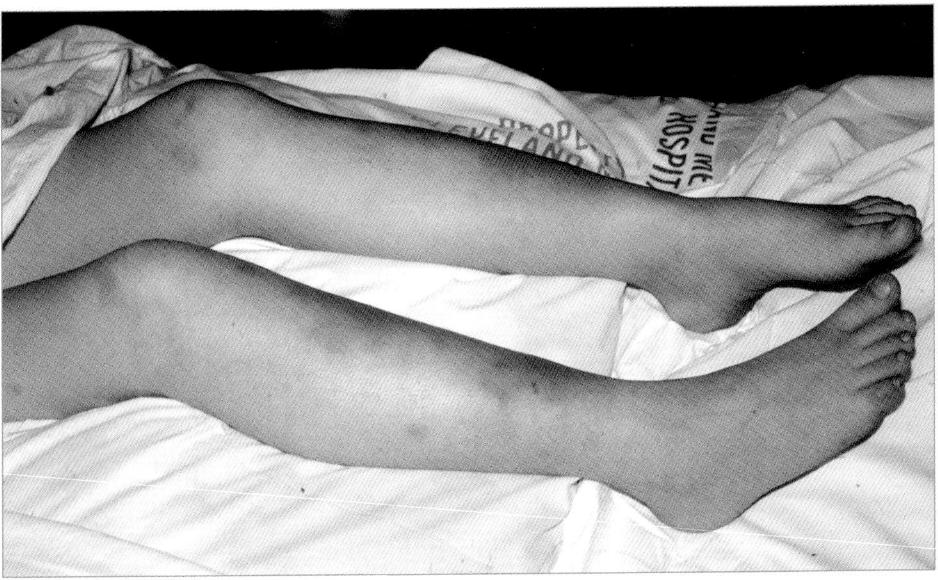

Image 155.3
Multiple erythema nodosum lesions over both lower extremities of a 10-year-old girl following a *Yersinia enterocolitica* infection. This immunoreactive complication may also occur in association with *Campylobacter jejuni* infections, tuberculosis, leprosy, coccidioidomycosis, histoplasmosis, and other infectious diseases. Courtesy of George Nankervis, MD.

Index

Page numbers followed by *f* indicate a figure.
Page numbers followed by *i* indicate an image.
Page numbers followed by *t* indicate a table.

A

B

C

D

E

F

G

H

I

J

K

L

M

N

O

P

Q

R

S

T

U

V

W

X

Y

Z

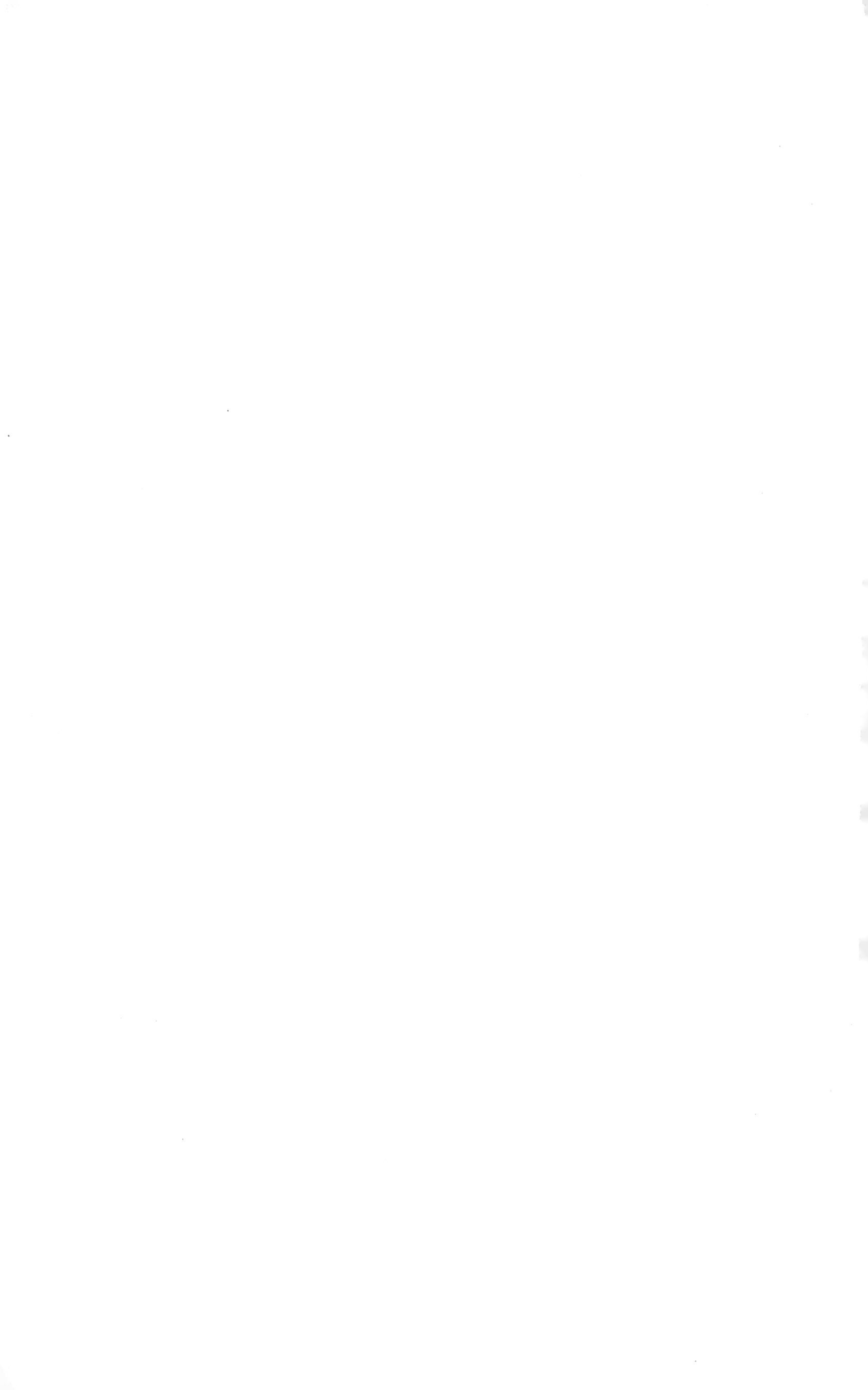